T0231393

Comprehensive Management of High Risk Cardiovascular Patients

Fundamental and Clinical Cardiology

Editor-in-Chief
Samuel Z. Goldhaber, M.D.
Harvard Medical School
and Brigham and Women's Hospital
Boston, Massachusetts, U.S.A.

Comprehensive Management of High Risk Cardiovascular Patients

edited by

Antonio M. Gotto, Jr.

Weill Medical College
Cornell University
New York, New York, U.S.A.

Peter P. Toth

Sterling Rock Falls Clinic
Sterling, Illinois, U.S.A.

University of Illinois College of Medicine
Peoria, Illinois, U.S.A.

Southern Illinois University School of Medicine
Springfield, Illinois, U.S.A.

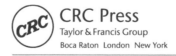

CRC Press
Taylor & Francis Group
Boca Raton London New York

CRC Press is an imprint of the
Taylor & Francis Group, an **informa** business

Informa Healthcare USA, Inc.
270 Madison Avenue
New York, NY 10016

© 2007 by Informa Healthcare USA, Inc.
Informa Healthcare is an Informa business

No claim to original U.S. Government works

International Standard Book Number-10: 0-8493-4066-7 (Hardcover)
International Standard Book Number-13: 978-0-8493-4066-6 (Hardcover)

This book contains information obtained from authentic and highly regarded sources. Reprinted material is quoted with permission, and sources are indicated. A wide variety of references are listed. Reasonable efforts have been made to publish reliable data and information, but the author and the publisher cannot assume responsibility for the validity of all materials or for the consequences of their use.

No part of this book may be reprinted, reproduced, transmitted, or utilized in any form by any electronic, mechanical, or other means, now known or hereafter invented, including photocopying, microfilming, and recording, or in any information storage or retrieval system, without written permission from the publishers.

For permission to photocopy or use material electronically from this work, please access www.copyright.com (http://www.copyright.com/) or contact the Copyright Clearance Center, Inc. (CCC) 222 Rosewood Drive, Danvers, MA 01923, 978-750-8400. CCC is a not-for-profit organization that provides licenses and registration for a variety of users. For organizations that have been granted a photocopy license by the CCC, a separate system of payment has been arranged.

Trademark Notice: Product or corporate names may be trademarks or registered trademarks, and are used only for identification and explanation without intent to infringe.

Library of Congress Cataloging-in-Publication Data

Comprehensive mamagement of high risk cardiovascular patients / edited by Antonio Gotto, Jr., Peter P. Toth.
    p. ; cm. -- (Fundamental and clinical cardiology ; v. 57)
    Includes bibliographical references and index.
    ISBN-13: 978-0-8493-4066-6 (hardcover : alk. paper)
    ISBN-10: 0-8493-4066-7 (hardcover : alk. paper)
    1. Cardiovascular system--Diseases. 2. Cardiovascular system--Patients. I. Gotto, Antonio M. II. Toth, Peter P. III. Series.
    [DNLM: 1. Cardiovascular Diseases--prevention & control. 2. Cardiovascular Diseases--diagnosis. 3. Cardiovascular Diseases--therapy. 4. Risk Factors. W1 FU538TD v.57 2006 / WG 120 C7375 2006]

RC669.C66 2006
616.1--dc22   2006046573

Visit the Informa Web site at
www.informa.com

and the Informa Healthcare Web site at
www.informahealthcare.com

*To my wife, Karen, and my daughters, Martha and Mary, for their
steadfast support and for giving me the energy and freedom to reach, and
to my patients for teaching me day in and day out about the experiences and
elements of our humanity that matter most.*

Peter P. Toth

*To my wife, Anita, and my daughters, Jennifer, Gillian, and Teresa,
for their love and support.*

Antonio M. Gotto, Jr.

Series Introduction

Informa Healthcare has developed various series of beautifully produced books in different branches of medicine. These series have facilitated the integration of rapidly advancing information for both the clinical specialist and the researcher.

My goal as Editor-in-Chief of the Fundamental and Clinical Cardiology Series is to assemble the talents of world-renowned authorities to discuss virtually every area of cardiovascular medicine. In the current monograph, Drs. Antonio Gotto and Peter P. Toth have written and edited a much-needed and timely book which addresses those risk factors for coronary arterycardiovascular disease patients which have until now received insufficient emphasis. Drs. Gotto and Toth have selected several risk factors for special emphasis, including, hemostatic risk factors, chronic infections, psychosocial factors, and clinical application of genotyping to risk stratification. They emphasize other issues which are becoming increasingly important, such as obesity, nutritional supplementation, diabetes, and metabolic syndrome. Contributing authors include world renowned authorities such as William B. Kannel, M.D., Stanley G. Rockson, M.D., and James T. Willerson, M.D. I know that I will bring this comprehensive volume to the office with me when I am evaluating my outpatients.

My goal as Editor-in-Chief of the Fundamental and Clinical Cardiology Series is to assemble the talents of world-renowned authorities to discuss virtually every area of cardiovascular medicine. Future contributions to this series will include books on molecular biology, interventional cardiology, and clinical management of such problems as coronary artery disease, venous thromboembolism, and ventricular arrhythmias.

Samuel Z. Goldhaber, M.D.
Professor of Medicine
Harvard Medical School
Boston, Massachusetts, U.S.A.

Foreword

In the first decade of the 20th century, approximately one of seven deaths in the United States and Western Europe were secondary to cardiovascular diseases. Although reliable numbers are not available, only about one-third of these deaths, i.e., about 5% of the total, were caused by atherosclerotic cardiovascular disease. During the next half century, as we transitioned from an agrarian, largely rural economy to an industrialized, largely urban one, the incidence of both total cardiovascular deaths and especially the fraction secondary to atherosclerosis—coronary, cerebral, and systemic vascular disease—rose steadily and sharply. By 1950, atherosclerotic cardiovascular disease had become the single most common cause of death, by far.

Although autopsy studies of middle-aged and older persons showed the presence of prominent and, in many cases, diffuse atherosclerosis, the enormous variability in the severity of this process among persons was a mystery. Furthermore, sudden cardiac death and massive acute myocardial infarction, the most dramatic and visible manifestation of coronary atherosclerosis, came like "bolts out of the blue" and often affected middle-aged males at the height of their professional lives and family responsibilities.

As a trainee in the 1950s, I remember being taught about the so-called coronary diathesis, which included male gender, age over 50 years, overweight, hypertension, and, sometimes, gout. The establishment of the Framingham Heart Study by the (then) National Heart Institute in 1949 was a historic event. This first prospective, observational, population-based study of heart disease established the concept of coronary risk factors. Clearly, the presence and severity of hypertension, serum cholesterol, smoking, and electrocardiographic evidence of left ventricular hypertrophy and, especially, combinations of these identified persons at high risk of being stricken by atherosclerotic vascular disease.

Although it seemed like a small step, conceptually, to move from the identification of risk to attempts to reduce it, cardiologists were at first not friendly to the concept of prevention. Instead, they focused on applying the rapidly developing technology to further refinements of cardiovascular diagnosis and to the treatment of the complications of the disease after they had occurred.

The first Surgeon General's Report on Smoking and Health in 1964 and the resultant antismoking campaign, the progressive improvement of well-tolerated and effective antihypertensive and lipid-reducing drugs, and the avalanche of clinical trials showing the benefit of using these agents, both in patients with established atherosclerotic cardiovascular disease and in those at risk but without overt disease, swung the balance of opinion. Cardiologists, the pharmaceutical industry, the press, and the government all became convinced that a vigorous approach to risk reduction was essential. Indeed, in the latter decades of the 20th century, a decline in coronary risk factors in the population became evident. Although cardiac prevention did not reduce the overall prevalence of atherosclerotic cardiovascular disease, it was well on its way to delaying it. Thus, the tide against this dread condition began to turn.

However, by the early 1990s, a new threat appeared. As we transitioned from an industrial to an information economy and as tasty "fast" foods became readily available and relatively inexpensive, the twin epidemics of obesity and type 2 diabetes mellitus became a serious threat to the prevention of atherosclerotic cardiovascular disease. These epidemics are now raging in the United States, are moving abroad, and are well on their way to becoming pandemics.

We must now engage in a battle to maintain and extend the gains in prevention made in the last half of the 20th century. A principal weapon in this battle is the education of the "front line officers," i.e., primary care physicians and cardiologists. Comprehensive Management of the High-Risk Cardiovascular Patient presents a logical "battle plan" by first providing contemporary evidence of the importance of individual risk factors and their combinations. It then provides a critical review of the evidence for the interventions intended to reduce risk and presents recommendations for what the title of this fine treatise reflects, i.e., comprehensive management. Moreover, it focuses on the unique problems presented by women and different racial groups.

The editors, Drs. Gotto and Toth, and their talented authors deserve our thanks for having provided such an authoritative and lucid book that will be of enormous interest to all of those who have the opportunity and responsibility to reduce the risk and extend the lives of a large segment of the population.

Eugene Braunwald, M.D.
Distinguished Hersey Professor of Medicine
Harvard Medical School
Boston, Massachusetts, U.S.A.

and

Chairman
TIMI Study Group
Brigham and Women's Hospital
Boston, Massachusetts, U.S.A.

Preface

In the new millennium, physicians worldwide face many new challenges. The past five decades have yielded extraordinary advances in the identification and management of a wide array of cardiovascular diseases. This work has sharply impacted average life expectancy for men and women and improved outcomes following disease onset. Considerable basic scientific and clinical research has revealed an extraordinarily detailed view of many of the most intimate biochemical and pathophysiologic mechanisms regulating cardiovascular disease. Despite the development of numerous pharmacologic and surgical interventions, cardiovascular disease remains the leading cause of death and disability in industrialized nations.

Many of the most important genetic backgrounds and risk factors for the development of cardiovascular disease have been well characterized in epidemiologic and clinical studies conducted throughout the world. Dyslipidemia, hypertension, obesity, insulin resistance, diabetes mellitus, and cigarette smoking are among the most important of these risk factors. The incidence of all these risk factors continues to increase and reach epidemic proportions throughout much of the world. As additional societies become progressively more industrialized and as the world population continues to grow older and more obese, the number of people affected clinically by the ravages of atherosclerotic disease will continue to rise. Much basic work using animal models and the completion of numerous human clinical trials have revealed much about the management of heart failure, cardiac arrhythmias, chronic kidney disease, noncoronary atherosclerotic disease, pulmonary hypertension, and stroke, among other clinical entities. Perhaps even more important than disease management is the increasing pressure on clinicians to identify risk factors for cardiovascular disease early and to intervene aggressively. Such measures are requisite to stemming the rising human and economic cost of cardiovascular disease.

This book is intended to help fill a large gap in the management of patients who have, or are at risk of developing, cardiovascular disease. Rather than being encyclopedic in scope, it is designed to serve as a resource for the busy, practicing clinician. The approach is evidence-based but practical. Conceptual development and the exploration of biochemical and physiological mechanisms are balanced by focused attention on the everyday issues of caring for patients with specific metabolic and cardiovascular disorders. Standards of care and challenging management issues are illustrated and reinforced by case studies. Pharmacotherapeutic choices are discussed in light of findings from clinical trials. Elements of care unique to women and people of different racial and ethnic groups are explored in detail. Lifestyle modifications and the risks and benefits of specific therapies are addressed. Comprehensive care in both primary and secondary prevention settings is stressed. Moreover, effort is made to remove the reluctance on the part of primary care providers to treat such disorders as atherosclerotic disease, congestive heart failure, severe hypertension, complex dyslipidemias, and chronic renal disease, among others.

It is our sincerest hope that this book will help ensure that the many lessons and the most important research findings of recent years will be more aptly and regularly applied to patients day in and day out, one precious life at a time.

Antonio M. Gotto, Jr.
Peter P. Toth

Acknowledgments

We wish to express our sincere gratitude to a number of people without whom we could not have brought this textbook to fruition. We are especially indebted to Mr. Jesse Y. Jou of the Weill Cornell Medical College for providing invaluable insights and assistance during every stage of this book's development. We thank Jennifer Moon for securing permission from publishers to reproduce many of the tables and figures contained herein. The formidable artistic abilities of Aaron Cormier, Patricia Kuharic, and Thom Graves of the Weill Cornell Medical College and Jude Gonzalez of the Sterling Rock Falls Clinic are greatly appreciated. We also thank Sandra Beberman, Vice President and Managing Director, and Vanessa Sanchez, Manager of Product Development and Production, of Informa Healthcare for sharing in our vision and helping to make this book possible.

Contents

Contributors

Annemarie Armani   Critical Pathways in Cardiology, Boston, Massachusetts, U.S.A.

Paul W. Armstrong   University of Alberta Hospital Heart Function Clinic, University of Alberta, Edmonton, Alberta, Canada

Stefano Bellosta   Department of Pharmacological Sciences, University of Milan, Milan, Italy

Deepak L. Bhatt   Department of Cardiovascular Medicine, Cleveland Clinic, Cleveland, Ohio, U.S.A.

Vera Bittner   Department of Medicine, Division of Cardiovascular Disease, University of Alabama at Birmingham, Birmingham, Alabama, U.S.A.

Herman Blomeier   Department of Medicine, Sections of Endocrinology and Cardiology, Feinberg School of Medicine, Northwestern University, Chicago, Illinois, U.S.A.

Yumei Cao   Department of Nutritional Sciences, The Huck Institute for Integrative Biosciences, Pennsylvania State University, University Park, Pennsylvania, U.S.A.

Adnan K. Chhatriwalla   Department of Cardiovascular Medicine, Cleveland Clinic, Cleveland, Ohio, U.S.A.

Alberto Corsini   Department of Pharmacological Sciences, University of Milan, Milan, Italy

Michael H. Davidson   Rush University Medical Center, Chicago, Illinois, U.S.A.

Emil M. deGoma   Division of Cardiovascular Medicine, Stanford University School of Medicine, Stanford, California, U.S.A.

Daniel A. Duprez   Cardiovascular Division, Rasmussen Center for Cardiovascular Disease Prevention and Cardiovascular Clinical Trial Center, University of Minnesota, Minneapolis, Minnesota, U.S.A.

Patrick Duriez   Department of Atherosclerosis, INSERM U545, University of Lille 2, Institut Pasteur de Lille, Lille, France

John A. Farmer   Baylor College of Medicine, Houston, Texas, U.S.A.

Keith C. Ferdinand   Association of Black Cardiologists, Atlanta, Georgia, U.S.A.

Jean-Charles Fruchart   Department of Atherosclerosis, INSERM U545, University of Lille 2, Institut Pasteur de Lille, Lille, France

David W. Gardner   Department of Internal Medicine, Diabetes, and Metabolism, Division of Endocrinology, Cosmopolitan-International Endocrinology and Diabetes Center, University of Missouri-Columbia, Columbia, Missouri, U.S.A.

Ronald Goldberg   Division of Endocrinology, Diabetes and Metabolism and the Diabetes Research Institute, University of Miami Miller School of Medicine, Miami, Florida, U.S.A.

Antonio M. Gotto, Jr.   Department of Medicine, Weill Medical College of Cornell University, New York, New York, U.S.A.

Gurushankar Govindarajan   Diabetes and Cardiovascular Disease Research Laboratory, Harry S. Truman Memorial VA Hospital, Columbia, Missouri, U.S.A.

Rowena Ivers   School of Public Health and Community Medicine, The University of New South Wales, Kensington, New South Wales, Australia

William B. Kannel   Department of Medicine and Public Health, Boston University School of Medicine and Framingham Heart Study, Framingham, Massachusetts, U.S.A.

Khurshid A. Khan   Department of Internal Medicine, Diabetes, and Metabolism, Division of Endocrinology, Cosmopolitan-International Endocrinology and Diabetes Center, University of Missouri-Columbia, Columbia, Missouri, U.S.A.

Nelson Kopyt   Department of Medicine, Temple University, Philadelphia, and Lehigh Valley Hospital, Allentown, Pennsylvania, U.S.A.

Penny M. Kris-Etherton   Department of Nutritional Sciences, The Huck Institute for Integrative Biosciences, Pennsylvania State University, University Park, Pennsylvania, U.S.A.

Bernardo Liberato   Stroke and Critical Care Division, The Neurological Institute, Columbia University, New York, New York, U.S.A.

Gérald Luc   Department of Atherosclerosis, INSERM U545, University of Lille 2, Institut Pasteur de Lille, Lille, France

John M. Palmer   Department of Internal Medicine, University of Missouri-Columbia, Columbia, Missouri, U.S.A.

Rodolfo Paoletti   Department of Pharmacological Sciences, University of Milan, Milan, Italy

Shyam Prabhakaran   Stroke and Critical Care Division, The Neurological Institute, Columbia University, New York, New York, U.S.A.

Charles Reasner   University of Texas Health Science Center and Texas Diabetes Institute, Zarzamora, San Antonio, Texas, U.S.A.

Robyn L. Richmond   School of Public Health and Community Medicine, The University of New South Wales, Kensington, New South Wales, Australia

Jennifer G. Robinson   Departments of Epidemiology and Medicine, College of Public Health, University of Iowa, Iowa City, Iowa, U.S.A.

Stanley G. Rockson   Division of Cardiovascular Medicine, Stanford University School of Medicine, Stanford, California, U.S.A.

Ralph L. Sacco   Stroke and Critical Care Division, The Neurological Institute, Columbia University, New York, New York, U.S.A.

Nicolas W. Shammas   Midwest Cardiovascular Research Foundation, Cardiovascular Medicine, P. C., Davenport, Iowa and University of Iowa Hospitals and Clinics, Iowa City, Iowa, U.S.A.

James R. Sowers   Department of Internal Medicine, Division of Nephrology, University of Missouri-Columbia, Columbia, Missouri, U.S.A.

Neil J. Stone   Department of Medicine, Sections of Endocrinology and Cardiology, Feinberg School of Medicine, Northwestern University, Chicago, Illinois, U.S.A.

Peter P. Toth   Department of Preventive Cardiology, Sterling Rock Falls Clinic, Sterling, University of Illinois College of Medicine, Peoria, and Southern Illinois University School of Medicine, Springfield, Illinois, U.S.A.

James T. Willerson   University of Texas Health Science Center and Texas Heart Institute, Houston, Texas, U.S.A.

Daniel J. Wilson   Hypertension Consultations, Rochester, Minnesota, and Pfizer, Inc., New York, New York, U.S.A.

Peter W. F. Wilson   Department of Medicine, Medical University of South Carolina, Charleston, South Carolina, U.S.A.

Jun Zhang   Department of Nutritional Sciences, The Huck Institute for Integrative Biosciences, Pennsylvania State University, University Park, Pennsylvania, U.S.A.

Nicholas Zwar   School of Public Health and Community Medicine, The University of New South Wales, Kensington, New South Wales, Australia

1 | Risk Factors for Cardiovascular Disease and the Framingham Study Equation

William B. Kannel
Department of Medicine and Public Health, Boston University School of Medicine and Framingham Heart Study, Framingham, Massachusetts, U.S.A.

Peter W. F. Wilson
Department of Medicine, Medical University of South Carolina, Charleston, South Carolina, U.S.A.

KEY POINTS

- Major risk factors for the atherosclerotic cardiovascular diseases (CVDs) have been identified and confirmed. These include: dyslipidemia, hypertension, glucose intolerance, insulin resistance, adiposity, cigarette smoking, physical inactivity, left ventricular hypertrophy, atrial fibrillation, and cardiomegaly, among others. Several of these have been selected to formulate CVD-specific multivariable risk profiles.
- Framingham Study multivariable risk formulations utilize ordinary office procedures and readily available blood tests to facilitate office estimation of the risk of coronary heart disease (CHD), stroke, peripheral artery disease, and heart failure outcomes.
- Because CVD risk factors usually cluster, and the risk imposed by each of them varies extensively in relation to this, multivariable CVD risk assessment is a necessity, especially now that near average risk factor levels are recommended for treatment.
- Novel risk factors deserve attention, but the standard CVD risk factors appear to account for as much as 85% of the CVD arising within the population.
- Because of shared modifiable risk factors, the CHD risk profile also predicts other atherosclerotic CVD outcomes. Measures taken to prevent any one outcome can be expected to also curb the others.
- Further improvement in the detection, evaluation, and control of the major identified risk factors through implementation of guidelines for primary and secondary CVD prevention is needed, particularly in the high multivariable risk segment of the population.

INTRODUCTION

Five decades of epidemiological research have provided significant information that has helped public health workers, scientists, physicians, and researchers increase their understanding of the factors predisposing to CVD. Identification of these modifiable *risk factors*, a term coined by the Framingham Study (1), stimulated an interest in preventive cardiology and made cardiovascular epidemiology its basic science. Awareness of major CVD risk factors, identified by the Framingham Study and corroborated by others, inspired public health initiatives against smoking in the 1960s, hypertension in the 1970s, and hypercholesterolemia in the 1980s (2).

Population appraisal of the evolution of CVD revealed that CHD is an extremely common and highly lethal disease that attacks one in five persons before they attain 60 years of age, that women lag men in incidence by 10 years, and that sudden death is a prominent feature of CHD mortality. One in every six coronary attacks was found to present with sudden death as the first, last, and only symptom (3). It also became evident that the disease can be asymptomatic in its most severe form, with one in three myocardial infarctions (MIs) going unrecognized (4). Because of this clinical profile, a preventive approach was deemed essential. Fortunately, epidemiological research was able to ascertain a number of modifiable predisposing factors, allowing the targeting of high-risk CVD candidates for preventive measures.

From the National Heart, Lung and Blood Institute's Framingham Heart Study, National Institutes of Health. Framingham Heart Study is supported by NIH/NHLBI Contract No. 01-HC-25195 and the Visiting Scientist Program, which is supported by Astra Zeneca.

In the United States, heart attacks occur every 20 seconds. Despite the identification of biologically plausible, major modifiable predisposing risk factors for development of CHD, it remains the largest single killer of Americans, accounting for one of every five deaths in 2001 (5). CVD imposes an economic burden of $300 billion/yr. Each year, 1.2 million Americans have a new (700,000) or recurrent (500,000) CHD event and 40% die as a result of it. There are 13.2 million Americans who have a history of CHD (MI or angina pectoris (AP) or both). During 2001, there were 922,000 deaths from CVD (38.5% of all deaths) and 6.2 million hospitalizations, more than for any other disease group (5). The need for a preventive approach is underscored by the fact that about 60% of cardiac deaths occur before the victims can reach a hospital.

LIFETIME RISKS

More than five decades of follow-up of the Framingham Study cohort permitted determination of the lifetime risk of coronary events. The lifetime risk of CHD for 40-year-old men in the Framingham Study was close to 49% and for women, 32% (Table 1) (6). This lifetime risk increases stepwise with the serum cholesterol (7) and also increases with the tertile of multivariable risk (8).

MULTIVARIABLE RISK ASSESSMENT

Multivariable analysis was initially employed to assess the contribution of suspected CHD risk factors in order to gain insight into the underlying atherogenic process. This analysis also generated a set of independent risk factors useful for crafting multivariable risk formulations to predict CVD events. Thus, a multivariable analysis of the influence of established and potential risk factors provides clues to the pathogenesis of CVD, estimates of the independent effect of risk factors, and the global risk of candidates for CVD events. The set of risk factors employed for gaining pathogenic insights is constrained by the hypothesis to be tested; that for multivariable risk assessment, by the availability of reliable noninvasive tests for selected risk factors, cost, and whether the risk factors used can be safely modified with the expectation of benefit. A number of efficient methods for combining the predictive information from a number of risk factors are now available, enabling estimation of the probability that persons with certain characteristics will develop CVD in a specified interval of time. This methodology implicitly recognizes that no known risk factor either inevitably leads to development of disease or confers absolute immunity. In considering multivariable risk formulations, one must understand that there is no unconditional probability of disease development, nor any conditional probability that will not alter if other factors are taken into consideration. Adding variables ordinarily increases the ability to estimate risk by designating more people at very high or low risk, but the three best risk factors will usually perform almost as well as a larger set, even though all may be independent predictors. The number of risk factors to include depends on the purpose for assigning risk and the costs entailed. It must be anticipated that a regression estimate will fit the data from which it is derived better than it will fit another data set.

Framingham Study multivariable risk profiles have been tested in a variety of population samples and were found to be reasonably accurate, except for those in areas where the CHD rates are very low (9–12). However, even in these areas, high-risk persons can be distinguished from those at low risk, and by adjusting the intercept, the true absolute risk can be estimated (12). Evolution of global CVD risk assessment has completed the necessary stages of identifying multiple independent contributing risk factors, defining risk categories, and developing preventive strategies.

TABLE 1   Lifetime Risk of Coronary Heart Disease: Framingham Heart Study

Age (yr)	Men (%)	Women (%)
40	49	32
70	35	24

Source: From Ref. 6.

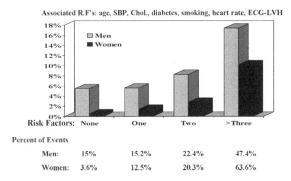

FIGURE 1 Risk of coronary attacks in the obese by burden of associated risk factors: Framingham Study (subjects ages 30–74 years). *Abbreviations*: RF, risk factor; SBP, systolic blood pressure; ECG-LVH, electrocardiogram-left ventricular hypertrophy. *Source*: From Ref. 16.

Risk factors are related to CVD occurrence in a continuous graded fashion, extending down into the perceived normal range, without indication of a critical value where normal leaves off. At any level of each risk factor, CVD risk varies widely in accordance with the burden of accompanying risk factors. National guidelines link treatment goals to global CHD risk (13). It has long been recognized that for any risk factor, predisposition to CVD is markedly influenced by the associated burden of other risk factors (14). It was recently postulated that an insulin resistance syndrome is the metabolic basis for other atherogenic risk factors to cluster with the major risk factors (15). Epidemiological investigation has long contended that atherosclerotic CVD is of multifactorial etiology. There are faulty lifestyles that promote atherogenic traits in susceptible persons, indicators of unstable lesions, and signs of a compromised arterial circulation that strongly indicate impending clinical events. CVD risk factors seldom occur in isolation of each other because they are metabolically linked, tending to cluster, the extent of which profoundly influences the CVD hazard of any particular risk factor. Weight gain leading to visceral adiposity promotes components of the cluster of risk factors characterized as the insulin-resistant *metabolic syndrome*. The hazard of obesity varies widely depending on the burden of atherogenic risk factors that accompany it (Fig. 1). In a patient with any particular CVD risk factor, it is essential to test for the others that are likely to coexist. Such coexistence can be expected 80% of the time. Now that guidelines for dyslipidemia, hypertension, and diabetes recommend treating modest abnormality, candidates for treatment are best targeted by global risk assessment so that the number needed to prevent one event is minimized.

All the major established risk factors contribute powerfully and significantly to CHD risk (Table 2). For atherothrombotic brain infarction, the relevant factors are hypertension, left ventricular hypertrophy, atrial fibrillation, and diabetes, whereas dyslipidemia *appears* to play a minor role (Table 3). For peripheral artery disease, glucose intolerance, cigarette smoking, and left ventricular hypertrophy are the most influential factors (Table 4). For heart failure, important factors are hypertension, diabetes, and reduced vital capacity, whereas serum total cholesterol appears unrelated (Table 5). The standard risk factors appear to influence CVD rates with different strengths in men and women. Diabetes operates more powerfully in women, eliminating their advantage over men for most atherosclerotic cardiovascular events (19,20). Cigarette smoking is more influential in men.

TABLE 2 Risk of Coronary Heart Disease According to Standard Risk Factors: Framingham Heart Study (36-Year Follow-Up)

	Risk ratio			
	35–64 yr		65–94 yr	
Risk factor	Men	Women	Men	Women
Cholesterol ≥ 240 mg/dL	1.9*	1.8**	1.2***	2.0*
Blood pressure ≥ 140/90 mmHg	2.0*	2.2*	1.6**	1.9*
Diabetes mellitus	1.5*	3.7*	1.6**	2.1*
ECG—left ventricular hypertrophy	3.0*	4.6*	2.7*	3.0*
Cigarette smoking	1.5**	1.1	1.0	1.2*

*$p < 0.001$, **$p < 0.01$, ***$p < 0.05$; risk ratios are age adjusted.
Source: From Ref. 17.

TABLE 3 Multivariate Risk Factors for Stroke from the Framingham Study (Subjects Aged 55–84 Years)

Risk factor	Multivariate risk ratio	
	Men	Women
Age (10 years)	1.66	1.93
Systolic blood pressure (10 mmHg)	1.91	1.68
Antihypertensive medication	1.39	–
Diabetes	1.40	1.72
Cigarette smoking	1.67	1.70
Cardiovascular disease	1.68	1.54
Atrial fibrillation	1.83	3.16
Left ventricular hypertrophy	2.32	2.34

Each relative risk is adjusted for the effects of the other risk factors.
Source: From Ref. 18.

Some of the standard risk factors—including glucose intolerance, smoking, dyslipidemia, and hypertension—tend to have lower risk ratios in advanced age, causing some to question the relevance of risk factors in later life. However, this reduced relative risk is offset by a higher absolute incidence of CVD and a large excess risk in advanced age. Thus, the standard risk factors continue to be important in the elderly (21). Atherosclerotic CVD events in the heart, brain, and limbs of the elderly can be predicted from identified risk factors.

Clinical categorical risk assessments according to the number of arbitrarily defined abnormalities present can identify high-risk persons, but epidemiological research points out that this approach tends to overlook persons at high risk because of multiple marginal abnormalities. Identification for treatment of persons with several borderline risk-factor values is important because such persons have a high risk and experience most of the cardiovascular events in the general population.

Epidemiological research has shown that prevention based on individual risk-factor assessment and treatment is inefficient and can be misleading. This approach often falsely reassures or needlessly alarms potential candidates for CVD because the risk of CVD for any particular risk factor varies widely, depending on the cluster of associated risk factors. Clusters of three or more risk factors occur at four to five times the expected rate.

A global risk assessment to estimate the multivariable risk is required to efficiently target candidates for aggressive preventive therapy. Substantial CHD risk for persons with mild to moderate risk factor levels is concentrated in those with coexistent risk factors such as hypertension, dyslipidemia, diabetes, and left ventricular hypertrophy. Major established risk factors have been synthesized into composite scoring algorithms based on Framingham Study data for the CVD outcomes of coronary disease, stroke, peripheral artery disease, and heart failure (18,22–26). Risk factors selected for this purpose are independent contributors to risk, are not highly intercorrelated, and are obtainable by ordinary office procedures and are reliable laboratory tests (Tables 2–5). The coronary risk factor scoring tool has been made available on the internet (Fig. 2) (27).

TABLE 4 Risk of Peripheral Artery Disease by Standard Risk Factors: Framingham Heart Study (36-Year Follow-Up)

Risk factors	Risk ratio (rate/1000)			
	Age 35–64 yr		Age 65–94 yr	
	Men	Women	Men	Women
Cholesterol ≥ 240 mg/dL	1.0	1.1	1.0	1.0
Hypertension ≥ 140/90 mmHg	5.7*	4.0*	2.0*	2.6*
Diabetes	3.0**	2.4***	1.6	2.9*
Electrocardiogram-left ventricular hypertrophy	5.1*	8.1*	3.6*	5.0*
Smoking	2.5**	1.0	1.4	1.9*

*$p < 0.001$, **$p < 0.01$, ***$p < 0.05$; biennial rates and risk ratios are age adjusted.
Source: From Ref. 17.

TABLE 5 Risk of Cardiac Failure by Standard Risk Factors: Framingham Heart Study (36-Year Follow-Up)

	Risk ratio			
	Age 35–64 yr		Age 65–94 yr	
Risk factors	**Men**	**Women**	**Men**	**Women**
Cholesterol ≥ 240 mg/dL	1.2	1.1	1.0	1.0
Hypertension ≥ 140/90 mmHg	4.0*	3.0*	1.9*	1.9*
Diabetes	4.4**	8.0*	2.0*	3.6*
ECG-LVH	15.0*	13.0*	4.9*	5.4*
Smoking	1.5*	1.1	1.0	1.3***

*$p<0.001$, **$p<0.01$, ***$p<0.05$; biennial rates and risk ratios are adjusted for age.
Source: From Ref. 17.

RISK FACTORS

Epidemiological, clinical, angiographic, and postmortem investigations have established a causal relationship between the major risk factors and occurrence of CHD and have demonstrated that altering risk factor levels substantially reduces the incidence of CVD (28,29). However, many novel risk factors are under investigation and that information may further enhance multivariable risk assessment.

Novel Risk Factors

It has been frequently claimed that only half the CHD incidence is explained by the standard major risk factors, but a recent report based on 120,000 patients enrolled in clinical CHD trials indicates that at least one major risk factor is present in 85% of men and 81% of women (30). Another report derived from three cohort studies of 400,000 persons indicates that among those who suffered fatal CHD events, 87% to 100% had had exposure to at least one major risk factor (31). Nevertheless, epidemiological research continues to find and evaluate additional risk factors that contribute to the occurrence of CVD and warrant further evaluation. Additional markers of CHD risk that enhance multivariable risk assessment or more precisely

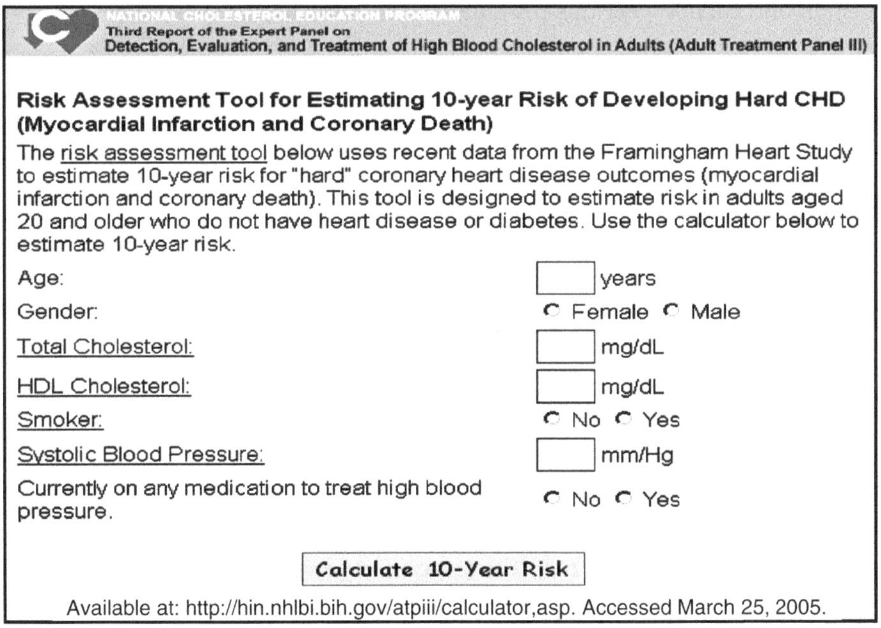

NATIONAL CHOLESTEROL EDUCATION PROGRAM
Third Report of the Expert Panel on
Detection, Evaluation, and Treatment of High Blood Cholesterol in Adults (Adult Treatment Panel III)

Risk Assessment Tool for Estimating 10-year Risk of Developing Hard CHD (Myocardial Infarction and Coronary Death)

The risk assessment tool below uses recent data from the Framingham Heart Study to estimate 10-year risk for "hard" coronary heart disease outcomes (myocardial infarction and coronary death). This tool is designed to estimate risk in adults aged 20 and older who do not have heart disease or diabetes. Use the calculator below to estimate 10-year risk.

Age: years
Gender: Female Male
Total Cholesterol: mg/dL
HDL Cholesterol: mg/dL
Smoker: No Yes
Systolic Blood Pressure: mm/Hg
Currently on any medication to treat high blood pressure. No Yes

Calculate 10-Year Risk

Available at: http://hin.nhlbi.bih.gov/atpiii/calculator,asp. Accessed March 25, 2005.

FIGURE 2 A cholesterol management implementation tool based on ATP III. *Abbreviations*: CHD, coronary heart disease; HDL, high-density lipoprotein; ATP, Adult Treatment Panel.

identify high-risk candidates are being sought. Most of those found have not greatly enhanced global risk assessment beyond the Framingham Study multivariable risk profile. Some factors have not been confirmed as playing an independent role.

Subgroups of high-density lipoprotein (HDL) and low-density lipoprotein (LDL) are associated with CHD, but the utility of these refinements over the standard lipoprotein determinations is not well established (32). Similarly, Lp(a) is associated with CHD and stroke in some studies (33). Only 6 of 10 large prospective studies found it to be an independent risk factor, and its importance is uncertain (34). Elevated triglyceride is consistently associated with increased CHD risk, but its predictive power is often lost or attenuated when HDL cholesterol or diabetes is taken into account. However a recent meta-analysis of 17 studies strongly suggests an independent incremental triglyceride CHD risk, particularly when the LDL or total/HDL cholesterol ratio is high (35).

Evidence linking plasma homocysteine to CVD is more convincing. An impressive 75 clinical and population studies have shown that it is associated with CVD (36). Homocysteine risk is also biologically plausible because it affects the coagulation system and the resistance of the endothelium to thromboembolism and may influence the vasodilator and antithrombotic effects of nitric oxide. Because thrombosis plays an important role in the development of atherosclerotic plaques and in precipitating acute coronary events, the Framingham Study tested the hypothesis that elevated homocysteine increases CVD risk by raising the potential for thrombus development (37). In the Framingham Offspring cohort an increase in homocysteine was found to be associated with higher levels of plasminogen activator inhibitor (PAI)-1, tissue plasminogen activator (tPA) antigen, von Willebrand factor, and level of fibrinogen. Significant associations between homocysteine and PAI-1 and tPA antigen persisted after adjustment for covariates, leading to the conclusion that increased homocysteine is associated with an impaired fibrinolytic potential. This finding offers the possibility that the use of folic acid or vitamin B_{12} to lower homocysteine may decrease excess CVD risk by reducing the thrombotic tendency (12).

Proteinuria and microalbuminuria are cited as important *new* risk factors for CVD. However, back in 1984, the Framingham Study reported that even a trace of proteinuria in casual urine specimens imparted a threefold excess mortality rate, and that proteinuria prevalence was three times more common in hypertensive persons and also occurred in excess in diabetics and persons with cardiac enlargement (38). Men with proteinuria reported increased ass-cause CVD mortality even when other contributing risk factors were taken into account. It was concluded that "proteinuria in the ambulatory general population is not benign and carries a serious prognosis. It appears to reflect widespread vascular damage."

Microalbuminuria predicts clinical proteinuria and early mortality in Type 2 diabetics, and increased urinary albumin excretion by sensitive immunoassay has been used for more than three decades to predict impending nephropathy in diabetics (39). Haffner et al. suggest that microalbuminuria should also be used as a CVD risk factor in *nondiabetics* (40). Increased urinary albumin excretion proportional to the size of the infarction is found in acute MI (41). It is also found after exercise-induced angina and intermittent claudication (42). The great sensitivity of the kidney to inflammatory conditions makes it difficult to establish an independent relationship of microalbuminuria to development of CVD. Valmadrid et al. recently established prospectively that microalbuminuria and gross proteinuria are independent risk factors for cardiovascular mortality in persons with Type 2 diabetes (43). Alterations in the fraction of plasma filtered by the glomerulus because of changes in blood pressure and intraglomerular pressure regulation produce large changes in urinary albumin excretion; this explains the correlation between microalbuminuria and blood pressure (44).

The recent Framingham Study investigation of the prognostic significance of casual dip stick proteinuria in older persons found, after adjusting for other CVD risk factors and serum creatinine, a hazard ratio of 1.3 for all-cause mortality associated with a trace or more of proteinuria in men. For women, trace proteinuria was associated with a hazard ratio of 1.6 for CVD death and 1.4 for all-cause mortality (45). The association between renal insufficiency and risk for adverse outcomes is apparently strongly related to the coexisting CVD and CVD risk factors (46).

A number of hemostatic and inflammatory factors are important promoters of occlusive atherogenic disease. Inflammatory markers such as leukocyte count, serum amyloid A, and

C-reactive protein (CRP) are the key markers that have been investigated in the population setting in relation to vascular outcomes in persons free of CVD at baseline. A high-normal leukocyte count is associated with increased CVD risk. Unfortunately, leukocyte counts need to be determined on fresh specimens, and current cigarette smoking can increase leukocyte counts, limiting the utility of the test. Similar to the CRP with which it is highly correlated, leukocyte count is not specific for vascular disease risk (47). A meta-analysis of seven studies by Danesh et al. estimates a 1.4-fold excess CHD risk for an elevated (upper third) leukocyte count compared with the bottom third of its distribution (48).

CRP is a confirmed risk factor for CHD along with other circulating markers of inflammation (49). Prospective studies of asymptomatic persons comparing people with low tertile CRP with those having top tertile values suggest a risk factor–adjusted odds ratio of 1.8 (95% confidence interval 1.6–2.0) for CHD among healthy persons or those with prior CHD (48). It would seem that these findings merit consideration of inflammatory markers for incorporation into CHD risk estimation algorithms. However, inflammatory and hematologic markers currently are not included in the roster of factors used to predict multivariable CVD risk in the population setting. Whether CRP enhances multivariable risk estimation based on the standard risk factors has been questioned (50).

Starting in the 1970s, elevated fibrinogen levels were shown to be a major independent risk factor for heart disease and stroke outcomes in several population studies (Fig. 3). CVD, CHD, and all-cause mortality are all increased in men and women with higher fibrinogen concentrations, and this excess mortality persists after adjusting for the standard risk factors. Higher fibrinogen levels enhance the CHD risk of hypertensive and dyslipidemic persons, cigarette smokers, and diabetics.

It seems likely that elevation of fibrinogen is a pathway by which CVD risk factors exert their thrombotic effect. Recent investigation of fibrinogen by the Framingham Study extends its interrelationship with risk factors to a number of additional ones (51). There were significant linear trends across fibrinogen tertiles ($p < 0.001$) for age, body mass index (BMI), smoking, diabetes mellitus, total cholesterol, HDL cholesterol, and triglycerides in men and women. Also, in both men and women, after adjustment for age, BMI, smoking, diabetes mellitus, total cholesterol, and triglycerides, fibrinogen was significantly higher in cases than noncases. The several mechanisms by which fibrinogen may increase cardiovascular risk include enhancement of platelet aggregation and promotion of fibrin formation, and as a major contributor to plasma viscosity. It is also an acute-phase reactant that is increased in inflammatory states.

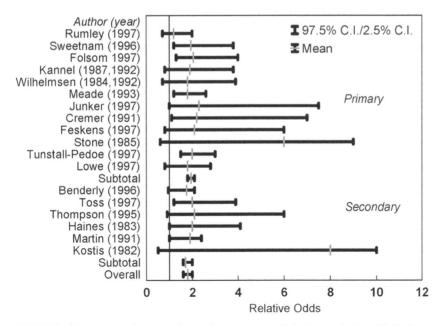

FIGURE 3 Fibrinogen and coronary heart disease meta-analysis (top vs. bottom third). *Source:* From Ref. 48.

Other hemostatic variables have also been shown to be related to established cardiovascular risk factors and prevalent CVD (52). Fibrinogen increases with age, smoking, waist/hip ratio, and LDL cholesterol and decreases in relation to educational level, physical activity, alcohol intake, and HDL cholesterol. Factor VII increases with BMI, waist/hip ratio, triglycerides, and HDL and LDL cholesterol. PAI-1 increases with BMI, waist/hip ratio, triglycerides, alcohol intake, and smoking and decreases with physical activity.

The increased risk of CVD associated with elevated LDL levels may be mediated in part through fibrinogen. Fibrinogen influences the risk of CHD at any level of LDL cholesterol. The Prospective Cardiovascular Munster study found that elevated LDL cholesterol imposes an ominous CHD risk when accompanied by a high fibrinogen (53).

Statins that reduce both LDL cholesterol and CRP appear to have a variable influence on CHD outcomes depending on the CRP level. Patients with a low CRP after statin therapy experience better clinical outcomes of MI or CHD mortality than those with higher CRP, regardless of resultant LDL cholesterol on treatment (54).

Thompson et al. (55) found fibrinogen to be a strong predictor of coronary events in patients with angina pectoris (AP). In subjects with high total cholesterol, a high fibrinogen level conferred added risk compared with those with low fibrinogen. Patients in the highest fibrinogen quintile had three times the risk of a coronary event than those in the lowest quintile.

Fibrinogen has not been widely adopted for risk stratification and prevention, partly because we lack interventions that consistently lower fibrinogen and reduce CHD events via this mechanism, although there is some evidence that therapy used for dyslipidemia is capable of lowering fibrinogen (56). However, the optimal fibrinogen assay for risk stratification is uncertain. In the Framingham Study, the immunoprecipitation test showed a stronger association with CVD than the Clauss method, suggesting that it may be a preferred screening tool to identify individuals at increased thrombotic risk of CVD (51).

HYPERTENSION

Blood pressure is deservedly a major component of multivariable cardiovascular risk profiles. Hypertension is a major, highly prevalent, and independent cause of vascular disease. Because CVD risk increases incrementally with the blood pressure (even within the high-normal range) and because moderate blood pressure elevation is so much more prevalent than severe hypertension, a large fraction of the CVD attributable to hypertension derives from seemingly innocuous levels of blood pressure elevation. Its high prevalence, powerful impact, and controllability give it a high priority for detection, risk stratification, and treatment.

The CVD risk hypertension imposes varies in relation to age, the degree of the blood pressure elevation, which blood pressure component is increased, the vital organ in jeopardy, and the burden of coexisting risk factors. Guidelines recently promulgated by the Seventh Joint National Committee on Hypertension (JNC VII) recommend consideration of lesser blood pressure elevations for treatment (28). Efficient treatment of blood pressure in the high-normal range that is now recommended requires multivariable risk stratification to be cost-effective and avoid needlessly alarming patients.

The JNC VII guidelines for detection, evaluation, and treatment of elevated blood pressure recognize that systolic blood pressure is more important than diastolic blood pressure, citing an incremental CVD risk extending down to what was previously regarded as the normal range, and defining a *prehypertensive* blood pressure category. Certain high-risk conditions are designated *compelling indications* that call for more stringent blood pressure goals (28). However, a notable omission among these is dyslipidemia, a condition that commonly accompanies hypertension and should also modify the blood pressure treatment goal because of its great influence on hypertensive CVD risk.

In agreement with most physicians who consider the maximum value of the blood pressure to be the most important consideration for treatment of hypertension, the British Hypertension Society guidelines assert that "the main determinant of benefit from blood pressure lowering is the achieved blood pressure, rather than the choice of therapy" (57). There is in fact, a continuous, graded influence of blood pressure on the incidence and mortality of CVD, but there is an unfortunate tendency for some clinicians to accept higher blood pressures as innocuous in the elderly; it is evident from prospective epidemiological data that at all

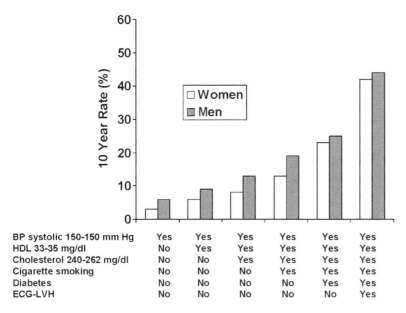

BP systolic 150-150 mm Hg	Yes	Yes	Yes	Yes	Yes	Yes
HDL 33-35 mg/dl	No	Yes	Yes	Yes	Yes	Yes
Cholesterol 240-262 mg/dl	No	No	Yes	Yes	Yes	Yes
Cigarette smoking	No	No	No	Yes	Yes	Yes
Diabetes	No	No	No	No	Yes	Yes
ECG-LVH	No	No	No	No	No	Yes

FIGURE 4 Risk of coronary disease in hypertension according to level of risk factors: Framingham Study (subject aged 42–48 years). *Source*: From Ref. 58.

ages, the hazard of CVD at any blood pressure is substantially greater if it is accompanied by other risk factors (Fig. 4). Furthermore, an examination of the systolic blood pressures at which CVD events occurred in Framingham Study male participants indicated that 45% occurred at systolic pressures below 140 mmHg, often designated as the threshold of *hypertensive* CVD risk.

The large Multiple Risk Factor Intervention Trial data set, which comprised more than 347,000 male screenees, provides a precise estimate of incremental CVD incidence at systolic blood pressures below 140 mmHg (59). These data confirm a continuous graded influence of systolic blood pressure on CHD mortality at pressures below 140 mmHg, with similar regression coefficients at all ages (Table 6). The Prospective Studies Collaboration meta-analysis of data from almost one million participants and 56,000 deaths also found blood pressure related to vascular mortality without a threshold down to 115/75 mmHg. Risk of stroke or coronary mortality doubles with every 20 mm increment in systolic blood pressure (or 10 mm diastolic) throughout the entire range (61). The Framingham Study documented this incremental risk at nonhypertensive blood pressures in age- and risk factor–adjusted analyses (62). Compared with optimal, high-normal blood pressure conferred a 1.6 to 2.5–fold risk of a "hard" CVD event (Fig. 5). Antecedent blood pressure within the normal range has also been shown to be a determinant of future hypertension in the Framingham Study, providing another reason for concern about even minimal blood pressure elevation. A prudent blood pressure for avoiding CVD is < 140/90 mmHg with no clearly defined critical blood pressure that distinguishes "normal" from abnormal. However, for cost-effective treatment

TABLE 6 Systolic Blood Pressure and Coronary Mortality (316,099 Screened for Multiple Risk Factor Intervention Trial)

Quintiles of systolic blood pressure (mmHg)	Number of CHD deaths	Crude CHD death rate per 10,000 person-years	Age-adjusted relative risk
<118	609	8.2	1.00 (referent)
118–124	763	10.4	1.2 ($p < 0.05$)
125–131	973	13.6	1.5 ($p < 0.05$)
132–141	1331	18.1	1.8 ($p < 0.05$)
≥142	2414	35.7	3.0 ($p < 0.05$)

Abbreviation: CHD, coronary heart disease.
Source: From Ref. 60.

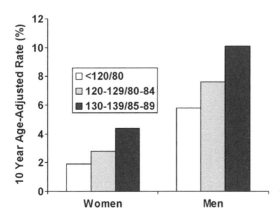

FIGURE 5 Relation of nonhypertensive blood pressure to cardiovascular disease (Framingham subjects aged 35–90 years). *Source*: From Ref. 63.

of *prehypertension* and stage 1 hypertension, multivariable risk stratification is needed, and the goal of therapy should be to improve the global CVD risk rather than to simply lower the blood pressure.

There appears to be lingering uncertainty about the CVD impact of the various components of the blood pressure. Medical concepts about the hazards of hypertension have been preoccupied with the diastolic blood pressure since the beginning of the 20th century. Only lately has the focus shifted to the systolic blood pressure and, most recently, to the pulse pressure. Framingham Study data, based on three decades of follow-up of subjects in relation to their pulse pressure, indicate a continuous, graded increase in CVD event rates of about 20% for each 10 mm increment in pulse pressure for persons aged 35 to 64 years. The incremental risk is somewhat lower (10.5% per 10 mmHg) in older women, but not for older men (61).

Vascular hemodynamics suggests that pulse pressure plays an important role in the development of CVD. Assessment of these pressure components individually in the Framingham Study indicated that increments of pulse pressure at particular systolic pressures are associated with greater CHD incidence than the converse. A major impediment to evaluating the net impact of the components of the blood pressure on the structure and function of the heart and other vital organs is their high correlation ($r = 0.9$) with each other. There is also an interaction with age. With increasing age, there is a shift in importance from diastolic to systolic and finally to pulse pressure for prediction of CHD. From age 60 on, diastolic pressure is negatively correlated with CHD incidence, so that pulse pressure becomes superior to systolic pressure (64). However, not all investigators agree about the relative importance of systolic and pulse pressure, even in the elderly.

In the past, because of the concept of *benign essential hypertension* and lack of the means for lowering blood pressure, emphasis was placed on identifying correctable causes of hypertension. Currently, extensive testing to identify causes of hypertension is not recommended unless there are findings pointing to secondary hypertension or that blood pressure control cannot be achieved. They account for only a small percentage of the hypertension encountered in clinical practice. A more common cause now being considered is the obesity-induced insulin-resistance or metabolic syndrome. The connection between abdominal adiposity, insulin resistance, and hypertension has received considerable attention, but there is uncertainty as to whether elevated blood pressure is an intrinsic feature of the metabolic syndrome or an associated condition. However, it is clear that when the blood pressure elevation is accompanied by features of the syndrome, its hazard is escalated.

Until very recently the dominant concept of hypertension pathogenesis overemphasized vascular resistance and underestimated the influence of arterial stiffness. Despite the demonstrated efficacy of treating *systolic* hypertension, the reported poor blood pressure control is overwhelmingly due to failure to control the systolic component (65). Guidelines now place greater emphasis on achieving specified *systolic* blood pressure goals.

The JNC VII report reflects upon a number of "special considerations" that require attention in the treatment of hypertension, including "compelling indications" and other "special situations." Among the latter are minority populations, obesity, the metabolic syndrome, left ventricular hypertrophy, peripheral artery disease, old age, postural hypotension, dementia, hypertension in women, children and adolescents, and hypertensive urgencies and emergencies (28).

Although the treatment recommended in minorities is similar for all demographic groups, there are socioeconomic and lifestyle barriers to blood pressure control in Mexican and Native Americans. The prevalence, severity, and impact of hypertension are greater in blacks, and they do not respond adequately to monotherapy. Left ventricular hypertrophy is an ominous feature of hypertension that independently escalates the risk of future CVD, equivalent to that of persons who already have overt atherosclerotic CVD. Peripheral artery disease is another condition equivalent to having CHD. Older persons, who have the bulk of hypertension in the population, have the poorest rate of blood pressure control. Interest in diabetes, an important component of hypertensive CVD risk, now focuses on lesser degrees of glucose intolerance as a component of an insulin-resistant metabolic syndrome.

The JNC VII notes a number of "compelling indications" that merit special attention and follow-up, and these conditions also require more stringent blood pressure targets. Included in this list are heart failure, post-MI status, high CHD risk (i.e., >20% hazard for 10 years), diabetes, chronic renal disease, and prior stroke. These have not been incorporated into multivariable risk profiles. However, different choices of antihypertensive therapy and blood pressure goals are advocated for each, based on trial data. Diabetic hypertension usually requires two or more drugs to achieve the recommended blood pressure goal of 130/80 mmHg. Renal disease requires aggressive blood pressure management, often needing the use of three drugs to reach the recommended target of <130/80 mmHg.

Elevated blood pressure seldom occurs in the absence of other CVD risk factors. More than 80% have one or more coexistent risk factors, and 55% of men and women have two or more, meeting the diagnostic criteria for the metabolic syndrome. Because the amount of risk factor clustering profoundly influences the CVD risk of elevated blood pressure, all hypertensive patients should be tested for other risk factors such as elevated total and LDL cholesterol, high triglycerides and glucose, increased BMI or waist girth, and reduced HDL cholesterol. These allow multivariable risk stratification of hypertension. Multivariable risk formulations for quantifying the impact of a set of risk factors for development of CVD have been developed from Framingham Study data. The composite risk factor score derived from the data corresponds to the probability of an event over 10 years. These estimated event rates when compared to the average risk for same-aged persons provide absolute and relative risks (Fig. 2). The Framingham point score system of risk estimation—recently adopted by the Adult Treatment Panel (ATP) III guidelines for assessment and treatment of dyslipidemia—linking the indication, intensity, and goal of therapy to the 10-year multivariable risk was not proposed for hypertension by JNC VII. This approach would appear to also be appropriate for persons with hypertension.

Hypertensive persons usually have dyslipidemia, abdominal obesity, and/or impaired glucose tolerance. These risk factors are components of the metabolic or insulin-resistance syndrome cited by the JNC VII as meriting special consideration. However, because most of the ingredients of the syndrome are also components of the Framingham multivariable risk formulation, the value of detecting persons with the metabolic syndrome applies more to therapeutic choices than to risk stratification. Hypertensive patients at high multivariable risk stand to benefit the most from treatment and the number needed to treat to prevent one event is lowest in this high-risk segment.

DIABETES

Type 2 diabetes is another accepted component of global risk assessment. The prevalence of Type 2 diabetes in the United States has been increasing, which is ominous because Type 2 diabetes is now regarded as a CHD equivalent in risk assessment (29). The CVD risk that diabetes imposes appears to antedate its overt appearance, residing in a *prediabetic* state of impaired glucose tolerance and insulin resistance that has been characterized as a metabolic syndrome (29). Increased risk of CHD has been reported in persons with impaired glucose tolerance, in the metabolic syndrome and in Type 2 diabetes (29). Hypertension is often a component of a metabolic syndrome composed of dyslipidemia, elevated blood pressure, and abdominal obesity. This entity has been defined by the National Cholesterol Education Program-ATP III as

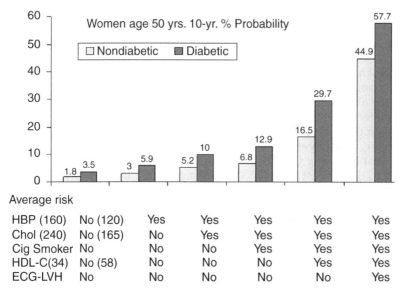

FIGURE 6 Risk of coronary disease by diabetic status according to level of risk factors: Framingham Study. *Abbreviations*: HBP, high blood pressure, HDL-c, high-density lipoprotein-c; ECG-LVH, electrocardiogram-left ventricular hypertrophy. *Source*: From Ref. 67, 68.

requiring the presence of three or more of the following: blood pressure $\geq 130/85$ mmHg, fasting glucose ≥ 110 mg/dL, reduced HDL-cholesterol (<40 mg/dL for men and <50 mg/dL for women), triglycerides ≥ 150 mg/dL, waist circumference >40 in men and >35 in for women (29). About 22% of American men and 24% of American women over 20 years of age have the syndrome. It imposes a threefold increased risk of CHD and fivefold risk of CVD mortality. It carries a lesser risk than overt diabetes, but because it is much more prevalent, it imposes a greater attributable risk for the general population.

The CVD risk in patients with Type 2 diabetes varies according to the amount of risk factor clustering that accompanies it (Fig. 6) (66). The cluster of risk factors that commonly accompany diabetes are chiefly those now designated as components of the metabolic syndrome. The CVD risk factors that comprise the syndrome are each predictors of the occurrence of diabetes itself, imposing a fivefold increased risk of Type 2 diabetes (2,69).

The approach to diabetes as a CVD risk factor now should be broadened to consider the insulin-resistance syndrome promoted by abdominal obesity and the cluster of risk factors that accompany it (29). A number of novel risk factors have been noted to accompany the syndrome and insulin-resistant state including small, dense LDL, endothelial dysfunction, CRP, and a pro-thrombotic tendency with elevated PAI-1 (70,71). The prevalence of the metabolic syndrome tends to increase with age, more steeply in women than in men. However, its prevalence in men exceeds that in women at all ages. Diabetes is found in only 16% of persons with the metabolic syndrome, whereas more than half the number of diabetics have the components of the metabolic syndrome. Because of its greater prevalence, substantial hazard, and greater population attributable risk, the metabolic syndrome should be routinely sought out in overweight elderly persons by periodically measuring the CVD risk factors that comprise it, and its components treated before the onset of overt Type 2 diabetes, which ensues and carries a greater risk of CVD. It now appears that for Type 2 diabetics, more emphasis should be placed on correcting the components of the metabolic insulin-resistance syndrome than on controlling the blood sugar.

DYSLIPIDEMIA

Because a causal association of dyslipidemia with the development of atherosclerotic CVD is established by epidemiological, clinical, angiographic, and postmortem investigations, it is a major component of multivariable risk assessment. It is established that treating dyslipidemia substantially reduces the CVD hazard it imposes (29). There is a substantial overlap of the

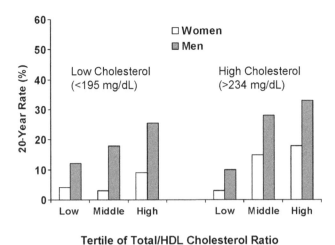

FIGURE 7 Coronary heart disease risk by total/HDL cholesterol ratio at low and high serum total cholesterol. *Abbreviation*: HDL, high-density lipoprotein. *Source*: Unpublished Framingham Study data.

distributions for all the lipids in cases and noncases and each of the blood lipids influences the risk of CHD in a continuous graded fashion, even within the range of lipid values that are considered normal. Population data and primary and secondary lipid-treatment prevention trials suggest that each 1% increase in total cholesterol, throughout its range, yields a 2% increment in CHD incidence. Similarly, comparable reduction in LDL-cholesterol however achieved, produces the same 2% reduction in initial or recurrent coronary events (29). Average lipid values at which CHD occurs is higher in women, decreases with age, and has been declining over the past five decades (72).

An efficient lipid profile for estimating CHD potential is the total/HDL cholesterol ratio, which affords a practical indication of the net effect of the cholesterol entering the arterial intima in the LDL and being removed in the HDL (73). This ratio determines the CHD risk whether the total cholesterol is above or below 240 mg/dL (Fig. 7). Optimal treatment of dyslipidemia at any age should improve this ratio to 3.5, a ratio that corresponds to half the high-average CHD risk. A high triglyceride (>150 mg/dL) in association with a reduced HDL-cholesterol (<40 mg/dL) signifies the presence of insulin resistance and more atherogenic small, dense LDL (71). Dyslipidemic CHD risk is also strongly influenced by the burden of associated risk factors (Table 7). Measurement of other risk factors such as blood pressure, blood glucose, and weight is important, because these usually cluster with dyslipidemia and profoundly influence the risk it imposes. These measurements allow multivariable risk stratification of dyslipidemia. Dyslipidemia also tends to cluster with thrombogenic risk factors such as PAI-1, and when associated with inflammatory markers such as CRP, it is especially dangerous (69,74). These covariates have not yet been widely accepted as components of multivariable risk profiles. It has been postulated that there is a metabolic basis for other atherogenic risk factors to cluster with dyslipidemia and hypertension (75).

High-risk coronary candidates cannot be identified based solely on their lipid values, making it necessary to evaluate dyslipidemia in the context of a multivariable risk assessment. Such global risk assessment is recommended by the ATP III guidelines for the evaluation and treatment of dyslipidemic risk using Framingham Study multivariable risk formulations to estimate the 10-year probability of developing CHD (29). Dyslipidemic persons at high global risk (>20% 10-year risk) are assigned more stringent LDL-cholesterol goals. Although epidemiological data show very little relationship between dyslipidemia and development of stroke, clinical trials indicate that statin therapy reduces stroke risk. It is postulated that this benefit derives from statin effects on platelet aggregation and endothelial dysfunction.

PREVENTIVE MANAGEMENT BASED ON RISK ASSESSMENT

Because of a continuous, graded relationship for all risk factors leading to CHD, and a substantial overlap of the distributions of their values in cases and noncases, it is not possible to select

TABLE 7   Twenty-Year Incidence of Coronary Heart Disease Associated with Elevated Lipids by Extent of Risk Factor Clustering: Framingham Offspring Cohort (Age-Adjusted Incidence Per 1000)

Number of risk factors	High cholesterol		High LDL cholesterol	
	Men	**Women**	**Men**	**Women**
None	126	51	159	8
One	158	84	167	12
Two or more	289	148	319	137

Note: Associated risk factors: high triglycerides, low HDL cholesterol, high BMI, high systolic BP, high blood glucose.
Abbreviations: LDL, low-density lipoprotein; HDL, high-density lipoprotein; BMI, body mass index; BP, blood pressure.
Source: Unpublished Framingham Study data.

critical risk factor values that definitively separate potential CHD cases from the rest of the population (59,72). Epidemiological population data and primary and secondary prevention trials suggest that each percentage increase in risk factor level, throughout its range, yields a corresponding percentage increment in CHD (76). Similarly, comparable reduction in risk factor levels, however achieved, produces similar percent reductions in initial or recurrent coronary events (76,77). The benefits of reducing the level of the major risk factors are well established for primary prevention of initial coronary events, and for secondary prevention in those already afflicted. However, in assessing the benefits, more attention needs to be paid to the *absolute* risk reduction attainable rather than the *relative* risk reduction, because the number needed to treat to prevent one case increases when the risk of the person treated decreases. Also, one must treat more to prevent one event when treating persons who have not yet sustained a cardiovascular event than persons who already are afflicted.

Hypertension, dyslipidemia, and diabetes promote accelerated atherogenesis, and correcting them stabilizes lesions and slows progression. Treatment is of proven benefit for initial and recurrent events without a penalty in overall mortality. The prevalence of these conditions in the general population is unacceptably high, and isolated occurrence of these major CVD risk factors is relatively uncommon. Because the average blood pressure, blood lipid, and glucose levels at which most coronary events occur is rather modest, multivariable risk assessment to target a high-risk subset is required.

Multivariable risk profiles for candidates for renal failure have not yet been crafted despite the identification of a number of predisposing risk factors. Persons in the general population who are at high risk for renal failure despite lack of a history of primary renal disease can be detected by screening for albuminuria, especially in hypertensive, obese, diabetic, or prediabetic persons with the metabolic syndrome (78). Therapies available to reduce albumin excretion include angiotensin-converting enzyme inhibitors, angiotensin receptor blockers, and statins, which if started early enough can reduce the likelihood of developing clinical renal disease and accompanying CVD.

It is likely that hemostatic and inflammatory indicators will soon be considered for inclusion in future versions of multivariable risk equations. Atherosclerotic cardiovascular events are commonly manifested via a thrombotic event. The process of clotting involves coagulation; it is limited and controlled by anticoagulation; and the counter-balancing process of fibrinolysis is limited by antifibrinolysis. Thrombosis clearly precipitates the acute manifestations of coronary, cerebrovascular, and peripheral artery disease. The role of hemostatic factors in the development of the *underlying atherosclerotic* lesions has been difficult to prove (79). There is the possibility that the association between hemostatic factors and CVD may be due to confounding by other risk factors or may result from the disease rather than causing it. It may also act as part of a causal pathway that requires interaction with other cardiovascular risk factors or already existing atherosclerotic disease. There are also issues about measurement of hemostatic factors that need to be resolved. Nevertheless, investigation has incriminated a number of coagulation factors such as fibrinogen, factor VII, factor VIII, and platelet aggregability. Fibrinolytic factors have also been implicated, including tPA PAI-1, Lp(a), and plasminogen or global fibrinolytic activity.

CONCLUSIONS

A preventive approach to atherosclerotic CVD is feasible and crucial because once clinically manifest, the disease is apt to progress with lethal consequences, and treatment can seldom cure or restore the patient to full function. Prevention is now feasible because epidemiological research has identified a number of modifiable predisposing lifestyles and personal attributes that, when corrected, have been shown to reduce the likelihood of the development of clinical atherosclerotic CVD. The Framingham Study and others have quantified several classes of cardiovascular risk factors—including atherosclerotic personal attributes, lifestyles that promote risk, signs of organ damage, and innate susceptibility. Those easy to ascertain during an office visit are a cigarette smoking history, blood lipids, glucose intolerance, blood pressure, and left ventricular hypertrophy as manifested on the electrocardiogram. To cost-effectively evaluate candidates for the major cardiovascular events, multivariable risk profiles have been formulated to facilitate targeting those at high risk for preventive measures. The American Heart Association and National Heart, Lung, and Blood Institute emphasize the importance of these risk profiles for motivating as well as reassuring patients, and to assist in selection of therapy. These scores direct health care professionals to look at the whole patient and to recognize the cumulative nature of risk factors.

Risk factor alteration significantly reduces the risk of initial and recurrent atherosclerotic CVD events. Hypertension, dyslipidemia, and diabetes are best regarded as ingredients of a CVD multivariable risk profile comprised of metabolically linked risk factors, because the hazard of each varies widely, contingent on the associated burden of risk factors. Maximum CVD risk reduction, even in diabetics, is best achieved by the concomitant control of the accompanying burden of risk factors that often constitute the metabolic syndrome (80).

Physicians treating the elderly should seek out more commonly encountered preclinical stages of the atherosclerotic diseases such as the abnormal Ankle Brachial Index, arterial vascular bruits, coronary artery calcification, left ventricular hypertrophy, a low ejection fraction, and silent MI, among others. High-risk candidates with an ominous multivariable risk profile indicating a 10-year risk of an event exceeding 20% deserve more aggressive risk factor modification. The goal of therapy concerning lipids, blood sugar, and blood pressure should be linked to the global level of risk. Physicians should more aggressively implement the guideline goals concerning management of patients at risk of atherosclerotic CVD.

Multivariable risk formulations are available for each of the major atherosclerotic CVD outcomes. Because of shared risk factors, the CHD multivariable risk formulation is likely to also be predictive of the other atherosclerotic CVD outcomes in aggregate. Health care providers should invoke multivariable risk assessment whenever a patient is evaluated or treated for obesity, diabetes, dyslipidemia, or hypertension. The laboratory to which blood samples are sent for testing of blood sugar, or blood lipids, should be encouraged to request the other ingredients of the CVD risk profile, including blood pressure and cigarette smoking history and provide a multivariable estimate of risk along with the lipid or glucose determination requested. Serial assessment of global risk should be undertaken in patients on treatment. Improvement in the multivariable risk score can be used to motivate the patient to continue with the recommended program. If treatment goals are unmet, additional resources may be required, including a dietician, a consultant, social workers to help with finances, and family support such as a concerned daughter.

The epidemic of CVD cannot be conquered solely by cardiologists caring for referred patients. The entire health care system has to be mobilized. Unfortunately, the U.S. health care system rewards provision of procedures more than preventive services. Despite means available to identify high-risk candidates and proof of the efficacy of modifying predisposing risk factors, goals for risk factor control are often unmet.

REFERENCES

1. Kannel WB, Dawber TR, Kagan A, et al. Factors of risk in development of coronary heart disease—six-year follow-up experience: the Framingham Study. Ann Intern Med 1961; 55:33–50.
2. Report of Intersociety Commission for Heart Disease. Resources for primary prevention of atherosclerotic disease. Circulation 1984; 70(suppl A):155A–205A.
3. Gordon T, Kannel WB. Premature mortality from coronary heart disease: the Framingham Study. JAMA 1971; 215:1617–1625.
4. Kannel WB, Abbott RD. Incidence and prognosis of unrecognized myocardial infarction: an update on the Framingham Study. N Engl J Med 1984; 311:1144–1147.

5. American Heart Association. Heart disease and stroke statistics: 2004 update. Dallas, TX: American Heart Association; 2003.

6. Lloyd-Jones DM, Larson MG, Beiser A, Levy D. Lifetime risk of developing coronary heart disease. Lancet 1999; 353:89–92.

7. Lloyd-Jones DM, Wilson PWF, Larson MG, et al. Lifetime heart disease by cholesterol levels at selected ages. Arch Intern Med 2003; 163:1966–1972.

8. Lloyd-Jones DM, Wilson PW, Larson MG, et al. Framingham risk score and prediction of lifetime risk for coronary heart disease. Am J Cardiol 2004; 94:20–24.

9. Brand RJ, Rosenman RH, Sholz RI, Friedman M. Multivariate prediction of coronary heart disease in the Western Collaborative Group Study compared to the findings of the Framingham Study. Circulation 1976; 53:348–355.

10. Leaverton PE, Sorlie PD, Kleinman JC, et al. Representativeness of the Framingham risk model for coronary heart disease mortality: a comparison with a national cohort study. J Chronic Dis 1987; 40:775–784.

11. McGee D, Gordon. The results of the Framingham Study applied to four other S.S.-based studies of cardiovascular disease. In: Kannel WB, Gordon T, eds. The Framingham Study: an Epidemiological Investigation of Cardiovascular Disease. Section 31. U.S. Dept of Health Education and Welfare Publication no. 76-1083. Bethesda, MD: U.S. Government Printing Office, 1976.

12. D'Agostino RB, Grundy S, Sullivan LM, Wilson P. For the CHD Risk Prediction Group. Validation of the Framingham risk prediction scores. Results of a multiple ethnic group investigation. JAMA 2001; 286:180–187.

13. Grundy SM. United States Cholesterol Guidelines 2001: expanded scope of intensive low-density lipoprotein lowering therapy. Am J Cardiol 2001; 88:23J–27J.

14. Kannel WB, Castelli WP, Gordon T. Cholesterol in the prediction of atherosclerotic disease. New perspectives based on the Framingham Study. Ann Intern Med 1979; 90:85–91.

15. DeFronzo RA, Ferrannini E. Insulin resistance: a multifaceted syndrome responsible for NIDDM, obesity, dyslipidemia, and atherosclerotic cardiovascular disease. Diabetes Care 1991; 14:173–194.

16. Kannel WB, Wilson PW, Nam BH, et al. Risk stratification of obesity as a coronary risk factor. Am J Cardiol 2002; 90:697–701.

17. Kannel WB, Wilson PW. Comparison of risk profiles for cardiovascular events: implications for prevention. Adv Intern Med 1997; 42:39.

18. Wolf PA, D'Agostino RB, Belanger AJ, et al. Probability of stroke: a risk profile from the Framingham study. Stroke 1991; 3:312–318.

19. Kannel WB, McGee DL. Diabetes and glucose tolerance as risk factors for cardiovascular disease: the Framingham Study. Diabetes Care 1979; 2:120–126.

20. Manson JE, Colditz GA, Stampfer MJ, et al. A prospective study of maturity-onset diabetes and risk of coronary heart disease and stroke in women. Arch Intern Med 1991; 151:1141–1147.

21. Kannel WB, D'Agostino RB. The importance of cardiovascular risk factors in the elderly. Am J Geriatr Cardiol 1995; 2:10–23.

22. Kannel WB, McGee DL, Gordon T. A general cardiovascular risk profile: the Framingham Study. Am J Cardiol 1976; 38:46–51.

23. Anderson KM, Wilson PWF, Odell PM, et al. An updated coronary risk profile: a statement for health professionals. Circulation 1991; 83:357–363.

24. Murabito JM, D'Agostino RB, Silberschatz H, Wilson PWF. Intermittent claudication: a risk profile from the Framingham Heart Study. Circulation 1997; 96:44–49.

25. Wilson PW, D'Agostino RB, Levy D, Belanger AM, Silbershatz H, Kannel WB. Prediction of coronary heart disease using risk factor categories. Circulation 1998; 97:1837–1847.

26. Kannel WB, D'Agostino RB, Silbershatz H, et al. Profile for estimating risk of heart failure. Arch Intern Med 1999; 159:1197–1204.

27. www.framinghamheartstudy.org.

28. Chobanian AV, Bakris GL, Black HR, et al. The seventh report of the Joint National Committee on prevention, detection, evaluation, and treatment of high blood pressure: the JNC 7 report. JAMA 2003; 289:2560–2572.

29. Executive Summary of the Third Report of the National Cholesterol Education Program (NCEP) Expert Panel on Detection, Evaluation, and Treatment of High Blood Cholesterol in Adults (Adult Treatment Panel III). JAMA 2001; 285:2486–2497.

30. Khot UN, Khot MB, Bajer CT, et al. Prevalence of conventional risk factors in patients with coronary heart disease. JAMA 2003; 290:898–904.

31. Greenland P, Knoll MD, Stamler J, et al. Major risk factors as antecedents of fatal and non-fatal coronary heart disease events. JAMA 2003; 290:891–897.

32. Wilson PWF. Relation of high-density lipoprotein subfractions and apolipoprotein isoforms to coronary disease. Clin Chem 1995; 41:165–169.

33. Ridker PM, Hennekens CH. Lipoprotein(a) and the risks of cardiovascular disease. Ann Epidemiol 1994; 4:360–362.

34. Nguyen TT, Elleform RD, et al. Lp(a) as a risk factor cardiovascular disease. Circulation 1997; 96:1390–1397.

35. Hokanson JE, Austin MA, Edwards KL. Hypertriglyceridemia as a cardiovascular risk factor independent of high-density lipoprotein: a meta-analysis of population-based prospective studies. J Cardiovasc Risk 1996; 3:213–219.

36. Stampfer MJ, Malinow MR, et al. A prospective study of plasma homocysteine and risk of myocardial infarction in US physicians. JAMA 1992; 24:877–881.
37. Tofler GH, D'Agostino RB, Jacques PF, et al. Association between increased homocysteine levels and impaired fibrinolytic potential: mechanism for cardiovascular risk. Thromb Haemost 2002; 88:799–804.
38. Kannel WB, Stampfer MJ, Castelli WP, Verter J. The prognostic significance of proteinuria: the Framingham Study. Am Heart J 1984; 108:1347–1352.
39. Mogensen CE. Microalbuminuria predicts clinical proteinuria and early mortality in maturity onset diabetics. N Engl J Med 1984; 310:66.
40. Haffner SM, Stein MB, Gruber KK, Hazuda HP, Mitchell BD. Microalbuminuria: potential marker for increased cardiovascular risk factors in non-diabetic subjects? Arteriosclerosis 1990; 10: 727–731.
41. Gosling P, Hughes EA, Reynolds TM, Fox JP. Microalbuminuria is an early response following acute myocardial infarction. Eur Heart J 1991; 123:508–513.
42. Horton RC, Gosling P, Reeves CN, Payne M, Nagle RE. Microalbuminuria excretion in patients with positive exercise electrocardiogram tests. Eur Heart J 1994; 15:1353–1355.
43. Valmadrid CT, Klein R, Moss SE, Klein BE. The risk of cardiovascular disease mortality associated with microalbuminuria and gross proteinuria in persons with older-onset diabetes mellitus. Arch Intern Med 2000; 160:1093–1100.
44. Hartland A, Gosling P. Microalbuminuria: yet another risk factor? Ann Clin Biochem 1999; 36:700–703.
45. Culleton BF, Larson MG, Parfrey PS, Kannel WB, Levy D. Proteinuria as a risk factor for cardiovascular disease and mortality in older people: a prospective study. Am J Med 2000; 109:1–8.
46. Culleton BF, Larson MG, Wilson PW, Evans JC, Parfrey PS, Levy D. Cardiovascular disease and mortality in a community-based cohort with mild renal insufficiency. Kidney Int 1999; 56;2214–2219.
47. Ernst E, Hammerschmidt DE, Bagge U, Matrai A, Dormandy JA. Leukocytes and the risk of ischemic diseases. JAMA 1987; 257:2318–2324.
48. Danesh J, Collins R, Appleby P, Peto R. Association of fibrinogen, C-reactive protein, albumin or leukocyte count with coronary heart disease; meta-analyses of prospective studies. JAMA 1998; 279:1477–1482.
49. Danesh J, Wheeler JG, Hirschfield GM, et al. C-reactive protein and other circulating makers of inflammation in the prediction of coronary heart disease. N Engl J Med 2004; 350:1387–1397.
50. Tall AR. C-reactive protein reassessed. Editorial. N Engl J Med 2004; 350:1450–1452.
51. Stec JJ, Silbershatz H, Tofler GH, et al. Association of fibrinogen with cardiovascular risk factors in the Framingham offspring population. Circulation 2000; 102:1634.
52. Scarabin PY, Aillaud MF, Amouyel P, et al. Association of fibrinogen, factor VII and PAI-1 with baseline findings among 10,500 male participants in a prospective study of myocardial infarction—the PRIME Study. Prospective Epidemiological Study of Myocardial Infarction. Thromb Haemost 1998; 80:749–756.
53. Heinrich J, Balleisen L, Schulte H, Assmann G, van de Loo J. Fibrinogen and factor VII in the prediction of coronary risk. Results from PROCAM study in healthy men. Arterioscler Thromb 1994; 14:54–59.
54. Ridker PM, Cannon CP, Morrow D, et al. Pravastatin or Atorvastatin Evaluation and Infection Therapy-Thrombolysis in Myocardial Infarction 22 (PROVE IT TIMI 22) Investigators. C-reactive protein levels and outcomes after statin therapy. N Engl J Med 2005; 6:352:20–28.
55. Thompson SG, Kienast J, Pyke SD, et al. Hemostatic factors and the risk of myocardial infarction or sudden death in patients with angina pectoris. European Concerted Action on Thrombosis and Disabilities Angina Pectoris Study Group. N Engl J Med 1995; 332:635–641.
56. Branchi A, Rovelini A, et al. Effects of three fibrate derivatives and of 3 HMG CoA reductase inhibitors on plasma fibrinogen levels in patients with primary hypercholesterolemia. Thromb Haemost 1993; 70:241.
57. Williams B, Poulter NR, Brown MJ, et al. British Hypertension Society Guidelines for management of hypertension: report of fourth working party of the British Hypertension Society. J Hum Hypertens BHS IV 2004; 18:139–185.
58. Wilson PWF. Coronary risk prediction in adults: the Framingham Heart Study. Am J Cardiol 1987; 59(G):91–94.
59. Kannel WB, Neaton JD, Wentworth D, et al, (for the Multiple Risk Factor Intervention Trial Research Group). Overall and coronary heart disease mortality rates in relation to major risk factors in 325, 348 men screened for the MRFIT. Am Heart J 1986; 112:825–836.
60. Neaton JD, Wentworth D. Serum cholesterol, blood pressure, cigarette smoking, and death from coronary heart disease. Overall findings and differences by age for 316,099 white men. Multiple Risk Factor Intervention Trial Research Group. Arch Intern Med 1992; 152:56–64.
61. Prospective Studies Collaboration. Age-specific relevance of usual blood pressure to vascular mortality: a meta-analysis of individual data for one million adults in 61 prospective studies. Lancet 2002; 360:1903–1913.
62. Kannel WB, Vasan R, Levy D. Is the relation of systolic blood pressure to risk of cardiovascular disease continuous and graded or are there critical values? Hypertension 2003; 453–456.

63. Vasan RS, Larson MG, Leip EP, et al. Impact of high-normal blood pressure on the risk of cardiovascular disease. N Eng J Med 2001; 345:1291–1297.

64. Franklin SS, Kahn SA, Wong ND, Larson MG, Levy D. Is pulse pressure useful in predicting risk for coronary heart disease? The Framingham Study. Circulation 1999; 100:354–360.

65. Lloyd-Jones DM, Evans JC, Larson MG, O'Donnell CJ, Rocella EJ, Levy D. Differential control of systolic and diastolic blood pressure: factors associated with lack of control in the community. Hypertension 2000; 36:595–599.

66. Wilson PW, Anderson KM, Kannel WB. Epidemiology of diabetes mellitus in the elderly. The Framingham Study. Am J Med 1986; 80 (suppl 5A):3–9.

67. Wilson PWF, Kannel WB. Clustering of risk factors, obesity, and syndrome X. Nutr In Clin Care 1998; 1(suppl 1):44–50.

68. Wilson PWF, Castelli WP, Kannel WB. Coronary risk prediction in adults: The Framingham Heart Study. Am J Cardiol 1987; 59(G):91–94.

69. Haffner SM. Insulin resistance, inflammation, and the prediabetic state. Am J Cardiol 2003; 92(suppl):18J–26J.

70. Ridker PM, Hennekens CH, Buring JE, Rifai N. C-reactive protein and other markers of inflammation in the prediction of cardiovascular disease in women. N Engl J Med 2000; 342:836–843.

71. Grundy SM. Small LDL. Atherogenic dyslipidemia, and the metabolic syndrome. Circulation 1997; 95:1–4.

72. Kannel WB. Range of serum cholesterol values in the population developing coronary artery disease. Am J Cardiol 1995; 76:69C–77C.

73. Kannel WB, Wilson PW. Efficacy of lipid profiles in prediction of coronary disease. Am Heart J 1992; 124:768–774.

74. Welty FK, Mittleman MA, Wilson PW, et al. Hypolipoproteinemia is associated with low hemostatic risk factors in the Framingham offspring population. Circulation 1997; 95:825–830.

75. Reaven GM. Insulin resistance, hyperinsulinemia, and hypertriglyceridemia in the etiology clinical course of hypertension. Am J Med 1991; 90:7S–12S.

76. Kwiterovitch PO Jr. State-of-the-art update and review: clinical trials of lipid-lowering agents. Am J Cardiol 1998; 82:3U–17U.

77. Grundy SM. Approach to lipoprotein management in 2001 national cholesterol guidelines. Am J Cardiol 2002; 90(suppl):11i–21i.

78. de Jong PE, Brenner BM. From secondary to primary prevention of progressive renal disease: the case for screening for albuminuria. Kidney Int 2004; 66:2109–2118.

79. Pearson TA, LaCava J, Weil HF. Epidemiology of thrombotic-hemostatic factors and their association with cardiovascular disease. Am J Clin Nutrition 1997; 65:1674S–1682S.

2 | Arterial Hypertension

Daniel A. Duprez

Cardiovascular Division, Rasmussen Center for Cardiovascular Disease Prevention and Cardiovascular Clinical Trial Center, University of Minnesota, Minneapolis, Minnesota, U.S.A.

Daniel J. Wilson

Hypertension Consultations, Rochester, Minnesota, and Pfizer, Inc., New York, New York, U.S.A.

KEY POINTS

- It is well established that lowering BP in patients with hypertension reduces CV morbidity and mortality. Yet, current hypertension control rates are disappointing. Many patients with elevated BP remained unaware their condition, or do not achieve recommended goals.
- Prevalence rates for hypertension appear to be increasing especially in younger patients in conjunction with the observed rises of obesity and sedentary behavior.
- In most cases of hypertension, there is no one dominant mechanism that can account for the development of high blood pressue. In most cases multiple mechanisms contribute to the pathogenesis and the progression of hypertension. Once present, hypertension if left untreated or poorly controlled will progress.
- BP classifications now recognize a new category of higher than normal BP: prehypertension, where SBP ranges from 120 to 139 mmHg and/or DBP is between 80 to 89 mmHg. Patients with prehypertension do not necessarily require antihypertensive medication, though they clearly have elevated CV risk, and are apt to develop future hypertension. Aggressive lifestyle modification is strongly encouraged for all patients with prehypertension, as well as for those with definite hypertension. Lifestyle modifications such as weight reduction in obese patients, dietary sodium reduction, increased physical activity, and moderation of alcohol consumption can effectively lower BP in these populations.
- Hypertension usually occurs in conjunction with other CV risk factors. The evaluation and treatment of hypertension should focus on lowering BP and reducing global CV risk, in an effort to maximize the potential reduction of CV and renal morbidity and mortality.
- The treatment of hypertension should be targeted and advanced to attain both systolic and diastolic goals. For most patients, goal BP is less than 140/90mmHg. Patients with multiple CV risk factors, established target organ damage, or specific comorbid conditions require lower BP goals. The target BP for high-risk patients with established CVD, diabetes, or renal insufficiency is below 130/80 mmHg. Multiple medications will be required to reach these goals.
- Antihypertensive therapy should be individualized. The selection of first line medication is predicated on a variety of factors including cost, target organ damage, compelling indications, and/or other factors. Goal attainment may be difficult, but is ofter achievable through the use of lifestyle modification and the use of multiple antihypertensive medications. In the absence of one of the above factors, Diuretics are considered to be the most cost-effctive first line modications on the basis of comparative clinical trial data. In patients with compelling indications, or high cardiovascular risk, a more expensive drug may be the most cost effective treatment. Several recently completed clinical trials emphasize the importance of prompt BP reduction in terms of reducing serious CV events.
- Drug-resistant hypertension appears to be an increasingly recognized phenomena which may be due to lifestyle changes, and more aggressive BP goals. True treatment resistance, however, is relatively rare. Secondary forms of hypertension, hypertensive emergencies, and urgencies do occur and may require clinical consultation or the expertise of the hypertension specialist.
- Poor control rates for hypertension are in large part related to patient and physician barriers to aggressive treatment as well as to shortcomings in national health care delivery. Improved hypertension control should be predicated on changes in patient as well as provider attitude and behavior
- New definitions for hypertension are emerging and may serve to better identify those patients who are at higher CV risk for hypertension, and who may be candidates for early intervention, including antihypertensive therapy. Future treatment algorithms for hypertension will likely change on the basis of recent and ongoing clinical trials.

- The outcomes from recent clinical trials challenge the concept that beta-blocker based regimens are equivalent to more contemporary antihypertensive therapy.
- The hypertensive patient is truly a high-risk patient for CVD. Improved control of hypertension should be a worldwide public health imperative.

INTRODUCTION

High blood pressure (BP) is a powerful cardiovascular (CV) risk factor that damages the arterial wall and which leads to serious CV events, such as cerebrovascular accidents and ischemic heart disease (1,2). In clinical practice, two specific and arbitrary points of the BP curve, peak systolic BP (SBP), and end-diastolic BP (DBP), are used to define this CV risk factor. Because the goal of anti-hypertensive is to prevent CV complications, it appears likely that the totality of the BP curve, not simply two specific and arbitrary points, should be considered. Therefore, there may be a need for further improvement in the definition of arterial hypertension (3).

DEFINITION

The strict definition of hypertension has been a source of some controversy for the past 40 to 50 years. Recent history has demonstrated that the definition, per se, has been in evolution and subject to change. BP, like many other risk factors, has a normal distribution across free-living populations. However, a curvilinear relationship without an apparent breakpoint exists between increasing levels of BP and heart attack and stroke. Throughout middle and old age, usual BP is strongly and directly related to vascular and overall mortality, without any evidence of a threshold down to at least 115/75 mmHg (4). Normal BP is widely considered to being less than 120/80 mmHg. Recent definitions for hypertension have been revised by national and international guidelines and on the basis of randomized clinical trial data, meta-analyses, and expert opinion.

Hypertension is now defined on the basis of SBP and DBP levels and classified into stages on the basis of the degree of elevation. The generally recognized cut point for hypertension is an average office BP of 140/90 mmHg or greater, which has been obtained by a recommended standard technique with an accurate manometer, and which has been confirmed on at least one other occasion. This general definition has been modified for the classification of hypertension in specific high-risk populations such as diabetes and chronic kidney disease (CKD). Blood pressures of 130/80 mmHg or more are now considered to be abnormal in patients with diabetes or in those with CKD.

Alternate definitions for hypertension exist for BP measurements made with ambulatory and home BP monitoring. Awake ambulatory BPs of more than 140/90 mmHg and sleep aver-aged BPs of more than 125/75 mmHg are now considered to be sufficient for the diagnosis of hypertension. Home BPs of more than 135/85 mmHg generally correlate well with office BPs of 140/90 mmHg or greater. Although pulse pressure (PP), the difference between SBP and DBP in mmHg, has been used to characterize CV risk in hypertension, it does not yet contribute to the definition of the hypertensive status.

Several expert groups now recognize prehypertension as a distinct clinical entity. The rational for this designation is heavily dependent on a recent secondary analysis of the Framingham Heart Study (5). A total of 6589 patients in this epidemiologic observation were classified as having high-normal, normal, or optimal BP on the basis of a baseline BP and were followed for 14 years. Men and women with high-normal BP at baseline had a higher incidence of cardiovascular disease (CVD) on follow-up and those with optimal BP. The rate of CV events in persons with optimal BP was low, but a continuous gradient of increasing risk was observed across the three BP categories. Thus, what was previously described as high-normal BP and which is now referred to as prehypertension, is associated with an increased risk of CVD. Those individuals with BPs between 120 and 139 mmHg systolic and 80 to 89 mmHg diastolic should now be advised that they have prehypertension and should be treated with lifestyle modifications in an effort to prevent progression to definite hypertension, and to reduce the risk of future CVD.

EPIDEMIOLOGY OF HYPERTENSION

Hypertension is considered to be the most common reversible or treatable CV risk factor. When defined as a BP of 140/90 mmHg, it affects 50 million residents of the United States, and an estimated one billion people worldwide. The population attributable risk due to elevated BP is large and present in all ethnic groups and regions of the world. It is not then surprising that hypertension has been identified as a condition which accounts for a substantial portion of total global disease burden (6). From a clinical perspective, there is one generally accepted cardinal principle that describes the hypertensive state and which has served to define the importance of hypertension to world health: hypertension begets hypertension. The presence of an elevated uncontrolled BP over time will lead to progression in the severity or stage of hypertension, the development, or worsening of target organ damage, and to increased CV morbidity and mortality. Given the relationship of hypertension to stroke, myocardial infarction, heart failure, and other vascular disease, the control of high BP will have a profound impact on individual well being and national healthcare costs.

The prevalence of hypertension varies depending on the population studied. Contrary to popular thought, the prevalence of hypertension is increasing in the United States. An analysis of the 1999 to 2000 National Health and Nutrition Examination Survey (NHANES), demonstrated that in both U.S. men and women, hypertension prevalence increased from earlier NHANES estimates in those aged 40 to 59 years and in those aged 60 years or older (7). Prevalence rates were highest in non-Hispanic blacks and lowest in Mexican-Americans. Current estimates are that overall 29% of U.S. residents have a BP of more than 140/90 mmHg and that this rate increases to 34% in the U.S. African-American population. Age continues to have a significant interaction on the prevalence of hypertension, with 65% of those in this NHANES analysis aged 60 years or more, after noted to have hypertension. While hypertension control rates have improved somewhat in recent surveys, they continue to be low.

Geographic variations in the worldwide prevalence of CV risk factors and CVD had been previously recognized. Such differences were confirmed for hypertension in a recent analysis of prevalence data on adults from six European countries, Canada, and the United States (Fig. 1) (8). An average BP of 136/83 mmHg was noted in the five European countries studied in men and women aged 35 to 74 years of age and the average BP was noted to be 127/77 mmHg in the Canadian and U.S. cohorts. The age- and sex-adjusted prevalence rate for hypertension was 44% in the European countries and 28% in North America. Hypertension prevalence was strongly correlated with stroke in this analysis, and more modest association was noted with total CVD. Thus, a 60% greater prevalence of hypertension was noted in the European cohort which included population data from Germany, Finland, Sweden, England, Spain, and Italy.

Elevated BP demonstrates a consistent, strong, and graded relationship with multiple CV events including CV death, myocardial infarction, stroke, heart failure, and renal dysfunction. The risk of CV mortality has been observed to double with each 20/10 mmHg increase in BP from 115/75 mmHg in adults aged from 40 to 69 years of age. This relationship between SBP and DBP elevation and CVD mortality is best described by the Prospective Studies Collaboration, a meta-analysis, which recorded 120,000 deaths among one million participants

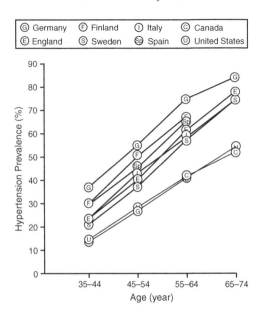

FIGURE 1 Hypertension prevalences in six European and two North American countries, men and women combined by age group. *Source:* From Ref. 8.

in 61 cohorts (4). Individuals with preexisting vascular disease were excluded from this meta-analysis. During 12.7 million person-years at risk, there were about 56,000 vascular deaths (12,000 stroke, 34,000 ischemic heart disease, 10,000 other vascular), which occurred in adults between 40 to 89 years of age. Throughout middle age as BP increases, each difference of 20 mmHg in the usual SBP (usual BP at the start of each decade) or/and approximately equivalent 10 mmHg usual difference in DBP was associated with a more than twofold increase in the stroke death rate. Because stroke is much more common in old age than in middle age, the absolute annual differences in stroke death associated with a given BP difference were greater in old patients. In addition, each 20-mmHg difference in usual SBP was associated with twofold differences in the death rate from ischemic heart disease. All of the proportional differences found in vascular mortality were reduced by half in the 80 to 89 year group. Age-specific associations for men and women were similar. Perhaps the most striking findings of this meta-analysis was that relatively small reductions in mean SBP would be associated with large absolute reductions in premature deaths and disabling strokes. Thus a 2-mmHg lower mean SBP could lead to a 7% lower risk of ischemic heart disease death and a 10% lower risk of stroke death.

Unfortunately, a gap continues to exist between hypertension and awareness and control worldwide. In the United States analysis of the 1999 to 2000 NHANES data, 69% of U.S. individuals were aware of their hypertension. A total of 58% were treated for their hypertension and 31% were controlled. Women, Mexican-Americans, and individuals 60 years of age or older had lower rates of control (7).

MECHANISMS OF HYPERTENSION
CV Hemodynamics

The pressure required to supply the different organs and tissues with blood through the circulatory bed is provided by the pumping action of the heart (cardiac output) and arterial tone (total peripheral vascular resistance). Each of these primary components is determined by the interaction of a complex series of factors. Arterial hypertension has been attributed to abnormalities in nearly every one of these factors (9,10).

Traditionally, the BP curve has been considered to contain a steady component, mean BP, and a pulsatile component, the PP. Hemodynamic research has shifted away from a steady flow approach toward a pulsatile flow approach, because the former is less predictive in relation to CV morbidity and mortality (11,12). The growing importance of pulsatile pressure indices paralleled the notion that not only increases in systemic vascular resistance but also increases in arterial stiffness are important in the pathophysiology of hypertension (13).

A current approach consists of considering the BP curve as the summation of a steady component, mean arterial pressure (MAP), and a pulsatile component, PP. MAP, the product of cardiac output multiplied by total peripheral resistance, is the pressure for the steady flow of blood and oxygen to peripheral tissues and organs. The pulsatile component, PP, is the consequence of intermittent ventricular ejection from the heart. PP is influenced by several cardiac and vascular factors, but it is the role of large conduit arteries, mainly the aorta, to minimize pulsatility. In addition to the pattern of left ventricular ejection, the determinants of PP (and SBP) are the cushioning capacity of arteries and the timing and intensity of wave reflections. The former is influenced by arterial stiffness, usually expressed in the quantitative terms of compliance and distensibility. The latter result from the summation of a forward wave coming from the heart and propagating at a given speed (pulse wave velocity, or PWV) toward the origin of resistance vessels and a backward wave returning toward the heart from particular sites characterized by specific reflection indices (14).

Wave reflections alter the ventricular–vascular coupling not only through increased arterial stiffness and changed timing but also through modifications in their amplitude. Such possibilities depend on the reflectance properties of the arterial tree, which arise from the distal part of the arterial tree. They are influenced by the geometry, number, structure, and function of smaller muscular arteries and arterioles. Thus, acute and active arterial and arteriolar constriction results in earlier aortic wave reflections at the aortic level and hence increased PP. It appears that elastic arteries buffer the pulsations, muscular arteries actively alter propagation velocity, and arterioles serve as major reflection sites. Each of these alterations (or their combination) enables a cross talk between the proximal and distal compartments of the arterial tree, which leads to the predominant or selective increases of SBP and PP observed in aged and/or hypertensive populations at high CV risk.

An increase in arterial tone has traditionally been viewed as the hallmark for an elevated BP. Although some have suggested that an increase in cardiac output with a normal vascular resistance is the initial hemodynamic abnormality in patients with hypertension (15), the chronic hypertensive state usually is associated with an increase in total systemic vascular resistance. This increase in resistance is generally attributed to an increase in vascular tone. Multiple mechanisms possibly contribute to this increase in systemic vascular resistance. Activation of the sympathetic nervous system and the renin–angiotensin–aldosterone system (RAAS), electrolyte changes, alterations in release of endothelial relaxing factor [nitric oxide (NO)], and increased release of endothelial constricting factors all have been implicated in the process (16). Neural and hormonal influences that alter tone of the arteriole, and thus the calculated systemic vascular resistance, also play a role in the larger conduit arteries. An increase in smooth muscle tone in the muscular arteries that represent most of the conduit vessels will alter the pressure-to-volume relationship in these vessels and result in a decrease in arterial compliance or elasticity (17).

Renal Mechanisms

The relationship between the development or pathogenesis of hypertension and the kidney is complex. The kidney through a variety of distinct renal mechanisms can cause or contribute to the development or to the progression of hypertension. On the other hand, hypertension per se, can contribute to progressive renal structural and vascular damage, which in turn may contribute to a worsening or perpetuation of the hypertensive state. In this vicious cycle, the role of the kidney in hypertension may be that of a culprit or a victim.

The proposal that the kidney plays a primary role in the pathogenesis of hypertension was championed by Guyton (18). On the basis of his animal experiments and clinical observations, he introduced a hypothesis that BP elevations can only persist if a key renal functional relationship between BP and renal sodium excretion was altered. A resetting of pressure–natriuresis relationship would be required to maintain hypertension no matter what mechanism initiated the BP elevation. He reasoned that an increase in BP could not persist unless the kidney shifts the normal relationship between BP and salt excretion to the right. Under normal circumstances a pressure-induced natriuresis should correct any type of hypertension by increasing sodium excretion, an action, which could be likened to that of a diuretic. On the basis of this hypothesis, BP can only rise if the kidney increases sodium reabsorption at any given BP level (18).

Renal functional and structural changes can promote sodium retention. Excessive sodium reabsorption can lead to plasma volume expansion, an increase in cardiac output and ultimately an increase in total peripheral resistance and BP. These mechanisms most certainly contribute to the BP elevation, which accompanies CKD and some cases of primary hypertension (19).

Several other renal factors have received attention as potential contributors to this vicious cycle that is characterized by development of hypertension and progressive renal damage. Most of these have been more closely associated with progression of hypertension in this setting and advancing CKD. Inappropriate or excessive activation of the RAAS in relationship to the sodium/volume balance may contribute to BP elevation, especially in the setting of renal parenchymal disease. In essence a "normal" renin concentration may be inappropriately high in reference to a specific sodium/volume balance. Increased release of aldosterone could further serve to advance hypertension and contributed to progression of renal disease in this setting (20).

Renal-mediated sympathetic nervous system overactivity may be a significant contributor to hypertension in patients with renal parenchymal disease. Activation of specific renal chemoreceptors or baroreceptors and the renal afferent nerves can disinhibit the integrative nuclei of the central nervous system, thereby activating sympathetic efferent pathways which can then raise BP. Sympathetic overactivity has been demonstrated in patients with uremia, and may in part be due to afferent renal nerve damage (21).

Decreased production or interference with nitric oxide (NO), reduced NO-mediated vasodilatation, and elevated endothelin (ET1) levels in patients with chronic renal disease suggests that the vascular endothelium may have a role in the pathogenesis of progression of hypertension in this setting. Insulin resistance, secondary hyperparathyroidism, and other mediators of oxidative stress can also potentially contribute to progression of the hypertension in patients with CKD. Thus, multiple renal mechanisms when activated, have the potential to simultaneously promote worsening of hypertension and renal disease.

Nephron mass at birth may also play a role in the patient's risk of developing primary hypertension. Brenner et al. recently proposed that "nephron underdosing" or the presence of a diminished number of glomeruli is a prerequisite for an increase in BP (21). A reduced number of nephrons could lead to glomerular hypertrophy, glomerular hyperfiltration, with resultant hypertension and accelerated loss of renal function.

Keller et al. tested this hypothesis when they compared the number and the volume of glomeruli in 10 hypertensive accident victims to 10 normotensive controls (22). Their observations support the above hypothesis in that the number of glomeruli was significantly lower, and the volume of glomeruli was significantly higher, in hypertensive individuals when compared with the normotensive controls. Such renal structural damage could serve as an initiating factor for the above-described multiple renal mechanisms which could promote or accelerate the hypertensive state.

Neurohumoral Mechanisms

The concept of hypertension as primarily a consequence of altered hemodynamics has changed. Many factors are now implicated in the development of hypertensive vascular disease, and the RAAS appears to be one of the most significant (Fig. 2). Angiotensin II, the principal effector peptide of the RAAS, has far-reaching effects on vascular structure, growth, and fibrosis, and is a key regulator of vascular remodeling and inflammation (23). Reactive oxygen species and a network of signaling pathways mediate angiotensin II and cellular mechanisms that promote remodeling and inflammation. The involvement of aldosterone in vessel wall and myocardial remodeling has also come under intensive research scrutiny. Treatments that block the pathologic effects of the RAAS at several points have been shown to limit target organ damage in hypertension and to decrease CV morbidity and mortality. Understanding the molecular and cellular mechanisms that participate in the early development of hypertensive vascular disease may lead to more targeted treatment and improved outcomes.

The RAAS is an important contributor to the regulation of BP, water and salt balance, and tissue growth. It functions both as a circulating endocrine system and as a tissue paracrine/autocrine system, most notably in the heart, brain, kidney, and vasculature. In the circulating system, renin is released by the kidneys and converts angiotensinogen into angiotensin I, which is then converted to angiotensin II by angiotensin-converting enzyme (ACE). Angiotensinogen is produced mainly by the liver, although there is also compelling evidence that adipose tissue secretes it (24). Under pathophysiological conditions, activation of components of the RAAS at the tissue level may contribute to the pathogenesis of CV and renal disease (25). Moreover, at the tissue level, enzymes (e.g., chymostatin-sensitive angiotensin II–generating enzyme, cathepsin G) other than ACE may contribute to angiotensin II synthesis. Inflammatory cells are also biochemically competent to contribute to the increase in angiotensin II (26).

The major effector peptide of the RAAS, angiotensin II is a powerful vasoconstrictor that triggers the release of aldosterone, causing the kidneys to increase the retention of

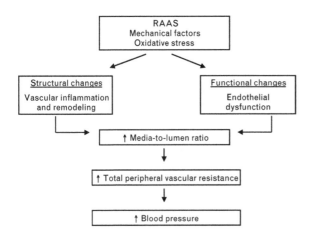

FIGURE 2 The pathological role of the renin–angiotensin II-aldosterone system (RAAS) extends beyond mechanical factors and oxidative stress to vascular remodeling and high blood pressure. *Source:* From Ref. 23.

sodium and water. This increases blood volume and maintains normal BP in hypotensive situations. In addition to its role in BP regulation, angiotensin II has a variety of actions that are associated with CV and renal pathology. Angiotensin II has been shown to contribute to vascular remodeling by activating signal transduction pathways that promote cell growth, inflammation, and fibrosis (27). The cytoskeleton is also involved in adaptive structural changes of the vasculature, and evidence shows that many of these changes can be induced by angiotensin II. Both angiotensin II and aldosterone are a major participant in profibrotic mechanisms. Platelet aggregation and activation have been added to the pathways that link angiotensin II to thrombotic events and to the development of CVD (28). It has been shown that angiotensin II exerts these various functions primarily through the generation of reactive oxygen species. An increase in the generation of reactive oxygen species leads to a reduction in NO synthesis and activity, with subsequent endothelial dysfunction (29). The AT_1 and AT_2 receptors have similar affinities for angiotensin II, but distinctly different effects. AT_1 is the major angiotensin II receptor expressed in adults. With some exceptions, most pathologic CV effects of angiotensin II are mediated through the AT_1 receptor: hypertension, coagulation, inflammation, and vascular smooth muscle cell growth (30). The role of angiotensin II in triggering vascular inflammation and fibrosis has been demonstrated in the heart and kidney, and has been observed in the development of atherosclerosis in large conduit vessels (31). The participation of angiotensin II in inflammation and remodeling of resistance arteries is beginning to be elucidated (32).

Aldosterone is the major mineralocorticoid hormone secreted by the adrenal cortex. Identification of mineralocorticoid receptors in the heart, vasculature, and brain has raised speculation that aldosterone may directly mediate its detrimental effects in these target organs, independent of angiotensin II and the regulatory role of aldosterone in kidney function and BP (33). Moreover, there is evidence for local biosynthesis of aldosterone in these same tissues (34). Increasing evidence suggests that aldosterone can act through nongenomic mechanisms in addition to genomic ones (35). Aldosterone is known to impair endothelium-related vasodilatation and contribute to inflammation and vascular and cardiac remodeling (36).

Baroreflexes

The arterial baroreflex is known to represent a mechanism of fundamental importance for short-term BP homeostasis in daily life. It is also deeply involved in the pathophysiology of several CVDs (37,38), where its impairment may contribute to the appearance of clinical complications (39,40). Reduced baroreflex sensitivity appears to characterize not only patients with established hypertension, but also normotensive offspring of hypertensive parents, who may display a slight BP increase and a decreased carotid elasticity. Arterial baroreceptor reflex control of renal sympathetic nerve activity has been proposed to play a role in long-term regulation of arterial pressure, but this concept has been recently challenged (41).

Effect of Aging

Available evidence suggests that the incidence of systolic hypertension is increasing in individuals over 50 years of age. The reasons for this evolution are quite simple (42). First, prolongation of the duration of life is responsible for an increased number of older individuals with increased SBP. Second, the goal for treatment of systolic–diastolic hypertension in middle-aged subjects has been based on the reduction of DBP. Because it is much easier to control DBP (less than 90 mmHg) than SBP (less than 140 mmHg), and because, with age, DBP tends spontaneously to be reduced and SBP to be enhanced, this situation contributes per se to increase the incidence of systolic hypertension in the elderly. Thus, there are multiple mechanisms involved in the pathogenesis of systolic hypertension. These include an altered vascular resistance, the classical hallmark of high BP, as well as changes in arterial stiffness and wave reflection, which occur in the conduit arteries, mainly the aorta and its principal branches.

Adaptations in the arterial vasculature play a critical role in influencing CV hemodynamics with advancing age (43). The generalized structural and functional changes in the arterial circulation contribute to alterations in regional blood flow, progression of atherogenesis, and the microvascular abnormalities that occur during senescence (44). In large arteries, aging results in progressive deposition of calcium salts, fraying and fragmentation of elastin, and an increase in the number and cross-linking of collagen fibers that alter the compliance characteristics of the vessel wall (45). A rigid aorta is less able to buffer the pulsatile output from the heart; it contributes to an increase in SBP and left ventricular afterload and a decrease in DBP and impaired coronary perfusion. Recent evidence suggests that an increase in PP is accompanied by progressive vessel wall damage and atherogenesis, and is associated with an increase in cardiac morbidity and mortality rates (46).

Sequential Vascular Changes in Hypertension

Abnormalities of the arterial vasculature that precede CV morbid events are likely to occur in a temporal sequence. The initial abnormalities appear to be functional, in large part related to endothelial dysfunction associated with decreased bioavailability of NO (47). A decrease in constitutive release of NO, which maintains low small artery tone, may be the initial abnormality, but it is soon accompanied by a decrease in stimulated release of endothelial vasodilators, as manifested by a reduction in flow-mediated dilation of conduit arteries (48,49). These functional abnormalities of the vasculature should precede and are mechanistic precursors of the structural alterations that are responsible for thickening of the conduit artery wall (50), increases in PP (51), and atherosclerotic plaque development (52). These structural changes may also result in additional functional abnormalities. But cross-sectional studies suggest that this sequence of vascular manifestations of vascular disease is not always detectable.

Functional and structural changes in the artery wall precede and accompany atherosclerosis and its obstructive and thrombotic events. These changes should alter the volume increment that occurs in the arterial bed during the systolic pressure increase with each cardiac cycle. An understanding of the sequential changes that occur in the arterial system is crucial in order to appreciate the temporal influence on the occurrence of CVD and its response to treatment (Fig. 3).

ETIOLOGY OF HYPERTENSION

The specific set of events that lead to progressive elevation of BP and the development of hypertension remains unknown. Depending on the clinical setting, 93% to 95% of hypertensives had no known cause for their hypertension. For that reason, most hypertension states was originally classified as essential hypertension. More recently, this conceptual term has been replaced by the moniker: primary hypertension.

Primary Hypertension

Although the pathogenesis of primary hypertension is uncertain, as previously noted, specific mechanisms appear to be involved in the development of primary hypertension: altered regulation of sympathetic nervous system, cell-membrane defects, renin secretion, salt sensitivity, as well as other vascular and hormonal factors. In addition to these multiple physiologic abnormalities, diet, environment, other lifestyle factors, and most certainly genetics frequently play a role in the development of hypertension.

Thus, the etiology of hypertension appears to be exceedingly complex. Irvine Page hypothesized that multiple factors, rather than a single underlying abnormality, are involved

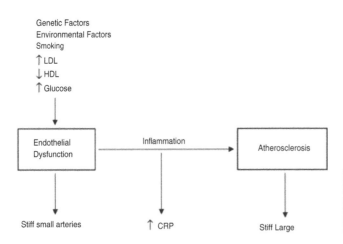

FIGURE 3 Sequential vascular changes in hypertension. *Abbreviations:* LDL, low-density lipoprotein; HDL, high-density lipoprotein; CRP, C-reactive protein. *Source:* From Ref. 55.

in the development of hypertension (53). This resulted in his conceptualization of a mosaic of interrelated factors, which may affect total peripheral resistance and result in the development of primary hypertension. Irrespective of the exact etiologic mechanism whereby patients develop hypertension, most patients seem to progress along a similar hemodynamic cascade which involves an early increase in cardiac output, followed by a subsequent rise in total peripheral resistance.

There still, however, is a possibility that our concept of primary hypertension is flawed and we are dealing with multiple distinct clinical syndromes (54). The majority of patients who develop primary hypertension do so between the ages 20 to 50 years of age. Most cases are diagnosed as part of routine examinations and generally in the absence of overt target organ damage at initial presentation. Few patients develop primary hypertension after age 50. The occurrence of new onset hypertension after age 50 can be used as a clue or indicator that a patient may have a secondary form of hypertension. Patients with primary hypertension are generally asymptomatic. Although some patients report symptoms related to hypertension such as headache, dizziness, fatigue, palpitations, and chest discomfort, these symptoms and their level of intensity generally do not correlate well with BP level. Thus, primary hypertension has no consistent symptoms or signs, except for the elevated BP itself.

A specific type of headache has, however, been reported to occur with elevated BP. Hypertensive headache is a clinical entity, which has been described as a diffuse morning headache, is generally associated with more severe stages of hypertension (stage II and III). In some circumstances these headaches may actually be associated with sleep apnea complicating arterial hypertension, rather than the BP itself.

Secondary Hypertension

Secondary causes of hypertension are uncommon, and account for less than 5% of all cases of high BP in an unselected hypertensive population. Although infrequent, secondary forms of hypertension account for many cases of drug-resistant hypertension. As a result of this finding, higher prevalence rates of secondary hypertension have been noted in specialized hypertension clinics. Secondary hypertension is usually associated with a specific organ and/or vascular abnormalities, a metabolic abnormality, or endocrine disorder. The diagnosis of these specific hypertensive conditions is important because of the potential for a permanent cure, or improvement in control of hypertension. If left undiagnosed, secondary hypertension may lead to progressive target organ damage, as well as CV and renal complications.

In secondary hypertension, the elevated BP may be the major presenting manifestation of an underlying process, or elevated BP may simply be one component of a complex group of signs and symptoms in a patient with a systemic disease. Secondary causes of hypertension are often nonspecific in their presentation and laboratory test and/or imaging studies are required for screening and confirmation of the diagnosis. Nevertheless, there are some well-recognized clinical presentations and clinical clues which deserve mention and which should raise a clinician's suspicion of a secondary cause of hypertension.

The documented early (less than age 30 years) or late (more than age 50 years) onset of hypertension is thought to raise the possibility of secondary form of hypertension. In pediatric populations, congenital renal or endocrine causes of secondary hypertension are more likely to result in elevated BP. Fibromuscular dysplasia of the renal artery(s) characteristically occurs in young white women, generally without a strong family history of hypertension. The most common cause of secondary hypertension in older patients, with associated vascular disease, is atherosclerotic renal artery stenosis. In obese patients, obstructive sleep apnea and Cushing's disease should be considered as potential causes of secondary hypertension.

A thorough search for secondary causes of hypertension is not considered cost-effective in most patients with hypertension. Expended workups should be considered with compelling clinical or laboratory evidence for a specific secondary cause, or when a patient presents with drug resistant or refractory hypertension, or hypertensive crisis. Causes of secondary hypertension are listed in Table 1.

Chronic Kidney Disease–Renal Parenchymal Hypertension

CKD or renal parenchymal disease is the most common form of secondary hypertension. Hypertension occurs in more than 80% of patients with chronic renal failure and is a major factor causing their increased CV morbidity and mortality seen in CKD. Any type of CKD, including

TABLE 1   Secondary Causes of Hypertension

Chronic kidney disease (renal parenchymal disease)
Renovascular hypertension
Atherosclerotic
Fibromuscular dysplasia
Renal artery aneurysm
Page kidney
Systemic vasculitis
Renin secreting tumor
Primary hyperaldosteronism
Aldosterone-producing adenoma
Idiopathic hyperaldosteronism
Glucocorticoid-remediable hyperaldosteronism
Pheochromocytoma
Cushing's disease/syndrome
Coarctation of the aorta
Hypothyroidism
Sleep apnea

acute or chronic glomerulonephritis, may be associated with hypertension. Hypertension is frequently the presenting feature of adult polycystic kidney disease. Clinically, affected patients may experience abdominal pain and hematuria, and the renal or associated hepatic cysts may be palpable on physical examination.

CKD should be suspected when the estimated glomerular filtration rate (eGFR) is less than or equal to 60 mL/min, or when 1+ or greater proteinuria and/or specific urinary sediment abnormalities are noted on urine analysis. The diagnosis can be confirmed either by the direct measurement of glomerular filtration rate (GFR) using a radioisotope or a 24-hour urine collection for a creatinine clearance showing a value of less than 60 mL/min. Proteinuria should be confirmed by a 24-hour urine, which should demonstrate a total protein excretion of more than 150 mg, or by a spot urine specimen showing microalbuminuria defined as a urine albumin-to-urine creatinine ratio between 30 and 300 mg/g.

In patients with mild or moderate renal insufficiency, stringent BP control is imperative to reduce the progression to end-stage renal disease and reduce the excessive CV risk associated with CKD. ACE inhibitors (ACEIs) have been showed to be effective in slowing the progression of developing renal disease in patients with Type-1 diabetes, and arteriolar or hypertensive nephrosclerosis in African-American patients. Angiotensin II antagonists have demonstrated similar benefits in those with Type-2 diabetes. In patients with far-advanced renal insufficiency, hypertension often becomes difficult to treat and may require intensive medical treatment using multiple classes of antihypertensive medications with a loop diuretic or loop/thiazide diuretic combinations. The initiation of chronic hemodialysis may be required for control of hypertension in an effort to reduce an expanded plasma volume and to restore the response to other antihypertensive medications.

The underlying mechanisms and management of hypertension and cystic kidney disease are unique, and deserves special comment. Hypertension is a recognized feature of adult polycystic disease (ADPKD) and may ultimately lead clinicians to the diagnosis of the disease. Hypertension is highly prevalent in ADPKD, and eventually occurs in 80% of affected patients. BPs may begin to rise in the second or third decade of life, well before renal function starts to decline. BP appears to correlate with renal size in ADPKD as renal volume is larger in hypertensive subjects than in matched normotensive subjects. Activation of the RAAS has long been associated with hypertension in ADPKD has been confirmed by the presence of an elevated plasma renin activity. Some studies suggest that intrarenal ischemia may occur in ADPKD as a result of large renal cysts. Compression of the renal vasculature and activation of the baroreflexes could also contribute to renal hypoperfusion. Such structural changes could lead to increased renin secretion and an upregulation of the RAAS in this clinical setting. In addition, high levels of active renin have been found in cyst fluid from patients with ADPKD. ACEIs are the mainstay of therapy in patients with ADPKD as they lower BP effectively, and result in a decrease in renal vascular resistance and increased in renal plasma flow in ADPKD.

Renovascular Hypertension

Renovascular hypertension may be the most common form of potentially curable hypertension. Current estimates indicate that is seen in 1% to 2% of a hypertensive population in general medical practice. There are two major causes: atheromatous disease and fibromuscular dysplasia of the renal artery and each is associated with a distinct clinical presentation. Less frequent causes of renovascular hypertension include renal artery aneurysm, systemic vasculitis, Page kidney (subcapsular renal with hematoma), and renin-secreting tumors. Renovascular hypertension frequently is associated with resistance to a multiple drug antihypertensive regimen. It is not surprising, therefore, that up to 30% of patients referred to some specialized hypertension clinics are found to have renovascular hypertension.

Several clinical clues occurring alone or in combination may point to the diagnosis of renovascular hypertension:

■ New onset or drug-resistant hypertension, before age 30 or after age 50
■ Accelerated or malignant hypertension
■ Lateralizing epigastric or upper quadrant systolic–diastolic abdominal bruit noted in a hypertensive patient
■ Progressive worsening of renal function in response to ACEI
■ Diffuse atherosclerotic vascular disease in the setting of severe hypertension
■ Unexplained pulmonary edema (flash pulmonary edema) generally associated with progressive renal insufficiency and occurring during antihypertensive therapy.

Elevated BP is but one of many pathophysiologic consequences that are associated with renal hypoperfusion. Critical or high-grade renal artery stenosis reduces renal blood flow, and leads to diminished renal perfusion and ischemia with a resultant increase in the secretion of renin. Unilateral renal artery stenosis leads to a reduction of tubular filtrate perfusing the juxtaglomerular cells of the affected kidney, which then promotes renin release and the development of a renin-dependent hypertension. Normal blood volume is maintained by the contralateral kidney. In contrast, bilateral renal artery stenosis and unilateral stenosis with a solitary kidney usually characterized as a volume-dependent type of hypertension, which may be accompanied by progressive renal failure. Renin promotes the conversion of angiotensinogen to angiotensin I, and converting enzyme then completes the transformation of angiotensin I to angiotensin II. Vasoconstriction then develops as a result of the direct pressor effect of angiotensin II. Other characteristics include angiotensin II-mediated aldosterone secretion, sodium retention, and potassium wasting. BP elevation in renovascular hypertension occurs as a result of this interaction between angiotensin-mediated vasoconstriction and the salt retaining effects of aldosterone. Other mechanisms can also contribute to the development of progressive hypertension in the setting of renovascular hypertension. Longstanding or accelerated hypertension can promote the development of structural changes such as arteriolar nephrosclerosis in a contralateral kidney in the case of unilateral renal artery stenosis. Associated renal parenchymal damage may also contribute further to BP elevation, and renal impairment.

The most common cause of renovascular hypertension is atherosclerotic renal artery stenosis, which generally affects the proximal renal arteries. Atherosclerotic renal artery stenosis is progressive and may lead to worsening hypertension, renal artery occlusion, ischemic nephropathy, and renal failure. The majority of these cases with atherosclerotic renal artery disease occur in the setting of other coronary, cerebrovascular, or peripheral vascular disease. These cases tend to be more frequently seen in men over 50 years of age with a long history of hypertension. Multiple reviews have reaffirmed these early observations. In one trial of older hypertensive patients undergoing diagnostic cardiac catheterization, with well-controlled BP and serum creatinines less than 2.0 mg/dL, aortography demonstrated that 47% of those studied had renal artery stenosis. A total of 19% had a stenosis of greater than 50%. Four percent of patients in this series had bilateral renal artery disease, while 7% of patients had a high-grade (> 70% stenosis) stenosis (56). Thus, the combination of progressive hypertension, vascular disease, and renal dysfunction raises a strong possibility of atherosclerotic renal artery disease and renovascular hypertension.

Fibromuscular dysplasia of the renal arteries is the most frequent cause of renovascular hypertension in young women (those under 50 years old). This disease occurs rarely in males, but may on occasion be seen in males with strong family histories of fibromuscular dysplasia.

Medial fibroplasia with aneurysms is the most common type of fibromuscular dysplasia seen and can easily be recognized by its classic "string of beads" appearance on the renal arteriogram. Typically, one or more fibrous bands partly occlude the lumen of the renal artery resulting in renal ischemia. On occasion, fibromuscular dysplasia may affect the iliac, mesenteric, or carotid arteries. Perimedial fibroplasia and intimal fibroplasia occur less frequently, though intimal fibroplasia appears to be more common in the pediatric population. The etiology of the fibromuscular dysplasias remains unknown.

The clinical suspicion and even the confirmed diagnosis of renovascular hypertension will frequently present clinicians with difficult diagnostic and therapeutic dilemmas. Individualized treatment decisions are currently required for the effective management and treatment of renovascular hypertension. The diagnostic evaluation and therapeutic strategy for patients with suspected renovascular hypertension is predicated on several factors including: the severity of hypertension, the presence of associated renal failure, or insufficiency, the type of renal artery lesion, the location of the stenotic lesion, the presence of concomitant CVD, a patients general health status, and the ability of a patient to tolerate multiple antihypertensive medications.

The work-up for renovascular hypertension should be predicated on the clinician's index of suspicion: low, suggestive, or high. No screening or work-up is recommended in patients with low likelihood of having renovascular hypertension, or in those patients, who because of other clinical conditions would not be candidates for a potential intervention. Patients with clinical presentations suggestive of renovascular hypertension can be screened with noninvasive studies and, if results are positive, confirmation of the diagnosis can be made with renal arteriography. If the index of suspicion for renovascular hypertension is high, renal arteriography and can be performed in the absence of noninvasive tests.

Noninvasive testing is frequently employed to diagnose or confirm the anatomical site of a renal artery lesion, or to examine the functional significance of a renal artery stenosis. Our ability to accurately and noninvasively detect renal artery stenosis has improved with new imaging techniques. Functional assessment of a hemodynamically significant renal artery lesion and of the viability of renal parenchyma is, however, still limited using the currently available noninvasive screening tests. Over the years, a variety of imaging techniques and diagnostic tests has been used as a screen for renovascular hypertension; hypertensive intravenous pyelograms with tomography, plasma renin activity, renal vein ratios, simple-timed renography and captopril renography, duplex renal artery sonography, magnetic resonance angiography, and computer-assisted tomographic angiography. These tests differ in diagnostic accuracy, safety, and cost. The implementation of a specific screening strategy for renovascular hypertension is frequently predicated on the institutional availability and expertise with a screening test and a patient's clinical presentation. Most specialized centers now favor duplex renal artery sonography for general screening or magnetic resonance angiography if cost is not a limitation. The specificity, sensitivity, and positive predictive value of these techniques vary and serve as a limiting factor in the diagnosis of renovascular hypertension.

Renal arteriography remains the "gold standard" for diagnosis of renal artery stenosis. Some experts feel that visualization of the renal arteries is required prior to even proceeding with a more complex drug therapy to rule out the possibility of bilateral high-grade renal artery stenosis. In situations where patients have impaired renal function, this can be accomplished with magnetic resonance angiography with gadolinium contrast. This latter approach may serve to provide the clinician with adequate vascular imaging as well as an estimate of kidney size and function.

Renal artery stenosis can be present without being the cause of a patient's hypertension. Clinicians need to be cognizant that the documentation of renal artery stenosis by arteriography in a hypertensive patient does not itself establish the diagnosis of renovascular hypertension. In the absence of renal ischemia or ischemic nephropathy, primary hypertension may account for the elevated BP in many patients with noncritical renal artery stenosis. Ideally, clinicians should look for some clinical or laboratory evidence of renal hypoperfusion before undertaking an intervention. With the advent of percutaneous renal artery interventions, renal vein renin levels have fallen out of favor, and are seldom used to determine the functional significance of a renal artery stenosis or for the prediction of potential for cure of hypertension. Most investigators now rely on the severity of the renal artery stenosis, and believe that a 70% or greater reduction in luminal diameter is required to cause renovascular hypertension and/or ischemic nephropathy.

Intensive medical therapy for renovascular hypertension is generally required for BP control and involves the use of ACEIs, in conjunction with multiple other medications. Treatment frequently involves the use of a calcium channel blocker (CCB), judicious use of diuretics, and occasionally the use of a sympathetic inhibitor. Renal function and serum potassium should be monitored regularly, as they can deteriorate with ACE inhibition or BP reduction alone. ACEIs should be withdrawn with moderate deterioration (>30%) in renal function, and/or if a patient becomes hyperkalemic. Angiotensin receptor blockers (ARBs) should be substituted in those patients who develop an ACEI cough or those who develop mild hyperkalemia with ACE inhibition. Medical management of renovascular hypertension includes intensive treatment of associated CV risk factors, with concomitant aggressive lipid lowering, smoking cessation, and the use of low dose aspirin.

Percutaneous renal artery angioplasty (PTRA) and stenting or surgical revascularization of the renal arteries should be considered in the setting of drug-resistant and worsening hypertension, in patients who develop progressive renal failure in response to medical therapy, and finally in those with high-grade bilateral renal artery stenosis. Preservation of renal function is currently the leading cited indication for intervention in patients with renal artery stenosis and renovascular hypertension. BP can frequently now be controlled with potent multidrug antihypertensive regimens. Revascularization, however, may prevent renal artery occlusion, progressive ischemic nephropathy, and renal atrophy.

Percutaneous and surgical procedures are not without risk. Patient selection and timing may be crucial to limit complications and maximize outcomes. Patients with creatinine levels more than 2.0 mg/dL face a 20% risk of progressive renal impairment following revascularization by either surgical or PTRA procedures (57). Looking at these data from a different perspective, renal function will stabilize in 52%, and may substantially improve in 28% of patients who undergo renal artery revascularization. Thus, treatment decisions must be highly individualized in older patients who present with generalized vascular disease, and renal artery stenosis, and renal impairment. Timing of a percutaneous or surgical procedure may be critical as outcomes are better if renal revascularization is performed before the development of advanced renal failure (serum creatinine ≥3 mg/dL). Further comparative clinical trials are needed to better define criteria for the prediction of potential long-term renal function improvement or stabilization, and for the proper timing of renal revascularization.

Percutaneous renal artery interventions have replaced surgery as the primary treatment of choice for BP reduction and preservation of renal function. Significant perioperative morbidity and mortality has limited the utilization of surgical procedures, but some experts suggest that perioperative complications may be reduced by patient selection and effective treatment of comorbid disease. Surgical renal artery revascularization has a proven record of long-term effectiveness, which has yet to be defined for other treatment modalities. Surgical renal artery revascularizations are now generally limited to those cases where aortic reconstruction is required, to some cases of high-grade bilateral renal artery stenosis, and to treat those patients who have had failed percutaneous procedures.

Technical improvements of diagnostic and interventional endovascular methods and tools have led to the widespread use of PTRA for the treatment of renovascular hypertension and have extended the indications for such therapy. Although there were early reports of prolonged BP improvement with PTRA, it has generally been replaced by angioplasty with stenting. The one exception to this trend is the continued high utilization of PTRA in the treatment of fibromuscular dysplasia. The high frequency of atherosclerotic aorto-ostial renal artery lesions is thought to limit the clinical utility of PTRA without stenting. Many of the proximal renal artery lesions seen in atherosclerotic renal artery stenosis are actually a result of an ingrowth of an aortic atherosclerotic plaque. Numerous single-center studies have reported the beneficial effect of PTRA. The impressive results of these early uncontrolled clinical trials with PTRA have been challenged by several recent comparative clinical trials. Small prospective randomized studies comparing medical management of renovascular hypertension with PTRA, have only demonstrated modest benefits in term of improved BP control following PTRA (58–60). Another randomized comparison of PTRA with PTRA plus stenting confirmed improved vascular patency with stents, but demonstrated remarkably little difference in the clinical outcomes in terms of BP control or renal function (61). Despite the absence of randomized studies, there appears to be sufficient evidence to consider PTRA with stenting in the properly selected patient as a treatment for a hemodynamically significant atherosclerotic renal artery stenosis given the potential impact on BP control, and renal function. Clinicians must continue to individualize therapy in patients with renovascular hypertension on the basis of clinical presentation, risk, and potential benefit as there is no general consensus on the most appropriate therapy for renovascular hypertension.

Primary Hyperaldosteronism

Primary hyperaldosteronism or Conn's syndrome is characterized by hypokalemia, hypertension, very low plasma or suppressed renin activity (PRA), and excessive aldosterone secretion.

Aldosterone binds with the mineralocorticoid receptor in the distal nephron and contributes to salt and water homeostasis and maintenance of plasma volume through this interaction. Excessive production of the hormone promotes an exaggerated renal Na^+–K^+ exchange, which usually results in hypokalemia. The diagnosis of primary hyperaldosteronism should be considered in any patient with severe refractory hypertension.

Traditionally, it was thought that 1% to 2% of patients with hypertension had primary hyperaldosteronism. The syndrome has been reported to be more common in females and may present with mild, moderate, or resistant hypertension. Several recent clinical investigations suggest a higher prevalence rate for primary hyperaldosteronism following the introduction of new screening tests and expanded screening strategies. Screening for primary hyperaldosteronism has often been restricted to individuals with resistant hypertension or hypokalemia. Some studies have suggested prevalence rates as high as 5% to 10% in patients with mild to moderate hypertension and up to 20% in those with resistant hypertension, others have suggested that the prevalence of primary hyperaldosteronism in a mild-to-moderate hypertensive population without hypokalemia is at most 3.2% (62).

Patients are generally asymptomatic, though symptoms such as muscle cramps, weakness, and paresthesias attributable to hypokalemia may predominate. Polyuria and polydipsia have also been reported. Many patients with primary hyperaldosteronism will present with severe, persistent, or refractory diuretic-induced hypokalemia. The best clinical clues to the diagnosis in patients with hypertension is either unprovoked hypokalemia with a serum K^+ less than 3.5 mmol/L in the absence of diuretic therapy, or the development of more profound hypokalemia during diuretic therapy with a serum K^+ less than 3.0 mmol/L.

There are multiple potential causes for primary hyperaldosteronism. These include aldosterone-producing adenoma (>60%), idiopathic hyperaldosteronism (>30%), glucocorticoid-suppressible hyperaldosteronism (<1%), and rarely an aldosterone-producing carcinoma (<1%). Aldosteronoma are benign tumors of the zona glomerulosa present in the adrenal cortex, which autonomously secrete an excess of aldosterone. Idiopathic hyperaldosteronism is a low renin hypertension, which demonstrates an excess of aldosterone secretion that is not associated with a tumor, and which may be related to bilateral adrenal hyperplasia. Laboratory testing is frequently required to differentiate between secondary hyperaldosteronism associated with diuretic use, renovascular hypertension, and renin secreting tumors. Accurate identification of specific cause of primary hyperaldosteronism will enable clinicians to individualize management and treatment: aldosterone antagonists vs. surgical resection of aldosterone-producing adenomas.

The plasma aldosterone to plasma renin activity ratio (ARR) is currently the most utilized screening test for primary hyperaldosteronism as it has a high negative predictive value even in the setting of ongoing antihypertensive therapy. Its specificity, however, is low and a high ARR, which is suggestive of primary hyperaldosteronism, still must be confirmed with other laboratory testing. A confirmatory test should demonstrate the presence of high levels aldosterone, and autonomous secretion. The most utilized confirmatory test is the urine aldosterone excretion rate, which involves the 24-hour collection of urine, under conditions of a high-salt load.

The plasma aldosterone–renin ratio can be drawn randomly from patients on most hypertensive medications. However, patients on the aldosterone antagonist spironolactone should have this medication withdrawn for three to four weeks prior to ARR testing. The test is calculated by dividing plasma aldosterone (mg/dL) by plasma renin activity (mg/mL/hr). ARR greater than 100 is considered elevated and is predictive of primary aldosteronism.

Following biochemical confirmation of hyperaldosteronism, clinicians should consider imaging studies to differentiate between the various causes of the syndrome. Adrenal computed tomography (CT) scans with 3-mm cuts should be used to localize adenomas or neoplasm. On occasion, it may be necessary to repeat a CT in one year if the initial scan is negative and the biochemical evidence for an adrenal adenoma is strong. Another imaging modality, available in selected centers, is adrenal scanning with iodocholesterol (NP-59) or 6-beta-iodomethyl-19-non-cholesterol. These radionuclide scans are performed after dexamethasone suppression. Aldosteronomas that take up and concentrate the tracer can be differentiated from idiopathic aldosteronism and adrenal carcinoma that do not.

Control of BP and hypokalemia can be obtained with antihypertensive regimens based on spironolactone, eplerenone or, on occasion, with amiloride. Multiple medications will be frequently required. Unilateral adrenalectomy is highly effective for reversing the metabolic consequences of hyperaldosteronism in patients with aldosterone-producing adenoma. Unilateral adrenalectomy normalizes hypertension and hypokalemia in 70% of patients with aldosterone-producing adenoma after one year, and follow-up studies have shown that 50% of patients remain normotensive after five years.

Glucocorticoid-remediable aldosteronism (GRA) is an autosomal dominant genetic form of hypertension, which occurs as a result of a specific genetic mutation. As a result of this specific mutation, aldosterone production becomes inappropriately linked to cortisol production. Although exceedingly rare, GRA is of great interest because it has been recognized as the first genetic form of hypertension for which a specific genetic mutation has been identified, although others have been subsequently discovered. Fewer than 100 cases of GRA have been reported. However, additional cases may likely go undetected or be misdiagnosed as bilateral adrenal hyperplasia. Clinically GRA presents in a similar fashion to an aldosterone-secreting tumor, with hypertension and hypokalemia. However, the increased aldosterone secretion is corticotrophin-dependent and thus is reversible by administration of dexamethasone.

Pheochromocytoma

Pheochromocytomas are rare catecholamine-producing tumors that originate from chromaffin cells of the adrenergic system. Majority of these tumors are benign and are located in the adrenal gland, but others can develop as functioning paraganglioma in a variety of extra-adrenal sites. Pheochromocytomas generally secrete both norepinephrine and epinephrine, though norepinephrine is usually the predominant amine.

Pheochromocytoma has a reported incidence of 0.05% in the general population with peak incidence occurring in the 30s and 40s. The rule of 10's has been used to characterize the clinical presentation of the tumor: approximately 10% of pheochromocytomas are extra-adrenal, 10% are malignant, 10% are familial, 10% occur in children, 10% are bilateral and affect both adrenals, and 10% are multiple. A family history or an early onset of pheochromocytoma may suggest an underlying genetic disorder such as multiple endocrine neoplasia Type II, Von Hippel-Lindau disease, or neurofibromatosis Type I.

Classic clinical presentations are characterized by hypertension, palpitations, headache, and hyperhidrosis. The hypertension can be severe and sustained (55%) or paroxysmal (45%). Pounding headaches, palpitations, and diaphoresis are prominent features of the syndrome and may occur together in a paroxysmal attack. Postural hypotension may occasionally be present as a result of low or constricted plasma volume. Hypertension associated with panic attack as well as other causes of neurogenic hypertension, including the BP elevations sometimes seen with sympathomimetic agents, and obstructive sleep apnea can be confused with pheochromocytoma.

Plasma-free metanephrines, if available, are a preferred screening test for excluding or confirming the diagnosis of pheochromocytoma. Plasma concentrations of normetanephrines more than 2.5 pmol/mL or metanephrine levels more than 1.4 pmol/mL indicate a pheochromocytoma with 100% specificity. Twenty-four hour urine collections for metanephrine (100% sensitive) are also useful for screening for the tumor. The accuracy of the 24-hour urine metanephrine may be improved by indexing urinary metanephrine levels by urine creatinine levels. A positive screening test should be reconfirmed if there is a suspicion of drug interference or a false positive test (63).

A variety of imaging studies can be used to localize pheochromocytoma. Abdominal CT scanning is useful in locating tumors more than 2.5 cm in diameter. Pheochromocytomas demonstrate a distinctive magnetic resonance imaging (MRI) appearance and MRI appears to be the diagnostic imaging modality of choice. Scintigraphy using the norepinephrine analog

^{131}I-MIBG, which localizes in adrenergic tissue, is particularly useful in locating extra-adrenal pheochromocytomas (64).

Laparoscopic or surgical removal of the tumor should be performed after a two-week period of stabilization. This involves the combination of phenoxybenzamine, a beta-blocker, and liberal fluid and salt intake starting 10 to 14 days before surgery. Metyrosine should be included in the medical regimen of patients with malignant pheochromocytoma. Volume expansion is done to prevent severe postoperative hypotension and vascular collapse. Phenoxybenzamine (Dibenzyline) 5 mg PO b.i.d. initially gradually increased to 10 mg q3d up to 50–100 mg b.i.d.; prazosin may be used when phenoxybenzamine therapy alone is not effective or not well tolerated. Clinicians should start beta-blockade with a nonselective beta-blocker only after the patient is on adequate alpha-blocker therapy. Propanolol in doses of 20 to 40 mg PO q6h is useful to prevent catecholamine-induced arrhythmias and tachycardia. The five-year survival rate is approximately 95% with benign disease and 40% for malignant pheochromocytoma.

Hypertensive crisis preoperatively and intraoperatively should be controlled with nitroprusside or phentolamine (Regitine) 2–5 mg IV q1-2h prn used in combination with beta-adrenergic blockers. On occasion, emerging surgery may be required for pheochromocytoma crisis unresponsive to parenteral medications.

COMPLICATED MANAGEMENT PROBLEMS IN HYPERTENSION
Resistant Hypertension

The prevalence of drug-resistant hypertension has not reliably been established. However, resistant hypertension is becoming an increasingly common problem with the national guidelines focusing on lower goal BPs (65).

True drug-resistant or refractory hypertension is relatively rare, but treatment failure is relatively common, frequently being secondary to nonadherence, socioeconomic factors, and lifestyle issues. Resistant hypertension is generally defined as the failure to achieve a therapeutic target of less than 140/90 mmHg in most hypertensive patients, or less than 130/80 mmHg in diabetics or patients with CKD on a well-designed three-drug antihypertensive medical regimen combined with intensive lifestyle modification. In most cases, resistant hypertension is now defined on the basis of a persistently high SBP level.

Before embarking on an expanded workup to determine the cause of drug-resistant hypertension, clinicians should be careful to rule out "pseudoresistance" secondary to BP measurement artifacts or errors, and "white-coat" hypertension. Out-of-office measurements, including home BPs, or 24-hour ambulatory BP monitoring (ABPM) may be required to establish a patient's actual BP. On rare occasions intraarterial BP measurements may be required to eliminate spurious BP artifacts related to arterial stiffness, or an alerting reflex. The absence of target organ damage in the setting of prolonged resistant or refractory hypertension should raise a clinician's suspicion regarding pseudoresistance.

Patients with resistant hypertension are older and commonly present with obesity, unrestricted or excessive dietary salt intake, and the clinical syndrome of sleep apnea. Common causes or resistant hypertension appear in Table 2. Current approaches to correction of drug resistance focus on evaluation and correction of potential contributing causes, the development of a more effective drug regimen, and identifying any unrecognized secondary causes of hypertension.

Recent efforts have focused on the use of hormone and hemodynamic measurements to specifically direct antihypertensive treatment. Clinical pathways based on plasma renin activity, aldosterone production, or hemodynamic measurements may be helpful in identifying a specific physiologic cause for drug resistance. Volume expansion plays a key role in drug resistance, and it cannot be adequately assessed with a clinical exam. Treatment should include a strong emphasis on lifestyle changes including weight loss, exercise, dietary, and salt restriction, all of which should be monitored. New multidrug antihypertensive regimens should incorporate the more potent vasodilator antihypertensive agents such a CCBs or direct acting vasodilators with adequate diuretic therapy, especially if intense vasoconstriction is suspected as the physiologic cause or culprit. Recent data indicate that aldosterone antagonists may be effective when added to existing antihypertensive regimens even in the absence of primary aldosterone (66). Consultation with a hypertension specialist should be considered if target BP cannot be achieved.

TABLE 2   Causes of Resistant Hypertension

Poor adherence to medical regimen
Poor adherence to lifestyle changes
   Obesity and weight gain
   Heavy alcohol intake
Improper BP measurement
   Improper cuff size
   Stress or office hypertension
   Pseudoresistance in the elderly
Volume overload
   Excess sodium intake
   Inadequate diuretic therapy
   Pseudotolerance
     Alpha methyldopa
     Direct acting vasodilators
   Progressive CKD
Drug-induced or other causes
   Inadequate doses of antihypertensive medication
   Inappropriate combinations of antihypertensive medications
   Drug interactions
     Nonsteroidal anti-inflammatory drugs
     Cocaine, amphetamines, other illicit drugs
     Sympathomimetics (decongestants, anorectics)
     Oral contraceptives Adrenal steroids
     Cyclosporine and tacrolimus
     Erythropoietin
   Licorice ingestion
Unsuspected secondary hypertension
   Sleep apnea

Hypertensive Emergencies and Urgencies

Hypertensive emergencies and urgencies present infrequently in medical practice. When they do occur, they require prompt evaluation and intervention. A hypertensive emergency can be defined as a sudden and/or severe elevation in BP which causes or contributes to pathologic disturbances in the central nervous system, the heart, the vascular system, or the kidneys and which requires prompt BP reduction in order to maintain the integrity of the CV system. Hypertensive emergencies are true medical emergencies, which require prompt recognition and thoughtful management in order to reduce the morbidity and mortality associated with severe hypertension. BP reduction typically is begun within minutes to hours of diagnosis and is frequently required to prevent worsening of an underlying clinical condition. The term "hypertensive urgency" refers to a clinical presentation of severe hypertension where the SBP is usually more than 200 mmHg and/or the DBP is usually more than 120 mmHg. These patients are generally asymptomatic and do not have evidence of acute target organ damage. BP lowering may occur over hours to days in the absence of acute target organ damage or serious comorbid disease.

The presence of severe hypertension alone is not sufficient to make the diagnosis of hypertensive emergency. The diagnosis of hypertensive emergencies ultimately depends on the clinical presentation rather than on the absolute level of the BP. Thus, these cases usually present with severe hypertension complicated by some cardiac, renal, neurologic, hemorrhagic, or obstetric manifestation. Hypertensive encephalopathy, acute aortic dissection, and pheochromocytoma crisis are well-recognized hypertensive emergencies. Some cases of accelerated or malignant hypertension, acute left ventricular failure, cerebral infarction, head injury, scleroderma, and acute myocardial infarction interaction can also present as hypertensive emergencies. Other causes for an acute symptomatic rise in BP include medications, noncompliance, and poorly controlled chronic hypertension.

The clinical history and physical examination should be highly focused in an attempt to determine the cause of a patient's severe hypertension and should attempt to exclude other clinical presentations which may mimic hypertensive emergencies or urgencies such as panic attack or postictal hypertension.

The choice of an appropriate oral or parenteral antihypertensive medication for treatment of severe hypertension depends upon the type of hypertensive emergency, the presence of associated target organ damage, and the specific hemodynamic properties and side effects of the emergency or urgency. When possible, clinicians should opt for a gradual controlled reduction of BP and avoid antihypertensive agents or methods that have been associated with rapid or precipitous reductions in BP. Cerebral, coronary, and renal autoregulatory mechanisms may be impaired in patients with severe hypertension. Chronic hypertension, vascular disease, and aging also interfere with normal autoregulation. Catastrophic side effects including acute myocardial infarction, cortical blindness, stroke, and death have been reported with rapid or precipitous reduction in BP in patients presenting with hypertensive urgency or emergency.

Treatment of hypertensive emergency needs to be tailored to each individual patient and presentation. Prompt and rapid reduction of BP under continuous surveillance is essential in patients who are symptomatic and have acute end-organ damage. Parenteral therapy, typically in a monitored bed in intensive care unit is recommended for the treatment of most hypertensive emergencies. Sodium nitroprusside is the "gold standard" for treating hypertensive emergencies, and the agent to which other parenteral agents are measured. Nitroprusside is metabolized to thiocyanate and cyanide, and may accumulate in patients receiving high doses, or prolonged infusions especially with CKD. Other attractive agents include fenoldopam mesylate, nicardipine, and labetalol. In pregnant women, magnesium and nifedipine are used commonly. A reduction in MAP of approximately 10% should occur during the first hour of therapy, and a further 10% to 15% during the next two to four hours. Precipitous falls, or normalization of BP can result in cerebral hypoperfusion with cardiac or neurologic symptoms. Oral antihypertensive therapy can usually be instituted after 6 to 12 hours of parenteral therapy (67).

Aortic dissection presents as a special circumstance in the treatment of hypertensive emergency. When severe hypertension complicates aortic dissection, the SBP target is set lower to less than 120 mmHg, is to be achieved during the first 20 minutes following diagnosis using a beta-blocker (intravenous esmolol) and a vasodilator to reduce shear stress on the aortic tear as well as BP. Repeated intravenous injections ("mini bolus" of 10–20 mg) of the combined alpha- and beta-adrenergic receptor-blocking agent labetalol can produce a prompt but gradual reduction of arterial BP without the induction of a reflex tachycardia. Labetalol appears to be a suitable alternative when BP reduction has to be initiated without the benefit of an intensive care unit or a monitored bed (68).

Hypertensive urgencies are usually treated with oral antihypertensive medications. Single oral agents or combinations of antihypertensive medications have been used to lower BP in this setting. Oral and sublingual nifedipine, although not approved by the Food and Drug Administration, has been long used for the treatment of hypertensive urgencies and some emergencies. Recent reports on the use of immediate-release nifedipine in hypertensive urgency and emergency have noted the development of nonanginal chest pain, "paradoxical" angina pectoris, hypotension, ischemic electrocardiographic changes, myocardial infarction, stroke, and death. Given these reports, clinicians should avoid using oral or sublingual nifedipine in the treatment of hypertensive urgency and emergency, especially in those patients with known or suspected coronary artery disease.

BLOOD PRESSURE MEASUREMENT

The problem of identifying an abnormality in arterial tone related to some neural or hormonal effect is compounded by the fact that during daily life, arterial tone and BP changes are continuously induced by alterations in neurohormonal activity. During exercise, emotional or temperature stress, and even during periods of standing, these systems may be activated and an alteration in regional or systemic vascular tone may result. Therefore, the dilemma in identifying individuals with elevated BP from the normal fluctuations of BP in normotensive individuals is intensified. Attempts to define the hypertensive state by the degree of BP elevation or the sustained nature of this elevation during 24-hour monitoring often serves as the only distinguishing feature between the "white-coat hypertensive" or the normotensive individual with fluctuations in arterial tone, and the hypertensive who is thought to be at risk for CV event (69).

Office Blood Pressure Measurement

The most common reason for an outpatient physician visit is for the diagnosis and treatment of hypertension. Standardized BP measurement is the basis for the diagnosis, management, treatment, epidemiology, and research of hypertension, and the decisions affecting these aspects of hypertension will be influenced, for better or worse, by the accuracy of measurement.

Acceptance by physicians of Riva-Rocci's mercury column sphygmomanometer for auscultatory BP measurement, brought to the United States by Harvey Cushing in 1901, was predicated in large part by its use being confined only to the physician's hands (70). Accurate BP measurement is well described by the Joint National Committee on Prevention, Detection, Evaluation and Treatment of High Blood Pressure (JNC-VII) (71). The World Health Organization– International Society of Hypertension (WHO/ISH) (72), and by the American Heart Association (AHA) (73). All of these guidelines are a synthesis of the methodology used in all the important epidemiologic and treatment trials of hypertension. Factors important in this methodology include: (*i*) resting for five minutes; (*ii*) sitting with back supported and feet on the floor (74,75); (*iii*) arm supported at heart level (76,77); (*iv*) appropriate size cuff applied (78–80); (*v*) use of the Korotkoff Phase I sound for SBP and Phase V for DBP; and (*vi*) using the mean of two or more BP measurements as the patient's BP (81). Failure to conform to all of these recommendations can result in significant errors in ausculted BP and misdiagnosis and mistreatment of the hypertensive patient. Certain groups of people merit special consideration for BP measurement. These include children; the elderly, who often have isolated systolic hypertension or autonomic failure with postural hypotension; obese people in whom the inflatable bladder may be too small for the arm size, leading to "cuff hypertension," patients with arrhythmias in whom BP measurement may be difficult and the mean of a number of measurements may have to be estimated; pregnant women in whom the disappearance of sounds (Phase V) is the most accurate measurement of diastolic pressure, except when sounds persist to zero, when the fourth phase of muffling of sounds should be used; and any individual during exercise (82).

Bilateral measurements should be made on first consultation and, if persistent differences greater than 20 mmHg for systolic or 10 mmHg for diastolic pressure are present on consecutive readings, the patient should be referred to a CV center for further evaluation with simultaneous bilateral measurement and the exclusion of arterial disease.

The second option for accurate BP measurement is the use of validated automated BP devices. The automated BP measuring devices use a proprietary oscillometric method. Each of these devices needs to be independently validated and then calibrated to each patient. Rarely, they do not sense BP accurately but more commonly, fail if the cardiac rhythm is very irregular (e.g., atrial fibrillation) (83). It is interesting to note that even with auscultatory BP measurement in elderly patients with atrial fibrillation, considerable observer variability is seen (84). It is critically important that if an automated BP-measuring device is used, it must have passed a recognized validation protocol.

Home BP

Home BP monitoring has become popular in clinical practice and several automated devices for home BP measurement are now recommendable. Home BP is generally lower than clinic BP, and similar to daytime ambulatory BP. Home BP measurement eliminates the white-coat effect and provides a high number of readings, and it is considered more accurate and reproducible than clinic BP. It can improve the sensitivity and statistical power of clinical drug trials and may have a higher prognostic value than clinic BP. Home monitoring may improve compliance and BP control, and reduce costs of hypertension management (85). Diagnostic thresholds and treatment target values for home BP remain to be established by longitudinal studies. Until then, home BP monitoring is to be considered a supplement. Home BP provides an opportunity for aditional monitoring of BP levels and its variability. The first international guidelines have established a consensus document with recommendations, including a proposal of preliminary diagnostic thresholds, but further research is needed to define the precise role of home BP monitoring in clinical practice.

Ambulatory BP

Ambulatory Blood Pressure (ABPM) provides automated measurements of brachial-artery pressure over a 24-hour period while patients are engaging in their usual activities. This method has been used for more than 30 years in clinical research on hypertension. These studies demonstrated that BP has a highly reproducible circadian profile, with higher values when the patient is awake and mentally and physically active, much lower values during rest and sleep, and an early-morning surge lasting three to five hours during the transition from sleep to wakefulness. In a patient with hypertension, 24-hour BP monitoring has substantial appeal. It yields multiple BP readings during all of the patient's activities, including sleep, and gives a far better representation of the "BP burden" than what might be obtained in a few minutes in the doctor's office (86).

Several prospective clinical studies, as well as population-based studies, have indicated that the incidence of CV events is predicted by BP as measured conventionally or with ambulatory methods, even after adjustment for a number of established risk factors (87–90). In some of these studies, ambulatory measurements of BP predicted CV events even after adjustment for conventional BP measurements (91–93). However, in most of these studies, the majority of data on ambulatory BP, which were used to predict end points, were recorded in initially untreated subjects or during a placebo run-in phase; in most cases, treatment was initiated afterward. The OvA study (Office vs. Ambulatory BP) addressed the issue whether ambulatory BP monitored in patients with treated hypertension could predict CV events and death even after adjustment for conventional office BP measurements (94). The OvA study showed that in patients with treated hypertension, a higher ambulatory SBP or DBP predicts CV events even after adjustment for classic risk factors including office measurements of BP. The next step will be to determine the role of ABPM in clinical practice and whether the cost–benefit ratio favors adding such monitoring to the standard care of patients with treated hypertension.

In clinical practice, measurements are usually made at 20- to 30-minute intervals in order not to interfere with activity during the day and with sleep at night. Measurements can be made more frequently when indicated. Whatever definition of daytime and nighttime is used, at least two-thirds of SBPs and DBPs during the daytime and nighttime periods should be acceptable. If this minimum requirement is not met, the ABPM should be repeated. A diary card may be used to record symptoms and events that may influence ABPM measurements, in addition to the time of drug ingestion, meals, and going to and arising from bed. If there are sufficient measurements, editing is not necessary for calculating average 24-hour, daytime, and nighttime values, and only grossly incorrect readings should be deleted from the recording. Normal ranges for ABPM are average daytime ABPM of less than 135/85 mmHg and average nighttime ABPM less than 120/70 mmHg, but even lower values are advocated, particularly in high-risk groups such as diabetic patients (Table 3) (82). ABMP is accepted as being of benefit in patients with the conditions listed in (Table 4).

ABPM has a number of advantages: it provides a profile of BP away from the medical environment, thereby allowing identification of individuals with a white-coat response; it shows BP behavior over a 24-hour period during usual daily activities, rather than when the individual is sitting in the artificial circumstances of a clinic or office. It can indicate the duration of decreased BP over a 24-hour period. ABPM can identify patients with blunted or absent BP reduction at night—the nondippers—who are at greater risk for organ damage and CV morbidity. It can demonstrate a number of patterns of BP behavior that may be relevant to clinical management, such as white-coat hypertension, isolated systolic hypertension, masked hypertension,

TABLE 3 Recommended Levels of Normality for Ambulatory Blood Pressure Monitoring in Adults

	Blood pressure value (mmHg)		
	Optimal	Normal	Abnormal
Awake	<130/80	<135/85	>140/90
Asleep	<115/65	<120/70	>125/75

Note: The evidence supporting the normal and abnormal demarcation values are based on a number of outcome studies; evidence is not yet available to make recommendations for the intermediate pressure ranges between the "normal" and "abnormal" values, or for recommendations lower than those given. It must be emphasized that these values are only a guide to "normal" and that lower "optimal" values may be more appropriate in patients whose total cardiovascular risk-factor profile is high, and in whom there is concomitant disease such as diabetes mellitus.
Source: From: Ref. 82

TABLE 4 Recommendations for the Use of Ambulatory Blood Pressure Monitoring in Clinical Practice[a]

Indication	JNC 7	WHO-ISH
White-coat hypertension	Yes	Yes
Labile hypertension	Yes	Yes
Resistant hypertension	Yes	Yes
Hypotensive episodes	Yes	Yes
Postural hypotension	Yes	No

[a]JNC 7 denotes the Seventh Report of the Joint National Committee on Prevention, Detection, Evaluation, and Treatment of High Blood Pressure (71), and WHO-ISH the World Health Organization-International Society of Hypertension (72).
Source: From Ref. 86

hypotension, and enhanced BP variability. In long-term outcome studies, ABPM has been shown to be a stronger predictor of CV morbidity and mortality than is office BP measurement (95).

Although the role of ABPM in the routine care of patients with hypertension remains uncertain, findings from these investigators and others support the broader use of ABPM in clinical practice. A suggested algorithm is shown in Figure 4 (96). Self-monitoring of the BP at home and at work can be used to assess whether there is a large disparity between the office and out-of-office BPs before ambulatory monitoring is considered. It is likely that many patients whose self-monitored BP is apparently normal will have elevated ambulatory BP and would benefit from antihypertensive therapy. For those whose ambulatory BP is truly normal (< 130/80 mmHg) despite an elevated office BP and in whom there is no evidence of other CV risk factors or target organ disease, avoidance of unnecessary drug therapy would be a clear benefit of the monitoring procedure (86,96).

Questions remain regarding the optimal use of ABPM in the diagnosis and management of hypertension. Research is needed to assess whether ambulatory monitoring can reduce the

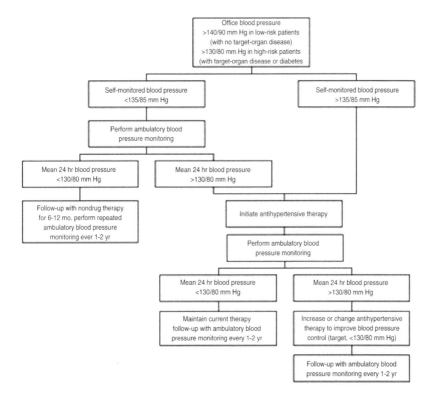

FIGURE 4 Algorithm for the use of ambulatory blood pressure monitoring in the management of hypertension.
Source: From Ref. 96.

overprescribing of drugs to patients who seem, in the office setting, to be resistant to therapy. Finally, it would be of great interest to determine whether CV outcomes could be improved by the use of ambulatory monitoring to assess and improve 24-hour BP control in high-risk patients whose office BP appears to be normal when they are at rest office normotension or during the time of the peak effect of their antihypertensive agents.

EVALUATION OF HYPERTENSION

Following the confirmation of hypertension, a targeted history and physical examination, and limited laboratory evaluation should be performed. The standard hypertensive work-up includes an assessment of CV risk, the identification of hypertensive target organ damage and is designed to rule out secondary hypertension. This examination should include information regarding a patient's habits and lifestyle, which could contribute to his or her hypertension. The identification of other CV risk factors or concomitant disorders may affect prognosis and guide treatment. The major CV risk factors and types of hypertension-associated target organ damage are listed in Table 5. The medical history and physical examination are also the most important components of a pretreatment evaluation in the differentiating between primary and secondary hypertension. The medical history should include detailed questioning which focuses on obtaining the following medical information:

- Family history of hypertension
- Family history of premature CVD, diabetes, or dyslipidemia
- Estimated duration of hypertension, current and previous hypertension stage, and drug therapy.
- Home BP measurements.
- Medical history, clinical signs, and symptoms of CV or renal disease.
- Medical history, clinical signs, and symptoms of comorbid disease, which may affect selection of drug therapy [asthma, chronic obstructive pulmonary disease (COPD)].
- Complete medication history including prescription, over-the-counter (OTC) medications, herbal remedies, and drug allergies.
- History of drug and alcohol abuse.

TABLE 5   Cardiovascular Risk Factors

Major risk factors
Hypertension
Cigarette smoking
Obesity (BMI $\geq$ 30)
Physical inactivity
Dyslipidemia
Diabetes mellitus
Microalbuminuria or estimated GFR < 60 mL/min
Age (>55 years for men, >65 years for women)
Family history of premature CVD (men < 55 years or women 65 years)
Target organ damage
Left ventricular hypertrophy
Angina or prior myocardial infarction
Coronary atherosclerosis
Prior coronary revascularization
Heart failure
Mild cognitive impairment
Stroke or transient ischemic attack
Chronic kidney disease
Peripheral arterial disease
Retinopathy

Note: BMI calculated as weight in kilograms divided by the square of height in meters.
Abbreviations: BMI, Body mass index; GFR, glomerular filtration rate.
Source: From Ref. 97.

The importance of the medication history cannot be overemphasized. A variety of drugs can elevate BP and interfere with the effect of antihypertensive medications. Corticosteroids, cyclosporine, tacrolimus, and oral contraceptives are well-recognized causes of BP elevation. Ephedrine, sympathomimetics, and amphetamine-like agents, available in OTC cough and sinus preparations, can increase peripheral resistance and interfere with BP control. Commonly used drugs such as nonsteroidal anti-inflammatory drugs (NSAIDs) can also cause hypertension or interfere with the effect of a variety of antihypertensive medications.

The initial physical examination should include the following:

- Vital signs, including body mass index (BMI).
- Sitting and standing BP and heart rates.
- BP measurement in the contralateral arm.
- Examination of optic fundi, neck, heart, lungs, and abdomen.
- Auscultation of the neck and abdomen for bruits.
- Palpation of peripheral pulses, and extremity check for edema.
- Neurological examination.

A limited laboratory evaluation is recommended at the time of initial diagnosis. This should include a complete blood count, chemistry (including Na, K, Ca, glucose, and uric acid), a complete lipid profile, and urinalysis. Electrocardiograms are recommended for most patients over 30 years of age. A chest X-ray, ABPM, echocardiography, and measurement and plasma renin activity are optional tests and are not recommended for most patients.

Recent trends have focused on better baseline assessment of renal function in hypertensive patients. Although not mandatory in most hypertensive patients, a measurement of urinary albumin excretion or albumin/creatinine ratio may be useful in diagnosing immanent renal disease or establishing future CV risk. A positive result could affect the intensity and type of antihypertensive therapy. Many reference laboratories now routinely calculate the eGFR, which can be used to identify or exclude CKD, or to monitor the effect of antihypertensive therapy on renal function. Additional laboratory and imaging tests may be required to quantify CV risk, to characterize target organ damage, or to screen for secondary hypertension in some complicated patients.

Given the high frequency of additional CV risk factors in hypertension, clinicians may want to use a risk assessment tool for determining a patient's 10-year risk for developing coronary heart disease (CHD). Such risk assessments may be useful for estimating global CV risk and in modifying patient behavior. Given the higher than expected frequency of hyperlipidemia with hypertension, clinicians could elect to use the risk-scoring calculator developed by The National Cholesterol Education Program (NCEP). The NCEP now recommends using a modification of the Framingham risk prediction model to estimate CV risk and adjust therapy in patients with dyslipidemia. The risk factors included in this Framingham calculation of 10-year risk are age, total cholesterol, high-density cholesterol, SBP, treatment for hypertension, and cigarette smoking. This modification of the Framingham point score does not account for all risk factors for CHD and should only be used in conjunction with NCEP guidelines. Separate NCEP Framingham risk calculators are available for men and women. Other risk factor calculators could be used for those patients who present without dyslipidemia (98).

TREATMENT

The stated goal for the treatment of hypertension is to prevent CV morbidity and mortality associated with high BP. Such a goal now requires the treatment of all identified reversible risk factors accompanying hypertension to maximize CV event reduction. The clinical goal is to lower BP to below 140/90 mmHg while controlling other CV risk factors. Further reductions in BP to a level less than 130/80 mmHg have been recommended in hypertensive patients with diabetes or renal disease. Reduction in BP to less than 130/80 mmHg can also be pursued with due regard in other populations, especially high-risk patients. Nondrug therapy should be employed in the management of all stages of hypertension and should also be implemented in individuals with prehypertension as a preventive strategy. The use of drug therapy is generally predicated on the stage of hypertension, the presence of high CV risk, comorbid conditions, and the documentation of target organ damage. For example, patients with prehypertension and specific comorbid conditions, such as a diabetes or hypertensive nephropathy, may benefit from early drug therapy.

Lifestyle modification may prevent or delay the onset of sustained hypertension, lower BP, and reduce the number of BP medications necessary for control in patients with established hypertension. Comprehensive lifestyle modification has been well studied and includes the following interventions:

- Weight reduction in those who are overweight or obese.
- Adoption of a Dietary Approaches to Stop Hypertension (DASH) diet—a low-fat diet rich in fruits, vegetables, and low-fat dairy products.
- Reduce sodium intake to 100 mmol/day (2.4 g sodium or 6 g sodium chloride).
- Limit alcohol intake to ~1 oz per day (24 oz of beer per day, or 8 oz of wine per day, or 2 oz of 100 proof whiskey per day).
- Regular aerobic exercise.
- Stop smoking and modify other known CV risk factors.

Adherence to one or several of these lifestyle modifications can result in substantial fall in BP, and aid in the management of hypertension. In general, weight loss and dietary changes have been observed to have the most dramatic effect on BP reduction (99,100), a 1600 mg sodium DASH eating plan has been shown to have effects on BP reduction similar to single drug therapy (101,102). Adoption of healthy lifestyles in both prehypertension and hypertension is critical for the prevention of future CVD.

Although the JNC-VII guideline recommends the use of pharmacologic therapy in patients with BPs greater than or equal to 140/90 mmHg, many clinicians continue to initiate a 3- to 6-month trial of comprehensive lifestyle modification in highly motivated patients who have uncomplicated Stage 1 hypertension. Drug therapy should be considered if BP remains greater than or equal to 140/90 mmHg after 3 to 6 months or if the patient is noncompliant with nondrug therapy.

Multiple drug classes, with different mechanisms of action and different side effects, are available for the treatment of hypertension (Table 6). Several classes of antihypertensives, including diuretics, calcium antagonists, ACEIs, and angiotensin receptor antagonists, are suitable for the initiation and maintenance of antihypertensive therapy. Beta-blockers and alpha-blockers are less favored by many clinicians and guidelines as first line therapy.

The selection of a specific medication for initial treatment of hypertension is complex and may depend on a variety of factors, including age and race, comorbid CV and non-CVD, and target organ damage. Potential drug-drug interactions with a patient's existing medical regimen may further limit therapeutic options. Repeated clinical observations have suggested that diuretics and CCBs may be more effective in standard doses in older patients and African-Americans, while beta-blockers and ACEIs appear to be more effective in younger and Caucasian populations. Gender has not been found to be a reliable predictor for drug response. For the majority of patients without a compelling indication for another class of an antihypertensive medication, a low dose of a thiazide diuretic is frequently recommended as the first choice of therapy.

On average, no more than 50% of a hypertensive population will be controlled by a single antihypertensive medication. In the antihypertensive and lipid-Lowering Treatment to Prevent Heart Attack Trial (ALLHAT), a population of older hypertensives with Stage I and II hypertension and high CV risk, BP was lowered to less than 140/90 mmHg in 66% of the population at five years, with an average of correct 2 ± 1 drugs. A total of 63% of the ALLHAT cohort were taking two or more medications at the end of the trial (103).

Physicians have been notably reluctant to change or to add medications in those patients whose BPs are not at recommended goals. This phenomenon, which is commonly seen in the management of hypertension is now referred to a clinical inertia. Clinical inertia is defined as the failure of healthcare providers to initiate or intensify therapy when indicated (104). Many physicians are still inclined to practice sequential monotherapy substituting individual agents in order to identify the most effective antihypertensive medication for a given patient and to limit the number of antihypertensive medications that a patient takes. The preferred strategy for the management of hypertension involves the use of multiple medications and utilizing the additive benefits of agents in combination. It is well recognized that the skillful use of two or more agents in combination can improve hypertension control rates to well above 80%.

TABLE 6 Oral Antihypertensive Medications

Medication class	Drug (trade name)	Usual dose	Daily frequency	Mechanism of action	Potential adverse reactions, side effects and complications	Comments and concerns
Thiazide diuretics	Chlorothiazide (Diuril)	125–500	1	Reduce plasma volume and cardiac output initially; in the long-term reduce TPR	Volume depletion	Inexpensive
	Chlorathalidone (generic)	12.5–25	1		Hypokalemia, hyperglycemia, hyponatremia, hyperuricemia, hypercalcemia,	Compelling indications in heart failure and diabetes
	Hydrochlorothiazide (Microzide, HydroDIURIL)	12.5–50	1		Dyslipidemia, photosensitivity	Ineffective when GFR ↓30 mL/min
	Polythiazide (Renese)	2–4	1			Insulin resistance
	Indapamide (Lozol)	1.25–2.5	1			New onset diabetes
	Metolazone (Mykrox)	0.5–1.0	1			Impotence
	Metolazone (Zaroxolyn)	2.5–5	1			Gout
						May potentate lithium and digitalis toxicity
Loop diuretics	Bumetanide (Bumex)	0.5–2	2	Reduce plasma volume and cardiac output initially; in the long-term reduce peripheral resistance	Volume depletion	Preferred in CKD or heart failure
	Furosemide (Lasix)	20–80	2		Hypokalemia, hyperuricemia, hyperglycemia	Except for torsemide, multiple daily doses required to prevent rebound sodium retention
	Torsemide (Demadex)	2.5–10	1			Ethacrynic acid use possible with sulfa or thiazide allergy
Potassium-sparing diuretics	Amiloride (Midamor)	5–10	1–2	Weak antikaluretic diuretics	Hyperkalemia	Adjunctive treatment with thiazide diuretics
	Triamterene (Dyrenium)	50–100	1–2	Sodium channel blockers, which interfere with distal renal tubular Na$^+$–K$^+$ exchange		Restores or prevents hypokalemia
						Contraindicated in advanced CKD
						Hyperkalemia risk with use in diabetics
						Hyperkalemia risk greater with ACE, or ARB
Aldosterone receptor blockers	Eplerenone (Inspra)	50–100	1–2	Specific pharmacologic antagonist of aldosterone	Hyperkalemia	Agents of choice for idiopathic hyperaldosteronism
	Spironolactone (Aldactone)	25–50	1–2	Competitive binding to aldosterone receptors in the distal tubule	Gynecomastia and impotence with spironolactone	May be useful in resistant hypertension
				Diuretic and antihypertensive activity	Metabolic acidosis	Spironolactone has heart failure indication

(Continued)

TABLE 6 Oral Antihypertensive Medications (*Continued*)

Medication class	Drug (trade name)	Usual dose	Daily frequency	Mechanism of action	Potential adverse reactions, side effects and complications	Comments and concerns
						Eplerenone has post MI indication antiproteinuric
						Contraindicated in advanced CKD
						Hyperkalemia risk with use in diabetics
						Hyperkalemia risk greater with ACE, or ARB
Beta blocker	Atenolol (Tenormin)	25–100	1	Blockade of beta adrenergic receptor, reduction in heart rate and cardiac output at rest and upon exercise	Bradycardia	Compelling indication in post MI, and heart failure
	Betaxolol (Kerlone)	5–20	1	Reduces renin release	Cold extremities	Cardioprotective effect with surgery
	Bisoprolol (Zebeta)	2.5–10	1		Bronchospasm	Avoid use in asthma and COPD
	Metoprolol (Lopressor)	50–100	1–2		Fatigue	Avoid abrupt withdrawal in patients with ischemic heart disease
	Metoprolol extended release (Toprol XL)	50–100	1		Dizziness	May interfere with symptoms of hypoglycemia
	Nadolol (Corgard)	40–120	1		Depression	Contraindicated in advanced heart block
	Propranolol (Inderal)	40–160	2		Lowers HDL	
	Propranolol long-acting (Inderal LA)	60–180	1		Triglyceride increase	
	Timolol (Blocadren)	20–40	2			
Beta blocker with Intrinsic sympathommetic activity	Acebutolol (Sectral)	200–800	2	Similar to beta blocker, but may reduce TPR as a result of a vasodilating effect	Similar to beta blocker	Less reduction in heart rate than beta-blockers without ISA
	Penbutolol (Levatol)	10–40	1			Approved for hypertension, no post MI or heart failure indications. Otherwise as above
	Pindolol (Visken)	10–40	2			May have less adverse effect on HDL and triglycerides
Combined alpha beta blocker	Carvedilol (Coreg)	12.5–50	2	Blockade of alpha and beta adrenergic receptors	Postural hypotension	Carvedilol indicated for heart failure and post-MI left ventricular dysfunction
	Labetalol (Normodyne, Trandate)	200–800	2	Reduction in TPR with little or no change in cardiac output heart rate	Similar to beta blocker	Intravenous Labetalol available for the treatment of hypertensive emergency. Similar to beta blocker
ACE inhibitors	Benazepril (Lotensin)	10–40	1–2	Blocks conversion of angiotensin I to angiotensin II	Cough	Compelling indications in high-risk post-MI, heart failure, diabetes, chronic renal disease

Class	Drug	Dose range	Freq	Mechanism	Side effect	Notes
	Captopril (Capoten)	25–100	2	Reduces aldosterone secretion	Angioedema	Antiproteinuric effect
	Enalapril (Vasotec)	2.5–40	1–2	Increases levels of brady kinin and prostaglandins	Rash	Hyperkalemia risk with use in diabetics and in CKD
	Fosinopril (Monopril)	10–40	1	Vasodilatation with reduction in TPR	Hyperkalemia	Monitor renal function in CKD and in renal artery stenosis
	(Lisinopril (Prinvil, Zestril)	10–40	1			Contra-indicated during pregnancy
	Moexipril (Univasc)	7.5–30	1			
	Perindopril (Aceon)	4–8	1–2			
	Quinapril (Accupril)	10–40	1			
	Ramipril (Altace)	2.5–20	1			
	Trandolapril (Mavik)	1–4	1			
Angiotensin II antagonists	Candesartan (Atacand)	8–32	1	Selectively blocks the AT 1 receptor, and the vasoconstrictor and aldosterone-secreting effects of angiotensin II	Angioedema	Compelling indications in heart failure, diabetes, and CKD
	Eprosartan (Tevetan)	400–800	1–2			Antiproteinuric effect
	Irbesartan (Avapro)	150–300	1		Excessive hypotension (rare)	Contraindicated in second and third semesters of pregnancy
	Losartan (Cozaar)	25–100	1–2			Monitor renal function in CKD and in renal artery stenosis
	Olmesartan (Benicar)	20–40	1			Contra-indicated during pregnancy
	Telmisartan (Micardis)	20–80	1			
	Valsartan (Diovan)	80–320	1			
Calcium antagonists – non dihydropyridine	Diltiazem extended release (Cardizem CD, DilacorXR, Tiazac)	180–420	1	Calcium ion influx inhibitors which selectively inhibit the transmembrane influx of ionic calcium into arterial smooth muscle as well as in conductile and contractile myocardial cells with resultant coronary and peripheral vasodilatation	Constipation	Compelling indication in high CV risk and diabetes
	Diltiazem extended release (Cardizem LA) Verapamil immediate release (Calan, Isoptin)	120–540	1		Headache Nausea	Antianginal Slow heart rate

(Continued)

TABLE 6 Oral Antihypertensive Medications (*Continued*)

Medication class	Drug (trade name)	Usual dose	Daily frequency	Mechanism of action	Potential adverse reactions, side effects and complications	Comments and concerns
	Verapamil long-acting (Calan SR, Isoptin SR)	80–320	2		Edema	Contraindicated in severe left ventricular dysfunction Second- or third-degree AV block and with atrial flutter or atrial fibrillation and an accessory bypass tract
	Verapamil-coer) (Covera HS, Verelan PM)	120–360	1–2		Elevated liver enzymes	Sick sinus syndrome, May affect digoxin, carbamazepine and cyclosporine levels
Calcium channel blockers–dihydropyridine	Amlodipine (Norvasc)	2.5–10	1	Calcium ion antagonists which inhibit the transmembrane influx of calcium ions into vascular smooth muscle and cardiac muscle	Edema	Compelling indication in high CV risk and diabet
	Felodipine (Plendil)	2.5–20	1	Primary arteriolar dilators	Dizziness	Antianginal
	Isradipine (Dynacirc CR)	2.5–10	2		Flushing	Amlodipine may be used for blood pressure control in the setting of NYHA class III, IV heart failure
	Nicardipine sustained release (Cardene SR)	60–120	2		Palpitation	Intravenous nicardipine available for treatment of hypertensive crisis
	Nifedipine long-acting (Adalat CC, Procardia XL)	30–60	1			Reports of gingival hyperplasia
	Nisoldipine (Sular)	10–40	1			
Alpha blockers	Doxazosin (Cardura)	1–16	1	Alpha-1-selective adrenoceptor blocking agents with vasodilatation of small arteries and arterioles reducing TPR	Syncope	May improve urine flow rates and reduce voiding symptoms in men
	Prazosin (Minipress)	2–20	2–3		"First" dose effect	Restricted to second- or third-line agent in hypertension
	Terazosin (Hytrin)	1–20	1–2		Postural hypotension	Doxazosin associated with higher rate of heart failure in ALLHAT
					Asthenia Palpitation Dizziness Nasal congestion	

Class	Drug	Dose range (mg)	Daily doses	Mechanism	Side effects	Comments
	Clonidine (Catapres)	0.1–0.8	2	Stimulate central alpha receptors, inhibit sympathetic outflow, ↓TPR and heart rate	Somnolence	Rebound hypertension may occur with abrupt withdrawal, with clonidine
	Clonidine patch (Catapres TTS)	0.1–0.3	1 wkly		Dry mouth Drowsiness Fatigue	Pseudo tolerance may occur when methyldopa is used without a diuretic
	Methyldopa (Aldomet)					
Centrally acting alpha agonists and peripheral sympatholytics	Reserpine (generic)	250–1000	2	Deplete sympathetic nerve terminals of norepinephrine, reducing reflex arterial and venous vasoconstriction	Postural dizziness Depression	Reserpine is contraindicated in patients with a prior history of depression or peptic ulcer disease. Combination with monoamine oxidase inhibitors may participate hypertensive crisis. Tricyclic antidepressants interfere with antihypertensive effects
	Guanfacine (generic)	0.5–2	1		Sexual dysfunction Postural hypotension Diarrhea	
Direct vasodilators	Hydralazine (Apresoline)	25–100	2	Direct relaxation of resistance vessels, primarily arteriolar vasodilatation	Tachycardia, flushing	Minoxidil remains useful in resistant hypertension
	Minoxidil (Loniten)	2.5–80	1–2		Headache	Pseudotolerance may occur as a result of reflex sympathetic nervous system activity, activation of the renin-angiotensin system, with resultant salt and water retention. Should be used with adrenergic inhibitor and a diuretic. Lupus-like reaction with hydralazine. Hair growth with minoxidil
					Fluid retention	

Abbreviations: TPR, total peripheral resistance; CKD, chronic kidney disease; ACE, angiotensin-converting enzyme; COER, controlled-onset extended-release; wkly, weekly.
Source: From Ref. 71.

SBP is the primary target for antihypertensive therapy. The Framingham Heart Study clearly demonstrated that poor BP control was overwhelmingly attributed to lack of SBP control (105). Among treated subjects, in this trial 85% had DBP less than 90 mmHg while fewer than 50% of participants had SBPs controlled less than 140 mmHg. In general, poor control rates for hypertension are driven by the failure to adequately treat and control SBP to recommended goals. These findings were confirmed in ALLHAT, where DBP was controlled and less than 90 mmHg in over 90% of the population, while SBP was less than 140 mmHg in only 67% (103).

GUIDELINES FOR TREATMENT OF HYPERTENSION
Joint National Committee VII Guidelines

Since 1977, and at nearly four-year intervals, the Joint National Committee (JNC) on the Prevention, Detection, Evaluation, and Treatment of Hypertension has published a consensus document for the U.S. clinicians treating patients with high BP. The JNC is a component of The National High Blood Pressure Education Program, which is funded by the National Heart, Lung and Blood Institute. The JNC VII report was purposely delayed until the results of the ALLHAT trial were concluded in 2002 (106). The therapeutic recommendations in JNC VII are in great part predicated on the findings of ALLHAT. The editor of the JNC VII, committee members, and writing teams were selected by the parent organization. The final report was reviewed by a group of 39 U.S. professionals, public, and volunteer organizations. The JNC VII summary was first published on May 21, 2003, and has had no updates following the publication of recent clinical trials such as Anglo-Scandinavian Cardiac Outcomes Trial (ASCOT), International Verapamil – Trandolapril Study (INVEST), Trial of Preventing Hypertension (TROPHY), or Valsartan Antihypertensive Long-term Use Evaluation (VALUE) (97).

The mandate of JNC VII was to provide an evidence-based approach to the prevention, detection, and management of hypertension and to highlight recent advances that have occurred in the field since JNC VI. The 2003 report introduced several new key messages which were emphasized in the document and supporting materials (107).

- In those older than age 50, SBP greater than or equal to 140 mmHg is a more important CVD risk factor than DBP.
- CVD risk doubles for each increment of 20/10 mmHg beginning at 115/75 mmHg.
- Even those who are normotensive at 55 years of age will have a 90% lifetime risk of developing hypertension.
- Individuals with prehypertension now defined as SBP 120 to 139 mmHg or DBP 80 to 89 mmHg require health-promoting lifestyle modifications to prevent the progressive rise in BP and CVD.
- In uncomplicated primary hypertension, thiazide diuretics should be used in drug treatment for *most*, either alone or combined with drugs from other classes.
- High-risk conditions which are generally defined by concomitant CVD are now recognized as compelling indications for the use of other antihypertensive drug classes (ACEIs, ARBs, beta-blockers, and CCBs).
- Two or more antihypertensive medications will be required to achieve goal BP (<140/90 mmHg, or <130/80 mmHg) for many patients with primary hypertension and those with diabetes and CKD.
- In patients whose BP is more than 20 mmHg above the SBP goal or more than 10 mmHg above the DBP goal, initiation of therapy using two antihypertensive agents, one of which usually will be a thiazide diuretic, should be considered.
- Hypertension will be controlled only if patients are motivated to stay on their treatment.

These themes were in part designed to correct persistent and prevalent misperceptions surrounding the treatment of hypertension, including the following: that most cases of hypertension can be controlled with one antihypertensive medication; that DBP is a better indicator than SBP for advancing or intensifying antihypertensive therapy; and that the age-related increase in SBP is normal.

A stated goal of JNC VII was to present clinicians with a streamlined, clear, and concise guideline for the classification and management of hypertension. As a result, the classification

TABLE 7 Classification and Management of Blood Pressure for Adults Aged 18 Years or Older

BP classifi-cation	Systolic BP, mmHg[a]		Diastolic BP, mmHg[a]	Lifestyle modifications	Management[a] Initial drug therapy Without compelling Indications	With compelling Indications[b]
Normal	<120	And	<80	Encourage		
Prehyper-tension	<120–139	Or	80–89	Yes	No antihypertensive drug indicated	Drug(s) for the compelling indications[c]
Stage 1 hypertension	140–159	Or	90–99	Yes	Thiazide-type diuretics for most; may consider ACE inhibitor, ARB, β-blocker, CCB, or combination	Drug(s) for the compelling indications Other antihypertensive drugs (diuretics, ACE inhibitor, ARB, β-blocker, CCB) as needed
Stage 2 hypertension	≥160	Or	≥100	Yes	2-Drug combination for most (usually thiazide type diuretic and ACE inhibitor or ARB or β blocker or CCB)[d]	Drug(s) for the compelling indications Other antihypertensive drugs (diuretics, ACE inhibitor, ARB, β-blocker, CCB) as needed

[a]Treatment determined by highest BP category.
[b]See Table 6.
[c]Treat patients with chronic kidney disease to BP goal of less than 130/80 mmHg.
[d]Initial combined therapy should be used cautiously in those at risk for orthostatic hypotension.
Abbreviations: ACE, angiotensin-converting enzyme; ARB, angiotensin-receptor blocker; BP, blood pressure; CCB, calcium channel blocker.
Source: From Ref. 97.

of hypertension, the integration of CV risk into the treatment paradigm, and treatment recommendations were simplified over those outlined in JNC-VI (108).

A notable difference between JNC-VII and JNC-VI is the new classification of hypertension. The current classification of hypertension is shown in Table 7. JNC-VII simplifies the classification of BP, and now defines three distinct categories across the BP continuum: normal, prehypertension, and hypertension. The definition of normal BP in JNC-VII has remained consistent with prior reports, and again is defined as a SBP less than 120 mmHg and DBP less than 80 mmHg. Prehypertension, is the most significant change in the new classification scheme and is defined as a SBP 120 to 139 mmHg or DBP 80 to 89 mmHg. The hypertension classification has also been revised and JNC-VII redefined Stage II hypertension. Stages II and III from JNC-VI are now combined into Stage II in JNC-VII.

The treatment goals in JNC-VII remain unchanged from JNC-VI. For patients with Stage I or II uncomplicated hypertension, the goal BP is less than 140/90 mmHg. In high-risk populations such as those with diabetes or CKD, a goal BP of less than 130/80 mmHg is recommended. Management principles and initial drug therapy recommendations appear in Table 7.

Lifestyle modification is now recommended for populations with prehypertension and hypertension. JNC-VII recognizes the importance of ACEIs, ARBs, beta-blockers, CCBs, and thiazide-type diuretics, in obtaining BP control and notes the ability of these agents to reduce CV complications. The report, however, focuses on the importance of thiazide diuretics as first line therapy in the treatment of hypertension and makes the point that in ALLHAT and other clinical trials, diuretics have been "virtually unsurpassed" in preventing the CV complications of hypertension.

Thus, in Stage I uncomplicated hypertension, thiazide-type diuretics are recommended in *most* patients, although ACEIs, ARBs, beta-blockers, or CCBs—or a combination therapy—are also recognized as suitable first line therapy (Table 7). JNC-VII indicates that about two-thirds of patients will ultimately require multiple drugs to control their hypertension. The addition of a second drug from a different class is indicated when a single drug is titrated to an adequate dose and fails to achieve the BP control. In patients with Stage II hypertension, treatment can be initiated with two drugs, one of which should be a diuretic.

High-risk patients who present with hypertension in conjunction with heart failure, diabetes, chronic renal disease, or other comorbid conditions are now recognized as having a compelling indication for specific antihypertensive medications. Antihypertensive therapy in these patients is introduced with those drugs, which have been shown on the basis of clinical trial data to be particularly beneficial for such conditions. Compelling indications with specific drug recommendations and the cited clinical trial support are listed in Table 8.

The JNC VII approach to hypertension control can best be summarized in the treatment algorithm in Figure 5. The essential elements of this approach to hypertension control are the establishment of a goal BP for each patient, aggressive treatment to that goal, and the use multiple medications if necessary. To improve BP control, JNC VII emphasizes the need for interaction between the physician and the patient, and for the physician empathy, which will likely build trust and increase motivation so as to improve patient adherence to therapy. Public health strategies involving lifestyle modification are recommended for the prehypertensive populations.

Controversy has surrounded the JNC VII report and limited its acceptance nationally and internationally. Most of the debate centers on the JNC VII definition of a prehypertensive state, the lack of an integrated CV risk assessment, and the strong recommendation for the preferential use of thiazide diuretics as first line therapy for hypertension control. As a result of these concerns, a writing group of the American Society of Hypertension (ASH) has recently proposed a new definition of hypertension, this defination is based on an assessment of the individual patient's global CV risk, such as age, sex, lipid levels, BMI, smoking, and family history of disease, as well as early markers of CVD, such as exaggerated BP responses to exercise or mental stress, microalbuminuria, or impaired glucose tolerance, and hypertensive target organ damage, measurable in the heart, arteries, kidneys, and eyes. The main aim of the new definition, however, is to urge physicians to look at overall CV risk rather than a patient's BP level in isolation. Thus, the new proposed ASH definition focuses on diagnosing hypertension on the basis of the presence or absence of hypertension-associated risk factors, early disease markers, and target organ damage, at any given BP level (3,110).

World Health Organization/ International Society of Hypertension Guidelines

The World Health Organization(WHO), International Society of Hypertension (ISH) guidelines address the following issues: (*i*) the ascertainment of overall CV risk to establish both

TABLE 8 Clinical Trial and Guideline Basis for Compelling Indications for Individual Drug Classes

High-risk conditions with compelling indications	Recommended drugs					
	Diuretic	B-Blocker	ACE Inhibitor	ARB	CCB	Aldosterone antagonist
Heart failure	●	●	●	●		●
Post-myocardial infarction		●	●			●
High coronary disease risk	●	●	●		●	
Diabetes	●	●	●	●	●	
Chronic kidney disease			●	●		
Recurrent stroke prevention	●		●			

Source: From Ref. 97. Abbreviations: ACE, angiotensin-converting enzyme; ARB, angiotensin-receptor blocker; CCB, calcium channel blocker.

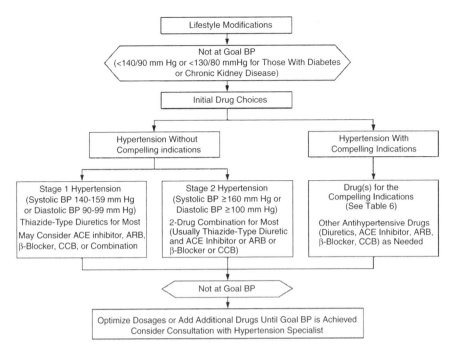

FIGURE 5 Algorithm for treatment of hypertension. *Source:* From Ref. 97.

the thresholds for initiation of treatment and the goals of treatment for people with hypertension in general and for various subgroups; (*ii*) the appropriate treatment strategies for both nondrug and drug therapies; and (*iii*) the cost-effectiveness of drug treatment (111).

Decisions about the management of hypertensive patients should not only take BP levels into account, but also the presence of other CV risk factors, target organ damage, and associated clinical conditions The risk stratification table from the 1999 WHO/ISH Guidelines (72) has been minimally amended to indicate three major risk categories with progressively increasing absolute likelihood of developing a major CV event (fatal and nonfatal stroke and myocardial infarction) within the next 10 years: (i) low risk—less than 15%; (ii) medium risk—15–20%; and (iii) high risk—greater than 20%. The simplicity of the method enables a rapid preliminary assessment of CV risk and provides a flexible risk stratification system that can be customized to a range of practice settings with varying levels of resources. However, the categorical method used is less accurate than those using continuous variables, and this is a limitation of this risk stratification chart.

The simplicity of the method enables a rapid preliminary assessment of CV risk and provides a flexible risk stratification system that can be customized to a range of practice settings with varying levels of resources. However, the categorical method used is less accurate than those using continuous variables, and this is a limitation of this risk stratification chart.

Observational data suggest that even low-risk patients with BP greater than or equal to 140 mmHg systolic and/or greater than or equal to 90 mmHg diastolic are likely to benefit from lower pressures. Although women are at lower absolute risk of CVD for a given level of BP, and randomized clinical trial evidence includes a greater proportion of men than women, the treatment threshold should be the same in both men and women.

Absolute risk of CVD for any given level of BP rises with age, but only limited evidence is currently available about the benefits of treating those over 80 years of age. For now, the treatment threshold should be unaffected by age at least up to the age of 80 years. Thereafter, judgment should be made on an individual basis and therapy should not be withdrawn from patients over 80 years of age. This is suggested by a meta-analysis of data from patients above 80 years of age in which the group on antihypertensive treatment showed a significant reduction in stroke incidence compared with the control group (112).

In patients with diabetes, reduction of DBP to about 80 mmHg and of SBP to about 130 mmHg was accompanied by a further reduction in CV events or diabetes-related microvascular complications, as compared with patients with less stringent BP control (113,114). Based on clinical trial evidence, and also on extrapolation from epidemiological studies, a target of less than 130/80 mmHg seems appropriate. There is no evidence of a need to modify these target BPs for female or older patients with hypertension.

The BP thresholds for treatment discussed above will result in as many as 25% of all adults—and more than 50% of those over the age of 65—in some populations requiring antihypertensive therapy. Further, less than half of all hypertensive patients will attain the BP targets recommended above with monotherapy (115,116). Most will need at least two antihypertensive drugs, and as many as 30% of patients will need three or more drugs in combination to attain target BP levels.

A variety of lifestyle modifications have been shown, in clinical trials, to lower BP (117) and to reduce the incidence of hypertension. These include weight loss in the overweight (118), physical activity (119), moderation of alcohol intake (120), a diet with increased fresh fruit and vegetables and reduced saturated fat content (100), reduction of dietary sodium intake, and increased dietary potassium intake (121–123). Other lifestyle changes have not been found in multiple clinical trials to have a significant or lasting antihypertensive effect. These include calcium (124) and magnesium supplements (125), reduction in caffeine intake (126), and a variety of techniques designed to reduce stress (127). In addition to their possible influence on BP, observational studies have found that other lifestyle modifications, in particular cessation of smoking; reduce CVD mortality (128). Moreover, weight reduction, dietary manipulation, and physical activity reduce the incidence of Type 2 diabetes and a low-saturated fat diet improves dyslipidemia (129–131). Therefore, regardless of the level of BP, all individuals should adopt appropriate lifestyle modifications. The protective effects of modifying lifestyle include a reduction in the incidence of hypertension, diabetes, and dyslipidemia, a reduction in mortality by cessation of smoking, and a lowering of BP that, in itself, is likely to reduce CV morbidity and mortality. Furthermore, unlike drug therapy, which may cause adverse effects and reduce the quality of life in some patients, nonpharmacological therapy has no known harmful effects, improves the sense of well-being of the patient, and is often less expensive.

The BP-lowering Treatment Trialists' Collaboration meta-analysis of data from randomized clinical trials comparing two newer classes, i.e., ACEIs and CCBs, against older classes, i.e., diuretics and beta-blockers, in almost 75,000 hypertensive patients showed no significant convincing differences between drug classes or between groups of old and new drugs (132). Despite these potential limitations, the available data conclusively documented the value of antihypertensive therapy and suggested that the benefits are largely derived from their reduction in BP.

For the majority of patients without a compelling indication for another class of drug, a low dose of a diuretic should be considered as the first choice of therapy on the basis of comparative trial data, availability, and cost. A diuretic is often available in single tablets combined with other classes of drugs. Where they are no more expensive, such combined formulations may be preferable, because they have advantages in terms of compliance and BP-lowering efficacy. Other combinations of drugs with complementary actions may be appropriate for patients' needs.

Most drugs used to treat hypertension have also been evaluated for a number of specific indications. These include ACEIs, ARBs, beta-blockers, CCBs, and diuretics in patients with concomitant diabetes, nephropathy, coronary and cerebrovascular disease, heart failure, and left ventricular hypertrophy (LVH). When studies have shown a greater reduction in various fatal and nonfatal major-disease endpoints with one or another type of drug class, that class is considered to have a compelling indication for its use.

Comparisons have been made between the ability of different classes of drugs to regress LVH and to slow the progression of nephropathies. For regression of LVH, CCBs, ACEIs, and ARBs have been found to be more effective than beta-blockers and diuretics (133–135). Multiple placebo-controlled trials have shown significant reductions in proteinuria and a slowing of progression of renal damage in both nondiabetic and Type 1 diabetic nephropathies with ACEIs (136) and in Type 2 diabetic nephropathy with ARBs (137,138).

In addition to these compelling indications, certain drugs may logically be chosen for other reasons. Thus, when used as monotherapy, a diuretic or CCB may lower BP more in African American and older patients than an ACEI or a beta-blocker (139,140) and an alpha-blocker will relieve symptoms of prostatism (141). Central alpha-agonists (e.g., clonidine), or peripheral adrenergic blockers (e.g., reserpine), may be used as inexpensive therapies in certain settings, despite the absence of outcome data.

RECENT LANDMARK HYPERTENSION TRIALS: IMPLICATIONS FOR EVIDENCE-BASED MEDICINE

A new series of trials has been completed, and several other trials started in efforts to further elucidate the effects of ACEIs, ARBs, CCBs, and other BP-lowering drugs on mortality and major CV morbidity in several populations of patients, including those with hypertension, diabetes mellitus, CHD, or renal disease.

The overview of placebo-controlled trials of ACEIs revealed 30% reductions in stroke, 20% in CHD, and 21% in major CV events. The overview of placebo-controlled trials of calcium antagonists showed 39% reductions in stroke and 28% in major CV events. In the overview of trials comparing BP-lowering strategies of different intensity, there were reduced risks of stroke (20%), CHD (19%), and major CV events (15%) with more intensive therapy (132).

Since 2000, several landmark trials in hypertension treatment have been published, providing more evidence-based medicine data regarding optimal treatment of hypertension to reduce CV morbidity and mortality.

Intervention as a Goal in Hypertension Treatment

The Intervention as a Goal in Hypertension Treatment (INSIGHT) study was a prospective, randomized, double-blind trial in 6321 patients, aged 55 to 80 years with hypertension (BP greater than or equal to 150/95 mmHg, or greater than or equal to 160 mmHg systolic) (142). Patients had at least one additional CV risk factor. Patients were randomly assigned to nifedipine 30 mg in a long-acting gastrointestinal transport system (GITS) formulation, or co-amilozide (hydrochlorothiazide 25 mg plus amiloride 2.5 mg). Dose titration was by dose doubling, and addition of atenolol 25 to 50 mg or enalapril 5 to 10 mg. The primary outcome was CV death, myocardial infarction, heart failure, or stroke. Analysis was done by intention to treat. Primary outcomes occurred in 200 (6.3%) of the patients in the nifedipine group and in 182 (5.8%) in the co-amilozide group (18.2 vs. 16.5 events per 1000 patient-years; relative risk 1.10 [95% CI 0.91–1.34], $p = 0.35$). Overall mean BP dropped from 173/99 to 138/82 mmHg. There was an 8% excess of withdrawals from the nifedipine group because of peripheral edema, but serious adverse events were more frequent in the co-amilozide group ($p = 0.02$). Deaths were mainly nonvascular (nifedipine 176 vs. co-amilozide 172; $p = 0.81$). Nifedipine once daily and co-amilozide were equally effective in preventing overall CV or cerebrovascular complications.

European Lacidipine Study on Atherosclerosis

The European Lacidipine Study on Atherosclerosis (ELSA) study was a randomized, double-blind trial in 2334 patients with hypertension that compared the effects of a four-year treatment based on either lacidipine or atenolol on an index of carotid atherosclerosis, the mean of the maximum intima-media thickness (IMT) in far walls of common carotids and bifurcations (CBMmax) (143). The yearly IMT progression rate was 0.0145 mm/yr in the atenolol-treated and 0.0087 mm/yr in the lacidipine-treated patients (completers, 40% reduction; $p = 0.0073$). Patients with plaque progression were significantly less common, and patients with plaque regression were significantly more common in the lacidipine group. Clinic BP reductions were identical in both treatments, but 24-hour ambulatory SBP/DBP changes were greater with atenolol ($-10/-9$ mmHg) than with lacidipine ($-7/-5$ mmHg). No significant difference between treatments was found in any CV events, although the relative risk for stroke, major CV events, and mortality showed a trend favoring lacidipine. The greater efficacy of lacidipine on carotid IMT progression and number of plaques per patient, despite a smaller ambulatory BP reduction, indicates an antiatherosclerotic action of lacidipine independent of its antihypertensive action.

Comparison of Amlodipine Versus Enalapril to Limit Occurrences of Thrombosis

The Comparison of Amlodipine versus Enalapril to Limit Occurrences of Thrombosis (CAMELOT) study was a double-blind, randomized, multicenter 24-month trial comparing amlodipine or enalapril with placebo in 1991 patients with angiographically documented coronary artery disease (CAD > 20% stenosis by coronary angiography) and DBP less than 100 mmHg (144). A substudy of 274 patients measured atherosclerotic progression by intravascular ultrasound (IVUS). Patients were randomized to receive amlodipine 10 mg, enalapril 20 mg, or placebo. IVUS was performed at baseline and study completion. The primary efficacy parameter was the incidence of CV events for amlodipine versus placebo. Other outcomes included comparisons of amlodipine versus enalapril and enalapril versus placebo. CV Event included CV death, nonfatal myocardial infarction, resuscitated cardiac arrest, coronary revascularization, hospitalization for angina pectoris, hospitalization for congestive heart failure, fatal or nonfatal stroke or transient ischemic attack, and new diagnosis of peripheral vascular disease. The IVUS substudy normalized end point was change in atheroma volume. Baseline BP averaged 129/78 mmHg for all patients; it increased by 0.7/0.6 mmHg in the placebo group and decreased by 4.8/2.5 mmHg and 4.9/2.4 mmHg in the amlodipine and enalapril groups, respectively ($p < 0.001$ for both vs. placebo). CV events occurred in 151 (23.1%) placebo-treated patients, in 110 (16.6%) amlodipine-treated patients [hazard ratio (HR), 0.69; 95% CI, 0.54–0.88 $p = 0.003$], and in 136 (20.2%) enalapril-treated patients HR, 0.85; 95% CI, 0.67–1.07 $p = 0.16$). Primary endpoint comparison for enalapril versus amlodipine was not significant (HR, 0.81; 95% CI, 0.63–1.04 $p = 0.10$). The IVUS substudy showed a trend toward less progression of atherosclerosis in the amlodipine group versus placebo ($p = 0.12$), with significantly less progression in the subgroup with SBPs greater than the mean ($p = 0.02$). Compared with baseline, IVUS showed progression in the placebo ($p < 0.001$), a trend toward progression in the enalapril group ($p = 0.08$), and no progression in the amlodipine group ($p = 0.31$). For the amlodipine group, correlation between BP reduction and progression was $r = 0.19$, $p = 0.07$. Administration of amlodipine to patients with CAD and normal BP resulted in a reduction of adverse CV events. Directionally similar, but smaller and nonsignificant treatment effects were observed with enalapril. For amlodipine, IVUS showed evidence of slowing of atherosclerosis progression.

Controlled Onset Verapamil Investigation of CV Endpoints

The Controlled Onset Verapamil Investigation of CV Endpoints (CONVINCE) trial was a randomized-trial, double-blind, actively controlled multicenter, international clinical trial designed to test the hypothesis of equivalence of two antihypertensive drug regimens, beginning either with controlled-onset, extended-release verapamil or the investigator's preselected choice of either atenolol or hydrochlorothiazide in reducing CV events (145). A total number of 16,602 hypertensive patients were enrolled with more than or equal to one additional CV risk factor. The primary objective was to compare the two regimens in preventing acute myocardial infarction, stroke, or CVD-related death. Major secondary outcomes included: (i) an expanded CVD endpoint (hospitalization for angina, cardiac revascularization or transplant, heart failure, transient ischemic attacks or carotid endarterectomy, accelerated or malignant hypertension, or renal failure in addition to primary outcome); (ii) all cause mortality; (iii) cancer; (iv) hospitalization for bleeding (excluding hemorrhagic stroke); and (v) incidence of primary endpoints occurring between 6:00 A.M. and noon (5). The overall results did not differ significantly by treatment group and the prespecified equivalence criteria were not met. In addition, treatment differences for the major endpoints were consistent for four geographical regions defined a priori—United States, Canada, Western Europe, and "other countries."

VALSARTAN ANTIHYPERTENSIVE LONG-TERM USE EVALUATION (VALUE) TRIAL

The Valsartan Antihypertensve Long-term Use Evaluation (VALUE) trial was designed to test the hypothesis that for the same BP control, valsartan would reduce cardiac morbidity and mortality more than amlodipine in hypertensive patients at high CV risk (146). A total number of 15,245 patients, aged 50 years or older with treated or untreated hypertension and high risk of cardiac events participated in a randomized, double-blind, parallel-group comparison of therapy based on valsartan or amlodipine. Duration of treatment was event-driven and the trial lasted until at least 1450 patients had reached a primary endpoint, defined as a composite of cardiac mortality and morbidity. Patients from 31 countries were followed up for a mean of 4.2 years. BP was reduced by both treatments, but the effects of the amlodipine-based regimen were more pronounced, especially in the early period (BP 4.0/2.1 mmHg lower in amlodipine than valsartan group after one month; 1.5/1.3 mmHg after one year; $p < 0.001$ between groups). The primary composite endpoint occurred in 810 patients in the valsartan group (10.6%, 25.5 per 1000 patient-years) and 789 in the amlodipine group (10.4%, 24.7 per 1000 patient-years; HR 1.04,

95% CI 0.94–1.15, $p = 0.49$). The main outcome of cardiac disease did not differ between the treatment groups. Unequal reductions in BP might account for differences between the groups in cause-specific outcomes. The findings emphasized the importance of prompt BP control in hypertensive patients at high CV risk. The VALUE trial was designed to test whether, for the same achieved BPs, regimens based on valsartan or amlodipine would have differing effects on CV endpoints in high-risk hypertension. But inequalities in BP, favoring amlodipine, throughout the multiyear trial limited the comparison of outcomes (147).

ANGLO-SCANDINAVIAN CARDIAC OUTCOMES TRIAL (ASCOT)

The apparent shortfall in prevention of CHD noted in early hypertension trials has been attributed to potential metabolic disadvantages of the diuretic and beta-blocker therapy. For a given reduction in BP, some suggested that newer agents would confer advantages over diuretics and beta-blockers. The aim of the Anglo-Scandinavian Cardiac Outcomes Trial (ASCOT) trial was to compare the effect on nonfatal myocardial infarction and fatal CHD of combinations of atenolol with a thiazide versus amlodipine with perindopril. The ASCOT trial was a multicenter, prospective, randomized controlled trial in 19,257 patients with hypertension who were aged 40 to 79 years and had at least three other CV risk factors (148). Patients were assigned either amlodipine 5 to 10 mg, adding perindopril 4 to 8 mg as required (amlodipine-based regimen; $n = 9639$), or atenolol 50 to 100 mg, adding bendroflumethiazide 1.25 to 2.5 mg and potassium as required (atenolol-based regimen; $n = 9618$). The primary endpoint was nonfatal myocardial infarction (including silent myocardial infarction) and fatal CHD. Analysis was by intention to treat. The study was stopped prematurely by the DSMI after 5.5 years' median follow-up and accumulated in total 106,153 patient-years of observation. Though not significant, compared with the atenolol-based regimen, fewer individuals on the amlodipine-based regimen had a primary endpoint (429 vs. 474; unadjusted HR 0.90, 95% CI 0.79–1.02, $p = 0.1052$), fatal and nonfatal stroke (327 vs. 422; 0.77, 0.66–0.89, $p = 0.0003$), total CV events and procedures (1362 vs. 1602; 0.84, 0.78–0.90, $p < 0.0001$), and all cause mortality (738 vs. 820; 0.89, 0.81–0.99, $p = 0.025$). The incidence of developing diabetes was less on the amlodipine-based regimen (567 vs. 799; 0.70, 0.63–0.78, $p < 0.0001$). The amlodipine-based regimen prevented more major CV events and induced less diabetes than the atenolol-based regimen.

CONDUIT ARTERY FUNCTION EVALUATION (CAFE) TRIAL

Different BP-lowering drugs could have different effects on central aortic pressures and thus CV outcome despite similar effects on brachial BP. The Conduit Artery Function Evaluation (CAFE) study, a substudy of the ASCOT, examined the impact of two different BP-lowering regimens (atenolol ± thiazide-based vs. amlodipine ± perindopril-based therapy) on derived central aortic pressures and hemodynamics. The CAFE study recruited 2199 patients in five ASCOT centers (149). Radial artery applanation tonometry and pulse wave analysis were used to derive central aortic pressures and hemodynamic indexes on repeated visits for up to four years. Most patients received combination therapy throughout the study. Despite similar brachial SBPs between treatment groups (Δ 0.7 mmHg; 95% CI, −0.4–1.7; $p = 0.2$), there were substantial reductions in central aortic pressures with the amlodipine regimen (central aortic SBP, Δ 4.3 mmHg; 95% CI, 3.3–5.4; $p < 0.0001$; central aortic PP, Δ 3.0 mmHg; 95% CI, 2.1–3.9; $p < 0.0001$). Cox proportional-hazards modeling showed that central PP was significantly associated with a post-hoc–defined composite outcome of total CV events/procedures and development of renal impairment in the CAFE cohort (unadjusted, $p < 0.0001$; adjusted for baseline variables, $p < 0.05$). BP-lowering drugs can have substantially different effects on central aortic pressures and hemodynamics despite a similar impact on brachial BP. Moreover, central aortic PP may be a determinant of clinical outcomes, and differences in central aortic pressures may be a potential mechanism to explain the different clinical outcomes between the two BP treatment arms in ASCOT.

TRIAL OF PREVENTION OF HYPERTENSION (TROPHY)

Prehypertension is considered a precursor of Stage I hypertension and a predictor of excessive CV risk. The Trial of Preventing Hypertension (TROPHY) studied whether pharmacologic treatment of prehypertension prevents or postpones Stage I hypertension (150).

Participants with repeated measurements of systolic pressure of 130 to 139 mmHg and diastolic pressure of 89 mmHg or lower, or systolic pressure of 139 mmHg or lower and diastolic pressure of 85 to 89 mmHg, were randomly assigned to receive two years of candesartan or placebo, followed by two years of placebo for all. When a participant reached the study endpoint of Stage I hypertension, treatment with antihypertensive agents was initiated. Both the candesartan group and the placebo group were instructed to make changes in lifestyle to reduce BP throughout the trial. A total of 409 participants were randomly assigned to candesartan, and 400 to placebo. Data on 772 participants (391 in the candesartan group and 381 in the placebo group; mean age, 48.5 years; 59.6% men) were available for analysis. During the first two years, hypertension developed in 154 participants in the placebo group and 53 of those in the candesartan group (relative risk reduction, 66.3%; $p < 0.001$). After four years, hypertension had developed in 240 participants in the placebo group and 208 of those in the candesartan group (relative risk reduction, 15.6%; $p < 0.007$). Over a period of four years, Stage I hypertension developed in nearly two-thirds of patients with untreated prehypertension (the placebo group). Treatment of prehypertension with candesartan appeared to be well tolerated and reduced the risk of incident hypertension during the study period. Thus, treatment of prehypertension appears to be feasible. However, we need to learn who should be treated, for how many years, and with which drug and at what dose. For now, a healthy lifestyle is the foundation for all therapies in persons with prehypertension. This is still true even after the lessons of the TROPHY study. Ultimately, another battle must be won—that of successful control of BP in millions of patients who have established hypertension (151).

REFERENCES

1. Cohn JN. Arteries, myocardium, blood pressure and cardiovascular risk towards a revised definition of hypertension. J Hypertens 1998; 16:2117–2124.
2. Lloyd-Jones DM, Leip EP, Larson MG, Vasan RS, Levy D. Novel approach to examining first cardiovascular events after hypertension onset. Hypertension 2005; 45:39–45.
3. Giles TD, Berk BC, Black HR, et al. Expanding the definition and classification of hypertension. J Clin Hypertens 2005; 7:505–512.
4. Lewington S, Clarke R, Quizilbash N, Peto R, Collins R. Age-specific relevance of usual blood pressure to vascular mortality: a meta-analysis of individual data for one million adults in 61 prospective studies. Lancet 2002; 360:1903–1913.
5. Vasan RS, Larson MG, Leip EP, et al. Impact of high-normal blood pressure on the risk of cardiovascular disease. N Engl J Med 2001; 345:1291–1297.
6. Ezzati M, Lopez AD, Rodgers A, et al. For the Comparative Risk Assessment Collaborating Group. Selected major risk factors and global and regional burden of disease. Lancet 2002; 360:1347–1360.
7. Hajjar I, Kotchen TA. Trends in prevalence, awareness, treatment, and control of hypertension in the United States, 1988–2000. JAMA 2003; 290:199–206.
8. Wolf-Maier K, Cooper RS, Banegas JR, et al. Hypertension prevalence and blood pressure levels in 6 European countries, Canada, and the United States. JAMA 2003; 289:2363–2369.
9. Freis ED. Studies in hemodynamics and hypertension. Hypertension 2001; 38:1–5.
10. Susic D, Frohlich ED. Hypertension and the heart. Curr Hypertens Rep 2000; 2:565–569.
11. Duprez DA, Kaiser DR, Whitwam W, et al. Determinants of radial artery pulse wave analysis in asymptomatic individuals. Am J Hypertens 2004; 17:647–653.
12. O'Rourke MF, Staessen JA, Vlachopoulos C, et al. Clinical applications of arterial stiffness; definitions and reference values. Am J Hypertens 2002; 15:426–444.
13. McVeigh GE. Pulse waveform analysis and arterial wall properties. Hypertension 2003; 41:1010–1011.
14. Cohn JN, Quyyumi AA, Hollenberg NK, Jamerson KA. Surrogate markers for cardiovascular disease: functional markers. Circulation 2004; 109(Suppl 1):IV31–IV46.
15. Messerli FH, Frohlich ED, Suarez DH, et al. Borderline hypertension: relationship between age, hemodynamics and circulating catecholamines. Circulation 1981; 64:760–764.
16. Clement DL, Duprez D. Circulatory changes in muscle and skin arteries in primary hypertension. Hypertension 1984; 6(6 Pt 2):III122–III127.
17. Duprez DA, De Buyzere ML, Verloove HH, et al. Influence of the arterial blood pressure and nonhemodynamic factors on regional arterial wall properties in moderate essential hypertension. J Hum Hypertens 1996; 10:251–256.
18. Guyton AC. Dominant role of the kidneys and accessory role of whole-body autoregulation in the pathogenesis of hypertension. Am J Hypertens 1989; 2:575–585.
19. Ritz E. The role of the kidney in cardiovascular medicine. Eur J Int Med 2005; 16:321–327.
20. Campese VM. Pathophysiology of renal parenchymal hypertension. In: Izzo JL, Black J, eds. Hypertension Primer: The Essentials of High Blood Pressure. Baltimore, MD: Lippincott Williams and Wilkins, 1999:135–137.

21. Brenner BM, Chertow GM. Congenital oligonephropathy and the etiology of adult hypertension and progressive renal injury. Am J Kidney Dis 1994; 23:171–175.
22. Keller G, Zimmer G, Mall G, Ritz E, Amann K. Nephron number in patients with primary hypertension. N Engl J Med 2003; 348:101–108.
23. Duprez DA. Role of the renin–angiotensin–aldosterone system in vascular remodeling and inflammation: a clinical review. J Hypertension 2006; 24:983–991.
24. Pantanetti P, Garrapa GGM, Mantero F, et al. Adipose tissue as an endocrine organ? A review of recent data related to cardiovascular complications of endocrine dysfunctions. Clin Exp Hypertens 2004; 26:387–398.
25. Pagliaro P, Penna C. Rethinking the renin–angiotensin system and its role in cardiovascular regulation. Cardiovasc Drugs Ther 2005; 19:77–87.
26. Suzuki Y, Ruiz-Ortega M, Lorenzo O, et al. Inflammation and angiotensin II. Int J Biochem Cell Biol 2003; 35:881–900.
27. Touyz RM, Tabet F, Schiffrin EL. Redox-dependent signaling by angiotensin II and vascular remodeling in hypertension. Clin Exp Pharmacol Physiol 2003; 30:860–866.
28. Duprez D. Angiotensin II, platelets, and oxidative stress. J Hypertens 2004; 22:1085–1086.
29. Watanabe T, Barker TA, Berk BC. Angiotensin II and the endothelium; diverse signals and effects. Hypertension 2005; 45:163–169.
30. Berk BC. Angiotensin type 2 receptor (AT2R): a challenging twin. Sci STKE 2003; 181:PE16.
31. Weiss D, Kools JJ, Taylor WR. Angiotensin-induced hypertension accelerates the development of atherosclerosis in apoE-deficient mice. Circulation 2001; 103:448–454.
32. Touyz RM. Molecular and cellular mechanisms in vascular injury in hypertension: role of angiotensin II. Curr Opin Nephrol Hypertens 2005; 14:125–131.
33. Rocha R, Rudolph AE, Frierdich GE, et al. Aldosterone induces a vascular inflammatory phenotype in the rat heart. Am J Physiol Heart Circ Physiol 2002; 283:H1802–H1810.
34. Duprez D, Buyzere M, Rietzschel ER, Clement DL. Aldosterone and vascular damage. Curr Hypertens Rep 2000; 2:327–334.
35. Funder JW. The nongenomic actions of aldosterone. Endocr Rev 2005; 26:313–321.
36. Struthers AD. The clinical implications of aldosterone escape in congestive heart failure. Eur J Heart Fail 2004; 6:539–545.
37. Bristow JD, Honour AJ, Pickering GW, Sleight P, Smyth HS. Diminished baroreflex sensitivity in high blood pressure. Circulation 1969; 39:48–54.
38. Sculati G, Giannattasio C, Seravalle G, et al. Early alterations of the baroreceptors control of heart rate in patients with acute myocardial infarction. Circulation 1990; 81:939–948.
39. La Rovere MT, Bigger TJ, Marcus FI, Mortara A, Schwartz PJ. For the ATRAMI (Autonomic Tone and Reflexes After Myocardial Infarction) investigators. Baroreflex sensitivity and heart rate variability in prediction of total cardiac mortality after myocardial infarction. Lancet 1998; 351:478–484.
40. Parati G, Di Rienzo M, Bertinieri G, et al. Evaluation of the baroreceptor-heart rate reflex by 24-hour intra-arterial blood pressure monitoring in humans. Hypertension 1988; 12:214–222.
41. Osborn JW, Jacob F, Guzman P. A neural set point for the long-term control of arterial pressure: beyond the arterial baroreceptor reflex. Am J Physiol 2005; 288:R846–R855.
42. Galarza CR, Alfie J, Waisman GD, et al. Diastolic pressure underestimates age-related hemodynamic impairment. Hypertension 1997; 30:809–816.
43. Lund-Johansen P. Twenty-year follow-up of hemodynamics in essential hypertension during rest and exercise. Hypertension 1991; 18(5 Suppl):III54–III61.
44. Pepe S, Lakatta EG. Aging hearts and vessels: masters of adaptation and survival. Cardiovasc Res 2005; 66:190–193.
45. Robert L. Aging of the vascular wall and atherogenesis: role of the elastin-laminin receptor. Atherosclerosis 1996; 123:169–179.
46. London GM. Role of arterial wall properties in the pathogenesis of systolic hypertension. Am J Hypertens 2005; 18(1 Pt 2):19S–22S.
47. McVeigh GE, Allen PB, Morgan DR, Hanratty CG, Silke B. Nitric oxide modulation of blood vessel tone identified by arterial waveform analysis. Clin Sci (Lond) 2001; 100:387–393.
48. Clarkson P, Celermajer DS, Powe AJ, et al. Endothelium-dependent dilatation is impaired in young healthy subjects with a family history of premature coronary disease. Circulation 1997; 96:3378–3383.
49. Anderson TJ, Uehata A, Gerhard MD, et al. Close relation of endothelial function in the human coronary and peripheral circulation. J Am Coll Cardiol 1995; 26:1235–1241.
50. Barenbrock M, Hausberg M, Kosch M, et al. Flow-mediated vasodilation and distensibility in relation to intima-media thickness of large arteries in mild essential hypertension. Am J Hypertens 1999; 12:973–979.
51. Lee KW, Blann AD, Lip GY. High pulse pressure and nondipping circadian blood pressure in patients with coronary artery disease: relationship to thrombogenesis and endothelial damage/dysfunction. Am J Hypertens 2005; 18:104–115.
52. Ross R. The pathogenesis of atherosclerosis: a perspective for the 1990s. Nature 1993; 362:801–809.
53. Page IH. The nature of arterial hypertension. Arch Intern Med 1963; 111:103–115.
54. Kannel WB. Risk stratification in hypertension: new insights from the Framingham Study. Am J Hypertens 2000; 13:3S–10S.

55. Dupres DA, Somasundaram PE, Sigurdsson G, et al. Relationship between C. reactive protein and arterial stiffness in an asymptomatic population. J Hum Hypertension 2005; 19:515–519.
56. Rihal CS, Textor SC, Grill DE, et al. Incidental renal artery stenosis among a prospective cohort of hypertensive patients undergoing coronary angiography. Mayo Clin Proc 2002; 77:309–316.
57. Textor SC, Wilcox CS. Renal artery stenosis: a common, treatable cause of renal failure? Annu Rev Med 2001; 52:421–442.
58. Webster J, Marshall F, Abdalla M, et al. Randomised comparison of percutaneous angioplasty vs. continued medical therapy for hypertensive patients with atheromatous renal artery stenosis. J Hum Hypertens 1998; 12:329–335.
59. van Jaarsveld BC, Krijnen P, Pieterman H, et al. The effect of balloon angioplasty on hypertension in atherosclerotic renal artery stenosis. N Engl J Med 2000; 342:1007–1014.
60. Plouin PF, Chatellier G, Dame B, et al. Blood pressure outcome of angioplasty in atherosclerotic renal artery stenosis: a randomized trial. Hypertension 1998; 31:822–829.
61. van de Ven PJ, Kaatee R, Bentler JJ, et al. Arterial stenting and balloon angioplasty in ostial atherosclerotic renovascular disease: a randomized trial. Lancet 1999; 353:282–286.
62. Williams JS, Williams GH, Raji A, et al. Prevalence of primary hyperaldosteronism in mild to moderate hypertension without hypokalaemia. J Hum Hypertens 2006; 20:129–136.
63. Lenders JW, Pacak K, Walther MM, et al. Biochemical diagnosis of pheochromocytoma, which test is best? JAMA 2002; 287:1427–1434.
64. Pacak R, Linehan WM, Eisenhofer G, Walther MM, Goldstein DS. Recent advances in genetics, diagnosis, localization, and treatment of pheochromocytoma. Ann Intern Med 2001; 134:315–329.
65. Taler SJ. Treatment of resistant hypertension. Curr Hypertens Rep 2005; 7:323–329.
66 Calhoun D. Use of aldosterone antagonists in resistant hypertension. Prog Cardiovasc Dis 2006; 48:387–396.
67. Elliott-William J. Clinical features in the management of selected hypertensive emergencies. Progr Cardiovasc Dis 2006; 48:316–325.
68. Cressman MD, Vidt DG, Gifford RW Jr., Moore WS, Wilson DJ. Intravenous labetalol in the management of severe hypertension and hypertensive emergencies. Am Heart J 1984; 107:980–985.
69. Duprez DA, Cohn JN. Monitoring vascular health beyond blood pressure. Curr Hypertens Rep 2006 (in press).
70. Crenner CW. Introduction of the blood pressure cuff into U.S. medical practice: technology and skilled practice. Ann Intern Med 1998; 128:488–493.
71. Joint National Committee on Prevention, Detection, Evaluation, and Treatment of High Blood Pressure. Seventh report of the Joint National Committee on Prevention, Detection, Evaluation, and Treatment of High Blood Pressure. JAMA 2003; 289:2560–2572.
72. World Health Organization–International Society of Hypertension Guidelines for the Management of Hypertension. Guidelines Subcommittee. J Hypertens 1999; 17:151–183.
73. American Heart Association. Recommendations for human blood pressure determination by sphygmomanometers. Report of a special task force appointed by the steering committee. Hypertension 1988; 11:210A–222A.
74. Cushman WC, Cooper KM, Horne RA, Meydrech EF. Effect of back support and stethoscope head position on seated blood pressure determinations. Am J Hypertens 1990; 3:240–241.
75. Netea RT, Smits P, Lenders JWM, Thien T. Does it matter whether blood pressure measurements are taken sitting or supine? J Hypertens 1998; 16:263–268.
76. Silverberg DS, Shemesh E, Iaina A. The unsupported arm: a cause of falsely raised blood pressure readings. BMJ 1977; 2:1331.
77. Webster J, Newnham D, Petrie JC, Lovell HG. Influence of arm position on measurement of blood pressure. BMJ 1984; 288:1574–1575.
78. Manning DM, Kuchirka C, Kaminski J. Miscuffing: inappropriate blood pressure cuff application. Circulation 1983; 68:763–766.
79. Iyriboz Y, Hearon CM, Edwards K. Agreement between large and small cuffs in sphygmomanometer: a quantitative assessment. J Clin Monit 1994; 10:127–133.
80. Linfors EW, Feussner JR, Blessing CL, et al. Spurious hypertension in the obese patient. Effect of sphygmomanometer cuff size on prevalence of hypertension. Arch Inter Med 1984; 144:1482–1485.
81. Souchek J, Stamler J, Dyer AR, Paul O, Lepper MH. The value of two or three versus a single reading of blood pressure at a first visit. J Chronic Dis 1979; 32:197–210.
82. O'Brien E, Asmar R, Beilin L, et al. On behalf of the European Society of Hypertension Working Group on Blood Pressure Monitoring. Practice guidelines of the European Society of Hypertension for clinic, ambulatory and self blood pressure measurement. J Hypertension 2005; 23:697–701.
83. Van Montfrans GA. Oscillometric blood pressure measurement: progress and problems. Blood Press Monit 2001; 6:287–290.
84. Sykes D, Dewar R, Mohanaruban K, et al. Measuring blood pressure in the elderly: does atrial fibrillation increase observer variability? BMJ 1990; 300:162–163.
85. Reims H, Fossum E, Kjeldsen SE, Julius S. Home blood pressure monitoring. Current knowledge and directions for future research. Blood Press 2001; 10:271–287.
86. Pickering TG, Shimbo D, Haas D. Ambulatory blood-pressure monitoring. N Engl J Med 2006; 354:2368–2374.

87. Perlofff D, Sokolow M, Cowan R. The prognostic value of ambulatory blood pressure. JAMA 1983; 249:2792–2798.
88. Ohkubo T, Imai Y, Tsuji I, et al. Prediction of mortality by ambulatory blood pressure monitoring versus screening blood pressure: a pilot study in Ohasama. J Hypertens 1997; 15:357–364.
89. Khattar RS, Swales JD, Banfield A, et al. Prediction of coronary and cerebrovascular morbidity and mortality by direct continuous ambulatory blood pressure monitoring in essential hypertension. Circulation 1999; 100:1071–1076.
90. Verdecchia P, Schillaci G, Borgioni C, et al. Ambulatory pulse pressure: a potent predictor of total cardiovascular risk in hypertension. Hypertension 1998; 32:983–988.
91. Sander D, Kukla C, Klingelhöfer J, Winbeck K, Conrad B. Relationship between circadian blood pressure patterns and progression of early carotid atherosclerosis: a 3-year follow-up study. Circulation 2000; 102:1536–1541.
92. Perloff D, Sokolow M, Cowan RM, Juster RP. Prognostic value of ambulatory blood pressure measurements: further analyses. J Hypertens Suppl 1989; 7:S3–S10.
93. Redon J, Campos C, Narciso ML, et al. Prognostic value of ambulatory blood pressure monitoring in refractory hypertension: a prospective study. Hypertension 1998; 31:712–718.
94. Clement DL, De Buyzere M, De Bacquer DA, et al. Prognostic value of ambulatory blood-pressure recordings in patients with treated hypertension. N Engl J Med 2003; 348:2407–2415.
95. Verdecchia P, Reboldi G, Porcellati C, et al. Risk of cardiovascular disease in relation to achieved office and ambulatory blood pressure control in treated hypertensive subjects. J Am Coll Cardiol 2002; 39:878–885.
96. White WB. Ambulatory blood-pressure monitoring in clinical practice. N Engl J Med 2003; 348:2377–2378.
97. Chobanian AV, Bakris GL, Black HR, et al. National High Blood Pressure Education Program Coordinating Committee. The Seventh Report of the Joint National Committee on Prevention, Detection, Evaluation, and Treatment of High Blood Pressure. The JNC 7 report. JAMA 2003; 289:3560–3572.
98. Expert Panel on Detection, Evaluation, and Treatment of High Blood Cholesterol in Adults. JAMA 2001; 285:2486–2497.
99. The Trials of Hypertension Prevention Collaborative Research Group. Effects of weight loss and reduction intervention on blood pressure and hypertension incidence in overweight people with high normal blood pressure. Arch Intern Med 1997; 157:657–667.
100. He J, Whelton PK, Appel LJ, Charleston J, Klag MJ. Long-term effects of weight loss and dietary sodium reduction on incidence of hypertension. Hypertension 2000; 35:544–549.
101. Sacks FM, Svetkey LP, Vollmer WM, et al. For the DASH-Sodium Collaborative Research Group. Effects on blood pressure of reduced dietary sodium and the Dietary Approaches to Stop Hypertension (DASH) diet. N Engl J Med 2001; 344:3–10.
102. Vollmer WM, Sacks FM, Ard J, et al. Effects of diet and sodium intake on blood pressure. Ann Intern Med 2001; 135:1019–1028.
103. Cushmann WC, Ford CE, Cutler JA, et al. Success and predictors of blood pressure control in diverse North American settings: the antihypertensive and lipid-lowering treatment to prevent heart attack trial (ALLHAT). J Clin Hypertens 2002; 4:393–404.
104. Phillips LS, Branch WT, Cook CB, et al. Clinical inertia. Ann Intern Med 2001; 135:825–834.
105. Hyman DJ, Pavlik VN. Characteristics of patients with uncontrolled hypertension in the United States. N Engl J Med 2001; 45:479–486.
106. ALLHAT Officers and Coordinators for the ALLHAT Collaborative Research Group. Major outcomes in high-risk hypertensive patients randomized to angiotensin-converting enzyme inhibitor or calcium channel blocker vs diuretic. The Antihypertensive and Lipid-Lowering Treatment to Prevent Heart Attack Trial (ALLHAT). JAMA 2002; 288:2981–2997.
107. US Department of Health and Human Services. JNC 7 Express. The Seventh Report of the Joint National Committee on Prevention, Detection, Evaluation, and Treatment of High Blood Pressure. (Available from http://www.nhlbi.nih.gov/guidelines/hypertension/jncintro.htm).
108. Joint National Committee on Prevention, Detection, and Treatment of High Blood Pressure. The sixth report of the Joint National Committee on Prevention, Detection, and Treatment of High Blood Pressure (JNC VI). Arch Intern Med 1997; 157:2413–2446.
109. Neaton JD, Wentworth D. For the Multiple Risk Factor Intervention Trial Research Group. Serum cholesterol, blood pressure, cigarette smoking, and death from coronary disease. Overall findings and differences by age for 316,099 white men. Arch Intern Med 1992; 152:56–64.
110. Kostis JB, Messerli F, Giles TD. Hypertension: definitions and guidelines. J Clin Hypertens 2005; 7:538–539.
111. World Health Organization, International Society of Hypertension Writing Group. 2003 World Health Organization (WHO)/International Society of Hypertension (ISH) statement on management of hypertension [Guidelines and recommendations]. J Hypertens 2003; 21:1983–1992.
112. Gueyffier F, Boutitie F, Boissel JP, et al. The effect of antihypertensive drug treatment on cardiovascular outcomes in women and men. Results from a meta-analysis of individual patient data in randomised controlled trials. Ann Intern Med 1997; 126:761–767.
113. Zanchetti A, Ruilope LM. Antihypertensive treatment in patients with type 2 diabetes mellitus: what guidance from recent randomized controlled trials? J Hypertens 2002; 20:2099–2110.

114. UKPDS Prospective Diabetes Study Group. Tight blood pressure control and risk of macrovascular and microvascular complications in type 2 diabetes: UKPDS 38. BMJ 1998; 317:703–713.
115. Hansson L, Zanchetti A, Carruthers SG, et al. Effects of intensive blood-pressure lowering and low-dose aspirin in patients with hypertension. Principal results of the Hypertension Optimal Treatment (HOT) randomized trial. Lancet 1998; 351:1755–1762.
116. Okano GJ, Rascati KL, Wilson JP, et al. Patterns of antihypertensive use among patients in the US Department of Defense database initially prescribed an angiotensin converting enzyme inhibitor or calcium channel blocker. Clin Ther 1997; 19:1433–1435.
117. Ebrahim S, Smith GD. Lowering blood pressure: a systematic review of sustained effects of non-pharmacological interventions. J Public Health Med 1998; 20:4441–4448.
118. Stevens VJ, Obarzanek E, Cook NR, et al. Long-term weight loss and changes in results of the Trials of Hypertension Prevention, Phase II. Ann Intern Med 2001; 134:1–11.
119. Hagberg JM, Park JJ, Brown MD. The role of exercise training in the treatment of hypertension: an update. Sports Med 2000; 30:193–206.
120. Xin X, He J, Frontini MG, et al. Effects of alcohol reduction on blood pressure: a meta-analysis of randomized controlled trials. Hypertension 2001; 38:1112–1117.
121. Cutler JA, Follmann D, Allender PS. Randomized trials of sodium reduction: an overview. Am J Clin Nutr 1997; 65(suppl):643S–651S.
122. Whelton PK, Appel LJ, Espeland MA, et al. Sodium reduction and weight loss in the treatment of hypertension in older persons: a randomized controlled trial of non-pharmacological interventions in the elderly (TONE). JAMA 1998; 279:839–846.
123. He J, Whelton PK. What is the role of dietary sodium and potassium in hypertension and target organ injury? Am J Med Sci 1999; 317:152–159.
124. Griffith LE, Guyatt GH, Cook RJ, Bucher HC, Cook DJ. The influence of dietary and non-dietary calcium supplementation on blood pressure. An updated meta-analysis of randomized controlled trials. Am J Hypertens 1999; 12:84–92.
125. Kawano Y, Matsuoka H, Takishita S, Omae T. Effects of magnesium supplementation in hypertensive patients. Assessment by office, home, and ambulatory blood pressures. Hypertension 1998; 32:260–265.
126. Jee SH, He J, Whelton PK, Suh I, Klag MJ. The effect of chronic coffee drinking on blood pressure. A meta-analysis of controlled clinical trials. Hypertension 1999; 33:647–652.
127. Spence JD, Barnett PA, Linden W, Ramsden V, Taenzer P. Lifestyle modifications to prevent and control hypertension. Recommendations on stress management. CMAs J 1999; 160(suppl 9):S46–S50.
128. Kawachi I, Colditz GA, Stampfer MJ, et al. Smoking cessation and time course of decreased risks of coronary heart disease in middle-aged women. Arch Intern Med 1994; 154:169–175.
129. Tuomilehto J, Lindström J, Eriksson JG, et al. Prevention of type 2 diabetes mellitus by changes in lifestyle among subjects with impaired glucose tolerance. N Engl J Med 2001; 344:1343–1350.
130. Knowler WC, Barrett-Connor E, Fowler SE, et al. Reduction in the incidence of type 2 diabetes with lifestyle intervention or metformin. N Engl J Med 2002; 346:393–403.
131. Stefanick ML, Mackey S, Sheehan M, et al. Effects of diet and exercise in men and postmenopausal women with low levels of HDL cholesterol and high levels of LDL cholesterol. N Engl J Med 1998; 339:12–20.
132. Blood Pressure Lowering Treatment Trialists' Collaboration. Effects of ACE inhibitors, calcium antagonists, and other blood-pressure-lowering drugs. Lancet 2000; 356:1955–1964.
133. Dahlöf B, Devereux RB, Kjeldsen SE, et al. Cardiovascular morbidity and mortality in the Losartan Intervention for endpoint reduction in hypertension study (LIFE). A randomized trial against Atenolol. Lancet 2002; 359:995–1003.
134. Schmieder RE, Schlaich MF, Klingbeil AU, Martus P. Update on reversal of left ventricular hypertrophy in essential hypertension. Nephrol Dial Transplant 1998; 13:564–569.
135. Devereux RB, Palmieri V, Sharpe N, et al. Effects of once-daily angiotensin-converting enzyme inhibition and calcium channel blockade-based antihypertensive treatment regimens on left ventricular hypertrophy and diastolic filling in hypertension. The prospective randomized enalapril study evaluating regression of ventricular enlargement (preserve) trial. Circulation 2001; 104:1248–1254.
136. Jafar TH, Schmid CH, Landa M, et al. Angiotensin-converting enzyme inhibitors and progression of nondiabetic renal disease. A meta-analysis of patient-level data. Ann Intern Med 2001; 135:138–139.
137. Parving HH, Lenhert H, Brochner-Mortensen J, et al. Irbesartan in patients with type 2 diabetes and Microalbuminuria Study Group. The effect of Irbesartan on the development of diabetic nephropathy in patients with type 2 diabetes. N Engl J Med 2001; 345:870–878.
138. Brenner BM, Cooper ME, de Zeeuw D, et al. For the RENAAL Study Investigators. Effects of Losartan on renal and cardiovascular outcome in patients with type 2 diabetes and nephropathy. N Engl J Med 2001; 345:861–869.
139. Cushman WC, Reda DJ, Perry HM, et al. Regional and racial differences in response to antihypertensive medication use in a randomized controlled trial of men with hypertension in the United States. Department of Veterans Affairs Cooperative Study Group on Antihypertensive Agents. Arch Intern Med 2000; 160:825–831.

140. Radevski IV, Valtchanova ZP, Candy GP, Hlatswayo MN, Sareli P. Antihypertensive effect of low-dose hydrochlorothiazide alone or in combination with quinapril in black patients with mild to moderate hypertension. J Clin Pharmacol 2000; 40:713–721.
141. Oesterling JE. Benign prostatic hyperplasia. Medical and minimally invasive treatment options. N Engl J Med 1995; 99:109.
142. Brown MJ, Palmer CR, Castaigne A, et al. Morbidity and mortality in patients randomized to double-blind treatment with a long-acting calcium-channel blocker or diuretic in the International Nifedipine GITS study: Intervention as a Goal in Hypertension Treatment (INSIGHT). Lancet 2000; 356:366–372.
143. Zanchetti A, Bond G, Hennig M, et al. Calcium antagonist slows down progression of asymptomatic carotid atherosclerosis. Principal results of the European Lacidipine study on atherosclerosis (ELSA), a randomised, double-blind, long-term trial. Circulation 2002; 106:2422–2427.
144. Nissen SE, Tuczu EM, Libby P, et al. Effect of antihypertensive agents on cardiovascular events in patients with coronary artery disease and normal blood pressure. The CAMELOT Study: a randomized controlled trial. JAMA 2004; 292:2217–2226.
145. Black HR, Elliott WJ, Grandits G, et al. Principal results of the Controlled ONset Verapamil INvestigation of Cardiovascular Endpoints (CONVINCE) trial. JAMA 2003; 289:2073–2082.
146. Julius S, Kjelden SE, Weber M, et al. Outcomes in hypertensive patients at high cardiovascular risk treated with regimens based on valsartan or amlodipine: the VALUE randomised trial. Lancet 2004; 363:2022–2031.
147. Weber MA, Julius S, Kjeldsen SE, et al. Blood pressure dependent and independent effects of antihypertensive treatment on clinical events in the VALUE Trial. Lancet 2004; 363:2049–2051.
148. Dahlöf B, Sever PS, Poulter NR, et al. Prevention of cardiovascular events with an antihypertensive regimen of amlodipine adding perindopril as required versus atenolol adding bendroflumethiazide as required, in the Anglo-Scandinavian Cardiac Outcomes Trial-Blood Pressure Lowering Arm (ASCOT-BPLA): a multicentre randomised controlled trial. Lancet 2005; 366:895–906.
149. Williams B, Lacy PS, Thom SM, et al. Differential impact of blood pressure-lowering drugs on central aortic pressure and clinical outcomes. Circulation 2006; 113:1213–1215.
150. Julius S, Nesbitt SD, Egan BM, et al. Feasibility of treating prehypertension with an angiotensin-receptor blocker. N Engl J Med 2006; 354:1685–1697.
151. Schunkert H. Pharmacotherapy for prehypertension-mission accomplished? N Engl J Med 2006; 354:1742–1744.

3 | Obesity and Lifestyle Modification

Herman Blomeier and Neil J. Stone

Department of Medicine, Sections of Endocrinology and Cardiology, Feinberg School of Medicine, Northwestern University, Chicago, Illinois, U.S.A.

KEY POINTS

- Waist circumference (WC) measured perpendicular to the floor at the level of the iliac crest in expiration is a practical way to estimate the state of abdominal or visceral fat. In the INTER-HEART study, waist/hip ratio showed a graded and highly significant association with risk of myocardial infarction in contrast to body mass index (BMI), which had a weaker and less consistent relationship across ethnic and other subgroups.
- For those who are overweight or obese, energy deficits obtained by a healthful diet and regular exercise can cause beneficial changes in insulin sensitivity, markers of inflammation, and standard risk factors that are not seen with liposuction. Indeed, all of the five metabolic risk factors in the metabolic syndrome [increased abdominal circumference, low high-density lipoprotein-cholesterol (HDL-C), elevated triglyceride, blood pressure, and/or blood glucose] improve with modest weight loss obtained through a healthful lifestyle.
- Evaluation of the patient with obesity should include a detailed history and an appropriate physical examination. Use of an appropriately wide blood pressure cuff is required for accurate assessment of blood pressure. For those with a BMI >35, waist circumference is much less informative than it is when measured in those whose BMI is lower than 35.
- Before recommending lifestyle change, it is useful to determine how urgent the need is for lifestyle change, the patients past experience with dietary change, the patient's current commitment to lifestyle change, and his/her perceived barriers to change.
- Use of behavioral techniques such as self-monitoring (diet and exercise records), stimulus control, goal setting, social support, encouraging problem solving, and frequent feedback can greatly enhance successful lifestyle change.
- Higher intensities of exercise will give increasing metabolic benefits, but for the most sedentary patients, just doing some physical activity on a daily basis will result in improvements in risk factors and coronary heart disease risk.

INTRODUCTION

The prevalence of overweight and obesity has reached epidemic proportions in the United States. Being reported to be over 60% and 30%, respectively (1). Moderate obesity has become commonplace, and primary physicians are likely to encounter it on an almost daily basis. This rising prevalence of obesity was a major stimulus for including a syndrome of metabolic risk factors designated as the metabolic syndrome in the Adult Treatment Panel (ATP) III guidelines of the National Cholesterol Education Program released in 2001 (2).

The aim of this chapter is to put assessment and treatment approaches into a thoughtful framework for those concerned with clinical management of this condition.

MEASURING OVERWEIGHT, OBESITY, AND BODY FAT

In 1998, the National Heart, Lung, and Blood Institute (NHLBI) published clinical guidelines on obesity to help clinicians assess patients and provide evidence-based support for comorbidities and treatment options (3). In 2001, the companion *Practical Guide to the Identification, Evaluation, and Treatment of Overweight and Obesity in Adults* was published by the NHLBI and the North American Association for the Study of Obesity (4). According to these guidelines, the primary classification of overweight and obesity is based on the measurement of body mass index (BMI). BMI can be calculated as weight (kg)/height-squared (m²). This descriptive statistic is designed to reduce the dependence of weight on height. A useful way to calculate BMI if weight and height are in pounds and inches, respectively, is to simply divide weight in pounds (lbs) by

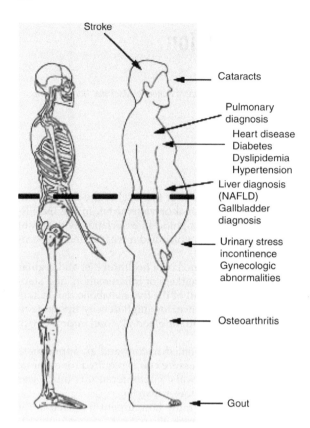

Stroke

Cataracts

Pulmonary
diagnosis

Heart disease
Diabetes
Dyslipidemia
Hypertension
Liver diagnosis
(NAFLD)
Gallbladder
diagnosis

Urinary stress
incontinence
Gynecologic
abnormalities

Osteoarthritis

Gout

FIGURE 1 Measuring tape position for waist (abdominal) circumference in adults, along with medical complications associated with obesity. *Source*: Adapted from Ref. 3.

height in inches-squared (in.^{2}) and then multiply this number by 703. A BMI of 25 to 29.9 is considered overweight, and 30 and higher is considered obesity. One of the limitations of the BMI measurement is that it does not distinguish muscle weight from fat weight. Thus, a very muscular person may have an elevated BMI despite having a very low body fat.

The tools for determining body fat are waist circumference (WC) and waist/hip ratio. WC should be measured at the level of the iliac crest (Fig. 1) at end-expiration, with the examiner at the patient's side, holding the tape perpendicular to the floor. WC is a practical way to evaluate the state of abdominal or visceral fat, which many believe has a higher health risk than peripheral or subcutaneous fat. Men are defined as having excess abdominal fat if they have a WC of 40 in. or more, and women 35 in. or more. ATP III in its original report noted that multiple metabolic risk factors that define the metabolic syndrome could occur with lower levels of WC, especially in certain populations. Recently, The International Diabetes Federation (IDF) proposed a new definition of the metabolic syndrome that emphasizes central adiposity as determined by ethnic group–specific thresholds of WC (Table 1) (5).

TABLE 1 Metabolic Syndrome (ATP III vs. IDF)

	ATP III	**IDF**	**Comments**
WC	Males ≥40 in.	Males >94 cm	In ATP III, WC is not mandatory; in IDF, WC is a mandatory criteria
	Females ≥35 in.	Females >80 cm	
HDL-C	Males <40 mg/dL	Males <40 mg/dL	In ATP III, 3 out of the 5 criteria listed are needed for diagnosis. In IDF, WC is mandatory and two more are required for diagnosis
	Females <50 mg/dl	Females <50 mg/dL	
Triglycerides	≥150 mg/dL	≥150 mg/dL	
Fasting blood sugar	≥100 mg/dL	≥100 mg/dL	
Blood pressure	>130 or >85	>130 or >85	

Abbreviations: WC, Waist circumference; ATP, Adult Treatment Panel; IDF, International Diabetes Federation; HDL-C, High-density lipoprotein-cheolesterol.

TABLE 2 Classification of Overweight and Obesity

	Body mass index	Obesity class
Normal	18.5–24.9[a]	
Overweight	25–29.9[a]	
Obesity	30–34.9[a]	Class I
	35–39.9	Class II
	≥40	Class III

[a]Increases disease risk for type 2 diabetes, hypertension and cardiovascular disease.
Source: Adapted from Ref. 3.

Many of these are lower than the 40 in. for men and 35 in. for women cut-offs for WC proposed by the initial ATP III report. An update in November 2005 from the American Heart Association (AHA) and the NHLBI suggested that lower WC thresholds are appropriate if either there is clinical evidence for insulin resistance or the patient belongs to an ethnic subgroup in whom the prevalence of insulin resistance is high (e.g., South Asians, Mexican-Americans) (2).

A suggested overview of the classification of overweight and obesity by BMI, WC, and associated risk of disease is summarized in Table 2. Insights into the predictive value for coronary heart disease (CHD) of these anthropomorphic measurements were evinced by the large-scale INTERHEART Study, which was a standardized case–control study of 15,152 cases of first myocardial infarction (MI) and 14,820 age-matched and sex-matched controls (6). A large cross section of ethnic populations was represented, because the study population came from 262 centers in 52 countries from Asia, Europe, the Middle East, Africa, Australia, North America, and South America. BMI showed a modest and graded association with MI that disappeared when adjusted for other risk factors. On the other hand, WC and waist-to-hip (W/H) ratio shows a graded and highly significant association with MI risk worldwide. The INTERHEART Study demonstrated clearly that the W/H ratio showed the strongest relation with the risk of MI globally. W/H ratio was a strong predictor of MI in men and women, across all age and ethnic groups, in smokers and in nonsmokers and in those with or without lipid abnormalities, diabetes, or hypertension. This was not true of BMI, whose relation to MI was weaker and less consistent across ethnic and other subgroups. WC and W/H ratio, but not BMI, were predictors of MI in those with a history of hypertension or a raised ApoB/ApoA ratio. Moreover, raised W/H ratio substantially increased the population attributable risk resulting from obesity by over threefold compared with BMI. The investigators concluded that the global burden of obesity has been underestimated by the reliance on BMI in previous studies. They further noted that because the measure of body fatness (w/h ratio) and not weight (BMI) remained significant after adjustment for other risk factors, it suggested that body fatness markers may act through mechanisms that differ from other risk factors. The importance of fatness and lack of fitness was emphasized by the Amsterdam Growth and Health Longitudinal Study which found that characteristics of those with metabolic syndrome as defined by ATP III included a trend toward higher energy intake, a decrease in cardiopulmonary fitness, and a more marked increase in total body fatness and subcutaneous trunk fat (7).

Clinical case: Dr. I.G. is a 38-year-old male of South Asian origin. He had a family history of premature CHD and diabetes on his father's side. His examination showed a blood pressure (BP) of 133/82.

Weight	Height	BMI
154	65.5	25.2

He had a WC of 38 in. His labs were:

Total Cholesterol	Triglyceride	High-density lipoproteins	Low-density lipoproteins	Non–high-density lipoproteins	Chemistries
232	342	39	125	193	FBS 99

He had criteria for the metabolic syndrome, with high triglyceride (TG) and low high-density lipoprotein (HDL-C) along with what we considered to be an increased WC. We considered his WC to be increased because he came from an ethnic group with a high prevalence of insulin resistance. He greatly improved his lipids and his waist with an intensive lifestyle change program of daily exercise, improved diet, and a modest weight loss.

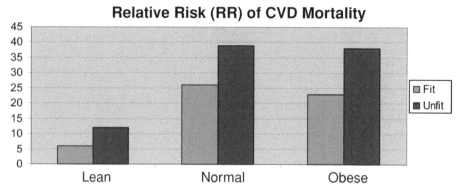

FIGURE 2   Relative risk of CVD mortality in fit and unfit men according to body type. Unfit men were the lowest quartile of oxygen uptake (as a measure of fitness). *Source*: Adapted from Ref. 8.

That our patient's attainment of fitness was likely to be helpful was suggested by the observational study of Lee et al. from the Cooper Institute in Houston, Texas (8). They followed for eight years 21,925 men, aged 30 to 83 years, who had a body-composition assessment and a maximal treadmill exercise test. They observed a direct relation between body fatness and all-cause and cardiovascular disease (CVD) mortality, but being fit decreased the high mortality seen in obese men. Likewise, being unfit increased the otherwise lower mortality seen in nonobese men (Fig. 2).

MAGNITUDE OF THE PROBLEM

Results from the 1999 to 2000 National Health and Nutrition Examination Survey indicate that an estimated 65% of U.S. adults are either overweight or obese (Fig. 3) (9). Obese adults aged 18 to 65 years have 36% higher health care costs compared with normal-weight individuals (10). Annual U.S. obesity-attributable medical expenditures are estimated at $75 billion in 2003, and approximately half of these expenditures are financed by Medicare and Medicaid (11). Another way to visualize this problem is to calculate lifetime risk, as was done in Framingham. Although these findings may not be generalizable to all populations, it is worth noting that after 30 years of follow-up, more than half of the women and men became overweight, while about one-third of the women and a quarter of the men became obese. Adults older than 50 years of age became overweight or obese less often than the younger adults (12).

This increasing burden of obesity is not limited to the United States. It is estimated that 10% of the world's school-aged children are carrying excess body fat and of those overweight, a quarter

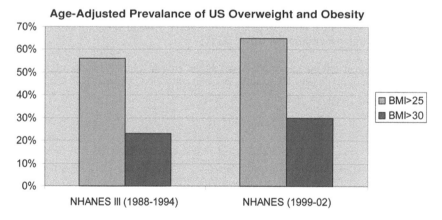

FIGURE 3   Age-adjusted prevalence of overweight and obesity among US adults, aged 20 years and over. Age-adjusted by the direct method to the year 2000 US Bureau of the Census estimates using the age groups 20–39, 40–59, and 60 years and over. *Source*: Redrawn from Ref. 9.

TABLE 3 The Facts of Less: What to Know About Weight Loss

1.	When fat weight is lost, it is usually due to the decreased size of fat cells
2.	An energy deficit of 3500 kcal causes more than 1 lb in body weight loss owing to the oxidation of lean tissue and associated water losses
3.	When we lose weight by dieting, 75% of the weight loss is fat and 25% come from fat-free mass
4.	When we add exercise training to diet (lifestyle change), there is a decreased percentage of weight loss as fat-free mass (usually by 1/2)
5.	Weight is not lost evenly; greater relative losses come from intraabdominal fat than from total body fat mass
6.	Those with increased intraabdominal fat, derive the most loss from intraabdominal fat with lifestyle change
7.	Removing the fat by liposuction does not provide the metabolic advantages of losing it through lifestyle change
8.	Diet-induced weight loss decreases intramyocellular and intrahepatic lipids

Source: From Ref. 14.

are obese (13). The problem of childhood obesity is worsening at an alarming rate, with increases in obesity-related problems (see below) occurring earlier in life than we have seen until now.

A BRIEF REVIEW OF WEIGHT LOSS PHYSIOLOGY

Counseling patients on weight loss requires knowledge of some of the basic facts of weight loss physiology (14). These are summarized in Table 3. The important points are that energy deficits need to be developed through a combination of diet and exercise to get the full metabolic advantages of weight loss. Cosmetic improvements obtained by surgical removal of adipose tissue do not significantly alter insulin sensitivity of muscle, liver, or adipose tissue (15). Indeed, liposuction did not reduce markers of inflammation (plasma concentrations of C-reactive protein, interleukin-6, tumor necrosis factor, and adiponectin were not improved) and did not significantly affect standard risk factors for CHD (blood pressure, plasma glucose, insulin, and lipid concentrations).

CLINICAL DISORDERS RELATED TO OBESITY

Weight gain leading to obesity has a significant health impact, being associated with diabetes risk (16,17), insulin resistance (18,19), atherogenic dyslipidemia [elevated TGs, low HDL-C, and small dense low-density lipoprotein (LDL)] (20,21), inflammation (22), impaired sleep as well as sleep apnea/hypoventilation syndrome (23), CHD, and stroke (24) and hepatobiliary disorders (25–27). Additionally, increased osteoarthritis (28) and some female cancers are associated with obesity (29,30). This increased prevalence of chronic health conditions related to elevated BMI is seen in all adult age groups and across racial and ethnic groups (31). A 10-year follow-up report of middle-aged women who were overweight (25–29.9) in the Nurses' Health Study and men who were overweight in the Health Professionals Follow-up Study clearly demonstrated that diabetes mellitus, hypertension, CHD, gallstones, colon cancer, and stroke (men only) increased with degree of overweight (32). Moreover, the dose–response relationship between BMI and the risk of developing chronic diseases showed no sharp cut-off as weight increased.

A more specific consequence of weight gain is abdominal obesity, manifested by increased WC, increased abdominal subcutaneous fat, and increased visceral fat. Indeed in young men, obesity as defined by BMI is associated with both fatty streaks and raised lesions in the right coronary artery (RCA) and with the microscopic grade of atherosclerosis and stenosis in the left anterior descending artery (33). The effect of BMI on RCA raised lesions was greater among men with a thick panniculus adiposus, a measure of a central pattern of obesity. Abdominal obesity is also shown to have an important association with insulin resistance, atherogenic dyslipidemia, and CHD. Quebec investigators found that in 185 healthy men with elevated insulin, apoB, and small dense LDL levels, more than 80% had WC values ≥90 cm and elevated TG levels (≥2.0 mmol/L) (34). Not surprisingly—to those who study metabolic causes of CHD—the same paper reported a subsequent validation study in 287 men with and without CHD that demonstrated that those with both elevated WC and elevated TG levels were at least three times more likely to have CHD compared with those with low WC and TG levels.

TABLE 4 Obesity Treatment Guidelines

Treatment	Body mass index (kg/m²)				
	25–26.9	27–29.9	30–34.9	35–39.9	≥40
Lifestyle: diet, exercise, behavior Tx	+	+	+	+	+
Pharmacotherapy		With comorbidities	+	+	+
Surgery				With comorbidities	+

The Framingham Study focused our attention on clustering of atherogenic risk factors such as BMI, cholesterol, TGs, HDL-C, glucose, and systolic blood pressure (35). It found that clusters of three or more occurred at twice the rate as predicted by chance. Indeed for those men and women so affected by multiple metabolic risk factors, the risk of CHD was 2.4 and 5.9 times greater than those not so affected. Thus, one reason the concept of metabolic syndrome was felt to be clinically so useful was its ability to easily define individuals at risk for obesity, diabetes, and CHD (all of the components can be measured during a routine office visit) (2,21) and for whom, lifestyle interventions (diet, exercise, and weight loss) could strongly be recommended as initial therapy, because the interventions were directed at the root causes of the syndrome.

MANAGEMENT OF THE OBESE PATIENT

A listing of therapies for obesity is given in Table 4. Before we discuss these therapies, it is important to remember that success requires a motivated patient, a physician/health care team that can recommend interventions that can improve the patient's overall health and also help him or her lose excess weight, and a system that provides for appropriate monitoring and feedback to prevent recidivism (36).

EVALUATION OF PATIENTS

In addition to standard items on a complete history and physical, the following areas should be carefully considered during the history taking (14).

- Weight history: prior attempts, what worked, and triggers that caused failure.
- Dietary history: an assessment tool is required for this; a diet diary is helpful.
- Physical activity and function history: again, an assessment tool such as a diary is helpful.
- Obesity-related health risks: age of onset of obesity, who in the family is obese, and medical complications related to obesity.
- Emotional assessment: especially psychiatric history or if patient would like some help in coping with life's stresses and strains.
- Assessment of ability to lose weight: are expectations realistic, and patient's limitations.

Physical examination can present challenges to the unprepared examiner. Can the scale in the room measure weight above 300 lb? Is there a large blood pressure cuff? Are the Korotkoff sounds weak and hard to hear? The latter point can be corrected. Raising the arm above the head and squeezing the hand three times relieves forearm venous congestion. Placing the arm then at heart level and taking the blood pressure will result in louder tones that make the readings more accurate and reproducible. If the patient has a BMI more than 35, a WC adds little to the information needed for treatment.

INITIATING DISCUSSIONS ABOUT MANAGEMENT WITH PATIENTS

A discussion of therapy for obesity almost always begins with trying to decide which diet is best. Interestingly, when four of the most popular diet therapies (Atkins, Ornish, Weight Watchers, and Zone) were compared, the amount of weight loss seen was significantly correlated with self-reported dietary adherence level ($r = 0.6$; $p = 0.001$) and not with diet type (37). Thus, we suggest that physicians ask four questions before initiating the discussion of lifestyle change. These could be handled on a questionnaire that the patient fills out before the visit:

- How urgent is the need for lifestyle change in this patient?
- What is the diet history? What kind of diet is the patient already on; what kinds of diets have failed?
- How committed is the patient to lifestyle change?
- What are the perceived barriers to change?

There are certain situations which, in our clinical experience, seem to require special emphasis. These include but may not be limited to:

- Life-cycle or drug/disease situations that make individuals prone to significant weight gain;
- Treating those at high risk for CHD (Framingham Risk score) and/or diabetes (personal characteristics and/or impaired fasting glucose/glucose tolerance);
- Those with chronic health conditions that are triggered by obesity or significantly worsened by weight gain. The shortlist would include diabetes, dyslipidemia, CHD, CVDs, sleep disorders, fatty liver, osteoarthritis, and, in some cases, the need for elective surgery in the future that would be made easier by weight loss;
- Those with the most severe level of obesity who have responded inadequately to lifestyle change and can be considered after appropriate evaluation by an expert team for surgical intervention.

The first two situations involve avoiding weight gain. While many physicians would not fail to recommend lifestyle change for those with risk factors for CHD and diabetes, it is distressing that in the presence of certain life milestones [adolescence (12), pregnancy (38), post–cigarette smoking cessation (39), menopause (40), and after institution of medications such as steroids, antidepressants, and even some antidiabetic drugs predictably associated with weight gain] we do not mount a more active intervention before the weight gain occurs. The last two situations are part of chronic disease management. Finally, we will briefly discuss surgical options in those with marked obesity (BMI $\geq$ 35 with multiple risk factors or BMI $\geq$ 40 who have had a limited response to medical therapy and require consideration for surgery).

One problem with the limited time that physicians have with their patients is that a diet history, including an evaluation of the current diet, is often not obtained. This can be invaluable to patient and physician alike. Some patients (perhaps most) cannot accurately describe their diet. Asking the patient to write down each day what they eat in a diet diary provides important information that can be used by the patient, the dietitian, or even the physician to great advantage. For example, when patients bring such diets back on a return visit, one can have the patient circle those items that they should have avoided. Noting what they circle and what they do not often can help enable patients to make improvements that specifically address their eating style. (For example, if you note donuts in the morning and French fries at noon on a daily basis in their diary, you could suggest that they substitute a whole wheat bagel for the donuts and a side of fruit or tomatoes for the French fries.) Sometimes the diet diary suggests that patients eat well at home but not when out, and this can provide a focus for referral to a dietitian.

Manson et al. published a call to action for clinicians to get involved with lifestyle change. Their review included a useful flowchart (Fig. 4) as well as their adaptation of the Stages of Change model for those who require weight loss, diet, and physical activity (Table 5) (41). We have found it useful to ask each patient before referring them to counseling or giving them lifestyle change materials to tell us where they stand on a scale of 1 to 10 where 1 to 3 is precontemplation (they do not intend to start) and 8 to 10 is a high commitment to change. When patients indicate that their likelihood for change is low, we simply indicate that others like them have been able to commit to change and when they are ready to change, we are prepared to help them.

DIET AS PART OF LIFESTYLE THERAPY

As noted above, both low carbohydrate and low fat diets can be successful in helping patients lose weight. Table 6 shows the numerous dietary/lifestyle programs available. On the other

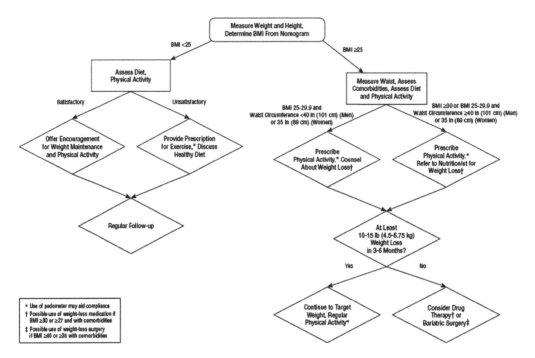

FIGURE 4 Additive effects of behavior and meal replacement therapy with pharmacotherapy for obesity. The use of pharmacotherapy alone is not as effective as pharmacotherapy given in conjunction with a comprehensive weight management program. The effect of adding behavior modification therapy and a portion-controlled diet with meal replacements to the pharmacologic treatment of obesity were compared in a one-year study of 53 obese women randomized to three treatment groups: (*i*) medication alone (sibutramine 10–15 mg daily), (*ii*) medication plus behavior modification therapy, or (*iii*) medication plus behavior modification plus a 1000 kcal/day portion-controlled diet (combined treatment group). *Source*: From Ref. 28.

hand, Table 7 shows that only a few long-term controlled studies (one year or more) in the obese patients are available to support evidence-based decisions.

In the studies of Foster et al. (44) and Stern et al. (45), carbohydrate restriction seemed to improve TGs and HDL-C, whereas in the study by McManus et al. (43), the best adherence was seen in the group with the more modest fat restriction. Knopp et al. examined the effect of progressive fat restriction on subjects with either high cholesterol or combined elevations in cholesterol and TGs (46). They found that lowering intake of fat below 25% of energy and carbohydrate intake above approximately 60% of energy yield no further LDL-C lowering in men with either high or combined elevations of lipids. Indeed, high carbohydrate and fat restrictive diets led to unwanted increases in TG and ApoB and a lowering of HDL-C.

Rather than restricting carbohydrates severely (this has always seemed unwise nutritionally), a popular approach has been to advocate limiting foods such as white bread and baked

TABLE 5 Stages of Change Model Adapted for Weight Loss and
Physical Activity

Stage	Losing weight	Physical activity	Comment
Precontemplation	No	No	Doesn't intend to start
Contemplation	No	No	Intends to start
Preparation	Considering	Considering	Intends to start
Action	Started	Started	Doing so for <6 mo
Maintenance	Yes	Yes	For ≥6 mo

Source: From Ref. 40.

TABLE 6 Avialble Dietary/Lifestyle Programs

Diet	Summary points
Low-carbohydrate diet (Atkins, Protein Power, Zone Diet)	Short-term weight loss Long term effects on CVD unknown Guide to initiate decreased energy intake
Glycemic index and diet (South Beach and Sugar Busters)	Unproven effects on CVD Guide to decreased consumption of energy-dense carbohydrates and initiate weight loss
Very low-fat diet	Possible decrease in cardiac events Concerns about universal applicability and sustainability
Mediterranean diet	Secondary prevention Prevention of sudden cardiac death Healthy overall approach to dieting Long-term sustainability
Dietary approaches to stop hypertension (DASH)	Decreased hypertension Similar to Mediterranean diet
Ornish lifestyle approach	Small study with angiographic endpoints Caused significant weight loss in the first year Strict dietary regimen (<10% fat) raises concerns about usefulness in general population; appears to require highly movitvated patients

Source: From Ref. 42.

goods, white potatoes, white rice, and sugars in juices and soda drinks. These foods are shown to have a high glycemic index (GI). The GI is a measure of the effect of dietary carbohydrates on a blood glucose scale from 0 to 100. Higher numbers correspond to substantial increases in glucose and insulin. Lower numbers are noted with foods such as whole grains, beans, nuts, and vegetables, which perhaps increase serum glucose and insulin less, because of a slower absorption. Glycemic load attempts to improve on GI by correcting for the amount of carbohydrate consumed. To date, clinical trial data showing a reduction in CHD/stroke endpoints from this kind of diet are lacking.

Sacks and Katan (47) have noted that the Dietary Approaches to Stop Hypertension (DASH) diet, which has only 27% of energy as fat (48), did not increase TGs compared with a typical U.S. diet with 37% fat. The DASH diet, which is an effective non-pharmacologic approach to hypertension, emphasizes fruit, vegetables, and low-fat dairy product. It also includes whole grains, poultry, fish, and nuts, and is low in high-GI foods. Indeed, in similar fashion, the ATP III report in 2001 suggested that a therapeutic diet derive 50% to 60% of calories from carbohydrates and that carbohydrate intake be predominantly from foods rich in complex carbohydrates including grains, especially whole grains, fruits, and vegetables (49).

Diets enriched in omega-3 fatty acids appear to reduce CHD mortality in a striking way. In the Lyon trial, free-living male and female survivors of MI were randomized to either a Mediterranean style diet or a more Western style diet (50). A highly significant reduction in cardiac events that was sustained over the course of the study was seen with the intervention diet. The diet given to the intervention group was high in fruits, vegetables, bread, other forms of cereals, potatoes, beans, nuts and seeds, and olive oil. Dairy products, fish, and poultry were consumed in low to moderate amounts. Little red meat was eaten, and eggs were eaten up to four times weekly. The diet was supplemented with a canola oil margarine that was rich in alpha linolenic acid. A sample of participants showed increased blood levels of omega-3 fatty acids on the intervention diet. Compared with the diet given, the therapeutic diet was low in saturated fat and dietary cholesterol as well as increased in fiber, monounsaturated fats (such as olive oil), and omega-3 fatty acids. In the GISSI trial, a similar early and pronounced effect on CHD mortality was seen in those MI survivors randomized to approximately 800 to 900 mg of omega-3 fatty acids given as a highly concentrated fish oil capsule (51). The beneficial effect did not appear to be mediated by changes in lipids (52). Although omega-3 fatty acid supplementation improved TGs and HDL-C, it actually raised LDL-C to a small degree.

There have been several critical reviews of diets and CVD. Schafer et al. at Tufts (53,54) reviewed data supporting the importance of both a low saturated fat diet and omega-3 fatty acids in CHD risk reduction. In addition, they felt that available evidence supports the restriction of sugars and carbohydrates having a high GI instead of total carbohydrate restriction as well as a

TABLE 7 Selected Controlled Studies of Weight Loss[a]

Name	Subjects, mean age, and mean BMI	Duration	% completed study	Interventions	Results
McManus et al. (2001)	101, 44 yr old, 33.5	18 mo	61/101; 20% in the low-fat group and 54% in the moderate fat group were still in the weight loss program after 18 mo ($p < 0.002$)	Moderate-fat diet (35% of energy) vs. low-fat diet (20% of energy)	A 7.0-kg weight change between the groups (95% CI 5.3, 8.7)
Foster et al. (2003)	63, 44 yr old, 33	1 yr	37/63 (59%)	High fat, low carbohydrate diet vs. calorie restricted, 25% fat diet	Nonsignificant changes in weight (-4.4 ± 6.7; vs. -2.5 ± 6.3) Significant improvement in TG and HDL-C
Stern et al. (2004)	132, 53 yr old, 42.9	1 yr	79/132	Low carbohydrate diet vs. calorie restricted conventional diet	Nonsignificant changes in weight (-5.1 ± 8.7; vs. 4.1 ± 8.4) Significant improvement in TG and HDL-C
Dansinger et al. (2005)	160, 49 yr old, 35	1 yr	Atkins (21/40, 53%) zone (26/40, 65%) Weight Watchers (26/40, 65%) Ornish (20/40, 50%)	Atkins, Zone, Weight Watchers, and Ornish diets	Amount of weight loss was significantly associated with self reported level of dietary. Adherence ($r = 0.60$; $P = 0.001$) but not with diet type ($r = 0.07$; $P = 0.40$). For each diet, decreasing levels of total/HDL-C, CRP, and insulin were significantly associated with weight loss (mean $r = 0.36$, 0.37, and 0.39, respectively) with no significant difference between diets

[a]With duration of one year and more than 50 subjects chosen because they were overweight/obese.
Abbreviation: BMI, body mass index; TG, triglyceride; HDL-C, high-density lipoprotein-cholesterol.

dietary plan with provision for increased intake of fiber and omega-3 fatty acids. Denke (55) emphasized the early onset of CHD reduction when omega-3 fatty acids were utilized. Parikh et al. (42) reviewed dietary studies and suggested that an optimal diet should encourage (i) a decreased carbohydrate intake, especially of refined and high-GI carbohydrates; (ii) increased consumption of fruits, vegetables, and whole grains; (iii) increased intake of polyunsaturated fats by increasing the consumption of plant oils and fish; (iv) and moderate intake of low-fat dairy products and nuts. Surprisingly, this review, published in 2005, characterized AHA and ATP III diets as low fat. This appears to ignore the 2001 recommendation of the ATP III panel that fat intake could range from 25% to 35% of total calories as part of the therapeutic lifestyle change (TLC) diet. This was done specifically to avoid a focus on quantity of fat and instead on quality of the diet, with the explicit recognition that those with metabolic syndrome/diabetes may benefit from a higher unsaturated fat and lower carbohydrate (see above) intake.

Finally, many physicians ask about how to use the Diet Pyramid in practice. Patients can learn about smart choices from every food group, find a balance between food and physical activity, and get the most nutrition out of their daily calories at the mypyramid Web site (56). The user can access the Tips and Resources Page on the home page. With another click, inquiring learners can find out how to:

- Make half their grains whole
- Vary their veggies
- Focus on fruit
- Get their calcium-rich foods
- Go lean with protein
- Find the balance between food and physical activity

Another click redirects the user to the guidelines page. Here the user can learn about the essentials of a healthy diet from Dietary Guidelines 2005. The Guidelines

- Emphasize fruits, vegetables, whole grains, and fat-free or low-fat milk and milk products;
- Include lean meats, poultry, fish, beans, eggs, and nuts in the diet; and
- Suggest a dietary plan low in saturated fats, trans-fats, cholesterol, salt (sodium), and added sugars.

Exercise as Part of Lifestyle Therapy

Using an overweight population, investigators in the Targeted Risk Reduction Interventions through Defined Exercise study have demonstrated that a relatively high amount of regular exercise—even in the absence of clinically significant weight loss—can significantly improve the overall lipoprotein profile (57). Although LDL-C levels were not improved substantially with exercise at a caloric equivalent of 17 to 18 mi (27.2–28.8 km) per week and an intensity equivalent to that of jogging at a moderate pace led to lipoprotein benefits that were substantial, with decreased small dense LDL and TG-rich particles and increased HDL. The authors noted that their data suggested that it was the amount and not the intensity of exercise that made the most difference in improving lipid and lipoprotein profiles. Jogging is not absolutely necessary. When postmenopausal women aged 50 to 79 either walked briskly or exercised vigorously at least 2.5 hr/wk, they demonstrated a relative CHD risk reduction of approximately 30% (58). Perhaps most telling was the substantial increase in CHD risk for those sedentary subjects who spent a prolonged time sitting. Although a large meta-analysis showed no statistically significant changes in HDL or TG alone ($p > 0.05$) with walking, the changes seen were in the direction of benefit (59). Regular walking was associated with decreases of 5% for LDL-C and 6% for the cholesterol/HDL-C ratio. One problem with meta-analyses is that they may not fully account for the time that may be needed to raise HDL-C by exercise. King et al. looked at group versus home training in 149 men and 120 postmenopausal women in the 50 to 65-year age group who were sedentary and free of CVD (60). It took up to the end of year two in subjects in the two home-based training conditions to show small but significant HDL-C increases over baseline ($p < 0.01$). An important observation was that the increases were especially pronounced for subjects in the lower-intensity condition, who required more frequent exercise sessions per week. For all exercise conditions, increases in HDL-C were associated with decreases in W/H ratio in both men and women ($p < 0.04$).

What kind of exercise should physicians prescribe? A recent study of 492 sedentary adults of whom almost two-thirds were female compared four randomly assigned exercise-counseling conditions with a physician advice comparison group (61). The duration (30 minutes) and type (walking) of exercise were held constant, while exercise intensity and frequency were manipulated to form four exercise prescriptions:

- Moderate intensity–low frequency
- Moderate intensity–high frequency (HiF)
- Hard intensity (HardI)–low frequency
- HardI–HiF

The control group received physician advice and written materials regarding recommended levels of exercise for health. The investigators demonstrated that exercise counseling with a prescription for walking (30 min/day) at either a moderate intensity for five to seven days/wk or a hard intensity three to four days/wk produced significant improvements in cardiorespiratory fitness that were observed at 6 months and maintained over 24 months.

Moreover, the HardI–HiF prescription was the only intervention that produced a significant improvement in HDL-C level (mean, 3.9%) compared with the physician advice group.

Thus, at each visit, we endorse a message regarding regular exercise. Most important is to go from completely sedentary to doing something on a daily basis. For those who can safely exercise in a high-intensity manner, three to four times per week may be all that is required. A useful way to get this message across is both to wear and recommend a pedometer so that patients can see how active (or inactive) they are.

Lifestyle Interventions

The 2001 ATP III guidelines suggested a lifestyle approach called TLC that included (i) reduced intakes of saturated fats and cholesterol, (ii) therapeutic dietary options to enhance LDL lowering (plant stanols/sterols and increased viscous fiber), (iii) weight control, and (iv) increased physical activity. This approach is consistent with the lifestyle regimens used in two studies of subjects with impaired glucose tolerance—the Finnish Diabetes Study and the Diabetes Prevention Program (DPP) (62,63). Both these trials of a high-fiber, low-saturated fat diet, regular exercise, and modest weight loss showed reductions in the progression to diabetes by almost 60%. This lifestyle approach worked in both genders and in each age group, and in the DPP, it was twice as effective as metformin therapy.

BEHAVIORAL APPROACHES

Many, if not all, patients require a set of skills to help them change unhealthy habits and reach their health goals, which often include a lower weight, improved lipids, and a better blood sugar. Behavioral experts recommend the use of self-monitoring (diet and exercise records), stimulus control, goal setting, frequent feedback, social support, and problem solving. Foster et al. (64) identified several questions (WHY? WHAT? and HOW?) that are recommended to help achieve adherence to a weight loss plan. We would add READY? as per the discussion earlier in the chapter (Table 8). We would underscore those program components with the "human touch," such as encouraging patients to seek social support, enabling patients by having them participate in choosing "achievable" goals, and helping them select those dietary and physical activity approaches that make sense for their lives.

TABLE 8 Questions to Ask Patients Who Require Behavioral Change

Question	Guidelines
Why?	Ask the patient if they know the rationale for changing the behavior
What?	Identify goals and a plan of action
How?	Identify facilitators and barriers
Ready?	Ask them to assess their readiness to change

Source: Adapted from Ref. 62.

INTEGRATING BEHAVIORAL APPROACH INTO LIFESTYLE CHANGE

A variety of strategies have been proposed for decreasing energy intake to assist in weight management in diabetic patients but they should be considered for all patients in whom weight control is an issue (65):

■ Lowering energy density of the diet by increasing fruit and vegetable intake and limiting foods that are high in fat [start by having the patient substitute high-fat items at breakfast (donuts, muffins) with lower fat choices]
■ Increasing portion control by reducing portion sizes; having patients simply eat half the calories at major meal times
■ Reducing total calories by eliminating snacks such as cereals and candy bars near bedtime (you have to have the patient bring in a diet diary or ask about bedtime eating specifically in many cases to find this out)
■ Advocating meal replacement products and following structured meal plans, for those who need extended training in portion control
■ Prescribing a lower-carbohydrate approach for obese diabetic patients, as suggested by ATP III (but avoiding carbohydrates such as fruits, vegetables, and whole grains is not supported by the literature)
■ Lowering fat in the diet for getting and maintaining weight loss.

This was illustrated by the findings of the Women's Health Initiative Dietary Modification Trial that randomized 19,541 women to an intervention diet and 29,294 to a control diet and followed them for 7.5 years (66). The intervention diet was lower in fat and higher in vegetables, fruit, and grains. Women with this dietary plan lost significantly more weight in the first year of the study and maintained the lower weight significantly better than control women over the 7.5 years of follow-up. In both groups, weight loss was greatest among women who decreased their percentage of energy from fat.

For those who need to increase energy expenditure, individualizing the kind of physical activity advocated can be useful. A small clinical trial of diet plus lifestyle activity to diet and structured aerobic activity in obese (mean BMI 32.9) women (21–60 years old) found no significant change in fat-free weight lost or improvement in lipids with either program; hence clinicians should try to make the exercise fit the person's life and not vice versa (67).

The National Weight Control Registry (NWCR) provides a description of how people have lost and maintained weight loss effectively (68–70). Participants enrolled in the registry must have maintained a weight loss of more than 30 lb for at least one year. On average, subjects have maintained almost a 70 lb weight loss for six years. The major behaviors reported by approximately 3000 NWCR participants were as follows:

■ Self monitoring with a daily food record and body weight checks at least once weekly
■ Restrict calories and fat in the diet (1300–1400 kcal/day and 20–25% as energy from fat)
■ Eat breakfast daily
■ Engage in physical activity consuming 2500–3000 kcal/wk

Unfortunately, those who lose weight successfully often regain their lost weight over time (71). It is noteworthy that despite regaining lost weight, those who have learned useful behaviors regarding diet and exercise are shown to gain less than their peers over that time (72). For those who turn to the use of pharmacotherapy to lose weight, attention to behavioral matters can provide extra benefit. In one randomized study, pharmacotherapy alone was not as effective as pharmacotherapy given in conjunction with behavior modification therapy and a portion-controlled diet with meal replacements. In addition to greater weight loss, subjects in the behavior modification group seemed more satisfied with the treatment outcome (73). In a recently completed study, those in the combined drug plus lifestyle group who frequently recorded their food intake lost more weight than those who did so infrequently (74).

CONCLUSIONS

A comprehensive approach to treating those with weight gain and especially those with health complications of weight gain is important. Although new medications and surgical approaches may capture the headlines, attention to lifestyle change will continue to be important to prevent weight gain, to help lose weight, and importantly to help avoid regaining weight that has been successfully lost. As an added bonus, lifestyle-induced weight loss improves the metabolic complications of abdominal obesity. Indeed, attention to these metabolic complications of obesity may prove especially helpful if we are to forestall an epidemic of diabetes and CHD that could result from obesity occurring at earlier ages than ever before. Indeed, a special challenge will be addressing the nutritional wants and needs of children. The Dietary Intervention Study in Children (DISC) was a randomized, controlled trial that extended beyond its original three-year intervention to exceed seven years of intervention and data collection (75). Investigators found that they had made a meaningful intervention of healthier foods, but that snack foods, desserts, and pizza contributed approximately one-third of total daily energy intake to both control and intervention subjects. Thus, in addition to further research into energy metabolism and genetic-environment interactions, we need more information on how to influence food choice beginning at the earliest ages, so that we can more easily turn frustration with weight control into success.

REFERENCES

1. Flegal KM, et al. Prevalence and trends in obesity among US adults 1999–2000. JAMA 2002; 288:1723–1727.
2. Grundy SM. Metabolic syndrome scientific statement by the American Heart Association and the National Heart, Lung, and Blood Institute. Arterioscler Thromb Vasc Biol 2005; 25:2243–2244.
3. National Heart, Lung, and Blood Institute. Clinical guidelines on the identification, evaluation, and treatment of overweight and obesity in adults. The evidence report. Obes Res 1998; 6(suppl 2):51S–209S.
4. National Heart, Lung, and Blood Institute, and North American Association for the study of obesity. Practical guide to the identification, evaluation, and treatment of overweight and obesity in adults. Bethesda, MD: National Institutes of Health, 2000 [Publication #NIH 00–4084].
5. Ford ES. Prevalence of the metabolic syndrome defined by the International Diabetes Federation among adults in the U.S. Diabetes Care 2005; 28(11):2745–2749.
6. Yusuf S, Hawken S, Ounpuu S, et al. Obesity and the risk of myocardial infarction in 27,000 participants from 52 countries: a case-control study. Lancet 2005; 366(9497):1640–1649.
7. Ferreira I, Twisk JW, van Mechelen W, Kemper HC, Stehouwer CD. Development of fatness, fitness and lifestyle from adolescence to age 36: determinants of the metabolic syndrome in young adults. The Amsterdam Growth and Health Longitudinal Study. Arch Intern Med 2005; 165:42–48.
8. Lee CD, Blair SN, Jackson AS. Cardiorespiratory fitness, body composition, and all-cause and cardiovascular disease mortality in men. Am J Clin Nutr 1999; 69:373–380.
9. Centers for Disease Control and Prevention, National Center for Health Statistics. Prevalence of overweight and obesity among adults: United States, 1999–2000. Available online at http://www.cdc.gov/nchs/products/pubs/pubd/hestats/obese/obse99htm. Accessed October 24, 2002.
10. Slurm R. The effects of obesity, smoking, and drinking on medical problems and costs. Health Aff (Millwood) 2002; 21:245–253.
11. Finkelstein EA, Fiebelkorn IC, Wang G. State-level estimates of annual medical expenditures attributable to obesity. Obes Res 2004; 12:18–24.
12. Vasan RS, Pencina MJ, Cobain M, Freiberg MS, D'Agostino RB. Estimated risks for developing obesity in the Framingham Heart Study. Ann Intern Med 2005; 143(7):473–480.
13. Lobstein T, Baur L, Uauy R. Obesity in children and young people: a crisis in public health. Obesity Rev 2004; 5(suppl 1):4–104.
14. Klein S, Burke LE, Bray GA, et al. Clinical implications of obesity with specific focus on cardiovascular disease: a statement for professionals from the American Heart Association Council on Nutrition, Physical Activity, and Metabolism. Circulation 2004; 110:2952–2967.
15. Klein S, Fontana L, Young VL, et al. Absence of an effect of liposuction on insulin action and risk factors for coronary heart disease. N Engl J Med 2004; 350:2549–2557.
16. Colditz GA, Willett WC, Rotnitzky A, Manson JE. Weight gain as a risk factor for clinical diabetes mellitus in women. Ann Intern Med 1995; 122:481–486.
17. Chan JM, et al. Obesity, fat distribution, and weight gain as risk factors for clinical diabetes in men. Diabetes Care 1994; 17:961–969.
18. Sharma AM, Chetty VT. Obesity, hypertension, and insulin resistance. Acta Diabetol 2005; 42(suppl 1): S3–S8.
19. McLaughlin T, Allison G, Abbasi F, Lamendola C, Reaven G. Prevalence of insulin resistance and associated cardiovascular disease risk factors among normal weight, overweight, and obese individuals. Metabolism 2004; 53(4):495–499.
20. Brown CD, Higgins M, Donato KA, et al. Body mass index and the prevalence of hypertension and dyslipidemia. Obes Res 2000; 8:605–619.

21. Tchernof A, Lamarche B, Prud'Homme D, et al. The dense LDL phenotype. Association with plasma lipoprotein levels, visceral obesity, and hyperinsulinemia in men. Diabetes Care 1996; 19:629–637.

22. Chambers JC, Eda S, Bassett P, et al. C-reactive protein, insulin resistance, central obesity, and coronary heart disease risk in Indian Asians from the United Kingdom compared with European whites. Circulation 2001; 104(2):145–150.

23. Vgontzas AN, Bixler EO, Tan TL, Kantner D, Martin LF, Kales A. Obesity without sleep apnea is associated with daytime sleepiness. Arch Intern Med 1998; 158(12):1333–1337.

24. Poirier P, Giles TD, Bray GA, et al. Obesity and cardiovascular disease: pathophysiology, evaluation, and effect of weight loss. An update of the 1997 American Heart Association scientific statement on obesity and heart disease from the Obesity Committee of the Council on Nutrition, Physical Activity, and Metabolism. Circulation 2006; 113(6):898–918.

25. Shiffman ML, Sugerman HJ, Kellum JH, Brewer WH, Moore EW. Gallstones in patients with morbid obesity. Relationship to body weight, weight loss, and gallbladder bile cholesterol solubility. Int J Obes Relat Metab Disord 1993; 17(3):153–158.

26. Matteoni C, Younossi ZM, McCullough A. Nonalcoholic fatty liver disease: a spectrum of clinical pathological severity. Gastroenterology 1999; 116:1413–1419.

27. Festi D, Colecchia A, Sacco T, Bondi M, Roda E, Marchesini G. Hepatic steatosis in obese patients: clinical aspects and prognostic significance. Obes Rev 2004; 5(1):27–42.

28. Felson DT, Anderson JJ, Naimark A, et al. Obesity and knee osteoarthritis. The Framingham Study. Ann Intern Med 1988; 109:18–24.

29. Shoff SM, Newcomb PA. Diabetes, body size, and risk of endometrial cancer. Am J Epidemiol 1998; 148:234–240.

30. Huang Z, Hankinson SE, Colditz GA, et al. Dual effects of weight and weight gain on breast cancer. JAMA 1997; 278:1407–1411.

31. Must A, Spadano J, Coakley EH, Field AE, Colditz G, Dietz WH. The disease burden associated with overweight and obesity. JAMA 1999; 282(16):1523–1529.

32. Field AE, et al. Impact of overweight on the risk of developing common chronic diseases during a ten-year period. Arch Intern Med 2001; 161:1581–1586.

33. McGill HC Jr., McMahan CA, Herderick EE, et al. Obesity accelerates the progression of coronary atherosclerosis in young men. Circulation 2002; 105:2712–2718.

34. Lemieux I, Pascot A, Couillard C, et al. Hypertriglyceridemic waist: a marker of the atherogenic metabolic triad (hyperinsulinemia; hyperapolipoprotein B; small, dense LDL) in men? Circulation 2000; 102:179–184.

35. Wilson PW, Kannel WB, Silbershatz H, D'Agostino RB. Clustering of metabolic factors and coronary artery disease. Arch Intern Med 1999; 159:1104–1109.

36. Stone NJ, Saxon D. Approach to treatment of the patient with metabolic syndrome: lifestyle therapy. Am J Cardiol 2005; 96(4A):15–21.

37. Dansinger ML, Gleason JA, Griffith JL, Selker HP, Schaefer EJ. Comparison of the Atkins, Ornish, Weight Watchers, and Zone Diets for weight loss and heart disease risk reduction: a randomized trial. JAMA 2005; 293:43–53.

38. Kaaja RJ, Greer IA. Manifestations of chronic disease during pregnancy. JAMA 2005; 294:2751–2757.

39. Davey Smith G, Bracha Y, Svendsen KH, Neaton JD, Haffner SM, Kuller LH; Multiple Risk Factor Intervention Trial Research Group. Incidence of Type 2 diabetes in the randomized multiple risk factor intervention trial. Ann Intern Med 2005; 142(5):313–322.

40. Kuller LH, Simkin-Silverman LR, Wing RR, Meilahn EN, Ives DG. Women's Healthy Lifestyle Project: a randomized clinical trial: results at 54 months. Circulation 2001; 103(1):32–37.

41. Manson JE, Skerrett PJ, Greenland P, VanItallie TB. The escalating pandemics of obesity and sedentary lifestyle. A call to action for clinicians. Arch Intern Med 2004; 164(3):249–258.

42. Parikh P, McDaniel MC, Ashen MD, et al. Diets and cardiovascular disease: an evidence-based assessment. J Am Coll Cardiol 2005; 45(9):1379–1397.

43. McManus K, Antinoro L, Sacks F. A randomized controlled trial of a moderate-fat, low-energy diet for weight loss in overweight adults. Int J Obesity 2001; 25:1503–1511.

44. Foster GD, Wyatt HR, Hill JO, et al. A randomized trial of a low-carbohydrate diet for obesity. N Engl J Med 2003; 348:2082–2090.

45. Stern L, Iqbal N, Seshadri P, et al. The effects of low-carbohydrate versus conventional weight loss diets in severely obese adults: one-year follow-up of a randomized trial. Ann Intern Med 2004; 140:778–785.

46. Knopp RH, Retzlaff B, Walden C, Fish B, Buck B, McCann B. One-year effects of increasingly fat-restricted, carbohydrate-enriched diets on lipoprotein levels in free-living subjects. Proc Soc Exp Biol Med 2000; 225(3):191–199.

47. Sacks FM, Katan M. Randomized clinical trials on the effects of dietary fat and carbohydrate on plasma lipoproteins and cardiovascular disease. Am J Med 2002; 113(9B):13S–24S.

48. Obarzanek E, Sacks FM, Vollmer WM, et al. Effects on blood lipids of a blood pressure-lowering diet: the Dietary Approaches to Stop Hypertension (DASH) Trial. Am J Clin Nutr 2001; 74:80–89.

49. Expert Panel on Detection, Evaluation, and Treatment of High Blood Cholesterol in Adults. Executive summary of the Third Report of the National Cholesterol Education Program (NCEP) Expert Panel on Detection, Evaluation, and Treatment of High Blood Cholesterol in Adults (Adult Treatment Panel III). JAMA 2001; 285:2486–2497.

50. De Lorgeril M, Renaud S, Mamelle N, et al. Mediterranean alpha-linolenic acid-rich diet in secondary prevention of coronary heart disease. Lancet 1994; 343:1454–1459.

51. GISSI-Prevenzione Investigators. Dietary supplementation with n-3 polyunsaturated fatty acids and vitamin E after myocardial infarction: results of the GISSI-Prevenzione trial. Lancet 1999; 354:447–455.

52. Leaf A. On the re-analysis of the GISSI-Prevenzione. Circulation 2002; 105:1874.

53. Schaefer EJ, Gleason JA, Dansinger ML. The Effects of low-fat, high-carbohydrate diets on plasma lipoproteins, weight loss, and heart disease risk reduction. Curr Atheroscler Rep 2005; 7(6):421–427.

54. Brousseau ME, Schaefer EJ. Diet and coronary heart disease: clinical trials. Curr Atheroscler Rep 2000; 2(6):487–493.

55. Denke MA. Diet, lifestyle, and nonstatin trials: review of time to benefit. Am J Cardiol 2005; 96(5A):3F–10F.

56. US Department of Agriculture. http://www.mypyramid.gov (accessed January 2, 2006).

57. Kraus WE, Houmard JA, Duscha BD, et al. Effects of the amount and intensity of exercise on plasma lipoproteins. N Engl J Med 2002; 347(19):1483–1492.

58. Manson JE, Greenland P, LaCroix AZ, et al. Walking compared with vigorous exercise for the prevention of cardiovascular events in women. N Engl J Med 2002; 347:716–725.

59. Kelley GA, Kelley KS, Tran ZV. Walking, lipids, and lipoproteins: a meta-analysis of randomized controlled trials. Prev Med 2004; 38(5):651–661.

60. King AC, Haskell WL, Young DR, Oka RK, Stefanick ML. Long-term effects of varying intensities and formats of physical activity on participation rates, fitness and lipoproteins in men and women age 50 to 65 years. Circulation 1995; 91:2596–2604.

61. Duncan GE, Anton SD, Sydeman SJ, et al. Prescribing exercise at varied levels of intensity and frequency: a randomized trial. Arch Intern Med 2005; 165(20):2362–2369.

62. Tuomilehto J, Lindstrom J, Eriksson JG, et al. Prevention of Type 2 diabetes mellitus by changes in lifestyle among subjects with impaired glucose tolerance. N Engl J Med 2001; 344:1343–1350.

63. The Diabetes Prevention Program Research Group. Reduction in the incidence of Type 2 diabetes with lifestyle intervention or metformin. N Engl J Med 2002; 346:393–403.

64. Foster GD, Makris AP, Bailer BA. Behavioral treatment of obesity. Am J Clin Nutr 2005; 82(suppl 1): 230S–235S.

65. Klein S, Sheard NF, Pi-Sunyer X, et al. Weight management through lifestyle modification for the prevention and management of type 2 diabetes: rationale and strategies: a statement of the American Diabetes Association, the North American Association for the Study of Obesity, and the American Society for Clinical Nutrition. Diabetes Care 2004; 27(8):2067–2073.

66. Howard BV, Manson JE, Stefanick ML, et al. Low-Fat dietary pattern and weight change over 7 years. The women's health initiative dietary modification trial. JAMA 2006; 295:39–49.

67. Andersen RE, Wadden TA, Bartlett SJ, Zemel B, Verde TJ, Franckowiak SC. Effects of lifestyle activity vs structured aerobic exercise in obese women: a randomized trial. JAMA 1999; 281(4):335–340.

68. Klem ML, et al. A descriptive study of individuals successful at long-term maintenance of substantial weight loss. Am J Clin Nutr 1997; 66:239–246.

69. Wyatt HR, et al. Long-term weight loss and breakfast in the National Weight Control Registry. Obes Res 2002; 10:78–82.

70. McGuire MT, et al. Long-term maintenance of weight loss: do people who lose weight through various weight loss methods use different behaviors to maintain their weight? Int J Obes Relat Metab Disord 1998; 22:572–527.

71. Klein S, Wadden T, Sugerman HJ. AGA technical review on obesity. Gastroenterology 2002; 123:882–932.

72. Field AE, Wing RR, Manson JE, Spiegelman DL, Willett WC. Relationship of a large weight loss to long-term weight change among young and middle-aged US women. Int J Obes Relat Metab Disord 2001; 25(8):1113–1121.

73. Wadden TA, Berkowitz RI, Sarwer DB, Prus-Wisniewski R, Steinberg C. Benefits of lifestyle modification in the pharmacologic treatment of obesity: a randomized trial. Arch Intern Med 2001; 161(2):218–227.

74. Wadden TA, Berkowitz RI, Womble LG, et al. Randomized trial of lifestyle modification and pharmacotherapy for obesity. N Engl J Med 2005; 353(20):2111–2120.

75. Van Horn L, Obarzanek E, Friedman LA. Children's adaptations to a fat-reduced diet: the dietary intervention study in children (DISC). Pediatrics 2005; 115:1723–1733.

4 | Effects of Nutrient Supplements and Nutraceuticals on Risk for Cardiovascular Disease

Yumei Cao, Jun Zhang, and Penny M. Kris-Etherton
Department of Nutritional Sciences, The Huck Institute for Integrative Biosciences, Pennsylvania State University, University Park, Pennsylvania, U.S.A.

KEY POINTS

- For primary prevention of cardiovascular disease, 500 mg/day of EPA + DHA is recommended, primarily via diet (consumption of two servings of fatty fish per week is advised). For secondary prevention of cardiovascular disease, 1 g/day is recommended. For triglyceride lowering, 2–4 g/day is indicated. Physician oversight is recommended for the latter two patient cohorts. Fish oil supplements will be necessary for triglyceride lowering and may be needed for secondary prevention of cardiovascular disease.
- Nicotinic acid (1–3 g/day) is recommended mainly to increase HDL-C levels, typically in patients with low HDL-C levels. Nicotinic acid often is prescribed with other pharmacologic agents to treat hypercholesterolemia and/or dyslipidemia (concomitant with low HDL-C).
- Sterols/stanols (2 g/day) and viscous fiber (10–25 g/day) are recommended as an additional dietary option for LDL-C lowering.
- There is no evidence of a beneficial effect of antioxidants and B-vitamins on cardiovascular disease morbidity and mortality. Despite recent evidence that B-vitamins (folic acid, vitamin B6 and vitamin B12) decrease homocysteine, there is no evidence of any benefits on cardiovascular disease morbidity and mortality (1,2).
- Although some botanical agents have been shown to have therapeutic benefits in small studies, further research is necessary to provide a sufficient evidence base to make sound recommendations for the prevention and treatment of cardiovascular disease.

INTRODUCTION

Nutrient supplements and nutraceuticals are growing in popularity in the United States and globally. Based on National Health and Nutrition Examination Survey (NHANES) 1999–2000 data (3), 52% of the adults in the United States reported taking a dietary supplement during the month prior to the survey, and had been doing so daily for at least two years. Thirty-five percent of the respondents reported taking a multivitamin/multimineral supplement. Other supplements taken (expressed as a percentage of respondents) were: vitamin E (12.7%), vitamin C (12.4%), calcium (10.4%), calcium/antacids (24.4%), and B-complex vitamins (5.2%). Sixty-three percent of the adults aged 60 years and above reported taking more than one supplement. Selected characteristics of supplement users can be listed as: female, older in age, well-educated, non-Hispanic whites, engaged in physical activity, and not overweight.

In a survey of 31,044 adults who participated in the 2002 National Health Interview Survey conducted by the National Center for Health Statistics (4), 18.9% reported herb use during the past 12 months. According to this survey, the most popular herbs were *Echinacea* (38.4%), ginseng (23%), ginkgo (20.1%), and garlic supplements (18.6%). Characteristics of herb users are: female, adults aged 45 to 64 years, individuals from multiple races rather than whites or blacks, and college graduates. Importantly, about one-third of the respondents reported telling their health care provider that they were taking herbs or supplements.

The widespread use of dietary supplements has resulted in sales that exceeded $20 billion in the United States in 2004. Multivitamins/mineral supplements, vitamins, and minerals accounted for the largest share of the market (about $9 billion), and herbs/botanicals accounted for about one-fifth of the total sales ($4.3 billion). The growing popularity of herbs has been the impetus to better understand what products are being used, and what their potential adverse effects may be [alone or in combination with nutrient supplements, other herbal products, and/or with prescription or over the counter (OTC) drugs]. The use of these products to promote health and treat disease is not consistent with food-based dietary guidance, which is widely endorsed by the scientific community (5). Consequently, it is important that we have a better understanding of the biological effects of these products and their interactions with prescription or OTC drugs for cardiovascular disease (CVD). This chapter will summarize the epidemiologic and clinical studies that assess the impact that vitamins and minerals, herbal products, and other nutrition supplements have on CVD risk. In addition, we will discuss adverse drug–nutrient interactions that are germane to CVD. There are some instances, however, where selected supplements should be used for the prevention and treatment of CVD. But, for many, there are no sufficient data to recommend their use. Moreover, for some, there is concern about drug–nutrient interactions. This chapter will also describe the evidence for making informed decisions about what supplements should be used for patients with CVD.

ANTIOXIDANT VITAMINS

The hypothesis that links antioxidant vitamins and CVD is based partly on the oxidative modification of low-density lipoprotein (LDL), and its role in the development and progression of atherosclerosis (6,7). Oxidation results in the production of reactive oxygen species (ROS) that impair vascular wall function (8), which results in a cascade of reactions that promote plaque development. Antioxidant vitamins have been shown to inhibit LDL oxidation (9,10), decrease ROS (11–13), and decrease LDL oxidative susceptibility (14). In addition, vitamin E may reduce platelet aggregability (15), reduce the expression of adhesion molecules (16), decrease the release of proinflammatory cytokines and chemokines (17), decrease plasminogen activator inhibitor (PAI-1) levels (17), and stimulate nitric oxide production (18). Epidemiologic and observational studies (19) have reported that diets rich in antioxidants (e.g., lots of fruits and vegetables), as well as specific antioxidants (i.e., vitamin E, vitamin C, and β-carotene), may have a beneficial effect on CVD risk. However, the data from clinical trials (both primary and secondary prevention studies) fail to support a beneficial effect of antioxidant vitamin supplements on CVD events, as reviewed in Ref. (20).

Epidemiologic Studies

Numerous observational studies have assessed the associations between various antioxidant vitamins (serum, food, and/or supplementation) and cardiac events (Table 1). The vitamins include carotenes/carotenoids, vitamin C, vitamin E, and various other vitamin combinations. The information about vitamin intake from diet or supplements is most often obtained from food-frequency questionnaires.

Carotenes

In the Lipid Research Clinics Coronary Primary Prevention Trial and Follow-up Study (LRC-CPPT) (24), after adjusting multiple coronary heart disease (CHD) risk factors, serum carotenoids were inversely related to CHD events. Compared with subjects in the lowest quartile (<2.33 μmol/L), subjects in the highest quartile of serum carotenoids (>3.16 μmol/L) had a relative risk (RR) of CHD 0.64 (95% CI 0.44–0.92; P for trend 0.01). This association was stronger among men who never smoked (RR: 0.28 for nonsmokers versus 0.78 for current smokers).

β-carotene intake was inversely associated with myocardial infarction (MI) events (30). Compared with the subjects in the lowest tertile of β-carotene intake (<1.13 mg/day), those in the highest tertile of dietary carotene intake (>1.57 mg/day) had an RR for MI 0.55 (95% CI 0.34–0.83; P for trend 0.013). In the Nurses' Health Study (36), both α- and β-carotene intake were inversely associated with total coronary artery diseases (CAD). The RRs of CAD for α- and β-carotene were 0.80 (P for trend 0.04) and 0.74 (P for trend 0.05), respectively. In contrast, no relationship was found between carotene levels and cardiac death in several studies (23,25–27), as well as carotene intake and carotid wall thickness (38).

TABLE 1 Epidemiologic Studies of Vitamin Intake on Relative Risks for Cardiac Events

Study and year	Population	Follow-up	Category	Outcome	Multivariate relative risk (95% CI) highest vs. lowest category
Rimm et al. (21) 1993	39,910 male U.S. health professionals age 40–75 Yr	4 yr	Median intake: VitE (IU/day): 6.4; 8.5; 11.2; 25.2; 419 Carotene (IU/day): 3969; 6019; 8114; 11653; 19034 VitC (mg/day): 92; 149; 218; 392; 1162	667 cases of CHD (fatal CHD, nonfatal MI, CABG, angioplasty)	CHD VitE: 0.60 (0.44–0.81); *P* for trend 0.01 Carotene: 0.71 (0.53–0.86); *P* for trend 0.03 VitC: 1.25 (0.91–1.71); *P* for trend 0.98 Taking ≥100 IU/day and ≥2 yrs: 0.63 (0.47–0.84)
Stampfer et al. (22)1993	87,245 female U.S. nurses, age 34–59 yr, with no history of cancer, angina, MI, stroke or other CVD	8 yr	Total VitE (IU/day) 1.2–3.5; 3.6–4.9; 5.0–8.0; 8.1–21.5; 21.6–1000 Dietary VitE (IU/day) 0.3–3.1; 3.2–3.9; 4.0–4.8; 4.9–6.2; 6.3–100	552 cases of major CHD (437 nonfatal MI or 115 CHD deaths)	Major CHD: Total intake: 0.66 (0.5–0.87) *P* for trend <0.001 Dietary intake: 0.95 (0.72–1.23) *P* for trend 0.99 Short term VitE supplements: 0.86 (0.52–1.43) Long term (>2yr) VitE supplements: 0.59 (0.38–0.91) VitE supplement only: 0.41 (0.18–0.93) Multivitamin only: 0.87 (0.69–1.09) Both: 0.50 (0.31–0.83)
Knekt et al. (23) 1994	5133 men and women in Finland, age 30–69yr	12–16 yr	VitC (age adjusted; mg/day) Men: ≤60; 61–85; >85 Women: ≤61; 62–91; >91 β-carotene (age adjusted; mg/d) Men: ≤147; 148–258; >258 Women: ≤182; 183–383; >383 VitE (age adjusted; mg/day) Men: ≤6.8; 6.9–8.9; >8.9 Women: ≤5.3; 5.4–7.1; >7.1	244 CHD deaths (male 186 and female 58	VitE—CHD mortality: Men: 0.68 (0.42–1.11); *P* for trend = 0.01 Women: 0.35 (0.14–0.88); *P* for trend <0.01 β-carotene—CHD mortality: Men: 1.02 (0.70–1.48); *P* for trend 1.02 Women: 0.62 (0.30–1.29); *P* for trend 0.60 VitC—CHD mortality Men: 1.00 (0.68–1.45); *P* for trend 0.94 Women: 0.49 (0.24–0.98); *P* for trend 0.06
Morris et al. (24) 1994	1899 men aged 40–59yr with type II-a hyperlipidemia and without known preexisting CHD, cancer, or other major illnesses	13 yr	Serum carotenoid (μmol/L) <2.33; 2.33–2.70; 2.71–3.16; >3.16	282 CHD events and 81 CHD death	CHD Total men: 0.64 (0.44–0.92), *P* for trend 0.01 Never smoked: 0.28 (0.11–0.73), *P* for trend 0.06 Quit: 0.63 (0.35–1.15); *P* for trend 0.30 Current smoking: 0.78 (0.44–1.34); *P* for trend 0.04
Pandey et al. (25) 1995	1,556 middle-aged men 40–55yr	24 yr	VitC (mg/day) 21–82; 83–112; 113–393 β-carotene (mg/day) 0.5–2.9; 3.0–4.0; 4.1–15.9	522 men died (231 CHD)	VitC—CHD death: Non-smoking: 0.58; *P* for trend 0.042 Smoking: 0.95; *P* for trend 0.818 All: 0.75; *P* for trend 0.063 β-carotene—CHD death: Nonsmoking: 0.70; *P* for trend 0.125 Smoking: 0.94; *P* for trend 0.417 All: 0.84; *P* for trend 0.094
Sahyoun et al.	254 elderly men and 471	12 yr	Cutoff value (lowest vs. highest	108 CVD deaths	Serum—heart disease mortality:

(Continued)

TABLE 1 Epidemiologic Studies of Vitamin Intake on Relative Risks for Cardiac Events

Study and year	Population	Follow-up	Category	Outcome	Multivariate relative risk (95% CI) highest vs. lowest category
(26) 1996	elderly women aged 60–101 yr		quartiles) Serum: VitC (mg/dL): 0.91 vs. 1.56; VitE (mg/dL): 0.94 vs. 1.72; Carotenoids (µg/dL): 93 vs. 168; Total intake VitC: 90 vs. 388; VitE: 2.6 vs. 35.1; Carotenoids: 1128 vs. 8582		VitC: 0.53 (0.27–1.06); P for trend 0.07; Carotenoids: 0.91 (0.42–1.99); P for trend 0.68; VitE: 1.51 (0.68–3.37); P for trend 0.15; Intake—heart disease mortality. VitC: 0.38 (0.19–0.75); P for trend 0.22; Carotenoids: 0.64 (0.33–1.27); P for trend 0.14; VitE: 0.75 (0.41–1.39); P for trend 0.40
Kushi et al. (27) 1996	34,486 Iowa postmenopausal women, age 55–69 yr	7 yr	Total intake (and dietary intake): VitA (IU/day) <7264 (≤6207); 7265–10748 (6208–8774); 10749–14572 (8775–11965); 14573–20332 (11966–16755); ≥20333 (≥16756) Carotenoid (IU/day) ≤4421 (≤4349); 4422–6087 (4350–5959); 6088–8856 (5960–8455); 8857–13464 (8456–13026); ≥13465 (≥13027) VitE (IU/day) <5.68 (<4.91); 5.69–7.82 (4.92–6.24); 7.83–12.18 (6.25–7.62); 12.19–35.58 (7.63–9.63); ≥35.59 (≥9.64) VitC (mg/day) ≤112.3 (≤87.3); 112.4–161.3 (87.4–120.5); 161.4–226.7 (120.6–151.7); 226.8–391.2 (151.8–196.2); ≥391.3 (≥196.3)	242 incident coronary deaths	CHD death Total intake: VitA: 1.22 (0.76–1.96); P for trend 0.89; Carotenoids: 1.03 (0.63–1.70); P for trend 0.71; VitE: 0.96 (0.62–1.51); P for trend 0.27; VitC: 1.49 (0.96–2.30); P for trend 0.2; Dietary intake: VitA: 1.25 (0.68–2.31); P for trend 0.83; Carotenoids: 1.19 (0.67–2.12); P for trend 0.89; VitE: 0.38 (0.18–0.80); P for trend 0.004; VitC: 1.43 (0.75–2.70); P for trend 0.47; Supplement VitA: 1.29 (0.70–2.39); P for trend 0.22; VitE: 1.09 (0.67–1.77); P for trend 0.39; VitC: 0.74 (0.30–1.83); P for trend 0.60
Nyyssonen. et al. (28) 1997	1605 men without symptomatic CHD or ischemia	Mean 5 yr	SAA (µmol/L): <11.4; 11.4–32.9; 33.0–49.9; 50.0–64.8; >64.8	70 men fatal or nonfatal MI	MI death Highest: 1.00; lowest: 2.08 (0.82–5.3)
Rimm et al. (26) 1998	80,082 female U.S. nurses, no previous history of CVD, cancer, DM or hypercholesterolemia	14 yr	Median folate intake (µg/L) 158; 217; 276; 393; 696; Median $VitB_6$ (mg/day) 1.1; 1.3; 1.7; 2.7; 4.6	658 cases of nonfatal MI and 281 coronary deaths	CHD Folate: 0.69 (0.55–0.87); P for trend 0.003; VitB6: 0.67 (0.53–0.85); P for trend 0.002

Study	Subjects	Duration	Exposure	Endpoints	Results
Klipstein-Grobusch et al. (30) 1999	4802 residents in the Netherlands, age 55–95 yr	3–7 yr	Dietary β-carotene (mg/day) <1.13; 1.13–1.57; >1.57; Dietary VitE (mg/day) <10.2; 10.2–14.2; >14.2; Dietary VitC (mg/day) <87, 87–126; >126	24 MI	MI β-carotene: 0.55 (0.34–0.83), P for trend 0.013; VitE: 1.21 (0.75–1.98); P for trend 0.528; VitC: 1.05 (0.65–1.67); P for trend 0.856
Loria et al. (31) 2000	3347 men and 3724 women	12–16 yr	SAA (μmol/L): Men: <28.4; 28.4–51.0; 51.1–73.7; ≥73.8; Women: <39.7; 39.7–68; 68.1–85.1; ≥85.2	791 men and 566 women died of CVD, cancer	CVD mortality: Men: highest quartile: 1.00; lowest quartile: 1.45 (0.90–2.32); P for trend 0.84; Women: highest quartile: 1.00; lowest quartile: 0.93 (0.57–1.53); P for trend 0.32
Simon et al. (32) 2001	8417 subjects age 30–75yr	Mean 14 yr	SAA (mg/dL) ≤0.4; 0.5–1.0; 1.1–2.7	561 CVD death	CVD death: 0.76 (0.54–1.06); P for trend 0.11
Mezzetti et al. (33) 2001	102 apparently healthy subjects age ≥80	47.4 mo	Serum VitE (μmol/L) <23; 23–30.6; 30.7–43.9; >43.9; VitC (μmol/L) <20.7; 20.7–24.8; 24.9–30.4; >30.4; β-carotene (μmol/L); <0.37; 0.37–0.47; 0.48–0.69; >0.69	32 CVD events	Cardiac event VitE: 0.10 (0.03–0.38); P for trend <0.000; VitC: 0.46 (0.13–1.63); ns; β-carotene: 0.73 (0.24–2.20); ns
Khaw et al. (34) 2001	19,496 men and women aged 45–79yr	4 yr	Mean SAA (μmol/L) Men: 20.8; 38.1; 48.1; 56.8; 72.6; Women: 30.3; 49.5; 59.1; 67.8; 85.1	180 died of CVD, 123 died of IHD	Men CVD mortality: 0.64 (0.51–0.78); P = 0.0001; IHD mortality: 0.63 (0.42–0.94); P = 0.022; Women CVD mortality: 0.81 (0.62–1.06); P = 0.13; IHD mortality: 0.56 (0.36–0.87); P = 0.009
Osganian et al. (35) 2003	85,118 female nurses	16yr	Total VitC intake (mg/day): ≤93; 94–132; 133–183; 184–359; ≥360; Dietary VitC intake (mg/day) ≤79; 80–108; 108–135; 135–173; ≥174	1,356 incident CHD	Total intake: CHD: 0.73 (0.57–0.94); P for trend 0.005; Dietary VitC: CHD: 0.86 (0.59–1.26); P for trend 0.52
Osganian et al. (36) 2003	73,286 female nurses	12 yr	Median β-carotene intake (μg/day) 1720; 2633; 3528; 4843; 7639; Median α-carotene intake (μg/day) 209; 341; 456; 711; 1518	998 cases of CAD	Total CAD β-Carotene: 0.74 (0.59, 0.93); P for trend 0.05; α-Carotene: 0.80 (0.65, 0.99); P for trend 0.04
Voutilainen et al. (37) 2004	1027 men aged 46–64yr	7.7 yr	Serum folate (nmol/L) <8.4; 8.4–11.3; >11.3; Serum total homocysteine (μmol/L) <9.55; 9.55–11.26; >11.26	37 definite and 17 possible AMI, 7 typical prolonged chest pain	Acute coronary events Folate: 0.39 (0.18–0.83); P for trend 0.016; Total homocysteine: 1.01 (0.55–1.87); P for trend 0.925

Abbreviations: CHD, coronary heart disease; MI, myocardial infarction; IHD, ischemic heart disease; CVD, cardiovascular disease; CAD, coronary artery disease; VitA, vitamin A; VitE, vitamin E; VitC, vitamin C; VitB$_6$, vitamin B$_6$; SAA, serum ascorbic acid; CABG, coronary artery bypass grafting; DM, diabetes mellitus.

Vitamin C

In some large cohort studies, higher vitamin C categories (i.e., higher dietary or plasma vitamin C levels) are usually associated with lower risk of ischemic heart disease (IHD) events (39) and CVD death (25–45% risk reduction) (31,32). However, after multivariate adjustment for age, gender, smoking, alcohol consumption, physical activities, diabetes, and hypertension, among others, there were no significant associations. In contrast, the European Prospective Investigation of Cancer—Norfolk Study (EPIC-Norfolk) (34) found that serum ascorbic acid (SAA) was inversely related to CVD and IHD mortality across quintiles. Mortality risk in the top quintile was half that in the lowest quintile. In the Kuopio Ischaemic Heart Disease Risk Factor Study, men with SAA below 11.4 μmol/L had a higher incidence of MI (RR 2.5, 95% CI 1.3–5.2, $P = 0.0095$) as against men with higher (SAA) concentrations (28).

In the NHANES I Epidemiologic Follow-Up Study (40), an increased vitamin C intake was associated with lower standardized mortality ratio (SMR) for all-cause and CVD deaths. The inverse relationship was stronger for males than for females (SMR of all CVD for males: 0.58, 95% CI 0.41–0.78; females: 0.75, 95% CI 0.55–0.99). In the Atherosclerosis Risk in Communities Study (ARIC) (38), an inverse relationship between vitamin C intake and average artery wall thickness was observed only among participants above 55 years of age. The average artery wall thickness differences between extreme quintiles of vitamin C intake for men and women aged 55 to 64 years were −0.032 mm ($P = 0.035$) and −0.022 mm ($P = 0.019$), respectively. However, these differences were not observed for men and women aged 45 to 54 years. The Western Electric Study (25) reported that dietary vitamin C was inversely associated with CHD death among nonsmoking men at entry (RR 0.58; P for trend 0.042), but not for current smokers. Similar findings were reported in the NHANES II Study.

Other observational studies reported no inverse association between vitamin C intake and serum levels and CHD mortality (27,41,42). Gale et al. (41) found that vitamin C status, as measured by either intake or SAA, was related to subsequent risk of death from stroke but not from CHD [RR 0.9 (95% CI 0.6–1.3); $P = 0.520$ and 0.8 (95% CI 0.6–1.2); $P = 0.595$, respectively]. In the Iowa Women's Health Study (WHS) (27), no significant associations were observed between vitamin C levels and CHD deaths (RRs were 1.49, 1.43, and 0.74, respectively, for total, diet, or supplementation vitamin C levels). In the Physicians' Health Study Screening Cohort (42), vitamin supplementation was not significantly associated with total CVD [0.88 (95% CI 0.7–1.12); P value 0.29] or CHD mortality [RR 0.86 (95% CI 0.63–1.18); P value 0.34]. In the Sahyoun et al. (26) study, subjects with SAA levels in the middle and high quintiles tended to have a lower overall mortality due to reduced heart disease mortality (RRs were 0.51 and 0.53, respectively; P for trend 0.07).

Vitamin E

In the Nurses' Health Study (22), vitamin E intake was inversely associated with risk of major coronary diseases. Long-term vitamin E supplementation (minimal 100 IU/day and more than two years) resulted in a 41% reduction in risk of major coronary diseases. Losonczy et al. (43) also found that vitamin E supplementation reduced the risk of all-cause and CHD mortality; RR for CHD mortality among subjects with vitamin E supplementation was 0.59 (95% CI 0.37–0.93). In the Health Professionals' Study (21), vitamin E supplementation (≥ 100 IU/day) for two years and above was also inversely related to reduced risk of coronary disease (RR 0.63, 95% CI: 0.47–0.84), compared to subjects not taking a vitamin E supplement. However, in the Iowa WHS (27) and the Physicians' Health Study Screening Cohort (42), no significant associations were observed between vitamin E supplementation and CHD death.

There are a number of other epidemiologic studies reporting beneficial associations of vitamin E intake and lower cardiac events. An inverse association was observed between dietary vitamin E intake and coronary mortality in both men (0.68; P for trend = 0.01) and women (0.35; P for trend <0.01) (23). In the study conducted by Kushi et al. (27), dietary vitamin E was associated with lower CHD death (RR 0.38, 95% CI 0.18–0.80; P for trend 0.004). In ARIC (38), an inverse relationship was reported between artery wall thickness and α-tocopherol intake for women aged 55 to 64 years. After multivariate adjustment and exclusion of subjects on special diets for five years or lesser, the differences of average artery wall thickness between the extreme quintiles for α-tocopherol intake in men and women aged 55 to 64 years were -0.007 mm ($P = 0.13$) and -0.028 mm ($P = 0.033$), respectively. In contrast, the Rotterdam

Study (30) reported no significant association between MI and dietary vitamin E intake (RR 1.21, 95% CI 0.75–1.98; *P* for trend 0.528).

Vitamin Combinations or Multivitamin Use

In the Established Populations for Epidemiologic Studies of the Elderly (43), concurrent use of vitamins E and C was associated with lower RRs: 0.58 of total mortality and 0.47 of CHD mortality. When Stampfer et al. (22) compared different vitamin E supplements, the RRs for CHD were—vitamin E supplement only: 0.41 {0.18–0.93}; multivitamin only: 0.87 {0.69–1.09}; both: 0.50 {0.31–0.83}. In the Cancer Prevention Study II (44), an inverse association was observed between vitamin supplementation and IHD: the RR for the antioxidant combination (15% lower than nonusers) was greater than for vitamin A, E, C only. In contrast, multivitamin use was not correlated with a significant decrease in total CVD or CHD mortality in the Physicians' Health Study (42). In addition, a cohort study in Finland (23) reported no significant association between antioxidant supplement use and coronary mortality (only 3% of the participants took the antioxidant supplement).

Randomized Controlled Clinical Trials

β-Carotene

Several large randomized, controlled clinical trials (45–49) have been conducted to evaluate the effects of β-carotene on cancer, CVD, and all-cause mortality (Table 2). The Physician's Health Study (PHS), the Skin Cancer Prevention Study (SCPS), and the Women's Health Study (WHS) found no evidence of the beneficial effects of β-carotene on CVD and/or cancer mortality.

The PHS (45) and WHS (48) provided 50 mg β-carotene on alternate days of treatment for 12 years (PHS) and 2.1 years (WHS). After 12 years of β-carotene supplementation, there was no effect on incidence of total malignant neoplasm (RR, 0.98; 95% CI, 0.91–1.06), CVD mortality (RR, 0.98; 95% CI, 0.91–1.06), or overall mortality in healthy men. Likewise, there were no effects of β-carotene supplementation in the WHS. Similarly, in the SCPS (46), 50 mg/day of β-carotene taken for 8.2 years did not reduce all-cause mortality (adjusted RR, 1.03; 95% CI, 0.82–1.30) or relative mortality rates due to CVD (adjusted RR, 1.16; 95% CI, 0.82–1.64).

Two studies found adverse effects of β-carotene on risk of cancer and CVD (47,49). In the β-Carotene and Retinol Efficacy Trial (CARET) (47), 50 mg/day of β-carotene was given to 4060 male asbestos workers, and 14,254 male and female current/former smokers for four years; and in the Alpha-Tocopherol-Beta-Carotene Cancer Prevention Study (ATBC) (49), 20 mg/day of β-carotene was given to 29,133 male smokers from Finland for 5.3 years. Both studies reported increased overall mortality (RR, 1.17; 95% CI, 1.03–1.33 in the CARET vs. RR, 1.08; 95% CI, 1.01–1.16 in the ATBC) in the β-carotene group. In addition, incidence of lung cancer was also increased (weighted analysis RR, 1.36; 95% CI, 1.07–1.73) in the CARET (47). Moreover, in a subgroup of ATBC, beta-carotene significantly increased fatal CHD in patients who had experienced a previous MI (multivariate-adjusted RR, 1.75; 95% CI, 1.16–2.64; *P* = 0.007) (66).

A recent meta-analysis of eight randomized trials of β-carotene treatment and seven of vitamin E treatment (each trial had 1000 or more subjects) evaluated the effect of supplementation on event rate. Vitamin E supplementation ranged from 50 to 800 IU daily and β-carotene ranged from 15 to 50 mg/day; follow-up duration was 1.4 to 12 years. There were no beneficial effects on mortality, cardiovascular death, or cerebrovascular events in the vitamin E supplement groups when compared with the control group. As shown in Figure 1, there were significant increases in all-cause mortality (RR, 1.07; 95% CI, 1.02–1.11; *P* = 0.003) and cardiovascular death (RR, 1.1; 95% CI, 1.03–1.17; *P* = 0.003) with β-carotene consumption (67).

Vitamin E

Primary-Prevention Trials

Randomized controlled clinical trials have not demonstrated the beneficial effects of vitamin E for primary prevention of coronary disease. The four major trials (ranging from 3 to 5.3 years) are the Microalbuminuria Cardiovascular Renal Outcomes (MICRO-HOPE) study (55), the Primary Prevention Project (PPP) (53), the Vitamin E Atherosclerosis Prevention Study (VEAPS) (50), and the Alpha-Tocopherol, Beta Carotene Cancer Prevention Study (ATBC) (49) (details of these studies are presented in Table 2).

TABLE 2 Effects of Antioxidant Supplements on Cardiovascular Disease: Summary of Clinical Trials

Primary-prevention trials

Name of trial	Study design	Participants	Intervention	Duration	Main end points and results
VEAPS 2002 (50)	Randomized, placebo-controlled	Men and women ≥ 40 years old with an LDL-cholesterol level - 3.37mmol/L (130 mg/dL)	DL-α-tocopherol: 400 IU/day Placebo	Mean 3 yr	IMT progression rates: Placebo: all subjects (0.0023 ± 0.0007mm/yr); men/women (0.0020 ± 0.0010/ 0.0026 ± 0.0009) Vitamin E: all subjects [0.0040 ± 0.0007mm/yr]; men/women [0.0044 ± 0.0011/0.0036 ± 0.0009] LDL oxidative susceptibility: Vitamin E/Control (61.8 ± 2.9/51.3 ± 2.9 9 minutes)
ATBC 1994 (49)	Double-blind, randomized, placebo controlled, 2 X 2 factorial	29,133 Finland male smokers aged 50-69 yr	α-Tocopherol: 50 mg/day β-Carotene: 20 mg/day both placebo	5-8 yr (median 6.1 yr)	CV events: Vitamin E group vs. placebo: 11 vs. 14 (P = 0.81) All-cause mortality: α-tocopherol RR, 1.02 (0.95-1.09); β-carotene RR,1.08↑ (1.01-1.16); MI: α-tocopherol RR, 1.04 (0.89-1.22), β-carotene RR, 1.06 (0.90-1.24) CVD: α-tocopherol RR, 0.98 (0.87-1.10), β-carotene RR, 1.03 (0.91-1.16) CVD Mortality: α-tocopherol RR, 0.90 (0.75-1.08), β-carotene RR, 0.99 (0.83-1.19)],
ATBC 1998 (51)		27,271 Finnish male smokers aged 50-69yr			Incident strokes: Subarachnoid hemorrhage: α-tocopherol RR, 1.50 (0.97-0.32) Cerebral infarction: α-tocopherol RR, 0.86 (0.75-0.99) Intracerebral hemorrhage: β-carotene RR, 1.62 (1.10-2.36)
ATBC 2000 (52)		28,519 Finnish male smokers aged 50-69yr		Same as above	Stroke mortality: Subarachnoid hemorrhage: α-tocopherol RR, 2.81 (1.37-5.79) Cerebral infarction: α-tocopherol RR, 0.81 (0.49-1.32)
CARET 1996 (47)	Randomized, double-blinded, placebo-controlled, multicenter	18,314 smokers, former smokers, and asbestos workers	30 mg β-Carotene + 25,000 IU retinol; placebo	5.5	All cause mortality: RR, 1.17 (1.03-1.33) CVD mortality: RR, 1.26 (0.99-1.61)
SCPS 1996 (46)	Randomized, controlled	1720 patients with skin cancer	50 mg β-carotene	8.2	All cause mortality: RR, 1.03 (0.82-1.30) CVD mortality: RR, 1.16 (0.82-1.64)
PHS 1996 (45)	Randomized, double-blinded, placebo-controlled	22,071 male healthy physicians	50 mg β-carotene on alternate days; placebo	12	CVD mortality: RR, 1.09 (0.93-1.27) CVD: RR, 1.00 (0.91-1.09) MI: RR, 0.96 (0.84-1.09)
PPP 2001 (53)	Randomized, controlled, open 2 × 2 factorial	4495 people at high risk of CVD	Aspirin: 100 mg/day No aspirin Vitamin E synthetic: 300mg/day No Vitamin E	3.6yr	CV death, nonfatal MI, and nonfatal stroke: Vitamin E RR, 1.07 (0.74-1.56) CVD mortality: Aspirin RR, 0.56 (0.31-0.99), Vitamin E RR, 0.86 (0.49-1.52) Non-fatal MI: Aspirin RR, 0.69 (0.38-1.23), Vitamin E RR, 1.01 (0.56-2.03) Non-fatal stroke: Aspirin RR, 0.84 (0.42-1.67),

Study	Design	Patients	Intervention/Dose	Duration	Results
ASAP 2000 (54)	Randomized, placebo-controlled, double-masked, 2 × 2 factorial	520 smoking and nonsmoking men and postmenopausal women aged 45–69 yr with serum cholesterol ≥ 5.0 mmol/L	RRR-AT: 136 IU twice a day Ascorbate: 250 mg twice a day both placebo	3 yr	Vitamin E RR, 1.56 (0.77–3.13) Peripheral-artery disease: Aspirin RR, 0.60 (0.33-1.08), Vitamin E RR, 0.54 (0.30–0.99) Average increase of the mean (common carotid artery mean intima-media thickness): Placebo: men/women (0.020/0.016 mm/yr) Vitamin E: men/women (0.018/0.015 mm/yr) Vitamin C: men/women (0.017/0.017 mm/yr) Vitamin C+E: men/women (0.011/0.016 mm/yr) ($P = 0.043$)
MICRO-HOPE 2002 (55)	Randomized, placebo-controlled, 2 × 2 factorial, multicenter	3654 patients with diabetes	Vitamin E (natural): 400 IU/day ramipril Vitamin E + Ramipril placebo	4.5 yr	A composite of MI, stroke, or CV death: RR, 1.03 (0.88-1.21) MI:RR, 1.01 (0.83–1.22) Stroke: RR, 1.21 (0.91–1.62) CV death:RR, 0.97 (0.77–1.23)
Secondary-prevention trials					
CHAOS 1996 (56)	Randomized, double blinded, placebo-controlled	2002 patients with angiographically proven coronary atherosclerosis	α-tocopherol: 800 IU/day or 400 IU/day placebo	510 day	Combination of CV death and nonfatal MI: RR, 0.53 [0.34–0.83] ($P = 0.005$) Nonfatal MI: RR, 0.23 [0.11–0.47] ($P = 0.005$) CV deaths: RR, 1.18 (0.62–2.27) ($P = 0.61$)
SPACE 2000 (57)	Randomized, placebo-controlled, multicenter	196 haemodialysis patients with pre-existing CVD aged 40–75 years yr	Vitamin E: 800 IU/day placebo	519 day	Composite CVD endpoints: Including sudden death: RR, 0.54 (0.33–0.89) ($P = 0.016$) Excluding sudden death: RR, 0.46 (0.27–0.78) ($P = 0.014$) MI: Including sudden death: RR,0.45 (0.20–0.99) ($P = 0.04$) Excluding sudden death: RR, 0.30 (0.10–0.80) ($P = 0.016$)
ATBC 1998 (58)	Randomized, placebo-controlled, 2 × 2 factorial	1795 male smokers aged 50–69 yr who had angina pectoris in the Rose chest pain questionnaire at baseline	Vitamin E: 50 IU/day β-Carotene: 20 mg/day both placebo	4 yr	Recurrences of angina pectoris: 2513 recurrences; Vitamin E RR, 1.06 (0.85–1.33); Vitamin E+ β-carotene RR, 1.02 (0.82–1.27); β-carotene RR, 1.06 (0.84–1.33)
ATBC 1997 (59)	Randomized, placebo-controlled, 2 × 2 factorial	1862 smokers with previous MI	Vitamin E: 50 IU/day β-Carotene: 20 mg/day both placebo	5.3 yr	Nonfatal MI: Vitamin E group RR, 0.62 (0.41–0.96) Fatal coronary heart disease: Vitamin E group: RR, 1.33 (0.86–2.05); vitamin E+ β-carotene group: RR, 1.58 (1.05–2.4); β-carotene group: RR, 1.75 (1.16–2.64)
GISSI 1999 (60)	Randomized, controlled, open-label, multicenter	11,324 patients with recent MI	Synthetic α-tocopherol: 300 mg/day N-3 PUFA: 1g/day Both None	3.5 yr	Death, non-fatal MI, and non-fatal stroke: Two way analysis: vitamin E/n-3 PUFA RR, 0.95 (0.86–1.05)/0.90 (0.82–0.99) Four way analysis: vitamin E/n-3 PUFA RR, 0.89 (0.77–1.03)/0.85 (0.74–0.98) vitamin E+n-3 PUFA RR, 0.86 (0.74–0.99) Cardiovascular death, non-fatal MI, and non-fatal stroke: Two way analysis: vitamin E/n-3 PUFA RR, 0.98 (0.87–1.10)/0.89 (0.80–1.01) Four way analysis: vitamin E/n-3 PUFA RR, 0.88 (0.75–1.04)/0.80 (0.68–0.95) vitamin E+n-3 PUFA RR, 0.88 (0.75–1.03)

(Continued)

TABLE 2 Effects of Antioxidant Supplements on Cardiovascular Disease: Summary of Clinical Trials

Name of trial	Study design	Participants	Intervention	Duration	Main end points and results
HATS 2001 (61)	Randomized, double-blind, controlled	160 patients with CVD, normal LDL-C and low HDL-C	Antioxidants: 800 IU/day vitamin E (D-α-tocopherol) + 1000 mg/day vitamin C+ 25 mg/day natural β-carotene + 100 µg/day selenium; antioxidant + simvastatin + niacin; Simvastatin + niacin; placebo	3.5 yr	Coronary stenosis progress: Placebo: 3.9%; simvastatin+niacin: 0.4%; antioxidant + simvastatin + niacin: 0.7%; antioxidants: 1.8% Frequency of the clinical end point (first cardiovascular event): Placebo: 24%; simvastatin + niacin: 3%; antioxidant + simvastatin + niacin: 14%; Antioxidants: 21%
WAVE 2002 (62)	Randomized, placebo-controlled, double-blind, 2 × 2 factorial, multicenter	423 postmenopausal women with CVD	HRT; Matching placebo; 400 IU vitamin E + 500 mg of vitamin C twice daily; HRT + vitamins; placebo	2.8	All cause mortality: HRT+vitamins group vs. vitamin placebo: HR, 2.8 (1.1–7.2) ($P = 0.047$)
IVUS 2002 (63)	Randomized, double-blind, controlled	40 patients after cardiac transplantation	500 mg vitamin C + 400 IU vitamin E, twice daily; placebo	1 yr	Intimal index: Treatment group: no change; placebo group: increase by 8% ($P = 0.008$)
Primary and secondary prevention trials					
HOPE 2000 (64)	Randomized, placebo-controlled, 2 × 2 factorial, multicenter	2545 women and 6996 men 55 years of age or older and at high risk of CVD	Vitamin E (natural): 400 IU/day ramipril vitamin E + ramipril placebo	4.5 yr	A composite of MI, stroke, or CV death: RR, 1.05 (0.95-1.16) MI: RR, 1.02 (0.90-1.15) Stroke: RR, 1.17 (0.95-1.42) CV death: RR, 1.05 (0.90-1.22)
HPS 2002 (65)	Randomized, placebo-controlled, 2 × 2 factorial, multicenter	20,536 U.K. adults (aged 40–80) with coronary disease, other occlusive arterial disease, or diabetes	Vitamin E: 600 IU/day + Vitamin C 250 mg/day + β-carotene Carotene:25 mg/day placebo	5 yr	Coronary cause of death: RR, 1.06 [0.95–1.18] Major coronary event: RR, 1.02 (0.94–1.11) Any major vascular event: RR, 1.00 (0.94–1.06) Any stroke: 0.99 (0.87–1.12)

Abbreviations: CCA-IMT, common carotid artery mean intima-media thickness; ASAP, Antioxidant Supplementation in Atherosclerocis Prevention study; ATBC, Alpha-Tocopherol-Beta-Carotene Cancer Prevention Study; CARET, Carotene and Retinol Efficacy Trial; IMT, intima-media thickness; CHAOS, Cambridge Heart AntiOxidant Study; CV, Cardiovascular; CVD, Cardiovascular disease; GISSI, Gruppo Italiano per lo Studio della Sopravvivenza nell' Infarto miocardico-prevenzione study; HATS, HDL-atherosclerosis Treatment Study; HDL, high-density lipoprotein; HPS, Heart Protection Study; IVUS, Intravacular Ultrasonography Study; LDL, low-density lipoprotein; MI, myocardial infarction; MICRO-HOPE, Microalbuminuria Cardiovascular Renal Outcomes Heart Outcomes Prevention Evaluation Trial; PHS, Physician's Health Study; PPP, Primary Prevention Project; PUFA, Polyunsaturated fatty acids; SCPS, Skin Cancer Prevention Study; VEAPS, Vitamin E Atherosclerosis Prevention Study; WAVE, Women's Angiographic Vitamin and Estrogen Study; RRR-AT, RRR-alpha tocopherol.

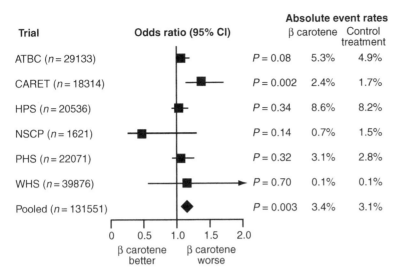

Breslow-Day test: *P* = 0.12

FIGURE 1   Odds ratios (95% CI) of cardiovascular death for individuals treated with beta-carotene or control therapy. *Abbreviations*: ATBC, Alpha-Tocopherol-Beta-Carotene Cancer Prevention Study; HPS, Heart Protection Study; PHS, Physician's Health Study; WHS, Women's Health Study. *Source*: From Ref. 67.

Vitamin E supplementation (400 IU/day of DL-α-tocopherol) in the VEAPS study did not affect the progression of intima-media thickness (IMT). The MICRO-HOPE study and the PPP study reported no significant differences in cardiovascular death, MI, and stroke in the vitamin E groups except for a beneficial effect (RR, 0.54; 95% CI, 0.30–0.99) of vitamin E supplementations in subjects with peripheral artery disease (in the PPP study). Of note is that vitamin E supplements increased the incidence of hemorrhagic stroke (66 subjects in vitamin E group vs. 44 subjects in the control group) and ischemic stoke in the ATBC study (49).

Collectively, vitamin E supplementation does not beneficially affect cardiovascular events. However, there is some evidence of a beneficial effect on markers of CVD risk, i.e., lowered oxidation of LDL (50). In contrast, there is some evidence that relatively small doses of vitamin E (50 IU/day) given over 5.3 years increase risk of hemorrhagic and ischemic stroke (49).

Secondary Prevention Trials
Several major secondary-prevention trials (60,64,65) have not demonstrated benefits of vitamin E supplements on CVD (Table 2). Subjects (*n* = 11,324) in the Gruppo Italiano per lo Studio della Sopravvivenza nell'Infarto miocardico (GISSI) (60) were given 300 mg of synthetic α-tocopherol/day for 3.5 years. In the HOPE Study (64), 2545 women and 6996 men were given 400 IU/day of vitamin E. These large studies with thousands of subjects provide compelling evidence-for not recommending vitamin E supplementation for secondary prevention of CVD despite some evidence of beneficial effect.

Several secondary-prevention trials (56,57,59,66) have reported effect of vitamin E supplementation on cardiovascular events (Table 2). The Cambridge Heart Antioxidant Study (CHAOS) (56) reported that vitamin E supplementation reduced risk by 77% (95% CI, −89 to −53%; *P* = 0.005) and 47% (95% CI, −66 to −17%; *P* = 0.005) for MI and all cardiovascular events (including nonfatal MI and cardiovascular death) in patients with established coronary artery disease. Similarly, in the Secondary Prevention with Antioxidants of Cardiovascular disease in End-stage renal disease (SPACE) Study, the vitamin E supplementation in 196 hemodialysis patients with-history of CVD resulted in a 64% significant reduction (RR, 0.46; 95% CI, 0.27–0.78; *P* = 0.014) in the composite CVD endpoint (fatal and nonfatal MI, ischemic stroke, peripheral vascular disease, and unstable angina). In the ATBC Study (59) of 1862 men with a previous MI, there was a significant reduction in nonfatal MI (38%; 95% CI, −4 to −59%) although no effects were shown for fatal coronary end points. Likewise, a subsequent report

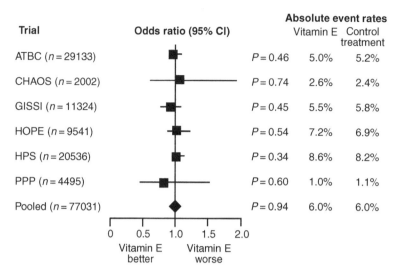

FIGURE 2 Odds ratios (95% CI) of cardiovascular; death for individuals treated with vitamin E or control therapy. Abbreviations: ATBC, Alpha-Tocopherol-Beta-Carotena Cancer Prevention study; HPS, Heart Protection Study; CHAOS, Cambridge Heart AntiOxidant Study; PPP, Primary Prevention Project; HOPE, Heart Outcomes Prevention Evaluation Trial. *Source:* From Ref. 67.

(66), which examined the effect of antioxidants on the incidence of angina pectoris, reported a 9% (95% CI, −1 to −17%; $P = 0.04$) reduction in the vitamin E supplement group.

Summary of Primary and Secondary Prevention Studies

Meta-analysis (67) or reviews of the literature (68,69) have also summarized the effects of vitamin E on CVD. In the meta-analysis conducted by Vivekananthan et al. (67), of 81,788 patients in two primary prevention and five secondary prevention trials, cardiovascular mortality in the vitamin E group (RR, 1.0; 95% CI, 0.94–1.06; $P = 0.94$) was not significantly decreased compared with the control group (Fig. 2). Of note is that although CHAOS demonstrated some favorable effects, there were no benefits on cardiovascular death. No improvements were associated with vitamin E treatment for all-cause mortality when primary (RR, 1.02; 95% CI, 0.97–1.06) and secondary (RR, 1.06; 95% CI, 0.93–1.25) prevention trials were analyzed separately. Similarly, reviews of randomized controlled trials (RCTs) did not show beneficial effects of vitamin E on cardiovascular mortality, and nonfatal MI (68,69). The Agency for Healthcare Research and Quality (AHRQ) report (70) reported that there is little evidence that vitamin E supplementation reduces cardiovascular mortality. In addition, pooled analyses showed no beneficial or adverse effect of vitamin E supplementation on risk of fatal and nonfatal MI.

Antioxidant Vitamin Combinations

Vitamin E and Vitamin C Supplements

Several clinical trials (54,62,63) have been conducted to evaluate the combination of vitamin E and C on CVD risk or risk factors. These trials used α-tocopherol 272 IU/day or 800 IU/day plus 500 or 1000 mg/day of vitamin C with study durations ranging from one to three years. The Antioxidant Supplementation in Atherosclerosis Prevention (ASAP) Study reported a 74% (95% CI, −36 to −89%; $P = 0.003$) reduction in atherosclerosis progression in men only in response to consumption of vitamin E and C together (54), while a study using intravascular ultrasonography (IVUS) found no significant increase in the intimal index (0.8%) in the vitamin E and C treatment group of cardiac transplanet patients (63). Although these two studies provided evidence of beneficial effects, the Women's Angiographic Vitamin and Estrogen (WAVE) Trial (62) reported an increase in all-cause mortality (HR, 2.8; 95% CI, 1.1–7.2) as a result of these two antioxidants.

Antioxidant Cocktails

The Heart Protection Study (HPS) (65) and the HDL-Atherosclerosis Treatment Study (HATS) (61) used three antioxidant vitamins (vitamin E, vitamin C, β-carotene, and Selenium) in combination to assess the effects on CVD. There was no effect on all-cause mortality (RR, 1.04; 95% CI, 0.97–1.12) and CVD mortality (RR, 1.05; 95% CI, 0.95–1.15) in the supplement group (600 mg/day of vitamin E, 250 mg/day of vitamin C, and 20 mg/day of β-carotene) in the HPS study. In the HATS study, the average stenosis progression in the antioxidant-alone group (800 IU/day of RRR-α-tocopherol, 1000 mg/day of vitamin C, 25 mg/day of β-carotene, and 100 μg/day of selenium) and the placebo group was not significantly different (1.8% vs. 3.9%, $P = 0.16$). (see Section "Niacin.")

B VITAMINS

In 1975, McCully and Wilson (71) introduced the homocysteine theory to explain, in part, the pathogenesis of arteriosclerosis. Many subsequent studies have reported that elevated homocysteine levels are associated with an increased risk of coronary atherosclerosis, cerebrovascular disease, peripheral vascular disease, and thrombosis (72,73). The evidence to explain the mechanisms of action includes endothelial damage resulting in impaired endothelial-dependent vasoreactivity and decreased endothelium thromboresistance (74). There is also evidence that vascular smooth muscle cell proliferation is stimulated in hyperhomocysteinemia (74).

In the Physicians' Health Study (75), subjects with higher levels of homocysteine were found to be at higher risk for an MI; a threefold increase in MI risk was found for homocysteine levels 12% above the upper normal range. Likewise, in a recent multicenter study (76), subjects in the highest quartile for homocysteine had an RR of 2.2 (95% CI, 1.6–2.9) compared with the rest of the population. A meta-analysis of observational studies (77) reported an odds ratio (OR) of 1.6 (95% CI, 1.4–1.7) for men and 1.8 (95% CI, 1.3–1.9) for women to coronary artery disease (CAD) for 5 μmol/L increase in fasting total homocysteine levels. Similarly, a recent review (78) reported that the OR for CHD was 1.06 (95% CI, 0.99–1.13) for two cohort studies and 1.7 (95% CI, 1.50–1.93) for 26 case-control studies for a 5 μmol/L increase in total homocysteine (tHcy).

An American Heart Association Science Advisory (73) recommends screening for homocysteine in high-risk patients (with strong family history of premature atherosclerosis, arterial occlusive diseases, or renal failure). However, routine screening for homocysteine is not recommended in the general population because of the inconsistent results from prospective studies, but for CHD patients without CHD risk factors as well as asymptomatic patients with a strong family history of premature CHD, homocysteine levels should be assessed (79,80).

Evidence for Lowering Homocysteine Level with B Vitamins

Folic Acid

A marked inverse relationship between folate status and plasma homocysteine concentration was reported in the Hordaland Homocysteine study (81). A meta-analysis (82) of 12 RCTs showed that supplements of 0.5–5.0 mg/day of folic acid significantly reduced tHcy by 25% (95% CI, 23–28%); adding 0.5 mg/day of vitamin B_{12} resulted in a further 7% (3–10%) reduction in blood homocysteine. There was no difference in the lowering of homocysteine within the range of 0.5 to 5.0 mg/day of folic acid. Patients with CVD may require more folate than is recommended for the general population to achieve normal homocysteine levels. In a randomized controlled trial conducted by Wald et al. (83), 151 patients with IHD were randomized to one of five doses of folic acid (0.2, 0.4, 0.6, 0.8, and 1.0 mg/day) for three months. In this study, 0.8 mg/day of folic acid was needed to maximally reduce serum homocysteine. The Recommended Dietary Allowance (RDA) of folate for healthy men and women 19 years of age and older, is 400 μg/day.

Based on a case-cohort study of 36,000 Dutch adults who did not have CVD at baseline (with a mean follow-up of 10.3 years) (84), the RR for the highest tertile of plasma folate concentration (9.5 nmol/L in women) versus the lowest tertile (6.1 nmol/L in women) was 0.22 (95% CI, 0.06–0.87) for fatal CHD. This study demonstrated the inverse association between a higher plasma folate concentration and the risk of CHD mortality in women but not in men. He et al. (85) found that subjects in the highest quintile of folate intake (936 μg/day) had a lower risk of ischemic stroke than those in the lowest quintile (237 μg/day) (RR, 0.68; 95% CI, 0.50–0.92; $p = 0.03$).

However, the same association was not found between folate intake and hemorrhagic stroke. Furthermore, vitamin B_{12}, but not vitamin B_6, intake had a similar effect.

Vitamin B_{12}

A meta-analysis (82) reported that vitamin B_{12} further reduced homocysteine levels in subjects who had been given a folic acid supplement. A mean intake of 0.5 mg/day of vitamin B_{12} resulted in an additional 7% reduction in homocysteine levels, in subjects who had also been given 0.5 to 5 mg/day of folic acid. Likewise, a recent cross-sectional analysis (86) of 140 elderly subjects reported that adequate folate and vitamin B_{12} synergistically decreased homocysteine levels.

Mann et al. (87) examined the effect of omnivorous and vegetarian diets on folate and vitamin B_{12} status on homocysteine concentration in 139 healthy men. In this study, vegetarians had lower plasma vitamin B_{12} and higher homocysteine levels compared with nonvegetarians. Consequently, vegetarians and the elderly (many of whom have a compromised vitamin B_{12} status), in general, require supplemental vitamin B_{12} to prevent hyperhomocysteinemia.

Vitamin B_6

A question has been raised about the effect that vitamin B_6 has on homocysteine levels compared to folic acid and vitamin B_{12}. In a meta-analysis (the Homocysteine Lowering Trialists' Collaboration), vitamin B_6 did not affect homocysteine levels, perhaps because the effect is masked by the greater effects of folic acid and vitamin B_{12} (82). In a recent randomized trial, healthy elderly subjects were given 1.6 mg/day of vitamin B_6 in conjunction with a folic acid supplement (400 µg/day) for six weeks. Supplementation with vitamin B_6 resulted in an additional 7.5% reduction ($p = 0.008$) in homocysteine levels beyond that observed for the folic acid supplement (which reduced homocysteine levels by 19.6%; $p < 0.001$) (88). It also has been reported that a low level (<20 nmol/L) of vitamin B_6 (OR, 4.6; 95% CI, 1.4–15.1; $P < 0.001$) rather than elevated homocysteine (OR, 0.92; 95% CI, 0.4–2.1) was strongly associated with the risk of stroke and transient ischemic attack (TIA) in a folate-repleted population (89). Kelly et al. (90) found a strong inverse relationship between blood levels of vitamin B_6 status and increased quartiles of C-reactive protein (CRP) distribution both in case (new ischemic stroke) and in control cohorts ($P = 0.001$ for each cohort).

Randomized Controlled Clinical Trials of B Vitamin Supplements

Despite the compelling evidence that B vitamins (folate, vitamin B_{12}, and/or vitamin B_6) lower tHcy, it is unclear whether decreasing tHcy levels with B vitamin supplements reduces cardiovascular morbidity and/or mortality. In the Vitamin Intervention for Stroke Prevention Study (VISP) (91), 3680 adults with nondisabling cerebral infarction were randomly assigned to receive a high-dose formulation of B vitamins (25 mg/day of pyridoxine, 0.4 mg/day of cobalamin, and 2.5 mg/day of folic acid) or a low-dose formulation (200 µg/day of pyridoxine, 6 µg/day of cobalamin and 20 µg/day of folic acid) for two years. There was a greater reduction of homocysteine, by 2 µmol/L, in the high-dose group than in the low-dose group; however, B vitamin therapy did not affect stroke, CHD events, or death.

In the Swiss Heart Study (92), 553 patients who had undergone successful angioplasty were randomized to receive 1 mg/day of folic acid, 400 µg/day of cyanocobalamin, and 10 mg/day of pyridoxine hydrochloride or placebo for six months. The composite endpoint of major adverse events including death, nonfatal MI, and need for repeat revascularization was significantly lower in patients on the B vitamin supplements (15.4% vs. 22.8%; RR, 0.68; 95% CI, 0.48–0.96; $P = 0.03$).

Liem et al. (93) studied the effect of folic acid supplementation in a secondary prevention study of patients with existing CAD. Subjects ($n = 300$) were randomly assigned to 0.5 mg/day folic acid for a 24-month follow-up. The RR for all-cause mortality and a composite of vascular events was 1.05 (95% CI: 0.63–1.75) for the folic acid supplementation group, which indicated no treatment effect on recurrent events.

Niacin

Numerous studies have shown that niacin (nicotinic acid) in gram doses increases high density lipoprotein cholesterol (HDL-C) and decreases triglycerides (TG), LDL-cholesterol (LDL-C), and lipoprotein (a) [Lp(a)] (94–100). Studies in both healthy subjects with hyperlipidemia

(97–100) and patients with Type-2 diabetes with dyslipidemia (101) have shown that 500 to 3000 mg/day of extended-release niacin is generally well tolerated and has a dose-related effect on the lipid profile [LDL-C was significantly decreased 6% and 14% while HDL-C was increased 17% and 23% by 1000 and 2000 mg/day, respectively (99); TG was decreased more as the dosage of extended release-niacin increased: 5% at 500 mg/day; 11% at 1000 mg/day, and 44% at 3000 mg/day (97)]. Greater lipid effects have been noted in some studies. For example, a 21% reduction in LDL-C levels has been reported by Goldberg et al. (97) and other investigators (98–100) with niacin alone. Goldberg et al. (97) also reported that 1 to 3 g/day of extended release-niacin can increase HDL-C levels by 30%. Capuzzi et al. (100) reported that niacin can decrease Lp(a) by as much as 40%. Backes and Gibson (102) demonstrated that niacin decreases small, dense LDL, especially in patients with mixed dyslipidemia or hypertriglyceridemia. The mechanism by which niacin exerts its effects on TG levels involves an inhibition of hepatic production of very-low-density lipoprotein (VLDL) (103). The increase in HDL-C is due to a decrease in HDL degradation (104).

Given that niacin significantly increases HDL-C, and decreases TG and Lp(a) levels, it is often prescribed with a statin for patients with low HDL-C and high LDL-C levels. There is a noted benefit of a combination of niacin and statin therapy on the lipid and lipoprotein profile; specifically, there is an improvement in TG-lowering and HDL-raising effects in combination therapy compared with statin monotherapy, which results only in a clinically significant LDL-C lowering effect (105).

The combination concept has been extended to include the addition of various antioxidant supplements. In a study conducted by Brown et al. (61) on 160 patients with CAD including 25 with diabetes mellitus, simvastatin (10–20 mg/day) plus niacin (1 g BID as tolerated) significantly decreased plasma cholesterol, TG, VLDL-C, LDL-C, and apo B by 25% to 57% and increased apo A-I and HDL_2 levels from 107 ± 15 to 128 ± 24 mg/dL and from 3.9 ± 1.7 to 6.6 ± 4.1 mg/dL, respectively (61,106). However, when an antioxidant cocktail (β-carotene 12.5 mg BID, vitamin C 500 mg BID, vitamin E 400 IU BID, and selenium 50 μg BID) was added to this pharmacologic treatment regimen, the beneficial effects on HDL were attenuated. The increases in HDL-C and HDL_2 were greater in the simvastatin + niacin group (25% and 42%, respectively) versus the simvastatin + niacin + antioxidant cocktail group (18% and 0%, respectively). Brown et al. (107) have shown that this may be due to a down-regulation of apoA-I, ATP binding cassette transmembrane transporter A1, and lecithin-cholesterol acyltransferase (LCAT) genes.

Clinical studies have also been conducted to evaluate the effects of niacin, either alone or combined with statin drugs, on CHD outcomes. The Coronary Drug Project evaluated the long-term efficacy and safety of lipid-influencing drugs (niacin is one of those) in 8341 men with previous MI. For patients with niacin therapy, recurrent nonfatal coronary events were decreased by 27% and cerebrovascular end points (strokes or TIA) by 24%; there was no reduction in total mortality (108). Nine years after conclusion of the study, all-cause mortality was 11% lower in the niacin group than in the placebo group ($p = 0.0004$) (109). The HATS study evaluated the relationship between changing lipids and lipoproteins and CHD outcomes (61). Simvastatin/niacin was the only treatment group that produced a regression in stenosis (by 0.4%; $P < 0.001$). Of note was that inclusion of the antioxidant cocktail with the drug regimen blunted the benefits of simvastatin/niacin treatment. Stenosis progressed by 3.9% in the placebo group, by 1.8% in the antioxidant cocktail group ($P = 0.16$ vs. the placebo group), and by 0.7% with simvastatin/niacin plus antioxidants ($P = 0.004$). In the simvastatin/niacin group there was 0.4 percent regression in stenosis ($P < 0.001$).

The RDAs for the antioxidant vitamins (vitamin A, vitamin C, and vitamin E) and B vitamins (vitamin B_6, vitamin B_{12}, folate, and niacin) are shown in Table 3. The Tolerable Upper Intake Levels (UL) and adverse effects are also reported. Dietary intake of selected vitamins for the U.S. population during 1999–2000 indicated that Americans' vitamin intake met most of the RDAs in the age group of 19 to 50; however, folate (male 60 years and above and female 19 years and above), vitamin B_6 (male 60 years and above), and vitamin E (all age groups) intakes were less than the amounts in RDA (129).

The UL for niacin is 35 mg/day, whereas of note is that the dose needed to achieve an HDL-C-raising effect is about 1 to 3 g. Typically, niacin is given as a prescription drug [immediate release nicotinic acid, extended nicotinic acid, and sustained release nicotinic acid (96)]. There are three OTC niacin products (immediate release, sustained release, and "no flush"); the no-flush preparation is the most expensive. Meyers et al. found that the

TABLE 3   Recommended Dietary Allowance (RDA) and Tolerable Upper Intake Levels for Selected Vitamins for Adults

| | RDA | | | | √UL | Adverse effects, |
| | Male | | Female | | (>19 yr) | |
Vitamins	19–50 yr	>50 yr	19–50 yr	>50 yr		toxicity, or contraindication
Vitamin C[a] (mg/day)	90	90	75	75	2000	Gastrointestinal disturbances; increased oxalate excretion and kidney stone formation; increased uric acid excretion; lower vitamin B_{12} levels. (110–113)
Vitamin E (mg/day)	15	15	15	15	1000	Hemorrhagic toxicity; abdominal pain; diarrhea; marginal signs of scurvy; those people who are taking anticoagulant drug or vitamin K deficiency should be closely monitored. (49,114,115)
Vitamin A (µg/day)	900	900	700	700	3000	Weakness; headache; vomiting; carotenodermia; lycopenodermia; inconsistent results of effects on lung cancer. (116, 117)
Vitamin B_6 (mg/day)	1.3	1.7	1.3	1.5	100	Sensory neuropathy; dermatological lesions. (118, 119)
Vitamin B_{12} (µg/day)	2.4	2.4	2.4	2.4	N/A	Low toxicity; people at risk for Leber's optic atrophy should not be given cyanocobalamin to treat vitamin B_{12} deficiency. (120)
Folate (µg/day)	400	400	400	400	1000	Neurological effects; excess intake may delay the diagnosis of vitamin B_{12} deficiency; mental changes; sleep disturbances; hypersensitivity; adversely effect intestinal zinc absorption. (121–124)
Niacin (mg/day)	16	16	14	14	35	Flushing; nonspecific gastrointestinal effects (especially with slow-release preparations); hepatoxicity; glucose intolerance (3 g/day). (123–126. 125–128)

Note: RDA is the average daily dietary intake level that is sufficient to meet the nutrient requirement of nearly all (97–98%) healthy individuals in a particular life stage and gender group.
[a]Increase by 35 mg for smokers.
Abbreviation: UL, upper intake levels; N/A, not available.

no-flush preparation does not contain free nicotinic acid and is not recommended for the treatment of dyslipidemia (130).

MINERALS

An adequate mineral status is important for the prevention of many chronic diseases such as heart disease, hypertension, metabolic syndrome, and for a normal profile of different biomarkers associated with these conditions.

Calcium

Blood Pressure

Meta-analyses of epidemiologic studies have shown that an increase in dietary calcium is associated with a blood pressure (BP) lowering response (131,132). Systolic blood pressure (SBP) decreased by 0.34 and 0.15 mmHg for each 100 mg/day increase in calcium intake for men and women, respectively. For diastolic blood pressure (DBP), the decrease was 0.22 and 0.051 mmHg for men and women, respectively.

In a meta-analysis of 42 studies (9 dietary and 33 supplement studies), there was a significant reduction in SBP by 1.44 mmHg and in DBP by 0.84 mmHg with an increase of calcium intake of 1 g/day after two weeks of intervention (133). In a comparison of dietary versus supplemental calcium sources, SBP tended to decrease by 2.10 and 1.09 mmHg ($P = 0.14$), respectively; and DBP by 1.09 and 0.87 mmHg ($P = 0.67$), respectively. Collectively, the data show that dietary and supplemental sources of calcium have comparable hypotensive effects.

Data from a cross-sectional study (134) conducted in Spain also supported the combination use of minerals for lowering BP. The results showed that the BP change was related to calcium and sodium intake and to the ratio of sodium to potassium. Controlling sodium intake (below 2400 mg/day) in combination with a calcium intake of more than 800 mg/day reduced BP by 44% in hypertensive patients on hypotensive drug therapy. In addition, BP was decreased by 30% and 52%, with moderate reduction sodium intake (<2400 mg/day) in normotensive and nonmedicated hypertensive subjects.

Magnesium
Blood Pressure
In the ARIC Study (135), Ma et al. assessed the association between dietary/serum magnesium levels and cardiac risk among different population groups. SBP was significantly inversely related to serum magnesium (except for African-American women; correlation coefficients were –0.06 to –0.08, $P \leq 0.01$). However, no significant associations were observed between serum magnesium and DBP levels. Dietary magnesium was inversely associated with both SBP and DBP among women (correlation coefficients were: –0.05 to –0.07, $P \leq 0.01$). Dietary magnesium was only significantly inversely related with DBP among African-American men (correlation coefficient was –0.09, $P \leq 0.01$). In another analysis of data from the ARIC Study (136), BP was inversely related to serum magnesium but not dietary magnesium. Compared with subjects with the lowest quartile serum magnesium (≤ 1.5 meq/L), women in the highest quartile (≥ 1.8 meq/L) had an OR of incident hypertension of 0.7 (P for trend 0.01). No inverse association was found between incident hypertension and either serum or dietary magnesium levels among men. In NHANES III (137), there was no association between magnesium intake and BP.

In a review conducted by Jee et al. (138) of 20 clinical studies, increasing magnesium intake had a very modest BP-lowering effect among hypertensive and normotensive subjects. The median magnesium dose was 15.4 mmol/day with median study intervention duration of 8.5 weeks. Magnesium supplementation resulted in a small reduction in BP. The pooled net estimates of BP change were –0.6 mmHg ($P = 0.051$) for SBP and -0.8 mmHg ($P = 0.142$) for DBP. However, there was an apparent dose-dependent effect of magnesium when limiting the analysis to data from double-blind studies. For each 10 mmol/day magnesium increase, SBP decreased significantly (-4.3 mmHg, $P < 0.001$); however, DBP did not change significantly (-2.3 mmHg, $P = 0.09$).

Glucose Homeostasis
Dietary magnesium is positively related to glucose homeostasis and improved insulin sensitivity. In the WHS (139), a significant inverse association was found between magnesium intake and risk of Type-2 diabetes, independent of age and body mass index (BMI). This inverse relationship was also reported in an analysis of data from the Health Professionals' Follow-up Study and the Nurses' Health Study (140). In the ARIC Study (141), the adjusted relative odds of incident Type-2 diabetes rose progressively across the lower serum magnesium categories. In another analysis of data from the Nurses' Health Study (142), higher magnesium intake was associated with lower fasting insulin concentrations among women without diabetes, compared with subjects with serum magnesium levels of 0.95 mmol/L or greater.

Potassium
In an analysis of randomical controlled trials (RCTs), potassium intake was found to be inversely related to BP (143). Potassium supplementation (31 trials with a dose of at least 60 mmol/day and a median intervention of five weeks) was associated with a significant reduction in SBP (-3.11 mmHg) and DBP (-1.97 mmHg), respectively. The effects of treatment were enhanced in studies when participants were concurrently exposed to a high sodium intake.

When calcium intake was increased in combination with magnesium and potassium in conjunction with a reduction in sodium intake, the hypotensive effect was more pronounced. In the Dietary Approaches to Stop Hypertension study (DASH) (144), participants were allocated to one of three treatments: a typical American diet, a diet rich in fruits and vegetables and a combination diet (i.e., "DASH" rich in fruits, vegetables and low-fat dairy products, characterized by higher contents of calcium, magnesium, potassium and fiber). Compared with the control diet, the DASH diet and the fruits and vegetable diet reduced SBP by 5.5 and 2.8 mmHg, respectively; and DBP by 3.0 and 1.1 mmHg, respectively. The DASH diet reduced SBP in the hypertensive participants by 11.4 mmHg and DBP by 5.5 mmHg. When comparing the DASH diet to the fruits-vegetables diet in hypertensive subjects, the DASH diet further decreased SBP by 4.1 mmHg and DBP by 2.6 mmHg.

Selenium

The association between selenium level and cardiac events is not conclusive. Some studies showed that higher selenium levels decreases coronary risk. In a large case-control study, the European Antioxidant MI and Breast Cancer (EURAMIC) Trial (145), toenail selenium was assessed in 683 subjects with a first nonfatal acute MI and in 729 controls less than 70 years of age. Median toenail selenium content was 0.55 µg/g for the cases and 0.59 µg/g for the controls. After adjustment for age, center, and smoking, the OR for acute MI in the highest quintile of toenail selenium compared with the lowest was 0.63 (95% CI 0.37–1.07, P for trend = 0.08). Likewise, selenium was protective in a study conducted in Finland (149). Mean serum selenium levels of subjects were 63.3 µg/L in eastern Finland and 47.5 µg/L in western Finland. The adjusted RR of CVD, CHD deaths and MI of men with serum selenium <45 µg/L were 1.6 ($p < 0.05$),1.3 and 1.1, respectively. However, there is some evidence that higher serum selenium increases risk of coronary disease. In a nested case-control study (Physicians' Health Study) (146), the mean levels of plasma selenium were 114 µg/g in the 251 MI cases, and 113 µg/g in 251 controls. Subjects in the highest quintile (median 134 µg/g) had an unajusted RR for MI of 1.27 (95% CI 0.71–2.29) and 1.53 (95% CI 0.61–3.84) after adjustment for other cardiovascular risk factors when compared with the lowest quintile (median 93 µg/g). There also is evidence of no association of selenium status and coronary risk. A longitudinal case-control study in Finland (147) reported that serum selenium concentration (50–105 µg/L) was not associated with development of CHD during five to seven years follow-up. In addition, Kok et al. (148) found between serum selenium and risk of CVD death at levels of >105.0 µg/L (lowest quinite <105.0 µg/L vs. highest quinite >153.0 µg/L) no significant relation.

There is some evidence, however, that serum selenium increases risk of coronary disease. In a study conducted in Finland (149), mean serum selenium levels of subjects were 63.3 µg/L in eastern Finland and 47.5 µg/L in western Finland. The adjusted RR of CVD, CHD deaths, and MI of men with serum selenium less than 45 µg/L were 1.6 ($P < 0.05$), 1.3 and 1.1, respectively.

Zinc
Coronary Mortality

In the Iowa WHS (151), an insignificant inverse relationship was observed between dietary zinc and CVD mortality. In a nested case-control prospective study (152), low serum zinc and high serum copper were significantly associated with an increased CVD mortality. Compared with the lowest tertiles of plasma zinc (<12.7 (M/L) and copper (<16.2 µmol/L) levels, subjects in the highest tertiles of zinc (>14.9 µM/L) and copper (>19.4 µmol/L) levels had RRs for CVD mortality of 0.64 (0.34–1.19; P for trend 0.01) and 3.38 (1.70–6.70; P for trend 0.06). In the Zutphen Study (153), serum zinc was significantly inversely related with resting heart rate.

Diabetes and Obesity

In a case-control study conducted by Konukoglu et al. (154), lower serum zinc levels were associated with obesity and diabetes. Compared with the control group, serum zinc level was 27.4% lower in nonobese diabetic subjects ($n = 35$) and 48% lower in obese diabetic subjects ($n = 45$). A similar trend has been observed in other case-control studies (155–157) of obese or diabetic subjects. However, in several studies of individuals with Type-1 diabetes, no relationship was observed (158–160). de Sena et al. (159) did not find significant differences in plasma zinc concentrations and erythrocytes between individuals with Type-1 diabetes and controls after four months of oral zinc supplementation (7.5 or 15 mg/day). These results are consistent with those reported by Ruiz et al. (160). In addition, in a study conducted by Anderson et al. (158), patients with diabetes were given 30 mg/day of zinc, or 400 µg/day of chromium or combined Zn/Cr supplementation or placebo for six months. Supplementation did not significantly modify HbA1C or glucose homeostasis.

TABLE 4 Dietary Reference Intakes for Selected Minerals for Adults

	Adequate intake				Upper intake level	
	Male		Female			Adverse effect or toxicity
Minerals	19–50 yr	>50 yr	19–50 yr	>50 yr	(>19 yr)	
Calcium	1000 mg/day	1200 mg/day	1000 mg/day	1200 mg/day	2500 mg/day	Nephrolithiasis; hypercalcemia and renal insufficiency (milk-alkali syndrome); interacts with iron, zinc, magnesium, and phosphorus
Potassium	4.7 g/day	4.7 g/day	4.7 g/day	4.7 g/day	N/A	GI discomfort; ulcer; Arrhythmia
Zinc	11 mg/day	11 mg/day	8 mg/day	8 mg/day	40 mg/day	Acute: epigastric pain, nausea, vomiting, loss of appetite, abdominal cramps, diarrhea, and headaches Chronic: immunologic response; lipoprotein and cholesterol; reduced copper status; zinc-iron interactions
Selenium	55 μg/day	55 μg/day	55 μg/day	55 μg/day	55 μg/day	Acute: severe gastrointestinal and neurological disturbances; acute respiratory distress syndrome; myocardial infarction; and renal failure Chronic: hair and nail brittleness and loss; gastrointestinal disturbances; skin rash; garlic breath odor; fatigue; irritability; and nervous system abnormalities
	Male 19–31 yr	Female >31 yr	19–30 yr	>31 yr		
Magnesium	400 mg/day	420 mg/day	310 mg/day	320 mg/day	350 mg/day	Diarrhea; nausea; abdominal cramping metabolic alkalosis; neurological and cardiac symptoms; paralytic ileus

Note: Adequate intake (AI): If sufficient scientific evidence is not available to calculate an EAR, a reference intake called AI is provided instead of RDA. AI is a value based on experimentally derived intake levels or approximations of observed mean nutrient intakes by a group (or groups) of healthy people. Tolerable upper intake level: is the highest level of daily nutrient intake that is likely to pose no risk of adverse health effects for almost all individuals in the specified life stage group.
Adverse effect references:
- Calcium: http://newton.nap.edu/books/0309063507/html/134.html
- Potassium: http://newton.nap.edu/books/0309091691/html/247.html
- Zinc: http://newton.nap.edu/books/0309072794/html/482.html
- Selenium: http://newton.nap.edu/books/0309069351/html/311.html
- Magnesium: http://newton.nap.edu/books/0309063507/html/242.html
Abbreviations: AI, adequate intake; RDA, recommended dietary allowance; UL, upper intake level; N/A, not available.

The Adequate Intake (AI) for calcium and potassium, the RDA for zinc, selenium and magnesium, the UL, and adverse effects of selected minerals are reported in Table 4. Based on NHANES 1999–2000 data (161), calcium, potassium, and magnesium intakes in adults were much lower than the AI or RDA [except the intake of calcium for men <60 years (969–1025 mg/day), which was close to the AI (1000 mg/day)]. In contrast, zinc and selenium among all adult groups were higher than the RDA. Elderly individuals (>60 years) usually have lower micronutrient intakes than people aged 20–59 years.

Fiber
Epidemiologic Studies on Heart Disease Risks
Several large cohort studies (Table 5) (162–169) have shown that dietary fiber intake is associated with a reduction in CHD risk. These epidemiologic studies were conducted typically on thousands of participants and followed up for several years. The endpoints included CHD, CVD, MI, coronary death, and others. The majority of the results showed that higher dietary fiber intake was inversely associated with risk of cardiac incidences, although this trend generally was attenuated or insignificant after multivariate adjustment. When comparing the different sources of fiber intake, fiber from cereal and fruits usually was associated with a lower risk of cardiac events than fiber derived from vegetable sources. Soluble fiber seemed to lower heart disease risk more than insoluble fiber.

TABLE 5 Epidemiologic Studies of Fiber Intake and Relative Risk of Cardiac Events

Study/yr	Subjects	Follow-up (yr)	Category (total) (low→high)	Cardiac incidence	RR (multivariate adjustment) highest vs. lowest category
Wolk et al. 1999 Nurses' Health Study (162)	68,782 female	10	Median (g/day): 11.5, 14.3, 16.4, 18.8, 22.9	591 CHD cases (429 nonfatal MI and 162 CHD deaths)	0.77 (95% CI, 0.57–1.04) for total CHD Cereal 0.63 (0.49–0.81), fruit 0.93 (0.74–1.16), vegetable 1.13 (0.77–1.64)
Pietinen et al. 1996 ATBC Cancer Prevention Study (163)	21,930 male	6.1	Median (g/day): 16.1, 20.7, 24.3, 28.3, 34.8	1399 major coronary events and 635 events mortality from CHD	Coronary death: total fiber 0.73 (0.56–0.95), soluble 0.68 (0.50–0.92), insoluble 0.75 (0.58–0.98), lignin 0.75 (0.58–0.97), cellulose 0.72 (0.54–0.97), cereal 0.74 (0.57–0.96), vegetable 0.88 (0.66–1.19), fruit 1.16 (0.80–1.67)
Jensen et al. 2004 Health Professionals' Follow-up Study (164)	42,850 male	14	Median (g/day): 3.5, 9.6, 16.0, 24.7, 42.4	1261 nonfatal MI and 557 fatal CHD	CHD: whole grain 0.82 (0.70–0.96), added bran 0.70 (0.60–0.82), added germ 0.95 (0.83–1.09)
Mozaffarian et al. 2003 Cardiovascular Health Study (165)	3588 subjects	8.6	<1.7, 1.7–3.3, 3.4–4.7, 4.8–6.3, >6.3 (g/day)	159 IHD deaths, 308 nonfatal MIs, 344 strokes	Incident CVD: total fiber 0.84 (0.66–1.07), cereal 0.79 (0.62–0.99), fruit 0.99 (0.78–1.25), vegetable 1.08 (0.86–1.36)
Liu et al. 2002 Women's Health Study (166)	38,480 female	6	Median (g/day): 12.5, 15.7, 18.2, 21.1 26.3	570 incident cases of CVD, including 177 MIs	MI: total fiber 0.68(0.39–1.22), cereal 0.91 (0.56–1.47), vegetable 0.89 (0.52–1.53), fruit 1.11 (0.62–1.96), soluble 0.83 (0.47–1.48), insoluble 0.74 (0.42–1.30)
Rimm et al. 1996 Health Professionals' Study (167)	43,757 male	6	Median (g/day): 12.4, 16.6, 19.6, 23.0, 28.9	734 MI cases (229 fatal CHD)	Total MI: total fiber: 0.64 (0.47–0.87), cereal: 0.71 (0.54–0.92), fruit: 0.81 (0.62–1.06), vegetable: 0.83 (0.64–1.08)
Jacobs et al. 1998 Iowa Women's Health Study (168)	34,492 female	10	Median (servings/wk): 0–3.5, 4.0–7.0, 7.5–10.0, 10.5–18.0, 18.5–84.5∂	438 IHD deaths	IHD death: total whole grain 0.70 (0.50–0.98)

Abbreviations: CHD, coronary heart disease; MI, myocardial infarction; IHD, ischemic heart disease; CVD, cardiovascular disease; ATBC, alpha tocopherol beta carotene; RR, relative risk.

Effects of Dietary Fiber on CVD Risk Factors

A number of studies have been conducted to evaluate the effects of dietary fiber on risk factors for CVD. Many studies have demonstrated cholesterol-lowering effects of dietary fiber. The response depends mainly on the type and amount of fiber in the diet. Also, there is some evidence of a BP lowering effect.

Brown et al. (170) conducted a meta-analysis of 67 studies that evaluated the blood-cholesterol lowering effects of oat products, psyllium, pectin, and guar gum. The average dose of soluble fiber was 9.5 g/day, which was given for an average of 49 days. Over a range of 2–10 g of soluble fiber per day, net reductions of total cholesterol (TC) and LDL-C were −0.045 and −0.057 mmol/L per gram of soluble fiber. Over a wider dose response range (2–30 g/day), the reductions were −0.028 mmol/L and −0.029 mmol/L per gram of soluble fiber. High fiber diets also significantly reduced HDL-C, but to a lesser extent (0.002 mmol/L per gram of soluble fiber). The soluble fiber from oats, psyllium, pectin, or guar gum significantly decreased TC and LDL-C levels; none significantly affected TG. One gram of soluble fiber from oats, psyllium, pectin, or guar gum produced changes in TC of −0.037, −0.028, −0.070, and −0.026 mmol/L, respectively, and for LDL-C of −0.032, −0.029, −0.055, and −0.033 mmol/L, respectively.

In a meta-analysis conducted by Anderson et al. (171), 10.2 g/day of psyllium lowered serum TC by 4%, LDL-C by 7%, and the ratio of Apolipoprotein (Apo) B to apoA-I by 6%, compared to subjects in the placebo group. No significant effects on serum HDL-C or TG concentrations were observed.

Two recent meta-analyses (172,173) reported BP lowering effects of dietary fiber. Streppel et al. (173), reported that fiber supplementation (average dose, 11.5 g/day) decreased SBP by 1.13 mmHg and DBP by 1.26 mmHg. The average BP reduction in these studies tended to be greater among elder population (>40 years) and in patients with hypertension (SBP: 5.95 mmHg, DBP: 4.20 mmHg), respectively.

FISH OIL SUPPLEMENTATION

In 1976 and 1980, Bang et al. published three articles that suggested that marine-derived omega-3 fatty acids (or *n*-3 fatty acids) were responsible for the low mortality from CHD in Greenland Eskimos (174–176). Since then, numerous epidemiologic studies (Table 6), clinical trials (Table 7), and animal experiments have consistently demonstrated that fatty fish or fish oil has a beneficial effect on CVD risk factors and reduces the risk of some cardiovascular events. Most of the epidemiologic literature pertains to studies evaluating fish consumption, whereas the controlled clinical studies have also evaluated fish oil supplements on CVD endpoints. The most recent guidelines from the American Heart Association supported the use of fish oil supplementation for patients with CHD (231).

Randomized Controlled Clinical Trials
Effects on Cardiac Events
The Diet and Reinfarction Trial (DART) (229) and the GISSI-Prevention study (60) are two important trials that examined the effects of a high fatty fish diet and fish oil supplements on secondary prevention of CVD; both showed protective effects (Fig. 3). The DART study was a randomized controlled trial with a factorial design where 2033 male MI survivors were randomly assigned to one of the three following treatment groups: type and amount of fat in the diet; fish advice (at least 200–400 g fatty fish per week); and fiber advice (increase of cereal fiber intake to 18 g/day) for two years. Subjects who selected not to eat fish were given a fish oil supplement (three "MaxEPA" capsules per day: 0.5 g). In this study, there was a 29% reduction in all-cause mortality in subjects who consumed fatty fish. An identical response was observed for subjects taking the fish oil supplement.

The GISSI-Prevention Study is the largest prospective randomized controlled trial to examine the efficacy of long chain *n*-3 fatty acids in over 11,000 recent MI survivors. Subjects were randomized to 300 mg/day of vitamin E, 850 mg/day of eicosapentenoic acid (EPA) + docosahexenoic acid (DHA), both, or none for 3.5 years. In the fish oil supplement group, there was a 15% significant reduction in the primary endpoint (death, nonfatal MI, and nonfatal stroke); RR was 0.85 (95% CI, 0.74–0.98; $P < 0.02$). In addition, there was a 20% reduction in all-cause mortality (RR, 0.80; 95% CI, 0.67–0.94; $P = 0.01$) as well as a 45% reduction in sudden death (RR, 0.55; 95% CI, 0.40–0.76; $P < 0.001$) for the fish oil group versus the control group (Fig. 4). Vitamin E did not confer any beneficial effect. In a meta-analysis of 10 studies that evaluated the effects of *n*-3 fatty acids' intake (DART used 200–400 g/wk of fatty fish; the other nine studies provide *n*-3 fatty acid supplements that ranged from 1 to 6 g/day), in 14,727 patients with angina or acute/recent MI, there was 16% decrease in all-cause mortality (RR 0.84, 95% CI: 0.76–0.94) and a 24% decrease in incidences of death due to MI (RR 0.76, 0.66–0.88) (232).

Some recent studies have not shown a beneficial effect of fish oil supplementation on CVD events. Nilsen et al. (204) conducted a study of 300 patients with acute MI who were given 3.5 g/day of EPA + DHA for 12 to 24 months, and there was no clinical benefit on cardiac events. Subsequently, it was suggested that the lack of beneficial effects of *n*-3 fatty acids may be due to a high habitual fish consumption of this Norwegian population (233). In another recent trial conducted by Burr et al. (230), 3114 men with angina were assigned to one of the following treatment groups: consume two portions of fatty fish per week or take three fish oil capsules (MaxEPA) per day; eat more fruits, vegetables, and oats; both; or no specific dietary advice except for guidance about weight loss for those subjects with a BMI greater than 30 kg/m^2. After three to nine years of follow-up, subjects who were advised to consume fish or fish oil had a higher cardiac death rate than subjects not on the fish/fish oil treatment (RR, 1.26; 95% CI, 1.00–1.58; $P = 0.047$). Moreover, the risk of sudden cardiac death was greater in the fatty fish/fish oil group (RR, 1.54; 95% CI, 1.06–2.23; $P = 0.025$). The subgroup taking fish oil

TABLE 6 Epidemiologic Studies of Fish Intake and Relative Risk of Cardiac Events

Selected study	Population	Follow-up (yr)	Categories	Cardiac incidences	Multivariate relative risks (95% CI) (highest vs. lowest category)
Ascherio et al. (177)	44895 men, (40–75 yr) free of CVD	6	<1 serving/mo; 1–3/mo; 1/wk; 2–3/wk; 4–5/wk; ≥6/wk	1543 total CHD events, 264 CHD death, 547 nonfatal MI and 732 coronary artery bypass or angioplasty procedures	Nonfatal MI: 0.96 (0.63–1.47, P for trend 0.62) Fatal CHD: 0.77 (0.41–1.44, P for trend 0.14) Any MI: 0.90 (0.63–1.28, P for trend 0.70) Any CHD 1.14 (0.86–1.51, P for trend 0.19)
Morris et al. (178)	21,185 U.S. male physicians aged 40–84 yr	4	<1 serving/wk; 1/wk; 2–4/wk and ≥5/wk	281 MI cases (259 nonfatal, 22 fatal), 121 CVD deaths and 525 combined important vascular events	Total MI: 0.9 (0.4–1.8, P for trend 0.72) Non-fatal MI: 0.8 (0.4–1.7, P for trend 0.79) CVD death: 2.2 (0.8–5.9, P for trend 0.35) Total CVD events: 0.9 (0.6–1.5, P for trend 0.65)
Daviglus et al. (179)	1822 men (40–55 yr)	30	0 g/day; 1–17 g/day; 18–34 g/day; ≥35 g/day	573 CVD death; 430 CHD deaths; 293 MI (196 sudden, 94 non-sudden, and 3 not classifiable)	MI death: 0.56 (0.33–0.93, P for trend 0.017) CHD death: 0.62 (0.40–0.94, P for trend 0.040) CVD death: 0.74 (0.52–1.06, P for trend 0.010) All-cause death: 0.85 (0.64–1.10, P for trend 0.175)
Albert et al. (180)	20551 male physicians (40–84 yr)	11	<1 serving/mo; 1–3/mo; 1–<2/wk; 2–<5/wk; (5/wk	133 sudden deaths (115 definite and 18 probable) 737 MI	Sudden death: 0.39 (0.15–0.96, P for trend 0.11) MI: 1.00 (0.62–1.60, P for trend 0.67) Nonsudden cardiac death: 1.19 (0.38–3.70, P for trend 0.33) CHD death: 0.81 (0.41–1.61, P for trend 0.49) CVD mortality: 0.81 (0.49–1.33, P for trend 0.50) Total mortality: 0.73 (0.55–0.96, P for trend 0.045)
Oomen et al. (181)	1088 Finnish men; 1097 Italian men; 553 Dutch men. total 2738 men (50–69yr)	20	0–19 g/day; 20–39 g/day; ≥40 g/day 0 g/day; 1–19 g/day; 20–39 g/day; ≥40 g/day 0 g/day; 1–19 g/day; ≥20 g/day	Finland: 242 CHD deaths (22.2%) Italy: 116 CHD deaths (10.6%) Netherlands: 105 (19%) CHD deaths.≈	CHD mortality Finland: 1.25 (0.89–1.76 P for trend 0.2); Italy: 0.67 (0.33–1.39 P for trend 0.33); Netherlands: 1.10 (0.68–1.79 P for trend 0.69)
Hu et al. (182)	84688 female nurses (34–59 yr)	16	<1 serving/mo; 1–3/mo; 1/wk; 2–4/wk; ≥5/wk	1513 CHD cases (484 CHD deaths and 1029 nonfatal MI)	Total CHD: 0.69 (0.52–0.93, P for trend 0.007) Fatal CHD: 0.55 (0.33–0.91, P for trend 0.01) Nonfatal MI: 0.77 (0.54–1.11, P for trend 0.10)

Study	Subjects	Duration (yr)	Intake	Cases	Results
Mozaffarian et al. (183)	3910 adults aged ≥65 years and free of known CVD	Mean 9.3	<1 serving/mo; 1–3/mo; 1/wk; 2/wk; ≥3/wk	247 IHD deaths (148 arrhythmic deaths), 363 incident nonfatal MI	Total IHD death: Tuna/other fish: 0.47 (0.27–0.82, P for trend 0.002); Fried fish/fish sandwich: 1.37 (0.48–3.9, P for trend 0.35); Arrhythmic IHD death: Tuna/other fish: 0.32 (0.15–0.70, P for trend 0.001); Fried fish/fish sandwich: 1.54 (0.82–2.90, P for trend 0.28); Nonfatal MI: Tuna/other fish: 0.67 (0.42–1.07, P for trend 0.10); Fried fish/fish sandwich: 1.93 (0.91–4.08, P for trend 0.11)
Osler et al. (184)	4513 men and 3984 women (30–70yr)	8–18	≈1 serving/mo, 2/mo, 1/wk, ≥2/wk	Total of 349 men and 142 women developed CHD; 168 and 79 were fatal events	All cause mortality: 1.06 (0.88–1.28, P for trend 0.02); CHD mortality and morbidity: 0.93 (0.68–1.27, P for trend 0.55); CHD mortality: 0.98 (0.62–1.52, P for trend 0.74)
Folsom et al. (185)	Iowa women aged 55–69yr	15	<0.5 serving/wk, 0.5–<1.0/wk, 1.0–1.5/wk,>1.5–<2.5/wk, ≥2.5/wk	4,653 deaths	Mortality in diabetic women: All causes: 0.92 (P for trend 0.78); CVD: 0.91 (P for trend 0.82); CHD: 1.16 (P for trend 0.68)
Mozaffarian et al. (186)	4815 adults ≥age 65 years	12	<1 serving/mo; 1–3/mo; 1–4/wk; ≥5/wk	980 cases of incident atrial fibrillation (AF)	AF incidence 0.69 (0.52–0.91, P = 0.008) and 31% lower risk
Mozaffarian et al. (187)	4,738 men and women aged ≥65Yr	12	Tuna/other fish: <1/mo; 1–3/mo; 1–2/wk; 3–4/wk; ≥5/wk Fried fish: <1/mo; 1–3/mo; ≥1/wk	955 incident CHF	CHF: Tuna/other fish: 0.65 (0.44–0.97) P for trend 0.003; Fried fish: 1.35 (1.12–1.62) P for trend 0.005
Frost et al. (188)	47,949 participants (22,528 men and 25,421 women) (mean age: 56 yr)	Mean 5.7	Mean n-3 PUFA from fish (g/day): 0.16, 0.36, 0.52, 0.74 and 1.29	Atrial fibrillation or flutter developed in 556 subjects (374 men and 182 women)	AF 1.34 (1.02–1.76) P for trend 0.006

Abbreviations: CHD, coronary heart disease; CVD, cardiovascular disease; MI, myocardial infarction; IHD, ischemic heart disease; CHF, chronic heart failure; PUFA, polyunsaturated fatty acids; AF, atrial fibrillation; CI, confidence interval.

TABLE 7 Randomized Controlled Clinical Trials of Fish Oil, EPA + DHA or Fatty Fish Consumption and Coronary Endpoints

Effects on progression of atherosclerosis, restenosis after PTCA

Study (yr)	Design	Patients	Regimen	Follow-up (months)	Results
Sacks et al. (1995) (189)	Randomized, double-blind, controlled, parallel	59 patients with CHD	Intervention: 2.88 g/day EPA + 1.92 g/day DHA + 1.2 g/day DPA; control: olive oil	28	Mean minimal diameter of atherosclerotic coronary arteries: Fish oil group: ↓ 0.104 mm; Placebo group: ↓ 0.138 mm ($P= 0.6$) Percent stenosis: Fish oil group: ↑2.4%; Placebo group: 2.6% ($P = 0.8$) Lipids: ↓ TG by 30% ($P = 0.007$)
Eritsland et al. (1996) (190)	Randomized, controlled, factorial 2 × 2	610 patients undergoing coronary artery bypass grafting	Intervention: 3.3 g/day EPA + DHA; control	12	Vein graft occlusion rates per distal anastomoses: Fish oil group: 27%; control group: 33%; OR, 0.77 [0.60, 0.90] ($P = 0.034$) Patients with 1 or more than 1 occluded vein graft(s): Fish oil group: 43%; control group: 51%; OR, 0.72 [051, 1.01] ($P = 0.05$) Lipids: ↓TG by 19%
Cairns et al. (1996) (191)	Randomized, controlled, factorial 2 × 2	814 patients undergoing PTCA	Intervention: 5.4 g/day fish oil; control: corn oil	4.5	Restenosis rates per patient: Fish oil group: 46.5%; control group: 44.7% Restenosis rates per lesion: Fish oil group: 39.7%; control group: 38.7% Mean minimal lumen diameters: Fish oil group: 1.12 mm; control group: 1.10 mm
von Schacky et al. (1999) (192)	Randomized, placebo-controlled double-blind, parallel	223 patients with angiographically proven CAD	Intervention: 1.06 g/day EPA + 0.65 g/day DHA for the first 3 mo then half dose; control: fatty acid mixture	24	Pairs of standardized coronary angiography were evaluated as global score: Placebo group: 35 changed out of 80 pairs Fish oil group: 35 changed out of 82 pairs Progression of coronary segments: Fish oil group showed less progression and more regression when compared with the placebo group ($P = 0.041$) Mean loss (±SD) of minimal luminal diameter per patient: Placebo group: 0.45±0.8 mm ($P = 0.07$) Fish oil group: 0.38±0.8 mm ($P = 0.023$) MI and stroke: Seven in placebo group vs. two in fish oil group ($P = 0.10$)
Johansen et al. (1999) (193)	Randomized, double-blind, placebo-controlled, parallel	500 patients undergoing PTCA	2.7 g/day EPA + 2.3 g/day DHA; placebo: olive oil	6	Incidence of restenosis: Fish oil group: 40.6%; Placebo group: 35.4% OR, 1.25[0.87–1.80] ($P = 0.21$) One or more Restenoses: Fish oil group: 45.9%; Placebo group: 44.8% OR, 1.05 [0.69–1.59] ($P = 0.82$)
Goodfellow et al. (2000) (194)	Randomized, placebo-controlled double-blind, parallel	30 subjects with confirmed hypercholes-terolemia	Intervention: 1 g marine *n-3* fatty acid twice daily; control: corn oil	4	FMD: Fish oil group: from 0.05±0.12 to 0.12±0.07 mm ($P<0.05$) Placebo group: no change Fish oil group: TG decreased from 2.07±1.13 to 1.73±0.95 mmol/L ($P<0.05$) Placebo Group: no change
Angerer et al.	Randomized, placebo-	223 patients with	Intervention:	24	Mean maximum intima-media thickness:

Study	Design	Population	Intervention	Duration	Results
(2002) (195)	controlled, double-blind	CAD who had >20% stenosis in ≥1 coronary vessel	3.33 g/day EPA + DHA first 3 mo then 1.65 g/day EPA + DHA; control: mixture of FAs		Fish oil group: ↑0.07(0.13 mm); Control group: ↑0.05(0.11 mm) ($P = 0.24$) Global change score: Fish oil group vs. control group: 38% vs. 35% showed progression
Maresta et al. (2002) (196)	Randomized, placebo-controlled double-blind, multicenter	339 patients before and after PTCA	Intervention: 3 g/day EPA + 2.1 g/day DHA for 2 mo then half dose; control: olive oil	8	Restenosis rates per vessel: By definitions I: 29.4% in the fish oil group and 39.6% in the control group ($P = 0.04$); By definitions II: 31.6% in the fish oil group and 35.4% in the control group ($P>0.05$) Restenosis rates per patient: By definitions I: 31.2% in the fish oil group and 40.9% in the control group ($P = 0.05$); By definitions II: 33.6% in the fish oil group and 37.1% in the control group ($P>0.05$)
Thies et al. (2003) (197)	Randomized, placebo controlled double-blind	188 patients awaiting carotid endarterectomy	Intervention: 1.4 g/day fish oil; 3.6 g/day sunflower oil; control: palm oil+ soybean oil	Median 1.5	Carotid plaque morphologic classification: Fish oil group differed with control ($P = 0.0234$) and sunflower oil group ($P = 0.0107$); fish oil group had 71.7% type IV and 15.1% type V Lipids: TG: 0.48 mmol/L ↓from baseline in fish oil group ($P = 0.0032$); 0.33 mmol/L lower than sunflower oil and control group ($P = 0.0294$ and 0.0347)

Effects on lipids and oxidation

Study	Design	Population	Intervention	Duration	Results
Silva et al. (1996) (198)	Randomized, controlled, double-blind	40 patients with hypertriglyc-eridaemia or mixed hyperlipidaemia	Intervention: 3.6 g/day fish oil; Control: soya oil	2	TG: Fish oil group: ↓27.8%; soya oil group:↑19.9% LDL-C: Fish oil group: ↑7.7%; soya oil group: 10% Glucose: 11% in fish oil group ($P = 0.0047$)
McGrath et al. (1996) (199)	Randomized, placebo-controlled double-blind, cross-over	23 patients with NIDDM	Intervention: 10 g/day fish oil control: olive oil	4.5	TBARS and vitamin E:↑ in the fish oil group ($P<0.001$ and $p<0.01$, respectively TG:↓ from 1.8 mmol/L to 1.4 mmol/L ($P = 0.07$)
Sirtori et al. (1997) (200)	Randomized, controlled, double-blind and open, multicenter	935 patients with hypertriglyc-eridemia type IIb or IV and at least one more CV risk factor	Intervention: 1530 mg EPA + 1050 mg DHA first 2 mo then 1020 mg EPA + 700 mg DHA; control: olive oil	First 6 for doubleblind (DB); Second 6 for open study	TG: In the double blind phase EPA + DHA group ↓21.5% ($P<0.0001$); in the open phase EPA + DHA group had a further ↓ from −21.5 to 25.2%, the control group ↓19.5% TC: In the open phase all patients had an overall 3.0%; 4.15% in the type IIB hyperlipoproteinemia subgroup
Nordy et al. (1998) (201)	Randomized, placebo-controlled double-blind	41 patients with defined hyperlipidemia	Intervention: 20 mg simvastatin + 4 g/day EPA + DHA;	5 wk	TG: Intervention group: ↓0.77 ± 0.19 mmol/L ($P<0.01$) TC: Intervention group:↓0.42±0.14 mmol/L ($P = 0.052$)

(Continued)

TABLE 7 Randomized Controlled Clinical Trials of Fish Oil, EPA + DHA or Fatty Fish Consumption and Coronary Endpoints

Study (yr)	Design	Patients	Regimen	Follow-up (months)	Results
Mori et al. (1999) (202)	Randomized, controlled	69 overweight, postmenopausal women receiving antihypertensive treatment	Control: 20 mg simvastatin + corn oil Intervention: daily fish meal (3.65 g/day n-3 FAs); weight-loss diet; both control: weight-maintaining diet	4	TG: Fish consumption ↓0.57 mmol/L (29%) and weight loss ↓0.51 mmol/L (26%), fish + weight loss group ↓38% ($P < 0.001$) HDL-C: fish consumption ↑ HDL_2–C 0.08 mmol/L (21%, $P = 0.004$) and ↓ HDL_3–C 0.04 mmol/L (5%, $P = 0.026$); fish + weight loss group ↑HDL_2–C 24% ($P = 0.04$)
Durrington et al. (2001) (203)	Randomized, controlled, double-blind multicenter	59 patients with established CHD	Intervention: 10–40 mg/day simvastatin + 2 g twice daily of n-3 FAs (Omacor) control: 10–40 mg/day simvastatin + corn oil	6	TG: Intervention group:↓20–30% ($P < 0.005$) VLDL-C: Intervention group:↓30–40% ($P < 0.005$)
Nilsen et al. (2001) (204)	Randomized, controlled, double-blind	300 patients with an acute MI	Intervention: 3.5 g/day EPA + DHA control: corn oil	12–24	TG: Intervention group: ↓ 1.30%/mo; corn oil group: ↑ 0.35%/mo ($P < 0.0001$) HDL-C: Intervention group: ↑ 1.11%; corn oil group: ↑ 0.55% ($P < 0.0001$)
Higdon et al. (2001) (205)	Randomized, controlled, blind, crossover	15 postmenopausal women	Intervention: sunflower oil: 12.3 g/day of oleate; SA: 10.5 g/day of linoleate; FO providing 2.0 g/day of EPA and 1.4 g/day of DHA	7–29 wks	LDL α-tocopherol depletion: More rapidly after FO supplementation than after SU ($P = 0.0001$) and SA ($P = 0.05$) Lag phase for phosphatidylcholine hydroperoxide (PCOOH) formation: Shorter after FO supplementation than after SU ($P = 0.0001$) and SA ($P = 0.006$) Lag phase for cholesteryl linoleate hydroperoxide (CE18:20OH) formation:Shorter after FO supplementation than in SU ($P = 0.03$) Maximal rates of PCOOH and CE18:20OH formation: Lower after FO supplementation than after SA ($P<0.05$ for both) Maximal concentrations of PCOOH and CE18:20OH: lower after FO supplementation than after SA ($P<0.05$ for both)
Finnegan et al. (2003) (206)	Randomized, placebo-controlled double-blind, parallel	150 moderately hyperlipidemic subjects	Intervention: 0.8 or 1.7 g/day EPA + DHA; 4.5 or 9.5 g/day ALA; control: placebo capsules	6	TG: mean change for 1.7- g/day EPA+DHA group is $-7.7 \pm 4.99\%$ and for 9.5- g/day ALA group is $10.9 \pm 4.5\%$ ($P<0.05$) LDL lag phase: Mean reduction for 1.7g/day EPA + DHA group is 9 ± 1.9 min; for the control group is 2 ± 1.8 min, for the 4.5- g/day ALA group1.9 ± 2.3 min, and for the 9.5-g/day ALA group is 0.3 ± 3.3 min ($P<0.05$)

Study	Design	Subjects	Intervention	Duration (wk)	Results
Mori et al. (2003) (207)	Randomized, placebo-controlled double-blind, parallel	59 subjects with treated-hypertensive and Type 2 diabetes	Intervention: 4 g/day EPA; 4 g/day DHA Control: olive oil	1.5	Urinary F_2-isoprostanes: EPA group: ↓19% ($P = 0.017$); DHA group: ↓20 b% ($P = 0.014$)
Mesa et al. (2004) (208)	Randomized, placebo-controlled double-blind, parallel	42 healthy subjects	Intervention: 9 g oil/day EPA-rich oil or a DHA-rich oil; control: olive oil	1	Formation of conjugated dienes during LDL oxidation: EPA-rich oil: significantly; DHA-rich oil: no effect LDL lag phase: Placebo group had a greater lag phase for oxidation than EPA or DHA rich oil

Effects on blood pressure

Study	Design	Subjects	Intervention	Duration (wk)	Results
Toft et al. (1995) (209)	Randomized, placebo-controlled double-blind	78 untreated hypertensive subjects	Intervention: 4 g/day EPA + DHA Control: corn oil	4	Systolic blood pressure: Fish oil group ↓3.8 mmHg more than control ($P = 0.04$) Diastolic blood pressure: Fish oil group↓ 2 mmHg more than control ($P = 0.10$) TG: Fish oil group ↓0.28 ± 0.08 mmol/L more than control ($P = 0.01$) VLDL-C: Fish oil group ↓0.13 ± 0.04 mmol/L more than control ($P = ↑ 0.01$)
Russo et al. (1995) (210)	Randomized, controlled	24 mild essential hypertensive sujects	Intervention: 3 g/day EPA + DHA Control	4	Systolic and diastolic blood pressure: No effect Heart rates: No effect
Gray et al. (1996) (211)	Randomized, placebo-controlled double-blind	21 men with suboptimally controlled blood pressure	Intervention: 4.5 g/day fish oil Control: placebo	2	Systolic and diastolic blood pressure: from 148/97 to 134/91 ($P<0.05$) in the fish oil group TG: 40.9% ($P<0.05$) in fish oil group, Platelet counts: ↓ 8.7% ($P<0.05$) in fish oil group LDL-C: 19.1% ($P<0.05$) in fish oil group
Bao et al. (1998) (212)	Randomized, controlled	69 overweight medication-treated hypertensive subjects	Intervention: a daily fish meal (3.65 g/day n-3 FAs); weight reduction; both Control regimen	4	Systolic and diastolic blood pressure: Fish group ↓ 6.0/3.0 mmHg; weight reduction group ↓ 5.5/2.2 mmHg; fish and weight reduction combined group 13.0/9.3 mmHg ($P<0.01$) Heart rates: Fish group ↓ 24-hour and awake (−3.1±1.4 bpm, $P = 0.036$), (−4.2 ± 1.6 bpm, $P = 0.013$) respectively
Leng et al. (1998) (213)	Randomized, controlled	120 patients with lower limb atherosclerosis	Intervention: 1.68 g/day Gamma-linolenic acid + 0.27 g/day EPA; Placebo: sunflower oil	24	Systolic blood pressure: Fatty acid group compared with baseline: 150 mmHg/161.8 mmHg, $P = 0.05$ Nonfatal coronary event: Fatty acid group: reduced from 15% to 10%, $P>0.05$
Woodman et al. (2002) (214)	Randomized, placebo-controlled double-blind, parallel	59 Type 2 diabetic patients with treated hypertension	Intervention: 4 g/day EPA; 4 g/day DHA; control: olive oil	1.5	Systolic and diastolic blood pressure: No significant effect Fasting glucose: EPA group 1.40 ± 0.29 mmol/L ($P = 0.002$); DHA group ↑ 0.98 ± 0.29 mmol/L ($P = 0.002$) TG: EPA group 19% ($P = 0.022$); DHA group ↓ 15% ($P = 0.022$) HDL_2-C: EPA group↑16% ($P = 0.026$);DHA group ↑12% ($P =0.05$)
Svensson et al. (2004) (215)	Randomized, controlled	64 patients with CRF	Intervention: 2.4 g/day of n-3 PUFAs; control: olive oil	2	Systolic and diastolic blood pressure: No significant effect HDL-C: n-3 PUFA group ↑ 8% ($P < 0.01$) TG: n-3 PUFA group ↓ 21% ($P < 0.02$)

(Continued)

TABLE 7　Randomized Controlled Clinical Trials of Fish Oil, EPA + DHA or Fatty Fish Consumption and Coronary Endpoints

Study (yr)	Design	Patients	Regimen	Follow-up (months)	Results
Dokholyan et al. (2004) (216)	Randomized, controlled	103 subjects with normal diastolic BP or stage 1 hypertension	Intervention: 0.48 g/day EPA + 0.12 g/day GLA; Control: olive oil	3	Incidental hypertension: 7 (13.2%) in the intervention group; five (10.0%) in the control group; RR, 1.4 [−0.4, 4.3] Systolic blood pressures: Intervention group: 1.23±0.91 (P = 0.1801); control group: ↓ 1.54 ± 0.92 (P = 0.1801) Diastolic blood pressures: Intervention group: ↓ 2.58 ± 0.62 (P = 0.0001); control group: ↓ 3.45 ± 0.63 (P = 0.0001)
Effects on hemostatic risk factors and endothelial cell markers					
Mori et al. (1997) (217)	Randomized, controlled	120 subjects with mildly elevated blood pressure and cholesterol	40% fat diet: Intervention: fish meal; fish meal + 6 g/day fish oil; fish meal + 12 g/day fish oil; control: placebo 30% fat diet: Intervention: fish meal Control:placebo	3	Collagen-stimulated platelet aggregation: ↓in groups taking fish meal or fish oil ($P<0.0001$) PAF-induced platelet aggregation: ↓in groups taking fish meal or fish oil ($P<0.05$); high fat fish meal group: ↓ 4.4% (P = 0.0544); high fat fish meal+ fish oil group: ↓ 4.6% (P = 0.0440); 6 g/day fish oil group: ↓ 9.7% ($P<0.0001$); 12 g/day fish oil group:↓8.5% (P = 0.0003)
Selieflot et al. (1998) (218)	Randomized, double-blind, placebo-controlled, 2 × 2 factorial	41 male smokers with hyperlipi-daemia	Intervention: 4.8 g/day n-3 FAs +antioxidant (150 mg VitC + 75 mg VitE + 15 mg β-carotene; n-3 FAs+ antioxidant placebo; antioxidant + n-3 FAs placebo Control: antioxidant placebo + n-3 FAs placebo	1.5	VWF and Thrombomodulin (sTM)(markers of endothelial injury): ↓in the fish oil group compare with placebo P = 0.034 and P 0.001, respectively E-selectin and VCAM-1: ↑ in the fish oil group compared with placebo P = 0.001 and 0.010, respectively
Johansen et al. (1999) (193)	Randomized, double-blind, placebo-controlled, parallel	500 patients undergoing PTCA	Intervention: 2.7 g/day EPA + 2.3 g/day DHA; Control: olive oil	6	Soluble E-selectin and soluble vascular cell adhesion molecule-1 (sVCAM-1): Increased in placebo group compared with fish oil group ($P<0.01$)
Pirich et al. (1999) (219)	Randomized, placebo-controlled, double-blind	26 patients with hyperchole-sterolemia	Intervention: 216 mg/day EPA + 140 mg/day DHA + 390 mg/day gamma-linolenic acid+ 3480 mg linoleic acid Control: placebo	1.5	Platelet survival: from 159±(14 hours to 164 ± 12 hours (P = 0.025) in the intervention group TXB_2: ↓from 225±16 to 212 ± 21 ng/mL (P = 0.003) in the intervention group MDA formation: ↓from 5.49±1.03 to 5.12 ± 1.05 nM/10^9 platelets (P = 0.005) in the intervention group

(Continued)

Study	Design	Subjects	Intervention	Duration	Results
Nordøy et al. (2000) (220)	Randomized, placebo-controlled, double-blind	41 subjects with combined hyperlipemia	Intervention: 20 mg simvastatin + 4 g/day EPA + DHA; Control: 20 mg simvastatin + corn oil	5 wk	Tissue factor pathway inhibitor antigen: ↓ in the n-3 FAs group ($P < 0.05$) Factor VIIa: ↓ in the n-3 FAs group;($P < 0.05$) during postprandial hyperlipemia
Finnegan et al. (2003) (221)	Randomized, placebo-controlled double-blind, parallel	150 moderately hyperlipidemic subjects	Intervention: 0.8 or 1.7 g/day EPA + DHA; 4.5 or 9.5 g/day ALA; Control: placebo capsules	6	Factors VIIa, VIIc, VIIag, XIIa, XIIag, fibrinogen concentrations, plasminogen activator inhibitor-1: No effects
Lindman et al. (2004) (222)	Randomized, controlled, 2 × 2 factorial	219 subjects with long-standing hyperlipidemia	Intervention: dietary advice + placebo; VLC n-3; VLC n-3 + dietary advice; Control: corn oil	6	FVIIag and FVIIa: ↓ 5.1% and 2.4 mU/ml, respectively, in the diet intervention group TG: ↓ in the VLC n-3 group ($P = 0.01$)
Seierstad et al. (2005) (223)	Randomized, controlled, double-blind, parallel	60 patients with angiographically verified CHD	700 g/wk differently fed salmon: 100% fish oil diet provides 2.9 g/day marine n-3 FAs; 50% fish oil/50% rapeseed oil diet provides 1.5 g/day marine n-3; 100% rapeseed oil diet provides 0.5 g/day marine n-3 FAs	1.5	sVCAM-1: ↓ from 447 to 391 ng/mL ($P < 0.001$) in the 100% fish oil diet group IL-6: ↓ from 4.38 to 2.98 ng/mL ($P = 0.053$) in the 100% fish oil diet group TNF-α: ↓ from 2.03 to 1.77 ng/mL ($P = 0.057$) in the 100% fish oil diet group Lipids: 100% fish oil group: TG ↓ from 1.75 to 1.27 mmol/L ($P = 0.002$); HDL-C ↑ from 1.22 to 1.32 mmol/L ($P = 0.042$)
Hjerkinn et al. (2005) (224)	Randomized, controlled	563 men with long-standing hyperlipidemia	Intervention: 2.4 g/day n-3 FAs; 2.4 g/day n-3 FAs + dietary counseling; dietary counseling+placebo; Control: no dietary counseling and placebo	36	sICAM-1: dietary counseling group: ↓ concentration ($P < 0.001$); n-3 FAs group: ↓ concentration ($P < 0.001$) sTM: dietary counseling group: ↓ concentration ($P = 0.004$); n-3 FAs group: ↓ concentration ($P = 0.006$) tPAag: dietary counseling group: ↓ concentration ($P < 0.001$)

Effect on heart rate and arrhythmia

Study	Design	Subjects	Intervention	Duration	Results
Christensen et al. (1996) (225)	Randomized, placebo-controlled, double-blind	49 patients with previous MI and had a ventricular ejection fraction below 0.40	Intervention: 5.2 g/day n-3 FAs Control: olive oil	3	Mean RR interval (ms): Intervention group: ↑ from 807 to 825 Control group: ↑ from 823 to 827 Standard deviation of all normal RR intervals in 24 hr Holter recording (ms): Intervention group: ↑ from 115 to 124 ($P = 0.04$ within group, $P = 0.01$ compared with control)

TABLE 7 Randomized Controlled Clinical Trials of Fish Oil, EPA + DHA or Fatty Fish Consumption and Coronary Endpoints

Study (yr)	Design	Patients	Regimen	Follow-up (months)	Results
Singer et al. (2004) (226)	Randomized, placebo-controlled, double-blind	65 patients with cardiac arrhythmias without CHD or heart failure	Intervention: 3 g/day fish oil Control: olive oil	6	Incidence of APC: Fish oil group: ↓ 46.9% ($P<0.01$) Incidence of VPC: ↓ 67.8% ($P<0.01$) Incidence of couplets: ↓ 71.8% ($P<0.01$)
Calò et al. (2005) (227)	Randomized, open-label, parallel	160 patients undergoing coronary artery bypass graft surgery (CABG)	Intervention: 2 g/day n-3 PUFA	5 days before surgery until discharged	Postoperative AF: Intervention group: 15.2% (12 of 79); control group: 33.3% (27 of 81) ($P = 0.013$) Length of hospital stay: Intervention group: 7.3 ± 2.1 days; control group: 8.2 ± 2.6 days ($P = 0.017$)
Raitt et al. (2005) (228)	Randomized, placebo-controlled, double-blind, multicenter	200 patients with an implantable cardioverter defibrillator (ICD) and a history of sustained ventricular tachycardia (VT) or ventricular fibrillation (VF).	Intervention: 1.8 g/day fish oil Control: placebo	Median: 24	Percentage of patients in each group had ICD therapy for VT/VF at 6, 12, and 24 months: Fish oil group: 46%, 51% and 65%, Control group: 36%, 41% and 59%; Recurrent VT/VF events: More common in the intervention group ($P<0.001$)

Effects on cardiovascular events

Study (yr)	Design	Patients	Regimen	Follow-up (months)	Results
Burr et al. (1989) (229)	Randomized, controlled, multicenter	2033 men recovered from MI	Intervention: fish advice at 200–400 g fatty fish twice weekly; fat advice at 30% of fat as total energy; fiber advice at 18 g/day intake of cereal	24	All-cause mortality: Fatty fish group has a 29% reduction compared with others Incidence of reinfarction and death: No difference in all three groups

Study	Design	Population	Intervention	Duration	Results
GISSI et al. (1999) (60)	Randomized, controlled, open-label, multicenter, factorial 2 × 2	11,324 patients with recent MI	Intervention: 0.3 g/day EPA + 0.6 g/day DHA; synthetic α-tocopherol: 300 IU/day; both; Control: none	42	Death, nonfatal MI, and nonfatal stroke (RR): Two way analysis: 0.90 [0.82–0.99] ($P = 0.048$). Four way analysis: 0.85 [0.74–0.98] ($P = 0.053$) Cardiovascular death, nonfatal MI, and nonfatal stroke (RR): Two way analysis: 0.89 [0.80–1.01] ($P = 0.023$) Four way analysis: 0.80 [0.68–0.95] ($P = 0.008$),
Burr et al. (2003) (230)	Randomized, controlled	3114 men with angina	Intervention: advised to eat twice fatty fish per week, or to take three fish oil per day; advised to eat more fruit, vegetables and oats; both; control: no advice	36–108	Cardiac death (RR): Fish advice group 1.26 [1.00–1.58] ($P = 0.047$) Sudden cardiac death: Fish advice group 1.54 [1.06–2.23] (↑$P = 0.025$)

Abbreviations: EPA, eicosapentaenoic acid; DHA, docosahexaenoic acid; CHD, coronary heart disease; TG, triglyceride; OR, odds ratio; CAD, coronary artery disease; TC, total cholesterol; LDL-C, low-density lipoprotein cholesterol; HDL-C, high-density lipoprotein cholesterol; VLDL-C, very-low-density lipoprotein cholesterol; RR, relative risk; TXB_2, thromboxane B_2; PAF, platelet activating factor; MDA, malondialdehyde; IL-6, interleukin 6; TNF-α, Tumor necrosis factor-α; APC, atrial premature complexes; VPC, ventricular premature complexes; MI, myocardial infarction; PTCA, percutaneous transluminal coronary angioplasty; AF, atrial fibrillation; BP, blood pressure; CABG, coronary artery bypass graft surgery; CV, cardiovascular; GISSI, Gruppo Italiano Studio della Sopravvivenza nell'Infarto miocardico; ICAM, intercellular adhesion molecule; ICD, implantable cardioverter defibrillator; NIDDM, non–insulin dependent diabetes mellitus; VCAM, vascular cell adhesion molecule; VF, ventricular fibrillation; VT, ventricular tachy cardia; CRF, chronic renal failure; (CVD) cardiovascular disease; DB double blind; FA, fatty acid; FMD, flow-mediated dilation; FO, fish oil; SA, safflower oil; PCOOH, phosphatidylcholine hydroperoxide; TBARS, thiobarbituric acid reacting substances; TM, thrombomodulin; VWF, von Willebrand factor.

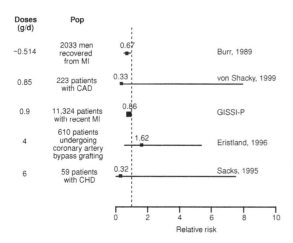

FIGURE 3 Effects of fish/fish oil supplements on fatal-MI.

capsules accounted largely for the excess risk. The most recent Cochrane Review does not recommend increased *n*-3 fatty acids (from both marine and plant sources) intake for angina patients without an MI (234).

A recent systematic review that was conducted by Studer et al. (235) compared lipid-intervention trials (statins, fibrates, resins, niacin, *n*-3 fatty acids, and diet) with regards to mortality from all, cardiac, and moncardiovascular causes. RRs for overall mortality in statins and *n*-3 fatty acids were 0.87 (95% CI, 0.81–0.94) and 0.77 (95% CI, 0.63–0.94), respectively, for the intervention compared with the control. The RRs were further reduced (0.78 in statins and 0.68 in *n*-3 fatty acids) with respect to cardiac mortality. They concluded that statins and *n*-3 fatty acids are the most potent lipid interventions in terms of reducing the risks of overall and cardiac mortality. This review included the Lyon Diet Heart Study (236) and some trials that were done by Singh; hence the results may differ produced if these trials are excluded. The heterogeneous tests for *n*-3 fatty acids were significant and primarily due to one trial (230). After excluding that trial, the heterogeneities were substantially reduced and the RRs for overall mortality and cardiac deaths were 0.75 (95% CI, 0.65–0.87), and 0.68 (95% CI, 0.52–0.90), respectively.

Effects on Progression of Atherosclerosis, Restenosis After Percutaneous Transluminal Coronary Angioplasty (PTCA)

Some evidence, albeit inconsistent, from controlled clinical studies supports the hypothesis that fish oil has a protective role in coronary atherosclerosis. Sacks et al. performed the first clinical trial (189) to examine this hypothesis in 59 patients with angiographically documented

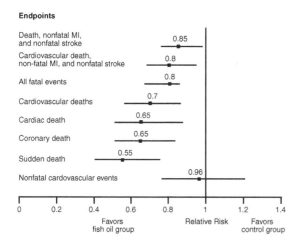

FIGURE 4 Effects of *n*-3 fatty acids on cardiac events and all fatal events in the GISSI trial. *Source*: from Ref. 232

CHD. After two years of fish oil supplementation (6 g/day n-3 fatty acids: 12.1 g capsule daily each contains 240 mg of EPA, 260 mg of DHA, and 100 mg of D-penicillanium), neither the mean minimal diameter of atherosclerotic coronary arteries ($P = 0.6$) nor the percent stenosis increase ($P = 0.8$) showed beneficial effects compared with the control group. In contrast, Eritsland et al. (190) found a beneficial effect. In this study, 610 patients undergoing coronary artery bypass grafting were given 3.3 g/day of EPA + DHA for one year to test graft patency as the primary endpoint. The OR for vein graft occlusion rates was 0.77 (95% CI, 0.60–0.99; $P = 0.05$) in the fish oil group versus the control group. But, recently, von Schacky et al. tested the antiatherogenic effects of fish oil concentrate in 223 patients with angiographically proven coronary artery disease and reported no statistically significant beneficial effect ($P > 0.10$) for changes in luminal diameter assessed by coronary angiography. In this study, 6 g/day of fish oil was provided for three months and then, 3 g/day for 21 months (192).

An earlier large trial (237) failed to demonstrate a reduction in the rate of restenosis after PTCA by 8 g/day supplemental omega-3 fatty acids. Similarly, in the EMPAR Study (Fish Oils and Low-Molecular-Weight Heparin for the Reduction of Restenosis After PTCA), 5.4 g n-3 fatty acids or plaubel patients were given before and after PTCA to 814 patients, and there was no reported reduction of PTCA restenosis (191). The Coronary Angioplasty Restenosis Trial (CART) showed the same trends on the incidence of restenosis when patients were supplemented with 5.1 g/day of n-3 fatty acids placebo patients for six months, started at least two weeks prior to coronary angioplasty (193). In contrast, a more recent trial started giving n-3 fatty acids (3 g/day of EPA and 2.1 g/day of DHA) to subjects one month before PTCA and continued for one more month, and reported a small but significant decrease in the restenosis rate compared with placebo (196). An earlier meta-analysis (238) concluded that fish oil supplementation reduced restenosis after coronary angioplasty. The ARHQ report demonstrated that there was an overall trend for a net reduction in coronary artery restenosis with fish oil supplementation, although the responses were variable (Fig. 5) (241).

Possible Mechanisms of Action

The mechanisms by which fish oil decreases the risk of subsequent coronary events, principally in patients who have had an MI, remain unclear. However, evidence suggests that there are multiple mechanisms that contribute to the effects noted, although a decrease in arryhythmia seems to account predominantly for the cardioprotective effect.

Arrhythmias

The primary beneficial effect of fish oil supplements appears to be antiarrhythmic. The decrease observed in all-cause mortality in the GISSI-Prevenzione trial (60) was mainly due to a reduction in sudden death. In the DART study (229), there was 29% reduction in all-cause mortality whereas there was no reduction in nonfatal MI. A previous study (249) of 334 patients who had experienced a primary cardiac arrest concluded that dietary intake of marine-derived n-3 polyunsaturated fatty acids (PUFA) was related to a reduced risk of primary cardiac arrest. In addition, the PHS (180) reported that the RR of sudden death was 0.48 (95% CI, 0.24–0.96; $P = 0.04$) for subjects who consumed one or more fish meals per week compared with those who consumed fish less than once per month.

Fish oil supplementation (4.3 g/day of EPA + DHA) (225) or one fish meal per week (250) increased heart rate variability in patients who survived an MI. Furthermore, Singer and Wirth (226) reported a reduced incidence of atrial and ventricular premature complexes in patients with cardiac arrhythmias who did not have CHD or heart failure. Calo et al. (227) found that the incidence of atrial fibrillation after coronary artery bypass graft surgery (CABG) was reduced after 850 to 882 mg/day of EPA+DHA consumption. However, a recent clinical trial in patients ($n = 200$) with an implantable cardioverter defibrillator (ICD) and a recent episode of sustained ventricular tachycardia (VT) or ventricular fibrillation (VF) did not find a beneficial effect on the incidence of VT or VF after two years of fish oil (1.8 g/day) or placebo (228). In the subset of patients that had an episode of sustained VT prior to enrollment, there was a significantly greater number of VT or VF events in the treatment group as against the control group, suggesting that fish oil could be proarrhythmic in this population. However, there was no increase in the risk of death for subjects taking fish oil. Based on this evidence, many are recommending that individuals with an ICD and a history of VT or VF not

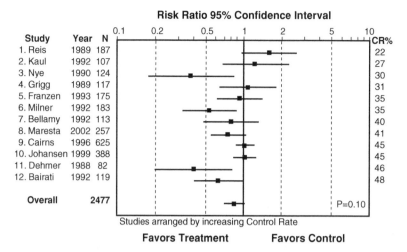

FIGURE 5 Random effects model of effect of fish oil on coronary artery restenosis following percutaneous trans-luminal coronary angioplasty. N = number of patients, except for two studies that reported number of lesions: Nye (239) had 35 patients on fish oil, 34 on control; Grigg (240) had 52 patients on fish oil, 56 on control. CR% = control rate, the restenosis rate in the control arm. *Source*: From Refs. 191, 193, 196, 239–248.

take fish oil supplements. Of note is that a recent study conducted by Leaf et al. reported that daily ingestion of fish oil by 402 patients with implanted ICDs showed antiarrhythmic benefit (251). Thus, additional research is needed in make n-3 fatty acids recommendations for patients with ICDs.

Blood Pressure
There is evidence that marine-derived *n*-3 fatty acids have a small, dose-dependent BP lowering effect (252). In a meta-analysis conducted by Morris et al. (253), of 31 placebo-controlled trials there was a significant reduction of -3.4/-2.0 mmHg in BP of hypertensive patients with 5.6 g/day of fish oil; no effect was observed for healthy subjects. Similarly, Appel et al. (254) reported a decrease of 5.5 and 3.5 mmHg in SBP and DBP in untreated hypertensive subjects who were taking more than 3 g/day of *n*-3 fatty acids. A recent meta-regression analysis (255) of 90 clinical trials reported a 1.7 and 1.5 mmHg reduction in SBP and DBP, respectively, after a median dose of 3.7 g/day of fish oil. There is one trial (216) that has evaluated a daily dose of 0.48 g of EPA + 0.12 g of Gamara linolenic acid on BP in patients with high normal DBP or Stage I hypertension, and found no significant effect.

Triglycerides
The triglyceride-lowering effect of marine-derived *n*-3 fatty acids is well established, especially in hypertriglyceridemic subjects. They have a dose-dependent triglyceride-lowering effect of about 25% to 30% for 4 g/day of *n*-3 fatty acids (256). Harris (256) also reported a 5% to 10% increase in LDL-C and a 1% to 3% increase in HDL-C in response to 4 g/day of marine-derived *n*-3 fatty acids. The GISSI-Prevenzione Study used a lower dose (1 g/day) of marine-derived *n*-3 fatty acids and found a smaller reduction (-3.4%) in triglyceride levels (60). As shown in Figure 6, the ARHQ report indicated a larger decrease in TG in subjects with higher baseline levels (241). Furthermore, there was a trend for a greater TG decrease at higher doses (Fig. 7) (241).

Inflammation, Thrombosis, and Vascular Homeostasis
n-3 fatty acids are a substrate for the *n*-3 family of eicosanoids, which exert a variety of anti-inflammatory effects. In addition, *n*-3 fatty acids suppress expression of cell adhesion molecules (257) that are part of a key biological process that promotes atherogenesis. Chin and Dart (258) suggested that dietary fish oils can improve endothelial function by reversing functional impairment of endothelium-dependent relaxation. There is evidence that marine-derived *n*-3 fatty acids enhance nitric oxide production in studies with humans (259) and animals (260).

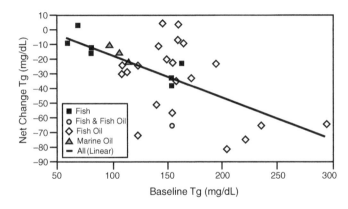

FIGURE 6 Meta-regression of baseline triglyceride (TG) level versus net changes in TG. Each point represents an individual study or study arm. Marine oils include non-fish animal sources including Minke whale and seal. Regression not adjusted for dose of omega-3 fatty acid of study size. *Source*: From Ref. 241.

This is important because nitric oxide promotes vascular homeostasis and, thereby, prevents adverse vascular atherosclerotic changes.

EPA inhibits the synthesis of thromboxane A_2 (platelet activator and vasoconstrictor) in platelets by acting as an alternative substrate, which in turn elicits an antithrombotic effect. Collagen-induced platelet aggregation is reduced significantly by a high fish diet (3.5–3.8 g/day of omega-3 fatty acids) or fish oil supplements (2.6 g/day of omega-3 fatty acids) (217,261), which favorably affects coagulation and fibrinolysis (262).

BOTANICAL AGENTS

The use of botanical dietary supplements is widespread and growing. There is limited research conducted to date on their safety and efficacy. Although there have been cardioprotective benefits reported for many botanical agents, the data are often limited because of a relatively small number of studies conducted and subjects studied. Thus, they fall short of the scientific standards required for clinical applications. Nonetheless, the available evidence for selected botanical agents (red yeast rice, garlic, ginkgo bilboa, ginseng, and tea) will be briefly discussed. As might be expected, the list of botanical agents with reported CV benefits continues to grow For example, a recent study conducted in China reported that 1g/d of Berberine administered to 63 hypercholesterolemic patients decreased TC and LDL-C by 29% ($P<0.0001$ and 25% ($P<0.001$), respectively moreover triglycerides were lowered by 35% ($P<0.0001$) (263). Abbreviated information about a variety of other botanical agents is listed in Table 8, and importantly includes adverse effects or contraindications. This is particularly important for individuals taking prescription medications and one or more botanical agents that may potentiate or antagonize the effects of the prescription drug.

Herbals on the market must meet the standard of the 1994 Dietary Supplement and Health Education Act (DSHEA), which requires the manufacturer to be responsible for the truthfulness

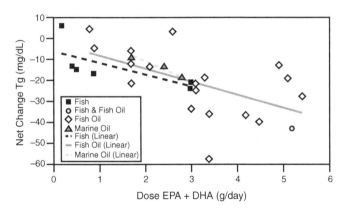

FIGURE 7 Meta-regression of dose of eicosapentenoic acid + docosahexenoic acid intake versus net change in triglyceride (TG). Each point represents an individual study or study arm. Separate simple regressions were performed for each oil source type (except for the individual study arm of combined fish and fish oil). Marine oils include non-fish animal sources including Minke whale and seal. Regression not adjusted for baseline TG or study size. *Source*: From Ref. 241.

TABLE 8   Selected Botanical Agents and Their Biological Effects on Cardiovascular Disease or CVD Risk Factors

Botanical agents	Other name(s)	Main constituent(s)	Biological effects	Adverse effects or contraindication
Arjuna bark	Terminalia arjuna	Tannins, triterpenoid saponins, flavonoids, gallic acid, ellagic acid, OPCs, phytosterols, calcium, magnesium, zinc, and copper	↓ Angina episodes; ↓ BP; improve cardiac functions	
Astragalus membranaceus	Huang-Qi	Formononetin, astraisoflavan, astrapterocarpan, 2'-3'-dihydroxy-7,4'-dimethooxyisoflavone and isoliquiritigenin	↑ Cardiac output; ↓ Heart rate	Relatively safe: 100 g/kg of the raw herb in rats with no adverse effect; LD50 of astragalus is about 40 g/kg if administer intraperitoneal injection; caution in organ transplantation, (increases T-lymphocytes, ADH inhibition)
Bitter melon or gourd	Momordica charantia		Antidiabetic activity; ↓ Cholesterol	
Black cumin seed	Nigella sativa	Thymoquinone, dithymoquinone, thymohydroquinone, thymol, carvacrol, tanethole and 4-terpineol	↓ BP (in animal studies)	
Chlorella pyrenoidosa	Chlorella	Chlorella growth factor	↓ BP; ↓ Cholesterol	
Danshen	Salvia Miltiorrhiza	Tanshinones, phenolic compounds	↓ Platelet aggregation; positive inotropic effect; dilate coronary arteries	Bleeding risk; inhibits platelet aggregation; clotting abnormalities; potentiate interaction with warfarin
European mistletoe	Viscum album	Flavonoids (quercitin, chalcone and flavone derivatives), amines, and terpenoids	↓ BP; diuretic effect; dilate arteries; cardiotonic effect; (all in animal studies)	
Fenugreek	Trigonella foenum graecum	Steroidal saponins	↓ Blood sugar; antioxidant and lipid lowering effect (in animal studies)	
Garlic	Allium sativum	Allicin	↓ Cholesterol; ↓ Platelet aggregation; anti-hypertensive; antiarrhythmic; ↓ Blood sugar	Prolonged clotting time; bleeding risk; potential interaction with warfarin
Guggul	Commiphora mukul	Guggulsterone	↓ Cholesterol; ↓ TG; ↓ LDL oxidation	Diarrhea, mild nausea, headache
Ginger	Zingiber officinale	Zingiberene and bisabolene	↓ Platelet aggregation; ↓ Cholesterol (in animal studies)	Flatulence; heartburn; potential interaction with warfarin

Common name	Scientific name	Constituents	Effects	Cautions/interactions
Ginkgo biloba		Flavonoids (quercetin, kaempferol, and isorhamnetin); terpenoids (ginkgolides A, B, and C and bilobalide)	Antioxidant; improvement in intermittent claudication; ↓ PAF-induced platelet aggregation	Potential interaction with aspirin or ibuprofen; contraindication for individuals with hypersensitivity to the plant or its products; stop taking ginkgo 36 hr before surgery to avoid the chance of bleeding
Ginseng	Ginseng radix	Panax ginseng: ginsenosides; Siberian ginseng: eleutherosides	Hypoglycemic activity; prevention of diabetes mellitus	Bleeding risk; decreased platelet aggregation; potential interaction with warfarin; panax ginseng: reported diuretic resistance; caution in organ transplantation (increased NK cell and CMI by panax ginseng and increased T-lymphocytes by siberian ginseng); should be avoided in children and in patients with hypertension, asthma, inflammation, infections with high fever, headaches, heart palpitations, insomnia, psychological imbalances, and pregnancy
Globe artichoke	Cynara scolymus	Coumarins, flavonoids, bitter lactones, and plant phenolic acid derivatives	↓ Cholesterol	Contraindication for those with bile duct obstruction
Garcinia cambogia	Citrin, gambooge	Hydroxycitric acid	↓ Fat synthesis (in animal studies)	
Hawthorne	Crataegus laevigata; crataegus oxycantha and monogyna	Flavonoids, catechins, triterpene saponins, amines, and OPCs	↑ Cardiac output; dilate coronary blood vessels; protection from ischemia; anti-arrhythmia (animal studies); ↓ Blood pressure	Nausea; headache; palpitations; may potentiate the effect of cardiac glycosides
Indian snakeroot	Rauwolfia serpentina	Ajmaline	↓ BP; antiarrhythmic effect	Severe hypertension if used with sympathomimetics; hypotension, depression; digoxin potentiates neuroleptics
Inula racemosa	Pushkarmoola	Alantolactone, isoalantolactone, dihydroalantolactone, and dihydroisoalantolactone	↓ Cholesterol; ↓ TG; improvement shown in ECG	
Ma huang	Ephedra sinica	Ephedrine	Promote weight loss	Headache; irritability tachycardia, hypertension; risk of MI, arrhythmia, and CVA; increased sympathomimetic effects with ephedrine, caffeine
Olive leaf	Olea Africana; Olea Europea	Oleuropein (a complex structure of flavonoids, esters, and multiple iridoid glycosides)	↓ BP; dilate arteries; antioxidant	

(Continued)

TABLE 8 Selected Botanical Agents and Their Biological Effects on Cardiovascular Disease or CVD Risk Factors

Botanical agents	Other name(s)	Main constituent(s)	Biological effects	Adverse effects or contraindication
Onion	Allium cepa	Sulphur containing volatile oil, and allyl propyl disulphide	↓ Blood sugar	Flatulence
Red yeast rice	Monascus purpureus	Monacolin K, sterols, isoflavones, isoflavone glycosides, and monounsaturated fatty acids	↓ Cholesterol; ↓ TG	One case reported rhabdomyolysis in a renal transplant recipient
Terminalia arjuna	Myrobalan	Tannins, triterpenoid saponins, flavonoids, gallic acid, ellagic acid, OPCS, phytosterols, calcium, magnesium, zinc, and copper	↑ Cardiac muscle function; ↓ Anginal episodes	
Tea	Camellia sinensis	Polyphenols, caffeine, alkaloids	↓ Cholesterol (in animal studies); ↓ Lipid oxidation	Excessive consumption of tea can cause typical caffeine effects; short term consumption may increase BP; End-Stage renal disease patients should not drink tea because it of high potassium content; potential interaction with warfarin
Yarrow	Achillea wilhelmsii	Flavonoids; sesquiter-penelactone	↓ BP; ↓ Cholesterol; ↓ TG; ↑HDL-C	

Abbreviations: CVD, cardiovascular disease; BP, blood pressure; TG, triglyceride; HDL-C, high-density lipoprotein-cholesterol; LDL, low-density lipoprotein-cholesterol; ECG, electrocardiogram; PAF, platelet-activating factor; NK, natural killer; CMI, cell-mediated immunity; ADH, antidiuretic hormone; CVA, cerebrovascular accident; MI, myocardial infarction; OPCS, oligomeric proanthocyanidins.

of claims made on the label, and to have evidence that the claims are supported. In contrast, drugs are regulated by the Federal Food, Drug and Cosmetic Act for efficacy and safety. Under DSHEA, a claim can be made about how a product affects the structure or function of the body. However, there can be no claim made about the prevention or treatment of a specific disease by the nutrient/herbal supplement. The manufacturer is responsible for product safety and quality control. Because of lack of rigorous regulatory oversight and a robust scientific evidence base for herbal products, clinicians should not prescribe or recommend such products to their patients (264). It is important, however, to inquire about herbal use to all patients, especially when unexplained health problems are present (264). Clinicians are in a unique position to inform patients about the potential hazards associated with the use of certain herbal products (264).

Chinese Red Yeast Rice (*Monascus purpureus*)

Red yeast rice, which is a traditional food in Asia, is produced by fermenting white rice with red yeast (*M. purpureus*). Monacolin K is the primary active ingredient in red yeast rice; in addition, *n*-3 fatty acids, isoflavones, plant sterols, and polyketides (monocolins) are also important components of red yeast rice. Monacolin K inhibits 3-hydroxy-3-methylglutaryl coenzyme A (HMG-CoA) reductase activity. Endo (265) reported that monacolin, in part, accounts for the cholesterol-lowering effect.

Animal and human studies (266–269) conducted in China have shown that consumption of red yeast rice reduces cholesterol by 11% to 32% and TG by 12% to 19%. Wang et al. (268) conducted a study in 324 hypercholesterolemic subjects who were given 1.2 g/day of Xuezhikang (which is a traditional Chinese Medical preparation of red yeast rice) for eight weeks. There was a 23% reduction in cholesterol levels, 37% decrease in TG, and a 20% increase in HDL-C. In another study, 101 hypercholesterolemic patients were given red yeast rice with 10 to 13 mg of monacolins (269), and similar results were reported.

In a double-blind, placebo-controlled clinical trial conducted in the United States, Heber et al. (270) evaluated the cholesterol-lowering effects of a 2.4 g/day red-yeast-rice supplement in 83 subjects with hyperlipidemia (TC, 5.28–8.74 mmol/L; LDL-C, 3.31–7.16 mmol/L; TG, 0.62–2.78 mmol/L; and HDL-C, 0.78–2.46 mmol/L). After eight weeks, there was a significant reduction in TC in the red yeast rice treatment group versus placebo (6.57 ± 0.93 mmol/L to 5.38 ± 0.80 mmol/L; $P < 0.001$). LDL-C was decreased by 17% and TG decreased by 12%; no changes were noted for HDL-C.

Garlic (*Allium sativum*)

Lipid-lowering effect: Both animal and humans studies have demonstrated lipid-lowering effects of garlic, which may be due to inhibition of HMG-CoA activity (271) and enhanced lipolysis of TG (272). In a meta-analysis, Warshafsky et al. evaluated the effects of garlic on total serum cholesterol in hypercholesterolemic individuals (>200 mg/dL) (273). Subjects treated with garlic (doses varied from 600 to 900 mg/day for the powder preparations and 1000 mg/day "dry weight of the active garlic components" for the aqueous extract) versus placebo had a 23 mg/dL reduction in TC (95%CI, 17–29 mg/dL; $P < 0.001$). A more recent meta-analysis of 13 randomized, double-blind, and placebo-controlled trials reported that garlic (daily dose ranged from 10 to 900 mg) significantly reduced TC ($P < 0.01$) by -0.41 mmol/L (95% CI, -0.66 to -0.15 mmol/L) (274). Moreover, a pooled analysis described in the AHRQ report indicated that LDL-C (range 0–13.5 mg/dL) and TG (range 7.6–34.0 mg/dL) were significantly reduced after three months of garlic consumption (with various garlic preparations) (275).

Ginkgo biloba

The *G. biloba* extract EGb 761 that is obtained from green leaves of the *G. biloba* tree contains a mixture of active compounds including flavonoids and terpenoids. The most common application of *G. biloba* is for the treatment of cerebrovascular and peripheral vascular diseases (276). In a meta-analysis of clinical trials, ginkgo extract was found to be effective in the treatment of cerebral insufficiency (277). Several clinical trials (278–282) reported beneficial effects of ginkgo extract (ranging from 40 mg/day to 320 mg/day) in patients with peripheral vascular disorder. Pittler and Ernst found that 120 mg or 160 mg daily dose of *G. biloba* extract significantly increased pain-free walking distance (weighted mean difference: 34 meters, 95% CI: 26–43 meters) for patients with intermittent claudication after *G. biloba* treatment (283). In another clinical trial (281) higher doses (*G. biloba* extract: 240 mg/day) increased pain-free walking distance compared with the lower doses (*G. biloba* extract: 120 mg/day).

Ginseng

American ginseng (*Panax quinquefolius*), Korean or Asian ginseng (*Panax ginseng*), and Siberian ginseng (*Eleutherococcus senticosus*) are derived from the roots of several species of plants. Ginseng is traditionally used as a tonic in oriental medicine and is also one of the top-selling herbal products in the United States. Chronic and acute hypoglycemic effects of ginseng have been reported in several studies (284–286). Ginseng therapy (100 or 200 mg for placebo for eight weeks) in 36 subjects with non–insulin-dependent diabetes mellitus (NIDDM) reduced fasting blood glucose (FBG) and the higher dose improved glycated hemoglobin (284). An acute oral glucose (25 g) challenge in the presence (3 g) or absence of ginseng was given to nine subjects with Type-2 diabetes mellitus and 10 healthy subjects (285). There was a significant reduction ($P < 0.05$) in incremental glycemia at 45 (1.7 ± 1.2 mmol/L vs. 2.8 ± 1.0 mmol/L, $P < 0.05$) and 60 minutes (0.1 ± 0.8 mmol/L vs. 0.8 ± 1.1 mmol/L, $P < 0.05$) compared with the placebo. Another short-term study has reported similar results, but in healthy individuals (286).

Tea (Camellia sinensis)

Tea made from the leaves of the plant *C. sinensis*, is one of the most common drinks in the world. It is a very good source of flavonoids, which are known for their antioxidant properties (287). Several epidemiologic studies have reported an inverse relationship between tea intake and risk of CVD (288–290) while others found no effects or even an adverse effect (291–293). The mechanisms that have been proposed to explain the beneficial effects include: inhibition of lipid peroxidation by the numerous polyphenolic compounds (294); upregulation of the LDL receptor resulting in favorable effects on LDL-C levels (295); and increased fecal bile acids and cholesterol excretion (296).

In an epidemiologic study of 9856 men and 10,233 women without a history of CVD or diabetes, serum cholesterol levels were lower (9.3 mg/dL for men and 5.8 mg/dL for women) in those who drank five or more cups of tea per day as against those who did not drink or drank less than one cup of tea (297). In addition, SBP was inversely related to tea consumption. Hertog et al. (298) examined the relationship between dietary intake of flavonoids (61% came from tea) and heart disease in 12,763 middle-aged men from seven countries. Flavonoid content of the diet was inversely correlated with the risk of CHD death and risk of nonfatal heart attack. A recent meta-analysis (299) assessed the relationship between tea consumption and stroke, MI, and all CHD in 10 cohort studies and seven case–control studies. Tea consumption (three cups per day vs. no tea) was associated with an 11% reduction in MI (RR, 0.89; 95% CI: 0.79–1.01). However, this study found that the risk for CHD in the United Kingdom and for stroke in Australia increased with increasing tea consumption, whereas risk decreased in Europe. One explanation is that the addition of milk to tea could result in milk proteins binding flavonoids (300), thereby attenuating their antioxidant effects (301).

Controlled clinical studies have evaluated the effects of tea consumption on lipids and lipoproteins in subjects with mild to moderate hypercholesterolemia. In a controlled clinical study (302), five servings/day of black tea reduced TC by 6.5% and LDL-C by 11% in moderately hypercholesterolemic adults. Interestingly, in this study, oxidative status was not affected by tea consumption. In a larger randomized controlled clinical trial (240 subjects with mild to moderate hypercholesterolemia), consumption (for 12 weeks) of a daily capsule containing 375 mg of theaflavin-enriched green tea extract lowered total cholesterol by 11%, LDL-C by 16%, HDL-C by 2% and TG by 3% (303). Collectively, the results of the clinical studies suggest that tea is an effective adjunct to a blood cholesterol-lowering diet.

OTHER NUTRITION SUPPLEMENTS AND CVD RISK
Coenzyme Q10

Coenzyme Q10 (ubiquinone), a lipid soluble provitamin, is an indispensable component of the respiratory chain in mitochondria, which provides ATP. Coenzyme Q10 also has important antioxidant functions. Although the clinical studies of coenzyme Q10 evaluated different cardiovascular endpoints, most results are limited because of the lack of tight control, unblinded study designs and number of subjects studied. The most recent AHRQ Report summarized study results on coenzyme Q10 supplements only in a narrative way because of the different study designs employed and outcomes measured to justify statistical pooling for meta-analysis. The selected studies described in the AHRQ Report each had at least 55 subjects and lasted for at least six months. The dose of coenzyme Q10 ranged from 100 to 300 mg/day. The selected studies evaluated the effects of coenzyme Q10 on heart failure, IHD, acute MI. Four of these studies showed either no (304,305) or a small clinical improvement in the endpoints measured [i.e., volume load (increased 8.7%); maximal exercise capacity (increased 6.4%) (306); QT interval (no prolongation after acute MI) (307)]. The results from two other studies reported improvements in clinical outcomes, including heart functional class (decrease of the patients in New York Heart Association class III) (308) and clinical symptoms (pulmonary edema, cardiac asthma and "arrhythmia appearance") (309).

A reduction in plasma coenzyme Q10 concentrations is thought to promote myotoxicity, an adverse effect that sometimes accompanies high-dose statin therapy. Statins primarily inhibit HMG CoA reductase and thus block the conversion from HMG CoA to mevalonate, a precursor of both cholesterol and coenzyme Q10. While it is clear that circulating coenzyme Q10 levels are decreased with statin therapy in many case–control studies, it is not clear whether tissue levels are affected. Furthermore, it has not been established that coenzyme Q10 supplementation increases tissue levels even though blood levels are increased. As recently reviewed by Nawarskas, there is insufficient evidence to support routine use of coenzyme Q10 as a means to prevent myotoxicity that can accompany statin therapy.

In summary, at this time there is insufficient evidence to justify recommending coenzyme Q10 supplements for CVD patients as well as those taking statin drugs.

Plant Stanols/Sterols

Plant-derived sterols are structurally similar to cholesterol. The most abundant plant sterols are sitosterol, campesterol, and stigmasterols. Stanols are saturated sterols that lack a delta, 5 double bond in their B-rings. Vegetable oils, nuts, soybeans, and seeds contain sterols. Plant sterols exist either in the free form or in combination with glycosides-or as esters with fatty acids. They displace intestinal cholesterol from the micelles, thereby reducing intestinal cholesterol absorption and blood cholesterol levels. To achieve a clinically meaningful cholesterol-lowering effect, a dosage of 2 g/day is needed. It is important to note that this level of intake is attainable only by consuming stanol or a supplement. The current recommendation of the National Cholesterol Education Program (NCEP) Adult Treatment Panel III (ATP III) is 2 g/day plant sterols/stanols as a therapeutic option to enhance LDL-C lowering effect. This recommendation is based on studies that show no further significant cholesterol lowering at doses higher than 2 to 3 g/day (Fig. 8) (311–316). Moreover, the majority of studies (Tables 9 and 10) (317–334) have shown that the LDL-C and TC-lowering effects are comparable irrespective of whether stanol or sterol is fed in either the free or the esterified form.

Stanols/Sterols-Statins

There is some evidence that stanols and/or sterols intake further improve cholesterol-lowering response to statin therapy. In a multicenter study (335), subjects with primary hypercholesterolemia (206 mg/dL) were randomized to four treatment groups: placebo plus regular margarine 25 g; placebo plus sterol-ester margarine (25 g/day; 2 g of plant sterol); cerivastatin (4000 μg plus 25 g/day regular margarine); and cerivastatin (400 μg plus 25 g/day sterol-ester margarine with 2 g of plant sterol). After four weeks, LDL-C was significantly reduced by 32% in the cerivastatin group (versus placebo) and by 8% in the sterol-ester margarine group (versus regular margarine). The combination of sterol-ester margarine plus cerivastatin lowered LDL-C by 39%, which is approximately additive to the independent treatment effects observed. Two other small studies (120,125) also demonstrated additive effects of stanol and statin on LDL-C lowering.

In the study conducted by Blair et al. (336) with a larger population 67 women and 100 men on statin therapy, doses of stains were not stated but with elevated LDL-C (130 mg/dL

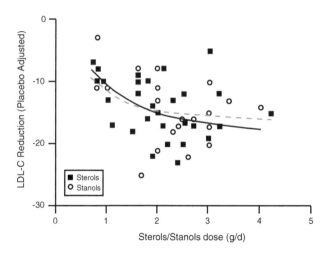

FIGURE 8 Effect of phytosterols on LDL-cholesterol lowering. Dashed curve is created for sterols studies using nonlinear regression with equation of one phase exponential association. Solid curve is created for stanols studies using the same method. *Source*: Data adapted from Ref. 310.

and above, subjects were given 5.1 g/day of plant stanol esters or placebo. Plant stanol esters reduced TC by 12% and LDL-C by 17% compared with 5% and 7% for the placebo, respectively. These results demonstrate that stanols can further reduce LDL-C beyond that achieved by statin therapy.

Conjugated Linoleic Acid

Conjugated linoleic acid (CLA) is a group of positional and geometric isomers of conjugated dienoic derivatives of linoleic acid. The major dietary sources of CLA are ruminant meats such as beef and lamb, and full-fat dairy products such as whole milk and cheese. The CLA supplement used in clinical studies usually contains a mixture of *cis-9 trans*-11 (c9t11) and *trans-10cis*-12 (t10c12) isomers.

The effects of CLA on lipid and lipoprotein levels are inconsistent. Noone et al. (337) reported that 3 g/day of a c9t11-t10c12 CLA isomeric mixture taken (for eight weeks) by normolipidemic subjects reduced fasting TG concentrations by 21%. However, CLA supplementation had no effect on LDL-C, or HDL-C. In a study conducted by Moloney et al. (338), individuals with Type-2 an diabetes who were given CLA (3.0 g/day; 1:1 mixture of c9t11 and t10c12 CLA isomers) for eight weeks had an 8% increase in HDL-C; this was due to an increase in HDL_2-C. Although there was an insignificant reduction of LDL-C by 8.8%, the ratio of LDL:HDL-C was significantly reduced by 14.5%. In a study by Tricon et al. (339), three doses (for eight weeks) of two CLA isomers [highly enriched c9t11 (0.59, 1.19, and 2.38 g/day) or t10c12 (0.63, 1.26, and 2.52 g/day)] were evaluated in healthy men. Mean plasma TG concentration was increased by 8.5% during supplementation with t10c12 CLA and decreased by 4% by c9t11 CLA, although there was no dose-response effect. There was no effect of either isomer on HDL-C. LDL:HDL-C and TC:HDL-C were elevated during supplementation with t10c12 CLA (2–13.3% and 1.5–9.2%, respectively) but reduced with c9t11 CLA (4.6–6.1% and 4.1–5.2%, respectively). The key outcome for this study was the divergent lipid and lipoprotein responses to the different CLA isomers. It is to be noted that there are some reports that claim that CLA increases LDL-C (340–341), and decreases HDL-C (343–347). Thus, the different CLA "effects" may reflect the isomer of mixture used in the study.

Arginine

Endothelial cell-derived nitric oxide plays an important role in the maintenance of vascular health. Inhibition of endothelial nitric oxide production leads to vasoconstriction and increases in adhesion molecule expression and smooth muscle cell proliferation. Since L-arginine is a substrate for the synthesis of nitric oxide, numerous studies have investigated the relationship between L-arginine intake and vasodilation and endothelial function.

Endothelial function can be assessed by measuring vascular tone. Brachial artery dilation in response to vasodilator stimuli and forearm blood flow provides a measure of endothelial health. Clinical trials of arginine supplementation have been conducted using randomized, placebo-controlled, double-blind, crossover or parallel designs in different population groups

TABLE 9 Randomized Controlled Trials of Stanol Effects on Total Cholesterol and Low-Density Lipoprotein Cholesterol

Selected studies	Stanols dosage	Total subject	Design	Stanols duration	TC changes (vs. control)	LDL-C changes (vs. control)
Miettinen et al. (317)	2.6 g/day or 1.8 g/day[a]	153	RCT, DB,[b]	1 yr	−10.3%	−13%
Gylling et al. (318)	3 g/day [a]	22	RCT, DB,[c]	7 wk	−8%	−15%
Plat et al. (319)	3.8 g/day (V)[a]	36	RCT, DB,[b]	8 wk	−8.6%	−14.6%
	4.0 g/day (W)[a]	34		8 wk	−8.1%	−12.8%
Hallikainen et al. (320)	2.2 g/day (V)[a]	20	RCT, DB,[b]	8 wk	−8.1%	−8.6%
	2.34 g/day (W)[a]	18		8 wk	−10.6%	−13.7%
Mensink et al. (321)	1.0 g/day[a]	60	RCT, DB,[b]	4 wk	−8.7%	−13.7%
Spilburg et al. (322)	0.625 g/day[d]	24	RCT, DB,[b]	4 wk	−10.1%	−14.3%
Cater et al. (323)	3 g/day[a]	13	RCT, DB,[c]	6 wk	−10%	−13%
Thuluva et al. (324)	2.0 g/day[e]	15	RCT, DB,[b]	4 wk	−11.8%	−11.7%

[a]Esterified form
[b]Parallel design
[c]Crossover design; V, vegetable-based stanols; W, wood-based stanols
[d]Non-esterified form
[e]Not specified in papers
Abbreviations: TC, total cholesterol; LDL-C, low-density lipoprotein cholesterol; RCT, randomized controlled trial; DB, double bind

(Table 11) (348–354). Some studies reported vasodilation in response to 3 to 20 g/day of arginine for two to four weeks (348–352) whereas others have not detected any beneficial effects (353,355).

Reductions in BP have been observed in some (356–358) but not all studies (348,353,359–363) in response to oral L-arginine supplementation. Siani et al. (356) reported a 5 to 7 mmHg reduction in both SBP and DBP in healthy subjects who consumed 10 to 14 g/day of L-arginine. A recent report by West et al. (364) found that giving L-arginine (12 g/day for three weeks) to hypercholesterolemic middle-aged men significantly decreased cardiac output (−0.4 L/m), DBP (−1.9 mmHg), and increased pre-ejection period (+3.4 msec). There is some

TABLE 10 Randomized Controlled Trials of Sterol Effects on Total Cholesterol and Low-Density Lipoprotein Cholesterol

Selected studies	Sterols dosage	Total subject	Design	Sterols duration	TC changes (vs. control)	LDL-C changes (vs. control)
Temme et al. (325)	2.075 g/day[a]	42	RCT, DB,[b]	4 wk	−7%	−10%
de Graaf et al. (326)	1.8 g/day[c]	70	RCT, DB,[d]	4 wk	−6.1%	−10.4%
Matvienko et al. (327)	2.7 g/day[e]	34	RCT, TB,[d]	4 wk	−7%	−10.3%
Mussner et al. (328)	1.82 g/day[a]	63	RCT, DB,[b]	3 wk	−3.4%	−5.4%
Cleghorn et al. (329)	2 g/day[a]	50	RCT, DB,[b]	4 wk	−4.3%	−6.8%
Hendriks et al. (330)	1.6 g/day[a]	185	RCT, DB,[d]	1 y	−4%	−6%
Varady et al. (331)	1.8 g/day[f]	84	RCT, DB,[d]	8 wk	−1.7% (E+S)	−5.4% (E+S)
Noakes et al. (328)	2.0 g/day[a]	39	RCT, SB,[b]	3 wk	−6 to −8%	−8 to −10%
Lee et al. (329)	3.2 g/day[a]	85	RCT, DB,[d]	12 wk	−5.5% (4 wk) [g]	−3.1% (4 wk) [g]
Lau et al. (330)	1.8 g/day[c]	29	RCT, DB,[b]	3 wk	−1% (DM) −1.8% (Non-DM)	−7.1% (DM) −8.4% (Non-DM)

[a]Esterified form
[b]Crossover design; S, sterols group; E, exercise group; DM, diabetes mellitus
[c]Non esterified form
[d]Parallel design
[e]Mixed form (2/3 esterified, 1/3 non-esterified form)
[f]Not specified in papers
[g]Only significant at the end of first 4 weeks
Abbreviations: TC, total cholesterol; LDL-C, low-density lipoprotein cholesterol; RCT, randomized controlled trial; SB, single bind; DB, doublebind; TB, triple bind

TABLE 11 Randomized Controlled Trials of L-Arginine Intervention and Vasodilation

Selected studies	Subjects	Dosage	Intervention duration	Design	Vasodilation (vs. baseline)
Clarkson et al. (348)	27 hypercholesterolemic subjects	21 g/day	4 wk	RCT, DB,[a]	FMD: ↑ 3.9%
Hambrecht et al. (349)	40 patients with severe heart failure	8 g/day	4 wk	RCT, DB,[b]	ACh induced vasodilation: L-arginine group: ↑ 6.6% handgrip exercise group: ↑ 6.5% combination group: ↑ 9.1% Maximal FMD: L-arginine group: ↑ 11.3% handgrip training group: ↑ 11.4% combination group: ↑ 15.5%
Lim et al. (350)	8 young cardiac transplant recipients	6 g/day	2 wk	RCT, DB,[a]	FMD: ↑ 7.5%
Boger et al. (351)	12 clinically asymptomatic, elderly subjects with elevated ADMA	3 g/day	3 wk	RCT, DB,[a]	Endothelium-dependent vasodilation: simvastatin alone (40 mg/day) no effect L-arginine: ↑ 3.8% Combination: ↑ 4.5%
Yin et al. (352)	31 stable CAD	10 g/day	4 wk	RCT, DB,[a]	FMD: L-Arginine: ↑ 4.87% VitC (500 mg/day): ↑ 3.17%
Chin-Dusting et al. (353)	26 healthy men	20 g/day	4 wk	RCT, DB,[b]	No effect on FBF responses to ACh, SNP, or L-NMMA
Blum et al. (354)	10 postmenopausal women	9 g/day	4 wk	RCT, DB,[a]	No effects on brachial artery diameters, FMD with hyperemia or nitroglycerin-induced dilation

[a]Crossover design
[b]Parallel design
Abbreviations: FMD, flow-mediated dilation; Ach, acetylcholine; FBF, forearm blood flow; CAD, coronary artery disease; SNP, sodium nitroprusside; L-NMMA, N(G)-monomethyl-L-arginine; ADMA, Asymmetric dimethylarginine; RCT, randomized controlled trial; DB, double-blind.

evidence that L-arginine (9 g/day for six months) improves coronary blood flow (149% vs. 6%) and epicardial coronary artery diameter (16% vs. −25.9%) in response to acetylcholine (ACh) (362). In a study conducted by Theilmeier et al. (365), oral L-arginine (7.0 g/day) for two weeks reduced monocyte adhesion by 53% in hypercholesterolemic subjects. Likewise, Chan et al. (366) found that oral L-arginine (14 or 21 g/day for 12 weeks) attenuated mononuclear cell adhesiveness. In the West et al. study (364), oral L-arginine did not significantly affect CRP levels. Blum et al. conducted three studies to evaluate L-arginine supplementation on soluble adhesion molecules (354,355,367). One study (367) reported that L-arginine intake (9 g/day) for three months significantly reduced plasma P-selectin (−10%), Interleukin (IL) 1-β (−31%), and IL-6 (−23%). However, the other two studies using the same dose but for only one month reported no effect of L-arginine on E-selectin, intercellular adhesion molecule-1 (ICAM-1), and vascular cell adhesion molecule-1 (VCAM-1). A recent study by Yin et al. (352) found that giving 10 g/day of L-arginine to individuals with stable coronary artery disease did not affect several circulating inflammatory markers [von Willebrand Factor (vWF), VCAM-1, ICAM-1, P-selectin and high-sensitivity C-reactive protein (hsCRP)]. The effects of arginine supplementation on platelet function and lymphocyte activation also have been evaluated. Wolf et al. (368) assessed the platelet function in conjunction with 8.4 g/day oral L-arginine supplementation for two weeks. The response to collagen-induced platelet aggregation did not differ between the treated and control groups. In another study by George et al. (369), patients with unstable angina received 6 g/day L-arginine for one month. The percentage of activated T lymphocytes (CD3+/human leukocyte antigen-DR+) was significantly increased (+43%) in the control subjects; however, in subjects given L-arginine there was a minor (approximately 5%) decrease in the number of activated T lymphocytes. A very recent paper (370) reported that when L-arginine was given (9 g/day for six months) to post-MI patients there was no improvement in vascular stiffness measurements or ejection fraction (EF). In fact, there was an increase in postinfarction mortality in the treatment group. As per this finding, the authors concluded that L-arginine should not be recommended following acute MI.

Carnitine

The primary role of carnitine is to shuttle long-chain fatty acids across the inner mitochondrial membrane for fatty acid β-oxidation and other physiological processes. Several large multicenter studies have evaluated the effects of L-carnitine treatment on heart disease endpoints. In an early multi center study (371), patients with exercise-induced stable angina were given 2 g/day of L-carnitine for six months. Compared with the control group, carnitine significantly reduced the number of premature ventricular contractions (PVC). Canale et al. (372) evaluated both healthy subjects and individuals with effort-induced angina. Participants were given 3 g/day of L-carnitine for 30 days. Compared with baseline in the L-carnitine group, there was a mean 0.5 mm improvement in ST-T segment depression in response to a bicycle ergometer exercise test. M-code echocardiography also showed beneficial changes in a number of ventricular function parameters in subjects with angina who were given an L-carnitine supplement.

In the L-Carnitine Ecocardiografia Digitalizzata Infarto Miocardico (CEDIM) trial (373), patients with a first acute MI were given 9 g/day of L-carnitine intravenously for five days and then 6 g/day orally for the next 12 months. There was no effect on death rate, ischemic events, and heart failure incidences. However, the adjusted differences for end-diastolic volume (EDV) and end-systolic volume (ESV) in the L-carnitine group were progressively improved at three months, six months, and 12 months. The results do not agree with a study performed by Iyer et al. (374) in post-MI patients who were given intravenous L-carnitine (6 g/day for the first seven days) followed by oral L-carnitine (3 g/day for three months). There were no differences in the EF, ESV and EDV observed for the two groups at admission, discharge, or after three months.

Soy Protein

Soy protein is produced from raw whole soybeans by removing the lipids and indigestible components and concentrating the protein. In addition to protein, other components include isoflavones, fiber, and saponins (375). Isoflavones, the most common form of phytoestrogens, are found in a variety of food sources, including fruits and vegetables, but are especially abundant in soy protein. Two of the major isoflavones are genistein and daidzein. Many studies have been conducted to elucidate the effects of soy protein and isoflavones on biomarkers of heart disease risk.

Lipids and Lipoproteins

In a meta-analysis of 38 controlled clinical trials, Anderson et al. (376) evaluated the effects of soy protein consumption on serum lipids and lipoproteins. The results showed that soy protein (47 g/day average) reduced TC by 9.3%; LDL-C by 12.9%; and TG by 10.5%, respectively. The changes in serum TC and LDL-C were directly related to the initial serum cholesterol concentration. The consumption of soy protein was associated with an insignificant 2.4% increase in HDL-C.

In a recent report from AHRQ, the effects of soy products on lipids and lipoproteins were systematically evaluated. The meta-analysis demonstrated that consumption of soy products had a small benefit on LDL-C and on TG (377). There was no effect on HDL-C. Among the 61 eligible studies in the AHRQ analysis, median soy protein intake was 38 g/day (14–113 g/day) and median soy isoflavone intake was 80 mg/day (10–185 mg/day). Across the studies, TC was decreased by 6 mg/dL (range, −33 to +7 mg/dL). This corresponds to a percentage change of −2.5% (−12% to +4%). Overall median change for LDC-C was −5 mg/dL (−32 to +13 mg/dL), which was equivalent to a 3% decrease (−21% to +9%).

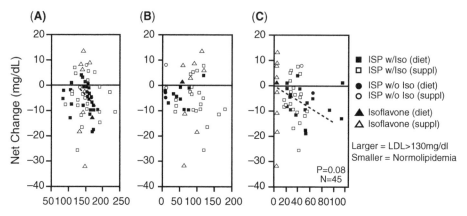

FIGURE 9 Low-density lipoprotein (LDL) change after soy products consumption. (**A**) Net change of LDL with soy product consumption compared to control, by baseline level. Isoflavone content and soy protein content. Studies without nonsoy control are not included. Studies without data on isoflavone or protein content are omitted from relevant graphs. (**B**) ISP w/Iso = soy protein with isoflavones; ISP w/o Iso = soy protein without isoflavones; suppl = supplement. (**C**) Dashed lines represent adjusted regressions for studies with sufficient data for regression. Regression lines are drawn only within the range of independent variable (*x*-axis) data examined. *P*-values and number of studies included in regressions are shown. Both regression lines drawn are for all studies with abnormal baseline LDL. *Source*: From Ref. 377.

Figure 9 (left panel) shows the changes in LDL-C levels in response to soy protein and soy isoflavones as a function of baseline LDL-C. Only soy protein at a high dose, but not soy isoflavones, decreased LDL-C significantly with a more pronounced effect in subjects with high LDL-C (Fig. 9 middle and right panel). For each additional 10 g/day of soy protein consumed, the reduction in LDL-C was 1.4 mg/dL. Soy products increased HDL-C 1 mg/dL in 56 studies, although the responses reported were highly variable (-4 to +13 mg/dL). TG was decreased by 3 mg/dL (-49 to +66 mg/dL) or 2%. An American Heart Association Science Advisory (378) that assessed the more recent work on soy protein and isoflavones concluded that LDL-C is only lowered by about 3%; in these studies (22 randomized trials; 1998–2005) soy protein intake was 50 g/day. Thus, there is a very modest effect of soy protein on LDL-C. In addition, soy isoflavones had no effect on LDL-C in the studies evaluated.

Vasodilation

There have been several clinical studies conducted to evaluate the effects of soy protein and isoflavones on vascular reactivity and BP. As noted in an AHA Science Advisory (378), soy protein has a very modest hypotensive effect (-1 mmHg SBP). Soy isoflavones did not affect BP. There is some evidence that soy isoflavones favorably affect arterial compliance (379,380) whereas other clinical studies (381–387) evaluating isoflavones (doses ranged from 54 to 118 mg/day; for 2–24 weeks) did not find significant effects on endothelial dependent or independent vasodilation. With respect to soy protein, there is some evidence that it improves endothelial function (388,391), whereas other evidence does not support a beneficial effect (390).

Inflammation Markers

In some studies, soy protein or isoflavone intake was associated with reduction in E-selectin (391), VCAM-1 (385), endothelin-1 (ET-1) (386), homocysteine (392) and an increase in nitrites/nitrates (386). However, a study performed by Jenkins et al. (393) did not find an effect of soy protein and isoflavones on markers of inflammation. No treatment differences were observed for CRP, serum amyloid A (SAA), or tumor necrosis factor–alpha (TNF-α) (393). To be noted is that a high intake of isoflavones appeared to increase serum IL-6 concentrations in women. In another study done by Steinberg et al. (387), plasma ET-1 or nitric oxide–derived products (i.e., total nitrate + nitrite concentration) did not differ among treatment groups or compared with baseline. No significant differences were observed in sVCAM-1 and soluble intracellular adhesion molecule-1 (sICAM-1) or in soluble E-selectin among the treatment groups.

DRUG–HERB INTERACTIONS

As previously discussed, herb use is prevalent in the United States (394). In addition, with the aging U.S. population requiring prescription and nonprescription medications for different medical conditions along with new treatment guidelines to decrease risk of many different diseases that recommend aggressive pharmacotherapy, many people are taking the necessary drugs. This is problematic for those who are combining certain drugs with specific herbs. In this section, the potential risks of cardiovascular pharmacotherapy and herbal interactions will be discussed. It is important for health professionals to be attentive to this because of possible adverse health effects.

Interactions with Anticoagulant Drugs or Platelet Aggregation Inhibitor Drugs

Clinical reports have demonstrated altered anticoagulation effects of warfarin when combined with herbs such as garlic, danshen, ginkgo, ginseng, green tea, and St. John's wort.

Because of the anti platelet effects of aspirin, use of these herbal supplements should be avoided. In the section that follows, much of the evidence comes from case reports rather than controlled clinical studies. While this presents limitations in providing guidance about herbal use with pharmacotherapy, the information is nonetheless of benefit to clinicians who encounter many patients who may be taking one or more herbal supplements.

Garlic

Garlic is associated with decreased platelet aggregation and prolonged bleeding episodes. One older study (395) found that 120 mg of garlic oil taken for 20 days was associated with a 9% decrease in platelet aggregation. Similar results were reported for six healthy subjects who consumed 25 mg garlic oil for five days (396). There were case reports (397,398) that garlic consumption causes postoperative bleeding and spontaneous spinal epidural hematoma. Two cases were reported of increased clotting time when warfarin and garlic extract were used (399).

Ginkgo biloba

Spontaneous bleeding may occur as the result of *G. biloba* consumption (400–405). A 33-year-old woman experienced bilateral subdural hematomas after taking 60 mg twice a day of ginkgo (402). A 72-year-old woman developed a left frontal subdural hematoma after taking 50 mg ginkgo for six months (403,404). Another patient experienced spontaneous bleeding of the anterior chamber of the eye after consuming 40 mg ginkgo twice daily for one week (405). In this case, the subject had been taking aspirin for three years. Two case reports (406,407) suggested that concomitant use of warfarin and ginkgo was associated with the development of an intracerebral hemorrhage. In addition, two case reports of a bleeding problem were associated with combined use of either aspirin (405) or ibuprofen (408) with ginkgo.

Ginseng

The International Normalized Ratio (INR, which reports the results of blood-clotting tests) was reduced in a patient taking warfarin and ginseng for five years. The patient's INR decreased from 3.1 to 1.5 after two weeks of taking ginseng and warfarin (409). In addition, when ginseng was stopped, INR returned to 3.3 within two weeks.

Green Tea

Because green tea is a great source of vitamin K, it has the potential to cause a drug interaction with warfarin. Inhibition of warfarin action by green tea has been reported (410) in a 44-year-old man who was receiving warfarin treatment. The INR decreased to about two, in response to consuming about one-half to one gallon of green tea per day for one week. After discontinuing tea drinking, the INR increased.

St. John's Wort

There is some evidence that St. John's wort increases the metabolism of warfarin by activating CYP1A2 (cytochrome P450 1A2) . A Swedish Medical Product Agency-reported (411) case shows that concomitant use of warfarin and St. John's Wort decreased the INR. A clinical trial

(411) has demonstrated that phenprocoumon, an anticoagulant chemically related to warfarin, concentration in plasma is reduced when administrated together with St. John's Wort.

Interactions with Cardiac Inotropic Drugs
Digoxin is a cardiac glycoside that can increase the contractility of the heart and thus is used in heart failure treatment.

St. John's Wort
A single-blind, placebo-controlled study in 25 healthy subjects demonstrated a decreased digoxin level after 10 days of co medication with St. John's Wort (413). There is evidence that St. John's Wort reduces efficacy of digoxin by inducing P-glycoprotein, which regulates the metabolism of digoxin.

Ginseng
A 74-year-old man who had been taking digoxin was found to have an elevated serum levels of digoxin without any toxic effects (414). The elevated levels were due to the concomitant intake of ginseng.

G. biloba
A recent randomized controlled trial (415) conducted with eight healthy human volunteers demonstrated that taking 80 mg ginkgo extract three times daily increased the area under the plasma digoxin curve by 212%.

Interactions with Statin Drugs is redunder for LDL-C Lowering
A reduction in plasma concentrations of simvastatin, but not pravastatin by repeated St. John's Wort treatment has been reported in a randomized controlled clinical trial (416). Simvastatin is metabolized to inactive metabolites by CYP3A4 in the intestinal wall and liver. The decreased concentration of simvastatin was caused by activation of CYP3A4 (the main drug-metabolizing enzyme which can be induced by St. John's Wort), which degrades simvastatin.

Interactions with Antihypertensive Drugs
Ginkgo is a peripheral vasodilator. Concomitant use of ginkgo and a thiazide diuretic results in a further decrease in BP (417). Verapamil reduces BP by inhibiting calcium ion influx into vascular smooth muscle cells. Recently, Tannergren et al. (418) reported that the bioavailability of verapamil was significantly reduced after repeated administration of St. John's Wort. Similar to simvastatin, the decrease in verapamil is possibly caused by induction of CYP3A4 by St. John's Wort.

SUPPLEMENTS RECOMMENDED FOR CVD RISK REDUCTION

As discussed herein, there is abundant evidence about the benefits of many nutrients for CVD risk reduction. There is widespread support for a food-based approach to meet nutrient needs because a dietary pattern delivers multiple nutrients/bioactive compounds and not just a single nutrient that typically targets just one CVD risk factor (419). Nonetheless, there are specific nutrient recommendations from federal agencies and health organizations with the expressed intent of targeting single CVD risk factors (Table 12). For example, nicotinic acid is recommended to increase HDL-C, and sterols/stanols are recommended as an adjunctive therapy for further reducing LDL-C. Consequently, supplements are necessary to meet certain nutrient recommendations that cannot be attained by diet exclusively. For some, physician oversight is required to monitor potential side effects. Table 12 summarizes the four nutrients that are widely recommended for the primary and secondary prevention of CVD—these include nicotinic acid, fish oil, sterols/stanols, and viscous (soluble) fiber. All of these can be gotten as a supplement or in fortified foods. Nicotinic acid and concentrated EPA and DHA are also available as a prescription drug, which in turn, requires physician oversight.

For nicotinic acid supplements, the prescription version is recommended. The main side effect of nicotinic acid is flushing. There is evidence that OTC sustained-release niacin, which contains free nicotinic acid may be hepatotoxic (130). There is a "no-flush" nicotinic acid supplement available without a prescription; however, it contains no free nicotinic acid and therefore, is not recommended for the treatment of dyslipidemia (130).

TABLE 12 Recommended Supplements/Pharmacologic Agents to Reduce CVD Risk[a]

	Biologic actions	Recommended dose for clinical benefits	Diet	Supplement/ fortified foods	Prescription drug
Niacin (nicotinic acid)	↑ HDL-C 15–35%; ↓TG 20–50%; ↓LDL-C 5–25%	Typically 1–3 g/day	Not possible to achieve clinically significant lipid/lipoprotein effects with diet only	Niacin supplements: immediate release; sustained release typically 500 mg/tablet or capsule	Crystalline nicotinic acid 1.5–3 g/day; sustained-release nicotinic acid 1–2 g/day; extended-release nicotinic acid (Niaspan®) 1–2 g/day
EPA + DHA: Primary Prevention	Antiarrhythmic; anti-inflammatory; ↓ CVD risk factors	About 500 mg/day stabilize plaque;	2 sv/fatty fish/wk	Fish oil supplement: about 110–500 mg/soft gel or packet	Omacor (840 mg/capsule: 465 mg EPA + 375 mg DHA)
Secondary Prevention		1 g/day	1 sv/fatty fish/day or fish oil supplement	Fortified foods-eggs, bread, juice, etc.	
TG lowering	↓ TG	2–4 g/day	Fish oil supplement		
Sterols/stanols	↓ LDL 6–15%	2 g/day	Not possible to achieve a clinical significant LDL-C lowering effect with diet only	Benecol: 2 softgels = 1.1 g stanol ester sterol/stanol fortified foods: margarine/spread; yogurt; orange juice; cereal bar, etc.	N/A
Viscous (soluble) fiber	↓ LDL-C 3–5% (for 5–10 g/day)	10–25 g/day	Cereal grain, fruits, vegetables, legumes (varies 1–5 g)	Psyllium (from dry seed or husk): about 4–10 g fiber/sv (powder) or 0.5–1.0 g fiber/capsule methylcellulose: about 0.5 g methylcellulose/capsule or 2 g methylcellulose/sv polycarbophil: about 500 mg polycarbophil/capsule Fortified foods-cereal, bread, etc.	N/A

[a]Physician monitoring of supplement use is recommended for all patients on an ongoing basis.
Abbreviation: CVD, cardiovascular disease; NA, not available; SV, serving.

The American Heart Association recommends two fatty fish meals per week for the primary prevention of CVD (231). This is equivalent to approximately 500 mg of EPA + DHA per day. For secondary prevention, 1 g/day is recommended. To obtain about 1 g/day, four fatty fish meals per week are required. For lowering triglyceride, a 2 to 4 g/day dose of EPA + DHA is recommended. For individuals who do not eat fish, for primary and secondary prevention, a fish oil supplement or omega-3 fortified foods are advised. For TG lowering, a fish oil supplement is required. Fish oil supplements that are available on the market contain negligible amounts of mercury and are free of other environmental contaminants (420,421). For individuals who elect to consume fish, there are FDA advisories that provide guidance for minimizing exposure to environmental contaminants. Thus, the risks associated with exposure to environmental contaminants can be minimized and the benefits of fish consumption can be realized.

Stanols/sterols are obtained from fortified foods (Table 12). Stanol ester supplements can be purchased online. With the increasing number of fortified foods available with sterol/stanol esters, meeting the 2 g/day recommendation of the NCEP ATP III is not difficult.

To achieve the upper end for the viscous fiber recommendation, there must be a major emphasis on fruits, vegetables, cereal grains, and legumes. Even so, it is challenging to consume 25 g of viscous fiber each day. Consequently, a lower viscous fiber dose (5–10 g/day) will still achieve a 3% to 5% LDL-C lowering. There are viscous fiber supplements available but it is important to note that some provide calories and many do not deliver the same nutrient-dense package that viscous fiber-rich foods do.

A vitamin supplement that is recommended for individuals over the age of 50 is the crystalline form of vitamin B_{12}, which is absorbed better than the naturally occurring form. The recommended dose of B12 is 2.4 µg/day.

SUMMARY

This chapter has reviewed the most impressive evidence of the cardiovascular benefits reported for many nutrients. The story has evolved in many different ways with regard to individual nutrients, their effects on CVD risk, and the recommendations that have been made. With respect to antioxidant vitamins, there was great promise based on findings from the epidemiologic literature that they would have beneficial effects on risk of CVD. However, the randomized controlled clinical trials conducted with various antioxidant supplements have not demonstrated efficacy, and, in fact, some have demonstrated adverse effects. The story for soy protein has changed over the years. The early studies demonstrated a hypocholesterolemic effect, whereas the more recent literature demonstrates only a small LDL-C lowering effect, most typically at high doses, and in subjects with hypercholesterolemia. In contrast, the story about marine-derived omega-3 fatty acids and stanols/sterols has been consistent over time, showing benefits on cardiovascular endpoints, as well as risk factors for CVD. Research on herbal products is in its infancy, and lacks robust scientific evidence to make recommendations about use of these products. For some nutrients that have a strong science base, specific nutrient-based recommendations can be made to decrease risk of CVD. Some of these cannot be "delivered" in sufficient quantities via food (i.e., EPA + DHA for triglyceride lowering; stanols/sterols); hence, supplements and/or fortified foods are warranted.

We have made impressive strides in developing food-based dietary recommendations that substantively reduce risk of CVD. Additional micronutrient-based research will clarify existing questions about the effects of individual nutrients and herbal products. As is always the case in science, additional evidence will better position us to make recommendations that further reduce risk of CVD.

■ Case Studies

Case 1: Patient with Dyslipidemia Treated with Fish Oil and Stanol-Fortified Foods

Initial Visit

ML is a 52-year-old male who is being seen for a routine physical examination. He has not seen his physician for the past two years. Since his last visit, he has gained 10 pounds. He has smoked one pack of cigarettes per day since he was 15 years old. He consumes a typical American diet, which is high in saturated fat, trans-fat and dietary cholesterol, and low in fruits, vegetables, whole grains, and dietary fiber. He is sedentary and has a high-stress management position, and typically works six days per week. ML has a family history of heart disease on his father's side of the family; his father passed away from an acute myocardial infarction when he was 71 years old. ML is not being treated for any medical condition. The results of his physical examination are as follows: BMI 28 kg/m^2; BP 135/85 mmHg; Pulse 82/min; fasting glucose 100 mg/dL; total cholesterol 210 mg/dL; LDL-C 138 mg/dL; triglycerides 195 mg/dL; HDL-C 43 mg/dL.

After learning that he has hypercholesterolemia and hypertriglyceridemia, ML is concerned about his health, and motivated to aggressively treat his dyslipidemia. ML has two children in high school and is the sole source of income for the family since his wife elects not to work outside the home. ML would first like to implement lifestyle behaviors (diet, physical activity, smoking cessation) to normalize his lipid profile before considering drug therapy.

Questions

1. *What diet and lifestyle changes would you recommend for ML?*

ML's estimated 10-year CHD risk (based on Framingham Risk Scoring as described in the Third Report of the National Cholesterol Education Program) is 16% (Table 13). The following diet and lifestyle modification intervention is recommended: a therapeutic lifestyle and diet changes along with weight loss, smoking cessation, and a program of regular physical activity (30 min/day of moderate intensity). In addition, to treat ML's elevated triglycerides, 3.0 g/day of fish oil is recommended.

2. *What would be the expected lipid and lipoprotein changes in response to the intervention described in question 1?*

Reducing saturated fat to lesser than 7% of calories would be expected to lower LDL-C by 8% to 10% and decreasing dietary cholesterol to less than 200 mg/day would result in a further LDL-C lowering of 3% to 5%. A 10-pound weight loss would be expected to decrease LDL-C by 5% to 8%. Weight loss will decrease triglyceride levels also. The fish oil supplementation would be expected to lower serum triglycerides level by 10% to 33%.

Second Visit

Two months later, ML returns to the doctor's office for a follow-up visit. He has lost four pounds. The lab results indicate that triglycerides were 156 mg/dL and HDL-C was 46 mg/dL. However, LDL-C increased slightly (to 145 mg/dL) as did total cholesterol (219 mg/dL).

3. *How would you manage the elevated total cholesterol and LDL-C by diet first before considering drug therapy?*

ML is encouraged to continue his program of diet and physical activity. ML is advised to implement therapeutic options to enhance lowering of LDL-C. These include: consumption of 2 g/day sterol/stanol esters (delivered in fortified foods such as spreads, yogurt, orange juice, cereal bars); and viscous (soluble) fiber (10–25 g/day).

4. *What would be the expected lipid and lipoprotein changes in response to the intervention described in Question 3?*

The sterol/stanol fortified foods would be expected to lower total cholesterol by 4% to 11% and LDL-C by 7% to 15% without changing HDL-C or triglycerides. A 5–10 g of viscous fiber per day is expected to lower LDL-C by 3% to 5% (Table 14).

Third Visit

After another two months, ML returns for a follow-up visit. Mike has successfully stopped smoking and has lost another four pounds. Lab results show that triglycerides are 140 mg/dL. There is no change of HDL-C level. Total cholesterol is reduced to 193 mg/dL and LDL-C is decreased to 126 mg/dL.

5. *What advice would you give Mike at this point about diet and lifestyle behaviors to implement?*

Mike should be encouraged to maintain his new diet and lifestyle program. In addition, he should schedule an appointment for another visit in six months. Since some studies have observed differences in plasma carotenoids in patients taking sterol/stanol esters, ML should be encouraged to consume recommended amounts of fruits and vegetables (at least five servings/day) to maintain normal plasma carotenoid levels.

TABLE 13 10-Year CHD Risk Estimation for Men (Framingham Point Scores)

	Age (52 yr)	TC (210 mg/dL)	HDL (43 mg/dL)	SBP (135 mmHg)	Smoking (yes)	Total point	10-yr risk
Points	6	3	1	1	3	14	16%

TABLE 14   Changes of Lipids and Other Risk Factors at Baseline and During Follow-Up

	TC	LDL-C	HDL-C	TG	Weight	Smoking
Baseline	210	138	43	195	190	Yes
2 mo (DHA + EPA)	219	145	46	156	186	Quit
4 mo (DHA + EPA + Sterol/Stanol esters)	193	126	46	140	182	Quit

Note: Data estimations are derived from NCEP ATP III Guideline, AHRQ report of omega-3 fatty acids and ADA Evidence Analysis Library of plant sterols and stanols.

Case 2: Patient Taking a Statin Drug + Niacin Followed by an Antioxidant Supplement

Initial Visit

ST is a 52-year-old male who is being seen for an annual physical examination. He has smoked one pack of cigarettes per day since he was 20, and has tried quitting many times. His BP is normal (125/80) and his BMI is 27 kg/m². His 56-year-old sister was diagnosed with angina two months ago. A lipid screen indicated the following: total cholesterol = 250 mg/dL, LDL-C = 145 mg/dL, triglycerides = 195 mg/dL and HDL-C = 31 mg/dL. ST's estimated 10-year CHD risk (based on Framingham Risk Scoring) was 20% (see Table below).

	Points
Age: 52	6
Total cholesterol: 250 mg/dL	4
Nonsmoker	3
HDL-C: 31 mg/dL	2
Systolic BP: 125 mmHg (untreated)	0
Total	15

ST has four major risk factors for CHD (age greater than 45 years; smoker; family history of premature CHD; low HDL-C. ST's physician prescribed 10 mg/day of simvastatin plus 1 g of niacin twice a day. In addition, a TLC diet and weight loss were prescribed along with a program of regular physical activity and smoking cessation.

Second Visit

Four months later, ST's lipid profile improved. His total cholesterol was 180 mg/dL and his LDL-C was 95 mg/dL. His triglyceride was 120 mg/dL and his HDL-C was 41 mg/dL. ST is adhering well to his diet, lifestyle and drug therapy treatment program. ST had not lost weight.

Third Visit

One year later, ST returned for routine lipid/lipoprotein screen. Total cholesterol, LDL-C, and triglyceride changes had been maintained since ST's last visit. However, his HDL-C dropped to 37 mg/dL. Upon questioning, ST indicated that he had started taking antioxidant supplements since he had heard that they might reduce risk of heart disease. ST shared that he has been taking 12.5 mg of β-carotene, 500 mg of vitamin C, 400 IU of vitamin E, and 50 mg of selenium twice a day.

Question

What would you do to address the reduction in HDL cholesterol since ST's last visit?

It is important to ask ST what changes he has made in his lifestyle. Factors that can decrease HDL-C include a low-fat diet, weight gain, decreased physical activity, cessation of alcohol consumption, cigarette smoking, antioxidants, and possibly other nutrient supplements including herbal products.

Since ST has not changed any of the factors except for the antioxidant supplements, this probably accounts for the reduction in HDL-C without any changes in other lipids and lipoproteins. ST should be advised to stop taking the antioxidant vitamin supplements since there is evidence from the HATS Study (106) that antioxidants blunt the HDL-increasing effect of niacin.

Fourth Visit

The blood lipid profile six months after the last visit is: total cholesterol = 180 mg/dL, LDL-C = 95 mg/dL, triglyceride = 120 mg/dL, and HDL-C = 41 mg/dL.

ST is to continue with the statin-niacin therapy. Follow-up visits should monitor cessation of antioxidant supplements.

RESOURCES

Agency for Healthcare Research and Quality – Clinical Reports: http://www.ahrq.gov/clinic/epcindex.htm#dietsup

American Dietetic Association Evidence Analysis Library:http://www.ebg.adaevidencelibrary.com/topic.cfm?cat=2662

American Heart Association Scientific Statements: http://www.americanheart.org/ presenter.jhtml?identifier=9181

Dietary Guidelines for Americans (2005):http://www.health.gov/dietaryguidelines/dga2005/document/

Dietary Reference Intakes from the Institute of Medicine of the National Academies: http://www.iom.edu/CMS/3788/4574.aspx

Dietary Supplement Health and Education Act: http://www.fda.gov/opacom/laws/dshea.html#sec5

National Center for Complementary and Alternative Medicine–National Institutes of Health: http://nccam.nih.gov/health/supplements.htm

National Cholesterol Education Program Adult Treatment Panel-III – National Heart, Lung and Blood Institute: http://www.nhlbi.nih.gov/guidelines/cholesterol/

US Food and Drug Administration – Health Claims and Dietary Supplements:
http://www.cfsan.fda.gov/~dms/lab-qhc.html
http://www.cfsan.fda.gov/~dms/lab-ssa.html
http://www.cfsan.fda.gov/~dms/supplmnt.html

REFERENCES

1. Bonaa KH, Njolstad I, Ueland PM, et al. NORVIT Trial Investigators. Homocysteine lowering and cardiovascular events after acute myocardial infarction. N Engl J Med 2006; 354:1578–1588.
2. Lonn E, Yusuf S, Arnold MH, et al. Heart Outcomes Prevention Evaluation (HOPE) 2 Investigators. Homocysteine lowering with folic acid and B vitamins in vascular disease. N Engl J Med 2006; 354:1557–1567.
3. Radimer K, Bindewald B, Hughes J, Ervin B, Swanson C, Picciano MF. Dietary supplement use by US adults: data from the national health and nutrition examination survey, 1999-2000. Am J Epidemiol 2004; 160:339–349.
4. Kennedy J. Herb and supplement use in the US adult population. Clin Ther 2005; 27:1847–1858.
5. Lichtenstein AH, Russell RM. Essential nutrients: food or supplements? Where should the emphasis be? JAMA 2005; 294:351–358.
6. Morel DW, DiCorleto PE, Chisolm GM. Endothelial and smooth muscle cells alter low density lipoprotein in vitro by free radical oxidation. Arteriosclerosis 1984; 4:357–364.
7. Steinberg D, Parthasarathy S, Carew TE, Khoo JC, Witztum JL. Beyond cholesterol. Modifications of low-density lipoprotein that increase its atherogenicity. N Engl J Med 1989; 320:915–924.
8. Diaz MN, Frei B, Vita JA, Keaney JF Jr. Antioxidants and atherosclerotic heart disease. N Engl J Med 1997; 337:408–416.
9. Jialal I, Vega GL, Grundy SM. Physiologic levels of ascorbate inhibit the oxidative modification of low density lipoprotein. Atherosclerosis 1990; 82:185–191.
10. Steinbrecher UP, Parthasarathy S, Leake DS, Witztum JL, Steinberg D. Modification of low density lipoprotein by endothelial cells involves lipid peroxidation and degradation of low density lipoprotein phospholipids. Proc Natl Acad Sci USA 1984; 81:3883–3887.
11. Frei B, England L, Ames BN. Ascorbate is an outstanding antioxidant in human blood plasma. Proc Natl Acad Sci USA 1989; 86:6377–6381.
12. Ingold KU, Webb AC, Witter D, Burton GW, Metcalfe TA, Muller DP. Vitamin E remains the major lipid-soluble, chain-breaking antioxidant in human plasma even in individuals suffering severe vitamin E deficiency. Arch Biochem Biophys 1987; 259:224–225.
13. Reilly M, Delanty N, Lawson JA, FitzGerald GA. Modulation of oxidant stress in vivo in chronic cigarette smokers. Circulation 1996; 94:19–25.
14. Nyyssonen K PE, Salonen R, Korpela H, Salonen JT. Increase in oxidation resistance of atherogenic serum lipoproteins following antioxidant supplementation: a randomized double-blind placebo-controlled clinical trial. Eur J Clin Nutr 1994; 48:633–642.
15. Mower R, Steiner M. Synthetic byproducts of tocopherol oxidation as inhibitors of platelet function. Prostaglandins 1982; 24:137–147.
16. Yoshikawa T, Yoshida N, Manabe H, Terasawa Y, Takemura T, Kondo M. alpha-Tocopherol protects against expression of adhesion molecules on neutrophils and endothelial cells. Biofactors 1998; 7:15–19.
17. Singh U, Jialal I. Anti-inflammatory effects of alpha-tocopherol. Ann N Y Acad Sci 2004; 1031:195–203.
18. Mitchinson MJ. The new face of atherosclerosis. Br J Clin Pract 1994; 48:149–151.

19. Tribble DL. AHA science advisory. Antioxidant consumption and risk of coronary heart disease: emphasison vitamin C, vitamin E, and beta-carotene: a statement for healthcare professionals from the american heart association. Circulation 1999; 99:591–595.

20. Kris-Etherton PM, Lichtenstein AH, Howard BV, Steinberg D, Witztum JL. Antioxidant vitamin supplements and cardiovascular disease. Circulation 2004; 110:637–641.

21. Rimm EB, Stampfer MJ, Ascherio A, Giovannucci E, Colditz GA, Willett WC. Vitamin E consumption and the risk of coronary heart disease in men. N Engl J Med 1993; 328:1450–1456.

22. Stampfer MJ, Hennekens CH, Manson JE, Colditz GA, Rosner B, Willett WC. Vitamin E consumption and the risk of coronary disease in women. N Engl J Med 1993; 328:1444–1449.

23. Knekt P, Reunanen A, Jarvinen R, Seppanen R, Heliovaara M, Aromaa A. Antioxidant vitamin intake and coronary mortality in a longitudinal population study. Am J Epidemiol 1994; 139:1180–1189.

24. Morris DL, Kritchevsky SB, Davis CE. Serum carotenoids and coronary heart disease. The Lipid Research Clinics Coronary Primary Prevention Trial and Follow-up Study. JAMA 1994; 272:1439–1441.

25. Pandey DK, Shekelle R, Selwyn BJ, Tangney C, Stamler J. Dietary vitamin C and beta-carotene and risk of death in middle-aged men. The Western Electric Study. Am J Epidemiol 1995; 142:1269–1278.

26. Sahyoun NR, Jacques PF, Russell RM. Carotenoids, vitamins C and E, and mortality in an elderly population. Am J Epidemiol 1996; 144:501–511.

27. Kushi LH, Folsom AR, Prineas RJ, Mink PJ, Wu Y, Bostick RM. Dietary antioxidant vitamins and death from coronary heart disease in postmenopausal women. N Engl J Med 1996; 334:1156–1162.

28. Nyyssonen K, Parviainen MT, Salonen R, Tuomilehto J, Salonen JT. Vitamin C deficiency and risk of myocardial infarction: prospective population study of men from eastern finland. Bmj 1997; 314:634–638.

29. Rimm EB, Willett WC, Hu FB, et al. Folate and vitamin B6 from diet and supplements in relation to risk of coronary heart disease among women. JAMA 1998; 279:359–364.

30. Klipstein-Grobusch K, Geleijnse JM, den Breeijen JH, et al. Dietary antioxidants and risk of myocardial infarction in the elderly: the rotterdam study. Am J Clin Nutr 1999; 69:261–266.

31. Loria CM, Klag MJ, Caulfield LE, Whelton PK. Vitamin C status and mortality in US adults. Am J Clin Nutr 2000; 72:139–145.

32. Simon JA, Hudes ES, Tice JA. Relation of serum ascorbic acid to mortality among US adults. J Am Coll Nutr 2001; 20:255–263.

33. Mezzetti A, Zuliani G, Romano F, et al. Vitamin E and lipid peroxide plasma levels predict the risk of cardiovascular events in a group of healthy very old people. J Am Geriatr Soc 2001; 49:533–537.

34. Khaw KT, Bingham S, Welch A, et al. Relation between plasma ascorbic acid and mortality in men and women in EPIC-Norfolk prospective study: a prospective population study. European prospective investigation into cancer and nutrition. Lancet 2001; 357:657–663.

35. Osganian SK, Stampfer MJ, Rimm E, et al. Vitamin C and risk of coronary heart disease in women. J Am Coll Cardiol 2003; 42:246–252.

36. Osganian SK, Stampfer MJ, Rimm E, Spiegelman D, Manson JE, Willett WC. Dietary carotenoids and risk of coronary artery disease in women. Am J Clin Nutr 2003; 77:1390–1399.

37. Voutilainen S, Virtanen JK, Rissanen TH, et al. Serum folate and homocysteine and the incidence of acute coronary events: the kuopio ischaemic heart disease risk factor study. Am J Clin Nutr 2004; 80:317–323.

38. Kritchevsky SB, Shimakawa T, Tell GS, et al. Dietary antioxidants and carotid artery wall thickness. the aric study. Atherosclerosis risk in communities study. Circulation 1995; 92:2142–2150.

39. Fehily AM, Yarnell JW, Sweetnam PM, Elwood PC. Diet and incident ischaemic heart disease: the caerphilly study. Br J Nutr 1993; 69:303–314.

40. Enstrom JE, Kanim LE, Klein MA. Vitamin C intake and mortality among a sample of the United States population. Epidemiology 1992; 3:194–202.

41. Gale CR, Martyn CN, Winter PD, Cooper C. Vitamin C and risk of death from stroke and coronary heart disease in cohort of elderly people. Bm j 1995; 310:1563–1566.

42. Muntwyler J, Hennekens CH, Manson JE, Buring JE, Gaziano JM. Vitamin supplement use in a low-risk population of US male physicians and subsequent cardiovascular mortality. Arch Intern Med 2002; 162:1472–1476.

43. Losonczy KG, Harris TB, Havlik RJ. Vitamin E and vitamin C supplement use and risk of all-cause and coronary heart disease mortality in older persons: the established populations for epidemiologic studies of the elderly. Am J Clin Nutr 1996; 64:190–196.

44. Watkins ML, Erickson JD, Thun MJ, Mulinare J, Heath CW Jr. Multivitamin use and mortality in a large prospective study. Am J Epidemiol 2000; 152:149–162.

45. Hennekens CH, Buring JE, Manson JE, et al. Lack of effect of long-term supplementation with beta carotene on the incidence of malignant neoplasms and cardiovascular disease. N Engl J Med 1996; 334:1145–1149.

46. Greenberg ER, Baron JA, Karagas MR, et al. Mortality associated with low plasma concentration of beta carotene and the effect of oral supplementation. Jama 1996; 275:699–703.

47. Omenn GS, Goodman GE, Thornquist MD, et al. Risk factors for lung cancer and for intervention effects in CARET, the Beta-Carotene and retinol efficacy trial. J Natl Cancer Inst 1996; 88:1550–1559.

48. Lee IM, Cook NR, Manson JE, Buring JE, Hennekens CH. Beta-carotene supplementation and incidence of cancer and cardiovascular disease: the women's health study. J Natl Cancer Inst 1999; 91:2102–2016.

49. The effect of vitamin E and beta carotene on the incidence of lung cancer and other cancers in male smokers. The alpha-tocopherol, beta carotene cancer prevention study group. N Engl J Med 1994; 330:1029–1035.

50. Hodis HN, Mack WJ, LaBree L, et al. Alpha-tocopherol supplementation in healthy individuals reduces low-density lipoprotein oxidation but not atherosclerosis: the Vitamin E atherosclerosis prevention study (VEAPS). Circulation 2002; 106:1453–1459.

51. Virtamo J, Rapola JM, Ripatti S, et al. Effect of vitamin E and beta carotene on the incidence of primary nonfatal myocardial infarction and fatal coronary heart disease. Arch Intern Med 1998; 158:668–675.

52. Leppala JM, Virtamo J, Fogelholm R, et al. Controlled trial of alpha-tocopherol and beta-carotene supplements on stroke incidence and mortality in male smokers. Arterioscler Thromb Vasc Biol 2000; 20:230–235.

53. de Gaetano G. Low-dose aspirin and vitamin E in people at cardiovascular risk: a randomised trial in general practice. Collaborative group of the primary prevention project. Lancet 2001; 357:89–95.

54. Salonen JT, Nyyssonen K, Salonen R, et al. Antioxidant supplementation in atherosclerosis prevention (ASAP) study: a randomized trial of the effect of vitamins E and C on 3-year progression of carotid atherosclerosis. J Intern Med 2000; 248:377–386.

55. Lonn E, Yusuf S, Hoogwerf B, et al. Effects of vitamin E on cardiovascular and microvascular outcomes in high-risk patients with diabetes: results of the HOPE study and MICRO-HOPE substudy. Diabetes Care 2002; 25:1919–1927.

56. Stephens NG, Parsons A, Schofield PM, Kelly F, Cheeseman K, Mitchinson MJ. Randomised controlled trial of vitamin E in patients with coronary disease: cambridge heart antioxidant study (CHAOS). Lancet 1996; 347:781–786.

57. Boaz M, Smetana S, Weinstein T, et al. Secondary prevention with antioxidants of cardiovascular disease in endstage renal disease (SPACE): randomised placebo-controlled trial. Lancet 2000; 356:1213–1218.

58. Rapola JM, Virtamo J, Ripatti S, et al. Effects of alpha tocopherol and beta carotene supplements on symptoms, progression, and prognosis of angina pectoris. Heart 1998; 79:454–458.

59. Rapola JM, Virtamo J, Ripatti S, et al. Randomised trial of alpha-tocopherol and beta-carotene supplements on incidence of major coronary events in men with previous myocardial infarction. Lancet 1997; 349:1715–1720.

60. Dietary supplementation with n-3 polyunsaturated fatty acids and vitamin E after myocardial infarction: results of the GISSI-Prevenzione trial. gruppo italiano per lo studio della sopravvivenza nell'infarto miocardico. Lancet 1999; 354:447–455.

61. Brown BG, Zhao XQ, Chait A, et al. Simvastatin and niacin, antioxidant vitamins, or the combination for the prevention of coronary disease. N Engl J Med 2001; 345:1583–1592.

62. Waters DD, Alderman EL, Hsia J, et al. Effects of hormone replacement therapy and antioxidant vitamin supplements on coronary atherosclerosis in postmenopausal women: a randomized controlled trial. Jama 2002; 288:2432–2440.

63. Fang JC, Kinlay S, Beltrame J, et al. Effect of vitamins C and E on progression of transplant-associated arteriosclerosis: a randomised trial. Lancet 2002; 359:1108–1113.

64. Yusuf S, Dagenais G, Pogue J, Bosch J, Sleight P. Vitamin E supplementation and cardiovascular events in high-risk patients. The heart outcomes prevention evaluation study investigators. N Engl J Med 2000; 342:154–160.

65. MRC/BHF heart protection study of antioxidant vitamin supplementation in 20,536 high–risk individuals: a randomised placebo–controlled trial. Lancet 2002; 360:23–33.

66. Rapola JM, Virtamo J, Haukka JK, et al. Effect of vitamin E and beta carotene on the incidence of angina pectoris. A randomized, double-blind, controlled trial. Jama 1996; 275:693–698.

67. Vivekananthan DP, Penn MS, Sapp SK, Hsu A, Topol EJ. Use of antioxidant vitamins for the prevention of cardiovascular disease: meta-analysis of randomised trials. Lancet 2003; 361:2017–2023.

68. Shekelle PG, Morton SC, Jungvig LK, et al. Effect of supplemental vitamin E for the prevention and treatment of cardiovascular disease. J Gen Intern Med 2004; 19:380–389.

69. Morris CD, Carson S. Routine vitamin supplementation to prevent cardiovascular disease: a summary of the evidence for the U.S. preventive services task force. Ann Intern Med 2003; 139:56–70.

70. Shekelle P, Morton S, Hardy ML. Effect of supplemental antioxidants vitamin C, vitamin E, and coenzyme Q10 for the prevention and treatment of cardiovascular disease. Evid Rep Technol Assess (Summ) 2003:1–3.

71. McCully KS, Wilson RB. Homocysteine theory of arteriosclerosis. Atherosclerosis 1975; 22:215–227.

72. Duell PB, Malinow MR. Homocyst(e)ine: an important risk factor for atherosclerotic vascular disease. Curr Opin Lipidol 1997; 8:28–34.

73. Malinow MR, Bostom AG, Krauss RM. Homocyst(e)ine, diet, and cardiovascular diseases: a statement for healthcare professionals from the nutrition committee, american heart association. Circulation 1999; 99:178–182.

74. Cook JW, Taylor LM, Orloff SL, Landry GJ, Moneta GL, Porter JM. Homocysteine and arterial disease. experimental mechanisms. Vascul Pharmacol 2002; 38:293–300.

75. Stampfer MJ, Malinow MR, Willett WC, et al. A prospective study of plasma homocyst(e)ine and risk of myocardial infarction in US physicians. Jama 1992; 268:877–881.

76. Graham IM, Daly LE, Refsum HM, et al. Plasma homocysteine as a risk factor for vascular disease. The european concerted action project. Jama 1997; 277:1775–1781.

77. Boushey CJ, Beresford SA, Omenn GS, Motulsky AG. A quantitative assessment of plasma homocysteine as a risk factor for vascular disease. Probable benefits of increasing folic acid intakes. Jama 1995; 274:1049–1057.

78. Ford ES, Smith SJ, Stroup DF, Steinberg KK, Mueller PW, Thacker SB. Homocyst(e)ine and cardiovascular disease: a systematic review of the evidence with special emphasis on case-control studies and nested case-control studies. Int J Epidemiol 2002; 31:59–70.

79. Grundy SM, Bazzarre T, Cleeman J, et al. Prevention conference v: beyond secondary prevention: identifying the high-risk patient for primary prevention: medical office assessment: writing Group I. Circulation 2000; 101:E3–E11.

80. Pearson TA. New tools for coronary risk assessment: what are their advantages and limitations? Circulation 2002; 105:886–892.

81. Brattstrom LE, Israelsson B, Jeppsson JO, Hultberg BL. Folic acid—an innocuous means to reduce plasma homocysteine. Scand J Clin Lab Invest 1988; 48:215–221.

82. Lowering blood homocysteine with folic acid based supplements: meta–analysis of randomised trials. homocysteine lowering trialists' collaboration. Bmj 1998; 316:894–898.

83. Wald DS, Bishop L, Wald NJ, et al. Randomized trial of folic acid supplementation and serum homocysteine levels. Arch Intern Med 2001; 161:695–700.

84. de Bree A, Verschuren WM, Blom HJ, Nadeau M, Trijbels FJ, Kromhout D. Coronary heart disease mortality, plasma homocysteine, and B-vitamins: a prospective study. Atherosclerosis 2003; 166:369–377.

85. He K, Merchant A, Rimm EB, et al. Folate, vitamin B6, and B12 intakes in relation to risk of stroke among men. Stroke 2004; 35:169–174.

86. Huerta JM, Gonzalez S, Vigil E, et al. Folate and cobalamin synergistically decrease the risk of high plasma homocysteine in a nonsupplemented elderly institutionalized population. Clin Biochem 2004; 37:904–910.

87. Mann NJ, Li D, Sinclair AJ, et al. The effect of diet on plasma homocysteine concentrations in healthy male subjects. Eur J Clin Nutr 1999; 53:895–899.

88. McKinley MC, McNulty H, McPartlin J, et al. Low-dose vitamin B-6 effectively lowers fasting plasma homocysteine in healthy elderly persons who are folate and riboflavin replete. Am J Clin Nutr 2001; 73:759–764.

89. Kelly PJ, Shih VE, Kistler JP, et al. Low vitamin B6 but not homocyst(e)ine is associated with increased risk of stroke and transient ischemic attack in the era of folic acid grain fortification. Stroke 2003; 34:e51–e54.

90. Kelly PJ, Kistler JP, Shih VE, et al. Inflammation, homocysteine, and vitamin B6 status after ischemic stroke. Stroke 2004; 35:12–15.

91. Toole JF, Malinow MR, Chambless LE, et al. Lowering homocysteine in patients with ischemic stroke to prevent recurrent stroke, myocardial infarction, and death: the vitamin intervention for stroke prevention (VISP) randomized controlled trial. Jama 2004; 291:565–575.

92. Schnyder G, Roffi M, Flammer Y, Pin R, Hess OM. Effect of homocysteine-lowering therapy with folic acid, vitamin B12, and vitamin B6 on clinical outcome after percutaneous coronary intervention: the swiss heart study: a randomized controlled trial. Jama 2002; 288:973–979.

93. Liem A, Reynierse-Buitenwerf GH, Zwinderman AH, Jukema JW, van Veldhuisen DJ. Secondary prevention with folic acid: effects on clinical outcomes. J Am Coll Cardiol 2003; 41:2105–2113.

94. Carlson LA. Nicotinic acid: the broad-spectrum lipid drug. A 50th anniversary review. J Intern Med 2005; 258:94–114.

95. Altschul R, Hoffer A, Stephen JD. Influence of nicotinic acid on serum cholesterol in man. Arch Biochem 1955; 54:558–559.

96. Executive summary of the third report of the national cholesterol education program (NCEP) expert panel on detection, evaluation, and treatment of high blood cholesterol in adults (adult treatment panel III). Jama 2001; 285:2486–2497.

97. Goldberg A, Alagona P Jr, Capuzzi DM, et al. Multiple-dose efficacy and safety of an extended-release form of niacin in the management of hyperlipidemia. Am J Cardiol 2000; 85:1100–1105.

98. Knopp RH, Alagona P, Davidson M, et al. Equivalent efficacy of a time-release form of niacin (Niaspan) given once-a-night versus plain niacin in the management of hyperlipidemia. Metabolism 1998; 47:1097–1104.

99. Morgan JM, Capuzzi DM, Guyton JR, et al. Treatment effect of niaspan, a controlled-release niacin, in patients with hypercholesterolemia: a placebo-controlled trial. J Cardiovasc Pharmacol Ther 1996; 1:195–202.

100. Capuzzi DM, Guyton JR, Morgan JM, et al. Efficacy and safety of an extended-release niacin (niaspan): a long-term study. Am J Cardiol 1998; 82:74U–81U; discussion 85U–86U.

101. Grundy SM, Vega GL, McGovern ME, et al. Efficacy, safety, and tolerability of once-daily niacin for the treatment of dyslipidemia associated with type 2 diabetes: results of the assessment of diabetes control and evaluation of the efficacy of niaspan trial. Arch Intern Med 2002; 162:1568–1576.

102. Backes JM, Gibson CA. Effect of lipid-lowering drug therapy on small-dense low-density lipoprotein. Ann Pharmacother 2005; 39:523–526.

103. Clark AB, Holt JM. Identifying and managing patients with hyperlipidemia. Am J Manag Care 1997; 3:1211–1219; quiz 1223–1225.

104. Kamanna VS, Kashyap ML. Mechanism of action of niacin on lipoprotein metabolism. Curr Atheroscler Rep 2000; 2:36–46.

105. Levy DR, Pearson TA. Combination niacin and statin therapy in primary and secondary prevention of cardiovascular disease. Clin Cardiol 2005; 28:317–320.

106. Cheung MC, Zhao XQ, Chait A, Albers JJ, Brown BG. Antioxidant supplements block the response of HDL to simvastatin-niacin therapy in patients with coronary artery disease and low HDL. Arterioscler Thromb Vasc Biol 2001; 21:1320–1326.
107. Brown BG, Cheung MC, Lee AC, Zhao XQ, Chait A. Antioxidant vitamins and lipid therapy: end of a long romance? Arterioscler Thromb Vasc Biol 2002; 22:1535–1546.
108. Clofibrate and niacin in coronary heart disease. Jama 1975; 231:360–381.
109. Canner PL, Berge KG, Wenger NK, et al. Fifteen year mortality in coronary drug project patients: long-term benefit with niacin. J Am Coll Cardiol 1986; 8:1245–1255.
110. Hoffer A. Ascorbic acid and toxicity. N Engl J Med 1971; 285:635–636.
111. Hughes C, Dutton S, Truswell AS. High intakes of ascorbic acid and urinary oxalate. J Hum Nutr 1981; 35:274–280.
112. Levine M, Conry-Cantilena C, Wang Y, et al. Vitamin C pharmacokinetics in healthy volunteers: evidence for a recommended dietary allowance. Proc Natl Acad Sci USA 1996; 93:3704–3709.
113. Herbert V, Jacob E. Destruction of vitamin B12 by ascorbic acid. Jama 1974; 230:241–242.
114. Bendich A, Machlin LJ. Safety of oral intake of vitamin E. Am J Clin Nutr 1988; 48:612–619.
115. Corrigan JJ Jr, Marcus FI. Coagulopathy associated with vitamin E ingestion. Jama 1974; 230:1300–1301.
116. Bendich A. The safety of beta-carotene. Nutr Cancer 1988; 11:207–214.
117. Lascari AD. Carotenemia. A review. Clin Pediatr (Phila) 1981; 20:25–29.
118. Schaumberg HH, Arezzo J, Otto DA, Eckerman DA. Neurotoxic chemical exposure scenarios and suggested solutions. Neurobehav Toxicol Teratol 1985; 7:351–353.
119. Schaumberg H, Berger A. Pyridoxine neurotoxicity. In: Clinical and Physiological Applications of Vitamin B6. New York: Alan R. Liss., 1988:403–414.
120. Foulds WS, Cant JS, Chisholm IA, Bronte-Stewart J, Wilson J. Hydroxocobalamin in the treatment of Leber's hereditary optic atrophy. Lancet 1968; 1:896–897.
121. Butterworth CE Jr, Tamura T. Folic acid safety and toxicity: a brief review. Am J Clin Nutr 1989; 50:353–358.
122. van der Westhuyzen J, Metz J. Tissue S-adenosylmethionine levels in fruit bats (rousettus aegyptiacus) with nitrous oxide-induced neuropathy. Br J Nutr 1983; 50:325–330.
123. Hunter R, Barnes J, Oakeley HF, Matthews DM. Toxicity of folic acid given in pharmacological doses to healthy volunteers. Lancet 1970; 1:61–63.
124. Sparling R, Abela M. Hypersensitivity to folic acid therapy. Clin Lab Haematol 1985; 7:184–185.
125. Schwartz M. Severe reversible hyperglycemia as a consequence of niacin therapy. Arch Intern Med 1993; 153:2050–2052.
126. Miller D, Hayes K. Vitamin excess and toxicity. In: Hatchcock JN, ed. Nutritional Toxicology, Vol. 1. New York: Academic Press, 1982.
127. McKenney JM, Proctor JD, Harris S, Chinchili VM. A comparison of the efficacy and toxic effects of sustained- vs immediate-release niacin in hypercholesterolemic patients. Jama 1994; 271:672–677.
128. Knodel LC, Talbert RL. Adverse effects of hypolipidaemic drugs. Med Toxicol 1987; 2:10–32.
129. Ervin RB, Wright JD, Wang CY, Kennedy-Stephenson J. Dietary intake of selected vitamins for the United States population: 1999–2000. Adv Data 2004:1–4.
130. Meyers CD, Carr MC, Park S, Brunzell JD. Varying cost and free nicotinic acid content in over-the-counter niacin preparations for dyslipidemia. Ann Intern Med 2003; 139:996–1002.
131. Cappuccio FP, Elliott P, Allender PS, Pryer J, Follman DA, Cutler JA. Epidemiologic association between dietary calcium intake and blood pressure: a meta-analysis of published data. Am J Epidemiol 1995; 142:935–945.
132. Birkett NJ. Comments on a meta-analysis of the relation between dietary calcium intake and blood pressure. Am J Epidemiol 1998; 148:223–228; discussion 232–233.
133. Griffith LE, Guyatt GH, Cook RJ, Bucher HC, Cook DJ. The influence of dietary and nondietary calcium supplementation on blood pressure: an updated metaanalysis of randomized controlled trials. Am J Hypertens 1999; 12:84–92.
134. Schroder H, Schmelz E, Marrugat J. Relationship between diet and blood pressure in a representative mediterranean population. Eur J Nutr 2002; 41:161–167.
135. Ma J, Folsom AR, Melnick SL, et al. Associations of serum and dietary magnesium with cardiovascular disease, hypertension, diabetes, insulin, and carotid arterial wall thickness: the ARIC study. Atherosclerosis risk in communities study. J Clin Epidemiol 1995; 48:927–940.
136. Peacock JM, Folsom AR, Arnett DK, Eckfeldt JH, Szklo M. Relationship of serum and dietary magnesium to incident hypertension: the atherosclerosis risk in communities (ARIC) study. Ann Epidemiol 1999; 9:159–165.
137. Hajjar IM, Grim CE, George V, Kotchen TA. Impact of diet on blood pressure and age-related changes in blood pressure in the US population: analysis of NHANES III. Arch Intern Med 2001; 161:589–593.
138. Jee SH, Miller ER III, Guallar E, Singh VK, Appel LJ, Klag MJ. The effect of magnesium supplementation on blood pressure: a meta-analysis of randomized clinical trials. Am J Hypertens 2002; 15:691–696.
139. Song Y, Manson JE, Buring JE, Liu S. Dietary magnesium intake in relation to plasma insulin levels and risk of type 2 diabetes in women. Diabetes Care 2004; 27:59–65.
140. Lopez-Ridaura R, Willett WC, Rimm EB, et al. Magnesium intake and risk of type 2 diabetes in men and women. Diabetes Care 2004; 27:134–140.

141. Kao WH, Folsom AR, Nieto FJ, Mo JP, Watson RL, Brancati FL. Serum and dietary magnesium and the risk for type 2 diabetes mellitus: the atherosclerosis risk in communities study. Arch Intern Med 1999; 159:2151–2159.

142. Fung TT, Manson JE, Solomon CG, Liu S, Willett WC, Hu FB. The association between magnesium intake and fasting insulin concentration in healthy middle-aged women. J Am Coll Nutr 2003; 22:533–538.

143. Whelton PK, He J, Cutler JA, et al. Effects of oral potassium on blood pressure. Meta-analysis of randomized controlled clinical trials. Jama 1997; 277:1624–1632.

144. Sacks FM, Obarzanek E, Windhauser MM, et al. Rationale and design of the dietary approaches to stop hypertension trial (DASH). A multicenter controlled-feeding study of dietary patterns to lower blood pressure. Ann Epidemiol 1995; 5:108–118.

145. Kardinaal AF, Kok FJ, Kohlmeier L, et al. Association between toenail selenium and risk of acute myocardial infarction in european men. The EURAMIC study. European antioxidant myocardial infarction and breast cancer. Am J Epidemiol 1997; 145:373–379.

146. Salvini S, Hennekens CH, Morris JS, Willett WC, Stampfer MJ. Plasma levels of the antioxidant selenium and risk of myocardial infarction among U.S. physicians. Am J Cardiol 1995; 76:1218–1221.

147. Miettinen TA, Alfthan G, Huttunen JK, et al. Serum selenium concentration related to myocardial infarction and fatty acid content of serum lipids. Br Med J (Clin Res Ed) 1983; 287:517–519.

148. Kok FJ, de Bruijn AM, Vermeeren R, et al. Serum selenium, vitamin antioxidants, and cardiovascular mortality: a 9-year follow-up study in the netherlands. Am J Clin Nutr 1987; 45:462–468.

149. Virtamo J, Valkeila E, Alfthan G, Punsar S, Huttunen JK, Karvonen MJ. Serum selenium and the risk of coronary heart disease and stroke. Am J Epidemiol 1985; 122:276–282.

150. Ringstad J, Thelle D. Risk of myocardial infarction in relation to serum concentrations of selenium. Acta Pharmacol Toxicol (Copenh) 1986; 59(Suppl 7):336–339.

151. Lee DH, Folsom AR, Jacobs DR Jr. Iron, zinc, and alcohol consumption and mortality from cardiovascular diseases: the iowa women's health study. Am J Clin Nutr 2005; 81:787–791.

152. Reunanen A, Knekt P, Marniemi J, Maki J, Maatela J, Aromaa A. Serum calcium, magnesium, copper and zinc and risk of cardiovascular death. Eur J Clin Nutr 1996; 50:431–437.

153. Kromhout D, Wibowo AA, Herber RF, et al. Trace metals and coronary heart disease risk indicators in 152 elderly men (the Zutphen study). Am J Epidemiol 1985; 122:378–385.

154. Konukoglu D, Turhan MS, Ercan M, Serin O. Relationship between plasma leptin and zinc levels and the effect of insulin and oxidative stress on leptin levels in obese diabetic patients. J Nutr Biochem 2004; 15:757–760.

155. Terres-Martos C, Navarro-Alarcon M, Martin-Lagos F, Lopez GdlSH, Perez-Valero V, Lopez-Martinez MC. Serum zinc and copper concentrations and Cu/Zn ratios in patients with hepatopathies or diabetes. J Trace Elem Med Biol 1998; 12:44–49.

156. Raz I, Havivi E. Trace elements in blood cells of diabetic subjects. Diabetes Res 1989; 10:21–24.

157. Di Martino G, Matera MG, De Martino B, Vacca C, Di Martino S, Rossi F. Relationship between zinc and obesity. J Med 1993; 24:177–183.

158. Anderson RA, Roussel AM, Zouari N, Mahjoub S, Matheau JM, Kerkeni A. Potential antioxidant effects of zinc and chromium supplementation in people with type 2 diabetes mellitus. J Am Coll Nutr 2001; 20:212–218.

159. de Sena KC, Arrais RF, das Gracas Almeida M, et al. Effects of zinc supplementation in patients with type 1 diabetes. Biol Trace Elem Res 2005; 105:1–9.

160. Ruiz C, Alegria A, Barbera R, Farre R, Lagarda J. Selenium, zinc and copper in plasma of patients with type 1 diabetes mellitus in different metabolic control states. J Trace Elem Med Biol 1998; 12:91–95.

161. Ervin RB, Wang CY, Wright JD, Kennedy-Stephenson J. Dietary intake of selected minerals for the United States population: 1999–2000. Adv Data 2004:1–5.

162. Wolk A, Manson JE, Stampfer MJ, et al. Long-term intake of dietary fiber and decreased risk of coronary heart disease among women. Jama 1999; 281:1998–2004.

163. Pietinen P, Rimm EB, Korhonen P, et al. Intake of dietary fiber and risk of coronary heart disease in a cohort of finnish men. The alpha-tocopherol, beta-carotene cancer prevention study. Circulation 1996; 94:2720–2727.

164. Jensen MK, Koh-Banerjee P, Hu FB, et al. Intakes of whole grains, bran, and germ and the risk of coronary heart disease in men. Am J Clin Nutr 2004; 80:1492–1499.

165. Mozaffarian D, Kumanyika SK, Lemaitre RN, Olson JL, Burke GL, Siscovick DS. Cereal, fruit, and vegetable fiber intake and the risk of cardiovascular disease in elderly individuals. Jama 2003; 289:1659–1666.

166. Liu S, Buring JE, Sesso HD, Rimm EB, Willett WC, Manson JE. A prospective study of dietary fiber intake and risk of cardiovascular disease among women. J Am Coll Cardiol 2002; 39:49–56.

167. Rimm EB, Ascherio A, Giovannucci E, Spiegelman D, Stampfer MJ, Willett WC. Vegetable, fruit, and cereal fiber intake and risk of coronary heart disease among men. Jama 1996; 275:447–451.

168. Jacobs DR Jr., Meyer KA, Kushi LH, Folsom AR. Whole-grain intake may reduce the risk of ischemic heart disease death in postmenopausal women: the iowa women's health study. Am J Clin Nutr 1998; 68:248–257.

169. Erkkila AT, Herrington DM, Mozaffarian D, Lichtenstein AH. Cereal fiber and whole-grain intake are associated with reduced progression of coronary-artery atherosclerosis in postmenopausal women with coronary artery disease. Am Heart J 2005; 150:94–101.

170. Brown L, Rosner B, Willett WW, Sacks FM. Cholesterol-lowering effects of dietary fiber: a meta-analysis. Am J Clin Nutr 1999; 69:30–42.

171. Anderson JW, Allgood LD, Lawrence A, et al. Cholesterol-lowering effects of psyllium intake adjunctive to diet therapy in men and women with hypercholesterolemia: meta-analysis of 8 controlled trials. Am J Clin Nutr 2000; 71:472–479.

172. Whelton SP, Hyre AD, Pedersen B, Yi Y, Whelton PK, He J. Effect of dietary fiber intake on blood pressure: a meta-analysis of randomized, controlled clinical trials. J Hypertens 2005; 23:475–481.

173. Streppel MT, Arends LR, van't Veer P, Grobbee DE, Geleijnse JM. Dietary fiber and blood pressure: a meta-analysis of randomized placebo-controlled trials. Arch Intern Med 2005; 165:150–156.

174. Bang HO, Dyerberg J, Hjoorne N. The composition of food consumed by greenland eskimos. Acta Med Scand 1976; 200:69–73.

175. Bang HO, Dyerberg J, Sinclair HM. The composition of the eskimo food in north western greenland. Am J Clin Nutr 1980; 33:2657–2661.

176. Bang HO, Dyerberg J. The bleeding tendency in greenland eskimos. Dan Med Bull 1980; 27:202–205.

177. Ascherio A, Rimm EB, Stampfer MJ, Giovannucci EL, Willett WC. Dietary intake of marine n-3 fatty acids, fish intake, and the risk of coronary disease among men. N Engl J Med 1995; 332:977–982.

178. Morris MC, Manson JE, Rosner B, Buring JE, Willett WC, Hennekens CH. Fish consumption and cardiovascular disease in the physicians' health study: a prospective study. Am J Epidemiol 1995; 142:166–175.

179. Daviglus ML, Stamler J, Orencia AJ, et al. Fish consumption and the 30-year risk of fatal myocardial infarction. N Engl J Med 1997; 336:1046–1053.

180. Albert CM, Hennekens CH, O'Donnell CJ, et al. Fish consumption and risk of sudden cardiac death. Jama 1998; 279:23–28.

181. Oomen CM, Feskens EJ, Rasanen L, et al. Fish consumption and coronary heart disease mortality in finland, italy, and the netherlands. Am J Epidemiol 2000; 151:999–1006.

182. Hu FB, Bronner L, Willett WC, et al. Fish and omega-3 fatty acid intake and risk of coronary heart disease in women. Jama 2002; 287:1815–1821.

183. Mozaffarian D, Lemaitre RN, Kuller LH, Burke GL, Tracy RP, Siscovick DS. Cardiac benefits of fish consumption may depend on the type of fish meal consumed: the cardiovascular health study. Circulation 2003; 107:1372–1377.

184. Osler M, Andreasen AH, Hoidrup S. No inverse association between fish consumption and risk of death from all-causes, and incidence of coronary heart disease in middle-aged, Danish adults. J Clin Epidemiol 2003; 56:274–279.

185. Folsom AR, Demissie Z. Fish intake, marine omega-3 fatty acids, and mortality in a cohort of postmenopausal women. Am J Epidemiol 2004; 160:1005–1010.

186. Mozaffarian D, Psaty BM, Rimm EB, et al. Fish intake and risk of incident atrial fibrillation. Circulation 2004; 110:368–373.

187. Mozaffarian D, Bryson CL, Lemaitre RN, Burke GL, Siscovick DS. Fish intake and risk of incident heart failure. J Am Coll Cardiol 2005; 45:2015–2021.

188. Frost L, Vestergaard P. n-3 Fatty acids consumed from fish and risk of atrial fibrillation or flutter: the danish diet, cancer, and health study. Am J Clin Nutr 2005; 81:50–54.

189. Sacks FM, Stone PH, Gibson CM, Silverman DI, Rosner B, Pasternak RC. Controlled trial of fish oil for regression of human coronary atherosclerosis. HARP research group. J Am Coll Cardiol 1995; 25:1492–1498.

190. Eritsland J, Arnesen H, Gronseth K, Fjeld NB, Abdelnoor M. Effect of dietary supplementation with n-3 fatty acids on coronary artery bypass graft patency. Am J Cardiol 1996; 77:31–36.

191. Cairns JA, Gill J, Morton B, et al. Fish oils and low-molecular-weight heparin for the reduction of restenosis after percutaneous transluminal coronary angioplasty. The EMPAR study. Circulation 1996; 94:1553–1560.

192. Von Schacky C, Angerer P, Kothny W, Theisen K, Mudra H. The effect of dietary omega-3 fatty acids on coronary atherosclerosis. A randomized, double-blind, placebo-controlled trial. Ann Intern Med 1999; 130:554–562.

193. Johansen O, Brekke M, Seljeflot I, Abdelnoor M, Arnesen H. n-3 fatty acids do not prevent restenosis after coronary angioplasty: results from the CART study. Coronary angioplasty restenosis trial. J Am Coll Cardiol 1999; 33:1619–1626.

194. Goodfellow J, Bellamy MF, Ramsey MW, Jones CJ, Lewis MJ. Dietary supplementation with marine omega-3 fatty acids improve systemic large artery endothelial function in subjects with hypercholesterolemia. J Am Coll Cardiol 2000; 35:265–270.

195. Angerer P, Kothny W, Stork S, von Schacky C. Effect of dietary supplementation with omega-3 fatty acids on progression of atherosclerosis in carotid arteries. Cardiovasc Res 2002; 54:183–190.

196. Maresta A, Balducelli M, Varani E, et al. Prevention of postcoronary angioplasty restenosis by omega-3 fatty acids: main results of the esapent for prevention of restenosis italian study (ESPRIT). Am Heart J 2002; 143:E5.

197. Thies F, Garry JM, Yaqoob P, et al. Association of n-3 polyunsaturated fatty acids with stability of atherosclerotic plaques: a randomised controlled trial. Lancet 2003; 361:477–485.

198. Silva JM, Souza I, Silva R, Tavares P, Teixeira F, Silva PS. The triglyceride lowering effect of fish oils is affected by fish consumption. Int J Cardiol 1996; 57:75–80.

199. McGrath LT, Brennan GM, Donnelly JP, Johnston GD, Hayes JR, McVeigh GE. Effect of dietary fish oil supplementation on peroxidation of serum lipids in patients with non-insulin dependent diabetes mellitus. Atherosclerosis 1996; 121:275–283.

200. Sirtori CR, Paoletti R, Mancini M, et al. n-3 fatty acids do not lead to an increased diabetic risk in patients with hyperlipidemia and abnormal glucose tolerance. Italian fish oil multicenter study. Am J Clin Nutr 1997; 65:1874–1881.

201. Nordoy A, Bonaa KH, Nilsen H, Berge RK, Hansen JB, Ingebretsen OC. Effects of Simvastatin and omega-3 fatty acids on plasma lipoproteins and lipid peroxidation in patients with combined hyperlipidaemia. J Intern Med 1998; 243:163–170.

202. Mori TA, Bao DQ, Burke V, Puddey IB, Watts GF, Beilin LJ. Dietary fish as a major component of a weight-loss diet: effect on serum lipids, glucose, and insulin metabolism in overweight hypertensive subjects. Am J Clin Nutr 1999; 70:817–825.

203. Durrington PN, Bhatnagar D, Mackness MI, et al. An omega-3 polyunsaturated fatty acid concentrate administered for one year decreased triglycerides in simvastatin treated patients with coronary heart disease and persisting hypertriglyceridaemia. Heart 2001; 85:544–548.

204. Nilsen DW, Albrektsen G, Landmark K, Moen S, Aarsland T, Woie L. Effects of a high-dose concentrate of n-3 fatty acids or corn oil introduced early after an acute myocardial infarction on serum triacylglycerol and HDL cholesterol. Am J Clin Nutr 2001; 74:50–56.

205. Higdon JV, Du SH, Lee YS, Wu T, Wander RC. Supplementation of postmenopausal women with fish oil does not increase overall oxidation of LDL ex vivo compared to dietary oils rich in oleate and linoleate. J Lipid Res 2001; 42:407–418.

206. Finnegan YE, Minihane AM, Leigh-Firbank EC, et al. Plant- and marine-derived n-3 polyunsaturated fatty acids have differential effects on fasting and postprandial blood lipid concentrations and on the susceptibility of LDL to oxidative modification in moderately hyperlipidemic subjects. Am J Clin Nutr 2003; 77:783–795.

207. Mori TA, Woodman RJ, Burke V, Puddey IB, Croft KD, Beilin LJ. Effect of eicosapentaenoic acid and docosahexaenoic acid on oxidative stress and inflammatory markers in treated-hypertensive type 2 diabetic subjects. Free Radic Biol Med 2003; 35:772–781.

208. Mesa MD, Buckley R, Minihane AM, Yaqoob P. Effects of oils rich in eicosapentaenoic and docosahexaenoic acids on the oxidizability and thrombogenicity of low-density lipoprotein. Atherosclerosis 2004;175:333–343.

209. Toft I, Bonaa KH, Ingebretsen OC, Nordoy A, Jenssen T. Effects of n-3 polyunsaturated fatty acids on glucose homeostasis and blood pressure in essential hypertension. A randomized, controlled trial. Ann Intern Med 1995; 123:911–918.

210. Russo C, Olivieri O, Girelli D, et al. Omega-3 polyunsaturated fatty acid supplements and ambulatory blood pressure monitoring parameters in patients with mild essential hypertension. J Hypertens 1995; 13:1823–1826.

211. Gray DR, Gozzip CG, Eastham JH, Kashyap ML. Fish oil as an adjuvant in the treatment of hypertension. Pharmacotherapy 1996; 16:295–300.

212. Bao DQ, Mori TA, Burke V, Puddey IB, Beilin LJ. Effects of dietary fish and weight reduction on ambulatory blood pressure in overweight hypertensives. Hypertension 1998; 32:710–717.

213. Leng GC, Lee AJ, Fowkes FG, et al. Randomized controlled trial of gamma-linolenic acid and eicosapentaenoic acid in peripheral arterial disease. Clin Nutr 1998; 17:265–271.

214. Woodman RJ, Mori TA, Burke V, Puddey IB, Watts GF, Beilin LJ. Effects of purified eicosapentaenoic and docosahexaenoic acids on glycemic control, blood pressure, and serum lipids in type 2 diabetic patients with treated hypertension. Am J Clin Nutr 2002; 76:1007–1015.

215. Svensson M, Christensen JH, Solling J, Schmidt EB. The effect of n-3 fatty acids on plasma lipids and lipoproteins and blood pressure in patients with CRF. Am J Kidney Dis 2004; 44:77–83.

216. Dokholyan RS, Albert CM, Appel LJ, Cook NR, Whelton P, Hennekens CH. A trial of omega-3 fatty acids for prevention of hypertension. Am J Cardiol 2004; 93:1041–1043.

217. Mori TA, Beilin LJ, Burke V, Morris J, Ritchie J. Interactions between dietary fat, fish, and fish oils and their effects on platelet function in men at risk of cardiovascular disease. Arterioscler Thromb Vasc Biol 1997; 17:279–286.

218. Seljeflot I, Arnesen H, Brude IR, Nenseter MS, Drevon CA, Hjermann I. Effects of omega-3 fatty acids and/or antioxidants on endothelial cell markers. Eur J Clin Invest 1998; 28:629–635.

219. Pirich C, Gaszo A, Granegger S, Sinzinger H. Effects of fish oil supplementation on platelet survival and ex vivo platelet function in hypercholesterolemic patients. Thromb Res 1999; 96:219–227.

220. Nordoy A, Bonaa KH, Sandset PM, Hansen JB, Nilsen H. Effect of omega-3 fatty acids and simvastatin on hemostatic risk factors and postprandial hyperlipemia in patients with combined hyperlipemia. Arterioscler Thromb Vasc Biol 2000; 20:259–265.

221. Finnegan YE, Howarth D, Minihane AM, et al. Plant and marine derived (n-3) polyunsaturated fatty acids do not affect blood coagulation and fibrinolytic factors in moderately hyperlipidemic humans. J Nutr 2003; 133:2210–2213.

222. Lindman AS, Pedersen JI, Hjerkinn EM, et al. The effects of long-term diet and omega-3 fatty acid supplementation on coagulation factor VII and serum phospholipids with special emphasis on the R353Q polymorphism of the FVII gene. Thromb Haemost 2004; 91:1097–1104.

223. Seierstad SL, Seljeflot I, Johansen O, et al. Dietary intake of differently fed salmon; the influence on markers of human atherosclerosis. Eur J Clin Invest 2005; 35:52–59.
224. Hjerkinn EM, Seljeflot I, Ellingsen I, et al. Influence of long-term intervention with dietary counseling, long-chain n-3 fatty acid supplements, or both on circulating markers of endothelial activation in men with long-standing hyperlipidemia. Am J Clin Nutr 2005; 81:583–589.
225. Christensen JH, Gustenhoff P, Korup E, et al. Effect of fish oil on heart rate variability in survivors of myocardial infarction: a double blind randomised controlled trial. BMJ 1996; 312:677–678.
226. Singer P, Wirth M. Can n-3 PUFA reduce cardiac arrhythmias? Results of a clinical trial. Prostaglandins Leukot Essent Fatty Acids 2004; 71:153–159.
227. Calo L, Bianconi L, Colivicchi F, et al. n-3 Fatty acids for the prevention of atrial fibrillation after coronary artery bypass surgery: a randomized, controlled trial. J Am Coll Cardiol 2005; 45:1723–1728.
228. Raitt MH, Connor WE, Morris C, et al. Fish oil supplementation and risk of ventricular tachycardia and ventricular fibrillation in patients with implantable defibrillators: a randomized controlled trial. Jama 2005; 293:2884–2891.
229. Burr ML, Fehily AM, Gilbert JF, et al. Effects of changes in fat, fish, and fibre intakes on death and myocardial reinfarction: diet and reinfarction trial (DART). Lancet 1989; 2:757–761.
230. Burr ML, Ashfield-Watt PA, Dunstan FD, et al. Lack of benefit of dietary advice to men with angina: results of a controlled trial. Eur J Clin Nutr 2003; 57:193–200.
231. Kris-Etherton PM, Harris WS, Appel LJ. Fish consumption, fish oil, omega-3 fatty acids, and cardiovascular disease. Circulation 2002; 106:2747–2757.
232. Yzebe D, Lievre M. Fish oils in the care of coronary heart disease patients: a meta-analysis of randomized controlled trials. Fundam Clin Pharmacol 2004; 18:581–592.
233. Nilsen DW, Harris WS. n-3 Fatty acids and cardiovascular disease. Am J Clin Nutr 2004; 79:166.
234. Hooper L, Thompson RL, Harrison RA, et al. Omega 3 fatty acids for prevention and treatment of cardiovascular disease. Cochrane Database Syst Rev 2004:CD003177.
235. Studer M, Briel M, Leimenstoll B, Glass TR, Bucher HC. Effect of different antilipidemic agents and diets on mortality: a systematic review. Arch Intern Med 2005; 165:725–730.
236. de Lorgeril M, Salen P, Martin JL, Monjaud I, Delaye J, Mamelle N. Mediterranean diet, traditional risk factors, and the rate of cardiovascular complications after myocardial infarction: final report of the lyon diet heart study. Circulation 1999; 99:779–785.
237. Leaf A, Jorgensen MB, Jacobs AK, et al. Do fish oils prevent restenosis after coronary angioplasty? Circulation 1994; 90:2248–2257.
238. Gapinski JP, VanRuiswyk JV, Heudebert GR, Schectman GS. Preventing restenosis with fish oils following coronary angioplasty. A meta-analysis. Arch Intern Med 1993; 153:1595–1601.
239. Nye ER, Ablett MB, Robertson MC, Ilsley CD, Sutherland WH. Effect of eicosapentaenoic acid on restenosis rate, clinical course and blood lipids in patients after percutaneous transluminal coronary angioplasty. Aust N Z J Med 1990; 20:549–552.
240. Grigg LE, Kay TW, Valentine PA, et al. Determinants of restenosis and lack of effect of dietary supplementation with eicosapentaenoic acid on the incidence of coronary artery restenosis after angioplasty. J Am Coll Cardiol 1989; 13:665–672.
241. Balk E, Chung M, Lichtenstein A, et al. Effects of omega-3 fatty acids on cardiovascular risk factors and intermediate markers of cardiovascular disease. Evid Rep Technol Assess (Summ) 2004; 1–6.
242. Reis GJ, Boucher TM, Sipperly ME, et al. Randomised trial of fish oil for prevention of restenosis after coronary angioplasty. Lancet 1989; 2:177–181.
243. Kaul U, Sanghvi S, Bahl VK, Dev V, Wasir HS. Fish oil supplements for prevention of restenosis after coronary angioplasty. Int J Cardiol 1992; 35:87–93.
244. Franzen D, Schannwell M, Oette K, Hopp HW. A prospective, randomized, and double-blind trial on the effect of fish oil on the incidence of restenosis following PTCA. Cathet Cardiovasc Diagn 1993; 28:301–310.
245. Milner MR, Gallino RA, Leffingwell A, et al. Usefulness of fish oil supplements in preventing clinical evidence of restenosis after percutaneous transluminal coronary angioplasty. Am J Cardiol 1989; 64:294–299.
246. Bellamy CM, Schofield PM, Faragher EB, Ramsdale DR. Can supplementation of diet with omega-3 polyunsaturated fatty acids reduce coronary angioplasty restenosis rate? Eur Heart J 1992; 13:1626–1631.
247. Dehmer GJ, Popma JJ, van den Berg EK, et al. Reduction in the rate of early restenosis after coronary angioplasty by a diet supplemented with n-3 fatty acids. N Engl J Med 1988; 319:733–740.
248. Bairati I, Roy L, Meyer F. Double-blind, randomized, controlled trial of fish oil supplements in prevention of recurrence of stenosis after coronary angioplasty. Circulation 1992; 85:950–956.
249. Siscovick DS, Raghunathan TE, King I, et al. Dietary intake and cell membrane levels of long-chain n-3 polyunsaturated fatty acids and the risk of primary cardiac arrest. Jama 1995; 274:1363–1367.
250. Christensen JH, Korup E, Aaroe J, et al. Fish consumption, n-3 fatty acids in cell membranes, and heart rate variability in survivors of myocardial infarction with left ventricular dysfunction. Am J Cardiol 1997; 79:1670–1673.
251. Leaf A, Albert CM, Josephson M, et al. Fatty acid antiarrhythmia trial investigators. Prevention of fatal arrhythmias in high-risk subjects by fish oil n-3 fatty acid intake. Circulation 2005; 112(18): 2762-2768.

252. Howe PR. Dietary fats and hypertension. Focus on fish oil. Ann N Y Acad Sci 1997; 827:339–352.
253. Morris MC, Sacks F, Rosner B. Does fish oil lower blood pressure? A meta-analysis of controlled trials. Circulation 1993; 88:523–533.
254. Appel LJ, Miller ER III, Seidler AJ, Whelton PK. Does supplementation of diet with 'fish oil' reduce blood pressure? A meta-analysis of controlled clinical trials. Arch Intern Med 1993; 153:1429–1438.
255. Geleijnse JM, Giltay EJ, Grobbee DE, Donders AR, Kok FJ. Blood pressure response to fish oil supplementation: metaregression analysis of randomized trials. J Hypertens 2002; 20:1493–1499.
256. Harris WS. n–3 fatty acids and serum lipoproteins: human studies. Am J Clin Nutr 1997; 65:1645S–1654S.
257. De Caterina R, Liao JK, Libby P. Fatty acid modulation of endothelial activation. Am J Clin Nutr 2000; 71:213S–223S.
258. Chin JP, Dart AM. How do fish oils affect vascular function? Clin Exp Pharmacol Physiol 1995; 22:71–81.
259. Harris WS, Rambjor GS, Windsor SL, Diederich D. N-3 fatty acids and urinary excretion of nitric oxide metabolites in humans. Am J Clin Nutr 1997; 65:459–464.
260. Lopez D, Orta X, Casos K, et al. Upregulation of endothelial nitric oxide synthase in rat aorta after ingestion of fish oil-rich diet. Am J Physiol Heart Circ Physiol 2004; 287:H567–H572.
261. Agren JJ, Vaisanen S, Hanninen O, Muller AD, Hornstra G. Hemostatic factors and platelet aggregation after a fish-enriched diet or fish oil or docosahexaenoic acid supplementation. Prostaglandins Leukot Essent Fatty Acids 1997; 57:419–421.
262. Knapp HR. Dietary fatty acids in human thrombosis and hemostasis. Am J Clin Nutr 1997; 65:1687S–1698S.
263. Kong W, Wei J, Abidi P, et al. Berberine is a novel cholesterol-lowering drug working through a unique mechanism distinct from statins. Net Med 2004; 10:1344–1351.
264. De Smet PA. Herbal remedies. N Engl J Med 2002; 347:2046–2056.
265. Endo A, Monacolin K. a new hypocholesterolemic agent produced by a monascus species. J Antibiot (Tokyo) 1979; 32:852–854.
266. Zhu Y, Li CL, Wang YY. Effects of Xuezhikang on blood lipids and lipoprotein concentrations of rabbits and quails with hyperlipidemia. Chin J Pharmacol 1995; 30:4–8.
267. Zhu Y, Li C, Wang Y, Zhu J, Chang J, Kritchevsky D. Monascus purpureus (red yeast): a natural product that lowers blood cholesterol in animal models of hypercholesterolemia. Nutr Res 1998; 18:71–81.
268. Wang J, Su M, Lu Z, et al. Clinical trial of extract of monascus purpureus (red yeast) in the treatment of hyperlipidemia. Chin J Exp Ther Prep Chin Med 1995; 12:1–5.
269. Shen Z, Yu P, Su M, et al. A prospective study on zhitai capsule in the treatment of primary hyperlipidemia. Nat Med J China 1996; 76:156–157.
270. Heber D, Yip I, Ashley JM, Elashoff DA, Elashoff RM, Go VL. Cholesterol-lowering effects of a proprietary chinese red-yeast-rice dietary supplement. Am J Clin Nutr 1999; 69:231–236.
271. Gebhardt R. Inhibition of cholesterol biosynthesis in primary cultured rat hepatocytes by artichoke (cynara scolymus L.) extracts. J Pharmacol Exp Ther 1998; 286:1122–1128.
272. Lawson LD. Garlic: a review of its medicinal effects and indicated active compounds. In: Lawson LK, Bauer R eds. Phytomedicines of Europe: Chemistry and Biological Activity. Washington DC: American Chemical Society, 1998:176–209.
273. Warshafsky S, Kamer RS, Sivak SL. Effect of garlic on total serum cholesterol. A meta-nalysis. Ann Intern Med 1993; 119:599–605.
274. Stevinson C, Pittler MH, Ernst E. Garlic for treating hypercholesterolemia. A meta-analysis of randomized clinical trials. Ann Intern Med 2000; 133:420–429.
275. Mulrow C, Lawrence V, Ackermann R, et al. Garlic: effects on cardiovascular risks and disease, protective effects against cancer, and clinical adverse effects. Evid Rep Technol Assess (Summ) 2000:1–4.
276. Curtis-Prior P, Vere D, Fray P. Therapeutic value of ginkgo biloba in reducing symptoms of decline in mental function. J Pharm Pharmacol 1999; 51:535–541.
277. Hopfenmuller W. Evidence for a therapeutic effect of ginkgo biloba special extract. Meta-analysis of 11 clinical studies in patients with cerebrovascular insufficiency in old age. Arzneimittelforschung 1994; 44:1005–1013.
278. Mouren X, Caillard P, Schwartz F. Study of the antiischemic action of EGb 761 in the treatment of peripheral arterial occlusive disease by TcPo2 determination. Angiology 1994; 45:413–417.
279. Thomson GJ, Vohra RK, Carr MH, Walker MG. A clinical trial of gingkco biloba extract in patients with intermittent claudication. Int Angiol 1990; 9:75–78.
280. Bauer U. 6-Month double-blind randomised clinical trial of ginkgo biloba extract versus placebo in two parallel groups in patients suffering from peripheral arterial insufficiency. Arzneimittelforschung 1984; 34:716–720.
281. Schweizer J, Hautmann C. Comparison of two dosages of ginkgo biloba extract EGb 761 in patients with peripheral arterial occlusive disease fontaine's stage IIb. A randomised, double-blind, multicentric clinical trial. Arzneimittelforschung 1999; 49:900–904.
282. Peters H, Kieser M, Holscher U. Demonstration of the efficacy of ginkgo biloba special extract EGb 761 on intermittent claudication—a placebo-controlled, double-blind multicenter trial. Vasa 1998; 27:106–110.
283. Pittler MH, Ernst E. Ginkgo biloba extract for the treatment of intermittent claudication: a meta-analysis of randomized trials. Am J Med 2000; 108:276–281.

284. Sotaniemi EA, Haapakoski E, Rautio A. Ginseng therapy in non-insulin-dependent diabetic patients. Diabetes Care 1995; 18:1373–1375.

285. Vuksan V, Sievenpiper JL, Koo VY, et al. American ginseng (panax quinquefolius L) reduces postprandial glycemia in nondiabetic subjects and subjects with type 2 diabetes mellitus. Arch Intern Med 2000; 160:1009–1013.

286. Vuksan V, Stavro MP, Sievenpiper JL, et al. American ginseng improves glycemia in individuals with normal glucose tolerance: effect of dose and time escalation. J Am Coll Nutr 2000; 19:738–744.

287. Kuhnau J. The flavonoids. A class of semi-essential food components: their role in human nutrition. World Rev Nutr Diet 1976; 24:117–191.

288. Sesso HD, Gaziano JM, Buring JE, Hennekens CH. Coffee and tea intake and the risk of myocardial infarction. Am J Epidemiol 1999; 149:162–167.

289. Geleijnse JM, Launer LJ, Hofman A, Pols HA, Witteman JC. Tea flavonoids may protect against atherosclerosis: the rotterdam study. Arch Intern Med 1999; 159:2170–2174.

290. Keli SO, Hertog MG, Feskens EJ, Kromhout D. Dietary flavonoids, antioxidant vitamins, and incidence of stroke: the zutphen study. Arch Intern Med 1996; 156:637–642.

291. Klatsky AL, Armstrong MA, Friedman GD. Coffee, tea, and mortality. Ann Epidemiol 1993; 3:375–381.

292. Woodward M, Tunstall-Pedoe H. Coffee and tea consumption in the scottish heart health study follow up: conflicting relations with coronary risk factors, coronary disease, and all cause mortality. J Epidemiol Community Health 1999; 53:481–487.

293. Hertog MG, Sweetnam PM, Fehily AM, Elwood PC, Kromhout D. Antioxidant flavonols and ischemic heart disease in a welsh population of men: the caerphilly study. Am J Clin Nutr 1997; 65:1489–1494.

294. Middleton E Jr., Kandaswami C, Theoharides TC. The effects of plant flavonoids on mammalian cells: implications for inflammation, heart disease, and cancer. Pharmacol Rev 2000; 52:673–751.

295. Bursill C, Roach PD, Bottema CD, Pal S. Green tea upregulates the low-density lipoprotein receptor through the sterol-regulated element binding Protein in HepG2 liver cells. J Agric Food Chem 2001; 49:5639–5645.

296. Yang TT, Koo MW. Inhibitory effect of chinese green tea on endothelial cell-induced LDL oxidation. Atherosclerosis 2000; 148:67–73.

297. Stensvold I, Tverdal A, Solvoll K, Foss OP. Tea consumption. Relationship to cholesterol, blood pressure, and coronary and total mortality. Prev Med 1992; 21:546–553.

298. Hertog MG, Kromhout D, Aravanis C, et al. Flavonoid intake and long-term risk of coronary heart disease and cancer in the seven countries study. Arch Intern Med 1995; 155:381–386.

299. Peters U, Poole C, Arab L. Does tea affect cardiovascular disease? A meta-analysis. Am J Epidemiol 2001; 154:495–503.

300. Hasalam E. Plant phenols: vegetable tannins revisited. Cambridge, United Kindom: Cambridge University Press 1989:154–219.

301. Serafini M, Ghiselli A, Ferro-Luzzi A. In vivo antioxidant effect of green and black tea in man. Eur J Clin Nutr 1996; 50:28–32.

302. Davies MJ, Judd JT, Baer DJ, et al. Black tea consumption reduces total and LDL cholesterol in mildly hypercholesterolemic adults. J Nutr 2003; 133:3298S–3302S.

303. Maron DJ, Lu GP, Cai NS, et al. Cholesterol-lowering effect of a theaflavin-enriched green tea extract: a randomized controlled trial. Arch Intern Med 2003; 163:1448–1453.

304. Watson PS, Scalia GM, Galbraith A, Burstow DJ, Bett N, Aroney CN. Lack of effect of coenzyme Q on left ventricular function in patients with congestive heart failure. J Am Coll Cardiol 1999; 33:1549–1552.

305. Khatta M, Alexander BS, Krichten CM, et al. The effect of coenzyme Q10 in patients with congestive heart failure. Ann Intern Med 2000; 132:636–640.

306. Hofman-Bang C, Rehnqvist N, Swedberg K, Wiklund I, Astrom H. Coenzyme Q10 as an adjunctive in the treatment of chronic congestive heart failure. The Q10 Study Group. J Card Fail 1995; 1:101–107.

307. Kuklinski B, Weissenbacher E, Fahnrich A. Coenzyme Q10 and antioxidants in acute myocardial infarction. Mol Aspects Med 1994; 15(Suppl:s1):43–47.

308. Di Somma S, Carati L. Efficacy of coenzyme Q10 in association with conventional therapy in the treatment of heart failure and ischemic heart disease. In: Folkers K, Yamamura Y, eds. Biomedical and Clincal Aspects of Coenzyme Q10. Amsterdam: Elsevier, 1991:257–265.

309. Morisco C, Trimarco B, Condorelli M. Effect of coenzyme Q10 therapy in patients with congestive heart failure: a long-term multicenter randomized study. Clin Investig 1993; 71:S134–S136.

310. Katan MB, Grundy SM, Jones P, Law M, Miettinen T, Paoletti R. Efficacy and safety of plant stanols and sterols in the management of blood cholesterol levels. Mayo Clin Proc 2003; 78:965–978.

311. Davidson MH, Maki KC, Umporowicz DM, et al. Safety and tolerability of esterified phytosterols administered in reduced-fat spread and salad dressing to healthy adult men and women. J Am Coll Nutr 2001; 20:307–319.

312. Tikkanen MJ, Hogstrom P, Tuomilehto J, Keinanen-Kiukaanniemi S, Sundvall J, Karppanen H. Effect of a diet based on low-fat foods enriched with nonesterified plant sterols and mineral nutrients on serum cholesterol. Am J Cardiol 2001; 88:1157–1162.

313. Hendriks HF, Weststrate JA, van Vliet T, Meijer GW. Spreads enriched with three different levels of vegetable oil sterols and the degree of cholesterol lowering in normocholesterolaemic and mildly hypercholesterolaemic subjects. Eur J Clin Nutr 1999; 53:319–327.

314. Hallikainen MA, Sarkkinen ES, Uusitupa MI. Plant stanol esters affect serum cholesterol concentrations of hypercholesterolemic men and women in a dose-dependent manner. J Nutr 2000; 130:767–776.

315. Mabley JG, Jagtap P, Perretti M, et al. Anti-inflammatory effects of a novel, potent inhibitor of poly (ADP-ribose) polymerase. Inflamm Res 2001; 50:561–569.

316. Homma Y, Ikeda I, Ishikawa T, Tateno M, Sugano M, Nakamura H. Decrease in plasma low-density lipoprotein cholesterol, apolipoprotein B, cholesteryl ester transfer protein, and oxidized low-density lipoprotein by plant stanol ester-containing spread: a randomized, placebo-controlled trial. Nutrition 2003; 19:369–374.

317. Miettinen TA, Puska P, Gylling H, Vanhanen H, Vartiainen E. Reduction of serum cholesterol with sitostanol-ester margarine in a mildly hypercholesterolemic population. N Engl J Med 1995; 333:1308–1312.

318. Gylling H, Radhakrishnan R, Miettinen TA. Reduction of serum cholesterol in postmenopausal women with previous myocardial infarction and cholesterol malabsorption induced by dietary sitostanol ester margarine: women and dietary sitostanol. Circulation 1997; 96:4226–4231.

319. Plat J, Mensink RP. Vegetable oil based versus wood based stanol ester mixtures: effects on serum lipids and hemostatic factors in non-hypercholesterolemic subjects. Atherosclerosis 2000; 148:101–112.

320. Hallikainen MA, Uusitupa MI. Effects of 2 low-fat stanol ester-containing margarines on serum cholesterol concentrations as part of a low-fat diet in hypercholesterolemic subjects. Am J Clin Nutr 1999; 69:403–410.

321. Mensink RP, Ebbing S, Lindhout M, Plat J, van Heugten MM. Effects of plant stanol esters supplied in low-fat yoghurt on serum lipids and lipoproteins, non-cholesterol sterols and fat soluble antioxidant concentrations. Atherosclerosis 2002; 160:205–213.

322 Spilburg CA, Goldberg AC, McGill JB, et al. Fat-free foods supplemented with soy stanol-lecithin powder reduce cholesterol absorption and LDL cholesterol. J Am Diet Assoc 2003; 103:577–581.

323. Cater NB, Garcia-Garcia AB, Vega GL, Grundy SM. Responsiveness of plasma lipids and lipoproteins to plant stanol esters. Am J Cardiol 2005; 96:23D–28D.

324. Thuluva SC, Igel M, Giesa U, Lutjohann D, Sudhop T, von Bergmann K. Ratio of lathosterol to campesterol in serum predicts the cholesterol-lowering effect of sitostanol-supplemented margarine. Int J Clin Pharmacol Ther 2005; 43:305–310.

325. Temme EH, Van Hoydonck PG, Schouten EG, Kesteloot H. Effects of a plant sterol-enriched spread on serum lipids and lipoproteins in mildly hypercholesterolaemic subjects. Acta Cardiol 2002; 57:111–115.

326. De Graaf J, De Sauvage Nolting PR, Van Dam M, et al. Consumption of tall oil-derived phytosterols in a chocolate matrix significantly decreases plasma total and low-density lipoprotein-cholesterol levels. Br J Nutr 2002; 88:479–488.

327. Matvienko OA, Lewis DS, Swanson M, et al. A single daily dose of soybean phytosterols in ground beef decreases serum total cholesterol and LDL cholesterol in young, mildly hypercholesterolemic men. Am J Clin Nutr 2002; 76:57–64.

328. Mussner MJ, Parhofer KG, Von Bergmann K, Schwandt P, Broedl U, Otto C. Effects of phytosterol ester-enriched margarine on plasma lipoproteins in mild to moderate hypercholesterolemia are related to basal cholesterol and fat intake. Metabolism 2002; 51:189–194.

329. Cleghorn CL, Skeaff CM, Mann J, Chisholm A. Plant sterol-enriched spread enhances the cholesterol-lowering potential of a fat-reduced diet. Eur J Clin Nutr 2003; 57:170–176.

330. Hendriks HF, Brink EJ, Meijer GW, Princen HM, Ntanios FY. Safety of long-term consumption of plant sterol esters-enriched spread. Eur J Clin Nutr 2003; 57:681–692.

331. Varady KA, Ebine N, Vanstone CA, Parsons WE, Jones PJ. Plant sterols and endurance training combine to favorably alter plasma lipid profiles in previously sedentary hypercholesterolemic adults after 8 wk. Am J Clin Nutr 2004; 80:1159–1166.

332. Noakes M, Clifton PM, Doornbos AM, Trautwein EA. Plant sterol ester-enriched milk and yoghurt effectively reduce serum cholesterol in modestly hypercholesterolemic subjects. Eur J Nutr 2005; 44:214–222.

333. Lee YM, Haastert B, Scherbaum W, Hauner H. A phytosterol-enriched spread improves the lipid profile of subjects with type 2 diabetes mellitus—a randomized controlled trial under free–living conditions. Eur J Nutr 2003; 42:111–117.

334. Lau VW, Journoud M, Jones PJ. Plant sterols are efficacious in lowering plasma LDL and non-HDL cholesterol in hypercholesterolemic type 2 diabetic and nondiabetic persons. Am J Clin Nutr 2005; 81:1351–1358.

335. Simons LA. Additive effect of plant sterol-ester margarine and cerivastatin in lowering low-density lipoprotein cholesterol in primary hypercholesterolemia. Am J Cardiol 2002; 90:737–740.

336. Blair SN, Capuzzi DM, Gottlieb SO, Nguyen T, Morgan JM, Cater NB. Incremental reduction of serum total cholesterol and low-density lipoprotein cholesterol with the addition of plant stanol ester-containing spread to statin therapy. Am J Cardiol 2000; 86:46–52.

337. Noone EJ, Roche HM, Nugent AP, Gibney MJ. The effect of dietary supplementation using isomeric blends of conjugated linoleic acid on lipid metabolism in healthy human subjects. Br J Nutr 2002; 88:243–251.

338. Moloney F, Yeow TP, Mullen A, Nolan JJ, Roche HM. Conjugated linoleic acid supplementation, insulin sensitivity, and lipoprotein metabolism in patients with type 2 diabetes mellitus. Am J Clin Nutr 2004; 80:887–895.

339. Tricon S, Burdge GC, Kew S, et al. Opposing effects of cis-9,trans-11 and trans-10,cis-12 conjugated linoleic acid on blood lipids in healthy humans. Am J Clin Nutr 2004; 80:614–620.

340. Riserus U, Berglund L, Vessby B. Conjugated linoleic acid (CLA) reduced abdominal adipose tissue in obese middle-aged men with signs of the metabolic syndrome: a randomised controlled trial. Int J Obes Relat Metab Disord 2001; 25:1129–1135.

341. Smedman A, Vessby B. Conjugated linoleic acid supplementation in humans—metabolic effects. Lipids 2001; 36:773–781.

342. Riserus U, Basu S, Jovinge S, Fredrikson GN, Arnlov J, Vessby B. Supplementation with conjugated linoleic acid causes isomer-dependent oxidative stress and elevated C-reactive protein: a potential link to fatty acid-induced insulin resistance. Circulation 2002; 106:1925–1929.

343. Gaullier JM, Halse J, Hoye K, et al. Conjugated linoleic acid supplementation for 1 y reduces body fat mass in healthy overweight humans. Am J Clin Nutr 2004; 79:1118–1125.

344. Mougios V, Matsakas A, Petridou A, et al. Effect of supplementation with conjugated linoleic acid on human serum lipids and body fat. J Nutr Biochem 2001; 12:585–594.

345. Blankson H, Stakkestad JA, Fagertun H, Thom E, Wadstein J, Gudmundsen O. Conjugated linoleic acid reduces body fat mass in overweight and obese humans. J Nutr 2000; 130:2943–2948.

346. Riserus U, Arner P, Brismar K, Vessby B. Treatment with dietary trans10cis12 conjugated linoleic acid causes isomer-specific insulin resistance in obese men with the metabolic syndrome. Diabetes Care 2002; 25:1516–1521.

347. Riserus U, Vessby B, Arnlov J, Basu S. Effects of cis-9,trans-11 conjugated linoleic acid supplementation on insulin sensitivity, lipid peroxidation, and proinflammatory markers in obese men. Am J Clin Nutr 2004; 80:279–283.

348. Clarkson P, Adams MR, Powe AJ, et al. Oral L-arginine improves endothelium-dependent dilation in hypercholesterolemic young adults. J Clin Invest 1996; 97:1989–1994.

349. Hambrecht R, Hilbrich L, Erbs S, et al. Correction of endothelial dysfunction in chronic heart failure: additional effects of exercise training and oral L-arginine supplementation. J Am Coll Cardiol 2000; 35:706–713.

350. Lim DS, Mooradian SJ, Goldberg CS, et al. Effect of oral L-arginine on oxidant stress, endothelial dysfunction, and systemic arterial pressure in young cardiac transplant recipients. Am J Cardiol 2004; 94:828–831.

351. Boger G, Maas R, Schwedhelm E, et al. Improvement of endothelium-dependent vasodilation by simvastatin is potentiated by combination with L-arginine in patients with elevated asymmetric dimethylarginine levels. J Am Coll Cardiol 2004; 43:A525.

352. Yin WH, Chen JW, Tsai C, Chiang MC, Young MS, Lin SJ. l-arginine improves endothelial function and reduces LDL oxidation in patients with stable coronary artery disease. Clin Nutr 2005; 24:988–997.

353. Chin-Dusting JP, Alexander CT, Arnold PJ, Hodgson WC, Lux AS, Jennings GL. Effects of in vivo and in vitro L-arginine supplementation on healthy human vessels. J Cardiovasc Pharmacol 1996; 28:158–166.

354. Blum A, Hathaway L, Mincemoyer R, et al. Effects of oral L-arginine on endothelium-dependent vasodilation and markers of inflammation in healthy postmenopausal women. J Am Coll Cardiol 2000; 35:271–276.

355. Blum A, Hathaway L, Mincemoyer R, et al. Oral L-arginine in patients with coronary artery disease on medical management. Circulation 2000; 101:2160–2164.

356. Siani A, Pagano E, Iacone R, Iacoviello L, Scopacasa F, Strazzullo P. Blood pressure and metabolic changes during dietary L-arginine supplementation in humans. Am J Hypertens 2000; 13:547–551.

357. Palloshi A, Fragasso G, Piatti P, et al. Effect of oral L-arginine on blood pressure and symptoms and endothelial function in patients with systemic hypertension, positive exercise tests, and normal coronary arteries. Am J Cardiol 2004; 93:933–935.

358. Rector TS, Bank AJ, Mullen KA, et al. Randomized, double-blind, placebo-controlled study of supplemental oral L-arginine in patients with heart failure. Circulation 1996; 93:2135–2141.

359. Adams MR, Forsyth CJ, Jessup W, Robinson J, Celermajer DS. Oral L-arginine inhibits platelet aggregation but does not enhance endothelium-dependent dilation in healthy young men. J Am Coll Cardiol 1995; 26:1054–1061.

360. Adams MR, McCredie R, Jessup W, Robinson J, Sullivan D, Celermajer DS. Oral L-arginine improves endothelium-dependent dilatation and reduces monocyte adhesion to endothelial cells in young men with coronary artery disease. Atherosclerosis 1997; 129:261–269.

361. Chin-Dusting JP, Kaye DM, Lefkovits J, Wong J, Bergin P, Jennings GL. Dietary supplementation with L-arginine fails to restore endothelial function in forearm resistance arteries of patients with severe heart failure. J Am Coll Cardiol 1996; 27:1207–1213.

362. Lerman A, Burnett JC Jr., Higano ST, McKinley LJ, Holmes DR Jr. Long-term L-arginine supplementation improves small-vessel coronary endothelial function in humans. Circulation 1998; 97:2123–2128.

363. Sydow K, Schwedhelm E, Arakawa N, et al. ADMA and oxidative stress are responsible for endothelial dysfunction in hyperhomocyst(e)inemia: effects of L-arginine and B vitamins. Cardiovasc Res 2003; 57:244–252.

364. West SG, Likos-Krick A, Brown P, Mariotti F. Oral L-arginine improves hemodynamic responses to stress and reduces plasma homocysteine in hypercholesterolemic men. J Nutr 2005; 135:212–217.

365. Theilmeier G, Chan JR, Zalpour C, et al. Adhesiveness of mononuclear cells in hypercholesterolemic humans is normalized by dietary L-arginine. Arterioscler Thromb Vasc Biol 1997; 17:3557–3564.

366. Chan JR, Boger RH, Bode-Boger SM, et al. Asymmetric dimethylarginine increases mononuclear cell adhesiveness in hypercholesterolemic humans. Arterioscler Thromb Vasc Biol 2000; 20:1040–1046.

367. Blum A, Porat R, Rosenschein U, et al. Clinical and inflammatory effects of dietary L-arginine in patients with intractable angina pectoris. Am J Cardiol 1999; 83:1488–1490, A8.

368. Wolf A, Zalpour C, Theilmeier G, et al. Dietary L-arginine supplementation normalizes platelet aggregation in hypercholesterolemic humans. J Am Coll Cardiol 1997; 29:479–485.

369. George J, Shmuel SB, Roth A, et al. L-arginine attenuates lymphocyte activation and anti-oxidized LDL antibody levels in patients undergoing angioplasty. Atherosclerosis 2004; 174:323–327.

370. Schulman SP, Becker LC, Kass DA, et al. L-arginine therapy in acute myocardial infarction: the vascular interaction with age in myocardial infarction (VINTAGE MI) randomized clinical trial. Jama 2006; 295:58–64.

371. Cacciatore L, Cerio R, Ciarimboli M, et al. The therapeutic effect of L-carnitine in patients with exercise-induced stable angina: a controlled study. Drugs Exp Clin Res 1991; 17:225–235.

372. Canale C, Terrachini V, Biagini A, et al. Bicycle ergometer and echocardiographic study in healthy subjects and patients with angina pectoris after administration of L-carnitine: semiautomatic computerized analysis of M-mode tracing. Int J Clin Pharmacol Ther Toxicol 1988; 26:221–224.

373. Iliceto S, Scrutinio D, Bruzzi P, et al. Effects of L-carnitine administration on left ventricular remodeling after acute anterior myocardial infarction: the L-carnitine ecocardiografia digitalizzata infarto miocardico (CEDIM) Trial. J Am Coll Cardiol 1995; 26:380–387.

374. Iyer R, Gupta A, Khan A, Hiremath S, Lokhandwala Y. Does left ventricular function improve with L-carnitine after acute myocardial infarction? J Postgrad Med 1999; 45:38–41.

375. Food labeling: health claims; soy protein and coronary heart disease. Food and drug administration, HHS. Final rule. Fed Regist 1999; 64:57700–57733.

376. Anderson JW, Johnstone BM, Cook-Newell ME. Meta-analysis of the effects of soy protein intake on serum lipids. N Engl J Med 1995; 333:276–282.

377. Balk E, Chung M, Chew P, et al. Effects of soy on health outcomes. Evid Rep Technol Assess (Summ) 2005:1–8.

378. Sacks FM, Lichtenstein A, Van Horn L, Harris W, Kris-Etherton P, Winston M. Soy Protein, isoflavones, and cardiovascular health. An american heart association science advisory for professionals from the nutrition committee. Circulation 2006.

379. Nestel PJ, Pomeroy S, Kay S, et al. Isoflavones from red clover improve systemic arterial compliance but not plasma lipids in menopausal women. J Clin Endocrinol Metab 1999; 84:895–898.

380. Nestel PJ, Yamashita T, Sasahara T, et al. Soy isoflavones improve systemic arterial compliance but not plasma lipids in menopausal and perimenopausal women. Arterioscler Thromb Vasc Biol 1997; 17:3392–3398.

381. Hodgson JM, Puddey IB, Beilin LJ, et al. Effects of isoflavonoids on blood pressure in subjects with high-normal ambulatory blood pressure levels: a randomized controlled trial. Am J Hypertens 1999; 12:47–53.

382. Hale G, Paul-Labrador M, Dwyer JH, Merz CN. Isoflavone supplementation and endothelial function in menopausal women. Clin Endocrinol (Oxf) 2002; 56:693–701.

383. Simons LA, von Konigsmark M, Simons J, Celermajer DS. Phytoestrogens do not influence lipoprotein levels or endothelial function in healthy, postmenopausal women. Am J Cardiol 2000; 85:1297–1301.

384. Teede HJ, Dalais FS, Kotsopoulos D, Liang YL, Davis S, McGrath BP. Dietary soy has both beneficial and potentially adverse cardiovascular effects: a placebo-controlled study in men and postmenopausal women. J Clin Endocrinol Metab 2001; 86:3053–3060.

385. Teede HJ, McGrath BP, DeSilva L, Cehun M, Fassoulakis A, Nestel PJ. Isoflavones reduce arterial stiffness: a placebo-controlled study in men and postmenopausal women. Arterioscler Thromb Vasc Biol 2003; 23:1066–1071.

386. Squadrito F, Altavilla D, Morabito N, et al. The effect of the phytoestrogen genistein on plasma nitric oxide concentrations, endothelin-1 levels and endothelium dependent vasodilation in postmenopausal women. Atherosclerosis 2002; 163:339–347.

387. Steinberg FM, Guthrie NL, Villablanca AC, Kumar K, Murray MJ. Soy protein with isoflavones has favorable effects on endothelial function that are independent of lipid and antioxidant effects in healthy postmenopausal women. Am J Clin Nutr 2003; 78:123–130.

388. Cuevas AM, Irribarra VL, Castillo OA, Yanez MD, Germain AM. Isolated soy protein improves endothelial function in postmenopausal hypercholesterolemic women. Eur J Clin Nutr 2003; 57:889–894.

389. Yildirir A, Tokgozoglu SL, Oduncu T, et al. Soy protein diet significantly improves endothelial function and lipid parameters. Clin Cardiol 2001; 24:711–716.

390. Hermansen K, Hansen B, Jacobsen R, et al. Effects of soy supplementation on blood lipids and arterial function in hypercholesterolaemic subjects. Eur J Clin Nutr 2005; 59:843–850.

391. Nikander E, Metsa-Heikkila M, Tiitinen A, Ylikorkala O. Evidence of a lack of effect of a phytoestrogen regimen on the levels of C-reactive protein, E-selectin, and nitrate in postmenopausal women. J Clin Endocrinol Metab 2003; 88:5180–5185.

392. Tonstad S, Smerud K, Hoie L. A comparison of the effects of 2 doses of soy protein or casein on serum lipids, serum lipoproteins, and plasma total homocysteine in hypercholesterolemic subjects. Am J Clin Nutr 2002; 76:78–84.

393. Jenkins DJ, Kendall CW, Connelly PW, et al. Effects of high- and low-isoflavone (phytoestrogen) soy foods on inflammatory biomarkers and proinflammatory cytokines in middle-aged men and women. Metabolism 2002; 51:919–924.

394. Brevoort P. The booming of U.S. botanical market: a new overview. Herbal Gram 1998; 44:33–46.

395. The effect of essential oil of garlic on hyperlipemia and platelet aggregation—an analysis of 308 cases. Cooperative group for essential oil of garlic. J Tradit Chin Med 1986; 6:117–120.

396. Bordia A. Effect of garlic on human platelet aggregation in vitro. Atherosclerosis 1978; 30:355–360.

397. Rose KD, Croissant PD, Parliament CF, Levin MB. Spontaneous spinal epidural hematoma with associated platelet dysfunction from excessive garlic ingestion: a case report. Neurosurgery 1990; 26:880–882.

398. Burnham BE. Garlic as a possible risk for postoperative bleeding. Plast Reconstr Surg 1995; 95:213.

399. Sunter W. Warfarin and garlic. Pharm J 1991; 246:722.

400. Vale S. Subarachnoid haemorrhage associated with ginkgo biloba. Lancet 1998; 352:36.

401. Benjamin J, Muir T, Briggs K, Pentland B. A case of cerebral haemorrhage-can Ginkgo biloba be implicated? Postgrad Med J 2001; 77:112–113.

402. Rowin J, Lewis SL. Spontaneous bilateral subdural hematomas associated with chronic ginkgo biloba ingestion. Neurology 1996; 46:1775–1776.

403. Gilbert GJ. Ginkgo biloba. Neurology 1997; 48:1137.

404. Lewis S, Rowin J. Ginkgo biloba (letter). Neurology 1997; 48:1775–1776.

405. Rosenblatt M, Mindel J. Spontaneous hyphema associated with ingestion of ginkgo biloba extract. N Engl J Med 1997; 336:1108.

406. Matthews MK Jr. Association of ginkgo biloba with intracerebral hemorrhage. Neurology 1998; 50:1933–1934.

407. Vaes LP, Chyka PA. Interactions of warfarin with garlic, ginger, ginkgo, or ginseng: nature of the evidence. Ann Pharmacother 2000; 34:1478–1482.

408. Meisel C, Johne A, Roots I. Fatal intracerebral mass bleeding associated with ginkgo biloba and ibuprofen. Atherosclerosis 2003; 167:367.

409. Janetzky K, Morreale AP. Probable interaction between warfarin and ginseng. Am J Health Syst Pharm 1997; 54:692–693.

410. Taylor JR, Wilt VM. Probable antagonism of warfarin by green tea. Ann Pharmacother 1999; 33:426–428.

411. Yue QY, Bergquist C, Gerden B. Safety of St. John's wort (hypericum perfotatum). Lancet 2000; 355:576–577.

412. Mauer A, Johne A, Bauer S, et al. Interaction of St. John's wort extract with phenprocoumon [abstract]. Eur J Clin Pharmacol 1999; 55:A22.

413. Johne A, Brockmoller J, Bauer S, Maurer A, Langheinrich M, Roots I. Pharmacokinetic interaction of digoxin with an herbal extract from ST John's wort (hypericum perfotatum). Clin Pharmacol Ther 1999; 66:338–345.

414. McRae S. Elevated serum digoxin levels in a patient taking digoxin and siberian ginseng. Cmaj 1996; 155:293–295.

415. Mauro VF, Mauro LS, Kleshinski JF, Khuder SA, Wang Y, Erhardt PW. Impact of ginkgo biloba on the pharmacokinetics of digoxin. Am J Ther 2003; 10:247–251.

416. Sugimoto K, Ohmori M, Tsuruoka S, et al. Different effects of St. John's wort on the pharmacokinetics of simvastatin and pravastatin. Clin Pharmacol Ther 2001; 70:518–524.

417. Shaw D, Leon C, Kolev S, Murray V. Traditional remedies and food supplements. A 5-year toxicological study (1991–1995). Drug Saf 1997; 17:342–356.

418. Tannergren C, Engman H, Knutson L, Hedeland M, Bondesson U, Lennernas H. St. John's wort decreases the bioavailability of R- and S-verapamil through induction of the first-pass metabolism. Clin Pharmacol Ther 2004; 75:298–309.

419. Lichtenstein AH, Appel LJ, Brands M, et al. Diet and Lifestyle Recommendations Rivision 2006: a scientific statement from the American Heart Association Nutrition Committee. Circulation 2006 114(1):82-96.

420. Foran SE, Flood JG, Lewandrowski KB. Measurement of mercury levels in concentrated over-the-counter fish oil preparations: is fish oil healthier than fish? Arch Pathol Lab Med 2003; 127:1603–1605.

421. Melanson SF, Lewandrowski EL, Flood JG, Lewandrowski KB. Measurement of organochlorines in commercial over-the-counter fish oil preparations: implications for dietary and therapeutic recommendations for omega-3 fatty acids and a review of the literature. Arch Pathol Lab Med 2005; 129:74–77.

5 | Type 1 Diabetes Mellitus

David W. Gardner and Khurshid A. Khan

Department of Internal Medicine, Diabetes, and Metabolism, Division of Endocrinology, Cosmopolitan-International Endocrinology and Diabetes Center, University of Missouri-Columbia, Columbia, Missouri, U.S.A.

Gurushankar Govindarajan

Diabetes and Cardiovascular Disease Research Laboratory, Harry S. Truman Memorial VA Hospital, Columbia, Missouri, U.S.A.

John M. Palmer

Department of Internal Medicine, University of Missouri-Columbia, Columbia, Missouri, U.S.A.

James R. Sowers

Department of Internal Medicine, Division of Nephrology, University of Missouri-Columbia, Columbia, Missouri, U.S.A.

KEY POINTS

- Based upon the outcome data from the DCCT and EDIC studies, there is clearly a great deal of benefit in prevention or slowing the progression of microvascular as well as macrovascular complications of T1DM, with tighter control of glycemic index.
- DSME is an integral component of diabetic management. The outcome of intensified insulin therapy is dependent upon the appropriateness of the insulin regimen used and the quality of the teaching process to empower patient to carry it out effectively and safely.
- Hallmarks of management of T1DM are as follows:
  - Tight glycemic control with HbA1C as close to normal as possible without exposing patient to any higher risk of hypoglycemic reactions
  - Early recognition and treatment of hypertension with goal blood pressure <130/80 mmHg
  - Identification of dyslipidemia and institution of drug therapy with statins if needed to achieve goal of LDL <70 mg/dL, HDL <45 mg/dL, triglycerides <150 mg/dL early enough in the course of the disease
  - Identification and treatment of insulin resistance with physical activity, weight maintenance and use of Insulin sensitizers in some cases
  - Recognition of proteinuria and microalbuminuria, and use of angiotensin-converting enzyme (ACE) inhibitors to delay the progression of renal dysfunction
  - Aspirin 81 mg qd in all Type 1 diabetic patients above 21 years of age

EPIDEMIOLOGY AND PREVALENCE

Type 1 diabetes mellitus (T1DM), previously referred to as insulin-dependent diabetes or juvenile diabetes, refers to diabetes that occurs as a result of the destruction of pancreatic beta-cells. According to the latest data, 1.4 million people in the United States and 10 to 20 million people worldwide have been diagnosed with Type 1 diabetes (T1D) (1), which comprises approximately 10% of all diagnosed cases of diabetes. In the United States, 30,000 new cases are diagnosed annually. Although these figures comprise a far smaller number of patients in comparison with Type 2 diabetes (T2D), Type 1 is the leading cause of blindness, end-stage renal disease (ESRD), cardiovascular disease (CVD), and premature death in the general population (2). The economic burden of this disease is substantial as well, because T1D accounts for about 30% of the total costs attributable to diabetes (3).

Although Type 1 is generally thought to be a disease of childhood, with 30% to 50% of all diagnosed patients showing clinical symptoms prior to 20 years of age (4,5), a growing number of older adults are being diagnosed with a newly classified type of T1DM. Latent autoimmune diabetes of adults (LADA) describes adult patients who have phenotype and immune markers of T1D but do not have complete beta-cell destruction at the time of diagnosis and still have insulin reserves for some years before progressing to complete insulin deficiency (6).

Through data collection from the DiaMond study and EURODIAB Study in Europe, it has been shown that geographical location plays a significant role in the variability of incidence rates (7,8). Areas such as Finland, Sweden, and Sardinia have the highest incidence rate. Areas such as the United States, Israel, and Spain have intermediate rates of incidence, and China and other Asian countries have the lowest documented rates. To put this geographic variability in perspective, an individual from Finland is nearly 400 times more likely to develop T1D than an individual from Japan or Korea. The geographical variance seen in incidence rates may be secondary to genetic and environmental factors. Prevalence also varies with racial groups as well. For example, in the United States, non-Hispanic whites are about 1.5 times more likely to develop T1D than are African-Americans or Hispanics (9).

PATHOGENESIS OF TYPE 1 DIABETES MELLITUS

The American Diabetes Association (ADA) has categorized T1D into two distinct groups, on the basis of immune-mediated factors. Type 1A has been defined as being immune mediated, and Type 1B (T1B) has been defined as being nonimmune-mediated, but with profound loss of insulin secretion (10). The vast majority of diagnosed Type 1 patients fall into the Type 1A group; hence immune-mediated aspects of the development of disease will be discussed here.

Type 1A diabetes results from autoimmune destruction of the pancreatic beta-cells in the islets of Langerhans, which are responsible for insulin secretion (11). The development and progression of disease is multifactorial, with a number of genetic and environmental factors playing important roles (12). Because overt disease is not clinically manifested until a large percentage of beta-cells have been destroyed, a prolonged period of latency is a hallmark of the disease and the focal point of research in regard to prevention and treatment.

Genetic Susceptibility

The lifetime risk of developing Type 1A diabetes has been shown to be greatly increased in those who have first-degree relatives affected by the disease. For example, the risk of development of Type 1A is about 2.5% and 1.5% in offspring of T1D-affected fathers and mothers, respectively. Furthermore, the risk in siblings has been found to range from 8.3% to 2.9 % (13) and in human leukocyte antigen (HLA)–identical siblings, the risk is increased to 33% (11). Although approximately 90% of Type 1A diabetes cases result spontaneously in patients without an affected first-degree relative, both familial and spontaneous cases of Type 1A diabetes have been shown to have strong patterns of inheritance, with susceptibility inherited from both the major histocompatibility complex (MHC) and the non-MHC genes.

Major Histocompatibility Genes

In order to understand the nature of genetic susceptibility in the pathogenesis of Type I diabetes, it is important to review some basic concepts pertaining to inherent immunologic responses. Several genes code for histocompatibility antigens, with the most important genes clustered on the short arm of chromosome 6 (6p21). This cluster of genes comprises the MHC, which is also referred to as the HLA complex. MHC genes are classified into three groups, on the basis of gene products. Class I antigens are expressed on nucleated cells as well as platelets. They are encoded on three separate loci, which have been designated HLA-A, HLA-B, and HLA-C. These molecules are heterodimers, which are made up of a polymorphic alpha or heavy chain, which is linked in a noncovalent bond to a smaller, nonpolymorphic peptide that has been designated beta 2 microglobulin, which is not encoded within the MHC. The extracellular region of the heavy chain is further subdivided into alpha 1, alpha 2, and alpha 3 subunits, respectively. Within the alpha 1 and alpha 2 domains, a structural cleft is present, which allows for the binding of peptides to the MHC molecule. Class I molecules bind to peptides, which are derived from proteins, and are recognized by CD8+ cytotoxic T cells. Class II antigens are coded within the region designated HLA-D, which has been further subdivided into three separate subdivisions, HLA-DP, HLA-DQ, and HLA-DR. The Class II molecule comprises heterodimer that consists of an alpha chain and beta chain that are noncovalently bonded. The extracellular portions of the alpha and beta chains have two separate domains, classified as alpha 1 and alpha 2, and beta 1 and beta 2. As in Class I molecules, an antigen-binding cleft is present as well, which allows for peptide binding. In contrast, however, the cleft in Class II molecules, is formed as a result of the interaction of alpha 1 and beta 1 domains of both chains, which allows for differences among Class II alleles. Each different sequence is given a number. Such differences are inherited in a Mendelian fashion and determine which peptides can be bound and presented. Thus, such inherited differences in HLA molecules between individuals can determine which antigen an individual can respond to, and importantly, which autoimmune disorder they are likely to develop. Class II molecules generally present exogenous antigens, which are recognized by CD4+ helper T cells (14). The importance of the differences within the HLA complex can be demonstrated through its association with Type I diabetes. Although a large number of genes that may enhance the risk of contracting T1D have been identified, about half of the genetic risk has been attributed to the products of the genes in the HLA complex found within the short arm of chromosome 6 (15). The association between the HLA genes and T1DM was first shown in the 1970s from studies that observed that Class I HLA B8, B15, and B18 alleles were more frequent in diabetics (16,17). Later, HLA Class II genes, in linkage disequilibrium with Class I antigens, were identified as the responsible agents in TID pathogenesis (18).

The major gene implicated in the development of T1D, labeled IDDM1, is located in the HLA region of chromosome 6p (19,20) and accounts for 35% of familial clustering in T1D (21). Genes from within this region code for MHC Class II molecules, which are displayed on the cell surface of antigen-presenting cells. There are three classes of HLA Class II molecules: HLA-DP, HLA-DQ, and HLA-DR. As discussed previously, the Class II proteins are dimeric in nature, composed of an alpha and a beta chain, and through the interaction of the two chains, a peptide-binding groove is formed, allowing antigens to bind (22). Ultimately, the complex presents to CD4 T-lymphocytes, resulting in T-cell activation and proliferation. A patient's individual HLA genotype affects to what extent the patient may respond to an antigen. In addition, substitutions within critical amino acid sequences of Class II alpha and beta chains will also affect the degree to which autoantigens are able to bind (23).

Within the Class II MHC, susceptibility or resistance to T1D is associated with various HLA-DR and HLA-DQ genotypes (24). The DR3- and DR4-containing haplotypes are known to confer a high risk for developing T1D (25), as 95% of patients with T1D have at least one of these HLA-DR antigens. Whereas the HLA-DR3 and -DR4 genotypes have been found to increase risk, those who carry the HLA-DR2 actually benefit from a protective effect, because this haplotype is negatively associated with T1D (26). The protection associated with HLA-DR2 is thought to be secondary to the HLA-DQA1*0102/DQB1*0602 phenotype, which confers protection against T1D (27), which occurs in 20% of the U.S. population (28,29), although it is found in less than 1% of individuals with T1D.

NONMAJOR HISTOCOMPATIBILITY GENES

While MHC susceptibility genes play a substantial role in the development of T1D, they alone are not sufficient in inducing the disease, because non-MHC genes account for only one-half of the overall genetic predisposition to T1D (30), thus suggesting a polygenic inheritance pattern (19). The insulin gene has been investigated for possible genetic susceptibility. It has been found that a variable tandem repeat (VNTR) within the insulin gene located in the upstream region is associated with T1D (31,32). It is thought that the increased expression of the VNTR in the thymus would, in fact, lead to a reduced risk of T1D, secondary to the deletion of high-affinity autoreactive T cells (33).

The Cytoxic T-lymphocyte–associated protein 4 has also been implicated in T1D, as it has been shown to play a major role in lymphocyte activation in mice, with possible diabetes development (34); though, the significance it plays in T1D patients is yet to be fully understood.

Other non-MHC genes that have been studied include interferon gamma, which is thought to play a primary role in injury to pancreatic beta-cells through cytotoxic T cells (35). Other factors that induce interferon gamma, including the cytokines interferon-gamma–inducing factor and interleukin-12 have also been shown to play roles of T1D susceptibility in mouse models (36).

Role of Autoimmunity

It has been found that during the development of T1D, antibodies are produced, which act against the pancreatic beta-cells (37), with resultant reduction in insulin production. We will discuss three autoantibodies that have emerged as important autoimmune agents in T1D. It is unclear whether these antibodies play a direct role in the disease process itself, or serve as markers of tissue damage.

Islet-cell autoantibodies (ICAs) were first discovered in the 1970s in patients with autoimmune disorders. Today, ICAs are detected by indirect immunofluorescence using pancreatic specific islet autoantigens for reaction. As research has progressed, it has now been documented that ICAs are present in 70% to 80% of all patients newly diagnosed with T1D (11). Furthermore, ICAs are found in only 0.5% to 4% of all nondiabetic individuals (37). ICA frequency decreases at the time of diagnosis, and less than 10% of T1D patients remain ICA-positive after 10 years (38). A certain group of adult patients who have been previously diagnosed with T2D have also been found to have ICAs present as well. This group has been described as the LADA, which is the progressive form of T1D that develops at a slower rate (6). Individuals from this group, mostly females, often present later in life, oftentimes in the fourth decade, generally maintain a lean body habitus, and have been diagnosed and treated as if they have T2D, often with inadequate control (39). The onset of Type 2-like diabetes in such patients is an indication for islet autoantibody testing, as it may aid in properly treating the patients with insulin initially (38).

Insulin antibodies (IA) are among the earliest markers to appear in children who develop T1D (40). At the time of diagnosis of T1D, IA have been detected in 35% to 60% of children, and several studies have shown that levels decrease with age (38). In fact, these antibodies can be detected shortly after birth, and levels of antibodies correlate inversely with the age at which TID develops (40). A genetic component for development of IA has also been found, as those who carry HLA-DR4 have an association with higher levels of IA (41).

Glutamic acid decarboxylase (GAD) is an enzyme that acts to catalyze the synthesis of gamma-aminobutyric acid, and has at least two separate isoforms in humans. GAD is not specific to the islet cells, or to the beta-cells, but rather, is predominantly found in the central nervous system, as well as the testes, ovary, pituitary, and thyroid (38,42). Antibodies to GAD have been found in up to 80% of patients with T1D (43). Because autoantibodies to GAD are generally more prevalent in older children and late-onset Type 1 diabetics, they are more persistent than ICAs after the diagnosis of T1D (44). Furthermore, because of the increased prevalence of these antibodies in older patients, antibody detection in those patients who have the characteristics of LADA may be of greater diagnostic value than ICAs (38).

Insulinoma-associated protein 2 (IA-2) is a neuroendocrine protein that acts as another autoantigen involved in T1D development. IA-2 is a protein tyrosine phosphate (37), which is expressed in cells of neuroendocrine origin which incudes beta, alpha, and delta cells in the pancreatic islets, pituitary cells, and cells in the adrenal medulla (45). Antibodies to IA-2 have been found in the serum of nearly 60% of patients at the time of diagnosis of T1D (46).

Environmental Factors

The influences of the environment, such as prenatal exposures, viral exposure, and dietary antigen exposure, play an important role in T1D development. Because of the low concordance rate of T1D among monozygotic twins (47), genetic risk factors may be necessary, but are not sufficient for the disease to occur. Thus, environmental exposures must play an important role in the disease process.

Several prenatal and perinatal factors have been associated with the development of T1D. The presence of jaundice at birth, especially related to ABO incompatibility and to a lesser extent Rh incompatibility, has shown increased risk of development of T1D (48). Fetal birth weight has been studied for possible links to later T1D development. A number of large trials have been done, which show weak, but significant associations between birth weight and T1D (49).

Low birth weight has also been considered a possible link in development of T1D. Some studies have shown a relationship between small-for-date births (50) and heavy-for-weight births (51). While these associations have been noted, several other studies have shown no definite causative link, casting some doubt as to the role weight at birth plays (52).

The role of breast feeding has also shown conflicting results as well. Some studies have shown a protective effect in children who primarily received breast milk (53), while others have shown an increased risk in those who were breast-fed (54). As a result, conclusive evidence has not been established as to the risk or benefit breast feeding provides.

Viral infections have been implicated in the development of T1D in genetically susceptible individuals, secondarily to triggering autoimmune reactions against beta-cells (55). Congenital rubella infections have been shown to have the strongest link to T1D in affected children (56). In addition, intrauterine enterovirus exposure has also been associated with an increased risk of the developing T1D (57). It is thought that molecular mimicry between the P2-C protein of Coxsackie virus and the GAD protein could be responsible for causing the development of autoantibodies to beta-cells (58). Along the same lines, recent concern has been raised with the potential risk of childhood vaccinations triggering T1D in genetically susceptible individuals. Despite the concerns, no distinct link has been established, and a study which considered the vaccinations for diphtheria, tetanus, pertussis, Hemophilus influenza type B, polio, measles, mumps, and rubella in a group of over 700,000 children showed that the incidence of T1D was not statistically different based on any number of the above vaccinations an individual received (59).

DIAGNOSTIC CRITERIA FOR TYPE 1 DIABETES MELLITUS

The criteria for diagnosis of diabetes was formulated by the National Diabetes Data Group of the United States in 1979 and the World Health Organization (WHO) Expert Committee on Diabetes Mellitus in the second report in 1980 (60,61). The diagnostic criteria of diabetes have undergone revision over the period of time with advances in understanding the etiology and pathogenesis of diabetes.

A minor modification was done to the diagnostic criteria by WHO in 1985 to coincide closely with the National Diabetes Data Group values.

In 1997, the ADA published yet another recommendation for the diagnosis and classification of diabetes mellitus (DM) to encompass the accumulated data and more information on etiology and to include the definition of the metabolic syndrome (62). The diagnostic criteria for normal fasting plasma glucose (FPG) and impaired fasting glucose (IFG) were updated in November 2003 (62,63).

It was strongly suggested that the diagnosis of diabetes be made on the basis of fasting blood glucose only, unlike the WHO criteria, which relied on oral glucose tolerance test (OGTT) for diagnosis. The ADA determined that OGTT is cumbersome and less reproducible (64). The WHO criteria were later updated in 1998 to reflect the 1997 ADA criteria (65). WHO agreed with the new ADA definitions, but suggested the continued use of the two-hour value on the OGTT for patients with blood glucose values in the range of IFG (detailed below) (65).

The diagnostic criteria was further revised by ADA and was published in 2003; it differed marginally from the 1997 report (62,63):

Normal was defined as fasting plasma glucose (FPG) <100 mg/dL (5.6 mmol/L).

IFG was defined as FPG between 100 and 125 mg/dL (5.6–6.9 mmol/L). This new cut-off for IFG decreased the discrepancies in the prevalence of impaired glucose tolerance (IGT) as proposed by the WHO criteria. Criteria for the diagnosis of DM were set as follows (Table 1). In the absence of unequivocal hyperglycemia, these criteria should be confirmed by repeat testing on a different day. The third measure (OGTT) is not recommended for routine clinical use (66).

The changes in diagnostic criteria likely contributed to changes in the prevalence of diabetes among populations studied, depending on the diagnostic criteria used (67,68). Obesity and age increased the proportion of the population with IFG/IGT or T2D (69). Both T1D and T2D are diagnosed in a similar way. T1D diagnosis in children and adolescents is easy when they present with classical symptoms of several weeks of polyuria, polydipsia, polyphagia, and weight loss, with hyperglycemia, glycosuria, ketonemia and ketonuria.

Hemoglobin A1c

There has been considerable interest in the use of hemoglobin A1C (HbA1C) values for screening and identification of IGT and diabetes (70,71). There are some data suggesting the use of HbA1C

TABLE 1 Criteria for the Diagnosis of Diabetes Mellitus, American Diabetes Association 2005

1. Symptoms of diabetes plus random plasma glucose concentration $\geq$200 mg/dL (11.1 mmol/L) or
2. FPG $\geq$ 126 mg/dL (7.0 mmol/L). Fasting is defined as no caloric intake for at least 8 or
3. 2 h Postload glucose $\geq$ 200 mg/dL (11.1 mmol/L) during an OGTT. The test should be performed as described by WHO, using a glucose load containing the equivalent of 75 g anhydrous glucose dissolved in water

Source: From Ref. 66.

in the diagnosis of diabetes, but the evidence is still lacking to recommend routine use of HbA1C in the diagnosis of diabetes. The latest ADA guidelines do not recommend routine use of HbA1C level for diagnostic purposes (66). However, with changing diagnostic criteria and the necessity for prompt and early diagnosis of diabetes, there may be value in measuring HbA1C along with FPG.

In the new classification, there is no distinction between the primary and secondary causes of diabetes (63). The terms Type 1 and Type 2 are to be used, whereas terms such as insulin-dependent, noninsulin-dependent, juvenile-onset, maturity-onset, adult-onset, maturity-onset diabetes of the young are to be eliminated. This change reflects an attempt to classify diabetes according to etiologic differences (as far as they are understood) and to move away from descriptions based upon age at onset or type of treatment (65,66).

T1D (previously defined as insulin-dependent or juvenile diabetes) is caused by beta-cell destruction, which leads to loss of insulin secretion and absolute insulin deficiency. This beta-cell destruction is immune-mediated most of the time and is classified as Type 1A diabetes (autoimmune) (55). Some T1D are nonimmune-mediated, but are characterized by absolute insulin deficiency (insulinopenia) and are classified as T1b (nonimmune-mediated) (72,73). Type 1A is by far the more common form of diabetes among Caucasian children and adolescents. It often has an acute presentation and patients require insulin for survival. The T1D in adult is less dramatic and the onset may not be as acute as in children and adolescents, and may be erroneously diagnosed as T2D resulting in delayed institution of insulin therapy. Type 1A diabetes, which is the predominant type, is due to autoimmune destruction of the pancreatic beta-cells. Testing for ICA or other autoantibodies (anti-GAD and anti-insulin) in serum may be helpful in establishing the diagnosis of T1D. Incidentally, Type 1A diabetes patients are also prone for other autoimmune disorders, such as Graves' disease, Hashimoto's thyroiditis, Addison's disease, vitiligo, celiac sprue, autoimmune hepatitis, myasthenia gravis, and pernicious anemia. However, patients with T1B diabetes have no evidence of autoimmunity and may not be identified by serological testing (74).

Besides the classical form of T1DM, other types considered in relation to T1DM are as discussed in the below section.

Latent Autoimmune Diabetes of Adults

With increased measurement of autoantibodies directed against pancreatic beta-cell antigens, it is being noted that numerous people who would have been wrongly diagnosed as T2D are being diagnosed as T1D. Studies indicate that among adults with apparent T2D, approximately 7.5 to 10 percent might have T1D as defined by the presence of circulating ICAs or antibodies to GAD (75–77). Among these autoantibodies, patients with antibody toward islet-cells, usually are thinner, have less endogenous insulin secretion, and respond poorly to drug therapy and require insulin therapy at diagnosis (76–79).

Thus, presence of anti-ICA or anti-GAD antibodies in this group of patients indicates that patients might actually have T1D and are less likely to respond to oral therapy, and require insulin for survival (80). Under new nomenclature, this type of diabetes has also been referred to as LADA.

Type 2 Diabetes in Youth

Diabetes in children was usually synonymous with T1D, but in the last decade, more and more cases of T2D have been reported in the youth across United States (81,82). This growing incidence of T2D in youth could be partly attributable to the epidemic of obesity (83) and change in lifestyle pattern (82).

Some of the characteristics that may be found in children and adolescents with T2D include the following:

1. Obesity: as many as 80% of youth may be overweight at the time of diagnosis.
2. Older than 10 years of age and in middle-to-late puberty, but cases of T2D in children as young as four years old have been documented.
3. Family history of T2D.
4. A member of a certain racial/ethnic group (African American, Hispanic/Latino and Native American descent) (81).

As the U.S. population is becoming increasingly overweight, researchers expect T2D to appear more frequently in younger, prepubescent children (82,83).

Flatbush Diabetes

Flatbush diabetics belong to non-T1D presenting as ketosis-prone diabetes. This group of diabetics has beta-cell insulin secretion and may or may not have autoimmune markers for T1D (84). This group of diabetic patients is more heterogenous and shares certain characteristics, such as positive family history of T2DM, overweight or obese, mostly nonwhite, and often presents with diabetic ketoacidosis (DKA) at diagnosis (85). However, recurrence of DKA is rare after the initial event and these patients can often initially be treated with diet or oral antidiabetic agents. This type of DM has been described globally by various names including "obese diabetes" or "T2DM with DKA."

TYPE 1 DIABETES MELLITUS AND CARDIOVASCULAR DISEASE

CVD constitutes the major cause of mortality and morbidity in both T1DM and T2DM diabetes patients (86). Advancement in the newer insulin treatment for persons with T1D has prolonged their lives significantly, along with its consequent increase in the CVD risk.

Persons with diabetes have about three times the risk of CVD. In the Multiple Risk Factor Intervention Trial, where about 5000 patients with diabetes were followed for 12 years, it was found that they had about three times higher risk of CVD when compared with controls, regardless of age, ethnicity, cholesterol profiles, systolic blood pressure (BP), or tobacco use (87). Most of the research and studies have focused mostly on T2D and CVD.

T1D is accompanied by long-term microvascular, neurologic, and macrovascular complications (88). Advancement in management of diabetes coupled with the advent of newer insulin for therapy has improved the life expectancy of patients with T1D and along with it, also increased the incidence of long-term complications, including retinopathy, nephropathy, neuropathy, and CVD (88,89).

Incidence of Coronary Artery Disease and Risk Factors

Coronary artery disease (CAD) is the main cause of death in persons with T1D and accounts for a large proportion of premature morbidity and mortality in the general population. CAD in T1D patients occurs earlier in life, affects women as often as men, and the associated mortality is dramatically higher than that in the general population (90–93). Women with T1D are 9 to 29 times more likely to die of CAD than nondiabetic women; the risk for men is increased four- to nine fold. If the diabetic patients develop proteinuria, they are at a 15 to 37 times increased risk of fatal CAD while the risk of those without proteinuria is three to fourfold, compared with the general population (90,94). While conventional CAD risk factors [hypertension (HTN), smoking, low high-density lipoprotein (HDL) cholesterol and high triglycerides (TGs)] increase the risk, the role of hyperglycemia, autonomic neuropathy, endothelial dysfunction, insulin resistance and diabetes duration is less established (95–98). In Type 1 diabetic patients, atherosclerosis is more diffuse (99,100), leading to higher case fatality, higher cardiac failure and restenosis rates, and shorter survival, compared with the general population. These poor outcomes emphasize the need for primary prevention of CAD in Type 1 diabetic patients.

The prevalence of CAD in T1D increases in patients rapidly with age, by their mid-40s; more than 70% of men and 50% of women with T1D have CAD, as indicated by the presence of coronary artery calcification, a surrogate indicator of atherosclerotic plaque (101).

Because of early onset of T1D, many patients develop early evidence of atherosclerosis. In one study, about 24% of asymptomatic T1D patients older than 35 years had ischemia diagnosed by noninvasive test such as exercise or pharmacological stress test and 10% had coronary stenosis greater than 50% by angiography (102). Early onset of atherosclerosis noted in T1D is strongly related to diabetes duration. Small clinical studies using high-resolution ultrasound to measure carotid intima-media thickness, a measure of atherosclerosis, showed significant atherosclerosis even at the age of 10 to 19 years (103,104). However, we have very little knowledge about the prevalence of subclinical CAD and risk factors for progression to clinical endpoints.

At all ages, ischemic heart disease mortality rate is much higher in T1D patients when compared with the general population (105). T1D shortens life expectancy; by age 55, 35% of T1D patients die of CAD in contrast to only 8% of nondiabetic men and 4% of women (90). Accelerated atherosclerosis and diabetic cardiomyopathy contribute to the excess mortality.

General Pattern of Atherosclerosis in T1D

Atherosclerosis occurs earlier in life in T1D (106) patients when compared with the general population. This is attributable to the duration of the disease. The disease process is more diffuse, resulting in higher case fatality, higher cardiac failure and restenosis rates, and shorter survival.

Cardioprotection normally afforded to young women is reduced in T1D and these patients are 9 to 29 times more likely to die of CAD than nondiabetic women; the risk for men is increased four- to ninefold (105). T1D patients with proteinuria have a 15 to 37 times increased risk of fatal CAD, whereas the risk for those without proteinuria is three- to fourfold compared with the general population (94). Chronic hyperglycemia seen in T1D confers increased risk of CVD and tighter glycemic control has been shown to decrease the progression of atherosclerosis (107).

Current Understanding of Type 1 Diabetes and Cardiovascular Disease

It is well know that CVD causes considerable mortality and expense in Type 2 diabetic patients (87,108,109). The risk of premature CAD in T1D may even exceed that of T2D, even when the traditional risk factors are absent (90,106). Relatively little is known about risks for CVD specific to T1D, except the substantial risk imparted by renal disease (90,110). Studies in T2D have demonstrated benefits of BP control, lipid lowering, and aspirin on CVD (87,111). Similarly, in T1D, intensive therapy has been shown to delay the progression of intima–media thickness, a measure of atherosclerosis, as well as other diabetic complications (88,107).

Factors Contributing to Atherosclerosis in Diabetic Patients

- Metabolic derangement, which includes hyperglycemia, increased free fatty acids, advanced glycation end products, and lipoprotein abnormalities
- Oxidative stress/glycoxidation
- Endothelial dysfunction and impaired endothelium-dependent vasodilation (112)
- Inflammation: atherosclerosis can be stated as fundamentally an inflammatory process exacerbated by diabetic dyslipidemia and other factors (113)
- Thrombosis/fibrinolysis
- Traditional risk factors, including smoking, HTN, and dyslipidemia

Besides the above-mentioned factors in the pathogenesis of atherosclerosis in diabetic patients, studies have shown that renal insufficiency is an independent predictor of progression of atherosclerosis in T1D (90). Potential intervention goals to prevent CAD in T1D are shown in Table 2.

Most of the aforementioned interventions in primary prevention of CAD in T1D patients comes from data gathered in general from diabetic patients and not particularly focused on T1D patients in particular, hence there remains a hindrance in clinical application as there is still lack of sufficient evidence demonstrating safety and long-term efficacy of these interventions. Existing observational studies provide more information regarding the pattern, progression, severity, associated comorbid conditions, and risk factors. In addition, research should

TABLE 2 Intervention Goals to Prevent Complications of Type 1 Diabetes Melitus

1. Tight glycemic control.
2. Early recognition and treatment of hypertension with goal Blood pressure <130/80 mmHg.
3. Identification of dyslipidemia and institution of drug therapy with statins if needed to achieve goal of LDL <70 mg/dL, HDL >45 mg/dL, triglycerides <150 mg/dL.
4. Identification and treatment of insulin resistance with physical activity, weight maintenance, and use of insulin sensitizers as needed in some cases.
5. Recognition of proteinuria and micro-albuminuria and use of angiotensin-converting enzyme inhibitors to delay the progression of renal dysfunction.
6. Aspirin 81 mg qd in all Type 1 diabetic patients above 21 years of age.

focus on expanding our knowledge of the pathogenesis of CVD in T1D and design clinical trials focusing on new interventions for CVD in T1D.

Management of T1DM

After more than 60 years of active debate and 10 years of study, the Diabetes Control and Complication Trial (DCCT) reported in 1993 the unequivocal effects of intensive DM management on the development and progression of the microvascular and neurologic complications of T1D (114). In DCCT, intensive treatment of T1D reduced the risk of retinopathy by 76%, nephropathy by 54% and neuropathy by 60% when compared with conventional treatment, as illustrated below (Table 3) (114).

On the basis of these results, the recommendation is to treat most patients with T1D with an intensive treatment regimen under the controlled supervision of a healthcare team consisting of a physician, nurses, nutritionist, and behavioral and exercise specialist, as needed. However, these recommendations of tighter glucose control may need to be modified for certain subgroups of diabetic patient where risk to benefit ratio may not be very favorable, e.g., children younger than 13 years, elderly people, and patients with advanced complications, such as ESRD, advanced CVD, or cerebrovascular disease.

TABLE 3 Risk of Microvascular Complications in Diabetes Control and Complication Trial Cohorts

Complications	Primary prevention			Secondary intervention			Both cohorts[b]
	Conventional therapy[a]	Intensive therapy % (95 CI)	Risk reduction	Conventional therapy[a]	Intensive therapy	Risk reduction % (95 CI)	Risk reduction % (95 CI)
≥3-step sustained rentinopathy	4.7	1.2	76 (62–85)[c]	7.8	3.7	54 (39–66)[c]	63 (52–71)[c]
Macular edema[d]	–	–	–	3.0	2.0	23 (−13–48)	26 (−8–50)
Severe nonproliferative or proliferative retinopathy[d]	–	–	–	2.4	1.1	47 (14–67)[e]	47 (15–67)[e]
Laser treatment[d,f]	–	–	–	2.3	0.9	56 (26–74)[c]	51 (21–70)[e]
Urinary albumin excretion (mg/24 hr)							
≥40	3.4	2.2	34 (2–56)[e]	5.7	3.6	43 (21–58)[c]	39 (21–52)[c]
≥300	0.3	0.2	44 (−124–86)	1.4	0.6	56 (18–76)[e]	54 (19–74)[e]
Clinical neuropathy at 5 Yr[g]	9.8	3.1	69 (24–87)[e]	16.1	7.0[c]	57 (29–73)[c]	60 (38–74)[c]

[a]Rates shown are absolute rates of the development and progression of complications per 100 patients-years. Risk reductions represent the comparison of intensive with conventional treatment, expressed as a percentage and calculated from the proportional-hazards model with adjustment for baseline values as noted, except in the case of neuropathy. CI denotes confidence interval.
[b]Stratified according to the primary-prevention and secondary-prevention cohorts.
[c]$P \leq 0.002$ by the two-railed rank-sum test.
[d]Too few events occurred in the primary-prevention cohort to all meaningful analyses of this variable.
[e]$P \leq 0.04$ by the two-tailed rank-sum test.
[f]Denotes the first episode of laser theraphy for macular edema or proliferative retinopathy.
[g]Excludes patients with clinical neuropathy at base line.
Source: From Ref. 114.

The pathogenetic effects of the level of hyperglycemia on the microvascular system persists for many years. This memory effect on the microvascular system lasts for years, even after good glycemic control. In DCCT (114), this time frame was three to four years, and in the United Kingdom Prospective Diabetes Study (UKPDS) (115), it was about nine years. The most proof of this memory effect has been elicited in the Epidemiology of Diabetes Interventions and Complications (EDIC) study, which is a long-term follow-up of some cohorts of DCCT patients (116). In the EDIC study, during seven years of follow-up of previously treated Type 1 diabetic patients from the DCCT cohort with intensive insulin treatment, the HgA1C went up to 8.0% from the previous level of 7.2%. In contrast, the mean HbA1C of the control cohort decreased to 8.0% from 9.0%. Despite the equal glycemic control over the past five years, the rate of development and progression of retinopathy and nephropathy was less than one-third in the previously intensively treated cohort compared with the previous control cohort.

In spite of abundant evidence demonstrating that aggressive risk factor management lowers the risk of vascular complications in diabetic patients, National Health and Nutrition Examination Survey (NHANES) 1999–2000, when compared with NHANES III (1988–1994) reported no improvement in the percentage of patients who achieved target goals for glycemia, BP, or serum cholesterol concentration (117).

GOALS OF THERAPY

The goals of treatment of diabetes are not only to control hyperglycemia, but also to take steps and institute measures to minimize the vascular inflammatory effects of diabetes and also to try to reduce the associated risk factors for microvascular and macrovascular complications. A complete medical evaluation should be performed to classify the patient, detect the presence or absence of diabetes complications, assist in formulating a management plan, and provide the basis for continuing care. A focus on the components of care and comprehensive examination will provide the health care team the information needed to ensure needed optimal management of patient with diabetes, as illustrated in Table 4.

The management plan should be formulated as an individualized therapeutic alliance among the patient and family, the physician, and other members of healthcare team. The plan should recognize diabetes self-management education (DSME) as an integral component of care. Implementation of the management plan requires that each aspect is understood and agreed on by the patient and the care providers, and the goals and treatment plans have to be reasonable.

In the next section, we will discuss the management of T1DM under the following headings:

1. Patient education
2. Glycemic control
3. Role of diet in diabetes management
4. Role of exercise in diabetes management
5. Insulin treatment
6. BP control
7. Lipid control
8. Screening for microvascular complications
9. Peripheral arterial disease
10. Management of acute complications of T1DM
11. Insulin pumps
12. Pancreatic and islet-cell transplantation

Patient Education

DSME is an integral component of diabetic management. At times, it can be quite challenging for the patient to get acquainted with the disease and how to manage it by both pharmacologic and nonpharmacologic interventions. The outcome of intensified insulin therapy is dependent upon the appropriateness of the insulin regimen used and the quality of the teaching process

TABLE 4 Components of Care and Comprehensive Examination in Type 1 Diabetes Mellitus

Medical history
- Symptoms, results of laboratory tests, and special examination results related to the diagnosis of diabetes
- Prior A1C records
- Eating patterns, nutritional status, and weight history; growth and development in children and adolescents
- Details of previous treatment programs including nutrition and diabetes self-management education, attitudes, and health beliefs
- Current treatment of diabetes, including medications, meal plan, and results of glucose monitoring and patients' use of data
- Exercise history
- Frequency, severity, and cause of acute complications such as ketoacidosis and hypoglycemia
- Prior or current infections, particularly skin, foot, dental, and genitourinary infections
- Symptoms and treatment of chronic eye, kidney, nerve, genitourinary (including sexual), bladder and gastrointestinal function (including symptoms of celiac disease in Type 1 diabetic patients), heart, peripheral vascular, foot, and cerebrovascular complications associated with diabetes
- Other medications that may affect blood glucose levels
- Risk factors for atherosclerosis: smoking, hypertension, obesity, dyslipidemia, and family history
- History and treatment of other conditions, including endocrine and eating disorders
- Assessment for mood disorder
- Family history of diabetes and other endocrine disorders
- Lifestyle, cultural, psychosocial, educational, and economic factors that might influence the management of diabetes
- Tobacco, alcohol, and/or controlled substance use
- Contraception and reproductive and sexual history

Physical examination
- Height and weight measurement (and comparison to norms in children and adolescents)
- Sexual maturation staging (during pubertal period)
- Blood pressure determination, including orthostatic measurements when indicated, and comparison to age-related norms
- Fundoscopic examination
- Oral examination
- Thyroid palpation
- Cardiac examination
- Abdominal examination (e.g., for hepatomegaly)
- Evaluation of pulses by palpation and with auscultation
- Hand/finger examination
- Foot examination
- Skin examination (for acanthosis nigricans and insulin-injection sites)
- Neurological examination
- Signs of diseases that can cause secondary diabetes (e.g., hemochromatosis and pancreatic disease)

Laboratory evaluation
- A1C
- Fasting lipid profile, including total cholesterol, HDL cholesterol, triglycerides, and LDL cholesterol
- Test for microalbum inuria in Type 1 diabetic patients who have had diabetes for at least five years and in all patients with Type 2 diabets; some advocate begining screening of pubertal children before five years of diabetes
- Serum creatinine in adults (in children, if proteinuria is present)
- TSH in all Type 1 diabetic patients; in Type 2 if clinically indicated
- Electrocardiogram in adults, if clinically indicated
- Urinalysis for ketones, protein, sediment, etc.

Referrals
- Eye exam, if indicated
- Family planning for women of reproductive age
- MNT, as indicated
- Diabetes educator, if not provided by physician or practice staff
- Behavioral specialist, as indicated
- Foot specialist, as indicated
- Other specialties and services, as appropriate

Abbreviations: LDL, low-density lipoprotein; HDL, high-density lipoprotein; TSH, thyroid-stimulating hormone; MNT, medical nutrition therapy.

to empower patient to carry it out effectively and safely. Furthermore, the success of diabetic treatment and teaching programs depends on the motivation and competence of the healthcare team and structural, organizational, and financial conditions.

Diabetes self-management refers to all of the activities in which a patient engages to care for his or her illness: promote health; augment physical, social, and emotional sources; and prevent long- and short-term effects of diabetes. Education is the essential first step in becoming an effective self-manager. Recent reviews and metanalyses have indicated that DSME is effective in improving metabolic and psychosocial outcomes. In addition, the DSME interventions that integrate the physiological, behavioral, and psychosocial aspects of diabetes are more effective than programs that focus strictly on knowledge (119).

It is important to ensure that newly diagnosed patients are well prepared, emotionally and physically, to treat symptoms: help them come to terms with the diagnosis, engage them in self-management plans, and show them how to gain some control of disease. These strategies not only will help them to achieve good glycemic control, but will also delay or prevent the onset of complications in the long run (115).

When designing any educational protocol, the curriculum should be based on the question "what do you want the patient to be able to do at the end of program," with the objectives set out in behavioral terms. At the end of program, the patient should be able to achieve a number of learning objectives as outlined below:

- Explain what diabetes is and how the disease progresses
- Describe a healthy diet
- Discuss the effects of exercise, alcohol, and smoking on diabetes
- List the possible long-term complications and ways to reduce the risk of these; that is, good glycemic and BP control, regular monitoring, foot care, and eye screening
- Describe the medical treatments for diabetes and how to overcome the potential side effects, e.g., hypoglycemia
- Discuss practical issues such as employment, driving, insurance, and prescription charges
- List the local and national services available, e.g., optometry, dietitians, hospital clinics, voluntary groups, and useful telephone numbers

An open approach is needed to encourage patients to participate in their own care. They should be given the opportunity and time to ask their questions, dispel myths, and discuss individual goals and objectives. Discussion replaces diktat, and informed self-management is the paradigm (120). Ewles and Simnet offer a good model of partnership, which includes the following (121):

- Promoting an atmosphere of trust and openness, so that patients are not intimated
- Active participation of patients, and carers are asked for their opinions and views, which are accepted and respected
- Informing people when health professionals learn something new from them
- Using informal, participative methods when involved in health education, drawing on experience and knowledge that patients bring with them

Glycemic Control

Monitoring of glycemic control is considered a cornerstone of diabetes care. Results of monitoring are used to assess the efficacy of therapy, and to guide adjustments in medical nutrition therapy (MNT), exercise, and medications to achieve the best possible glucose control. The past two decades resulted in major advances in monitoring, including the development and refinement of methods for self-monitoring of blood glucose (SMBG) and for assessment of chronic glycemia with glycated protein assays (glycated HbA1C). As mentioned earlier, prospective randomized clinical trials such as the DCCT have shown that improved glycemic control is associated with sustained decreased rate of retinopathy, nephropathy, and neuropathy (114). Epidemiological studies support the role of intensive glycemic control in reduction of CVD (122). The recommended glycemic goals for nonpregnant individuals with DM, according to the ADA, are shown in Table 5 (118).

A major limitation of the available data is that they do not identify the optimum level of control for a particular patient, as there are individual differences in the risk of hypoglycemia,

TABLE 5 Summary of Recommendations for Adults with Diabetes

Glycemic control	
A1C	<7.0%[a]
Preprandial plasma glucose	90–130 mg/dL (5.0–7.2 mmol/l)
Postprandial plasma glucose[b]	<180 mg/dL (<10.0 mmol/L)
Blood pressure	<130/80 mmHg
Lipids[c]	
LDL	<100 mg/dL (<2.6 mmol/L)
Triglycerides	<150 mg/dL (<1.7 mmol/L)
HDL	>40 mg/dL (>1.1 mmol/L)[d]

Key concepts in setting glycemic goals:
- Goals should be individualized
- Certain populations (children, pregnant women, and elderly) require special considerations
- Less intensive glycemic goals may be indicated in patients with severe or frequents hypoglycemia
- More stringent glycemic goals (i.e., a normal A1C, <6%) may further reduce complications at the cost of increased risk of hypoglycemia (particularly in those with type 1 diabets)
- Postprandial glucose may be targeted if A1C goals are not met despite reaching preprandial glucose goals

[a]Referenced to a nondiabetic range of 4.0% to 6.0% using a DCCT-based assay.
[b]Postprandial glucose measurements should be made one to two hours after the beginning of the meal, generally peak levels in patients with diabetes.
[c]Current NCEP/ATP III guidelines suggest that in patients with triglycerides 200 mg/dL, the non-HDL cholesterol (total cholesterol minus HDL) be utilized. The goal is 130 mg/dL (61).
[d]For women, it has been suggested that the HDL goal be increased by 10 mg/dL.
Abbreviations: LDL, low-density lipoprotein; HDL, high-density lipoprotein; DCCT, Diabetes Control and Complications Trial. NCEP/ATP-III, National Cholestrol Education Program/Adult Treatment Panel III.

weight gain, and other adverse effects. There are no clinical trials data to show optimum glycemic control in the elderly (≥65 years of age), young children (<13 years of age), or patients with advanced complications. Less stringent treatment goals may be appropriate for the very young or very old, individuals with comorbidities or in patients with limited life expectancy. More strict treatment goals can be considered in individual patients based on the epidemiological analysis that suggests that there is no lower limit of HbA1C at which lowering does not reduce the risk of complications. In every individual case, the risks of hypoglycemia should be weighed carefully against the benefits of better glycemic control (123).

Glycemic control in patients with gestational DM has to be more stringent because of higher risk of fetal complications and increased mortality associated with high blood glucose readings. In gestational DM, the target for FPG level is ≤ 105 mg/dL (5.8 mmol/L) or one hour postprandial plasma glucose ≤155 mg/dL (8.6 mmol/L) or two hours postprandial plasma glucose ≤130 mg/dL (7.2 mmol/L).

The ADA recommends that patients with T1DM should monitor blood glucose at least three times daily (124). The best way to monitor T1DM is by SMBG along with periodic HbA1C testing. In DCCT (113), a minimum requirement of "four" daily glucose testings (preprandial and bedtime) was implemented. In addition, 90 minutes postprandial tests were performed when HbA1C tests did not reach the target range despite preprandial blood glucose levels in the target range (70–120 mg/dL). A weekly "3.00 A.M." (or mid-sleep) blood glucose measurement was also required as a safety check to guard against unrecognized nocturnal hypoglycemia. A value of <65 mg/dL (<3–6 mmol/L) required a repeat mid-sleep test the next day; if the repeat value was the same, the insulin regime was adjusted.

In difficult and complex cases, continuous glucose monitoring (CGM) can be done. Different modalities for CGM are GlucoWatch; CGM system (CGMS) and implantable subcutaneous glucose sensors. Both GlucoWatch and CGMS are approved by Food and Drug Administration (FDA) (125).

To check for control of diabetes for the preceding two to three months, HbA1C is the standard test (126). The DCCT found an inverse relationship between the HbA1C value and the incidence of developing diabetic retinopathy in patients with T1D.

The risk of retinopathy was near its lowest level in patients with HbA1C values of approximately 7% to 7.5%. There was a slight further improvement at lower HbA1C values between 5.5% and 7% but at the risk of significantly increased risk of hypoglycemia in many patients, as illustrated below in Figure 1.

(A)

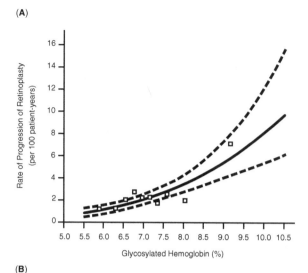

(B)

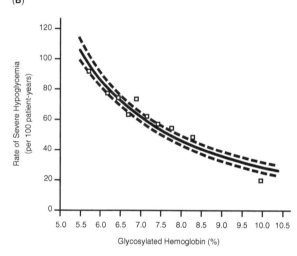

FIGURE 1 (**A**) Risk of sustained progression of retinopathy and (**B**) rate of severe hypoglycemia in the patients receiving intensive therapy, according to their mean glycosylated hemoglobin values during the trial (1). *Source*: From Ref. 114.

The ADA recommends HbA1C of <7.0% in diabetic patients for good control, while according to recommendations from the American Association of Clinical Endocrinologists, for good control, HbA1C level should be <6.5% in diabetic patients. According to the ADA, measurement of the HbA1C should be done every three months to determine the patient's metabolic control, even though it needs to be individualized, and frequency of testing A1C should be dependent on the clinical situation, the treatment regimen used, and the judgment of the clinician. In a stable well-controlled case of diabetes, A1C can be done twice a year. Correlation between A1C levels and mean plasma glucose levels is shown in Table 6 (127).

TABLE 6 Serum Glucose vs. Hemoglobin A1C

A1C (%)	Mean plasma glucose	
	mg/dL	mmol/L
6	135	7.5
7	170	9.5
8	205	11.5
9	240	13.5
10	275	15.5
11	310	17.5
12	345	19.5

Role of Nutrition in Glycemic Control

The biggest challenge associated with translating nutrition research into clinical practice involves making modifications and recommendations sufficiently reasonable so that they fit into the lifestyle of an average person. Results of the DCCT (114) and other studies reinforce the importance of nutrition therapy in the intensive management of T1DM. Food and eating are deeply rooted in our cultural, emotional, and physiological well being. There is no longer an ADA diet that applies to everyone with diabetes. An ADA diet can only be defined as an individualized food/meal plan based on assessment, therapy goals, and use of approaches that meet patient needs. Diet sheets or one-time diet instructions are rarely sufficient to change eating habits. Adherence to an individually prescribed nutrition plan improves glycosylated hemoglobin levels in adults (128) and has repeatedly been identified as the single behavior most positively correlated with good blood glucose control in children (129). Within two to three months of initiating MNT, HbA1C levels fall by 1% to 2%. Additionally, MNT is also effective in lowering BP, improving lipid profile, and lowering weight in some cases (130).

Individuals with T1DM respond to nutrient modifications differently from those with Type 2 DM. Genetics, insulin secretion capacity, age, duration of DM and the presence of complications are only a few of the factors that contribute to individual metabolic response to nutrient modifications (131). Because of the complexity of nutrition issues, it is recommended that a registered dietician, knowledgeable and skilled in implementing nutrition therapy in diabetic management and education, be the team member providing MNT. Implementing a successful nutrition plan requires an accurate assessment of usual food intake, including individual macronutrient consumption and pattern of consumption. Dramatic alterations in usual eating patterns are often unnecessary and produce large lifestyle changes that almost certainly result in failure to adhere to the meal plan. In fact, dietary modification should be driven by desired medical outcomes. Nutrition-related desired medical outcomes in T1DM, in order of priority, are to achieve near normal blood glucose levels, to achieve normal serum lipid levels, and to achieve normal BP. Implementation of nutrition plan can be elicited as the following (131):

1. Assess food intake
   a. Calories
   b. Carbohydrate, protein, fat
   c. Alcohol
   d. Supplements
   e. Pattern of intake
2. Develop nutritional goals
   a. Optimal blood glucose levels
   b. Normal growth
   c. Weight gain, maintenance, reduction
   d. Normal serum lipids
   e. Reduced proteinuria
   f. Normal BP
3. Implement nutrition strategies
   a. General guidelines, food pyramid
   b. Exchange system
   c. Carbohydrate exchanges
   d. Carbohydrate counting
4. Evaluate outcome
   a. Blood glucose testing
   b. Glycemic control
   c. Serum lipids
   d. Proteinuria
   e. Body weight
   f. Frequency of reactions

Caloric Intake

For youth with T1D, goals of MNT are to provide adequate calories to ensure normal growth and development, integrate insulin regimens into usual eating and physical activity habits.

Because most individuals with T1DM are thin adults or children, there is less of a need to focus on calories as there is in Type 2 DM. The theoretically ideal caloric intake can be determined from different formulas that take into account the patient's age, sex, height, weight, and usual level of activity. The results obtained should be adjusted upward for patients who are very active and in special circumstances such as pregnancy. How much emphasis is given to calorie intake depends upon how close the patient is to his or her desirable body weight. If patient has been close to ideal weight for several months or years, his or her current caloric intake is probably appropriate and few, if any, alterations need to be made. The majority of clinicians agree that the best way to estimate daily caloric needs is by monitoring body weight and adjusting food intake up or down by small increments of 200 to 300 kcal/day (132). In one report, for example, unmeasured diets were compared with "exchange" diets among lean adults with diabetes. There were no significant differences in body weight, serum cholesterol, fasting blood glucose, or number of hypoglycemic episodes during two years of follow-up (133).

Carbohydrates and Diabetes

As recommended by the ADA, carbohydrates and monounsaturated fat together should provide 60% to 70% of energy intake (134). Current ADA nutrition recommendations for persons with diabetes do not advocate sugar restriction for the purpose of blood glucose control. Foods containing carbohydrates from whole grains, fruits, vegetables, and low-fat meats should be included in a healthful diet. With regard to the glycemic effects of carbohydrates, the total amount of carbohydrate in meals or snacks is more important than the source or type. As sucrose does not increase glycemia to a greater extent than isocaloric amounts of starch, sucrose and sucrose-containing food do not need to be restricted by people with diabetes; however, they should be restricted for other carbohydrate sources, or if added, covered with insulin or other glucose-lowering medications. Individuals receiving intensive insulin therapy should adjust their premeal insulin doses on the basis on the carbohydrate content of meals.

Although use of low-glycemic index foods may reduce postprandial hyperglycemia, there is not sufficient evidence of long-term benefit to recommend use of low-glycemic index diet as a primary strategy in food/meal planning. As with the general public, consumption of dietary fiber is to be encouraged; sucrose and sucrose-containing foods should be eaten in the context of a healthful diet.

Protein and Diabetes

Proteins should account for 15% to 20% of average energy intake. For persons with diabetes, there is no evidence to suggest that usual protein intake of 15% to 20% of total daily energy should be modified if renal function is normal.

The long-term effects of diets high in protein and low in carbohydrate are unknown. Although such diets may produce short-term weight loss and improve glycemia, it has not been established that weight loss is maintained long term. The long-term effect of such diets on plasma LDL cholesterol is also a concern.

Dietary Fat and Diabetes

Less than 10% of energy should be derived from saturated fats. Some individuals (i.e., persons with LDL cholesterol ≥100 mg/dL) may benefit from lowering saturated fat intake to <7% of energy intake. Dietary cholesterol intake should be <300 mg/day. To lower LDL cholesterol, energy derived from saturated fat can be reduced if weight loss is desirable or replaced with either carbohydrate or monounsaturated fat when weight loss is not a goal. Intake of trans-unsaturated fatty acids should be minimized. Reduced-fat diets when maintained long term, contribute to modest loss of weight and improvement in dyslipidemia. Two to three servings of fish per week provide dietary *n*-3 polyunsatruated fat and can be recommended. Polyunsaturated fat intake should be approximately 10% of energy intake.

Alcohol and Diabetes

If individuals choose to drink alcohol, no more than two alcohol-containing drinks per day for adult men and no more than one drink per day for adult women is recommended. One drink is defined as 12 oz of beer, 5 oz of wine, or 1.5 oz of distilled spirits, each of which contains approximately 15 g of alcohol (132). Alcohol can have both hypoglycemic and hyperglycemic effects in people with diabetes. The effects are determined by the amount of alcohol acutely ingested, if consumed with or without food and if use is chronic and excessive. In studies using moderate amounts of alcohol ingested with food in diabetic patients, alcohol had no acute effect on blood glucose or insulin levels.

Carbohydrate Counting (Concept of Carbs)

In DCCT, carbohydrate counting was used as one of the four meal-planning approaches and was found to be effective in helping people achieve glycemic control while allowing flexibility in their food choices (114). Because carbohydrate rich foods have the greatest impact on postprandial blood glucose response, the primary strategy in control of T1DM is balancing carbohydrate intake and insulin dose. Implementing such a carbohydrate-monitored nutrition plan is usually accomplished either by carbohydrate counting or by an exchange system that focuses on carbohydrate-containing foods only. In basic carbohydrate counting, goals are to encourage people to eat consistent amounts of carbohydrates at meals and snacks at similar times each day. Advanced carbohydrate counting is appropriate for people who use multiple daily injections (MDI) of insulin or continuous subcutaneous insulin infusion (CSII) via an insulin pump. The goal is to match the amount of rapid-acting insulin to the amount of carbohydrate they plan to eat for their meal. This is done by selecting insulin to carbohydrate ratio empirically, which is calculated on the basis of individual insulin needs and metabolic responses to carbohydrates. Carb is a term, which is commonly used in carbohydrate counting and 15 g of carbohydrate make up 1 carb. Carbohydrate counting can be accomplished for any individual patient as follows (131):

- Determine goal for grams of carbohydrate to be eaten at each meal or snack
- Discuss how to approximate goal
  - Using food label
  - Using exchange list for carbohydrate foods
- Estimate insulin-to-carbohydrate ratio
  - Approximately 10g to 15g of carbohydrate/unit of rapid-acting insulin
  - Less in children under 100lbs (20–30g/unit of rapid-acting insulin)
- Collect SMBG records for two-hour postprandial testing
- Adjust insulin ratio to optimize glucose response
  - Decrease grams of carbohydrate/unit of insulin if blood glucose level higher than goal
  - Increase grams of carbohydrate/unit of insulin if blood glucose level lower than goal
- Teach patient how to increase or decrease insulin in relation to changes in carbohydrate intake

Exercise and T1DM

Regular physical exercise is recognized to have several benefits in T1DM as listed below (135).

- Lower blood glucose concentration during and after exercise (136)
- Improve insulin sensitivity and decrease insulin requirement
- Improve lipid profile
  - Decrease TGs
  - Slightly decrease LDL cholesterol
- Increase HDL cholesterol
- Improve mild to moderate HTN
- Increase energy expenditure
  - Adjustment to diet for weight reduction
- Increase fat loss
- Prevent loss of lean body mass
- Cardiovascular (CV) conditioning
- Increase strength and flexibility
- Improve sense of well being and enhance quality of life

Insulin Therapy

Insulin is the sine quo non for the treatment of T1DM. Insulin became available for clinical use in the early 1920s. Major advances have been made in the last 30 years in management of T1DM, especially in the way insulin therapy is used in clinical practice. Much of this progress has been made possible because of the following reasons:

1. A change in the philosophy of diabetes management, such that patient self-management and flexibility in life style have come to drive contemporary treatment approaches.
2. The emphasis on SMBG by patient and using this as a guide for treatment changes
3. The development of insulin analogs that have time action profiles aligned with physiological insulin secretion.

Characteristics of Currently Available Insulin Preparation

There are four major characteristics of insulin preparations:

1. Species of insulin
2. Purity of insulin
3. Concentration of insulin
4. Onset and duration of action

Species of Insulin

Human insulin is now produced by recombinant DNA technologies (biosynthetic human insulin). Eli Lilly and Novo Nordisk dispense human insulin as regular (R) and NPH (N). Three analogs of human insulin—two rapidly acting (insulin lispro and insulin aspart) and one very long-acting (insulin glargine) are now available for clinical use. A limited supply of mono-species pork insulin (illectem II) remains available for use by select group of patients.

Purity of Insulin

Improvements in purification techniques for insulin have reduced or eliminated contaminating insulin precursors that were capable of inducing anti-insulin antibodies. "Purified" insulin is defined by the FDA as containing less than 10 ppm of proinsulin.

Concentration of Insulin

At present, insulins in the United States are available only in a concentration of 100 units/mL (U100). For use in rare cases of severe insulin resistance in which large quantities of insulin are required, a limited supply of 500 units/mL (U500) regular insulin is available from Eli Lilly.

Onset and Duration of Action of Insulin

The time course of action falls into five general categories (137).

1. Rapid-acting, including the genetically engineered insulin analogs insulin lispro, insulin aspart, and insulin glulisine.
2. Short-acting specifically regular insulin (also know as soluble insulin).
3. Intermediate acting, including NPH insulin (also know as isophane insulin).
4. Long-acting insulin analogs including insulin glargine and insulin detemir.
5. Preparation of mixtures of regular and NPH insulin and also insulin analogs (insulin lispro and insulin aspart) mixed with insulin aspart protamine.

Please refer to Table 7 for more details of above-mentioned insulin subtypes available in market (138).

Insulin Regimens in T1DM

In people without DM, normal homeostasis is maintained by following two modes of insulin secretion (139).

1. Basal insulin secretion, which is the insulin secreted continuously by the pancreas 24 hours a day to maintain blood glucose levels in normal range, regardless of food intake
2. Prandial insulin secretion, which is the insulin secreted by the pancreas during meal times to control meal-related glucose excursions

TABLE 7 Different Types of Insulin and Timings of Their Actions

Insulin preparation	Onset of action	Peak action	Effective duration of action
Rapid-acting insulin analogs			
Insulin lispro	5–15 min	30–90 min	3–5 h
Insulin aspart	5–15 min	30–90 min	3–5 h
Insulin glulisine	5–15 min	30–90 min	3–5 h
Short-acting insulin			
Regular	30–60 min	2–3 h	5–8 h
Intermediate-acting insulin			
NPH	2–4 h	4–10 h	10–16 h
Lente	3–4 h	4–12 h	12–18 h
Long-acting insulin			
Ultralente	6–10 hr	10–16 h	18–24 h
Insulin glargine	2–4 hr	Peakless	20–24 h
Insulin detemir	2–4 hr	6–14 h	16–20 h
Insulin mixtures			
70/30 human mix (70% NPH, 30% regular)	30–60 min	Dual	10–16 h
75/25 lispro analog mix (75% intermediate, 25% lispro)	5–15 min	Dual	10–16 h
70/30 aspart analog mix (70% intermediate, 30% as apart)	5–15 min	Dual	10–16 h
50/50 human mix (50% NPH, 50% regular)	30–60 min	Dual	10–16 h

Source: Adapted from Ref. 138.

Basal insulin secretion restrains hepatic glucose utilization, keeping it in equilibrium with basal glucose utilization by brain and other tissues that are obligate glucose consumers.

After meals, meal-related prandial insulin secretion stimulates glucose utilization and storage while inhibiting hepatic glucose output. Patients with T1D lack both basal and meal-related insulin secretion. The goal in T1DM management is an insulin regimen that gives patient insulin coverage for both basal and prandial times (140).

Common types of insulin regimens currently being used in T1DM are as follows:

1. Intensive insulin therapy with MDI of insulin
2. CSII
3. Twice-daily insulin and other regimes

Intensive Multiple Daily Injections of Insulin
Prandial Insulin Therapy. The best way to initiate an insulin regimen is to give injections of short-acting insulin before meals. With insulin analogs (insulin lispro and insulin aspart), injection has to be given about 10 to 15 minutes before the meal, and with regular insulin, injection should be about 30 minutes before the meal. Ideally, carbohydrate in the meal should be counted and insulin dose should be calculated according to the ratio of insulin to carbohydrates values from one individual to another depending upon multiple factors but usually one unit of insulin for each 15 g of carbohydrate (1 carb) is a good start. This regimen allows a lot of flexibility in meal timing. Patients may consume any number of meals per day—one, two, three, or more—taking meal-related prandial insulin with each meal; the dose should be determined by meal content.

Basal Insulin Therapy. Basal insulin coverage is best accomplished by giving one or two daily injections of long-acting insulin (insulin glargine or insulin detemir). These insulin analogs reach a steady state within one to two hours of injection and do not have any peaks effect; the aforementioned feature minimizes the chances of hypoglycemia with these types of insulin activity (141). Insulin glargine has action for up to 24 hours and can be given once daily although occasionally may have to be divided in two doses in some patients depending upon individual response. Insulin detemir almost always has to be given twice daily. In the past, lente and ultralente insulin were also used for the same purpose but are not available on the market anymore. Basal insulin replacement can also be accomplished with intermediate-acting

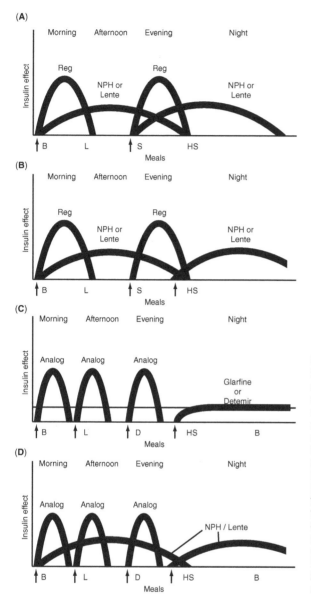

FIGURE 2 (**A**) Insulin effect provided by an insulin regimen consisting of two injections per day (*arrows*) of short-acting regular insulin (reg) and intermediate-acting insulin (NPH or lente). (**B**) Insulin effect provided by an insulin regimen consisting of injections (*arrows*) of short-acting regular insulin (reg) and intermediate-acting insulin (NPH or lente) before breakfast, short-acting insulin (reg) before the evening meal and intermediate-acting insulin (NPH or lente) at bedtime. (**C**) Idealized insulin effect provided by flexible multiple dose insulin regimen (*arrows*) with insulin analog as bolus insulin and insulin glargine as basal insulin. (**D**) Idealized insulin effect provided by flexible multiple dose insulin regimen (*arrows*) with insulin analog as bolus insulin and NPH insulin as basal insulin. *Abbreviations*: B, breakfast; L, lunch; S, supper; HS, bedtime snack. *Source*: From Ref. 138.

insulin (NPH insulin) injections twice a day, but this is far less optimal because NPH does not have flat insulin profile, but rather clear peaks of activity. The major problem with NPH is nocturnal hypoglycemia, which can be minimized somewhat by using NPH at bedtime to match the peak effect with time period of relative insulin resistance during early morning hours, also called Dawn's phenomenon. Oftentimes combining NPH with regular insulin works well, compared with NPH and short-acting insulin analogs (Fig. 2).

Figures 2A–D are illustrations of different types of insulin regimen and their glycemic effects as adapted from Skyler et al. (138).

Intensive Insulin Therapy Using Insulin Pumps

CSII by portable battery-operated "open loop" devices currently provides the most flexible approach, allowing the setting of different basal rates throughout the 24 hours and permitting patients to delay or skip meals and vary meal size and composition. The dosage is usually based upon providing 50% of the estimated insulin dose as basal and the remainder as intermittent boluses prior to meals (142). The meal bolus would depend on the carbohydrate content of the meal and pre-meal blood glucose value. One unit per 15 g of carbohydrate plus 1 unit for each 50 mg/dL of blood glucose above a target value (e.g., 120 mg/dL) is a good starting point. Most patients use the ultrashort-acting insulin analogs (analogs lispro and aspart) in the pump. Patients using regular insulin should use buffered insulin preparation (Velosulin) to minimize the risks of precipitation of the insulin in the pump tubing.

Other Insulin Programs/Regimens

Intensive multiple dose insulin therapy in Type 1 diabetic patients gives good insulin coverage for prandial and basal needs. However, such an approach requires a motivated, educated patient who carefully monitors blood glucose several times a day. In the absence of motivation, education, or frequent blood glucose monitoring, an alternative approach is to maintain day-to-day consistency; both of activity and of timing and quantity of food intake and this permits prescription of a relatively constant insulin dose (143). This can be accomplished by: twice-daily administration of mixtures of short-acting insulin (regular insulin, insulin asapart, insulin lispro) plus intermediate-acting insulin (NPH).

Blood Pressure Control in Type 1 Diabetes Mellitus

Both HTN and DM have been shown to be predisposing risk factors for the development of CVD and renal disease (144). HTN frequently coexists with DM, as the prevalence of HTN in patients with Type 2 DM is three times greater than in age and sex-matched patients without DM (109,145,146). Furthermore, patients with documented HTN are 2.5 times more likely to have DM than are their normotensive counterparts (147). It is the coexistence of HTN and DM together that synergistically promotes the development of CVD and renal disease (148). When HTN coexists with DM, the risk for CVD is increased by 75%, which further contributes to the overall morbidity and mortality of an already high-risk population (148). Even relatively small increases in BP have been proven to be detrimental in the diabetic population, as a 10 mmHg increase in systolic BP leads to a 15% increase in mortality related to diabetes, 11% increase in acute myocardial infarctions, 19% increase in strokes, and 12% increase in episodes of congestive heart failure (146,149). In addition, when these two conditions are present, the risk for developing ESRD is increased five to six times in comparison to those patients who have been diagnosed with HTN, but are not diabetic (146).

The treatment of HTN begins with alterations in lifestyle. According to the latest JNC VII recommendations, dietary and exercise habits are pivotal for the prevention and treatment of HTN. Patients who have been diagnosed with T1D should be encouraged to improve their dietary and exercise habits as the initial step of therapy.

The benefits of adopting a healthier lifestyle through improved diet and exercise have been shown in a number of clinical trials. In the Dietary Approaches to Stop Hypertension Study, patients who were placed on a dietary regimen that emphasized foods low in saturated fats and rich in fruits, vegetables, and low-fat dairy products, with or without sodium restrictions, were shown to significantly reduce BP. In addition, reductions were significantly greater in hypertensives than in normotensives (150). Increased physical activity also plays a beneficial role in therapy. In the Finnish Diabetes Prevention Study, overweight patients with glucose intolerance who received intensified lifestyle intervention, which consisted of diet and moderate exercise for at least 30 minutes per day, showed not only a marked reduction in the risk of developing T2D, but also a significant drop in BP (151). It is also important to note that for patients who find weight loss to be difficult to obtain, exercise and dietary changes that act to lower BP and improve lipid levels will also improve insulin resistance, even in the absence of weight loss (152).

Angiotensin-Converting Enzyme Inhibitors

Angiotensin II (Ang-II) plays a significant role in insulin resistance and the progression of HTN and CVD. There is significant evidence that interruption of the Renin-Angiotensin Aldos terone System (RAAS) can provide significant cardioprotective properties. Data from trials such as the Captopril Prevention Project (CAPP), Heart Outcomes Prevention Evaluation (HOPE) trial and its substudy, the Micro-HOPE, have all shown the CVD benefits that ACE Inhibitors (ACEI) can provide (153–155). In addition to these CVD benefits, there are also increasing data suggesting that agents that disrupt the RAAS have direct effects on improving insulin sensitivity (153–156), and may prevent development of diabetes in hypertensive patients as compared with other medications such as beta-blockers (BBs) (157). A 14% reduction in the risk of new onset diabetes was observed in the CAPP trial compared with conventional therapy with either a beta-blocker, diuretic or both. A 34% relative risk reduction for developing diabetes was also observed in the HOPE trial.

In addition, ACEIs also are renal-protective, by decreasing the membrane permeability to albumin, as well as decreasing intraglomerular pressure (158,159). Ultimately, this reduction in Microalbuminuria (MAU) helps prevent the progression to Chronic Kidney Disease (CKD), and meta-analyses had shown this antiproteinuric effect is independent of BP reduction (160).

When initiating therapy, renal function and serum potassium levels should be monitored carefully. While a slight increase in serum creatinine (Cr) may be seen secondary to intravascular depletion (161), an increase in Cr levels of greater than 30%, or levels that increase continuously during the first two months of therapy, may point to underling pathology such as renal artery stenosis or chronic volume depletion (158,161). Oftentimes, the elevated Cr levels are secondary to underlying volume depletion, and will normalize with correction of volume status (161).

Angiotensin Receptor Blockers

Angiotensin receptor blockers (ARBs) offer another group of medications that provide RAAS blockade. Specifically, these agents act to block the AT-1 receptor, which is responsible for the effects of Ang-II (156,162,163). Moreover, ARBs offer a more complete RAAS blockade, as ACEI may not completely block the conversion of Ang-I to Ang-II secondary to alternative pathway activation (164). In addition, the antihypertensive efficacy of ARB is similar to that of ACEI, while having an improved side effect profile, most notably significant lower rates of cough (165). As with ACEI, recent data have shown that ARBs reduce the risk of new onset diabetes. In the Losartan Intervention for Endpoint Reduction in Hypertension, a 25% reduction in the risk of new onset diabetes was observed in the Losartan group compared with beta blocker–based therapy (166). Similar results were also seen in the Candesartan in Heart Failure Assessment of Reduction in Mortality and Morbidity trial, which reported a 22% reduction in the risk of new onset diabetes in patients with heart failure when treated with candesartan (167).

Like ACEI, ARBs also offer significant renal protection as well. In the Reduction of Endpoint in NIDDM with Losartan, as well as the Irbesartan in Diabetic Nephropathy Trial, significant reductions in renal disease progression was seen, as well as reduction in albuminuria and Cr doubling time (156,162). Furthermore, combined ACEI and ARB therapy has shown greater reduction in albuminuria, as displayed in the Candesartan and Lisinopril Microalbuminuria trial (168).

As with ACEI, patients who started on ARB therapy should be monitored closely after initiation of therapy. Again, serum potassium and renal function indices should be followed. Because ARBs have similar effects on the vasculature, the possibility of worsening of renal function exists in those who may have underlying renal stenosis or who are chronically volume depleted.

Thiazide Diuretics

While thiazide diuretics are among the oldest available antihypertensive agents, they still play a significant role in the management of HTN, especially in the cardiometabolic syndrome (CMS). In the Antihypertensive and Lipid-Lowering Treatment To Prevent Heart Attack Trial (ALLHAT), it was shown that thiazide diuretics, when compared with ACEI and calcium channel blockers (CCB), comparably reduced all-cause mortality such as stroke, CAD, and heart failure (169). Moreover, results from ALLHAT show thiazides should be considered as firstline therapy for many hypertensive patients, including those with DM and the CMS (158,159).

Thiazides, at high doses, can lead to electrolyte disturbances, as well as worsening of insulin resistance, and can have adverse effects on lipid metabolism (169–171). Moreover, the efficacy of thiazides are limited by a reactive increase in renin and Ang-II levels in response to reduced plasma volume, leading to sodium and water retention and vasoconstriction (172). This adverse effect may be overcome with combination therapy with either an ACEI or an ARB secondary to RAAS blockade, and the combination potentiates the antihypertensive efficacy of each agent alone.

Calcium Channel Blockers

Through data compiled through clinical studies, 65% of all hypertensive patients require at least two, and often three, antihypertensive agents to achieve target BP of less than 130/80 mmHg (173,174). CCBs offer a proven, second-line therapy as adjuncts to the previously mentioned agents (175). In addition to their role in control of HTN, CCB have also been shown to reduce insulin resistance or new onset diabetes among people with the metabolic syndrome (159,176). Furthermore, CCB have also been shown to have renal protective qualities as well. While these agents do not offer the same degree of renal protection as ACEI when used in head to head monotherapy, combination therapy has been shown to have additive effects in reducing albuminuria (177). Findings from ALLHAT and Reduction of Endpoints in Noninsulin dependent diabetes mellitus with the Angiotensin II Antagonist Losartan (RENAAL) both showed that dihydropyridine calcium antagonists, such as amlodipine and nifedipine, are renoprotective when used in combination with the agents that block the RAAS (159,163). The nondihydropyridine calcium antagonists, such as verapamil and diltiazem, have also been shown to have additional benefits of reducing proteinuria, when used in combination with the RAAS blockers (178). Another added benefit of CCB therapy is their effect on lipid metabolism, as a 7% to 10% increase in HDL cholesterol above baseline has been shown in patients with metabolic syndrome (179).

Beta-Blockers

BBs have also been shown to be effective antihypertensive agents in the diabetic population, as demonstrated in the UKPDS, which showed that atenolol was comparable to captopril in reduction of BP and CV outcomes (180). Nonetheless, their use has often been complicated with their associated adverse effects on glucose and lipid profiles, as well as their implication in new-onset diabetes in obese patients (148,181). Further complicating their use is the propensity for vasospasm, and subsequent peripheral vasculature compromise. However, nonselective BBs such as carvedilol, which have been shown to induce vasodilatation, have a role in therapy in the CMS, as they not only benefit in HTN control, but they also have been shown to have favorable effects on CVD outcomes (182), as well as improvement in insulin sensitivity (182–184). Furthermore, agents such as carvedilol and atenolol have renal protective qualities, because they have demonstrated reductions in albuminuria, especially when used in conjunction with a RAAS-blocking agent (184).

Lipid Control in Type 1 Diabetes Mellitus

Coronary heart disease (CHD) is the leading cause of morbidity and mortality in the United States, accounting for approximately 500,000 deaths per year and an associated annual morbidity cost of more than $200 billion (185). The coexistence of diabetes and hyperlipidemia further increases the risk for CHD and its ill effects (186). Despite the numerous studies, which have documented the deleterious effect coexistence of diabetes and hyperlipidemia has, many patients are not adequately managed. In fact, one study, which gathered data from a managed care organization, showed only 15.8% of 6586 patients achieved their Intermediate-density liporotein (LDL)-cholesterol goal of <100 mg/dL (187). While those with T1D who maintain adequate glycemic control tend to have normal levels of lipoproteins, T1D patients who are overweight or obese may have a lipid profile very similar to that seen in T2D (188).

Screening for hyperlipidemia should be considered shortly after the time of diagnosis. According to the most recent ADA guidelines, children older than two years of age should have a fasting lipid profile performed at the time of diagnosis if they have a family history of hypercholesterolemia, defined as a total cholesterol level >240 mg/dL; a history of a CV event before age 55 years; or if family history is unknown. If one of these three criteria is not met, the first lipid screening should be performed at 12 years of age and older. If values fall within the accepted risk levels, an LDL <100 mg/dL, a lipid profile should be repeated every five years. For patients who are diagnosed after the age of 12, a fasting lipid profile should be performed at the time of diagnosis, and like their younger counterparts, should be repeated every five years if LDL values are less than 100 mg/dL. If lipid levels are abnormal, annual monitoring is recommended in either age group.

The target lipid goals for patients with T1D include LDL-cholesterol level of <100 mg/dL, HDL-cholesterol levels <40 mg/dL and TG levels <150 mg/dL. For those without preexisting

CVD, the current ADA recommendations for starting pharmacological therapy are an LDL-cholesterol level of 130 mg/dL with a goal of <100 mg/dL. As with the treatment of glycemia, lifestyle modifications should be the cornerstone of lipid therapy. However, for those Type 1 patients who have dyslipidemia, pharmacologic therapy in the way of lipid-lowering drugs will be necessary. Goals of therapy should be set according to individual lipid profiles.

3-hydroxy-3-methyl glutaryl coenzyme A reductase inhibitors are the first line in therapy as they are the most potent LDL-cholesterol-lowering medications. A number of clinical trials have established the benefits statin therapy has on CAD (189). While a subgroup analysis of the Heart Protection Study considered primarily the patients with T2D, the small group of T1D patients who were studied showed evidence of parallel benefit from statin therapy, and furthermore, evidence shows CVD in persons with T1D begins around age 40 years, suggesting that statins should be initiated by age 30 in T1D groups (90). In addition, while the majority of data obtained at this time regarding statin therapy pertains to the T2D population, it seems logical that the benefits from statin therapy can be extrapolated from the Type 2 population and applied to T1D.

Often, statin therapy alone may not be enough to reach target goals established. One possible loss of agents, which can be used in combination therapy, is treatment with fibrates. A series of clinical trials have shown fibrate therapy reduces the risk of CHD. One such study was the Veterans Affairs HDL Intervention Trial, which included subjects with elevated TG (<150 mg/dL) levels and low HDL cholesterol (<40 mg/dL), with entry-level LDL levels of about 140 mg/dL. Patients who were started on gemfibrozil reduced CV events by 35%, without changing LDL levels (190), showing the benefits of treating TG as well as HDL levels for risk reduction. In addition, while fibrates may not reduce levels of LDL, they do increase expression of the gene lipoprotein lipase, which decreases levels of dense, more artherogenic LDL (191). When used in combination, statins and fibrates offer additive benefits as demonstrated in a clinical trial that, compared simvastatin therapy versus simvastatin and fenofibrate together; the combination therapy with fenofibrate increased HDL cholesterol by 16% versus simvastatin alone, while significantly lowering very-low-density lipoprotein VLDL + Intermediate-density lipoprotein cholesterol and VLDL + Intermediate-density lipoprotein apolipoprotein B by 36% and 32%, respectively (192). When using combination therapy with statins and fibrates, the risk of myopathy from statins may be increased, and prescribers must consider the risks prior to initiation of therapy. When initiating either statin or combination therapy, both muscle and liver indices should be followed closely, especially in the first few months of therapy.

Other potential agents for treatment include niacin, which has been shown to be beneficial in CAD outcomes in monotherapy (193) or in combination with statins (194). Recently niacin and lovastatin were compared with simvastatin and atorvastatin, and the benefits of combination therapy with the two agents were demonstrated with reductions in LDL cholesterol and TG of 47% and 41%, respectively, while increasing HDL cholesterol by 30% (195). As with combination therapy with fibrates, the risk of statin-induced myopathy has been reported to be increased with niacin; however, no cases of myopathy were reported in the niacin/lovastatin combination trial. Nevertheless, close monitoring is necessary when initiating therapy.

Frequency of Nephropathy and Retinopathy Screening

These are some of the microvascular complications of T1DM, and DCCT (114) has established beyond a doubt that better glycemic control has favorable outcome on these complications.

Diabetic Nephropathy

Diabetic nephropathy occurs in 20% to 40% of patients with diabetes and is the single leading cause of ESRD. Persistent albuminuria in the range of 30 to 299 mg/24 hr (microalbuminuria) has been shown to be the earliest sign of nephropathy in T1D. Microalbuminuria is also a well-established risk factor for increased CVD (196). Patients with microalbuminuria (≥300 mg/24 hr) are likely to progress to ESRD over a period of years (197,198).

Screening for microalbuminuria can be performed by these methods:

1. Measurement of albumin to Cr ratio in a random spot collection (preferred method) (199,200)

2. 24-hour urine collection, with Cr measurement
3. Timed (e.g., four hours or overnight) collection

At least two of three tests measured within a six-month period should show elevated levels before a patient is designated as having microalbuminuria. Perform annual testing for the presence of microalbuminuria in Type 1 diabetic patients with diabetes duration of more than or equal to five years. Once microalbuminuria is diagnosed, the role of annual microalbuminuria assessment is less clear after institution of ACE inhibitor or ARB therapy and BP control. Most experts, however, recommend continued surveillance to assess both response to therapy and progression to disease. Consider referral to a physician experienced in the care of diabetic renal disease either when the glomerular filtration rate has fallen to <60 mL/min/1.73 m^2 or if difficulties occur in the management of HTN or hyperkalemia (201).

Diabetic Retinopathy
The prevalence of retinopathy is strongly related to the duration of diabetes and this is highly specific vascular complication of T1DM.

Better glycemic control prevents and or/delays the onset of retinopathy (114). The pressure of nephropathy is associated with retinopathy. High BP is an established risk factor for retinopathy. During pregnancy and one-year postpartum, retinopathy may be transiently aggravated (202); laser photocoagulation surgery may minimize this risk (203).

Patients with T1D should have an initial dilated and comprehensive eye examination by an ophthalmologist or optometrist within three to five years after the onset of diabetes. Subsequent eye exams should be repeated annually by an ophthalmologist or optometrist who is knowledgeable and experienced in diagnosing the presence of diabetic retinopathy and is aware of its management. Less frequent exams (every two to three years) may be considered with the advice of an eye care professional in the setting of a normal eye exam (204,205). Examination will be required more frequently if retinopathy is progressing. One of the main motivations for the screening for diabetic retinopathy is the established efficacy of laser photocoagulation surgery in preventing visual loss (206–210). When planning pregnancy, women with preexisting diabetes should have a comprehensive eye examination and should be counseled on the risks of development and/or progression of diabetic retinopathy.

Diabetic Neuropathy
Amputation and foot ulceration are the most common consequences of diabetic neuropathy and major cause of morbidity and disability in people with diabetes. All individuals with diabetes should receive an annual foot examination to identify high-risk foot conditions. This examination should include assessment of protective sensations, foot structure and biomechanics, vascular status, and skin integrity. People with neuropathy should have a visual inspection of their feet at every visit with a health care professional. Evaluation of neurological status in low-risk groups should include a quantitative somatosenory threshold test, using the Semmes-Weinstein 5.07 (10 g) monofilament. The skin should be assessed for integrity, especially between the toes and under the metatarsal heads.

Insulin Pumps
Several small portable "open loop" devices for the delivery of insulin are on the market. Theses devices contain an insulin reservoir and an pump programmed to deliver regular insulin subcutaneously. With improved methods of SMBG at home, these devices are becoming increasingly popular. The great advantage of CSII is that it allows for establishment of a basal profile tailored to the patient. The patient can therefore eat with less regard to timing because the basal insulin infusion should maintain a constant blood glucose level between meals. These pumps are small (about the size of a pager) and easy to program. They have many features including the ability to record a number of different basal rates throughout a 24-hour period and adjust the time over which the bolus doses are given. They are also able to detect pressure build up if the catheter is kinked. Improvements have also been made in the infusion sites. The catheter connecting the insulin reservoir to the subcutaneous cannula can be discontinued, so that patient can remove the pump temporarily (e.g., while bathing).

CSII therapy is appropriate for patients who are motivated, mechanically adept, and educated about diabetes and monitor their blood glucose four to six times a day. Potential candidates for pump therapy include the following (142):

1. Patients who have hypoglycemia unawareness or a history of recurring hypoglycemia episodes.
2. Patients who have HbA1C levels greater than 7%.
3. Patients who have difficulty maintaining glycemic control with MDIs.
4. Patients who are planning to become or are already pregnant.
5. Patients who experience "dawn phenomenon" (defined as abrupt increases in fasting levels of plasma glucose concentrations between 5 and 9 AM, in the absence of antecedent hypoglycemia).
6. Patients who have metabolic instability, early neuropathy, retinopathy, nephropathy, gastroparesis, and rental transplantation.

The dosage is usually based on providing 50% of the estimated insulin dose as basal and the remainder as intermittent boluses prior to meals. Ultrashort-acting insulin analog are the most commonly used insulins in CSII. Patients using regular insulin should use the buffered insulin preparation (Velosulin) to minimize the risk of precipitation of insulin in the insulin pump.

The following scheme can be utilized for establishment of initial basal and bolus insulin doses, when switching patient from subcutaneous insulin injection to insulin pump treatment (Fig. 3) (142).

Hypoglycemia

Insulin regimens are unphysiological and lead to peripheral hyperinsulinemia. This is thought to result in defective counter-regulation and various syndromes of absent to delayed warning symptoms in response to hypoglycemia. Hypoglycemia is one of the main factors limiting glycemic control to prevent long-term complications of diabetes (211). In DCCT (114), rates of hypoglycemia were 61.2 per 100 patient years versus 18.7 per 100 patient years in the intensive and conventional groups, respectively, with a relative risk of 3.28.

Definition of Hypoglycemia

Hypoglycemia can be defined as a blood glucose level <50 mg/dL (<3.1 mmol/L). People with DM experience symptoms with varying level of glucose concentration, and Whipple's triad is the best way to diagnose hypoglycemia in diabetics. Whipple's triad consists of symptoms compatible with hypoglycemia, a low blood glucose level and relief of symptoms after blood glucose is raised.

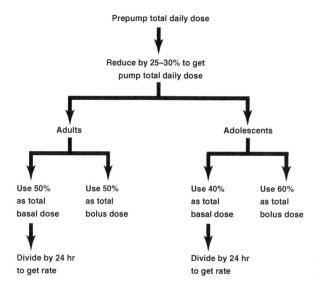

FIGURE 3   Establishment of initial basal and bolus insulin doses. *Source*: From Ref. 142.

Signs and Symptoms of Hypoglycemia

The signs and symptoms of hypoglycemia could be because of the following reasons:

1. Autonomic hyperactivity: This could be because of activation of adrenergic system (tachycardia, palpitations, sweating, and tremulousness) and parasympathetic system (nausea, hunger). In normal people, autonomic hyperactivity starts at blood glucose level of <60 mg/dL (<3.3 mmol/L).
2. Neuroglycopenia: Signs and symptoms of neuroglycopenia could include mental confusion with impaired abstract and later concrete thought process; this may be followed by bizarre antagonistic behavior, stupor, and coma, and even death may occur with profound hypoglycemia. In normal people, these symptoms start at blood glucose level <50 mg/dL (<3.1 mmol/L).

Hypoglycemia Unawareness

Patient with T1D uniformly loose their ability to secrete glucagons in response to acute insulin-induced hypoglycemia within a few years after developing diabetes. Thereafter, they are totally dependent upon triggered androgenic responses to counteract an impending hypoglycemia crisis as well as for early warning. With advanced age or with autonomic neuropathy, the autonomic responses may be blunted considerably and may become absent. In these circumstances, reduced awareness of hypoglycemia can lead to potential life-threatening sequels from neuroglycopenia convulsions or coma (212).

Causes of Hypoglycemia in Type 1 Diabetes Mellitus

Conventional wisdom suggests that hypoglycemia results from absolute or relative excess of insulin due to inability of most insulin regimens to mimic physiological insulin secretion. Conditions of relative or absolute insulin excess can occur because of the following reasons (213):

1. The insulin dosage is excessive or improperly timed.
2. Access to exogenous glucose is decreased during an overnight fast.
3. A meal is delayed or missed, or the meal has insufficient carbohydrates.
4. Gastric emptying is delayed because of high fat content of the meal or the presence of gastroparesis in autonomic neuropathy or episodes of gastroenteritis.
5. Glucose utilization is increased during exercise.
6. Insulin sensitivity is increased during the night or after prolonged exercise and during regular physical training, weight loss, recovery from infections, postpartum, lactation, and menopause.
7. Hepatic glucose production is decreased because of inhibited gluconeogenesis caused by excessive alcohol intake.
8. Insulin clearance is decreased as in renal failure.

Other causes of insulin excess can be related to daily variations in the insulin absorption from the subcutaneous sites. On any given day, there may be a 20% to 30% variation in the rate of absorption depending on body or ambient temperature, blood flow, anatomical site, or depth of injection among other factors.

DIABETIC KETOACIDOSIS

DKA is an acute complication of diabetes characterized by absolute or relative insulin deficiency aggravated by ensuing hyperglycemia, volume depletion, and altered level of consciousness. DKA is more common in T1D. The most common causes of DKA are underlying infection, disruption of insulin treatment, and new onset of diabetes.

Pathophysiology

Many of the underlying pathophysiologic disturbances in DKA are directly measurable by the clinician and need to be followed throughout the course of treatment. Close attention to clinical lab data allows the emergency physician not only to track the underlying acidosis and hyperglycemia but also to prevent common potentially lethal complications such as hypoglycemia, hyponatremia, and hypokalemia.

The absence of insulin and excess of counterregulatory hormones such as glucagon, growth hormone, corticosteroids, and catecholamines results in development of DKA. These hormonal changes cause decreased uptake of glucose in tissues such as skeletal muscle, fat, and liver and enhance TG breakdown into free fatty acids and gluconeogenesis, and ketone body formation resulting in hyperglycemia and ketosis. Overall, metabolism in DKA shifts from the normal fed state characterized by carbohydrate metabolism to a fasting state characterized by fat metabolism. This primary metabolic derangement leads to other changes that result in clinical and laboratory findings noted in DKA. The bicarbonates neutralize these ketone bodies produced by beta-oxidation of free fatty acids. As bicarbonate stores are depleted, anion gap metabolic acidosis ensues.

Lactic acidosis due to tissue hypoperfusion also contributes to acidosis. The hyperglycemia-induced osmotic diuresis depletes sodium, potassium, phosphates, and water as well as ketones and glucose. Hence, DKA patients have depleted total body water, total body potassium deficit, and other electrolytes changes like hypophosphatemia. Acidosis drives the intracellular potassium into the serum and may mask the total body potassium deficit. The potassium level can drop precipitously once rehydration and insulin treatment start. Urinary loss of ketoanions with brisk diuresis and balance should be maintained on a flowchart for easy review and evaluation. Intact renal function may also lead to a component of hyperchloremic metabolic acidosis. Please refer to Table 8 for summary of clinical manifestations and laboratory findings in DKA.

Treatment

The principle for management of DKA treatment in diabetes consists of the following:

1. Replenishing circulatory volume and tissue perfusion.
2. Insulin administration to overcome an insulin deficient state.
3. Correction of hyperglycemia and osmolar gap toward normal levels.

TABLE 8   Manifestation and Laboratory Findings in Diabetic Ketoacidosis

Symptoms
  Nausea/vomiting
  Thirst/polyuria/nocturia
  Abdominal pain
  Altered mental function
  Shortness of breath (Kussmaul's breathing)
  Malaise/lethargy
  Generalized weakness
  Change in appetite
  Symptoms related to associated infection such as fever, abdominal pain, chills, dysuria, shortness of breath

Physical findings
  Tachycardia
  Signs of dehydration-dry mucous membrane/reduced skin turgor
  Hypotension
  Dyspnea /Kussmaul respiration
  Abdominal tenderness
  Fever
  Altered mental status

Laboratory findings
  Hyperglycemia
  Metabolic acidosis: serum bicarbonate is frequently less than 10 mmol/L and arterial pH rages between 6.8 and 7.3, depending on the severity of the acidosis
  Hyperosmolality
  Hyperlipidemia
  Electrolyte disturbances
  Renal insufficiency–elevated Blood-urea-nitrogen creatinine ratio as a result of dehydration
Urine analysis shows glycosuria, ketonuria

4. Correction of acidosis.
5. Correcting electrolyte imbalances.
6. Identifying and treating precipitating events or agents (214).

Close monitoring and frequent assessment is the key to successful management of DKA. Most errors in management occur because of lapse in monitoring, and result in a "lag behind" situation or over treatment. Blood glucose needs to be monitored hourly; this provides information regarding the adequacy on insulin therapy. Serum electrolytes and ketones should be monitored every two hours, and this should include measurement of serum phosphorus. Frequent monitoring of the acid–base imbalance and correction of the same toward normal range is of paramount importance in the success of the therapy.

Fluid Replacement
Fluid loss in adults with DKA averages 5 to 7 L and may sometimes may be as much as 10% to 15% of the body weight. In adults, once the diagnosis of DKA is made, a rapid infusion of isotonic saline is given and then reduced gradually if the BP is stable and urine flow is adequate. For adults, in first two hours 2 L of isotonic saline is infused, and this can be followed by 2 L in next four hours and then two more liters over the next eight hours to replace the fluid loss. Fluid replacement should be modified according to the ongoing assessment of volume replacement needs and serum sodium level. Once the patient is hemodynamically stable with adequate BP to maintain tissue perfusion, 0.45% sodium chloride solution with potassium added is commonly used to provide free water and initiate potassium replacement. The potassium deficit is approximately 300–1000 mmol. In most patients, the initial serum K is high normal or elevated, and the initiation of potassium replacement usually can be deferred for two hours, using hourly serum measurements as a guide. Because insulin will shift K into cells, in patients who presently are normokalemic or hypokalemic, potassium replacement is started with initiation of insulin therapy.

Insulin Therapy
Initial intravenous (IV) bolus administration 10 to 20 units of regular insulin is followed by continuous IV infusion of 5 to 10 units/hr in 0.9% sodium chloride solution. Such treatment is adequate in most adults, but others who do not show adequate response in two to four hours require significantly higher doses. In most children a bolus IV injection of regular insulin (0.1 U/kg) is given, followed by a continuous IV infusion of regular insulin in 0.9% sodium chloride solution at a rate of 0.1 U/kg/hr; the insulin infusion should be adjusted based on response to therapy. The plasma glucose should be monitored hourly to assess the efficacy of the insulin regimens and to make appropriate adjustments to induce a gradual decline in plasma glucose. Insulin infusion should cause blood glucose to fall at a rate of about 75 mg/dL/hr. The rate of insulin infusion should be continued if the fall in blood glucose level is appropriate. When serum glucose falls to 230 to 300 mg/dL (13.88–16.65 mmol/L), 5% glucose is started through the IV fluids to reduce the risk of hypoglycemia. The insulin dosage can then be reduced, but the continuous IV infusion of regular insulin should be maintained until plasma and urine are consistently negative for ketones. Resolution of ketosis should be monitored using a combination of the anion gap, bicarbonate measurement, and if necessary, arterial blood gas pH measurement. With appropriate therapy, ketone levels will be corrected within several hours. Plasma pH and bicarbonate usually improve significantly within six to eight hours, but the plasma bicarbonate levels may take 24 hours to reach normal range. Once ketosis has cleared, and if the patient is able to tolerate oral diet, patient may then be switched to subcutaneous insulin. Subcutaneous insulin is started at least 30 minutes before the insulin infusion is stopped. Any lapse in insulin therapy during the recovery for DKA may result in a rapid resurgence of hyperketonemia and failure of therapy.

Pancreatic Transplantation and Pancreatic Islet-Cell Transplantation
A successful pancreatic transplant is an effective treatment option for T1DM and eliminates the acute complications related to T1DM, such as hypoglycemia or hyperglycemia, and removes dietary restriction and could delay the progression of renal and CV complication related to diabetes. Pancreatic transplantation for diabetes treatment is a century old concept

but the earlier approach was fraught with excessive patient morbidity and hence did not find favor among the medical community. Advent of newer immunosuppressive regimens, especially cyclosporine and anti–T-cell agents, improved surgical technique and proper selection of patient donor and recipient resulted in better outcomes (215). The number of pancreatic transplantation done in recent times continues to increase (216). Pancreatic transplantations in diabetic patients are done either alone [Pancreatic transplantation alone (PTA)] or simultaneously with kidney transplant [Simultaneous Pancreas Kindney (SPK)] or after kidney transplant [Pancreas after kidney (PAK)]. Most pancreatic transplantations in diabetic patients with chronic kidney disease are performed at the same time as or after kidney transplantation. Success rate for PTA is lower and this may be attributed to lack of a marker to detect pancreas rejection. Hence, rejection can go undiagnosed and delay the antirejection therapy. Pancreatic transplantation can be considered in diabetic patients with imminent or established ESRD who have had or plan to have a kidney transplant. In diabetic patients with no indications for kidney transplantation, pancreas transplantation should only be considered a therapy in patients who exhibit frequent, acute, and severe metabolic complications, and incapacitating clinical and emotional problems associated with use of exogenous insulin (217).

Pancreatic islet-cell transplantation is a newer and novel method of beta-cell replacement in that it does not involve major surgery, involves lesser degree of immunosupression and lower cost. The pancreatic beta-cell is harvested from healthy pancreas from a brain-dead donor with a beating heart. The purified harvested beta-cells are then transplanted into the donor liver through percutaneous catheter (218). Pancreatic islet-cell transplants hold significant potential advantages over whole-gland transplants. However, at this time, islet-cell transplantation is an experimental procedure, and should be performed only within the setting of controlled research studies. Pancreatic islet-cell transplantation also requires lifelong immunosuppression with drugs.

■ Case Illustrations

Case No. 1

A 40-year-old Caucasian male presents to the clinic with complaints of polyuria, polydipsia, and weight loss for the last couple of weeks. He denies any other symptoms. Review of systems is totally unremarkable except for as mentioned above. Patient has no significant medical history. No family history of diabetes. He is 71 in. tall and has a weight of 156 lbs with body mass index (BMI) 22 kg/m². On physical examination, his pulse is 78 bpm, BP is 135/84 mmHg, respiratory rate is 16 breaths per minute, and he is afebrile. Rest of the physical examination is unremarkable. A basic metabolic panel done in the clinic was as follows:

■ Glucose 360 mg/dL (70–100)
■ Sodium 142 mEq/L (136–148)
■ Potassium 4.5 mEq/L (3.7–5.4)
■ Chloride 104 mEq/L (96–111)
■ CO_2 25 mEq/L (23–33)
■ Anion gap 13 mEq/L (10–16)
■ Blood-urea nitrogen BUN 20 mg/dL (10–20)
■ Cr 1 mg/dL (0.4–1.5)
■ Complete blood counts done on this patient was within normal limits
■ Urinary ketones were 3+

Diagnosis of T1DM was made and his blood was sent for GAD antibodies, fasting lipid profile, thyroid-stimulating hormone, and HbA1C. Urine microalbuminuria was also ordered.

He was started on MDIs of insulin. His insulin dose for 24 hours was calculated to be 36 units based upon 0.5 units/kg/day. Fifty percent of this dose was given to him in the form of long-acting insulin for basal coverage and rest of the 50% was divided in three equal doses to be given for bolus coverage before his meals. He was started on insulin glargine 18 units subcutaneous at bedtime and insulin lispro 6 units tid before his meals. The patient was also advised to take aspirin 81 mg qd. He was referred for a DSME program and for evaluation by an ophthalmologist for baseline fundoscopic eye examination. He was counseled on the signs and symptoms of hypoglycemia and how to manage it. The patient was also encouraged to come involved in regular physical activity. He was instructed to do home glucose monitoring before meals and at bedtime and come back to clinic for reevaluation in one week.

Discussion

This is the case of a 30-year-old male who was diagnosed with T1D based upon his presentation, 3+ urine ketones, normal BMI and absence of family history of T2DM. In this patient, GAD antibodies came back positive. In the past, T1D was considered as juvenile onset only, but lately we are diagnosing more and more cases of T1D in fourth and even in fifth decade of life. Therefore, age of presentation is not relevant anymore in diagnosing the type of diabetes. Except for the complaints of polyuria and polydipsia, our patient was asymptomatic. He was able to eat and drink and was hemodynamically stable. Even though he was positive for ketones, blood tests did not show any acidosis or increased anion gap and his electrolytes were in the normal range. Therefore, it was appropriate to manage him as an outpatient. Patients with T1D have absolute insulin deficiency and they should preferably be on intensive insulin regimen with MDI of insulin rather than just twice a day insulin injections. Anyone above 21 years of age with diabetes should be on aspirin 81 mg qd. Need for diabetic education for these patients cannot be overemphasized. It is very important that patients on MDI of insulin learn the concept of carbohydrate counting because carbohydrate counting will not only help manage their diabetes appropriately but will also give patients some flexibility in their day to day routine. Other important factors in management of these patients are aggressive control of BP to levels <130/80 mmHg and treatment of their dyslipidemia. Usually these patients initially tend to have hypertriglyceridemia because of insulin deficiency but once their T1D is controlled, TG tend to become normal in these patients. On the basis of the fact that these patients also have high risk of CVD, LDL goal in them should be <100 mg/dL. Testing for microalbuminuria is very important in these patients to diagnose diabetic nephropathy early enough. In lieu of recent trials, progression of diabetic nephropathy can be slowed down or even improved if these patients can be started on ACEI or ARBs early enough. They should be evaluated by an ophthalmologist at baseline and annually thereafter. Patient should also be encouraged to engage in physical activity on a regular basis. These patients need close follow-up and monitoring.

Case No. 2

A 23-year-old female was referred to an endocrine clinic because of uncontrolled T1D. She had a medical history of T1D for the last 13 years. Currently she is on NPH insulin 12 units and regular insulin 8 units bid. She takes her insulin injections before her breakfast and dinner. She checks her blood glucose about a couple of times a day and tends to have blood glucose around 200 before breakfast and before dinner. A couple of times a week, she gets hypoglycemia—usually during her sleep around 2:00 AM. Sometimes she gets hypoglycemia before her lunch also. She has not visited an ophthalmologist in the last five years. She has a BMI of 20 kg/m^2. On physical examination, it was found that she has BP of 138/76 mmHg. She has abnormal 10 g monofilament test on distal extremities and callous on each foot on the plantar surface. Review of records from phencyclidine office shows multiple BP readings in last one year, and her systolic BP has ranged between 132 and 140 mmHg.

Her recent labs done before the visit are as follows:

- Glucose 210 mg/dL; reference ranges (70–100)
- Sodium 136 mEq/L (136–148)
- Potassium 4.7 mEq/L (3.7–5.4)
- Chloride 99 mEq/L (96–111)
- CO_2 24 mEq/L (23–33)
- BUN 19 mg/dL (10–20)
- Cr 1.7 mg/dL (0.4–1.5)
- HgA1C 8.6% (4.0–6.0)
- Urine microalbumin 180 mcg/mg of Cr
- Total cholesterol 170 mg/dL (140–200)
- LDL cholesterol Unable to calculate because of high TGs
- HDL cholesterol 54 mg/dL (32–72)
- TGs 453 mg/dL (30–150)

Discussion

The above mentioned patient has T1D for the last 13 years with poor control and has diabetic neuropathy and nephropathy and has not visited an ophthalmologist in the last five years. Besides the above complications, the major problem with this patient is the frequency of hypoglycemic episodes along with uncontrolled DM. This case illustrates prime example of maldistribution of insulin. She is on NPH insulin, which peaks at four to six hours after injection. Therefore, her NPH dose from dinnertime peaks during her sleeptime to cause hypoglycemia and same thing happens before lunchtime from the NPH injected before breakfast. This kind of situation makes it very hard to control blood glucose without causing significant hypoglycemic episodes. Some times, frequency of hypoglycemia can be minimized by having the patient to take mid-morning and bedtime snacks ands increase insulin dose gradually. Switching the evening dose of NPH from suppertime to bedtime can also be helpful. But in such patients, the best approach is to put them on a basal insulin which does not have a peak action, i.e., insulin glargine and for bolus/prandial dose cover them with an ultrashort-acting insulin analog, i.e., insulin lispro or insulin aspart three times a day before their meals. This patient's BP persistently has been <130/80 mmHg in the last one year. For diabetic patients, the target is BP < 130/80 mmHg. Our patient also has diabetic nephropathy. ACEI or ARBs have been shown to slow the progression of diabetic nephropathy. Therefore, for BP management, ACEI or ARBs will be the first choice of drugs in diabetic hypertensives with nephropathy. With mild chronic kidney disease, the Cr can go up by 20% to 30% in the short run after these patients go on ACEI or ARB but in the long run in this subset of patients these drugs have renoprotective effect and should be used liberally. The patient has hypertriglyceridemia and this could be because of uncontrolled diabetes and insulin deficiency. Once her T1D is well controlled, she should have fasting lipid profile done, and if her TGs are still high, she would need to be on lipid-lowering treatment. Target TG and LDL in patients with diabetes is less than 150 and 100 mg/dL, respectively. In presence of CAD, the goal for LDL should be preferably less than 70 mg/dL. She should also start using aspirin 81mg qd. She has diabetic neuropathy and calluses on feet, and should be referred to podiatrist for foot care and diabetic shoes. She needs to be referred to a DSME program for diabetic education and carbohydrate counting. She also needs evaluation by an ophthalmologist. Most likely, she has some degree of retinopathy at this time because it is rare for diabetic nephropathy to develop before retinopathy in T1D.

REFERENCES

1. Rewers M, La Porte RE, King H, et al. Trends in the prevalence and incidence of diabetes: insulin-dependent DM in childhood. World Health Stat Q 1988; 41:179–189.
2. Diabetes Am 1995; 2.
3. Songer TJ. The economics of diabetes care. In: Alberti KGMM, Defranzo RA, Keen H, Zimmat P, eds. The International Textbook of Diabetes Mellitus. Chichester, U.K: Wiley, 1992:1643–1654.
4. Laakso M, Pyörälä K. Age of onset and type of diabetes. Diabetes Care 1985; 8:114–117.
5. Molbak AG, Christau B, Marner B, Borch-Johnsen K, Nerup J. Incidence of insulin dependent diabetes mellitus in age groups over 30 years in Denmark. Diabetes Med 1994; 11:650–655.
6. Tuomi T, Groop LC, Zimmet PZ, Rowley MJ, Knowles W, Mackay IR. Antibodies to glutamic acid decarboxylase reveal latent autoimmune diabetes mellitus in adults with a non–insulin-dependent onset of disease. Diabetes 1993; 42:359–362.
7. Green A, Gale EAM, Patterson CC. Incidence of childhood-onset insulin-dependent diabetes mellitus: the EURODIAB ACE Study. Lancet 1992; 339:905–909.
8. Karvonen M, Viik-Kajander M, Moltchanova E, Libman I, LaPorte R, Tuomilehto J. Incidence of childhood type 1 diabetes worldwide. Diabetes Mondiale (DiaMond) Project Group. Diabetes Care 2000; 23:1516–1526.
9. Diabetes Epidemiology Research International Group. Geographic patterns of childhood insulin dependent diabetes mellitus. Diabetes 1988; 37:1113–1119.
10. American Diabetes Association. Diagnosis and classification of diabetes mellitus. Diabetes care 2004; 27(suppl 1):S5–S10; S5–S10.
11. Atkinson MA, Maclaren NK. The pathogenesis of insulin-dependent diabetes mellitus. N Engl J Med 1994; 331:1428.
12. Dorman J. The WHO DiaMon Molecular Epidemiologie Sub-Project Group: molecular epidemiology of insulin-dependent diabetes mellitus. WHO Diamon Project. Gac Méd Méx 1997; (suppl 1):151–154.
13. Wagener DK, Sacks JM, LaPorte RE, MacGregor JM. The Pittsburgh study of insulin-dependent diabetes mellitus: risk for diabetes among relatives of IDDM. Diabetes 1982; 31:136–44; Allen C, Palta M, D'Alessio DJ. Risk of diabetes in siblings and other relatives of IDDM subjects. Diabetes 1991; 40:831–836.
14. Eisenbarth SC. Type 1 diabetes: molecular, cellular, and clinical immunology. Chapter 1. Primer immunology and Autoimmunity. Online edition version 2.5. http://www.uch.sc.edu/misc/diabetes/eisenbrook.html.
15. Bach JF, Garchon HJ, van Endert P. Genetics of human type 1 diabetes mellitus. Curr Dir Autoimmun (Basel, Karger) 2001; 4:4.
16. Nerup J, Platz P, Anderson OO, et al. HLA antigens and diabetesmellitus, Lancet 1974; 2:864–866.
17. Singal DP, Blajchman MA. Histocompatibility antigens, lymphocytotoxic antibodies and tissue antibodies in patients with diabetes mellitus. Diabetes 1973; 22:429–432.
18. Neopom GT. HLA and type 1 diabetes. Immunol Today 1990; 11:314–315.
19. Davies JL, Kawaguchi Y, Bennett ST, et al. A genome-wide search for human type 1 diabetes susceptibility genes. Nature 1994; 371:130.
20. Tisch R, McDevitt H. Insulin-dependent diabetes mellitus. Cell 1996; 85:291.
21. Todd JA. Genetic analysis of type 1 diabetes using whole genome approaches (Rev). Proc Natl Acad Sci USA 1995; 92:8560–8565.
22. Rudensky AJ, Prston-Hurlburt P, Hong S, Barlow A, Janeway CA Jr. Sequence analysis of peptides bound to MHC class II molecules. Nature 1991; 353:622–627.
23. Khalil I, d'Auriol L, Gobet M, et al. A combination of HLA-DQb Asp57-negative and HLA DQa Arg52 confers susceptibility to insulin-dependent diabetes mellitus. J Clin Invest 1990; 85:1315.
24. Todd JA, Bain SC. A practical approach to identification of susceptibility genes for IDDM. Diabetes 1992; 41:1029–1034.
25. Cisse A, Chauffert M, Chevenne D, et al. Distribution of HLA-DQA1 and -DQB1 alleles and DQA1-DQB1 genotypes among Senegalese patients with insulin-dependent diabetes mellitus. Tissue Antigens 1996; 47:333–337.
26. Kawabata Y, Ikegami H, Kawaguchi Y, et al. Age-related association of MHC class I chain-related gene A (MICA) with type 1 (insulin-dependent) diabetes mellitus. Hum Immunol 2000; 61:624–629.
27. NEJM, Pugliese AE, Kawasaki M, Zeller, et al. Sequence analysis of the diabetes-protective human leukocyte antigen-DQB1*0602 allele in unaffected, islet cell antibody-positive first-degree relatives and in rare patients with type 1 diabetes. J Clin Endocrinol Metab 1999; 84:1722–1728.

28. Pugliese A, Gianani R, Moromisato R, Awdeh ZL, Alper CA, Erlich HA, et al. HLA-DQB1*0602 is associated with dominant protection from diabetes even among islet cell antibody-positive first-degree relatives of patients with IDDM. Diabetes 1995; 44(6):608–613.

29. Pugliese A, Kawasaki E, Zeller M, Yu L, Babu S, Solimena M, et al. Sequence analysis of the diabetes-protective human leukocyte antigen-DQB1*0602 allele in unaffected, islet cell antibody-positive first degree relatives and in rare patients with type 1 diabetes. J Clin Endocrinol Metab 1999; 84(5):1722–1728.

30. Chervonsky AV, Wang Y, Wong FS et al. The role of Fas in autoimmune diabetes. Cell 1997; 89:17–24.

31. DiSanto JP, Muller W, Guy-Grand D, et al. Lymphoid development in mice with a targeted deletion of the interleukin-2 receptor gamma chain. Proc Natl Acad Sci USA 1995; 92:377–381.

32. Dai Z, Arakelov A, Wagener M, et al. The role of the common cytokine receptor gamma-chain in regulation IL-2-dependent, activation induced CD 8+ T-cell death. J Immunol 1999; 163:3131–3137.

33. Diez J, Park Y, Zeller M, Brown D, et al. Differential splicing of the IA-2 mRNA in pancreas and lymphoid organs as a permissive genetic mechanism for autoimmunity against the IA-2 type 1 diabetes autoantigen. Diabetes 2001; (4):895–900.

34. Oosterwegel MA, Grrenwald RJ, Mandelbrot DA, et al. CTLA-4 and T-cell activation. Curr Opin Immunol 1999; 11:294–300.

35. von Herrath MG. Oldstone MBA. Interferon is essential for destruction of cells and development of insulin-dependent diabetes mellitus. J Exp Med 1997; 185:531–540.

36. Nakahira M, Ahn HJ, Park WR, et al. Synergy of IL-12 and IL-18 for IFN-gene expression: IL-12–induced STAT4 contributes to IFN-promoter activation by up-regulating the binding activity of IL-18–induced activator protein 1. J Immunol 2002; 68:1146–1153.

37. Scriver C, Beaudet A, Sly W, Valle D. The Metabolic and Molecular Bases of Inherited Disease. 7th ed. New York: McGraw-Hill Inc, 1995:859–863.

38. William EW, Neil H, Desmond S. Immunological markers in the diagnosis and prediction of autoimmune type 1a diabetes. Clin Diabetes 2002; 4(6):817–839.

39. Tan HH, Lim SC. Latent autoimmune diabetes in adults (LADA): a case series. Singapore Med J 2001; 42(11):513–516.

40. Pietropaolo M, Eisenbarth GS. Autoantibodies in human diabetes. In: von Herrath MG, ed. Molecular Pathology of Type 1 Diabetes mellitus. Basel: Karger, (Curr Dir Autoimmun) 2001; 4:252–282.

41. Ziegler AG, Standl E, Albert E, Mehnert H. HLA-associated insulin autoantibody formation in newly diagnosed type I diabetic patients. Diabetes 1991; 40:1146–1149.

42. Baekkeskov S, Aanstoot HJ, Christgau S, et al. Identification of the 64K autoantigen in insulin-dependent diabetes as the GABA-synthesizing enzyme glutamic acid decarboxylase. Nature 1990; 347:151.

43. Verge CF, Gianani R, Kawasaki E, et al. Prediction of type 1 diabetes mellitus in first-degree relatives using a combination of insulin, glutamic acid decarboxylase and ICA512/bdc/IA-2 autoantibodies. Diabetes 1996; 45:926–933.

44. Lohmann T, Kellner K, Verlohren HJ, et al. Titre and combination of ICA and autoantibodies to glutamic acid decarboxylase discriminate two clinically distinct types of latent autoimmune diabetes in adults (LADA). Diabetologia 2001; 44:1005–1010.

45. Solimena M, Dirkx R Jr, Hermel JM, Pleasic-Williams S, Shapiro JA. Caron L & Rabin DU ICA 512, an autoantigen of type I diabetes, is an intrinsic membrane protein of neurosecretory granules. EMBO J 1996; 15:2102–2114.

46. Ellis, TM, Schatz, DA, Ottendorfer, EW, et al. The relationship between humoral and cellular immunity to IA-2 in IDDM. Diabetes 1998; 47:566.

47. Dahlquist G. Non-genetic risk determinants of type 1 diabetes. Diabetes Metab 1994; 20(3):251–257.

48. Dahlquist G, Källén B. Maternal-child blood group incompatibility and other perinatal events increase the risk for early onset type 1(insulin-dependent) diabetes mellitus. Diabetologia 1992; 35:671–675.

49. Stene, LC, Magnus P, Lie RT, et al. Birth weight and childhood onset type 1 diabetes: population based cohort study. BMJ 2001; 322:889.

50. Dalquist G, Bennich SS, Kallen B. Intrauterine growth pattern and risk of childhood onset insulin dependent (type 1) diabetes: population based case-control study. BMJ 1996; 313:1174–1177.

51. Lawler-Heavener J, Cruikshank KJ, Hay WW, Gay EC, Hamman RF. Birth size and risk of insulin dependent diabetes mellitus (IDDM). Diabetes Res Clin Pract 1994; 24:153–159.

52. McKinney PA, Parslow R, Gurney KA, et al. Perinatal and neonatal determinants of childhood type 1 diabetes. A case-control study in Yorkshire, U.K. Diabetes Care 1999; 22.

53. Mayer ES, Hamman RF, Gay EC, Lezotte DC, Savitz DA, Klingensmith GJ. Reduced risk of IDDM among breast-fed children: The Colorado IDDM Registry. Diabetes 1988; 37:1625–1632.

54. Nigro G. Breast feeding and insulin-dependent diabetes mellitus (Letter). Lancet 1985; 1:467.

55. Atkinson MA, Eisenbarth GS. Type 1 diabetes: new perspectives on disease pathogenesis and treatment. Lancet 2001; 358:221–229.

56. Forrest JM, Menser MA, Burgess JA. High frequency of diabetes mellitus in young adults with congenital rubella. Lancet 1971; ii:332–334.

57. Dahlquist G, Ivarsson S, Lindberg B, Forsgren M. Maternal enteroviralinfection during pregnancy as a risk factor for childhood IDDM. Diabetes 1995; 44:408–413.

58. Kaufman DL, Erlander MG, Clare-Salzler M, Atkinson MA, Maclaren NK, Tobin AJ. Autoimmunity to two forms of glutamate decarboxylase in insulin dependent diabetes mellitus. J Clin Invest 1992; 89:283–292.

59. Hviid A et al. Childhood vaccination and type 1 diabetes. N Engl J Med 2004; 350:1398–1404.
60. National Diabetes Data Group. Classification and diagnosis of diabetes mellitus and other categories of glucose intolerance. Diabetes 1979; 28(12):1039–1057.
61. WHO Expert Committee on Diabetes Mellitus. Second Report. Geneva: WHO, 1980. Technical Report Series 646, 1980.
62. Report of the Expert Committee on the Diagnosis and Classification of Diabetes Mellitus. Diabetes Care 1997; 20(7):1183–1197.
63. Genuth S, Alberti KG, Bennett P, et al. Follow-up report on the diagnosis of diabetes mellitus. Diabetes Care 2003; 26(11):3160–3167.
64. Riccardi G, Vaccaro O, Rivellese A, Pignalosa S, Tutino L, Mancini M. Reproducibility of the new diagnostic criteria for impaired glucose tolerance. Am J Epidemiol 1985; 121(3):422–429.
65. Alberti KG, Zimmet PZ. Definition, diagnosis, and classification of diabetes mellitus and its complications. Part 1: diagnosis and classification of diabetes mellitus provisional report of a WHO consultation. Diabetes Med 1998; 15(7):539–553.
66. American Diabetes Association. Diagnosis and classification of diabetes mellitus. Diabetes Care 2005; 28(suppl 1):S37–S42.
67. DECODE Study Group on behalf of the European Diabetes Epidemiology Study Group. Will new diagnostic criteria for diabetes mellitus change phenotype of patients with diabetes? Reanalysis of European epidemiological data. BMJ 1998; 317(7155):371–375.
68. Dinneen SF, Maldonado D 3rd, Leibson CL, et al. Effects of changing diagnostic criteria on the risk of developing diabetes. Diabetes Care 1998; 21(9):1408–1413.
69. Harris MI. Impaired glucose tolerance in the U.S. population. Diabetes Care 1989; 12(7):464–474.
70. Peters AL, Davidson MB, Schriger DL, Hasselblad V. A clinical approach for the diagnosis of diabetes mellitus: an analysis using glycosylated hemoglobin levels. Meta-analysis Research Group on the Diagnosis of Diabetes Using Glycated Hemoglobin Levels. JAMA 1996; 276(15):1246–1252.
71. Rohlfing CL, Little RR, Wiedmeyer HM, et al. Use of GHb (HbA1C) in screening for undiagnosed diabetes in the U.S. population. Diabetes Care 2000; 23(2):187–191.
72. Bottazzo GF, Florin-Christensen A, Doniach D. Islet-cell antibodies in diabetes mellitus with autoimmune polyendocrine deficiencies. Lancet 1974; 2(7892):1279–1283.
73. Imagawa A, Hanafusa T, Miyagawa JI, Matsuzawa Y, The Osaka ISG. A novel subtype of type 1 diabetes mellitus characterized by a rapid onset and an absence of diabetes-related antibodies. N Engl J Med 2000; 342(5):301–307.
74. Libman IM, Pietropaolo M, Trucco M, Dorman JS, LaPorte RE, Becker D. Islet cell autoimmunity in white and black children and adolescents with IDDM. Diabetes Care 1998; 21(11):1824–1827.
75. Harris MI, Robbins DC. Prevalence of adult-onset IDDM in the U.S. population. Diabetes Care 1994; 17(11):1337–1340.
76. Landin-Olsson M, Nilsson KO, Lernmark A, Sundkvist G. Islet cell antibodies and fasting C-peptide predict insulin requirement at diagnosis of diabetes mellitus. Diabetologia 1990; 33(9):561–568.
77. Niskanen LK, Tuomi T, Karjalainen J, Groop LC, Uusitupa MI. GAD antibodies in NIDDM. Ten-year follow-up from the diagnosis. Diabetes Care 1995; 18(12):1557–1565.
78. Kobayashi T, Itoh T, Kosaka K, Sato K, Tsuji K. Time course of islet cell antibodies and beta-cell function in non–insulin-dependent stage of type I diabetes. Diabetes 1987; 36(4):510–517.
79. Falorni A, Gambelunghe G, Forini F, et al. Autoantibody recognition of COOH-terminal epitopes of GAD65 marks the risk for insulin requirement in adult-onset diabetes mellitus. J Clin Endocrinol Metab 2000; 85(1):309–316.
80. Zimmet P, Turner R, McCarty D, Rowley M, Mackay I. Crucial points at diagnosis. Type 2 diabetes or slow type 1 diabetes. Diabetes Care 1999; 22(suppl 2):B59–B64.
81. Rosenbloom AL, Joe JR, Young RS, Winter WE. Emerging epidemic of type 2 diabetes in youth. Diabetes Care 1999; 22(2):345–354.
82. Botero D, Wolfsdorf JI. Diabetes mellitus in children and adolescents. Arch Med Res 2005; 36(3):281.
83. Kuczmarski RJ, Flegal KM, Campbell SM, Johnson CL. Increasing prevalence of overweight among US adults. The National Health and Nutrition Examination Surveys, 1960 to 1991. JAMA 1994; 272(3):205–211.
84. Maldonado M, Hampe CS, Gaur LK, et al. Ketosis-prone diabetes: dissection of a heterogeneous syndrome using an immunogenetic and {beta}-cell functional classification, prospective analysis, and clinical outcomes. J Clin Endocrinol Metab 2003; 88(11):5090–5098.
85. Kitabchi AE. Ketosis-prone diabetes—a new subgroup of patients with atypical type 1 and type 2 diabetes? J Clin Endocrinol Metab 2003; 88(11):5087–5089.
86. Diabetes Mellitus: A Major Risk Factor for Cardiovascular Disease. A Joint Editorial Statement by the American Diabetes Association; the National Heart, Lung, and Blood Institute; the Juvenile Diabetes Foundation International; the National Institute of Diabetes and Digestive and Kidney Diseases; and the American Heart Association. Circulation 1999; 100(10):1132–1133.
87. Stamler J, Vaccaro O, Neaton JD, Wentworth D. Diabetes, other risk factors, and 12-yr cardiovascular mortality for men screened in the Multiple Risk Factor Intervention Trial. Diabetes Care 1993; 16(2):434–444.

88. The Diabetes Control and Complications Trial Research Group. The effect of intensive treatment of diabetes on the development and progression of long-term complications in insulin-dependent diabetes mellitus. N Engl J Med 1993; 329(14):977–986.
89. Deckert T, Poulsen JE, Larsen M. Prognosis of diabetics with diabetes onset before the age of thirty-one. I. Survival, causes of death, and complications. Diabetologia 1978; 14(6):363–370.
90. Krolewski AS, Kosinski EJ, Warram JH, et al. Magnitude and determinants of coronary artery disease in juvenile-onset, insulin-dependent diabetes mellitus. Am J Cardiol 1987; 59(8):750–755.
91. Moss SE, Klein R, Klein BE. Cause-specific mortality in a population-based study of diabetes. Am J Public Health 1991; 81(9):1158–1162.
92. Dorman JS, Laporte RE, Kuller LH, et al. The Pittsburgh insulin-dependent diabetes mellitus (IDDM) morbidity and mortality study. Mortality results. Diabetes 1984; 33(3):271–276.
93. Manson JE, Colditz GA, Stampfer MJ, et al. A prospective study of maturity-onset diabetes mellitus and risk of coronary heart disease and stroke in women. Arch Intern Med 1991; 151(6):1141–1147.
94. Borch-Johnsen K, Kreiner S. Proteinuria: value as predictor of cardiovascular mortality in insulin dependent diabetes mellitus. Br Med J (Clin Res Ed) 1987; 294(6588):1651–1654.
95. Martin FI, Hopper JL. The relationship of acute insulin sensitivity to the progression of vascular disease in long-term type 1 (insulin-dependent) diabetes mellitus. Diabetologia 1987; 30(3):149–153.
96. Orchard TJ, Dorman JS, Maser RE, et al. Factors associated with avoidance of severe complications after 25 yr of IDDM. Pittsburgh Epidemiology of Diabetes Complications Study I. Diabetes Care 1990; 13(7):741–747.
97. Orchard TJ. From diagnosis and classification to complications and therapy. DCCT. Part II? Diabetes Control and Complications Trial. Diabetes Care 1994; 17(4):326–338.
98. Lloyd CE, Kuller LH, Ellis D, Becker DJ, Wing RR, Orchard TJ. Coronary artery disease in IDDM: gender differences in risk factors but not risk. Arterioscler Thromb Vasc Biol 1996; 16(6):720–726.
99. Crall FV, Jr, Roberts WC. The extramural and intramural coronary arteries in juvenile diabetes mellitus: analysis of nine necropsy patients aged 19 to 38 years with onset of diabetes before age 15 years. Am J Med 1978; 64(2):221–230.
100. Valsania P, Zarich SW, Kowalchuk GJ, Kosinski E, Warram JH, Krolewski AS. Severity of coronary artery disease in young patients with insulin-dependent diabetes mellitus. Am Heart J 1991; 122(3 Pt 1):695–700.
101. Dabelea D, Kinney G, Snell-Bergeon JK, et al. Effect of type 1 diabetes on the gender difference in coronary artery calcification: a role for insulin resistance? The Coronary Artery Calcification in Type 1 Diabetes (CACTI) Study. Diabetes 2003; 52(11):2833–2839.
102. Koistinen MJ. Prevalence of asymptomatic myocardial ischaemia in diabetic subjects. BMJ 1990; 301(6743):92–95.
103. Yamasaki Y, Kawamori R, Matsushima H, et al. Atherosclerosis in carotid artery of young IDDM patients monitored by ultrasound high-resolution B-mode imaging. Diabetes 1994; 43(5):634–639.
104. Kanters SD, Algra A, Banga JD. Carotid intima-media thickness in hyperlipidemic type I and type II diabetic patients. Diabetes Care 1997; 20(3):276–280.
105. Laing SP, Swerdlow AJ, Slater SD, et al. Mortality from heart disease in a cohort of 23,000 patients with insulin-treated diabetes. Diabetologia 2003; 46(6):760.
106. Libby P, Nathan DM, Abraham K, et al. Report of the National Heart, Lung, and Blood Institute-National Institute of Diabetes and Digestive and Kidney Diseases Working Group on Cardiovascular Complications of Type 1 Diabetes Mellitus. Circulation 2005; 111(25):3489–3493.
107. The Diabetes Control and Complications Trial/Epidemiology of Diabetes Interventions and Complications Research Group. Intensive diabetes therapy and carotid intima-media thickness in type 1 diabetes mellitus. N Engl J Med 2003; 348(23):2294–2303.
108. Nichols GA, Brown JB. The impact of cardiovascular disease on medical care costs in subjects with and without type 2 diabetes. Diabetes Care 2002; 25(3):482–486.
109. Sowers JR, Epstein M, Frohlich ED. Diabetes, hypertension, and cardiovascular disease: an update. Hypertension 2001; 37(4):1053–1059.
110. Tuomilehto J, Borch-Johnsen K, Molarius A, et al. Incidence of cardiovascular disease in Type 1 (insulin-dependent) diabetic subjects with and without diabetic nephropathy in Finland. Diabetologia 1998; 41(7):784–790.
111. Tuomilehto J, Lindstrom J, Qiao Q. Strategies for the prevention of type 2 diabetes and cardiovascular disease. Eur Heart J 2005; (suppl 7) (suppl D):D18–22.
112. Eckel RH, Wassef M, Chait A, et al. Prevention conference VI: diabetes and cardiovascular disease: Writing Group II: Pathogenesis of atherosclerosis in diabetes. Circulation 2002; 105(18):138–143.
113. Libby P. Inflammation in atherosclerosis. Nature 2002; 420(6917):868–874.
114. DCCT Research Group. The effect of intensive treatment of diabetes on the development and the progression of long-term complications in insulin dependent diabetes mellitus. N Engl J Med 1993; 329:977.
115. UKPDS Study Research Group. The Lancet 1998; 352:837–853.
116. Epidimiology of Diabetes Intervention and Complications Research Group. Effect of intensive therapy on the microvascular complications of type 1 diabetes mellitus. JAMA 2002; 287:2563–2569.
117. Saydah SH, Fradkin J, Cowie CC. Poor control of risk factors for vascular disease among adults with previously diagnosed diabetes. JAMA 2004; 291:335.

118. American Diabetes Association: position statement. Diabetes care 2004; 27.
119. Anderson RM, Funnell MM. The role of physician in patient education. Pract Diabetol 1990; 9:10–12.
120. Keen H. A diabetes overview: occasion for jubilee? Br J Diab Vasc Dis 2002; 2:419–422.
121. Ewles L, Simnett I. Promoting Health: A Practical Guide. 5th ed, 2005. Bailliere Tindall, Edinburgh. Promoting Health: A practical guide. 4th ed, 1999.
122. Lawson ML, Gerstein HC, Tsui E, Zinman B. Effect of intensive insulin therapy on early macrovascular disease in young individuals with type 1 diabetes. Diabetes Care 1999; 22 (suppl 1):B35–B39.
123. www.accordtrial.org
124. Goldstein DE, Lorenz RA, et al. Tests of glycemia in diabetes. Diabetes Care 2004; 27(suppl 1):S91.
125. Crawford LM Jr. From the Food and Drug Administration. JAMA 2002; 288:1579.
126. Sacks DB, Burns DE, Goldstein DE, MacLaren NK, McDonald JM, Parrot M. Guidelines and recommendation for the lab analysis in the diagnosis and management of diabetes mellitus. Diabetes Care 2002; 25:750–786.
127. Rohlfing CL, Weidmeyer HM, Little RR, England JD, Tennill A, Goldstein DE. Defining the relationship between plasma glucose and HbA1C in the Diabetes Control and Complications Trial. Diabetes Care 2002; 25:275–278.
128. Delahanty L, Halford B. The role of diet behaviors in achieving improved glycemic control in intensively treated patients in the diabetes control and complications trial. Diabetes Care 1993; 16:1453.
129. Charron-Prochownik D, Becher MH, Brown MB, et al. Understanding young children's health benefits and diabetes regimen adherence. Diabetes Educator 1993; 19:409.
130. American Diabetes Association: Nutrition principles and recommendation in diabetes. Diabetes Care 2004; 27:S36–S46.
131. Christine Beebe. Diet therapy in type 1 diabetes mellitus. Diabetes Mellitus—A Fundamental and Clinical Text. 2nd ed, Lippincott Williams and Wilkins, Philadelphia, 2000 pp.471–481.
132. US Department of Agriculture. Report of dietary guidelines advisory committee, on dietary guidelines for Americans, to the Secretary of Health and Human Services and the Secretary of Agriculture. Washington, D.C.: USDA, 1995.
133. Abraira C, de Bartolo M, Myofski JW. Comparison of unmeasured versus exchange diabetic diets in lean adults. Body weight and feeding patterns in a two years prospective pilot study. Am J Clin Nutr 1980; 33:1064.
134. American Diabetes Association Position Statement. Nutrition principles and recommendations. Diabetes Care 2004; 27:S38.
135. Horton ES. Exercise in patients with type 2 diabetes mellitus. In Diabetes Mellitus—A fundamental and clinical text. 2nd ed., Lippincott Williams and Wilkins, Philadelphia, pp.765–769.
136. Kemmer FW, Berchtod P, Berger M, et al. Exercise-induced fall of blood glucose in insulin-treated diabetics unrelated to alteration of insulin mobilization. Diabetes 1979; 28:1131.
137. Gerich JE. Novel insulins: expanding options in diabetes management. Am J Med 2002; 113:308–316.
138. Skyle JS. Insulin treatment therapy for diabetes mellitus and related disorders: 4th ed. 2004; 208.
139. Dewitt, Hirsch. Outpatient insulin therapy in type 1 and type 2 diabetes mellitus: scientific review. JAMA 2003; 289:2254–2264.
140. Hirsch IB, Farkas-Hirsch R, Skylar JS. Intensive insulin therapy for treatment of type 1 diabetes. Diabetes Care 1990; 13:1265–1283.
141. Porcellati F, Rossetti P, Pampanelli S, Bolli GB, et al. Better long term glycemic control with the basal insulin glargine as compared to NPH in patients with type 1 diabetes mellitus given mealtime lispro insulin. Diabetes Med 2006.
142. Bode BW, Tamborlane WV, Davidson PC. Insulin pump therapy in 21st century: strategies for successful use in adults, adolescents, and children with diabetes. Postgrad Med 2002; 111:69–77.
143. Skyle JS. Insulin therapy in type 1 diabetes mellitus. In: DeFronzo RA, ed. Current Therapy of Diabetes Mellitus. St. Louis: MO: Mosby, 1998:36–49.
144. Kitagawa T, Owada M, Urakami T, Tajima N. Epidemiology of type 1 (insulin-dependent) and type 2 (non–insulin-dependent) diabetes mellitus in Japanese children. Diabetes Res Clin Pract 1994; 24(suppl):S7–S13.
145. Neel JV. Diabetes mellitus: a thrifty genotype rendered detrimental by 'progress'? Am J Hum Genet 1962; 14:353–362.
146. Sowers JR. Treatment of hypertension in patients with diabetes. Arch Intern Med 2004; 164:1850–1857.
147. Sowers JR, Williams M, Epstein M, Bakris G. Hypertension in patients with diabetes: strategies for drug therapy to reduce complications. Postgrad Med 2000; 107:47–54.
148. Gress TW, Nieto FJ, Shahar E, Wofford MR, Brancati FL. Hypertension and antihypertensive therapy as risk factors for type 2 diabetes mellitus. N Engl J Med 2000; 342:905–912.
149. El-Atat F, McFarlane SI, Sowers JR. Diabetes, hypertension, and cardiovascular derangements: pathophysiology and management. Curr Hypertens Rep 2004; 6:215–223.
150. Sacks FM, Svetkey LP, Vollmer WM, Appel LJ, Bray GA, et al. The DASH-Sodium Collaborative Research Group. Effects on blood pressure of reduced dietary sodium and the dietary approaches to stop hypertension (DASH) diet. N Engl J Med 2001; 344:3–10.
151. Tuomilehto J, Lindstrom J, Eriksson JG, et al. Prevention of type 2 diabetes mellitus by changes in lifestyle among subjects with impaired glucose tolerance. N Engl J Med 2001; 344:1343–1350.

152. Duncan GE, Perri MG, Theriaque DW, Hutson AD, Eckel RH, Stacpoole PW. Exercise training, without weight loss, increases insulin sensitivity and postheparin plasma lipase activity in previously sedentary adults. Diabetes Care 2003; 26:557–562.
153. Effects of Ramipril on cardiovascular and microvascular outcomes in peoples with diabetes mellitus; results of the HOPE study and MICRO-HOPE substudy. Lancet 2000; 355:253–259.
154. Hansson L, Lindholm LH, Niskanen L, et al. Effect of angiotensin-converting-enzyme inhibition compared with conventional therapy on cardiovascular morbidity and mortality in hypertension; the Captopril Prevention Project (CAPP) randomized trial. Lancet 1999; 353:611–616.
155. Yusuf S, Sleight P, Pogue J, Bosh J, Davies R, Dagenais G. Effects of an angiotensin-converting enzyme inhibitor, ramipril, on cardiovascular events in high-risk patients: the Heart Outcomes Prevention Evaluation. N Engl J Med 2000; 342:145–153.
156. Brenner BM, Cooper ME, de Zeeuw D, et al. Effects of losartan on renal and cardiovascular outcomes in patients with type 2 diabetes and nephropathy. N Engl J Med 2001; 345:861–869.
157. Dahlof B, Devereux R, Kjeldsen S, Julius S, Beevers G, Faire U. Cardiovascular morbidity and mortality in the Losartan Intervention For Endpoint Reduction in Hypertension Study, a randomised trial against atenolol. Lancet 2002; 359:995–1003.
158. Chobanian AV, Bakris GL, Black HR, et al. Seventh report of the Joint National Committee on Prevention, Detection, Evaluation, and Treatment of High Blood Pressure. Hypertension 2003; 42:1206–1252.
159. Major outcomes in high-risk hypertensive patients randomized to angiotensin-converting-enzyme inhibitor or calcium channel blocker vs diuretic: The Antihypertensive and Lipid-Lowering Treatment to Prevent Heart Attack Trial (ALLHAT). JAMA 2002; 288:2981–2997.
160. Bohlen L, de Courten M, Weidmann P. Comparative study of the effect of ACE inhibitors and other antihypertensive agents on proteinuria in diabetic patients. Am J Hypertens 1994; 7(pt 2): 84S–92S.
161. Bakris GL, Weir MR. Angiotensin-converting enzyme inhibitor associated elevations in serum creatinine: is this a cause for concern? Arch Intern Med 2000; 160:685–693.
162. Lewis EJ, Hunsicker LG, Clarke WR, Berl T, Pohl MA, Lewis JB, et al. Renoprotective effect of the angiotensin-receptor antagonist irbesartan in patients with nephropathy due to type 2 diabetes. N Engl J Med 2001; 345:851–860.
163. Bakris GL, Weir MR, Shanifar S, et al. Effects of blood pressure level on progression of diabetic nephropathy: results form the RENAAL study. Arch Inter Med 2003; 163:1555–1565.
164. Deedwania PC. Hypertension and diabetes: new therapeutic options. Arch Intern Med 2000; 160(11):1585–1594.
165. Larochelle P, Clack JM, Marbury TC, Sareli P, Kreiger EM, Reeves RA. Effects and tolerability of irbesartan versus enalapril in patients with severe hypertension. Am J Cardiol 1997; 80:1613–1615.
166. Lindholm LH, Ibsen H, Dahlof B, et al (for the LIFE Study Group). Cardiovascular morbidity and mortality in patients with diabetes in the Losartan Intervention For Endpoint reduction in hypertension study (LIFE): a randomised trial against atenolol. Lancet 2002; 359(9311):1004–1010.
167. Pfeffer MA, Swedberg K, Granger CB, et al. CHARM Investigators and Committees. Effects of candesartan on mortality and morbidity in patients with chronic heart failure: the CHARM-Overall programme. Lancet 2003; 362(9386):759–766.
168. Mogensen CE, Neldam S, Tikkanen I, et al. Randomized controlled trial of dual blockade of rennin-angiotensin system in patients with hypertension, microalbuminuria, and non-insulin dependent diabetes: the candersartan and lisinopril microalbuminuria (CALM) study. Br Med J 2000; 321:1440–1444.
169. Murphy MB, Lewis PJ, Kohner E, Schumer B, Dollery CT. Glucose intolerance in hypertensive patients treated with diuretics: a fourteen-year follow-up. Lancet 1982; ii:1293–1295.
170. Bengtsson C, Blohme G, Lapidus L, et al. Do antihypertensive drugs precipitate diabetes? BMJ 1984; 289:1495–1497.
171. Ames RP. A comparison of blood lipid and blood pressure responses during the treatment of systemic hypertension with indapamide and with thiazides, Am J Cardiol 1996; 77(6):12B–16B.
172. Lacourcière Y. A new fixed-dose combination for added blood pressure control: Telmisartan plus hydrochlorothiazide. J Int Med Res 2002; 30(4):366–379.
173. McFarlane S, Gizycki HV, Winer N, et al. Control of cardiovascular risk factors in patients with diabetes and hypertension at Urban Academic Medical Centers. Diabetes Care 2002; 25:718–723.
174. Black HR, Elliot WJ, Neaton JD, et al. Baseline characteristics and early blood pressure control in the Convince Trial. Hypertension 2001; 37:12–18.
175. American Diabetes Association. Hypertension management in adults with diabetes: clinical practice recommendations. Diabetes Care 2004; 27(suppl 1):S65–S67.
176. Koyama Y, Kodama K, Suziki M, Harano Y. Improvement of insulin sensitivity by a long-acting nifedipine preparation (nifedipine-CR) in patients with essential hypertension. Am J Hypertens 2002; 15:927–931.
177. Bakris GL, Weir MR, DeQuattro V, McMahon FG. Effects of an ACE inhibitor/calcium antagonist combination on proteniuria in diabetic nephropathy. Kidney Int 1998; 54:1283–1289.
178. Birkenhager WH, Staessen JA, Gasowski J, de Leeuw PW. Effects of antihypertensive treatment on endpoints in the diabetic patients randomized in the Systolic Hypertension in Europe (Syst-Eur) trial. J Nephrol 2000; 13(3):232–237.

179. Bakris GL, Smith AC, Richardson DJ, et al. Impact of an ACE inhibitor and calcium antagonist on microalbuminuria and lipid subfractions in type 2 diabetes: a randomized, multi-centre pilot study. J Hum Hypertens 2002; 16:185–191.

180. UKPDS Group. UK Prospective Diabetes Study 38: tight blood pressure control and risk of macrovascular and microvascular complications in type 2 diabetes. BMJ 1998; 317:703–717, 27, 48.

181. Mykkanen L, Kuusisto J, Pyorala K, Laakso M, Haffner SM. Increased risk of non–insulin-dependent diabetes mellitus in elderly hypertensive patients. J Hypertens 1994; 12:1425–1432.

182. Jacob S, Balletshofer B, Henriksen EJ, et al. Beta-blocking agents in patients with insulin resistance: effects of vasodilating beta-blockers. Blood Press 1999; 8:261–268.

183. Jacob S, Rett K, Wickelmayr M, Aggarwal B, Augustin HJ, Dietze GJ. Differential effect of chronic treatment with two beta-blocking agents on insulin sensitivity: the carvedilol-metoprolol study. J Hypertens 1996; 14:489–494.

184. Giugliano D, Acampora R, Marfella R, et al. Metabolic and cardiovascular effects of carvedilol and atenolol in non–insulin-dependent diabetes mellitus and hypertension. A randomised, controlled trial. Ann Inter Med 1997; 126:955–959.

185. American Heart Association. Heart and stroke statistical update. Dallas: American Heart Association, 1997.

186. Grundy SM, Balady GJ, Criqui MH, et al. Primary prevention of coronary heart disease: guidance from Framingham: a statement for healthcare professionals from the AHA Task Force on Risk Reduction. Circulation 1998; 97:1876–1887.

187. Straka RJ, Taheri R, Cooper SL, Tan AWH, Smith JC. Assessment of hypercholesterolemia control in a managed care organization. Pharmacotherapy 2001; 21:818–827.

188. American Diabetes Association: Clinical Practice Recommendation 2006. Diabetes Care 2006; 29: S41–S42.

189. National Cholesterol Education Program Expert Panel on Detection, Evaluation, and Treatment of High Blood Cholesterol in Adults (Adult Treatment Panel III). Third Report of the National Cholesterol Education Program (NCEP) Expert Panel on Detection, Evaluation, and Treatment of High Blood Cholesterol in Adults (Adult Treatment Panel III) final report. Circulation 2002; 106:3143–3421.

190. Rubins HB, Robins SJ, Collins D. The Veterans Affairs High-Density Lipoprotein Intervention Trial: baseline characteristics of normocholesterolemic men with coronary artery disease and low levels of high-density lipoprotein cholesterol. Am J Cardiol 1996; 78:572–575.

191. Tilly-Kiesi M, Tikkanen M. Low density lipoprotein density and composition in hypercholesterolaemic men treated with HMG CoA reductase inhibitors and gemfibrozil. J Intern Med 1991; 229:427–434.

192. Vega GL, Ma PT, Cater NB, et al. Effects of adding fenofibrate (200 mg/day) to simvastatin (10 mg/day) in patients with combined hyperlipidemia and metabolic syndrome. Am J Cardiol 2003; 91:956–960.

193. Canner PL, Berge KG, Wenger NK, et al. (for the Coronary Drug Project Research Group). Fifteen-year mortality in Coronary Drug Project patients: long-term benefit with niacin. J Am Coll Cardiol 1986; 8:1245–1255.

194. Brown BG, Zhao XQ, Chait A, et al. Simvastatin and niacin, antioxidant vitamins, or the combination for the prevention of coronary disease. N Engl J Med 2001; 345:1583–1592.

195. Bays HE, McGovern ME. Once-daily niacin extended release/lovastatin combination tablet has more favorable effects on lipoprotein particle size and subclass distribution than atorvastatin and simvastatin. Prev Cardiol 2003; 6(4):179–188.

196. Garg J, Bakris GL. Microalbuminuria: marker of vascular dysfunction, risk factor for cardiovascular disease. J Vasc Med 2002; 7:35–43.

197. Gall MA, Hougaard P, Borch-Johnsen K, Parving HH. Risk factors for development of incipient and overt diabetic nephropathy in patients with non-insulin dependent diabetes mellitus: prospective, observational study. BMJ 1997; 314:783–788.

198. Ravid M, Lang R, Rachmani R, Lishner M. Long-term renoprotective effect of angiotensin-converting enzyme inhibition in non-insulin-dependent diabetes mellitus: a 7-year follow-up study. Arch Intern Med 1996; 156:286–289.

199. Eknoyan G, Hostetter T, Bakris GL, et al. Proteinuria and other markers of chronic kidney disease: a position statement of the National Kidney Foundation (NKF) and the National Institute of Diabetes and Digestive and Kidney Diseases (NIDDK). Am J Kidney Dis 2003; 42:617–622.

200. K/DOQI Clinical Practice Guidelines for Chronic Kidney Disease: Evaluation, Classification, and Stratification. Kidney disease outcome quality initiative. Am J Kidney Dis 2002; 39(suppl 2):S1–S246.

201. American Diabetes Association. Nephropathy in diabetes (position statement). Diabetes Care 2004; 27(suppl 1):S79–S83.

202. Aiello LP, Gardner TW, King GL, et al. Diabetic retinopathy (technical review). Diabetes Care 1998; 21:143–156.

203. The Diabetes Control and Complications Trial Research Group. Effect of pregnancy on microvascular complications in the Diabetes Control and Complications Trial. Diabetes Care 2000; 23:1084–1091.

204. Klein R. Screening interval for retinopathy in type 2 diabetes. Lancet 2003; 361:190–191.

205. Younis N, Broadbent DM, Vora JP, Harding SP. Incidence of sight-threatening retinopathy in patients with type 2 diabetes in the Liverpool Diabetic Eye Study: a cohort study. Lancet 2003; 361:195–200.

206. The Diabetic Retinopathy Study Research Group. Preliminary report on effects of photocoagulation therapy. Am J Ophthalmol 1976; 81:383–396.

207. The Diabetic Retinopathy Study Research Group. Four risk factors for severe visual loss in diabetic retinopathy: the third report of the Diabetic Retinopathy Study. Arch Opthalmol 1979; 97:654–655.

208. The Diabetic Retinopathy Study Research Group. Design, methods, and baseline results: DRS report no. 6. Invest Ophthalmol Vis Sci 1981; 21:149–209.

209. The Diabetic Retinopathy Study Research Group. Photocoagulation treatment of proliferative diabetic retinopathy: clinical application of Diabetic Retinopathy Study (DRS) findings: DRS report number 8. Opthalmology 1981; 88:583–600.

210. The Diabetic Retinopathy Study Research Group. Indications for photocoagulation treatment of diabetic retinopathy: DRS report no. 14. Int Opthalmol Clin 1987; 27:239–253.

211. Cryer PE. Hypoglycemia is the limiting factor in the management of diabetes. Diabetes Metab Res Rev 1999; 15:42.

212. Clarke WL et al. Multifactorial origin of hypoglycemic symptom unawareness in IDDM. Diabetes 1991; 40:680.

213. Skyle JS. Therapy for diabetes mellitus and related disorders: Hypoglycemia in patients with type 1 diabetes 2004; 2680.

214. Kitabchi AE, Umpierrez GE, Murphy MB, et al. Management of hyperglycemic crises in patients with diabetes. Diabetes Care 2001; 24(1):131–153.

215 Sutherland DE. Report from the International Pancreas Transplant Registry. Diabetologia 1991; 34(suppl 1):S28–S39.

216. Sutherland DE, Gruessner A, Moudry-Munns K. Report on results of pancreas transplantation in the United States October 1987 to October 1991 from the United Network for Organ Sharing Registry. Clin Transpl 1991; 31–38.

217. Pancreas Transplantation in Type 1 Diabetes. Diabetes Care 2004; 27(90001):105S

218. Robertson RP. Islet transplantation as a treatment for diabetes—a work in progress. N Engl J Med 2004; 350(7):694–705.

6 | Type 2 Diabetes

Ronald Goldberg

Division of Endocrinology, Diabetes and Metabolism and the Diabetes Research Institute, University of Miami Miller School of Medicine, Miami, Florida, U.S.A.

KEY POINTS

- CVD is responsible for at least 50% to 60% of deaths in diabetes.
- In 1991, the six-year post-MI survival in diabetes was 50% in men and 40% in women.
- The prevalence of clinical CHD, stroke, and PVD is 40%, 10%, and 10% to 20%, respectively, in middle-aged diabetic subjects.
- Diabetic subjects without clinical CHD have 70% to 100% the MI risk of nondiabetic subjects with evident CHD.
- Approximately 20% to 25% of all subjects with CHD/stroke have known diabetes; a further 20% have undiagnosed diabetes, and an additional 20% to 40% have IGT.
- Atherogenesis is accelerated in subjects with type 2 diabetes, probably for years if not decades prior to diagnosis
- Pathophysiologic pathways, especially increased reactive oxygen species, drive accelerated atherogenesis by producing
    - an activated, dysfunctional endothelium
    - up-regulation of inflammatory pathways in endothelial, monocyte/macrophage, and smooth muscle cells
    - an increase in MMP activity
    - a procoagulant state
- Implicated, though not clinically established, cardiovascular risk factors in diabetes
    - insulin resistance
    - obesity and altered adipocytokine release
    - increased FFA and lipotoxicity
    - hyperglycemia (controversial as to whether this is an established risk factor or not)
    - proinflammatory factors
    - hyperhomocysteinemia
- Clinically established cardiovascular risk factors in diabetes
    - dyslipidemia
    - hypertension and increased arterial stiffness
    - hypercoagulability
    - cardiac dysfunction and dysautonomia
    - renal disease and microalbuminuria
    - smoking
- A meta-analysis of epidemiologic studies demonstrated that hyperglycemia was a significant predictor of CVD.
- Although modest reduction of hyperglycemia using sulfonylurea agents and insulin did lower the incidence of MI in the UKPDS, this was not significant.
- Intensive insulinization in subjects presenting with acute MI reduces CVD events and mortality (DIGAMI).
- A small substudy in the UKPDS found that modest reduction of hyperglycemia with metformin in obese diabetic subjects was accompanied by a significant reduction in MI incidence presumably independently of the antihyperglycemic effect.
- The most vasoactive of the antihyperglycemic agents is the TZD, and pioglitazone was found to reduce CVD events when added to preexisting therapy in subjects with diabetes and CVD (PROactive).
- Targeting prediabetes may reduce future CVD risk; lifestyle intervention reduced progression to diabetes by 58% and to the metabolic syndrome by 33% in DPP. Acarbose reduced progression to diabetes by 25% and to CVD by 49% in STOP-NIDDM.
- The target for antihyperglycemic therapy is a GHb of 6% to 7% and a fasting or preprandial blood glucose of <100 to 120 mg/dL.

- Combination oral agent therapy with the addition of insulin if goals are not achieved with oral agents is necessary to reach targets.
- Approximately 60% of diabetic subjects have triglyceride levels >150 mg/dL, and about 60% have HDL-C levels <40 mg/dL in men or <50 mg/dL in women. Small dense LDL may be found in 40%, and over 75% have LDL-C levels >100 mg/dL. These abnormalities are thought to be due to the expanded plasma triglyceride pool resulting from increased VLDL secretion due to insulin resistance and hyperglycemia.
- In a large epidemiologic study of newly diagnosed type 2 diabetic subjects, LDL-C was the most powerful predictor of CVD, followed closely and independently by HDL-C.
- There is robust evidence that lowering LDL-C levels in diabetic subjects by 30% to 40% will reduce CVD by approximately 25% to 30%, and this appears to be independent of the starting LDL-C level. In diabetic groups with average LDL-C of 120 to 130 mg/dL, lowering LDL-C to <100 mg/dL with statins will safely reduce CVD by 25% to 30%. In addition, in diabetic subjects with CVD, additional benefit is obtained in lowering LDL-C from 100 mg/dL down to 70 mg/dL, on average. Therapeutic lifestyle change is an essential component in the therapeutic plan.
- Fibrates reduce CVD events in diabetic subjects; for gemfibrozil this was demonstrated in a cohort with CHD and for fenofibrate in a cohort without CVD. Fenofibrate is preferred because in combination therapy with statins, it appears to be safer than gemfibrozil.
- Niacin is the most effective HDL-C raising agent, appears to reduce CHD or its surrogates, and may be used with care in subjects that do not have brittle diabetes or severe hyperglycemia, mainly as a second-line drug in statin-treated subjects.
- Ezetemibe, bile sequestrants, and high-dose niacin (2000 mg/day) all have second line LDL-C–lowering action.
- Approximately 50% to 60% of subjects with type 2 diabetes have hypertension.
- Sodium retention, increased vascular wall A-II activity, increased sympathetic activity and reduced vascular compliance are thought to be causes of the increased prevalence of hypertension in diabetes.
- Although advantages of certain antihypertensives over others have been demonstrated in clinical trials with CVD outcomes in diabetic subjects, thiazides, beta blockers, CCBs ACEIs and ARBs have all been demonstrated to reduce CVD events, and a recent meta-analysis shows little advantage of any one over another in prevention of CVD in diabetes.
- Clinical trials demonstrate benefit in lowering BP down to about 80 mmHg in diabetic subjects. This has led to widespread agreement for a treatment target of 130/80.
- ACEIs and ARBs are more effective than other antihypertensives in the prevention of renal disease.
- The fact that most hypertensive diabetic subjects require two antihypertensive agents and many require three or four, tends to reduce the significance of any single drug advantage.
- The most important objective in successful antihypertensive treatment is to reach the BP target. Surveys show that most treated patients do not achieve this.

INTRODUCTION

Type 2 diabetes is one of the major risk factors for cardiovascular disease (CVD), and atherosclerotic vascular diseases constitute the most important group of complications leading to hospital admission and mortality in people with diabetes (1,2). For years the gap in our understanding between elevated blood glucose values and increased CVD risk constituted a significant barrier to connecting diabetes with macrovascular disease, but thanks to advances in our knowledge of the etiopathogenesis of both diabetes and vascular disease, and a clearer appreciation of the epidemiology of diabetes and its complications, CVD is now widely regarded as the most important threat to health in people with diabetes. This has led to the notion that all therapeutic decisions, whether they be directed at improving glycemic control, lowering blood pressure (BP), and preventing retinal or renal disease, as well as of course managing classical CVD risk factors such as dyslipidemia, smoking, and hypercoagulability, need to be viewed in the context of whether that decision reduces the risk of CVD. In the final analysis, because the glycemic definition for diabetes is probably of limited value per se in defining risk of CVD complications, taken to its logical conclusion this approach leads to the concept that prevention of diabetes itself may ultimately be the optimal path to the amelioration of the risk of CVD in prospectively diabetic individuals, and in recent years evidence to support this point of view has begun to emerge. Thus effective identification and management of CVD in type 2 diabetes is not only of great importance for the health and survival of the 194 million subjects currently estimated by the International Diabetes Federation to have diabetes worldwide, but a full understanding of the topic may pave the way to the prevention of CVD in up to an estimated 300 additional million individuals with impaired glucose tolerance (IGT) at significant risk for the disease (3,4). In order to allow the reader to appreciate both developing concepts and therapies as well as established management approaches to the problem, familiarity with the epidemiology and etiopathogenesis of CVD in diabetes is required. These two sections will then be followed by a section on evaluation and management of CVD risk.

EPIDEMIOLOGY OF CARDIOVASCULAR DISEASE IN TYPE 2 DIABETES
Mortality
CVD is the most important cause of mortality in type 2 diabetes, accounting in the WHO International Study (5) for 54% of deaths in men, and 49% of women with this disease. Although men with diabetes have higher absolute rates of CVD mortality (by one-third to twice the rate in women), the excess risk of mortality compared to nondiabetic subjects tends to be greater in women so that the male to female mortality ratio is significantly lower in diabetic subjects. Most of the excess CVD mortality in diabetes is due to coronary heart disease (CHD), and it is important to recognize that in men the majority of deaths due to myocardial infarction (MI) occur before hospitalization (64%), emphasizing the importance of prevention, with a further 24% occurring in the first 28 days after hospitalization, whereas most deaths in women (52%) occurred in the first 28 days following hospitalization (Fig. 1) (6). The one-year mortality rate in diabetic men presenting with their first MI was 44% (nondiabetic men 33%), and in diabetic women it was 37% (nondiabetic women 20%); the male-to-female mortality ratio among subjects with diabetes was 2.7 to 1 versus 5.3 to 1 among those without diabetes. Causes of the excess post-MI mortality in those with diabetes include cardiogenic shock, sudden death, and congestive heart failure (7). In 1985 (8), the six-year risk of death in diabetic subjects after MI was 40%, and was significantly greater than in nondiabetic subjects (survival in diabetic subjects vs. nondiabetic subjects; 50% vs. 65% in men and 40% vs. 60% in women) (Fig. 2).

Prevalence
From the standpoint of prevalence, CVD has been shown in surveys from the 1970s to 1980s to be at least twice as frequent in diabetic subjects compared to those without diabetes (2). Overall, subjects with established diabetes have been reported to have a CHD prevalence rate of about 40% in middle-aged to older adults, with an age-adjusted risk ratio compared to nondiabetic subjects of approximately 2 in men and 3 in women (2). The risk ratio is higher in younger individuals, but the prevalence is lower. At initial presentation approximately 20% to 25% of subjects with type 2 diabetes are reported to manifest cardiac abnormalities (9,10). For stroke, the prevalence rates in comparable populations are about 10% (with approximately a 50% fatality rate) and the risk ratio compared to nondiabetic individuals was about 2.5 in both sexes (11). For peripheral vascular disease (PVD) in diabetes a prevalence of about 10% to 20% based on findings in diabetic individuals with missing pedal pulses was recorded, although this measure may not be particularly sensitive (12). In the Framingham study the risk ratio for

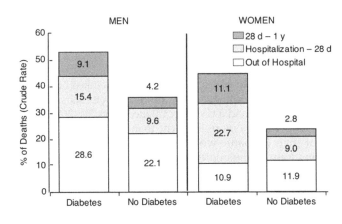

FIGURE 1 In-hospital versus out-of-hospital cardiovascular deaths in diabetic and nondiabetic individuals.

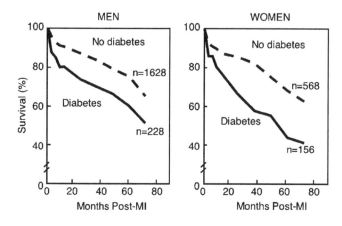

FIGURE 2 Survival post myocardial infarction in men and women with and without diabetes from the Minnesota Heart Survey.

diabetic versus nondiabetic individuals with PVD was approximately 4 for men and 8 for women (Fig. 3) (13). The prevalence of CVD in diabetic subjects is, however, dependent upon many factors, such as age, gender, and ethnicity. In addition the definitions, sensitivities, and specificities of methods used to detect CVD and diabetes have not been standardized. Furthermore as time has gone by, definitions and methodologies for diagnosis and therapeutic approaches to both diseases have advanced, and we are sorely in need of systematic, carefully collected, up to date prevalence studies. There is concern over the fact that the decline in CHD mortality experienced in the United States by the general population was not detected in men with diabetes, and that women with diabetes were found to have an increase in CHD during the observation period (14). This issue needs urgent verification and more widespread study in view of the projected increase in diabetes prevalence in the decade to come.

More recent prevalence data come from the Cardiovascular Health Study, which evaluated an elderly population with diabetes aged on average 65 years, and found that 29.7% had clinical CVD, of whom 68.1% had CHD mostly without any other type of CVD accompanying it, 11.5% had cerebrovascular disease, and 4.5% had PVD (15). Most individuals with cerebrovascular or PVD had concomitant CHD. Similarly data from the Centers of Disease Control and Prevention (CDCP) in the United States indicates that in 2003, approximately 38% of diabetic subjects >35 years of age were reported as having been diagnosed with CVD; CHD was present in 22.3% and stroke in 9.0%. Among those 35 to 64 years of age the prevalence of clinical CVD was 30%, whereas it was 48% in those aged 65 to 74 years, and 58% in those aged 75 years and older (16). This, not surprisingly, indicates a significant age effect on prevalence of CVD in diabetes. However little is known about the prevalence of CVD in subjects under the age of 50 years, which includes about half of all diabetic subjects (15). In a prospective observational study (16) of the incidence of macrovascular disease in 7844 newly diagnosed diabetic subjects in a large health maintenance organization (mean follow-up, 3.9 years), individuals diagnosed before the age of 45 years (mean age at diagnosis was 38 years) had an MI incidence of 4.6% as compared to 23.4% in those diagnosed after 45 years of age (mean age, 60 years). The respective incidences of stroke were 1.6% and 11.1%. This study does suggest, again not surprisingly, that at diagnosis the younger cohort had a significantly lower risk of CVD than the older subjects. Although not the subject of this review, it may be relevant that juvenile onset type 1 diabetic subjects begin to experience a significant increase in CVD events by the age of 40 years irrespective of whether the onset of their disease was in the first or second decade of life (18).

Another issue of increasing importance as the global explosion of diabetes takes hold and with the expansion in numbers of immigrants and minority groups is the effect of ethnicity. Again, the data are limited. In the CDCP data set White men had a CVD prevalence of 38.7% (26% more frequent than White women), Black men 31.3% (7.6% more frequent than Black women), and Hispanic men 29.9% (26% more frequent than Hispanic women). In a 20-year cohort study reported in 1996 from London (United Kingdom), compared to Europeans, Afro-Caribbean diabetic subjects had a risk ratio for CVD of 0.33 and for CHD of 0.37 (19), and in two studies from the Netherlands, both Moroccan and Turkish immigrants with diabetes had significantly lower CVD mortality rates than did diabetic subjects in the indigenous population (20,21). In the United States,

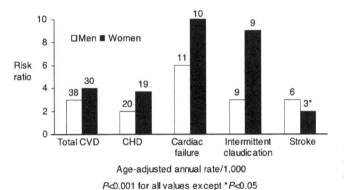

FIGURE 3 Excess risk of cardiovascular complications in diabetic men and women as compared to nondiabetic subjects in the Framingham Heart Study.

earlier data had suggested that despite greater rates of obesity and diabetes, Mexican Americans had lower CVD mortality rates than did non-Hispanic Whites, giving rise to the so-called "Hispanic paradox." However this was likely due to migration factors and selection, because a more recent study indicated that Mexican American diabetic subjects born in the United States had higher CVD mortality rates than Mexican born individuals and indigenous non-Hispanic Whites (22). It is also well recognized that in the United States, Black subjects have a higher risk of stroke than do Whites, but this does not appear to be the case for diabetic individuals (23).

The utilization in more recent surveys of subclinical measurements including electrocardiography (ECG), duplex ultrasound, and ankle/brachial BP measurements to identify CVD has led to the recognition that prevalence rates of CVD are unsurprisingly considerably greater than that indicated by CVD events. In the Cardiovascular Health Study for example, of the 70% of subjects without clinical evidence of CVD, 60.7% had positive tests of subclinical CVD, indicating that the overall prevalence of CVD in this population was >70% (15). Of subjects only with positive subclinical measures, CHD by ECG constituted 16.2%, a positive carotid Doppler was found in 52.2%, and a positive ankle-brachial index in 3.1%. Combining the 22% of subjects with clinically established CHD and those with ECG evidence alone provides an overall CHD prevalence estimate of about 30%. Based on the proportion of individuals with any coronary calcium, in a study of middle-aged to elderly men (average age, 61 years) with diabetes, the prevalence of CHD was 90% (24). In two recent studies using ankle/brachial indices to assess prevalence of PVD in diabetic subjects respectively >40 years and >50 years of age, abnormal tests were found in 20% and 29% (25,26). Thus in older diabetic subjects, CVD prevalence appears to exceed 70%. There is insufficient information available to assess its prevalence in younger individuals or in those with a recent diagnosis.

Is Diabetes a Coronary Heart Disease Equivalent?

The advent of the National Cholesterol Education Program's Adult Treatment Panel guidelines for management of hypercholesterolemia did more than any other program to promote a risk-based approach to the problem of CVD and its prevention (27). In particular the concept of a CHD risk equivalent state introduced the idea that high-risk individuals deserve more aggressive lowering of their low-density lipoprotein (LDL) cholesterol levels than do those at lower risk. While this approach has not formally been accepted for management of other risk factors such as hypertension, the results of clinical intervention trials in subjects with CHD with statins have led to widespread support for this approach as far as LDL-cholesterol levels, and the decision to treat or not is concerned. Thus the report from Finland in 1998 that diabetic subjects without CHD had essentially the same risk of MI as did nondiabetic subjects who had already experienced an MI (28) prompted the National Cholesterol Education Panel (NCEP) Adult Treatment Panel III (ATP III) to label essentially all diabetic subjects as having a CHD equivalent risk (27). This finding garnered support quite soon from the Organization to Assess Strategies for Ischemic Syndromes study (29), although an Australian study found that the risk for CHD in diabetic individuals without CHD was significantly lower than that in nondiabetic subjects with CHD (30). Since then there have been at least five reports indicating that men and women with diabetes but no evident CHD have approximately a third to a quarter less relative risk for CHD than do nondiabetic individuals with established CHD (30–35). The reason for these discrepancies are unknown, but likely have to do with differences in the diabetic populations being surveyed, including factors such as age, severity, and duration of diabetes (31,33). The implications of these differences may be important for public health policy decisions, but they do not significantly minimize concern for the heightened risk of CVD in diabetic subjects.

Prevalence of Diabetes in Subjects with Cardiovascular Disease

Assessment of the overall contribution of diabetes as a determinant of CVD is a complex subject for several reasons. First, at least a third of all diabetic subjects are undiagnosed (36), so that relying on a medical history will miss a large proportion of diabetic subjects, and even a single fasting glucose or HbA1C level often obtained under highly stressed conditions is unreliable, because many undiagnosed diabetic subjects have isolated postprandial hyperglycemia (37). Second, the direct relationship between elevated glucose levels and CVD risk is still unclear. Third how one defines CVD constitutes yet another variable. Finally given the fact there is evidence that the relationship between glucose levels in epidemiologic studies is continuous, and that studies of subjects with IGT have demonstrated an increased risk of CVD compared to euglycemic individuals (38), a full picture may only emerge from carefully conducted assessments of glucose tolerance. Thus although approximately only about 20% of subjects with an acute MI give a medical history of diabetes (39), 25% of nondiabetic subjects with an acute MI were found to have diabetes on oral glucose tolerance testing that was verified three months after admission, suggesting that the actual prevalence of diabetes in this group of patients is close to 40% (40). Using fasting glucose measurements only, the prevalence of undiagnosed diabetes was only 10%. In addition a further 40% of those without a medical history of diabetes had IGT, yielding a projected total prevalence of abnormal glucose tolerance in subjects with an acute MI of about 70% (40). For stroke, approximately 20% of subjects give a medical history of having diabetes (41), but the frequency of undiagnosed diabetes or IGT on follow-up oral glucose tolerance testing in a hospitalized population of subjects without a history of diabetes who had experienced a transient ischemic attack or nondisabling stroke was 24% and 28%, respectively (42), suggesting that at least 50% of these individuals have abnormal glucose tolerance. A medical history of diabetes was found to be present in 40% of subjects with PVD followed in a vascular surgery clinic (43), but there are no data testing prevalence with oral glucose tolerance tests (OGTTs) in this population. Overall the majority of subjects with CVD have an abnormality of glucose tolerance. The etiopathogenic and therapeutic implications of these findings will be discussed in the sections below.

ETIOPATHOGENESIS OF CARDIOVASCULAR DISEASE IN DIABETES

The past decade has witnessed substantial advances in our understanding of the pathogenesis of atherosclerosis. It has become clear that there are multiple overlapping biochemical pathways leading to the development of a clinically threatening lesion (44). As a result it is becoming possible to explore the fundamental influences of putative diabetes–associated pathogenic factors on these processes, and this should lead to more effective approaches to treatment and prevention of CVD. To appreciate the impact of these pathogenic factors on atherosclerosis in diabetes, a modern understanding of atherogenesis is required (44).

Atherogenesis

The earliest detectable vascular abnormalities in the pathway to atherosclerosis involve dysfunction of endothelium in response to injurious stimuli. Healthy endothelium is antithrombotic, antiproliferative, antioxidant, anti-inflammatory, and antivasoconstrictive, and injury to the endothelium alters the normal pattern of functional regulation. The mechanisms for initial injury remain poorly understood, but there is evidence that excessive production of reactive oxygen species may play a central role in turning on pathways leading to a reactive endothelium that is labeled dysfunctional, activating vascular wall inflammatory activity, and many of the subsequent steps in the development of the atherosclerotic plaque. Key among the initial changes that occur is a reduced capacity for nitric-oxide (NO)–induced vasodilatation and an increased vasoconstrictive tendency in response to angiotensin II (A-II) and endothelin. Second, endothelial dysfunction is characterized by the increased expression of inflammatory molecules, including IL-6 and IL-8, the release of monocyte chemotactic factors, e.g., monocyte chemotactic protein-1 (MCP-1) as well as chemotactic factors for lymphocytes, granulocytes, and mast cells, and expression of cell surface adhesion molecules such as E-selectin, Vascular cell adhesion molecule-1 (VCAM-1), and Intercellular adhesion molecule-1 (ICAM-1) that comprise mechanisms for the access and entry of inflammatory cells into the subendothelial space. The transcription agent nuclear factor kappa-b (NF-κB) is considered to be a key cellular switch in the development of this inflammatory state, and factors that increase its activity enhance progression and intensity of the proinflammatory state. One such factor is the receptor for advanced glycosylation endproducts (AGE) on endothelial cells known as RAGE, which is activated by increased formation of AGE. Subendothelial monocytes are activated by the endothelial cytokine, macrophage colony stimulating factor which transforms them into inflammatory macrophages. These cells now increase their expression of the proinflammatory CD40 ligand pathway, and scavenger receptors for oxidized LDL such as CD36, as well as releasing inflammatory cytokines such as tumor recrosis factor-alpha (TNF-α) and molecules such as tissue factor and matrix metalloproteinases (MMPs). Endothelial injury and macrophage activation thus set in motion both procoagulant changes involving increased tissue factor formation, plasminogen activator inhibitor 1 (PAI-1) deposition, and platelet activation, as well as smooth muscle proliferation (driven by increased A-II and decreased NO) accompanied by increased secretion of extracellular matrix and MMPs—the digestive enzymes allowing for proliferation of cells through matrix. Circulating endothelial progenitor cells may home in to the area in an effort to repair damaged endothelium. In addition, an excess of either anti- or proinflammatory molecules from adipose tissue and other distant sites may localize to the inflammatory lesion and modulate its activity. Adipocytes release the adipocytokine adiponectin, which stimulates NO production, inhibits cell adhesion molecule expression, and down-regulates scavenger receptor expression. In the obese state the production of adiponectin is decreased, and in this condition the adipose tissue release of increased free fatty acids (FFA), PAI-1, angiotensinogen, TNFα, and leptin collectively has been shown to have proinflammatory and prothrombotic effects on the vascular wall (45). In addition, increased hepatic production of C reactive protein (CRP) in response to increased levels of the messenger cytokine IL-6 may bind to sites in the vascular lesion and may contribute to inflammatory activity, although this remains controversial (46). There is considerable evidence that CRP may be a useful circulating marker of the level of vascular inflammatory activity, given its association with vascular events (48). In addition several of these molecules have soluble, circulating forms, including MCP-1, sICAM and sVCAM, PAI-1, TNFα, IL-6, MMPs, and adiponectin that may constitute markers of the activity of the pathways in which they are involved, and therefore constitute potential targets for monitoring and intervention in atherosclerosis.

Uptake of cholesterol from LDL and other apo B–containing lipoproteins is thought to require prior chemical modification, such as peroxidation or immune complex formation, and if the pace of entry of cholesterol into the cell exceeds rates of efflux of cholesterol to HDL, accumulation of cholesteryl esters in macrophages occurs. This leads to foam cell formation, and if unrelieved, eventually leads to cell necrosis through apoptosis, and the deposition of extracellular cholesterol into the subendothelial space. Activation of certain protein kinase C isoforms may stimulate differentiation, proliferation, or apoptotic pathways. Proliferation of smooth muscle cells into the neointima walls off the developing atheroma in a protective fashion from the vessel surface by forming a fibrous cap, the integrity of which is critical in protecting the highly thrombogenic core of the atheroma, rich in tissue factor, from activated platelets in the bloodstream. Clinical events appear to occur in several ways, all related to conversion of a subclinical, silent plaque to a clinically evident obstruction as a result of acute thrombosis, usually rather suddenly. The most common mechanism is the rupture of a vulnerable plaque, so-called because of its thin, fibrous cap, which is susceptible to lysis by the effects of enhanced MMP and rupture through sheer-stress forces. About a quarter of acute coronary events are due to superficial erosions of endothelium in which platelets are activated by exposed collagen or von Willebrand factor. In addition intraplaque rupture of microvessels developing as a result of angiogenic stimuli may cause a sudden expansion or disruption of the plaque.

The Impact of Diabetes on Atherogenesis

A key development in this area was the recognition that there are many factors associated with diabetes that contribute to an enhanced pace of development of occlusive atherosclerosis, and as time has gone by the list has expanded. They include hyperglycemia, increased FFA, visceral obesity, insulin resistance, increased oxidative stress, a proinflammatory, procoagulant state, dyslipidemia, hypertension, renal disease, and hyperhomocysteinemia. Information is also beginning to develop on how the atherosclerotic plaque in diabetic subjects differs from that in nondiabetic individuals. In addition the pathways by which these processes influence CVD is being increasingly understood. Also important has been a better appreciation of the natural history of type 2 diabetes and its pathophysiology, which has helped provide perspective on the processes involved (Fig. 4).

Effects of Diabetes on the Morphology of the Human Atherosclerotic Plaque

Although the greater extent and severity of atherosclerosis in diabetic versus nondiabetic individuals has been recognized for decades, there have been few pathologic studies comparing atherosclerotic plaque between diabetic and nondiabetic subjects. Recently, in a series of 270 autopsied hearts from patients with sudden coronary death, 66 with a history of type 1 or type 2 diabetes were studied, and plaque morphology was compared with plaque from nondiabetic subjects (48). There was a considerably greater plaque burden in subjects with type 2 diabetes than in controls, especially in distal coronary arteries. There were also more fibrous cap atheromas and healed plaque ruptures than in controls although somewhat surprisingly no increase in thin-capped lesions. Calcified matrix area, macrophage plaque area, and percent necrotic core were all significantly greater in the type 2 diabetic subjects. For cases with type 1 diabetes, the total plaque burden was slightly increased above controls, with similar increases to that in type 2 diabetes in macrophage area and necrotic core percentage. Both of these latter changes correlated with CVD risk factors including glycohemoglobin (GHb), although for similar total cholesterol levels, macrophage area and necrotic core size were significantly greater for cases with diabetes than for controls. The finding of an enhanced expression of the receptor for AGE (RAGE) and an increase in apoptosis in smooth muscle and macrophage cells in the vascular wall from diabetic subjects provides support for the importance of the RAGE pathway in atheroma formation, and increased apoptosis may contribute to necrotic core formation, thinning of the fibrous cap, and plaque instability. These findings generally support the notion that there is a greater pace of atherogenesis in lesions from subjects with type 2 diabetes, with heightened levels of inflammation and, as will be discussed below, of prothrombotic activity (49).

Relevance of the Natural History of Type 2 Diabetes to the Development of Cardiovascular Disease

It is now believed that the clinical diagnosis of diabetes is preceded by an extended period of increasing risk for CVD. First, it is estimated that diabetes is typically present undiagnosed for on average four to seven years prior to clinical diagnosis (50). Second, subjects developing diabetes spend varying periods of time (typically years) in a prediabetic state (51) in which either

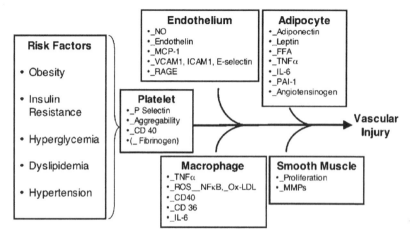

FIGURE 4 Biochemical pathways to atherogenesis in type 2 diabetes.

fasting or postprandial plasma glucose abnormalities can be demonstrated. Prior to the phase of abnormal glucose tolerance, normoglycemic prediabetic individuals have been demonstrated to manifest the earliest discernible defect associated with type 2 diabetes, namely insulin resistance, and this may emerge as early as in childhood (52). Glucose intolerance does not occur until the beta cell dysfunction characteristic of type 2 diabetes becomes significant, in the face of ongoing insulin resistance. The significance of this pathophysiological sequence for CVD emerged from studies demonstrating an association between insulin resistance and CVD even in subjects with normal glucose tolerance (53). This suggested a mechanism for enhanced risk for CVD that begins with the early origins of a disease that is only later characterized by hyperglycemia (Fig. 5).

Insulin Resistance, the Metabolic Syndrome, and Cardiovascular Disease

A considerable effort is being expended in attempting to dissect out the nature of the relationship between insulin resistance and CVD. It has become recognized that not only are risks for CVD events increased in insulin, resistant subjects, but that these individuals can be shown to manifest more subtle abnormalities relevant to the development of future clinical CVD. These include endothelial dysfunction (54), a proinflammatory and a procoagulant state (45), and increased carotid intimal-medial thickness (55), which is a surrogate for CHD and cerebrovascular disease. The pathways that link insulin resistance to vascular disease are still being clarified. It is clear that subjects with insulin resistance have an increased frequency of proatherogenic lipoprotein abnormalities, elevated BP, inflammatory and procoagulation markers, and visceral obesity, in addition to their predisposition to hyperglycemia (56), and etiologic roles for insulin resistance in the pathogenesis of these comorbidities are being increasingly elucidated (see below). Because each of these factors has been associated with increased risk for CVD, it is possible that insulin resistance relates to atherosclerosis mainly by virtue of its effects on classic CVD risk factors such as dyslipidemia, hypertension, hyperglycemia, and hypercoagulability (56). From a natural history standpoint these abnormalities can be identified in normoglycemic prediabetic individuals, years before they are diagnosed with diabetes (57). In this formulation, obesity may be a major contributor to the development or worsening of insulin resistance as well perhaps as also aggravating the same cluster of CVD risk factors as does insulin resistance (54,58). These clustering risk factors have been codified into a clinical syndrome, the metabolic syndrome. It is of interest and perhaps some controversy that the NCEP and the more recent International Diabetes Federation definitions of the key CVD risk factors making up the metabolic cluster predicting CVD beyond LDL-cholesterol excluded a measure of insulin resistance (27,59), unlike the WHO definition, which includes such a measure (60).

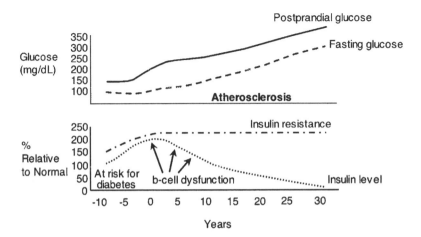

FIGURE 5 Natural history of type 3 diabetes demonstrating the presence of insulin resistance and increased metabolic risk for atherosclerosis in the prediabetic phase, decades prior to development of criteria for diabetic hyperglycemia.

It has been argued that because >80% of type 2 diabetic subjects have the metabolic syndrome (61), this syndrome is of little diagnostic value in diabetic individuals. It may, however, turn out that the metabolic syndrome does not explain all of the relationship between insulin resistance and CVD, or for that matter, between diabetes and CVD. First, nondiabetic subjects with the metabolic syndrome are not as insulin resistant as are subjects with type 2 diabetes (61). Second, there is evidence that diabetic subjects with the metabolic syndrome have a greater risk for CVD than nondiabetic subjects with the metabolic syndrome (61). Third, though insulin resistance is strongly linked to the metabolic syndrome, it is associated with wide ranging abnormalities that extend beyond identification of clinical metabolic syndrome components, including increased FFA release, which is thought to lead to excessive lipotoxic effects in many tissues (62) and the induction of a dysfunctional vascular endothelial response through reduction of NO-mediated vasodilatation (54). Insulin has also been shown to inhibit the generation of reactive oxygen species and to inhibit NF-κB activation (45). The proinflammatory effects directly associated with insulin resistance are thought to result from reduced insulin signaling through the PI3 kinase/Akt pathways, supporting a direct effect of insulin resistance on inflammatory pathways important for atherogenesis. In addition the mitogenic pathway of insulin action through MAP kinase is thought to remain intact in the insulin resistant state, raising the possibility that the hyperinsulinemia that is frequently found in insulin resistance may enhance protein kinase C and proliferative activity in the vascular wall (63). The roles of insulin resistance in the development of dyslipidemia, elevated BP, and hypercoagulability, and the overall impact of the metabolic syndrome on CVD in diabetic subjects will be discussed under the subsections devoted to these established CVD risk factors below.

Obesity

Most patients with type 2 diabetes are either overweight or obese, and excess adiposity has long been associated with an increased risk for CVD, especially when it is expressed in terms of central or abdominal obesity (64). Because of the difficulty of establishing an independent role for obesity as a CVD risk factor epidemiologically, it has been concluded that the increased prevalence of CVD in obese individuals is related to the fact that obese individuals have increased frequencies of dyslipidemia, glucose intolerance, hypertension, and hypercoagulability, which are considered more direct atherogenic risk factors (27). Because waist circumference and insulin resistance are closely correlated (65) these comorbidities could primarily be the consequences of insulin resistance. However there is increasing evidence for independent effects of obesity on pathways leading to atherosclerosis (66,67) since the discovery that adipose tissue is an active secretory organ, releasing several cytokines such as adiponectin, TNFα, IL-6, and MCP-1, as well as certain metabolites and proteins such as FFA, angiotensinogen, leptin, PAI-1, and CRP. These factors have all been identified to influence vascular wall processes either directly or indirectly for example through induction or aggravation of hypertriglyceridemia by elevated FFA (68). Importantly, the pattern of release of these factors, especially in those with visceral obesity, exhibits a proatherogenic pattern (69) suggesting a direct role for visceral fat in atherogenic processes.

Hyperlipacidemia-Increased Free Fatty Acids

The combination of an expanded visceral fat mass and insulin resistance conspires to produce elevated FFA (70) in diabetic subjects, and these abnormalities can be identified early on in the course of development of type 2 diabetes (71). Raised FFA have not only been incriminated in the development and worsening of insulin resistance (72) and beta cell dysfunction (73), but have been shown to have adverse effects on the vasculature. The most well-known effect is an indirect one, via increased production of triglyceride-rich lipoproteins in the liver. However, direct effects on the vascular wall have been described as well. These include reduction in NO-induced vasodilatation, induction of adhesion molecule expression, cytokine expression and apoptosis in endothelial cells, an increase in cholesterol uptake and a reduction in cholesterol efflux in macrophages, and an increase in arterial smooth muscle cell proliferation and migration (74,75). Multiple mechanisms may be involved, including activation of protein kinase C isoforms, increased ceramide formation leading to apopotosis, and increased production of reactive oxygen species through increased mitochondrial uncoupling and beta oxidation (76–78).

Hyperglycemia

One of the long-standing debates in this area is whether hyperglycemia contributes directly to CVD, in contrast to its well-recognized association with microvascular complications in diabetes. Most epidemiological studies indicate a significant positive relationship both in known diabetic subjects and in population studies (79–81). Using GHb measurements, which provide a more stable test of glycemia than do fasting or postprandial glucose measurements, a recently published meta-analysis of 10 studies considered suitable for evaluation (82) found that for each 1% increase in GHb, the relative risk for CVD was 1.18 (CI, 1.10–1.26). The discovery that chronic hyperglycemia leads to nonenzymatic glycation of proteins (83), to produce AGEs that were found to alter key structural and functional constituents of the vascular wall or external proteins capable of influencing vascular wall function, such as apo B (84), provided a rather compelling mechanism for the observed relationship between glycemia and CVD. Since then our understanding of the mechanisms by which hyperglycemia damages tissues has expanded significantly (85). Increases in polyol pathway activity, hexosamine synthesis, protein kinase C expression, and in the formation of AGEs that bind to an AGE receptor, RAGE, have each been shown to lead to abnormalities in vascular integrity. A unifying hypothesis posits that hyperglycemia directly increases generation of mitochondrial superoxide, leading to increased reactive oxygen species, which accelerates each one of these pathways, as well as having other deleterious effects on the vascular wall (76). In recent years there has also been substantial interest in the concept that acute spikes of hyperglycemia, such as occur postprandially, may be more damaging to the vascular wall than chronically elevated but lower levels of glycemia, such as occur overnight and preprandially in diabetic subjects. The idea was fueled by epidemiologic observations that postprandial glucose levels are better predictors of CVD than are fasting levels (38). Further exploration of this idea has led to the recognition that postprandial spikes of hyperglycemia are accompanied by surges of oxidative stress, fitting nicely with all of the evidence supporting a central role for increased generation of reactive oxygen species in the development of vascular damage (86). The paradox as to why it has not been possible to demonstrate in a convincing manner that improving hyperglycemia in diabetic subjects reduces rates of CVD and therefore what our therapeutic strategy should be is dealt with in a section to follow.

Proinflammatory Factors

Early studies in experimental models of insulin resistance or obesity demonstrating increased levels of proinflammatory cytokines paved the way to the first observation that type 2 diabetes was associated with increases in inflammatory markers (87). This was followed by a report that inflammatory markers predicted the development of type 2 diabetes (88), which has now been widely confirmed. Reports indicating that the presence of genetic polymorphisms of TNF-α and IL-6 independently increase the likelihood of development of diabetes (89) together with experimental evidence that inflammatory cytokines or induction of NF-κB may induce insulin resistance (90) suggest a pathogenic role for inflammation in the development of insulin resistance and type 2 diabetes. On the other hand, as discussed above, insulin has a direct anti-inflammatory effect, so that a reduction in the insulin signal is likely associated with acceleration of proinflammatory pathways. Whichever the initial stimulus is, the presence of insulin resistance, obesity, elevated FFA, and hyperglycemia likely combine to accelerate the inflammatory state associated with type 2 diabetes. This would of course be expected to aggravate atherogenic processes in the vascular wall of these subjects (91). Because traditional risk factors such as hypertension and dyslipidemia have also been documented to lead to endothelial dysfunction and stimulate inflammatory pathways in nondiabetic subjects, a similar question to that posed earlier for insulin resistance may be asked regarding inflammation and vascular disease; is the role for inflammation in the development of CVD in diabetic subjects simply explained by the effects of insulin resistance, obesity, hyperglycemia, dyslipidemia, and hypertension on inflammatory pathways? Because circulating high sensitivity CRP levels are thought to reflect subclinical inflammatory activity, CRP measurements may provide some insight in this area. CRP levels have been demonstrated to be higher in diabetic subjects than in obese nondiabetic subjects (92). In another study the presence of hypertension was the only independent positive predictor of CRP levels in a cohort with diabetes after age and body mass index were taken into account (93), although the effects of comorbidities other than obesity were not evaluated. There have been two published studies examining the relationship between CRP and CVD in diabetic subjects, one of which found diabetic subjects with CHD to have higher CRP levels than did those without CVD (94), whereas the other did not (95). More information is needed on this issue.

Homocysteinemia
Interest in hyperhomocysteinemia stems from genetic and epidemiologic studies as well as evidence that it induces oxidative stress and therefore may be damaging to the vascular wall (96). Although there is little evidence that homocysteine levels are increased in subjects with type 2 diabetes (97), it is possible, given the heightened predisposition of diabetic individuals to CVD, that homocysteine may be playing a pathogenic role in the genesis of vascular disease in diabetic subjects (98).

Established Cardiovascular Risk Factors in Type 2 Diabetes and Cardiovascular Disease
Dyslipidemia
Nature and Prevalence of Diabetic Dyslipidemia
Diabetic dyslipidemia is characterized by moderate elevation in triglyceride levels, reduced high-density lipoprotein (HDL-C) values, and increased small dense LDL particles. Other abnormalities include increased triglyceride-rich lipoproteins in the postprandial state (postprandial lipemia), increased remnant lipoproteins, increased apolipoprotein B 100 (apo B) concentration, and an increase in small dense HDL particles (99–101). LDL-C and Lp(a) levels in type 2 diabetic subjects are generally similar to those found in the general population (99,102). The prevalence of dyslipidemia in individuals with diabetes depends on the criteria used to define it. Overall, 30% to 40% of patients with diabetes have triglyceride levels >200 mg/dL and 10% >400 mg/dL (61). Sixty-two percent of diabetic participants in National Health and Nutrition Examination Survey (NHANES) III aged 50 years and older had triglyceride levels >150 mg/dL and 60% had low HDL-C levels (<40 mg/dL in men and <50 mg/dL in women) (103). In the United Kingdom Prospective Diabetes Study (UKPDS), baseline HDL-C levels were 9% lower in newly diagnosed diabetic men and 23% lower in diabetic women compared to nondiabetic controls (104). Triglyceride levels were 50% higher in diabetic subjects than in controls while LDL-C values were similar in diabetic men and higher in diabetic women compared to their nondiabetic controls (Fig. 6). As a comparison, in subjects with IGT, 46% had triglyceride levels >150 mg/dL, 57% had HDL-C <40 mg/dL in men <50 mg/dL in women, and 41% of men and 25% of women had the small dense LDL phenotype (105).

Pathogenesis of Diabetic Dyslipidemia and Its Impact on the Vascular Wall
An increased flux of FFA associated with insulin resistance and abdominal obesity has been implicated in the enhanced production of very low-density lipoprotein (VLDL) by the liver (Fig. 7) (106). Added to this, the effects of hyperglycemia and increased de novo lipogenesis combine to increase hepatic triglyceride production and increased VLDL apo B and triglyceride secretion (107). In addition, the enrichment of VLDL with apo C–III is thought to retard its clearance, and this may contribute to reduced remnant clearance (108) and further contribute to hypertriglyceridemia. Deficiency of lipoprotein lipase due to insulin deficiency may also interfere with clearance, but this has been difficult to demonstrate unequivocally in the typical

	MEN		WOMEN	
	Type 2	Control	Type 2	Control
Number of Pts	2139	52	1574	143
TC (mg/dl)	213	205	224	217
LDL-C (mg/dl)	139	132	151*	135
HDL-C (mg/dl)	39**	43	43*	55
TG (mg/dl)	159*	103	159*	95

* P<0.001, ** P<0.02 comparing type 2 vs. control

FIGURE 6 Lipid and lipoprotein values in newly diagnosed type 2 diabetic subjects from UKPDS compared to control values.

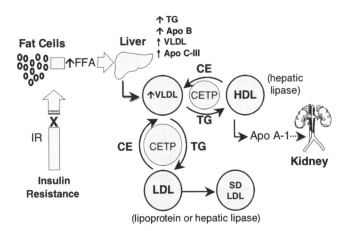

FIGURE 7 Pathophysiology of diabetic dyslipidemia.

patient with type 2 diabetes (108,109). Accumulation of triglyceride-rich lipoproteins is generally more severe postprandially when chylomicron triglyceride is added to unsuppressed VLDL triglyceride output (110). The expanded circulating triglyceride pool increases exchange of triglyceride for cholesterol mediated by the action of cholesteryl ester transfer protein between VLDL and HDL and between VLDL and LDL particles. Triglyceride enrichment of LDL and HDL is followed by hydrolysis of their triglyceride by hepatic lipase, considered to be up-regulated in type 2 diabetes (108), resulting in the formation of small, relatively cholesterol- and lipid-poor, and therefore dense HDL and LDL particles (108,111). The frequency of LDL phenotype B (preponderance of small dense LDL particles) in diabetic subjects is two fold higher than in the rest of the population (112). Many of these abnormalities are not directly reflected in the standard lipid profile, and this has given rise to several advanced lipoprotein testing methods that are able to identify particle size and distribution. These have mostly served to strengthen the observations previously described, although the nuclear magnetic resonance spectroscopy technique has an advantage of being able to provide a measure of particle number, and in one report using this technique, subjects with type 2 diabetes clearly had increased numbers of LDL particles that correlated with the degree of insulin resistance (113). The basis for that association is not fully understood.

From the perspective of atherogenesis, LDL and varying degrees of oxidized LDL have been well demonstrated to interfere with endothelial function, to induce inflammatory effects in the vascular wall, and to contribute to the development of the foam cell (114,115). This is important because as mentioned in diabetes, oxidized stress is increased, and this would be predicted to increase LDL peroxidation. However this has not been consistently demonstrated (116). Also of interest in a mouse model are findings suggesting that while hyperglycemia alone increases monocyte recruitment, glucose-induced LDL oxidation induces their proliferation (117). Small dense LDL appears to be more susceptible to peroxidation (118), is more likely to traverse the intimal layer of the arterial wall (119), and has a more prolonged residence time in the circulation, due to retarded LDL-receptor–mediated clearance compared to larger less dense LDL (120). Furthermore there is evidence that triglyceride-rich lipoproteins such as VLDL may induce endothelial dysfunction, promote inflammatory activity, induce protein kinase C, cause lipid accumulation without prior oxidation, and in an apparently unique effect among lipoproteins, induce the synthesis of PAI-1 (114,115). In addition apo B 48 receptors have been identified on macrophages providing a pathway for vascular wall lipid accumulation from postprandial apo B 48–containing triglyceride-rich lipoproteins (121). There is also evidence that retention of lipoproteins in the vascular wall involves proteoglycans, which may be modified in diabetes (122). HDL protects against plaque formation by enhancing cholesterol efflux, acting as an antioxidant, by inhibiting inflammatory pathways, interfering with the activating effect of LDL on platelets, and inhibiting lipoprotein lipid uptake (114,115,123). Although there is some evidence that cellular cholesterol efflux to HDL is reduced in diabetes this may have as much to do with primary cellular defects in the efflux process as it has to do with abnormal HDL (108). Subjects with type 2 diabetes do have reduced paraoxonase activity, and in vitro studies have shown that glycation impairs the activity of this HDL-associated enzyme, which may imply a reduction in HDL antioxidant capacity (124). Another important question is the role glycation plays in dysregulated lipoprotein metabolism; clearly AGE formation is associated with increased generation of reactive oxygen species, which would be expected to increase LDL oxidation, but in addition AGE-LDL and ox-LDL have been also shown to be immunogenic, and capable of promoting inflammatory activity (125). There is also evidence that AGE products in LDL per se promote excess lipid accumulation in macrophages (126).

Lipoproteins and Cardiovascular Events in Type 2 Diabetes

In the general population, a curvilinear relationship exists between the total cholesterol or LDL-C and CHD events. Similarly in a large population of male diabetic subjects evaluated in Multiple Risk Factor Intervention Trial (MRFIT), total cholesterol was shown to be strongly related to CHD mortality (127). Although hypertriglyceridemia predicts CHD, its importance as an independent CVD risk factor is controversial due to its close associations with other CVD risk factors such as HDL-C, obesity, insulin resistance, and glucose intolerance. The Paris Prospective Study suggested that the association between hypertriglyceridemia and CVD appears to be restricted to individuals with increased LDL-C (or increased numbers of apo B–containing particles) (128). Few prospective studies in diabetic subjects have been performed in which the relationships between lipoprotein levels and CVD outcomes have been fully assessed. In a seven-year study of 313 Finnish diabetic subjects, VLDL triglyceride was positively correlated with CHD rates, and HDL-C was inversely associated. LDL-C showed no relationship to outcomes, and in multivariate analysis, HDL-C remained the only independent predictor of CHD risk among lipoproteins (129). By contrast in the UKPDS, LDL-C was a powerful predictor of CHD among newly diagnosed diabetic subjects, followed closely by HDL-C (Fig. 8) (130). The NCEP ATP III introduced non–HDL-cholesterol (non–HDL-C = total cholesterol-HDL-C) as a secondary therapeutic goal after LDL-C, with the expectation that this measure would provide additional predictive value for CVD in hypertriglyceridemic subjects. In a recent pooled analysis of subjects from the Framingham, MRFIT and Lipid Research Clinics studies, it was found that non–HDL-cholesterol was a superior predictor of CVD compared to LDL-C in diabetic subjects (131).

Hypertension and Arterial Stiffness

Prevalence of Hypertension

Approximately 50% to 60% of diabetic subjects were found to have hypertension in NHANES II, which is twice the prevalence in the general population (Fig. 9) (103). There is evidence that mean BP is as high in previously undiagnosed diabetic subjects or individuals with IGT as it is in those with established diabetes (103). In a large group with IGT, 50% were found to have hypertension (132). Mean systolic BP increased from 126 mmHg in subjects with type 2 diabetes aged 20 to 44 years to 150 mmHg in those >65 years in NHANES II, was higher in men than women, and higher in Blacks versus Whites (103). These surveys, which are often quoted, are from the 1970s, however, and utilize dated cutpoints for hypertension. Interestingly though, Behavioral Risk Factor Surveillance System data from the CDCP in 2003, using self-reporting in telephone surveys, which is regarded as having moderate sensitivity, indicate a total hypertension prevalence among diabetic subjects of 52.5% in the United States after age adjustment, which represents a relatively small approximate 5% increase over the previous eight years (133). The prevalence in the 18- to 44-year-old group was 39.3% and in those aged 65 to 74 years was 69.7%. Overall men and women had a similar frequency of reported hypertension (53.3% and 51.7%), while Black

Position in Model	Variable	P Value
First	Low-Density Lipoprotein Cholesterol	<0.0001
Second	High-Density Lipoprotein Cholesterol	0.0001
Third	Hemoglobin A_{1c}	0.0022
Fourth	Systolic Blood Pressure	0.0065
Fifth	Smoking	0.056

FIGURE 8 Stepwise selection of risk factors for coronary artery disease in 2693 newly diagnosed type 2 diabetic subjects in UKPDS.

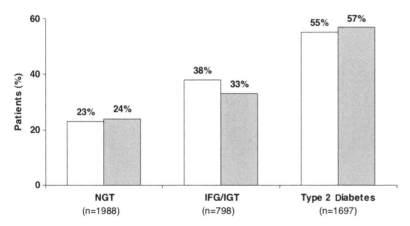

FIGURE 9   Prevalence of dyslipidemia (*white bars*) and hypertension (*grey bars*) according to glucose tolerance status in Finland and Sweden (Botnia Study).

subjects (63.6%) continued to have a higher prevalence than Whites (51.8%) or Hispanics (48%) (133). Approximately 10% of subjects <50 years of age with essential hypertension have diabetes and among those aged 50 to 74 years, the prevalence was 20% (134). In a recent survey in the United States and Canada, the prevalence in diabetic subjects was about 50% (135). Diabetic subjects also have an increased prevalence of isolated systolic hypertension (136).

Pathogenesis of Hypertension in Diabetes and Its Impact on Vascular Disease
The basis for the increased prevalence of hypertension in diabetes has been attributed to effects of obesity, insulin resistance, hyperglycemia, and renal disease, but the mechanisms involved are still far from clear. There is unequivocal evidence for an increased sodium content in diabetic subjects (137) in part related to increased reabsorption of glucose and ketones leading to hypervolemia, to which are added the effects of the renin–angiotensin–aldosterone system (RAAS), insulin resistance and obesity, hyperglycemia, abnormal sympathovagal balance, and genetic factors. Although the systemic RAAS appears to be suppressed in type 2 diabetes, it may be inappropriately elevated for the degree of increased exchangeable sodium, and be absolutely enhanced in the vascular wall itself (138). A-II has been increasingly recognized to play a critical role in atherogenesis. By interacting with its AT_1-receptor, it has been shown to enhance the activity of vascular wall NAPDH oxidase, thereby increasing oxidative stress and subsequent inflammatory and proliferative pathways as outlined above (139). The importance of this pathway to vascular disease is emphasized by studies of angiotensin converting enzyme inhibitors (ACEIs) or A-II receptor blockers (ARBs) in rodent models of diabetic atherosclerosis (140,141), which were shown to attenuate the development of atherosclerosis associated with reduced activity of some of the key protagonists in these pathways (e.g., MCP-1, VCAM-1, and platelet derived growth factor–B) whereas a calcium channel blocker (CCB) was ineffective. It is well established that endothelial dysfunction is a hallmark of hypertension and is thought to be characterized by impaired NO bioactivity resulting from increased reactive oxygen species (142). Indeed NO generation has been shown to be a net contributor to increased superoxide as a result of depletion of its cofactor tetrahydrobiopterin in hypertensive subjects (143). Accompanying the loss of endothelial vasodilatation is an apparent up-regulation of the endothelin receptor (144), which may contribute to the vasoconstrictor tendency, but perhaps more important are the observations that increased endothelin receptor activation (145) and reduced NO bioavailability contribute to increased arterial stiffness (146). It is important to appreciate that impaired endothelium-dependent vasodilatation is often portrayed as a causal mechanism of the increase in BP, or maintenance of hypertension, but this is unlikely because endothelial dysfunction is not specific to essential hypertension and because there is dissociation between the degree of endothelial dysfunction and BP values (142).

Perhaps more important is reduced vascular compliance. Until recently, arterial stiffness was thought to depend largely upon structural components within the arterial wall, such as elastin and collagen, and the distending pressure. However, it is now recognized that arterial

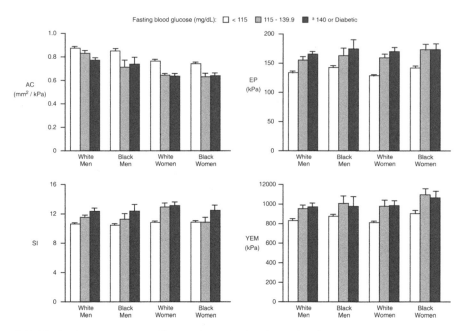

FIGURE 10   Race- and sex-specific associations in the atherosclerosis risk in communities study of arterial compliance (AC), stiffness index (SI), pressure-strain elastic modulus (EP), and Young's elastic modulus (YEM) with fasting glucose level. Bars depict means and SEMs.

smooth muscle also regulates vessel stiffness and that a number of locally derived and circulating factors, including NO, endothelin-1, and the natriuretic peptides, contribute to the short-term or functional regulation of large artery stiffness (147). In addition increased AGE formation has been related to increasing arterial stiffness, and this may reflect effects on both endothelial dysfunction and inflammation as well as physicochemical changes on structural proteins such as collagen (148). It has long been recognized that diabetes is associated with increased arterial stiffness (149,150), and a community study has confirmed this and demonstrated a relationship between a measure of arterial stiffness and fasting glucose levels (Fig. 10) (151). The loss of arterial compliance is associated with an increase in systolic BP, a fall in diastolic BP, and a widening of the pulse pressure. In fact, a widened pulse pressure is an independent predictor of CVD risk, more potent than either systolic or diastolic BP alone (152). The increased stiffness of the arterial wall contributes to isolated systolic hypertension, which, as mentioned, is increased in subjects with diabetes. Increased systolic pressure in turn produces an increased workload on the left ventricle, resulting in increased left ventricular mass. A reduction in arterial wall compliance has been linked to increased CVD risk in type 1 and type 2 diabetics and has been reported to occur early in the course of diabetes before vascular disease is clinically apparent (153,154).

Based on these considerations it is likely that arterial wall changes associated with obesity and insulin resistance contribute to this pathophysiology and may be important reasons for the increased prevalence of hypertension not only in diabetes but in prediabetic and in normoglycemic insulin resistant individuals. There is also a theory that the hyperinsulinemia associated with insulin resistance may play a pathogenic role, particularly because insulin increases renal reabsorption of sodium and activates the sympathetic nervous system, but there is little hard evidence to support this view. More important may be the effects of hyperglycemia, which as already mentioned increase AGE formation and oxidative stress. Oxidative stress has been associated with increased vascular smooth muscle proliferation (155).

Impact of Hypertension in Diabetes on CVD Events
The excess prevalence of hypertension in diabetes has powerful effects on morbidity and mortality from CVD; as for serum cholesterol, the MRFIT study demonstrated in men with diabetes that the impact of a rising BP on CHD mortality, though parallel to that in nondiabetic subjects was much magnified among the 6000 diabetic men (127); CHD mortality was increased in diabetic over nondiabetic individuals whose systolic BP was <120 mmHg. The UKPDS studied the

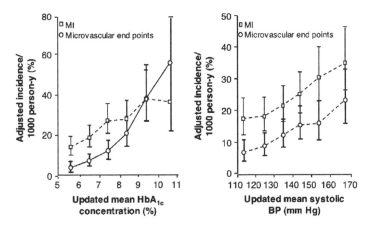

FIGURE 11 Comparison between the relationships of glycemic control and systolic blood pressure with micro vascular complications and myocardial infarction in UKPDS. *Source*: Ref. 156. Reproduced with permission from the BMJ Publishing Company.

effect of hypertension over a 10-year period on 3642 newly diagnosed subjects with type 2 diabetes and documented a direct relationship between systolic BP and all-cause, diabetes-associated, and cardiovascular mortality, as well as with individual outcomes, such as MI, stroke, lower extremity amputation, and heart failure (156). Unlike hyperglycemia, hypertension had a similar impact on macrovascular disease as it had on microvascular disease, demonstrating about a two- to threefold increase in risk for each outcome over the range of systolic BP from <120 to >160 mmHg (Fig. 11). The impact on stroke and amputation was even greater than threefold. Hypertension is a risk factor for diabetic nephropathy and a contributor to its progression (157), which increases risk for CVD (see below).

Hypercoagulability
Multiple abnormalities in platelet function, coagulation, and fibrinolysis have been described in diabetic subjects as well as in experimentally induced diabetes, and it is their concurrence that is responsible for the procoagulant state that is present in those with type 2 diabetes. The best-recognized abnormalities include increased platelet stickiness and aggregability, an increase in fibrinogen and factor VII levels, and an increase in the concentration of PAI-1.

Platelets
Platelets from diabetic subjects are hyperactive (158), and given that platelets provide amplification surfaces on which the coagulation system complexes are formed, this has importance in the precipitation of acute coronary syndromes. It appears that oxidative stress may be at least in part responsible for this hyperactivity, because peroxidation of arachidonic acid leads to the production of isoprostanes (159), which may activate the platelet through increased thromboxane synthesis in response to hyperglycemia (160). Subjects with diabetes have been shown to have increased populations of platelets that express activation-dependent adhesion molecules such as glycoprotein IIb/IIIa, consistent with the enhanced fibrinogen binding noted in platelets from diabetic subjects (161). Hyperglycemia appears to be important because incubation of whole blood samples with glucose leads to activation of platelet glycoprotein IIb/IIIa and P-selectin perhaps related to the osmolar effect (162). In addition platelet NO generation, which normally inhibits aggregability and cell surface attachment, is impaired in people with type 2 diabetes as a result of hyperglycemia and oxidative stress (163). Platelets from diabetic subjects have reduced membrane fluidity (164) probably resulting from increased glycation of membrane proteins. Decreased fluidity has been shown to occur when platelets are incubated in media that contain concentrations of glucose similar to those seen in blood from people who have poorly controlled diabetes. Altered membrane fluidity may change accessibility to membrane receptors, which could explain how reduced membrane fluidity contributes to platelet hypersensitivity in diabetic subjects. Accordingly, improved glycemic control is expected to

decrease glycation of membrane proteins, increase membrane fluidity, and decrease platelet hypersensitivity (165). Finally the platelet from diabetic subjects has been shown to be more resistant to aspirin than platelets from nondiabetic subjects (166).

Coagulation Factors
Measurement of the levels of the fibrinogen cleavage product following thrombin generation, namely fibrinopeptide A, and levels of thrombin–antithrombin complexes and of prothrombin-fragment 1.2, a cleavage fragment released in the conversion of prothrombin to thrombin, are all increased in subjects with type 2 diabetes, especially if they have CVD, consistent with a hyperactivated state of coagulation (167–169). Increased Factor Xa, a key component of the pro-thrombinase complex, as well as levels of fibrinogen, Factor VII, and von Willebrand factor have also been found to be increased in diabetic subjects (170–172), and are likely to be important factors in the generation of the procoagulant state, with fibrinogen levels being most closely correlated among these with CVD events (171,173). Observational studies have also demonstrated that serum fibrinogen is an independent predictor of CVD mortality (174). Furthermore most increased coagulation factor concentrations are not improved by treatment of hyperglycemia, may be found in normoglycemic relatives of diabetic subjects, and because fibrinogen levels correlate better with insulin levels than GHb, it has been suggested that these abnormalities may be more closely tied to insulin resistance (175). By contrast, levels of antithrombotic factors such as antithrombin 3 and protein C, which have been shown to be decreased in diabetic individuals and therefore may predispose to thrombosis, respond to improvement in glycemic control (176,177).

Fibrinolysis
It has been known for many years that fibrinolysis is reduced in diabetes (178). This impairment, which results from increased circulating PAI-1 (178), may contribute to acceleration of athero-sclerosis that is mediated by persistence of microthrombi and the impact of clot-associated mitogens on and within vessel walls. It also may predispose to acute thrombotic events, such as those that underlie precipitation of acute coronary syndromes. In addition PAI-1 can inhibit migration of vascular smooth muscle cells from the tunica media to the neointima by inhibit-ing vascular smooth muscle surface urokinase activity (179).
Contributors to the Procoagulant State in Diabetes
    A paucity of such cells in the neointima may limit elaboration of thick fibrous caps on developing atheroma, thereby increasing plaque vulnerability. Many factors associated with insulin resistance and type 2 diabetes, including cytokines, such as TGFβ, TNFα, and IL-1, increased visceral fat, A-II, hyperglycemia, insulin and proinsulin, VLDL, FFA, and hyper-glycemia, increase PAI-1 expression or levels (175). PAI-1 levels have been shown to be predic-tive of CHD and stroke (180,181).

1. *Hyperaggregable platelets* (somewhat responsive to glycemic control)
   ■ Increased oxidative stress may increase thromboxane synthesis
   ■ Increased expression of activation-dependent adhesion molecules, e.g., glycoprotein IIb/IIIa and P-selectin
   ■ Decreased NO generation
   ■ Altered membrane fluidity
2. *Increased fibrin formation* (apparently unresponsive to glycemic control)
   ■ Increased thrombin generation
   ■ Increased Factor Xa, fibrinogen, Factor VII, and von Willebrand factor
   ■ Decreased antithrombin 3 and Protein C (improve with glycemic control)
3. *Increased fibrinolysis* (somewhat responsive to glycemic control)
   ■ Increased PAI-1

Cardiac Dysfunction and Dysautonomia
Subjects with type 2 diabetes have been shown to have increased left ventricular mass (182) a known risk factor for CHD, attributable to increased myocardial fibrosis, and leading to both systolic and diastolic dysfunction. Other myocardial abnormalities that have been identified include microangiopathy, myocyte hypertrophy, perivascular fibrosis, increased collagen, and increased fat and most recently, increased myocyte monofilament dysfunction. The cause of

these abnormalities are not understood but might be explained by phenomena such as glycation of structural proteins, increased fatty acid uptake and altered energy supply, increased cytokine release, increased A-II activity, and chronically raised catecholamines and oxidative stress (183). Diabetic subjects have an increased risk of unexplained congestive heart failure (184), and the findings of left ventricular dysfunction in subjects without evidence of significant coronary artery obstruction or significant hypertension (185) have led to the idea that there is a distinctive diabetic cardiomyopathy, which may contribute to the poor prognosis of diabetic subjects with heart disease (183). A small study suggested an association between left ventricular dysfunction and number of metabolic syndrome components in a group of recently diagnosed, asymptomatic, normotensive men with diabetes and no known heart disease (186). Unfortunately without definitive diagnostic criteria for diabetic cardiomyopathy, the entity remains poorly characterized.

Reduced vagal tone and increased sympathetic activity as reflected by an increased pulse rate and reduced heart rate variability are well-established features of diabetes (187). They have usually been related to effects of hyperglycemia and hyperinsulinemia (188). In a recent study of heart rate variability in a mixed population of adults without heart disease, reduced activity was related to blood glucose, presence of diabetes, smoking, CRP, and white count, raising the possibility that subclinical inflammation could also contribute to altered sympathovagal tone or vice versa (189). Altered sympathovagal tone may be responsible for increased rates of hypertension, QT interval prolongation, and increased QT dispersion in patients with type 2 diabetes (190). Cardiac autonomic neuropathy has been shown to contribute to the high mortality rate in diabetic patients after MI (191) as well as being associated with changes in common CHD risk factors and with progression of CHD, and contrary to general belief it is found to occur early in the course of diabetes (192).

Renal Disease and Microalbuminuria

Type 2 diabetes is the most important cause of renal disease (193) and this is a well-known risk factor for CVD. In fact with more effective renal replacement therapy, CVD is by far the most important cause of death in advanced diabetic nephropathy (194). In the carefully studied Pima Indian population, subjects in renal failure receiving renal replacement therapy, had a ninefold excess of CVD deaths compared to those without renal disease, whereas those with clinical proteinuria had a 3.5-fold excess (195). The advent of sensitive urine albumin assays makes it possible to identify albuminuria at an early phase of glomerular damage, and prospective studies quite soon demonstrated that the urine albumin excretion rate predicted CVD events, and that the presence of microalbuminuria approximately doubles the risk of CVD in diabetic subjects (196). This meant that the well-known effect of established renal disease as a CVD risk factor originates years or even decades earlier in association with the development of elevated urine albumin excretion. The explanation for this finding is that elevated urine albumin is probably a marker of generalized endothelial dysfunction, not simply a feature of glomerular dysfunction (197), and is therefore a subclinical indicator of both micro- and macrovascular disease, because endothelial dysfunction is common to both. Increased urinary albumin excretion may therefore have value as an integrated marker of CVD risk. Microalbuminuria is not specific to established diabetes, being present in approximately 10% to 15% of the general population (198), about 15% to 20% of newly diagnosed diabetic subjects (199), and approximately 20% to 40% of individuals with established type 2 diabetes (200). Furthermore urine albumin values begin to predict an increased risk for CVD when only slightly elevated, and below the cut-points for microalbuminuria. For example, in the Heart Outcome Prevention Evaluation (HOPE) study (201), compared to those in the lowest quartile of urinary albumin/creatinine values, those in the third quartile (range, 0.58–1.62 mg/mmol or 6–18 mg/g) experienced a significant increased risk of MI, stroke, and CVD death (odds ratio 1.38, $p < 0.002$). Microalbuminuria predicts CVD independently of the Framingham score (202). It also appears that the glomerular filtration rate independently and inversely predicts CVD (203). This is important because at least 10% of renal disease in diabetic subjects is thought to be due to causes other than diabetic nephropathy.

Smoking

National surveys indicate that smoking habits in diabetic subjects are no different from those in nondiabetic individuals. Approximately 25% of diabetic individuals smoke. Cigarette smoking has been shown to aggravate insulin resistance (204) and thereby worsen glycemic control (205) as well as increasing the risk for development of diabetes in nondiabetic subjects by about 50% (206). Smokers have higher levels of FFA, triglycerides, postprandial lipemia, small dense LDL particles, fibrinogen and PAI-1, and lower HDL-C values than nonsmokers (207–209). Smoking increases the risk of microangiopathy, erectile dysfunction, and as in nondiabetic subjects, of CVD (206). This risk for CVD is not surprising given the evidence that cigarette smoking impairs vasodilation function in both macrovascular and microvascular beds, increases arterial wall inflammation and oxidative stress promoting LDL oxidation, and by enhancing MMP activity, activating platelet reactivity, and increasing fibrinogen, tissue factor, and PAI-1 levels, smoking exacerbates the risk of acute plaque rupture (210). This has been well shown for CHD, cerebrovascular disease, and PVD (211–213) as well as for total mortality in subjects with diabetes (214). CVD risk falls with smoking cessation, being still 50% higher than nonsmokers in years 1 to 9 following cessation, and still 25% higher after that (215).

EVALUATION AND MANAGEMENT OF CVD RISK FACTORS
Hyperglycemia

Despite the evidence that the degree of hyperglycemia correlates with the development and the severity of diabetic vascular complications, the rationale for intensive glucose lowering and especially the definition of cutpoints and targets requires evidence for benefit of this treatment. The demonstration in clinical trials in several different diabetic populations that lowering of elevated glucose levels clearly reduced the likelihood or severity of microvascular complication (216,217) provided that rationale and has shaped the targets for management of hyperglycemia. Unfortunately in none of these studies was glucose lowering demonstrated to unequivocally reduce CVD events.

Clinical Trials Targeting Hyperglycemia
Insulin and Insulin Secretagogues (Sulfonylureas and Glitinides)

The study that came closest to demonstrating that improving hyperglycemia per se reduced CVD events was the UKPDS, which, beginning in 1979, randomized 3867 newly diagnosed type 2 diabetic subjects either into conventionally or intensively treated cohorts (216). In the main study, diet management was maintained until the fasting glucose reached 270 mg/dL (15 mM/L) whereupon participants received sulfonylurea or metformin treatment, and insulin was used only in the event of severe hyperglycemia despite oral agent treatment. The intensively treated cohort had sulfonylurea or insulin therapy (in an approximately 3:2 ratio) instituted once their blood glucose values exceeded 108 mg/dL (6 mM/L), and the sulfonylurea-treated subjects had either metformin or/and insulin added if despite sulfonylurea treatment glucose levels rose significantly. In those relatively early days of intensive glucose management, before it was recognized that type 2 diabetes is characterized by progressive beta cell failure, physicians had not yet appreciated the constant effort required to boost treatment in order to keep up with worsening beta cell function and recurrent hyperglycemia. Thus, by the end of the study, although the intensively treated group had a median GHb over 10 years that was 0.9% less than in those conventionally treated (7.9% vs. 7.0%), their median GHb was as high as 8.1% in the last years of the study, indicating that their glycemic control was by no means satisfactory in modern terms. Despite this, in the intensively treated group, microvascular complications were reduced by 25%, a number which fitted well with the earlier observation in the Diabetes Control and Complications Trial (DCCT) in type 1 diabetes, which found that microangiopathy rates could be reduced by ~25% per 1% GHb lowering at any baseline GHb level (217). This is an important principle in the management of hyperglycemia, because it implies that lowering glucose levels by a fixed amount will lead to the same relative benefit for microangiopathy at whatever blood glucose level this is initiated. Whether this is true for macrovascular disease is unknown. A key CVD endpoint in the study was MI, and this was reduced by 16% ($p = 0.052$) in the intensively treated group (17.4% vs. 14.7%, 10-year rate). This result did not achieve statistical significance, and may be taken to mean that lowering glucose levels does not reduce CVD events significantly. However the effect size is worth noting and had there been a larger number of subjects studied together with more effective glucose lowering, a significant result might have been obtained. In the epidemiological analysis comparing GHb values in all UKPDS subjects with

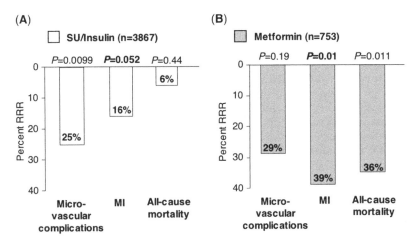

FIGURE 12 Effect of intensive versus conventional glycemic control on microvascular complications and myocardial infarction in UKPDS. (**A**) Intensive treatment with sulfonylurea/insulin. (**B**) Intensive treatment with metformin.

MI rates there was a twofold increase in MI over the entire GHb range (218) but for a given amount of glucose lowering, the effect on CVD prevention was significantly less impressive than that on microangiopathy (Fig. 11). This has left physicians uncertain as to the benefits of glucose lowering for CVD prevention; on the other hand prevention or amelioration of microvascular disease mandates that physicians strive for euglycemia in any event, so to some extent the issue as far as CVD prevention is concerned is rather academic (Fig. 12A).

Looking at the UKPDS results from the current perspective of the etiopathogenesis of CVD discussed above, improvement in hyperglycemia per se should have improved vascular dysfunction, even though clinical event rates were not reduced significantly. There is little evidence that sulfonylurea treatment has direct effects on the vascular wall, and its antihyperglycemic potency is limited. Furthermore in the admittedly flawed UGDP study, sulfonylurea treatment was found to increase CVD events (219). In addition, first and second generation agents such as glyburide and glipizide are potent inhibitors of cardiac K/ATP channels and inhibit myocardial ischemic preconditioning (which could aggravate myocardial ischemia in susceptible individuals), and perhaps these agents should not be used in patients with unstable CHD (220,221). It was therefore reassuring to see that intensive treatment with sulfonylurea and insulin in the UKPDS was associated with a net reduction in events. There were no apparent differences between first and second generation sulfonylureas, which were both tested in UKPDS on CHD. However a recent one-year study in a group of type 2 diabetic subjects comparing the rapidly acting insulin secretagogue, repaglinide, which targets postprandial hyperglycemia, with the sulfonylurea glyburide, demonstrated that despite similar GHb levels and better postprandial but higher fasting glucose levels compared to glyburide repaglinide was associated with a significantly reduced progression of carotid intimal-medial thickness. This is evidence, using a surrogate marker for CHD, for potential CVD benefit derived from an insulin secretagogue targeting postprandial hyperglycemia (222).

It is conceivable though that much of the effect seen in UKPDS was related to improvement in glycemic control per se, to which insulin treatment contributed significantly. Insulin, unlike sulfonylurea therapy, has almost unlimited antihyperglycemic potential and offers the opportunity for most patients to achieve normalization or near normalization of hyperglycemia if the dose is advanced sufficiently. Insulin treatment has been shown to improve endothelial NO production, reduce oxidative stress, and inhibit NF-κB activity (44), and with its superior antihyperglycemic properties could well have more powerful vasculoprotective effects than do the insulin secretagogues. Several clinical trials are evaluating the effects of intensive treatment with insulin in both established (223) and new-onset, Outcome Reduction with an Initial Glargine Intervention (ORIGIN) type 2 diabetic subjects. The only completed intervention trial that investigated the effects of intensive treatment with insulin on macrovascular endpoints was the DCCT, conducted in type 1 diabetic subjects. Even though intensive insulin treatment lowered

the GHb to 7% for the duration of the study as compared to 9% in the group treated conventionally with insulin, there were too few CVD events to assess the treatment effect because a
relatively young population was studied. However after six years of follow-up, in which all
participants went off study treatment onto their own preferred insulin regimens, and glycemic
control in the two groups respectively rose or fell to reach very similar mean GHb values by five
years (7.9% in the intensive group and 8.0% in the conventionally treated group), carotid wall
intimal-medial thickness progressed significantly less in those who were in the intensively
treated group (224). In addition, presentation of the 10-year follow-up results at the American
Diabetes Association (ADA) Scientific Sessions in June 2005, revealed the important finding of a
significant reduction of hard CVD events in the original intensively treated cohort compared to
the original conventionally treated group despite similar mean GHb values in the two groups
over the most recent five years. These data demonstrate that a 10-year period of improved
glycemic control was associated with a significant inhibition of the acceleration of atherosclerosis
in type 1 diabetes. Whether this will apply to type 2 diabetic subjects in whom obesity, insulin
resistance, and dyslipidemia are significantly more prominent remains to be determined.

Intensive Insulinization for Acute Myocardial Infarction
The Diabetes Mellitus, Insulin Glucose Infusion in Acute Myocardial Infarction (DIGAMI)
study demonstrated in subjects with acute MI that randomization to an intensive insulinization strategy beginning on admission to the intensive care unit was associated with a 25%
reduction in mortality within three months despite the fact that there was more hypoglycemia, compared to maintenance of the prior antihyperglycemia regimen according to
standard care (225). Further follow-up during which the insulinized group was maintained
on intensive insulin outpatient treatment demonstrated that this benefit persisted through
three years with an 11% reduction in mortality (226). The benefit was greatest in those with
relatively low cardiac risk. In addition the finding that beta blocker use did not have a significant effect in predicting post-MI event rates in the intensively treated group as it did in
the conventionally treated subjects raised the possibility that intensive insulinization was
operating on pathways through which beta blockers typically improve morbidity and mortality post-MI, namely the reduction of FFA in favor of glucose oxidation (227). A second
DIGAMI study (DIGAMI 2), aimed at dissecting out the effects of the acute intensive insulinization to the long-term intensive insulinization in explaining the benefits in DIGAMI 1, was
unsuccessful in confirming the results of DIGAMI 1. Because outcomes continued to be
strongly predicted by GHb, the investigators concluded that lower admitting GHb values
and significantly smaller differences in GHb between intensive and conventionally treated
groups in DIGAMI 2 as compared to the earlier study could explain failure to find
a beneficial effect of intensive insulinization in this study (228). As the potential benefits
of acute glucose lowering emerged from a better understanding of the deleterious effects of
hyperglycemia, intensive insulinization has been shown to improve outcomes in severely ill,
hyperglycemic patients admitted to intensive care and surgical care units without a previous
diagnosis of diabetes (229–231).

Antihyperglycemic Agents with Independent Vascular Effects
Metformin.   This agent has been demonstrated to have modest beneficial effects on the lipid
profile, and in some studies to decrease insulin resistance moderately (232,233). Metformin also
has an anorectic effect, increases fat oxidation, may be associated with weight loss, and reduces
PAI-1 levels (234). Metformin improves endothelial dysfunction, but has little effect on inflammatory markers (235,236). Another biguanide, phenformin, was shown earlier in the UGDP trial
to be associated with an increased risk of CHD, but this agent had a significantly greater tendency than metformin to cause lactic acidosis. In a substudy from the UKPDS, a smaller group
of overweight newly diagnosed diabetic subjects were randomized to metformin first ($n = 753$)
instead of sulfonylurea for the intensive treatment strategy (237). In similar fashion to the main
study, microangiopathy rates in the metformin substudy were reduced 29% in association with
a 0.6% reduction in GHb values in the intensively treated cohort (7.4% vs. 8.0%) although there
was insufficient statistical power to demonstrate significance. Despite this and in contrast to the
main study, however, MI rates were decreased by 39% in the metformin-treated subjects ($p < 0.01$),
and all cause mortality was reduced by 36% (Fig. 12B). These results suggested that metformin
treatment was associated with a rather impressive reduction in CHD, which appeared to be

associated at least in part with factors beyond glycemic control. These surprisingly impressive findings were rendered less robust by the findings of a secondary analysis of subjects in UKPDS who received combined treatment of metformin and sulfonylurea, in whom MI rates were inexplicably 96% higher than those in the conventionally treated group. It is difficult to justify completely dismissing the latter findings as a statistical quirk, while accepting the former, and the small number of patients involved further complicates interpretation. Although there has been a subsequent retrospective database review supporting the findings that regimens with metformin were associated with fewer CVD events than those with sulfonylureas (238), some uncertainty surrounding the beneficial effect of metformin on CHD remains. Finally because of the tendency for metformin to cause lacticacidosis in certain predisposing situations, it is prudent to avoid the use of metformin in subjects with overt congestive heart failure although analysis of the same database appeared to indicate that there were fewer clinical outcomes in subjects with heart failure on metformin as compared to sulfonylurea treatment (239).

Thiazolidinediones (TZDs). The addition of the TZD group of drugs to our therapeutic armamentarium brings the promise of a new group of antihyperglycemic agents that have been demonstrated to have significant anti-inflammatory and vascular effects (240,241). These agents improve hyperglycemia to the same degree as do metformin and sulfonylureas. They do this by reducing insulin resistance through activation of peroxisome proliferator-activated receptor-gamma (PPARγ) in at least two ways; first they lower FFA by promoting adipocyte differentiation and triglyceride storage, reducing the inhibitory effects of FFA on insulin-mediated glucose uptake and storage (242), and second, TZDs reduce TNFα (243) and increase the release of the adipocytokine adiponectin, which enhances insulin sensitivity as well as inhibiting early steps in vascular inflammatory activity by reducing adhesion molecule expression (244). TZDs decrease vascular reactive oxygen species production (245), and this is the likely reason that they decrease NF-κB expression and the downstream activation of inflammatory pathways, including reduction in CD40/CD 40 ligand and RAGE activities. In addition the TZDs increase NO release and inhibit thrombin-stimulated endothelin release, which may explain the basis for the finding that they increase vascular flow-mediated vasodilatation (246). The TZDs are antithrombotic, decreasing PAI-1 expression and platelet aggregability (247), and through increasing oxidized LDL uptake and enhancing ATP-binding cassette transporter A1 mediated cholesterol efflux, TZDs increase sequestration of oxidized LDL while limiting foam cell formation (248). By reducing IL-6, CRP levels are decreased significantly by TZDs, although the clinical significance of this is yet to be determined. Other clinically relevant properties of the TZDs demonstrated in subjects with type diabetes include lowering of BP, reducing urinary albumin excretion—a risk factor for both diabetic nephropathy and CVD, reduction of silent ischemia, and reducing progression of carotid intimal-medial thickness [reviewed in Ref. (241)]. Studies in atherosclerosis-susceptible mice have also shown that TZDs reduce the size of atheromatous plaques (249). It appears that most of these apparent vasculoprotective effects are class properties of the TZDs. One exception appears to be their actions on the lipid profile, where pioglitazone has triglyceride lowering and greater HDL-C raising effects compared to rosiglitazone (250). In addition TZDs have PPAR-independent effects on calcium fluxes and the cell cycle, and pioglitazone and troglitazone may have some PPARα activity. Currently several new agents with combined PPARα/γ effects are in clinical trials evaluating both their glucose-lowering properties and their effects on CVD risk factors (251). In the final analysis, clinical outcomes are needed to assess whether these agents reduce risk of CVD. The recent report of the Prospective Pioglitazone Clinical Trial in Macrovascular Events (PROactive) provides some evidence to support this contention (252). This trial compared add-on pioglitazone versus placebo treatment to the antihyperglycemic medical regimens (metformin, sulfonylurea, and/or insulin in all combinations) of 5238 type 2 diabetic subjects with established CVD, in centers in the United Kingdom and in Europe. At the predetermined stopping point of 760 first primary endpoint events, which occurred after an average follow-up of three years, there was 10% relative risk reduction for the primary endpoint ($p = 0.0951$), which was a composite of both "hard" and "softer" CVD events, and a 16% relative risk reduction for the secondary endpoint ($p = 0.0273$), which consisted only of all-cause mortality, non-fatal MI, and stroke (Fig. 13). Despite the fact that the majority of participants were on ACEIs, lipid-modifying agents, and antiplatelet drugs, the placebo rate of the secondary endpoint was a very high 4.6% per year, which illustrates the sheer size of the risk for recurrent CVD in

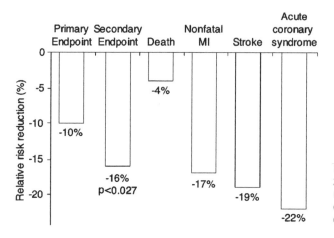

FIGURE 13 Effects of addition of pioglitazone to standard antihyperglycemic treatment on cardiovascular outcomes in type 2 diabetic subjects with established cardiovascular disease on PROactive,

diabetic subjects with established CVD, despite what are regarded as effective cardioprotective therapies. GHb, systolic blood pressure (SBP), triglyceride levels, and the LDL/HDL ratio were significantly lower and HDL-C significantly higher in the pioglitazone-treated versus the placebo-treated group, indicating several possible mechanisns through which the TZD might lower CVD event rates in addition to other unmeasured effects of the agent. These rather modest positive findings provide some initial support for the notion that TZDs—in this case pioglitazone—may reduce CVD events, although it has been argued that given the lack of a significant finding for the primary endpoint, caution should be exercised in interpreting the positive findings (253). They were further complicated by the finding that there were 41 more hospitalizations for congestive heart failure in the pioglitazone-treated group compared to the placebo group (the rates were 5.7% vs. 4.1%), although there were no increases in mortality from heart failure in pioglitazone-treated subjects.

The finding of an increased frequency of heart failure in subjects treated with pioglitazone is a concern and is in support of previous observations (254,255) although not all (256). It is known that these agents increase fluid retention at least in part by increasing capillary permeability and salt and water retention, and that this effect is greater when the agents are used in conjunction with sulfonylurea and especially insulin. Pedal edema may occur in up to 15% of patients. There is no evidence that these agents depress myocardial function, and it is likely that by increasing fluid retention in subjects with established or borderline heart failure they aggravate symptoms. Of greater concern is the possibility that they may precipitate congestive heart failure in subjects without apparent significant left ventricular dysfunction (257), although little is known about the frequency of this problem. Careful analysis of the 149 pioglitazone-treated subjects in PROactive will be informative in this regard. Although it has been suggested that authorities have been overly restrictive in the use of oral agents in subjects with heart disease (258), it can be argued that a safe alternative exists, namely insulin treatment, for which there is evidence for benefit in treatment of heart failure (259). A further concern regarding the extensive use of TZDs is their weight-promoting effect. Typically the weight gain is in the 5 to 10 lb range although occasionally the increase can be extreme. It tends to parallel the improvement in the GHb and to level off after six months. Although fluid retention may contribute, most of the weight gain is due to the effect of PPARγ activation on adipogenesis. However it is interesting to note that the weight gain associated with both troglitazone and pioglitazone has been shown to occur predominantly in subcutaneous depots, with an actual reduction in visceral fat mass, possibly representing a less hazardous arrangement of excess body fat (260).

Preventing CVD by Targeting Prediabetes
Although not as great as CVD risk in established diabetes, subjects with prediabetes, defined collectively as those with impaired fasting glucose [IFG = fasting glucose 100–125 mg/dL (5.6–7.0 mM/L), no glucose challenge employed] or IGT [IGT = fasting glucose <126 mg/dL (<7.0 mM/L) + two-hour post challenge glucose between 140 and 199 mg/dL (7.8–11.1 mM/L)], have an increased risk for CVD compared to the general population

(37,261–263). This has been attributed to metabolic abnormalities of a similar though generally milder nature to those that cluster in diabetes and which can be identified even before prediabetic glucose abnormalities arise in response to the development of insulin resistance and obesity (262). It may be that most of those with prediabetes who develop CVD in observational studies had progressed to subclinical diabetes by the time they had their MI, because follow-up OGTTs were usually not performed in these studies. In the largest survey of subjects with IGT, 50% of subjects in the Diabetes Prevention Program (DPP) were found to have the metabolic syndrome at baseline (264). Thirty percent of the group had hypertension, and 45% had the BP component of the metabolic syndrome ($\geq$130/85); 46% had triglyceride levels >150 mg/dL, 57% had HDL-C <40 mg/dL in men/<50 mg/dL in women, and 41% of men and 25% of women had the small dense LDL phenotype (264–266). Significant heterogeneity existed between participants in regard to their complement of CVD risk factors, indicating that predicted CVD risk may vary considerably among subjects with IGT, and this may be of importance for their future morbidity and mortality. Overall, the degree of insulin resistance was found to be a major factor associated with these abnormalities—especially the lipid abnormalities (262). DPP demonstrated that progression to diabetes in the standard care group occurred at a rate of 11% per year, and this was reduced 58% by intensive lifestyle modification, consisting of weight reduction and increased physical activity, while metformin treatment reduced the progression rate by 31%. Of those who did not have the metabolic syndrome at baseline in the standard care group, approximately 50% of those in the standard care group had developed the syndrome by study end (264), and the frequency of hypertension increased from 30% to 40% in the placebo and metformin groups (Fig. 14) (266). Because diabetic subjects have a more adverse risk factor profile than prediabetic individuals, presumably the risk factor profile in those that progress to diabetes deteriorates as diabetes evolves. Thus, the development of CVD in diabetic subjects may be viewed as a time-dependent exposure of intensifying atherogenic influences that originate years, if not decades, prior to clinical presentation with hyperglycemia.

Based on this concept, it follows that CVD prevention in prediabetic subjects should begin before waiting for diabetic hyperglycemia to develop. In DPP, triglyceride levels fell more, HDL-C increased to a greater degree, and the prevalence of hypertension did not increase in the lifestyle group as compared to the metformin or placebo groups (266). The Study To Prevent Noninsulin-Dependent Diabetes Mellitus (STOP NIDDM) trial demonstrated in subjects with IGT that the glucosidase inhibitor acarbose, which slows glucose absorption post-prandially, reduced the progression rate to diabetes by 25% compared to placebo (267). In addition in the acarbose group compared to placebo, the development of new cases of hypertension was reduced by 34%, and strikingly, the relative risk for CVD events was reduced by 49% ($p = 0.03$)—a surprisingly large decrease in events, that has been attributed to the effect of the agent on reducing postprandial hyperglycemia (268). These results should give impetus to the need to identify at least the most high-risk prediabetic subjects, e.g., those with the metabolic syndrome, for more intensive CVD prevention measures.

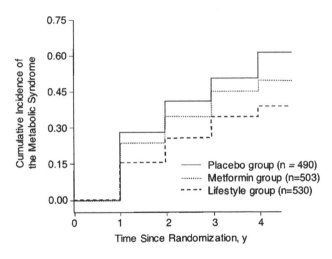

FIGURE 14 Comparison between lifestyle intervention and metformin treatment with standard care on development of the metabolic syndrome in the diabetes prevention program.

Diagnosis of Glucose Intolerance (The American Diabetes Association/WHO Criteria) (304)

Prediabetes.   This is defined as a state of glucose intolerance not thought to be associated with diabetes-specific microangiopathy that is associated with an increased risk for development of diabetes. IFG was more recently defined to obviate the need for performance of an OGTT, but it has become clear that subjects with IFG overlap only partially with IGT.

1. IFG: fasting plasma glucose 100 to 125 mg/dL (5.6–6.9 mmol/L)
2. IGT: fasting plasma glucose <100 mg/dL (<5.6 mmol/L) two-hour postload glucose 140 to 199 mg/dL (7.8–11.1 mmol/L)

Diabetes:
1. Symptoms of diabetes plus casual plasma glucose concentration $\geq$200 mg/dL ($\geq$11.1 mmol/L). Casual is defined as any time of day without regard to time since last meal. The classic symptoms of diabetes include polyuria, polydipsia, and unexplained weight loss
or
2. Fasting plasma glucose $\geq$126 mg/dL (7.0 mmol/L). Fasting is defined as no caloric intake for at least eight hours
or
3. Two-hour postload glucose $\geq$200 mg/dL (11.1 mmol/L) during an OGTT. The test should be performed as described by WHO, using a glucose load containing the equivalent of 75 g anhydrous glucose dissolved in water

In the absence of unequivocal hyperglycemia, these criteria should be confirmed by repeat testing on a different day. The third measure (OGTT) is not recommended by the ADA for routine clinical use, but some have argued that although more cumbersome than a fasting glucose measure the OGTT is more efficient in diagnosing diabetes. The GHb (HbA1c) is not used to diagnose diabetes, because it is not a precise measure of a given fasting or two-hour glucose value. It cannot, for example, distinguish reliably between prediabetes and diabetes as currently defined, although there is an argument that the GHb may be more valuable long term in predicting diabetic complications. It does of course correlate with average glucose values over the past two to three months, and a value $\geq$7.0% with few exceptions reflects diabetic hyperglycemia.

Therapeutic Guidelines

The findings of the DCCT, the UKPDS, and a smaller Japanese study of type 2 diabetes (269) constituted the principal clinical evidence supporting the recommendations of most official organizations. Following the initial report of the UKPDS results in 1998, the ADA published its guidelines governing glycemic control. Mindful of the fact that hypoglycemia was a potentially serious complication as elevated glucose levels were lowered toward normal in type 1 diabetes, and without clear significant benefit having being demonstrated to accrue between normal GHb levels (<6.0%) and 7.0%, the ADA guidelines initially recommended a GHb goal of <7.0%, with an endorsement of action required for values >8.0%, and preprandial fingerstick glucose goals of 80 to 120 mg/dL. It dropped the recommendation for action at a GHb >8.0% in 2003 and instead emphasized the need to individualize targets (270). The Canadian Diabetes Association (271) categorized GHb levels into ideal ($\leq$100% of the upper limit of normal, which is usually 4.0–6.0%), optimal ($\leq$115%, approximately <7%), suboptimal (116–140%), or inadequate (>140%, which is a GHb value of approximately 8.4%). The European Policy Diabetes Policy Group, endorsed by the International Diabetes Federation (272), and the American Association of Clinical Endocrinology favor a lower GHb target of <6.5% (273), while the guidelines of the European and Other Societies on Cardiovascular Disease Prevention in Clinical Practice (which incorporates the European Association for the Study of Diabetes) recommend a GHb target of >6.1% (Fig. 15) (274). Although the differences between these recommendations are small, the issue involved is an important one, in that it reflects differences in expert opinion on the importance of achievement of a normal versus a near normal GHb. Until the Action to Control Cardiovascular Risk in Diabetes (ACCORD) trial is complete in 2010 there will have been no study assessing whether achievement of normal GHb values provides significant benefit over near normal target values. Although it may appear self-evident that normal plasma glucose values are preferable to near normal values, abnormalities other than

	ADA	AACE	IDF	
			Arterial Risk	Microvasc
HbA$_{1c}$	<7	<6.5	≥6.5	≥7.5
Fasting/preprandial glucose (mg/dL)	80–120	<110	≥100	≥110
Postprandial glucose (mg/dL)	100–180	<140	≥135	≥160
Bedtime glucose (mg/dL)	100–140	100–140		

FIGURE 15 Glycemic targets according to the American Diabetes Association, The Association of American Clinical Endocrinologists and the International Diabetes Federation.

elevated glucose levels may be more important in defining health outcomes in this range of glucose intolerance, and together with the expense and side-effects of antihyperglycemic therapy, the requirement for more extensive treatment might not be demonstrated to provide an overall advantage.

Therapeutic Interventions
Medical Nutrition Therapy and Physical Activity
The goals of medical nutrition therapy in the management of type 2 diabetes are aimed at attaining and maintaining optimal metabolic targets, improving health, and preventing the development of progression of chronic complication and comorbidities of diabetes in an individualized manner (275). Key dietary issues are management of carbohydrate intake and, in most patients, initiation and achievement of weight reduction. Dietary fat recommendations are dealt with below in the Dyslipidemia section. With respect to dietary carbohydrate, it is important that the patient understands that it is almost solely the amount and type of carbohydrate ingested that determines the effect of food on blood glucose levels. Thus monitoring the total amount of carbohydrate consumed whether by food exchanges or by carbohydrate counting remains a key strategy in achieving glycemic control. This does not mean that carbohydrate intake should be low but rather that antihyperglycemic therapy be matched to carbohydrate intake in an individualized manner. It is recommended that carbohydrate calories comprise 45% to 65% of total calories, and there is some evidence that less refined carbohydrate, which has a richer content of fiber and a lower glycemic index, induces less postprandial hyperglycemia (276).

Moderate weight loss improves glycemic control, reduces CVD risk, and can prevent the development of type 2 diabetes in those with prediabetes. Therefore, weight loss is an important therapeutic strategy in all overweight or obese individuals who have type 2 diabetes or are at risk for developing diabetes. The primary approach for achieving weight loss, in the vast majority of cases, is medical nutrition therapy, which includes a reduction in energy intake and an increase in physical activity, both of which are more likely to be facilitated in the setting of a behavior modification program. A moderate decrease in caloric balance (500–1000 kcal/day) will result in a slow but progressive weight loss (1–2 lb/wk). For most patients, weight loss diets should supply at least 1000 to 1200 kcal/day for women and 1200 to 1600 kcal/day for men, and very low calorie diets are not recommended for the most part. A low-fat diet is the conventional approach to initiating weight reduction because these have shown long-term success (277). However, as discussed further below, there is a recent interest in the use of low-carbohydrate hypocaloric diets, and in the short term they may result in greater weight loss and better glycemic control than conventional weight reducing diets (278). Additional research is needed to clarify the long-term efficacy and safety of low-carbohydrate diets, particularly in patients with diabetes. Physical activity is an important component of a comprehensive weight management program (276). Regular, moderate intensity, physical activity enhances long-term weight maintenance. Regular activity also improves insulin sensitivity, glycemic control, and selected risk factors for CVD (i.e., hypertension and dyslipidemia), and increased aerobic fitness decreases the risk of CHD. Initial physical activity recommendations should be modest, based on the patient's willingness and ability, gradually increasing the duration and frequency to 30 to 45 minutes of moderate aerobic activity three to five days per week, when possible (279). Greater activity levels of at least one hour per day of moderate (walking) or 30 min/day of vigorous (jogging) activity may be needed to achieve successful long-term weight loss; however exercise testing should be performed at the discretion of the primary care physician before vigorous exercise, particularly in patients with diabetes.

The role of weight loss medications and bariatric surgery in the management of obesity in diabetes has not been well defined. While there is clinical trial evidence showing that the two currently available prescription medications with an indication for weight reduction, sibutramine and orlistat plus dietary recommendations do increase weight loss, reduce GHb, and improve lipids in subjects with type 2 diabetes compared to placebo and diet (280,281) the question as to whether or when patients should receive these medications long term given their side effects, expense and unproven benefit except in short-term studies, is unknown. Similarly while bariatric surgery is reported to lead to withdrawal of antihyperglycemic medications in approximately 60% of cases and to reductions of medicines in many others, most of these procedures are performed for reasons other than for management of diabetes (282). However most reports have been uncontrolled or inadequately controlled, and what is needed are long-term controlled clinical trials with the primary objective of assessing whether bariatric surgery is more efficacious, safe, and cost effective in the management of diabetes compared to standard medical therapy.

Approach to the Use of Antihyperglycemic Agents

Suggested approach to management of hyperglycemia:

1. *GHb <7.5% in an untreated patient.* Initiate medical nutrition therapy and home glucose monitoring. Obese subjects not responding adequately to medical nutrition therapy could be considered for weight loss pharmacotherapy with sibutramine or orlistat.
2. *GHb >6.5%/7.0% despite three to six months lifestyle change or GHB >8.0% in an untreated patient* requires oral monotherapy (metformin or a TZD is preferred if available and unless contraindicated).
3. *GHb >6.5%/7.0% despite two to three months of oral monotherapy* or sooner in the case of metformin or secretogogues if the fasting blood glucose is significantly and consistently above the target of 120 mg/dL requires dual oral therapy. Early addition of insulin or exenatide instead of an additional oral agent may be considered.
4. *GHb >6.5%/7.0% < 8.5% despite three months of dual oral monotherapy* requires triple oral therapy. Addition of insulin or exenatide instead of an additional oral agent may be considered.
5. *GHb >8.5% despite dual agent therapy or >6.5%/7.0% despite triple agent therapy* including exenatide treatment requires insulin.
6. *Initial insulin strategy* consists of basal insulin treatment (nonmeal targeted) using either bedtime intermediate-acting insulin (e.g., Neutral Protamine Hagedorn (NPH) or glargine insulin beginning with a relatively small dose (10–20 units) followed by up-titration based on the morning fingerstick blood sugar by medical staff or through the use of a titration algorithm by the patient.
7. If *intermediate-acting insulin is chosen*, dosing may be divided into morning and evening units once up-titration of bedtime insulin reaches 30 to 40 units without achievement of GHb goals.
8. Recognize that the average insulin-requiring patient requires a total of 40 to 100 units of insulin per day.
9. *If despite 100 units of insulin per day glycemic targets are not reached* with persistent hyperglycemia, the patient is considered to be severely insulin resistant and will likely require very high insulin doses. The patient is best managed with a basal–bolus strategy incorporating premeal rapid-acting insulin plus basal insulin. This generally requires the input of a diabetologist or other physician with significant experience in the use of basal–bolus insulin treatment.
10. *If the patient has significant meal-related glucose spiking* this is likely to be due to a significantly depleted meal-related insulin secretory capacity. The patient is best managed with a basal–bolus strategy.

Although a detailed discussion of their pharmacologic properties and clinical decision making in the use, choice, and monitoring of oral and injectable antihyperglycemic agents is beyond the scope of this chapter, some of their key advantages and disadvantages are summarized in the table (Fig. 16).

	Glucose lowering (GHb)	Weight	Hypo-glycemia	Other side effects	Expense
Sulfonylureas	1-1.5%	↑ ↑	Yes	Few	+
Meglitinides	0. 5-1.5%	↑ to ↑ ↑	Yes	Few	++ to +++
Metformin	1-1.5%	-	-	GI, MALA*	++
Acarbose	0.5-1.0%	-	-	GI++	+++
TZDs	0.5-1.5%	↑ ↑	-	Edema, hemodilution	++++
Insulin	Unlimited	↑ ↑	Yes	Edema	++ to +++

*Metformin Associated Lactic Acidosis

FIGURE 16 Characteristics of antihyperglycemic agents.

The principle issues governing their implementation are summarized below. Although there is little formal evidence to support the benefits of home blood glucose monitoring, this reflects the difficulties of designing an appropriate clinical trial. There can be little doubt than in an informed patient, "closing the loop" by assessing the impact of a given antihyperglycemic treatment using home glucose monitoring will enhance the ability to modify existing therapy and hence improve the efficiency of management. To be truly successful, this approach requires the closure of a second loop—that from the patient providing information back to the clinician for further recommendations.

- Oral agents are generally the initial choice after medical nutrition therapy has been given an adequate trial, or in those with presenting with relatively severe hyperglycemia, administered together with medical nutrition therapy.
- After medical nutrition therapy has produced its full effect, each oral agent (sulfonylurea, glitinide, metformin, glucosidase inhibitor, or TZD) will lower the GHb 0.5% to 1.5% in proportion to how high the baseline GHb is. Then either monotherapy or dual therapy with oral agents should be initiated. Addition of oral agents is undertaken as soon as it is clear that current therapy will be inadequate to reach targets (from one to eight weeks). In a minority of cases that have severer degrees of insulin deficiency, perhaps 5% to 10%, typically normal weight subjects of European extraction, oral agents will not be effective, and the decision to change to insulin treatment is taken early on.
- Metformin has taken over from sulfonylurea agents as first choice for antihyperglycemic therapy; sulfonylurea agents, glitinides, TZDs, and glucosidase inhibitors usually constitute second and third choices. Recently pramlintide, which slows gastric emptying, and exenatide, which boosts prandial insulin release through an incretin effect, have become available; both are administered subcutaneously, and their place in therapy is still being evaluated.
- Insulin therapy is typically initiated when combination oral therapy is insufficient to reach glycemic targets. Reasonable arguments have been made to support the continued use of current oral agent therapy when insulin is added, with the case for maintenance of oral agents probably weakest for sulfonylureas and glitinides overall. Insulin therapy is usually initiated at a starting dose of ~0.1 to 0.2 units/kg body weight and is based on two principles:
  - The first is that most type 2 diabetic subjects initiating insulin treatment may be effectively controlled with basal insulin, i.e., one or two shots of NPH or Lente or a single shot of glargine insulin, which has a daylong action. This approach, so-called basal therapy, may be viewed as providing supplementary insulin, widely distributed over the 24-hour period, and having little ability to boost insulin action with meals. The assumption here is that the patient produces enough postprandial insulin, which together with their oral antihyperglycemic medication can deal with postprandial glucose surges.
  - The second principle is that early on in some patients, later in others, a mixed insulin regimen is required, consisting of both long-acting insulin for interprandial and overnight

management of hyperglycemia, and quick-acting insulin to correct postprandial glucose spikes, so-called basal/bolus therapy. This approach is employed when it is clear that postprandial glucose surges are not controlled with basal insulin plus oral agents alone. Rapid-acting analogues (lispro insulin, insulin aspart) mimic physiological meal-related patterns of insulin release better than do regular insulin, but are more expensive. This approach requires up to four shots of insulin daily, typically quick-acting insulin before meals and basal insulin at bedtime or twice daily. In an attempt to simplify basal/bolus therapy premixed combinations of NPH and quick-acting insulin given twice a day provide bolus therapy for at least two of the meals as well as basal coverage in a relatively simple manner. Their major disadvantage is that the fixed nature of the combination limits the ability of this regimen to achieve good glycemic goals in an individualized manner .

■ The eventual insulin dose required to achieve glycemic targets may vary typically from 20 to 100 units per day, but occasionally may exceed 200 units per day. In general insulin-requiring type 2 diabetic subjects tend to be underdosed with insulin for many reasons, and practitioners are urged to refer such patients to an endocrinologist if glycemic targets are not reached within 6 to 12 months.

▦ Case Discussion 1

A 56-year-old obese woman (height 5 ft 4 in., weight 185 lb) who had not seen a doctor for at least five years was admitted to the coronary care unit with an acute coronary syndrome. Her mother had been treated with insulin for many years, and although she was not known to have diabetes, her plasma glucose on admission was found to be 346 mg/dL. There was no other significant history and the physical examination apart from the obesity, and a BP of 135/85 was unremarkable. The hyperglycemia initially was treated with regular insulin according to a sliding scale based on four to six hourly fingerstick glucose measurements, and an 1800 cal ADA diet was prescribed. Following the admission, her fingerstick glucose values varied between 187 and 286 mg/dL during the hospital stay with a total daily insulin requirement of approximately 60 units. No myocardial damage appeared to have been sustained, and she was discharged with a diagnosis of unstable angina, after being shown how to do fingerstick measurements of blood glucose and an otherwise uneventful recuperation, on glyburide 10 mg twice daily and aspirin and atorvastatin 10 mg daily. She was seen in the cardiologist's office several weeks later. Her cardiac status was stable and unchanged, and her only complaint was of tiredness. She had not been testing her blood glucose. Her fasting glucose level was 288 mg/dL, and the GHb result was 8.8%. The LDL-C was 101 mg/dL, triglyceride 165 mg/dL, and the HDL-C was 43 mg/dL. Metformin 500 mg twice daily was added to the antihyperglycemic regimen, the atorvastatin dose was increased to 40 mg, and she was told to reduce her intake of carbohydrate.

She was then referred for further care to a primary care physician. When seen in the office several months later the fasting plasma glucose value was 227 mg/dL, the GHb was 8.4%, and she had gained 5 lb in weight. A diabetologist was consulted. On physical examination bilateral background diabetic retinopathy was identified. No home glucose monitoring results were available. After review, the metformin dose was increased to 1000 mg twice daily together with rosiglitazone 8 mg in a combination tablet. The diabetologist emphasized to the patient the importance of daily home glucose monitoring and the need for weight reduction, referring her to dietician. She returned three months later having gained 5 lb, much to her frustration, but did report that her prebreakfast fingerstick tests had improved to an average of 160 mg/dL range. A two-hour postprandial values in the diabetologist's office were 278 mg/dL. Glargine insulin 15 units in the evening was then added to her treatment regimen.

Commentary.   The finding of undiagnosed hyperglycemia in patients presenting with an acute coronary syndrome is very common. Undoubtedly the severity of the hyperglycemia on admission was aggravated by stress. At that point the cardiac diagnosis was unclear, and a more intensive insulin regimen (e.g., an intravenous insulin drip) should probably have been initiated, because of the evidence that morbidity and mortality are reduced in diabetic subjects admitted with an acute MI. This case illustrates the challenges in reaching recommended glycemic targets, which in many patients is never achieved. In this case treatment was eventually successful when the patient was referred to the diabetologist. However there are not enough diabetologists to provide care to all people with type 2 diabetes, and therefore nondiabetologists need to be more assertive in their efforts. The initial handling of the patient's diabetes prior to discharge from hospital could have been more effective. First the hospitalization offered an opportunity to immediately enroll the patient into a formal diabetes education class, so the nature of the disease, its demands on the patient, and therapeutic strategies and targets are made clear. Second a referral to a dietician to initiate weight reduction while the patient is maximally motivated is more likely to be taken seriously. Third, the severity of hyperglycemia (GHb 8.8%), the ineffective, relatively large insulin dose required during the hospitalization, and the presence of retinopathy all point to fairly long-standing undiagnosed diabetes and the likely need for multiple antihyperglycemic agents and possibly insulin. A minimum requirement for initial pharmacotherapy of the hyperglycemia would be full doses of two agents, with likely requirement of a third agent or insulin. The failure of 60 units of insulin per day to significantly lower the blood glucose in the hospital should have signified to the physician the presence of severe insulin resistance and the likely need for a third drug or insulin at the first assessment visit. It is difficult for even experienced diabetologists to be able to predict how much treatment will eventually be needed to achieve good glycemic targets, and therefore a proactive approach is required. While the threat of hypoglycemia is always to be taken seriously, it should not prevent significant improvement in glycemic control. Pioglitazone may be preferred to rosiglitazone because of the former would lower the mildly elevated triglyceride moderately, and the glyburide could be changed to glimepiride because the latter has less action on myocardial K/ATPase channels and inhibits ischemic preconditioning less. There is also evidence that glucose control in diabetic patients who are not adequately controlled on oral agents will be better if insulin is added to the oral agents than if they are discontinued. In the final analysis while it is unclear how much benefit achievement of good glycemic values has for CVD, there has been no clinical trial assessing this strategy except that performed in subjects with acute MI. The possibility that such treatment might reduce CVD events and the fact that microvascular disease risk is markedly reduced make achievement of glycemic targets mandatory in diabetes. A good general rule is if glycemic targets are not achieved within 6 to 12 months, the patient should be referred to an endocrinologist.

Dyslipidemia

Until recently most of the data indicating benefit of treatment of dyslipidemia in diabetic subjects were derived from post hoc subgroup analyses of four intervention trials using statins. Collectively these trials suggested that the relative cardiovascular benefits of such treatment are similar among diabetic and nondiabetic participants. Recently the results of the Heart Protection Study (HPS) with its large predefined diabetes subgroup and the Collaborative Atorvastatin Diabetes Study (CARDS) trial, which was designed exclusively to test the effect of atorvastatin in diabetic subjects without overt heart disease, were published and added significantly to the robustness of the earlier data. There are fewer studies using fibrates or niacin. All of these studies unequivocally confirm the higher risk of CVD events in diabetic subjects compared to nondiabetic individuals.

Clinical Trial Evidence in Support of Statin Treatment
Scandinavian Simvastatin Survival Study, Cholesterol and Recurrent Events Trial,
Long-Term Intervention with Pravastatin in Ischemic Disease, and Anglo-Scandinavian
Cardiac Outcomes Trial–Lipid-Lowering Arm
In the Scandinavian Simvastatin Survival Study (4S), simvastatin treatment resulted in a 42% reduction in major CHD events (CHD death or nonfatal MI) compared to placebo in the 486 diabetic subjects (both diagnosed and previously undiagnosed) with established CHD and with a baseline LDL-C of 185 mg/dL that were included in the whole cohort of 4444 participants (283). The Cholesterol and Recurrent Events Trial demonstrated a 25% reduction in coronary events with pravastatin compared to placebo among the 586 diabetic participants with preexistent CHD and more typical baseline LDL-C levels (mean value of 136 mg/dL) (284). In the Long-Term Intervention with Pravastatin in Ischemic Disease study, treatment with pravastatin compared to placebo resulted in a 21% reduction in cardiovascular events in the 1077 diabetic subjects with history of CHD and a mean baseline LDL-C of 143 mg/dL (285). Primary prevention trials such as the West of Scotland Coronary Prevention Study and the Air Force/Texas Coronary Atherosclerosis Prevention Study included only a small number of diabetic participants and were thus unable to provide any conclusion on the benefit of lipid-lowering therapy in primary prevention of CVD in diabetic individuals (286,287). Two recent studies in hypertensive patients, the Antihypertensive and Lipid-Lowering Treatment to Prevent Heart Attack Trial (ALLHAT) and the Anglo-Scandinavian Cardiac Outcomes Trial-Lipid-Lowering Arm (ASCOT-LLA), each included a large number of diabetic individuals most of who did not have evident CVD, and did not show significant benefit for statin therapy for the primary outcome, CVD death plus nonfatal MI. The lack of effect in ALLHAT was

probably because the small effect size due to modest statin therapy coupled with "drop-in" statin therapy in the placebo group (↓9% in LDL-C). It has been suggested that there was insufficient power in ASCOT-LLA, although the number of diabetic subjects ($n = 2532$) was very similar to that in CARDS (below), which showed significant beneficial effect (288,289). Event rates were relatively low in ASCOT, perhaps due to effective BP lowering related to the BP-lowering component (see below).

The Heart Protection Study and Collaborative Atorvastatin Diabetes Study

Strong evidence for the beneficial effect of cholesterol lowering with statins in diabetic individuals with and without evidence of CVD and average cholesterol values come from the HPS (291). The effect of 40 mg of simvastatin compared to placebo was evaluated in 14,573 nondiabetic individuals with occlusive vascular disease and in 5963 diabetic individuals; of the subgroup with diabetes, 2912 had no clinical features of CVD. Treatment with simvastatin lowered LDL-C about 25% (~1 mmol/L or 39 mg/dL) and reduced the risk of the first major cardiovascular event by 33% in the diabetic subjects without CVD and by 18% in those with preexisting CVD (no significant difference in effect size in these two groups). These effects appeared to be independent of the age (all subjects were >40 years of age), gender, diabetes duration, type of diabetes, level of glycemic control, triglyceride, and HDL-C levels. Furthermore, the relative benefit of statin therapy in diabetic individuals whose baseline LDL-C was <3.0 mmol/L (<116 mg/dL) at entry was similar to that obtained in those with LDL-C >3.0 mmol/L (27% vs. 20% relative risk reduction in first major CVD event). Indeed, there were sufficient individuals among the combined diabetic and nondiabetic cohorts with baseline LDL-C <2.6 mmol/L (<100 mg/dL) to show that the proportional reduction in CVD event risk in these individuals was similar to that in those with LDL-C >3.5 mmol/L (>130 mg/dL). The investigators concluded that "statin therapy should be considered routinely for diabetic patients at sufficiently high risk of major vascular events, irrespective of their initial cholesterol levels." Many would argue that most diabetic subjects above the age of 40 years fit with this description.

The CARDS was the first statin trial conducted only in diabetic subjects (292). The investigators randomized 2383 individuals [mean age 62 years; mean LDL-C 3.0 mmol/L (118 mg/dL)] with diabetes but no CVD and at least one risk factor (hypertension, smoking, retinopathy and micro or macro-albuminuria) to atorvastatin 10 mg/day versus placebo. Treatment with atorvastatin resulted in a 36% reduction in acute CHD events and a 48% reduction in stroke after a median 3.9 years of follow-up when the study was prematurely ended because of the early positive results. The mean LDL-C in the atorvastatin group had fallen to 78 mg/dL, and the beneficial effect of atorvastatin was similar in subjects with LDL-C above and below 3.1 mmol/L (120 mg/dL) (Tables 1 and 2).

Clinical Trial Evidence in Support of Fibrate Therapy

There have been three clinical intervention trials using fibrate monotherapy that included a subgroup of diabetic individuals and a fourth conducted only in type 2 diabetic subjects (293–296). In the Helsinki Heart Study, gemfibrozil was associated with a 60% reduction in cardiovascular events in the 135 diabetic individuals included in the study but was underpowered to demonstrate a statistical difference (293). In the Bezafibrate Infarction Prevention study, 309 type 2 diabetic subjects with CHD were included among the 3088 participants with mean LDL-C values of 149 mg/dL. Bezafibrate (Table 2) treatment did not significantly reduce events in this study, except in a secondary analysis of a subgroup with triglyceride values >200 mg/dL (294). The Veterans Affairs Cooperative Studies Program High-Density Lipoprotein Cholesterol Intervention Trial (VA HIT) evaluated the effect of gemfibrozil, 1200 mg daily on major CHD events in 2531 men with CHD and low HDL-C without high LDL-C values (295). Twenty-five percent of the participants were diabetic. Treatment with gemfibrozil reduced the risk of CHD death, nonfatal MI, or confirmed stroke by 24% in both the diabetic and nondiabetic subsets. The only lipid measure that predicted the CVD benefit was the small increase in HDL-C on treatment. A recent subgroup analysis including 769 individuals with diagnosed and undiagnosed diabetes (fasting glucose >126 mg/dL) found that gemfibrozil in diabetic subjects resulted in a significant 32% lower risk of the combined end point (CHD death, nonfatal MI, or stroke), a 41% lower risk of CHD death and a 40% risk reduction in stroke compared to placebo (296). The risk reduction in these endpoints among

TABLE 1 Key Features of Clinical Trials Using Statins or Fibrates in Diabetic Subjects

Study	Number of subjects		Intervention	Baseline lipids[a] (mg/dL)		
	Diabetes	Total		LDL-C	HDL-C	TG
Statins						
Primary prevention						
CARDS (292)	2838		Atorvastatin 10 mg	117	54	151
Secondary prevention						
4S[b] (283)	483	4444	Simvastatin 20–40 mg	186	40	153
CARE (284)	586	4159	Pavastatin 40 mg	136	38	164
LIPID (285)	1077	9014	Pravastatin 40 mg	143	33	168
Primary + secondary prevention						
ALLHAT (288)	3635	10357	Pravastatin 40 mg	129	45	154
ASCOT-LLA (289)	2532	10305	Atorvastatin 10 mg	128	47	169
HPS (290)	5963	20536	Simvastatin 40 mg	124	41	203
Fibrates						
Primary prevention						
FIELD (296)	9795		Fenofibrate 200 mg	120	39	172
Secondary prevention						
VA HIT (295)	627	2531	Gemfibrozil 1200 mg	108	31	164
VA HIT[b] (297)	769	2531	Gemfibrozil 1200 mg			

[a]Baseline lipids in the diabetic subgroups except for Scandinavian Simvastatin Survival Study and Antihypertensive and Lipid-Lowering Treatment to Prevent Heart Attack Trial where baseline lipids are given for the treatment group of the entire cohort.
[b]Includes diagnosed and undiagnosed (fasting glucose >126 mg/dL).
Abbreviations: CARDS, Collaborative Atorvastatin Diabetes Study; 4S, Scandinavian Simvastatin Survival Study; CARE, Cholesterol and Recurrent Events; LIPID, Long-Term Intervention with Pravastatin in Ischemic Disease; ALLHAT, Antihypertensive and Lipid-Lowering Treatment to Prevent Heart Attack Trial; ASCOT-LLA, Anglo-Scandinavian Cardiac Outcomes Trial-Lipid-Lowering Arm; HPS, Heart Protection Study; FIELD, Fenofibrate Intervention and Event Lowering in Diabetes; VA-HIT, Veterans Affairs High-Density Lipoprotein Intervention Trial.

those without diabetes was not significant (18%, 3%, and 10%, respectively). These results suggest that fibrates are particularly effective in reducing CHD events and stroke in diabetic subjects with below average LDL-C levels.

The recently reported Fenofibrate Intervention and Event Lowering in Diabetes (FIELD) trial was a multinational randomized controlled trial of fenofibrate versus placebo over five years in 9795 subjects with type 2 diabetes (mean age 62 years; duration five years; GHb 6.9%; 22% having a history of CVD), not on statin therapy and with an LDL-C of 124 mg/dL (3.1 mmol/L), triglyceride 154 mg/dL (1.73 mmol/L), and HDL-C 44 mg/dL (1.1 mmol/L) (296). Although the hazard rate for the primary endpoint of nonfatal MI plus CHD death was reduced by 11%, this did not reach significance due to a nonsignificant increase in the rate of CHD death (19%). However nonfatal MI, a prespecified secondary outcome, was significantly decreased by 24% ($p = 0.01$), as was total CVD events (11%, $p = 0.035$) and coronary revascularization (21%, $p = 0.003$), and interestingly there were less albuminuria progression (2.6%, $p = 0.002$) and less retinopathy needing laser therapy (1.6%, $p = 0.003$) (Fig. 17). Fenofibrate was safe despite a concomitant statin "drop in" rate of 7% in fenofibrate-allocated individuals without CHD, with only a slight increase in subjects with pulmonary embolism (1%) and pancreatitis (0.8%) compared to placebo treatment. This finding suggests that fenofibrate is safe and effective in preventing nonfatal CHD events, but not CHD mortality, which differs from the findings with gemfibrozil, which did reduce CHD death (40%) as well as stroke (41%) in a smaller group of diabetic subjects with more advanced CHD and lower HDL-C levels (31 mg/dL). Either one has to postulate that the two fibrates are very different or that the differences in patient population or perhaps a detracting effect of drop-in statin use in FIELD (14% in the fenofibrate versus 23% in the placebo groups with prior CHD) explained much of the differences in findings. Although there was a minimal increase in elevated serum creatinine levels, participants could not enter the trial if they had an elevated creatinine, because fenofibrate is more likely to raise serum creatinine levels than is gemfibrozil and should be avoided in patients with diabetic nephropathy.

Three studies have evaluated the effect of fibrates on angiographic progression of CHD and demonstrated a beneficial effect of these agents on the vascular wall. One of these, the

TABLE 2 Subgroup Analysis of Cardiovascular Outcomes in Clinical Trials Evaluating Effects of Statins or Fibrates in Diabetes as Compared to Analysis in Nondiabetic Subjects

Study	CVD outcome	% with event Diabetes placebo	Diabetes treatment	RR diabetes (95% CI)	% with event Non-diabetes placebo	Non-diabetes treatment	RR non-diabetes (95% CI)
CARDS (292)	Acute coronary events	5.5	3.6	0.64[a] (0.45–0.91)			
	Stroke	2.8	1.5	0.52[a] (0.31–0.89)			
4S	Total mortality	24.7	14.3	0.57 (0.30–1.08)	10.9	7.9	0.71[a] (0.58–0.87)
	Major CHD event	45.4	22.9	0.45[a] (0.27–0.74)	27.7	19.2	0.68[a] (0.60–0.77)
	Any atherosclerotic event	62.8	43.8	0.63[a] (0.43–0.92)	45.2	35.4	0.74[a] (0.68–0.82)
4S (283)	Total mortality	16.4	12.8	0.79 (0.49–1.27)	10.4[b]	7.7[b]	0.72[a] (0.57–0.90)
	Major CHD event	37.5	23.5	0.58[a] (0.41–0.80)	26.2[b]	18.6[b]	0.68[a] (0.59–0.79)
	Revascularizations	21.1	11.6	0.52[a] (0.32–0.82)	16.6[b]	11.5[b]	0.67[a] (0.55–0.80)
CARE (284)	Major CHD event	20.3	17.7	0.87	11.9	9.1	0.74[a]
	Expanded end-point	36.8	28.7	0.75[a]	24.6	19.6	0.77[a]
LIPID (285)	Major CHD event	23.4	19.6	0.81	14.5	11.3	0.77[a]
	Any cardiovascular event	52.7	45.2	0.79[a]	38.5	34.5	0.87[a]
ALLHAT (288)	Major CHD event			0.89 (0.71–1.10)			0.92 (0.76–1.10)
ASCOT-LLA (289)	Major CHD event	3.0	3.6	0.84 (0.55–1.29)	2.8	1.6	0.56[a] (0.41–0.77)
	Total CV events and procedures	11.9	9.2	0.77[a] (0.61–0.98)	8.7	7.0	0.80[a] (0.68–0.94)
HPS (290)	Major CHD event	12.6	9.4	0.73[a] (0.62–0.85)	8.5	11.5	0.73[a] (0.66–0.81)
	Any major vascular event	25.1	20.2	0.78[a] (0.70–0.87)	25.2	19.6	0.76[a] (0.70–0.81)
FIELD (296)	CHD death	2.0	2.0	1.19 (0.90–1.57)			
	Nonfatal MI	4.0	3.0	0.76[a] (0.62–0.94)			
VA HIT (295)	CHD death, stroke or MI	36.5	28.4	0.76[c] (0.57–1.00)	22.5	17.8	0.76[a] (0.70–0.94)
VA HIT (297)	CHD death, stroke or MI			0.68[a] (0.53–0.88)			0.82 (0.67–1.02)
	Nonfatal MI			0.78			0.79
	CHD death			0.59[a] (0.39–0.91)			0.97
	Stoke			0.60[a] (0.37–0.99)			0.90

Note: RR: relative risk is the hazard ratio (treatment/placebo).
[a]Statistically significant compared to placebo. Major CHD event: CHD death or nonfatal myocardial infarction.
[b]% with event in individuals with normal fasting glucose.
[c]$p = 0.05$.
Abbreviations: CARDS, Collaborative Atorvastatin Diabetes Study; 4S, Scandinavian Simvastatin Survival Study; CARE, Cholesterol and Recurrent Events; LIPID, Long-Term Intervention with Pravastatin in Ischemic Disease; ALLHAT, Antihypertensive and Lipid-Lowering Treatment to Prevent Heart Attack Trial; ASCOT-LLA, Anglo-Scandinavian Cardiac Outcomes Trial-Lipid-Lowering Arm; HPS, Heart Protection Study; FIELD, Fenofibrate Intervention and Event Lowering in Diabetes; VA HIT, Veterans Affairs High-Density Lipoprotein Intervention Trial; CHD, coronary heart disease; MI, myocardial infarction; CVD, cardiovascular disease; RR, risk ration.

Diabetes Atherosclerosis Intervention Study was performed specifically in a diabetic population (298) and tested the effect of fenofibrate compared to placebo on angiographic endpoints in 418 individuals with type 2 diabetes and dyslipidemia. The fenofibrate group showed significantly less angiographic progression than the placebo group, and although the

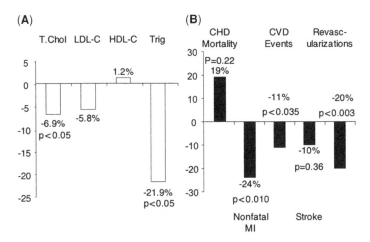

FIGURE 17 Effects of fenofibrate versus placebo treatment in the Fenofibrate Intervention and Event Lowering in Diabetes (FIELD) trial on (**A**) lipids and lipoproteins (**B**) cardiovascular outcomes.

study did not have enough power to identify differences in clinical endpoints, there were fewer cardiovascular events in the fenofibrate compared to the placebo group (18% vs. 23%).

Clinical Trial Evidence in Support the Use of Niacin

The only study that has evaluated the effect of niacin monotherapy on cardiovascular events is the Coronary Drug Project, published in 1975 (299). In this study, 1119 men with a history of MI were allocated to treatment with niacin 1 to 3 g/day, and 2789 participants received placebo. The mean baseline total cholesterol and triglyceride values were 250 and 177 mg/dL, respectively. Despite a lack of benefit on total mortality, the risk of recurrent non-fatal MI was reduced by 27% with niacin. A recent reanalysis showed that the benefit of niacin treatment on recurrent MI was similar in patients at all levels of blood glucose, including those with fasting blood glucose >126 mg/dL (Fig. 18) (300). Evidence for a beneficial effect arising from the addition of niacin therapy to statin treatment was suggested by the HDL Atherosclerosis Treatment Study (HATS) (301). In this trial the effect of combination therapy with simvastatin and niacin compared to placebo on angiographic end points was evaluated in 160 individuals with prior CHD and low HDL-C levels of whom 16% had diabetes. Simvastatin plus niacin resulted in a significant angiographic benefit with actual regression of lesions, an effect that has not clearly been documented with statin therapy alone. Furthermore, despite the small sample size, treatment with niacin plus simvastatin was associated with a significant 60% reduction in cardiovascular events (CHD death, non-fatal MI, stroke, or revascularization for worsening ischemia), which is a numerically greater

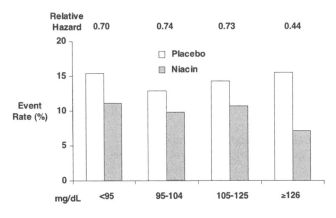

FIGURE 18 Effects of niacin monotherapy treatment versus placebo on cardiovascular events in the coronary drug project by fasting glucose categories.

	NCEP	ADA	IDF
LDL-C	<100	<100	<115
- Optional	<70	<70	
- Minimal lowering	30-40%	30-40%	
Triglyceride	>200	>150	>150
HDL-C	<40	<40 (<50 in women)	<46

FIGURE 19 Targets for lipid modification treatment according to the National Cholesterol Education 1 Panel, the American Diabetes Association and the International Diabetes Federation.

effect than has been demonstrated in monotherapy trials with the exception of the 4S diabetes subgroup.

Therapeutic Guidelines (Fig. 19)
National Cholesterol Education Panel Adult Treatment Panel III Guidelines
In the NCEP ATP III guidelines, diabetes is considered a CHD equivalent; and therefore, the lipid targets for individuals with diabetes are the same as those for individuals with established CHD (27). The primary target is an LDL-C <100 mg/dL. In a recently published update (302) the ATP III panel lowered the cut point for pharmacologic intervention, based in part on the HPS results, from >130 to >100 mg/dL, and in addition provided an optional lower target of 70 mg/dL for very high-risk subjects such as those with diabetes and heart disease. Along with these modifications, ATP III also proposed that if a statin is to be used, a dose that achieves at least 30% to 40% LDL-C lowering should be chosen. These recommendations have recently found support in the results of the Treatment to New Targets Study, which compared the effects of greater LDL-C lowering with atorvastatin 80 mg to atorvastatin 10 mg (mean on-treatment LDL-C 77 mg/dL vs. 101 mg/dL, respectively) in 10,003 subjects with CVD, 15% of whom had diabetes (303).

For individuals with triglyceride levels >200 mg/dL, the secondary lipid target is the non–HDL-C (total cholesterol–HDL-C). Non–HDL-C correlates well with apo B and includes all atherogenic lipoproteins that contain apo B, namely, LDL, Lp(a), intermediate-density lipoprotein, and VLDL. The goal for non–HDL-C is 30 mg/dL higher than the LDL target (<130 mg/dL for diabetic subjects). When triglyceride values are ≥500 mg/dL, the first priority is to lower triglyceride levels because of concerns about the risk of pancreatitis. HDL-C is the third lipid target and HDL-C–raising strategies may be considered in "high-risk" individuals with HDL-C levels <40 mg/dL. However, in the guidelines HDL-C target levels were not established.

American Diabetes Association Guidelines
The desirable LDL-C, HDL-C, and triglyceride levels considered by the ADA are <100 mg/dL, >40 mg/dL in men/>50 mg/dL in women, and <150 mg/dL, respectively (305). The primary treatment strategy as in NCEP is LDL-C lowering to <100 mg/dL. The recommended LDL-C level to start pharmacological therapy is >100 mg/dL in individuals with established CHD and >130 mg/dL in those without CHD. However, the 2005 recommendations now also state that "statin therapy to achieve an LDL-C reduction of ~30% regardless of baseline LDL-C levels may be appropriate." The second lipid strategy is HDL-C raising and the third is triglyceride lowering. However, specific treatment targets were not set. The ADA guidelines also emphasize the importance of glycemic control and lifestyle interventions such as weight loss, exercise and smoking cessation in the management of hypertriglyceridemia, and low HDL-C levels.

European Diabetes Policy Group and International Diabetes Federation
The International Diabetes Federation guidelines specify three categories of risk for each lipid/lipoprotein measure, namely low risk, at risk, and high risk (272). For total cholesterol these are <4.8 mmol/L (185 mg/dL), 4.8 to 6.0 mmol/L (230 mg/dL), and >6.0 mmol/L (>230 mg/dL), for LDL-C <3.0 mmol/L (<115 mg/dL), 3.0 to 4.0 mmol/L (115–155 mg/dL) and

>4.0 mmol/L (>155 mg/dL), for HDL-C >1.2 mmol/L (>46 mg/dL), 1.0 to 1.2 mmol/L (39–46 mg/dL), and <1.0 (<39 mg/dL), and triglyceride <1.7 mmol/L (<150 mg/dL), 1.7 to 2.2 mmol/L (150–200 mg/dL) and >2.2 mmol/L (>200 mg/dL).

Third Joint Task Force of European and Other Societies on Cardiovascular Prevention in Clinical Practice Guidelines

As in NCEP, the Task Force recommends that diabetes be considered a high-risk state, equivalent to established CVD and therefore warranting lower total cholesterol and LDL-C targets, i.e., for total cholesterol a target of <4.5 mmol/L (<175 mg/dL) and for LDL-C <2.5 mmol/L (<100 mg/dL) (274). No specific treatment goals are defined for HDL-C and triglycerides, but an HDL-C of <1.0 mmol/L (40 mg/dL) in men and <1.2 mmol/L (46 mg/dL) in women and a fasting triglyceride of >1.7 mmol/L (>150 mg/dL) serve as markers of risk and additional guides to choice of drug therapy.

Canadian Lipid Working Group on Hypercholesterolemia and Other Dyslipidemias Guidelines

These guidelines also consider diabetes as a CHD risk equivalent and recommend an LDL-C target of <2.5 mmol/L. In addition a total cholesterol/HDL-C ratio of <4.0 is recommended, and an apo B target of <0.9 g/L is suggested as an alternative to the LDL-C, particularly in monitoring statin-treated subjects (305).

Therapeutic Interventions

Lifestyle Modification

Nutrition therapy is essential in the management of diabetic dyslipidema. Both NCEP and ADA guidelines concur in reducing the intake of saturated fatty acids and trans-saturated fatty acids to lower LDL-C levels (27,306). ATP III recommends limiting the intake of saturated fat to less than 7% of the daily calories and the intake of cholesterol to less than 200 mg/day. This diet, also known as the Step 2 diet, has been shown in a meta-analysis to be associated with a 16% LDL-C reduction (307). Additional dietary options to lower LDL-C include increasing the amount of soluble dietary fiber to 10 to 25 g daily, adding 2 g daily of plant stanols/sterols, and including soy protein in the diet. These interventions have been associated with a 5% to 15% reduction in LDL-C values (308–310).

The distribution of macronutrients in the diet is a matter of debate particularly in individuals with diabetic dyslipidemia. Low-fat, high-carbohydrate (>60% of total caloric intake) diets have been associated with an increase in triglyceride and a fall in HDL-C levels (312). When monounsaturated fat is substituted for saturated fat in the diet, the LDL-lowering effect is similar to that obtained with a low-fat, high-carbohydrate diet without the rise in triglyceride and the fall in HDL levels (313). Therefore, ATP III recommends limiting the intake of carbohydrates to less than 60% in individuals with the metabolic syndrome and type 2 diabetes. Furthermore, for individuals with elevated triglyceride and low HDL-C levels, even lower-carbohydrate intake (i.e., 50% of calories) could be considered. The ADA also recommends replacing saturated fat with carbohydrates or monounsaturated fat (306). Low-carbohydrate diets have been used for many years and have recently become even more popular. Although these diets may have short-term beneficial effects on serum lipids, fasting glucose, and weight reduction, these apparent benefits have not been shown to persist over a more lengthy period (314). Furthermore low-carbohydrate diets have not been adequately evaluated in individuals with diabetes and hyperlipidemia and their long-term safety and efficacy remain unknown.

Exercise and pharmacologic approaches to weight loss in overweight individuals with diabetes are also important strategies in the management of atherogenic dyslipidemia. The predominant effect of exercise seems to be on maintaining or achieving weight reduction targets, and its most consistent effect on lipids is to raise HDL-C.

Pharmacologic Interventions

Improved Glycemic Control and Antihyperglycemic Agents. Improved glycemic control regardless of type of treatment is associated with improved lipid values in individuals with moderate to severe hyperglycemia. In the Veterans Affairs Cooperative Study in type II diabetes, intensive glycemic control with insulin therapy, in which hemoglobin A1C was reduced from 9.3% to 7.2%, was associated with a 31% reduction in triglyceride levels after one year, and 23% reduction at two years (315). LDL-C and HDL-C did not change significantly from baseline in the intensive treatment group. As mentioned above treatment with metformin and TZDs has been associated with beneficial effects on lipids. Metformin has been shown to lower triglycerides between 10% and 29% with beneficial changes of lesser magnitude in LDL-C and HDL in some but not all studies (316). Both rosiglitazone and pioglitazone raise HDL-C and LDL-C and increase the size of LDL; pioglitazone, but not rosiglitazone, lowers triglyceride and apo C–III, and rosiglitazone raises non–HDL-C (250).

Pharmacologic Lipid-Modifying Strategies.
LDL LOWERING.   All guidelines give priority to the achievement of LDL-C targets, essentially recommending LDL-lowering therapy with statins for all diabetic subjects with LDL-C levels >100 mg/dL, although the ADA expresses this in terms of a recommendation aimed at achieving at least a 30% to 40% LDL-C lowering at whatever the baseline LDL-C for those without heart disease. In individuals deemed to be at high or very high risk, the NCEP set an optional goal of 70 mg/dL. Because almost 80% of subjects who have diabetes have an LDL-C level more than 100 mg/dL, these proposals and the robustness of clinical trial data support the initiation of lipid-lowering pharmacotherapy with at least a moderate dose of a statin and frequently more treatment in most diabetic subjects. Initiating a statin in patients with a baseline LDL-C <100 mg/dL or lowering the LDL-C target to 70 mg/dL is now considered a reasonable therapeutic decision by the NCEP in patients that are still at very high absolute risk for future CVD events. This would clearly include diabetic subjects with CVD. Other high-risk subgroups among diabetic subjects without CVD are the elderly, especially with multiple additional risk factors, and those with hypertension and renal disease. Unfortunately old age and renal disease are also risk factors for statin side effects. Furthermore, based on the results of the CARDS trial, in subjects (>40 years of age) who have a low LDL cholesterol and who do not have heart disease a case can be made for initiating statin therapy as long as they have at least one major risk factor. A more potent statin is generally chosen to increase the likelihood that optimal lowering of both LDL-C and non–HDL-C (see below) is achieved. When the LDL-C target is not achieved with a statin alone, or where statins are not tolerable, most would recommend combination therapy with ezetimibe, bile acid sequestrants, or relatively high-dose niacin.

One exception to these recommendations is in severely hypertriglyceridemic individuals (>500 mg/dL) where fibrates are more effective than statins in reducing pancreatitis risk. Another possible exception might be those diabetic subjects whose CVD risk is deemed not to be high within the forthcoming decade, such as diabetic subjects under the age of 30 years. While this seems reasonable based on studies in type 1 diabetic subjects (18), there are no data describing risks of CVD in the increasingly important type 2 diabetic subgroup in this age category.

BEYOND LDL LOWERING   Near-routine prescription of a statin for diabetic patients creates a dilemma in regard to the place of fibrates and to a lesser extent of niacin, both of which have demonstrated CVD benefit in monotherapy trials in subjects who had CHD. One option is to use these agents in combination with statins. However, these drugs may interact with statins occasionally causing serious complications, and there is no available evidence in the case of fibrates that combination therapy adds further benefit over monotherapy so it is difficult to justify using these combinations routinely. On the other hand it should be remembered that the risk of CVD in diabetic subjects is increased two- to fourfold that in nondiabetic subjects. In comparison, statin trials typically demonstrate a 30% risk reduction, which means that despite adequate statin therapy, many diabetic subjects remain at significantly increased risk for CVD, and in them a reasonable case can be made for combination therapy. Furthermore the fact that statins, fibrates, and niacin have differing effects on lipoproteins, that the beneficial effect on CVD of gemfibrozil was found to be independent of LDL-C, and that niacin has a much more robust HDL-raising effect than statins do makes it likely that their effects are additive.

Non–HDL-C is the focus of the secondary therapeutic strategy proposed by ATP III in the management of dyslipidemia once the LDL-C goal is achieved and when triglyceride levels are ≥200 mg/dL. The ADA guidelines recommend lowering triglyceride levels presumably to low-risk targets i.e. <150 mg/dL but it is not known to this point whether prospective lowering of non–HDL-C or of triglyceride levels per se leads to added CVD benefit. Although gemfibrozil lowered triglyceride levels significantly in the VA HIT in the absence of a change in LDL-C, this did not correlate with the CVD benefit (317). Fibrates lower non–HDL-C in hypertriglyceridemic subjects and may therefore help reach the non–HDL-C target. Statins are the most effective agents for the lowering of non–HDL-C levels because in addition to lowering LDL-C, they also reduce VLDL- and IDL-C, probably by enhancing their removal rates via the LDL receptor. It has been suggested that at high doses, statins may reduce VLDL secretion as well (318). Therefore, even if LDL-C are at target levels on statin therapy, increasing the dose of statin or switching to a more potent statin would achieve greater non–HDL-C and triglyceride lowering and help achieve secondary lipid-lowering goals. Furthermore, if significant triglyceride lowering is achieved with high-dose statins, there is evidence that an increase in LDL particle size may be achieved (319). In addition, treatment with statins also results in a greater reduction of the total number of LDL particles and apo B concentration than other agents. It is being argued that apo B may be a better marker of dyslipidemia than non–HDL-C (320,321); in either case, statin therapy would appear to be a first choice in pharmacotherapy.

On the other hand, clinical data to support the use of fibrates in diabetic patients with prior CAD and dyslipidemia without elevated LDL-C come from the VA HIT showing a significant risk reduction in CAD events with gemfibrozil in subjects whose mean LDL-C level was <130 mg/dL and mean triglyceride values were <200 mg/dL and that this effect seems to be connected with the presence of diabetes and insulin resistance (297). On this basis NCEP ATP III recommends the use of a fibrate or niacin to lower non–HDL-C if triglyceride levels are ≥200 mg/dL and the LDL-C is less than 100mg/dL. Fibrate therapy might be preferred in individual patients with significantly elevated triglyceride, e.g., >350 mg/dL and at-goal LDL-C values. The use of high-dose omega-3 fatty acids (3–8 g/day) is another intervention that has shown to lower triglyceride levels by 15% to 30% in diabetic subjects in short-term studies without adverse effects on GHb or HDL-C and only a slight increase in LDL-C values, and the availability of omega-3 concentrates improves the tolerability of this treatment (322,323). However there is as yet no evidence that high-dose omega-3 fat reduces CVD. There is however clinical trial evidence to show that low-dose omega-3 fat (0.3–1.0 g/day) reduces CVD mortality in populations with CVD, although there are no specific data in diabetes (324).

Combination Therapy. The strategy underlying the addition of a second or third agent is to optimize improvements in the lipid profile achieved by initial (usually statin) therapy. In terms of the NCEP and ADA guidelines this means lowering LDL-C to <100 mg/dL, reducing non–HDL-C values to <130 mg/dL, and/or according to ADA, reducing triglyceride values to <150 mg/dL and raising HDL-C levels to >40 mg/dL (or >46–50 mg/dL in women). This strategy is based on the empirical assumption that further improvement in the lipid profile beyond that initially achieved will yield additional CVD benefit. However there are as yet no controlled trials with clinical outcomes. Recently a trial of add-on extended-release niacin 1000 mg daily versus placebo in statin-treated subjects with CVD revealed a lack of progression of carotid intimal-medial thickness in the niacin group as compared to the placebo group in which significant progression of carotid intimal-medial thickness was observed (325). It has been clearly shown that the addition of ezetimibe to a statin will lower LDL-C to goal in more individuals than a statin alone will do (326). Ezetimibe an intestinal inhibitor of cholesterol absorption has been associated with an additional 15% to 20% reduction in LDL-C levels in individuals with hypercholesterolemia and is well tolerated. Bile acid sequestrants may also help lower LDL-C but should be used with caution as they have a triglyceride-raising effect in hypertriglyceridemic subjects (327).

It is also clear that achievement of all three lipid goals is more likely with statin + fibrate or statin + niacin combinations (Fig. 20) (328,329). However the added complexity and risks of combination therapy in the absence of persuasive clinical trial evidence for additional CVD benefit should place some limitations on the use of these combinations. The presence of CVD should clearly be an indication, and in those without evident CVD it would seem appropriate for subjects above the age of 40 years and/or with another major CVD risk factor, such as hypertension. The presence of renal disease is a relative contraindication to statin–fibrate combinations.

Statin–Niacin Combination Therapy. The addition of niacin to statin therapy has significant lipid-modifying benefit because niacin lowers triglycerides by 20% to 50%, reduces LDL-C by 5% to 25%, raises HDL-C by 15% to 35%, and will lower non–HDL-C moderately. Thus addition of niacin to a statin may be helpful in achieving LDL-C and non–HDL-C goals. Niacin increases

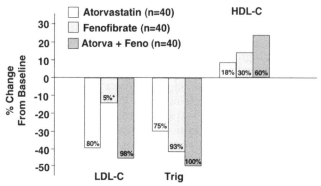

FIGURE 20 Effects of treatment with atorvastatin and fenofibrate alone and in combination on lipids and lipoproteins in type 2 diabetic subjects.

* Proportion meeting ADA LDL-C and desirable triglyceride and HDL-C goals

HDL-C to a greater extent than any other agent. Although pharmacological agents that affect HDL-C values also have effects on other lipoproteins, making it difficult to tease out what the benefits of raising HDL-C are, the VA HIT and HATS studies are supportive of this strategy (301,317) and a European Consensus Panel has supported this approach in subjects with diabetes (330). At high doses, niacin can lower lipoprotein Lp(a) up to 30% (331). Treatment with niacin also results in a shift in LDL and HDL particle density from small dense to larger, more buoyant particles (332). However niacin has significant adverse effects. Hepatotoxicity is the most important of these, particularly with "long-acting" or "sustained release" niacin preparations using doses >2000 mg daily. The extended-release once-a-day preparation of niacin (Niaspan) has been found to be effective and safe with a low incidence of hepatotoxicity. Myopathy has been reported with the combined use of niacin and lovastatin, but has not been described in studies of Niaspan and lovastatin in a single tablet formulation. The incidence of myopathy associated with the combination of niacin and statins appears to be significantly lower than with statins and gemfibrozil (333). Past use of niacin in diabetic patients has been limited because of concerns that this agent may lead to deterioration in glucose control. Recent studies have shown only modest increases in GHb values in fairly well-controlled diabetic patients receiving up to 3000 mg of immediate-release niacin (334) and up to 1500 mg of Niaspan (335). Nevertheless care should be exercised when using this agent in diabetic subjects, and it is probably unwise to increase the niacin dose above 1000 mg daily if the GHb level is >8.0%. In addition to these safety concerns, niacin may not be well tolerated by a significant proportion of patients, particularly at higher doses. However doses as low as 1000 mg/day may have moderate HDL-C raising effects (336).

Suggested Approach to the Management of Dyslipidemia

1. *The recommended diet* should contain <10% of calories as saturated fat and <200 mg cholesterol/day with <1% trans fats and unrefined carbohydrates, are preferred. Plant sterols and eating fish are recommended. The overweight patient should be on a hypocaloric diet. Obese subjects not responding adequately to medical nutrition therapy could be considered for weight loss pharmacotherapy with sibutramine or orlistat.
2. *If the triglyceride level is ≥400 mg/dL* , initiate pharmacotherapy with a fibrate. If the triglyceride level remains >400 to 500 mg/dL add high-dose fish oil (≥3 g of omega-3 fat/day) or and niacin (≥1500 mg/day—caution is required with higher doses in subjects with poor glycemic control).
3. *If the triglyceride level is <400 mg/dL, initiate statin therapy* irrespective of baseline LDL-C, with an initial objective to achieve 30% to 40% LDL-C lowering in the average patient (maximum dose lovastatin, pravastatin, or fluvastatin, or matching doses of more potent statins).
4. *The initial LDL-C target should be <100 mg/dL for subjects with an LDL-C >130 mg/dL*; in subjects with LDL-C >160 mg, greater degrees of LDL-C lowering than 30% to 40% may be required using either high doses of the more potent statins or the addition of ezetimibe.
5. *A lower LDL-C target of 70 mg/dL* should be considered in very high-risk subjects, such as those with CVD, or with multiple, inadequately controlled CVD risk factors, e.g., hypertension, smoking, albuminuria, and advancing retinopathy. This will usually require high-dose potent statins often with added ezetemibe. Add-on bile sequestrants, e.g.,

colesevelam, or high-dose niacin may be needed (especially in patients who do not tolerate statins generally or at high doses).

6. *Once the LDL-C is at goal, if the triglyceride level is ≥200 mg/dL*, reduce the non–HDL-C (total cholesterol—HDL-C) to <130 mg/day (<100 mg/dL in very high-risk subjects) either by up-titration of statins, addition of secondary LDL-C–lowering agents, and/or addition of fibrates and/or niacin (>1000 mg/day).

7. *If HDL-C is <50 mg/dL in women or <40 mg/dL in men* in subjects at the LDL-C and non–HDL-C goals, consider adding a fibrate or niacin (1000 mg/day is the minimal effective dose). This is especially recommended in very high-risk patients.

Statin–Fibrate Combination Therapy. The addition of a fibrate to statin treatment has been shown to achieve ADA goals in most diabetic subjects administered the combination (337). However combination treatment with a statin and a fibrate should be used with caution, as the risk of myopathy is increased, particularly in individuals with predisposing conditions such as renal failure (338). Myopathy and rhabdomyolysis have been reported with simvastatin, cerivastatin, lovastatin, and atorvastatin in combination with gemfibrozil (339–341). However, several short-to-medium-term studies (*n* = 81–420 subjects) evaluating the efficacy and safety of different statin–fibrate combinations in patients with combined hyperlipidemia have shown a very low incidence of clinically significant myopathy and no cases of rhabdomyolysis (342–345). Additionally, gemfibrozil and fenofibrate differ in their effects on statin pharmacokinetics. Gemfibrozil has been shown to significantly inhibit the glucuronidation of statins, an important but previously unrecognized metabolic pathway of statin catabolism, whereas fenofibrate has little effect (346,347). This probably explains why plasma statin levels are significantly increased with gemfibrozil treatment and not with fenofibrate. In addition analysis of national databases in the United States found fewer case of rhabdomyolysis associated with fenofibrate compared to gemfibrozil therapy in combination with statin treatment (348). Fenofibrate has thus been preferred to gemfibrozil for use in combination therapy with statins, but not in the presence of renal insufficiency (349).

■ Case Discussion 2

An obese 45-year-old male office worker (height 5 ft 9 in. and weight 255 lb) was admitted to the intensive care unit with an acute abdomen, vomiting, and severe hypovolemia. He had been feeling well until a recent family gathering, but had begun to develop abdominal symptoms the day after. Work up revealed the presence of pancreatitis. He was given analgesia and intravenous fluids, and no oral intake was permitted, and over a week his symptoms improved. His initial fasting chemistry results also indicated hyperglycemia and severe hypertriglyceridemia. He gave no history of either condition, although he had a strong family history of diabetes on the maternal side, and elevated cholesterol and CHD in his father, grandfather, and paternal uncle. He had a five-year history of hypertension, which was treated with amlodipine 10 mg daily. The fasting glucose was 339 mg/dL, triglyceride 4870 mg/dL, and cholesterol 546 mg/dL. He was started on a sliding scale of regular insulin as per four hourly fingerstick testing of blood glucose, and he received a total of approximately 55 units/day with blood glucose values varying between 178 and 276 mg/dL at this time. After one week of nothing by mouth, a repeat triglyceride level was 1700 mg/dL. Oral intake was then gradually recommenced and a low saturated fat diet prescribed; diabetes education and dietary teaching were commenced, and treatment with gemfibrozil 600 mg and metformin 500 mg each twice daily was initiated, following which he was discharged back to his primary care physician. When seen in the office a month later, he was without abdominal pain. A left-sided carotid bruit was heard and subsequent carotid ultrasound demonstrated a 40% stenosis on that side. Home glucose monitoring revealed that prebreakfast values ranged between 230 and 300 mg/dL. The fasting glucose was 285, the GHb 9.2%, the triglyceride 742 mg/dL, the total cholesterol 298 mg/dL, and the HDL-C was 32 mg/dL. A combination medication consisting of metformin 1000 mg twice daily and pioglitazone 15 mg twice daily was prescribed, and later when glycemic control was not found to be at targets, glipizide 10 mg was added in a slow-release preparation. On this regimen his GHb was lowered to 7.2%. At this time the fasting triglyceride was 338, the LDL-C, 165 mg/dL, and the HDL-C was 36 mg/dL. Simvastatin 40 mg in the evening was added and on follow-up testing the triglyceride level was 289 mg/dL, the LDL-C was 121 mg/dL, and the HDL-C, 38 mg/dL. The primary care physician was pleased with the results despite the fact that the patient had gained a few pounds. He was referred back to the dietician.

Commentary. This patient likely has the genetic lipid disorder known as familial combined hyperlipidemia, based on the facts that after control of his hyperglycemia, he is seen to consistently demonstrate a combined pattern of hyperlipidemia; there is a family history of hyperlipidemia and CHD on his father's side; and he has diabetes. Insulin resistance is a feature of familial combined hyperlipidemia, although he probably inherited a type 2 diabetes trait as well from his mother. His hyperlipidemia was exacerbated by worsened glycemic control, excessive food, and alcohol intake, on a background of obesity and sedentary living, into severe hypertriglyceridemia and pancreatitis. The management of his diabetes and hyperlipidemia in hospital and the final lipid profile achieved as an outpatient could be significantly improved. First, the evidence that intensive insulinization improves outcomes in intensive care unit patients is strong. This would have rapidly removed the effect of hyperglycemia. Second, the reinstituted diet should have been hypocaloric and restricted in all fat groups, because of the chylomicronemia that continued to be present with the recommencement of oral feeding; triglyceride values >1000 mg/dL indicate persistent chylomicronemia and restriction of all fats, not just saturated fat, are required for reduction of chylomicron formation. Third, it is preferable to initiate treatment with fenofibrate rather than gemfibrozil, because in the event that statins are to be added, as indeed was the case, this fibrate is safer in combination than gemfibrozil. Fourth, the most potent statins should have been utilized, namely atorvastatin or rosuvastatin, because at least 40% LDL-C lowering would be required to reach an LDL-C goal of <100 mg/dL, and simvastatin 40 mg is unlikely to achieve this amount of LDL-C lowering, especially in hypertriglyceridemic subjects where the LDL-C–lowering effect of statins is reduced. There is a strong possibility that a second-line LDL-C–lowering agent such as ezetemibe would be necessary to reach a target well below 100 mg/dL, which could be argued would be important in him with his multiple risk factors, asymptomatic carotid stenosis, and strongly positive family history. Furthermore high-dose atorvastatin or rosuvastatin therapy has a greater triglyceride-lowering effect than simvastatin. If his HDL-C remains at the current level, extended-release niacin 1000 mg at bedtime would likely be tolerable, and could increase his HDL-C by up to 20% while being unlikely to adversely affect glycemic control. Multiple lipid-modifying pharmacotherapies coupled with excellent glycemic control and lifestyle change are likely to significantly reduce his risk for CVD.

Hypertension

Modern Clinical Trials Demonstrating That Antihypertensive Agents Reduce Cardiovascular Disease in Diabetes

Earlier clinical trials in the 1990s were focused mostly at determining whether newer antihypertensive agents were effective in preventing CVD compared to prior standard antihypertensive in the 1980s diabetic subjects. All of these trials were conducted in large populations where those with diabetes were usually predefined subgroups for analysis and all began with the specific antihypertensive agent as the initial intervention, but inevitably many individuals would require second and third agents to achieve targets. Thus one may only conclude from these studies that any significant effect on CVD was due to antihypertensive regimens in which the targeted agent was the primary drug. The drugs tested included the thiazide, chlorthalidone (350), the dihydropyridine CCBs, felodipine (351) and nitrendipine (352), and the ACEI, ramipril (353). The Systolic Hypertension in the Elderly (SHEP) study was the first to demonstrate that treatment of isolated systolic hypertension was beneficial. In SHEP, 583 type 2 diabetic subjects >60 years of age with isolated systolic hypertension (>160/<90 mmHg) out of a total of 4736 study participants were randomized to active treatment, receiving clorthalidone 12.5 to 25.0 mg/day, to which could be added atenolol and then reserpine, or to usual care by their physicians (350). Both the nondiabetic and diabetic subjects in the active treatment group had a 34% lower rate of CVD, although as is typical in intervention trials in diabetic subjects, the absolute risk reduction in diabetic subjects was twice that in nondiabetic group because of the higher absolute rate of CVD events in subjects with diabetes. In a similarly designed study, the Systolic Hypertension in Europe Trial, 492 subjects with type 2 diabetes >60 years of age and with BP 160 to 219/<95 mmHg who were randomized either to the CCB nitrendipine (10–40 mg/day) or placebo, with add-on enalapril or hydrochlorthiazide (351). Active treatment for the entire study population (*n* = 4695) was found to reduce overall mortality by 55%, and CVD mortality by 76%, while in the diabetes subgroup, active treatment reduced all CVD events combined by 62%, fatal and nonfatal strokes by 69%, and all cardiac events combined by 57%. In the group of patients receiving active treatment, reductions in overall mortality and CVD mortality and events were significantly larger among the diabetic patients than among the nondiabetic patients.

The large HOPE study randomized 9541 participants >55 years of age who had either CVD or diabetes plus at least one CVD risk factor, to ramipril 10 mg/day versus placebo (with a separate randomization to 400 IU vitamin E or placebo, which showed no difference for CVD outcomes). In the diabetes substudy, there were 3577 subjects of whom 56% had hypertension (group mean BP 140/80) and 60% had CVD (329). Ramipril lowered the risk of the combined primary outcome by 25%, MI by 22%, stroke by 33%, CVD death by 37%, total mortality by 24% (Fig. 21), revascularisation by 17%, and overt nephropathy by 24%. Clinical trials evaluating the effects of antihypertensive agents on CVD do not always show a significant benefit for reduction in the rate of MI. The HOPE trial was the first study to demonstrate this in diabetic subjects. After adjustment for the changes in systolic (2.4 mmHg) and diastolic (1.0 mmHg) BPs, ramipril still lowered the risk of the combined primary outcome by 25% and it was felt that the benefit obtained could not be adequately explained by the modest degree of BP lowering. This led to the proposal that diabetic subjects >55 years of age with CVD or at least one CVD risk factor should receive ramipril treatment (or an ACEI) irrespective of whether they had hypertension or not. In point of fact, the HOPE trial did not require participants to be hypertensive, and therefore strictly does not qualify as a hypertension intervention study. However the study has been interpreted to indicate that inhibition of the renin–angiotensin system in high-risk subjects is cardioprotective, a conclusion that is supported by the Losartan Intervention For Endpoint reduction (LIFE) trial (see below). However there are several caveats to this interpretation. First, all of the benefit could be explained by the highest-risk subjects, i.e., those with CVD. This leaves less clear the issue as to whether diabetic subjects without CVD should qualify for routine ACEI therapy. Second, it was noted in a small substudy of ambulatory blood pressure (ABP) lowering in HOPE participants, that because the ramipril was given in the evening, there was thus substantial reduction of overnight ABP (17/8 mmHg) but less of a reduction in the daytime (6/2 mmHg = nonsignificant), which is when the outpatient BP measurements in the main study were taken (354). Thus the benefit may be completely explained by BP lowering, rather than some direct vasculoprotective hypothesis. Furthermore as discussed below [see Hypertension Optimal Treatment (HOT) trial], as the mean BP of the group was 140/80, more than 50% of subjects would have systolic hypertension by current ADA guidelines, and thus would be expected to benefit from BP lowering, so there is no need to postulate a special effect of ramipril or ACEIs on CVD prevention based on this study.

Clinical Trials Comparing the Cardiovascular Benefits of Different Antihypertensive Agents (Table 3)

The UKPDS is still the only long-term BP-lowering study conducted solely in diabetic subjects and was the first to compare two different antihypertensive regimens (355). The trial compared more intensive antihypertensive treatment ($n = 758$) using either atenolol or captopril to more conventional treatment with older antihypertensive drugs ($n = 390$), in newly diagnosed (mean age 56 years) type 2 diabetic subjects with a mean BP of 160/94 mmHg. The intensively treated group achieved a mean BP of 144/82 and showed a significant reduction in stroke (44%), in diabetes-related deaths (32%) and in retinopathy, but not in MI, compared to the conventional group (mean achieved BP 154/87). There was no difference in any endpoint between the ACEI and the beta-blocker, supporting the concept that the primary benefit was due to BP lowering and not the specific effect of one or other agent (356). A similar result was observed in the STOP 2 trial (357), but an advantage for ACEI over diuretics or beta blockers was found

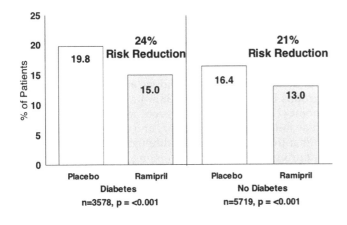

FIGURE 21 Effects of ramipril treatment versus placebo on cardiovascular events among diabetic and nondiabetic subjects in the HOPE trial.

TABLE 3 Summary of Recent Major Trials of Active Intervention with Specific Antihypertensive Agents and of Trials Demonstrating Significant Differences Between Compared Regimens, in Which Subgroup Analyses for Diabetes Were Performed

Study	Primary or comparative drugs	N-diabetes/ total group	Baseline BP	BP in comparison group	BP in active study group	Out-come	Relative risk reduction (%)
SHEP (350)	Chlorthalidone	583/4736	~170/76	Diff was 10/2	SBP ~155 vs. 145	CVD events	44[S]
						Stroke	22[NS]
						MI and CHD death	56[S]
SYS EUR (352)	Nitrendipine	446/4695	175/85	~161/82	~153/78	CVD events	62[a]
						Stroke	69[b]
						Cardiac	57
HOT (351)	Felodipine	1501/18,790	170/95	#DBP = 85	#DBP = 81	CVD events	RR = 2.06[S]
						MI	RR = 2.0[S]
						Stroke	RR = 1.43[NS]
HOPE (353)	Ramipril	3577/9541	~142/80	~142/77	140/77	Combined	25[a]
						MI	22[a]
						Stroke	33[a]
UKPDS (355)	Intensive vs. conventional	1148	160/94	154/87	144/82	Stroke MI	44
LIFE (364)	Losartan vs. atenolol	1195/7998	177/96	146/79	148/79	Combined	24[S]
						MI	17[NS]
						Heart failure	41[S]
ASCOT (366)	Amlodipine + perindopril vs. thiazide + atenolol	5145/19,257	164/95	138/79	136/77	CVD events	13[S]

[a] $p < 0.01$.
[b] $p < 0.05$.
Abbreviations: SHEP, Systolic Hypertension in the Elderly; SYS EUR, Systolic Hypertension in Europe; HOT, Hypertension Optimal Treatment; HOPE, Heart Outcome Prevention Evaluation; UKPDS, United Kingdom Prospective Diabetes Study; LIFE, Losartan Intervention For Endpoint reduction; ASCOT, Anglo-Scandinavian Cardiac Outcomes Trial; BP, blood pressure; CHD, coronary heart disease; MI, myocardial infarction; CVD, cardiovascular disease; NS, not significant; S, significant.

in the Captopril Prevention Project Trial for cardiovascular mortality but not stroke (358) and ACEI were found to lead to a lower CVD event rate in elderly men compared to diuretics in a family practice based clinical trial in Australia (359).

The ALLHAT was by far the largest clinical trial comparing antihypertensive treatments, and among the 31,512 randomized subjects with hypertension plus one other CVD risk factor were 13,101 subjects with diabetes (360). Their mean age was 67 years, 36% had prior CVD, their mean baseline BP was 147/83 mmHg, and they were randomized originally to chlorthalidone, lisinopril, amlodipine, and doxazocin. Previous studies with small numbers of diabetic subjects, underpowered to detect changes in CVD outcomes, had suggested that ACEI therapy reduced CVD events more than did dihydropyridine CCBs or diuretics (361,362). There was no superiority of either lisinopril or amlodipine over chlorthalidone either in BP lowering (mean last visit BP varied in the three groups between 133 and 138/74 and 76 mmHg) or in the primary combined CHD event endpoint (22.6–23.8% six-year event rate). Chlorthalidone appeared to be associated with less cardiac failure than amlodipine, and fewer strokes, coronary revascularizations, and cases of angina than was lisinopril, although the BP was somewhat less effectively reduced in the lisinopril group, particularly among African Americans. The alpha-blocker doxazosin was discontinued early mainly because of an increased prevalence of heart failure in that group (363). The investigators thus concluded that thiazide-type diuretics should be strongly considered as first-step agents for therapy in patients with hypertension and diabetes because they are efficacious, have been evaluated in many trials, and are the least expensive medications to prescribe.

In contrast to the UKPDS findings of no differences in outcomes comparing an ACEI with atenolol, the more recent LIFE trial (364) demonstrated that the ARB losartan, led to a significantly reduced CVD morbidity and mortality in comparison to atenolol among the subgroup with diabetes despite similar improvements in BP in the two treatment groups (mean last visit BP in the losartan and atenolol groups were 146/79 and 148/79 mmHg, respectively). This study randomized 1195 type 2 diabetic subjects (mean age 67 years) with hypertension (mean BP 177/96) and ECG evidence of left ventricular hypertrophy (35% had established vascular disease) out of a total of 9193 study participants, to either losartan- or atenolol-based treatment, followed by thiazide treatment and then other agents. First cardiovascular deaths, MIs and strokes collectively occurred in 103 losartan-treated subjects and 139 atenolol-treated participants, equating to a still very high 39% versus 54% 10-year event rate respectively, and this amounted to a 24% relative risk reduction by losartan—mainly due to stroke reduction. Losartan interestingly was more effective in reducing left ventricular hypertrophy as well as sudden death than atenolol in these patients (365). The investigators proposed that the added benefit of losartan over atenolol could be attributed to its effective inhibition of A-II action on vascular tissue.

In each of these primary antihypertensive agent-based clinical trials, the majority of participants received two or more drugs, especially as guidelines and targets were lowered and this is especially true for diabetes, such that it has been recommended that dual therapy be considered at the onset of treatment so as to reach BP goals more rapidly and effectively. Traditionally the most frequently used combination has been a thiazide plus beta-blocker, but as additional classes of antihypertensive agents were introduced other combinations became possible. The Anglo-Scandinavian Cardiac Outcomes Trial–Blood Pressure–Lowering Arm (ASCOT-BPLA) was the first study to compare a thiazide plus beta-blocker combination to a more "modern" combination, namely a CCB, amlodipine, plus an ACEI, perindopril (366). In ASCOT investigators randomized 19,257 patients with hypertension and at least three CVD risk factors but no established CHD, either to amlodipine 5 to 10 mg adding perindopril 4 to 8 mg as required, or to atenolol 50 to 100 mg adding bendroflumethiazide 1.25 to 2.5 mg and potassium as required. Their mean age was 63 years, mean baseline and close-out BP measurements were 164/95 and 137/78 mmHg respectively, and 27% of the population had type 2 diabetes ($n = 5145$). On average the amlodipine-based treatment group had a lower BP (by 2.7/1.9 mmHg) than the atenolol-based group. Although there was a 10% nonsignificant reduction by the amlodipine-based treatment group in the primary outcome (nonfatal MI and fatal CHD), this group had a significant 23% reduction in stroke, 22% reduction in total CVD events and an 11% reduction in all-cause mortality ($p = 0.025$). Although a detailed report in the subgroup with diabetes has not yet been published, subgroup analysis in those with diabetes demonstrated a significant 13% reduction in total CVD events, having an absolute 10-year rate of 33% versus 39%. As has been noted in previous trials with ACEIs and ARBs alone or versus beta-blockers or thiazides (e.g., HOPE and LIFE) the development of new diabetes in those without diabetes at baseline was significantly reduced in the amlodipine-based treatment group. Whether this advantage in nondiabetic subjects has meaning for treatment of diabetic individuals with A-II inhibitors is not known. In an accompanying paper, the ASCOT investigators argue that the added benefit seen in the amlodipine-based treatment group could not be fully explained by the slightly better BP-lowering effect, and attributed some of the difference to the lower glucose, triglyceride, creatinine levels and body weight, and higher HDL-C and serum potassium values in the amlodipine-based treatment group (367), although others consider the difference to be mainly related to superior BP lowering (368).

Evidence for Additional Benefit Resulting from Treatment to a Lower Target Than 140/90 mmHg

The HOT trial advanced the field significantly, because it was the first study and still the only study to demonstrate that further cardiovascular benefit would derive from treatment to yet lower targets than 140/90 in those with diabetes (351). In this large international study in 18,790 hypertensive individuals (mean age 62 years, mean baseline BP 170/105) of whom 1501 had type 2 diabetes, and 16% had pre-existing CVD, felodipine, a dihydropyridine CCB was used as the primary agent, followed by a stepped algorithm incorporating dose escalation, and addition of an ACEI, beta blocker, and thiazide. The study population was divided into three groups whose diastolic BP targets were respectively set at 90, 85, and 80 mmHg, with attained values of 85, 83, and 81 mmHg, respectively. The group with a diastolic target of 80 mmHg had a significantly reduced risk for cardiovascular death and major CVD events compared to that with a target of 90 mmHg in diabetic subjects, although interestingly there was no such effect noted in the larger nondiabetic cohort. The HOT trial also incorporated a secondary randomization to aspirin (75 mg/day) versus aspirin placebo and found that aspirin significantly reduced CVD events by 15%, with no excess bleeding risk associated with hypertension (Fig. 22).

Therapeutic Guidelines and Interventions
Suggested Approach to the Management of Hypertension

1. *The recommended diet* should include a low salt diet that should be hypocaloric if the subject is overweight. Obese subjects not responding adequately to medical nutrition therapy could be considered for weight loss pharmacotherapy with orlistat; because sibutramine may increase BP, use with caution.
2. *If the BP is >130/80<140/90 mm/Hg,* reassess after three months of medical nutrition therapy. The target is a BP of <130/80 mmHg. In elderly patients with significantly elevated SBP, e.g., with isolated systolic hypertension, BP lowering should be gradual.
3. *If despite medical nutrition therapy, BP is >130/80 mmHg or if >140/90 whether on medical nutrition therapy or not,* initiate pharmacotherapy. Initial dual therapy can be considered in patients with a systolic BP > 150 mmHg.
4. *If albuminuria is present* the initial agent should be an ACEI or an ARB titrated up to maximal doses.
5. *If there is no albuminuria* a diuretic, ACEI, ARB, or a CCB may be used to initiate therapy.
6. *The majority of subjects will require at least two agents.* At least one half of subjects will require >3 agents to achieve the goal.
7. A beta-blocker or alpha/beta-blocker may be added if the pulse rate is >84/min.
8. A centrally acting alpha blocker is usually used if four drugs are insufficient or not adequately tolerated.

    Based on these studies the ADA (304), the Joint National Committee on Prevention, Detection, Evaluation and Treatment of High Blood Pressure (JNC VII) (369), the European Society of Hypertension (370), the National Kidney Foundation (371), and the American College of Physicians (372) all agree that the target BP in diabetic subjects should be <130/<80. While the diastolic target is solidly evidence based as discussed above, the systolic target is less so, although the MRFIT study clearly demonstrated that the CVD risk associated with systolic BP increased curvilinearly above a systolic BP of 120 mmHg among diabetic men (127). As to the initial drug choice, authorities differ. The ADA simply recommends using a drug from a class that has been shown to reduce CVD, but also indicates that all hypertensive diabetic subjects should be on an ACEI or ARB for their additional renoprotective benefit. A recently published

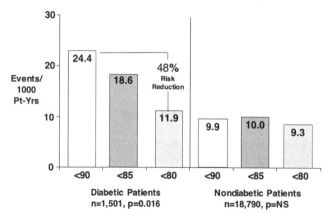

FIGURE 22 Effects on cardiovascular outcomes of treatment of blood pressure to three different diastolic blood pressure targets in diabetic and nondiabetic subjects in the hypertension optimal treatment (HOT) trial.

metaanalysis by the Blood Pressure–Lowering Treatment Trialists Collaboration examined 22 comparative trials in which participants with diabetes could be identified for their relative efficacy in preventing CVD events and concluded that clinicians may reasonably choose from a wide range of BP-lowering agents and that with respect to three to five years CVD outcomes there was no evidence of superiority of any single agent (373). The ADA also recommends against introducing immediate pharmacotherapy for subjects with a BP >130/80 but <140/90, proposing the use of lifestyle/behavioral modification for at least three months first, whereas above a BP of 140/90, drug treatment should coincide with lifestyle approaches. The importance of lifestyle modification especially weight reduction and decreased sodium intake should not be underestimated for its effect not only on BP but also on left ventricular hypertrophy (374). All guidelines emphasize the fact that most diabetic patients require multiple drug therapy, and efficient stepping up of antihypertensive therapy is key to the achievement of BP targets.

Renal Disease

Although not the focus of this review, as pointed out above, progressive renal disease is a major risk factor for CVD in diabetic subjects. To the extent that antihypertensive agents may prevent or delay progression of renal disease, this may add to their cardioprotective effects. Earlier work in type 1 diabetes demonstrated a powerful protective effect of BP lowering on progression of established diabetic nephropathy. Subsequently, that an ACEI was more effective than a beta blocker in this action established ACEIs as the preferred first choice for the treatment of hypertension or microalbuminuria in type 1 diabetic subjects. From these observations and because ACEIs consistently reduce albuminuria, this group of agents had been promoted as the first line antihypertensive agent in all diabetic subjects. The RENAAL study (375) in which the ARB losartan was demonstrated to significantly slow progression of diabetic nephropathy compared to atenolol, is the only long-term study to demonstrate an advantage of any antihypertensive over another on progression of overt nephropathy in type 2 diabetic subjects. All other studies have examined surrogate end-points such as albuminuria, in which ACEIs or ARBs show superiority over agents which do not directly impact the renin-angiotensin system, but which does not necessarily translate into delaying progression of nephropathy (376). The ADA recommends ACEIs and ARBs as first choice for hypertensive subjects with microalbuminuria or with overt renal disease (304).

■ Case Discussion 3

A 65-year-old overweight man presents at the office seeking continuity of care after relocation from another area. He has no complaints and he gives a history of having had a three-vessel coronary artery bypass approximately 7 year prior and soon after the procedure was found to have type 2 diabetes which has been well managed with insulin, metformin, and a TZD, with few insulin reactions. He has had no further cardiac problems except at a recent pharmacy visit when he found his BP to be in the 170 range systolic. His GHb is 7.1%, the LDL-C is between 70 and 80 mg/dL, triglyceride 190 mg/dL, and the HDL-C is 40 mg/dL, maintained on atorvastatin 40 mg plus ezetemibe 10 mg daily. He also has hypertension, apparently well controlled on enalapril 10 mg and hydrochlorothiazide 25 mg in a single tablet combination. He takes a baby aspirin and multiple vitamins including folic acid, flax-seed oil, calcium, and coenzyme Q10. His office BP was 170/92 mmHg and his pulse rate 78/min. He has mild pedal edema, but normal heart sounds, clear lung fields, and a normal abdominal examination. His serum creatinine is 1.5 mg/dL, electrolytes are normal, his urine albumin/creatinine ratio is 56, and he takes aspirin. The physician adds amlodipine 5 mg to his antihypertensive regimen. He returns two months later complaining of severe ankle swelling.

Commentary. This case illustrates the challenges inherent in managing the polypharmacy of multipronged antihyperglycemic and cardiopreventive therapy typical of most subjects with type 2 diabetes. The most compelling issue currently is the patient's hypertension and his worsening ankle edema. He has mainly systolic hypertension with a widened pulse pressure signifying reduced arterial compliance. His pedal edema is likely due to the addition of amlodipine which probably aggravated ankle edema already present; this is a common finding in diabetic subjects treated with combination insulin plus TZD treatment and does not necessarily mean that the patient is developing congestive heart failure, although this possibility must be borne in mind. The thiazide is unlikely to be effective at a serum creatinine level of 1.5 mg/dL and the patient has a reached a range of renal dysfunction where the metformin should be discontinued. Over-rapid reduction in BP in older subjects can interfere with cerebral perfusion and should be embarked on gradually. On the other hand simply increasing the dose of a single antihypertensive is unlikely to lower the BP more than 5 mmHg systolic. The presence of microalbuminuria signifies the likelihood that he has diabetic nephropathy aggravated by hypertension and merits consideration of more aggressive angiotensin-inhibitor treatment, because microalbuminuria is a valid target of therapy. Again, care needs to be exercised in this regard, because increasing the dose of ACEIs or ARBs may aggravate azotemia by decreasing renal perfusion especially in subjects with established renal dysfunction, and induce hyperkalemia particularly in diabetic subjects with hyporenninemic hypoaldosteronism. Some would favor the use of an ACEI with more inhibitory activity against tissue ACE, such as ramipril, perindopril or quinapril, but there is little clinical evidence to support this. An argument can also be made that the ACEI should be replaced by an equivalent dose of an ARB, which has been shown to slow the progression of diabetic nephropathy in contrast to simply slowing the progression of microalbuminuria as has been demonstrated for ACEI therapy. The amlodipine, thiazide, and metformin should be discontinued, and a higher dose of ACEI or ARB should be tried. The presence of a mild tachycardia and wide pulse pressure would also favor addition of a moderate dose of a beta blocker. The patient is asked to purchase his own BP monitor and to call in the results of five consecutive BPs and home blood glucose assessments over the next week to evaluate his response and the need for an increase in the insulin dose. Because fibrates are relatively contraindicated in renal insufficiency, low-dose niacin may be considered. The flax seed oil should be replaced with a fish oil capsule, because there is evidence to support the benefit of fish oil in preventing sudden death, or even better, eating several fish meals per week regularly. The recent report of negative results with folic acid in a controlled clinical trial raises serious questions about the ongoing use of this treatment.

Hypercoagulability

Based on the procoagulant abnormalities described in type 2 diabetes, a logical approach to antithrombotic therapy in diabetes would be targeted at hyperreactive platelets, increased concentrations of coagulation factors and the relatively inhibited fibrinolytic system characteristic of this disease. Although procoagulant predictors of CVD such as fibrinogen and PAI-1 have been demonstrated in epidemiological studies in patients with diabetes as independent predictors of CVD, there is a dearth of well characterized therapeutic interventions available aimed at lowering levels of procoagulant or antifibrinolytic risk factors such as fibrinogen and PAI-1. Lifestyle change has been clearly demonstrated to lower elevated PAI-1 levels and possibly, fibrinogen as well (377). In the case of PAI-1, weight reduction appears to be the most important factor, while treatment of hyperglycemia, especially with metformin or TZDs lowers elevated PAI-levels (378, 379). Weight reduction has less clearly been demonstrated to reduce fibrinogen levels (380); there is evidence that extended periods of exercise will lower fibrinogen, as do certain pharmacologic agents such as pentoxyfillin, ticlodipine, bezafibrate, and fenofibrate (380).

Clinical Trial Evidence in Support of Antiplatelet Therapy

Pharmacotherapy for hypercoagulability has focused mainly on aspirin, well recognized for decades to be a potent inihibitor of platelet aggregability and which has therefore constituted the mainstay of therapy in this area. There have been four trials of aspirin therapy in diabetic subjects involving low, medium, and high doses of aspirin (166,351,381,382). Although aspirin treatment was not always found to produce significant reductions in endpoints, these studies all tended to support the findings from the larger population-based trials that aspirin therapy is effective in reducing CHD and stroke in diabetic subjects. The Antithrombotic Trialists conducted a meta-analysis of published antiplatelet intervention trials (287 studies involving 135,000 high-risk subjects) and reported a mean 34% reduction in nonfatal MI and a 25% reduction in nonfatal stroke (362). From 9 trials with identified diabetic subjects ($n = 5126$) of which most of the subjects came from the Early Treatment of Diabetic Retinopathy Study and in which the majority of patients did not have prior CVD, received 650 mg of aspirin per day, and experienced a significant 28% reduction in MI (382), aspirin therapy was found to reduce vascular events by only 7%, which was not significant. An analysis of the subgroup with diabetes ($n = 1031$) from the Primary Prevention Project (in which 100 mg aspirin per day was associated with a 41% reduction in major CVD events in the entire cohort) also noted only a 10% nonsignificant reduction in relative risk for events (166). Although the study was not powered for significance in the subgroup with diabetes, the investigators suggested that the apparent reduced efficacy of aspirin in diabetic subjects compared to nondiabetic individuals might be due to an increased prevalence of "aspirin resistance" in diabetic subjects. This may result from increased activity of platelet activating pathways in diabetes that do not respond to aspirin, such as increased ADP release from compromised erythrocytes, increased binding of fibrinogen to the GPIIb/IIIa receptor, or increased release of PGG2 and PGH2 from activated macrophages and damaged endothelium which serve as substrates for platelet thromboxane synthesis even in the presence of aspirin-induced platelet cyclo-oxygenase 1 inhibition (384). These pathways will not be affected by higher doses of aspirin, nor did the Antithrombotic Trialists meta-analysis demonstrate any benefit of higher compared to lower doses of aspirin.

Accordingly interest has turned toward alternative antiplatelet agents. The glycoprotein IIb/IIIa inhibitors when used for acute coronary syndromes appear to have the greatest benefit in diabetic patients (385) but are not appropriate for chronic therapy. There has been interest in the use of clopidogrel, an inhibitor of the ADP pathway of platelet activation, either in monotherapy or in combination with aspirin in subjects with diabetes (386). In the Clopidogrel versus Aspirin in Patients at Risk for Ischemic Events (CAPRIE) trial, a post-hoc analysis comparing the responses of the subgroup with diabetes ($n = 3866$) found that the relative risk reduction in the clopidogrel group was 12.6% versus 6.1% in the aspirin group, a significantly greater reduction by clopidogrel, which was similar in relative terms to the result in the nondiabetic cohort and there was no difference in adverse events between the two agents (387). These findings also raised the possibility that combining the two antiplatelet drugs might have additive or synergistic effects. This had already been observed in the setting of unstable angina among the cohort with diabetes ($n = 2840$) in the Clopidogrel in Unstable Angina to Prevent Recurrent Events (CURE) trial, in which acute addition of clopidogrel to aspirin treatment reduced CVD death, nonfatal MI, or stroke by approximately a similar amount as it did in the entire cohort (not quite reaching significance), in which events were decreased by 20% (388). Whether the same advantage for combined antiplatelet therapy pertains in patients without unstable CHD is the topic of an ongoing study, the Clopidogrel for High Atherothrombotic Risk and Ischemic Stabilization, Management, and Avoidance (CHARISMA) trial (389). The fact that platelet aggregation in diabetic subjects on clopidogrel plus aspirin remained greater than in nondiabetic subjects with CHD or that the response to clopidogrel in diabetic subjects is said to be smaller compared to nondiabetic subjects (390), raises the possibility that still further therapies, e.g the thromboxane inhibitor picotamide, with which initial studies appear promising (391), may be required for a multifaceted approach for optimal reduction of hypercoagulability, such as is the case for treatment of hypertension.

Therapeutic Guidelines

The ADA (392) recommends aspirin at a dose of 75 to 162 mg/day as a secondary-prevention strategy in men and women with diabetes and established CVD, and as a primary-prevention strategy in those with increased CVD risk, which would include those over 40 years of age, or who have additional risk factors (family history of CVD, hypertension, smoking, dyslipidemia, or albuminuria). No formal recommendations are made for use of other antiplatelet agents except in individuals with aspirin allergy or a bleeding tendency on aspirin. The American Heart Association and the US Preventive Services Task Force recommend aspirin therapy for diabetic and nondiabetic individuals with a 10 year CHD risk $\geq$10% (393,394).

Smoking Cessation

Although the methods recommended for discontinuation of cigarette smoking are not discussed here, it is of utmost importance that diabetic subjects who smoke should discontinue. If the primary care clinician is unsuccessful in this endeavor, the patient should be referred to a specialist stop-smoking program.

Other CVD Risk Factors

A number of putative and novel CVD risk markers have been identified as possible determinants of CVD in diabetes and some of these may provide an opportunity for intervention, such as heightened inflammatory activity, endothelial dysfunction, hyperhomocysteinemia and elevated Lp(a), and for which therapeutic guidelines have not been developed because of the lack of strong evidence for benefit of interventions.

Inflammation and Endothelial Dysfunction

Although there have been no published formal clinical trials directly testing therapeutic approaches to these abnormalities, lifestyle change, statin and fibrate therapy, and treatment with TZDs have all been shown to reduce markers of inflammation and improve endothelial dysfunction. Whether these effects provide therapeutic benefit beyond the traditionally indicated usefulness of these therapeutic modalities is unknown, although it has been proposed that the benefits of statin therapy are greater in subjects with higher levels of the inflammatory marker high-sensitivity CRP (395), and that in subjects with an acute coronary syndrome, CVD benefits are associated both with the LDL-C–lowering effects and the CRP-lowering effect of statin therapy (396). It is however premature at this time to initiate pharmocotherapy purely on the basis of the finding of an elevated CRP. Furthermore far less is known about the meaning of an elevated CRP in type 2 diabetes than in the general population, and there are many factors contributing to inflammation in diabetes, including obesity, hyperglycemia, atherosclerosis, and insulin resistance, which complicate the design of a treatment rationale directed at increased inflammatory activity. On the other hand, these associations should strengthen and support the incorporation of lifestyle change as a critical therapeutic modality.

Hyperhomocysteinemia

Elevated serum homocysteine levels (>10.0 mmol/L) have been considered to increase risk for CVD based on epidemiologic surveys (96) and experimental studies have shown that homocysteine may increase oxidative stress with deleterious effects on the vascular wall (397). Furthermore there is some but not universal evidence that hyperhomocysteinemia is associated with insulin resistance, possibly because of an inhibitory action of insulin on cystathionine synthase which converts homocysteine to cystathione (398). These observations may mean that hyperhomocysteinemia may exert a greater vasculopathic effect in diabetic as compared to nondiabetic individuals. High-dose folic acid, vitamin B12 and vitamin B_6 have been used to lower homocysteine levels, but evidence for CVD benefit is weak. A recent report at the European Society of Cardiology Congress (September 2005, Stockholm yet to be published), described the results of the Norwegian Vitamin Trial (NORVIT) trial. In this study, in which 3749 subjects with elevated homocysteine levels on average (~10% with diabetes) were randomized in a 2 × 2 factorial design to folic acid, vitamin B_6, both, or neither, no significant effect on CVD was found in the monotherapy groups and a 21% increased risk of MI in the combined treatment group occurred ($p < 0.03$), despite a 28% lowering of homocysteine levels (399). The investigators concluded that homocysteine was an "innocent marker" of disease, that high doses of B vitamins should not be used in subjects with CVD, and that folate treatment has no beneficial effect on the risk of CVD.

Lipoprotein (a)

Lp(a) has been incriminated as a novel CVD risk factor and a metaanalysis of 27 prospective studies demonstrated a clear association between Lp(a) that appeared to be independent of other risk factors such as diabetes (400). Studies in diabetic subjects have differed in regard to whether Lp(a) is useful in predicting CHD or not (401,402). There have been no clinical trials of treatment, because Lp(a) levels are relatively impervious to interventions. One view is to treat subjects with elevated Lp(a) levels more aggressively for dyslipidemia and possibly other treatable CVD risk factors than would otherwise be indicated.

The Evidence Base for Prevention of Peripheral Vascular Disease

There is a dearth of clinical evidence to determine whether CVD risk factor interventions have benefit for PVD because there have been no clinical trials whose primary objective was to evaluate the effect of interventions on the progression of PVD, unlike for CHD and stroke. The absence of specific information on what is effective intervention for PVD contributes to a tendency among clinicians to overlook this very serious complication of diabetes. PVD is probably present in 20% to 30% of older diabetic subjects and is associated with a 20% nonfatal MI and stroke incidence, and a 30% fatality rate over five years (403). The single most important modifiable risk factor is cigarette smoking and smoking cessation is absolutely essential. The evidence for benefit from other forms of risk factor modification is however equivocal. In a metaanalysis of participants with PVD from seven eligible randomized statin trials ($n = 698$), lipid lowering produced a marked (odds ratio 0.21) though nonsignificant reduction in mortality, but little change in nonfatal events (404). In two of these, significant overall reduction of disease progression on angiography was noted and statin treatment was shown to reduce the severity of claudication. ATP III considers PVD a CHD equivalent (27). Similarly, the HOPE trial showed that subjects with PVD received a similar benefit in terms of CVD reduction to those without PVD. However neither treatment of hyperglycemia (UKPDS) nor aspirin therapy (Antiplatelet Trialist's, Collaboration) demonstrated any significant benefit for these interventions on PVD. Despite these findings, the ADA recommends aggressive approaches to hyperglycemia, hypertension, and dyslipidemia, and the use of antiplatelet agents (403).

Combined Effects of Vasculo-Preventive Treatment Strategies

By their very nature, therapeutic clinical trials are required to restrict their purpose to as narrow a focus as possible. Clinical practice recommendations on the other hand advocate a broad multi-faceted approach to CVD prevention. Clinicians as well as public health officials need to know what the combined impact of all of these interventions are, because clearly each one has only a limited 10% to 30% effect on relative risk reduction of CVD prevention. If the effects from each therapeutic intervention are truly additive, effective treatment of hyperglycemia, dyslipidemia, hypertension, and hypercoagulability might collectively reduce relative risks for CVD by 50% to 100%, which would represent a substantial reduction in the risk of CVD in diabetic subjects, bringing rates of CHD and stroke closer to that in nondiabetic individuals. The Steno-2 Study provides the best evidence that there are additive effects of a multipronged approach driven by ambitious targets for the prevention of vascular disease in type 2 diabetes. Beginning in 1992, 160 patients were randomized to either conventional multifactorial treatment by general practitioners following national guidelines ($n = 80$), or intensified multifactorial intervention integrating both behavior modification and polypharmacy by a diabetes team consisting of a doctor, nurse, and a clinical dietitian at Steno Diabetes Center in Copenhagen (405). Targets for blood glucose, glycated Hb, systolic and diastolic BP, and fasting values of serum total cholesterol, LDL-C, and triglycerides were lower in the intervention group than with conventional therapy. A stepwise, target-driven approach for drug treatment was used in order to achieve these goals. Endpoints were microvascular disease at four years and a composite of CVD events at eight years. There was a 53% reduction (20% absolute risk reduction) in the relative risk of the CVD endpoint in the intensified intervention group ($p < 0.008$) as well as significant reductions in the development or progression of retinopathy, nephropathy, and autonomic neuropathy. These differences were accompanied by significantly lower GHb, BP, and lipid levels in the intensified intervention group. The absolute risk reduction corresponded fairly well with what might be expected from clinical trials of hyperglycemia (UKPDS), antihypertensive treatment (HOT), and statin trials, suggesting that multiple risk factor interventions have additive effects. The investigators conclude with the statement that "the challenge for now is to ensure that the trial experiences are widely adopted in daily clinical practice" (Fig. 23).

Estimates of Efficacy of Cardiovascular Intervention Strategies in National Surveys

The most recent surveys in Europe and the United States place the challenges of translating clinical trials into clinical practice into perspective. In the United States the NHANES 1999–2000, a cross-sectional survey of a nationally representative sample of the noninstitutionalized civilian US population found that only 37.0% of participants with previously diagnosed diabetes achieved the target GHb goal of <7.0%, and 37.2% of participants were above the recommended "take action" level of >8.0% (406); these percentages did not change significantly from NHANES III (conducted 1988–1994). Only 35.8% of participants achieved the target of systolic BP <130 mmHg and diastolic BP < 80 mmHg, and 40.4% had hypertensive BP levels (SBP ≥140 or DBP ≥90 mmHg). These percentages also did not change significantly from NHANES III. Over half (51.8%) of the participants in NHANES 1999–2000 had total cholesterol levels of 200 mg/dL or greater (vs. 66.1% in NHANES III; p < 0.001). In total, only 7.3% adults with diabetes in NHANES 1999–2000 attained recommended goals of GHb level less than 7%, BP less than 130/80 mmHg, and total cholesterol level less than 200 mg/dL. The only improvements in mean risk factor levels between the

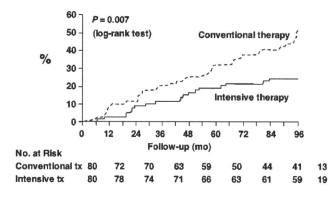

No. at Risk
Conventional tx 80   72   70   63   59   50   44   41   13
Intensive tx   80   78   74   71   66   63   61   59   19

FIGURE 23 Effects of intensive multifactorial versus conventional treatment on cardiovascular events in the Steno-2 study. *Source*: Ref. 405. Copyright © 2003 Massachusetts Medical Society. All rights reserved.

two surveys was a 3 mmHg lower mean SBP (138 vs. 135) and a 14 mg/dL lower mean total cholesterol (223 vs. 209) in NHANES 1999–2000 compared to NHANES III. GHb values did not improve (7.6% vs. 7.8%).

The Swedish National Diabetes Registry, a voluntary sub-national registry of diabetes and primary care clinics reported on changes in risk factors in registered diabetic subjects from 1996 through 2003. Although there was a fall in mean GHb from 7.8% to 7.2%, and a reduction in BP from 150/82 to 143/78 (total cholesterol was unavailable in 1996 but was 198 mg/dL in 2003), the new European treatment targets of GHb <6.1%, BP <130/80 mmHg and total cholesterol <175 (<4.5 mmol/L) were only attained by 16%, 13% and 28% of the patients in 2003, respectively, and only 36% of subjects were taking aspirin (407).

These data indicate that despite the substantial advances in our understanding of the causes of the heightened CVD risk in diabetes, it has not been possible to demonstrate any decrease in the incidence of the major cause of death in diabetes, despite the evidence that current preventive therapies if efficiently applied will markedly reduce the occurrence of these complications. It is hoped that this review will help move forward the global effort to reduce the risk of CVD in diabetes.

CONCLUSION

CVD is the major contributor to mortality and morbidity in diabetes, and glucose intolerance is present in up to 70% of subjects with CVD. Understanding the nature of the relationship between diabetes and CVD is therefore key to the prevention of the most common and important threat to health in Western countries and an increasingly important health concern throughout the rest of the world. The fact that the risk for CVD in subjects with diabetes is so much greater than in the rest of the population and that almost one half of CVD deaths in subjects with diabetes occur outside the hospital, means that ambulatory care physicians, by recognizing that the prevention of CVD is the foremost priority in their therapeutic strategy in patients with diabetes, bear a major responsibility in educating patients about their high level of risk for CVD, and need to ensure that all treatment targets are achieved efficiently. Although the interventions demonstrated to be effective in reducing CVD have not changed in the last decade, namely those directed at hyperglycemia, lipid abnormalities, hypertension, and hypercoagulability, targets have been lowered significantly and therapeutic advances have improved in parallel. Despite these developments, the majority of patients with diabetes do not get treated to any of the therapeutic targets. Although there are many reasons for this, from the clinician's standpoint, the use of combination therapy that is essential to reaching targets in many patients is probably significantly underutilized. Improved understanding of the pathophysiology of CVD, especially elucidations of the pathways that drive vascular inflammation and plaque rupture and erosion in diabetes will undoubtedly provide new diagnostic and therapeutic approaches to CVD prevention in diabetes; this may be of great importance because the initial evidence suggests it may not be possible using existent therapeutic approaches to reduce the excess CVD risk in diabetic subjects by more than one quarter to one half.

REFERENCES

1. Kannel WB, McGee DL. Diabetes and cardiovascular disease. The Framingham Study. JAMA 1979; 241:2035–2038.
2. Wingard DL, Barret-Connor E. Heart disease and diabetes. In: Harris, ed. Diabetes in America. 2nd ed. Bethesda: MD, National Institute of Health.
3. Diabetes Atlas. 2nd ed. International Diabetes Federation, 2003.
4. Zimmet P. Epidemiology of diabetes mellitus and associated cardiovascular risk factors: focus on human immunodeficiency virus and psychiatric disorders. Am J Med 2005; 118(suppl 2):3S–8S.
5. Morrish NJ, Wang SL, Stevens LK, Fuller JH, Keen H. Mortality and causes of death in the WHO multi-national study of vascular disease in diabetes. Diabetologia 2001; 44 (suppl 2):S14–S21.
6. Miettinen H, Lehto S, Salomaa V, et al. Impact of diabetes on mortality after the first myocardial infarction. Diabetes Care 1998; 21:69–75.
7. Fava S, Azzopardi J, Muscat HA, Fenech FF. Factors that influence outcome in diabetic subjects with myocardial infarction. Diabetes Care 1993; 16:1615–1618.
8. Sprafka JM, Burke GL, Folsom AR, McGovern PG, Hahn LP. Trends in prevalence of diabetes mellitus in patients with myocardial infarction and effect of diabetes on survival. The Minnesota Heart Survey. Diabetes Care 1991; 14:537–543.
9. UKPDS Group. UK Prospective Diabetes Study 6: complications in newly diagnosed type 2 diabetic patients and their association with different clinical and biochemical risk factors. Diabetes Res 1990; 13:1–11.
10. Harris MI. Undiagnosed NIDDM: clinical and public health issues. Diabetes Care 1993; 16:642–652.
11. Kuller LH. Stroke and diabetes. In: Harris, ed. Diabetes in America. 2nd ed. Bethesda: MD, National Institute of Health.
12. Palumbo PJ, Melton LJ. Peripheral vascular disease and diabetes. In: Harris, ed. Diabetes in America. 2nd ed. Bethesda: MD, National Institute of Health.
13. Kannel WB, Skinner JJ Jr, Schwartz MJ, Shurtleff D. Intermittent claudication. Incidence in the Framingham Study. Circulation 1970; 41:875–883.
14. Gu K, Cowie CC, Harris MI. Diabetes and decline in heart disease mortality in US adults. JAMA 1999; 281:1291–1297.
15. Barzilay JI, Spiekerman CF, Kuller LH, et al. Cardiovascular health study. Prevalence of clinical and isolated subclinical cardiovascular disease in older adults with glucose disorders: the cardiovascular health study. Diabetes Care 2001; 24:1233–1239.
16. Centers for Disease Control and Prevention (CDC), National Center for Health Statistics, Division of Health Interview Statistics, data from the National Health Interview Survey. http://www.cdc.gov/diabetes/statistics/age/source.htm
17. Hillier TA, Pedula KL. Complications in young adults with early-onset type 2 diabetes: losing the relative protection of youth. Diabetes Care 2003; 26:2999–3005.
18. Krolewski AS, Kosinski EJ, Warram JH, et al. Magnitude and determinants of cronary artery disease in juvenile-onset, insulin-dependent diabetes mellitus. Am J Cardiol 1987; 59:750–755.
19. Chaturvedi N, Jarrett J, Morrish N, Keen H, Fuller JH. Differences in mortality and morbidity in African Caribbean and European people with non-insulin-dependent diabetes mellitus: result of 20-year follow-up of a London cohort of a multinational study. BMJ 1996; 313:848–852.
20. Dijkstra S, Klok M, Hoogenhuyze van D, Sauerwein HP, Berghout A. Ischaemic heart disease in Turkish migrants with type 2 diabetes mellitus in the Netherlands: wait for the next generation? Neth J Med 2002; 60:21–24.
21. Weijers RNM, Goldschmidt, HMJ, Silberbusch J. Vascular complications in relation to ethnicity in non-insulin-dependent diabetes mellitus. Eur J Clin Invest 1997, 27:182–188.
22. Hunt KJ, Williams K, Resendez RG, Hazuda HP, Haffner SM, Stern MP. All-cause and cardiovascular mortality among diabetic participants in the San Antonio Heart Study: evidence against the "Hispanic Paradox." Diabetes Care 2002; 25:1557–1563.
23. Kittner SJ, White LR, Losonczy KG, Wolf PA, Hebel JR. Black-white differences in stroke incidence in a national sample. The contribution of hypertension and diabetes mellitus. JAMA 1990; 264:1267–1270.
24. Reaven PD, Sacks J. Investigators for the VADT. Coronary artery and abdominal aortic calcification are associated with cardiovascular disease in type 2 diabetes. Diabetologia 2005; 48:379–385.
25. Elhadd TA, Jung RT, Newton RW, Stonebridge PA, Belch JJ. Incidence of asymptomatic peripheral arterial occlusive disease in diabetic patients attending a hospital clinic. Adv Exp Med Biol 1997; 428:45–48.
26. Hirsch AT, Criqui MH, Treat-Jacobson D, et al., Peripheral arterial disease detection, awareness, and treatment in primary care. JAM 2001; 286:1317–1324.
27. Expert Panel on Detection, Evaluation, and Treatment of High Blood Cholesterol in Adults. Executive summary of the third report of the National Cholesterol Education Program (NCEP). Expert Panel on detection, evaluation, and treatment of high blood cholesterol in adults (Adult Treatment Panel III). JAMA 2001; 285:2486–2497.
28. Haffner SM, Lehto S, Rönnemaa T, et al. Mortality from coronary heart disease in subjects with type 2 diabetes and in nondiabetic subjects with and without prior myocardial infarction. N Engl J Med 1998; 339:229–234.

29. Malmberg K, Yusuf S, Gerstein HC, et al. Impact of diabetes on long-term prognosis in patients with unstable angina and non-Q-wave myocardial infarction: results of the OASIS (Organization to Assess Strategies for Ischemic Syndromes) Registry. Circulation 2000; 102:1014–1009.

30. Simons LA, Simons JS. Diabetes and coronary heart disease. N Engl J Med 1998; 339:1714–1716.

31. Hu FB, Stampfer MJ, Solomon CG, et al. The impact of diabetes mellitus on mortality from all causes and coronary heart disease in women: 20 years of follow-up. Arch Intern Med 2001; 161:1717–1723.

32. Lotufo PA, Gaziano M, Chae CU, et al. Diabetes and all-cause and coronary heart disease mortality among US male physicians. Arch Intern Med 2001; 161:242–247.

33. Cho E, Rimm EB, Stampfer MJ, et al. The impact of diabetes mellitus and prior myocardial infarction on mortality from all causes and from coronary heart disease in men. J Am Coll Cardiol 2002; 40:954–960.

34. Lee CD, Folsom AR, Pankow JS, Brancati FL. Atherosclerosis risk in communities (ARIC) study investigators. Cardiovascular events in diabetic and nondiabetic adults with or without history of myocardial infarction. Circulation 2004; 109:855–860.

35. Hu G, Jousilahti P, Qiao Q, Peltonen M, Katoh S, Tuomilehto J. The gender-specific impact of diabetes and myocardial infarction at baseline and during follow-up on mortality from all causes and coronary heart disease. J Am Coll Cardiol 2005; 45:1413–1418.

36. Diabetes in America. Epidemiology and scope of the problem. Diabetes Care 1998; (suppl 3):C11–C14.

37. Isolated postchallenge hyperglycemia and the risk of fatal cardiovascular dsease in older women and men. The Rancho Bernardo Study. Diabetes Care 1998; 21:1236–1239.

38. DECODE Study Group, the European Diabetes Epidemiology Group. Glucose tolerance and cardiovascular mortality: comparison of fasting and 2-hour diagnostic criteria. Arch Intern Med 2001; 161:397–405.

39. Malmberg K, Ryden L. Myocardial infarction in patients with diabetes mellitus. Eur Heart J 1988; 9:259–264.

40. Norhammar A, Tenerz A, Nilsson G, et al. Glucose metabolism in patients with acute myocardial infarction and no previous diagnosis of diabetes mellitus: a prospective study. Lancet 2002; 359:2140–2144.

41. Stig-J̄rgensen H, Nakayama H, Raaschou HO, Olsen TS. Stroke in patients with diabetes: the copenhagen stroke study. Stroke 1994; 25:1977–1984.

42. Kernan WN, Viscoli CM, Inzucchi SE, Brass LM, Bravata DM, Shulman GI, McVeety JC. Prevalence of abnormal glucose tolerance following a transient ischemic attack or ischemic stroke. Arch Intern Med 2005; 24(165):227–233.

43. Sukhija R, Yalamanchili K, Aronow WS, Kakar P, Babu S. Clinical characteristics, risk factors, and medical treatment of 561 patients with peripheral arterial disease followed in an academic vascular surgery clinic. Cardiol Rev 2005; 13:108–110.

44. Libby P. Inflammation in atherosclerosis. Nature 2002; 420:868–874.

45. Ritchie SA, Ewart MA, Perry CG, Connell JM, Salt IP. The role of insulin and the adipocytokines in regulation of vascular endothelial function. Clin Sci (Lond) 2004; 107:519–532.

46. Venugopal SK, Devaraj S, Jialal I. Effect of C-reactive protein on vascular cells: evidence for a proinflammatory, proatherogenic role. Curr Opin Nephrol Hypertens 2005; 14:33–37.

47. Ridker PM, Buring JE, Cook NR, Rifai N. C-reactive protein, the metabolic syndrome, and risk of incident cardiovascular events: an 8-year follow-up of 14 719 initially healthy American women. Circulation 2003; 107:391–397.

48. Burke AP, Kolodgie FD, Zieske A, et al. Morphologic findings of coronary atherosclerotic plaques in diabetics: a postmortem study. Arterioscler Thromb Vasc Biol 2004; 24:1266–1271.

49. Moreno PR, Fuster V. New aspects in the pathogenesis of diabetic atherothrombosis. J Am Coll Cardiol 2004; 44:2293–2300.

50. Harris MI, Klein R, Welborn TA, Knuiman MW. Onset of NIDDM occurs at least 4-7 yr before clinical diagnosis. Diabetes Care 1992; 15:815–819.

51. Edelstein SL, Knowler WC, Bain RP, et al. Predictors of progression from impaired glucose tolerance to NIDDM: an analysis of six prospective studies. Diabetes 1997; 46:701–710.

52. Srinivasan SR, Frontini MG, Berenson GS, Bogalusa Heart Study. Longitudinal changes in risk variables of insulin resistance syndrome from childhood to young adulthood in offspring of parents with type 2 diabetes: the bogalusa heart study. Metabolism 2003; 52:443–450.

53. Insulin and cardiovascular disease. Paris Prospective Study. Diabetes Care 1991; 14:461.

54. Dandona P, Aljada A and Bandyopadhyay A. Inflammation: the link between insulin resistance, obesity and diabetes. Trends in Immunology 2004; 25:4–7.

55. Howard G, O'Leary DH, Zaccaro D, et al. The Insulin Resistance Atherosclerosis Study (IRAS) Investigators. Circulation 1996; 93:1809–1817.

56. Reaven GM. Banting lecture 1988. Role of insulin resistance in human disease. Diabetes 1988; 37:1595–1607.

57. Haffner SM, Stern MP, Hazuda NP, Mitchell BD, Patterson JK. Cardiovascular risk factors in confirmed prediabetic individuals. Does the clock for coronary heart disease start ticking before the onset of clinical diabetes? JAMA 1990; 263:2893–2898.

58. Grundy SM. Obesity, metabolic syndrome, and cardiovascular disease. J Clin Endocrinol Metab 2004; 89:2595–2601.

59. Holt RI. International Diabetes Federation re-defines the metabolic syndrome. Diabetes Obes Metab 2005; 7:618–620.

60. Balkau B, Charles MA. Comment on the provisional report from the WHO consultation. European Group for the Study of Insulin Resistance (EGIR). Diabet Med 1999; 16:442–443.

61. Alexander CM, Landsman PB, Teutsch SM, Haffner SM. Third National Health and Nutrition Examination Survey (NHANES III); National Cholesterol Education Program (NCEP). NCEP-defined metabolic syndrome, diabetes, and prevalence of coronary heart disease among NHANES III participants age 50 years and older. Diabetes 2003; 52:1210–1214.

62. Unger RH. Minireview: weapons of lean body mass destruction: the role of ectopic lipids in the metabolic syndrome. Endocrinology 2003; 144:5159–5165.

63. Montagnani M, Golovchenko I, Kim I, et al. Inhibition of phosphatidylinositol 3-kinase enhances mitogenic actions of insulin in endothelial cells. J Biol Chem 2002; 277:1794–1799.

64. Clinical guidelines on the identification, evaluation, and treatment of overweight and obesity in adults—the evidence report. National Institutes of Health. Obes Res 1998; 2(suppl 6):51S–209S.

65. Nieves DJ, Cnop M, Retzlaff B, et al. The atherogenic lipoprotein profile associated with obesity and insulin resistance is largely attributable to intra-abdominal fat. Diabetes 2003; 52:172–179.

66. Abbasi F, Brown BW Jr, Lamendola C, McLaughlin T, Reaven GM. Relationship between obesity, insulin resistance, and coronary heart disease risk. J Am Coll Cardiol 2002; 40:937.

67. Grundy SM. What is the contribution of obesity to the metabolic syndrome? Endocrinol Metab Clin North Am 2004; 33:267–282.

68. Egusa G, Beltz WF, Grundy SM, Howard BV. Influence of obesity on the metabolism of apolipoprotein B in humans. J Clin Invest 1985; 76:596–603.

69. Rajala MW, Scherer PE. Minireview: the adipocyte—at the crossroads of energy homeostasis, inflammation, and atherosclerosis. Endocrinology 2003; 144:3765–3773.

70. Wyne KL. Free fatty acids and type 2 diabetes mellitus. Am J Med 2003; 115(suppl 8A):29S–36S.

71. Perseghin G, Ghosh S, Gerow K, Shulman GI. Metabolic defects in lean nondiabetic offspring of NIDDM parents: a cross-sectional study. Diabetes 1997; 4:1001–1009.

72. Dresner A, Laurent D, Marcucci M, et al. Effects of free fatty acids on glucose transport and IRS-1-associated phosphatidylinositol 3-kinase activity. J Clin Invest 1999; 103:253–259.

73. Lee Y, Hirose H, Ohneda M, Johnson JH, McGarry JD, Unger RH. β-Cell lipotoxicity in the pathogenesis of non-insulin-dependent diabetes mellitus of obese rats: impairment in adipocyte-β-cell relationships. Proc Natl Acad Sci U S A 1994; 91:10878–10882.

74. Davda RK, Stepniakowski KT, Lu G, Ullian ME, Goodfriend TL, Egan BM. Oleic acid inhibits endothelial nitric oxide synthase by a protein kinase C-independent mechanism. Hypertension 1995; 26:764–770.

75. Oram JF, Bornfeldt KE. Direct effects of long-chain non-esterified fatty acids on vascular cells and their relevance to macrovascular complications of diabetes. Front Biosci 2004; 9:1240–1253.

76. Evans JL, Goldfine ID, Maddux BA, Grodsky GM. Oxidative stress and stress-activated signaling pathways: a unifying hypothesis of type 2 diabetes. Endocr Rev 2002; 23:599–622.

77. Carlsson C, Borg LA, Welsh N. Sodium palmitate induces partial mitochondrial uncoupling and reactive oxygen species in rat pancreatic islets in vitro . Endocrinology 1999; 140:3422–3428.

78. Yamagishi SI, Edelstein D, Du XL, Kaneda Y, Guzman M, Brownlee M. Leptin induces mitochondrial superoxide production and monocyte chemoattractant protein-1 expression in aortic endothelial cells by increasing fatty acid oxidation via protein kinase A. J Biol Chem 2001; 276:25096–25100.

79. Fuller JH, Shipley MJ, Rose G, Jarrett RJ, Keen H. Mortality from coronary heart disease and stroke in relation to degree of glycaemia: the Whitehall study. Br Med J (Clin Res Ed) 1983; 287:867–870.

80. Coutinho M, Gerstein HC, Wang Y, Yusuf S. The relationship between glucose and incident cardiovascular events. A metaregression analysis of published data from 20 studies of 95,783 individuals followed for 12.4 years. Diabetes Care 1999; 22:233–240.

81. Khaw KT, Wareham N, Luben R, Bingham S, Oakes S, Welch A, et al. Glycated haemoglobin, diabetes, and mortality in men in Norfolk cohort of European prospective investigation of cancer and nutrition (EPIC–Norfolk). BMJ 2001; 322:5–8.

82. Selvin E, Marinopoulos S, Berkenblit G, et al. Meta-analysis: glycosylated hemoglobin and cardiovascular disease in diabetes mellitus. Ann Intern Med 2004; 141:421–431.

83. Brownlee M, Cerami A. The biochemistry of the complications of diabetes mellitus. Annu Rev Biochem 1981; 50:385–432.

84. Cerami A, Vlassara H, Brownlee M. Role of nonenzymatic glycosylation in atherogenesis. J Cell Biochem 1986; 30:111–120.

85. Brownlee M. Biochemistry and molecular cell biology of diabetic complications. Nature 2001; 414:813–820.

86. Ceriello A. Postprandial hyperglycemia and diabetes complications: is it time to treat? Diabetes 2005; 54:1–7.

87. JC Pickup, Mattock MB, Chusney GD, Burt D. NIDDM as a disease of the innate immune system: association of acute-phase reactants and interleukin-6 with metabolic syndrome X. Diabetologia 1997; 40:1286–1292.

88. MI Schmidt, Duncan BB, Sharrett AR, et al. Markers of inflammation and prediction of diabetes mellitus in adults (atherosclerosis risk in communities study): a cohort study. Lancet 1999; 353:1649–1652.

89. A Kubaszek, Pihlajamaki J, Komarovski V, et al. Finnish Diabetes Prevention Study. Promoter polymorphisms of the TNF-α (G-308A) and IL-6 (C-174G) genes predict the conversion from impaired glucose tolerance to type 2 diabetes: the Finnish diabetes prevention study. Diabetes 2003; 52:1872–1876.

90. Cai D, Yuan M, Frantz DF, et al. Local and systemic insulin resistance resulting from hepatic activation of IKK-beta and NF-kappaB. Nat Med 2005; 11:183–190.

91. Fernandez-Real JM, Ricart W. Insulin resistance and chronic cardiovascular inflammatory syndrome. Endocr Rev 2003; 24:278–301.

92. Ford E. Body mass index, diabetes, and C-reactive protein among U.S. adults. Diabetes Care 1999; 22:1971–1977.

93. Tsunoda K, Arita M, Yukawa M, et al. Retinopathy and hypertension affect serum high-sensitivity C-reactive protein levels in Type 2 diabetic patients. J Diabetes Complications 2005; 19:123–127.

94. Bahceci M, Tuzcu A, Ogun C, Canoruc N, Iltimur K, Aslan C. Is serum C-reactive protein concentration correlated with HbA1c and insulin resistance in Type 2 diabetic men with or without coronary heart disease? J Endocrinol Invest 2005; 28:145–150.

95. Best LG, Zhang Y, Lee ET, et al. C-Reactive Protein as a Predictor of Cardiovascular Risk in a Population With a High Prevalence of Diabetes. The Strong Heart Study. Circulation 2005; 112:1289–1295.

96. Welch GN and Loscalzo J. Homocysteine and atherothrombosis. N Engl J Med 1998; 338:1042–1050.

97. Munshi MN, Stone A, Fink L, Fonseca V. Hyperhomocysteinemia following a methionine load in patients with non-insulin-dependent diabetes mellitus and macrovascular disease. Metabolism 1996; 45:133–135.

98. Kark JD, Selhub J, Bostom A, Adler B, Rosenberg IH. Plasma homocysteine and all-cause mortality in diabetes. Lancet 1999; 353:1936–1937.

99. Goldberg RB, Capuzzi D. Lipid disorders in type 1 and type 2 diabetes. Clin Lab Med 2001; 1:147–172.

100. Sniderman AD, Scantlebury T, Clanfone K. Hypertriglyceridemic hyperapoB: the unappreciated atherogenic dyslipoproteimemia in type 2 diabetes mellitus. Ann Intern Med 2001; 135:447–459.

101. Rivellese AA, De Natale C, Di Marino L, et al. Exogenous and endogenous postprandial lipid abnormalities in type 2 diabetic patients with optimal blood glucose control and optimal fasting triglyceride levels. J Clin Endocrinol Metab 2004; 89:2153.

102. Haffner SM, Morales PA, Stern MP, Gruber MK. Lp (a) concentrations in NIDDM. Diabetes 1992; 41:1267–1272.

103. Cowie CC, Harris ML. Physical and metabolic characteristics of persons with diabetes. Diabetes in America. 2nd ed. National Institutes of Health 1995:117–164.

104. Manley SE, Frighi V, Stratton E, et al. For the U.K. Prospective Diabetes Study Group. U.K. Prospective Diabetes Study 27. Plasma lipids and lipoproteins at diagnosis of NIDDM by age and sex. Diabetes Care 1997; 20:1683–1687.

105. The Diabetes Prevention Program Research Group. Lipid, lipoproteins, C-reactive protein and hemostatic factors at baseline in the Diabetes Prevention Program. Diabetes Care 2005; 28:2472–2479.

106. Sniderman AD, Cianflone K. Substrate delivery as a determinant of hepatic apoB secretion. Arterioscler Thromb 1993; 13:629–636.

107. Adiels M, Boren J, Caslake MJ, et al. Overproduction of VLDL1 driven by hyperglycemia is a dominant feature of diabetic dyslipidemia. Arterioscler Thromb Vasc Biol 2005; 25:1697–1703.

108. Borggreve SE, De Vries R, Dullaart RP. Alterations in high-density lipoprotein metabolism and reverse cholesterol transport in insulin resistance and type 2 diabetes mellitus: role of lipolytic enzymes, lecithin: cholesterol acyltransferase and lipid transfer proteins. Eur J Clin Invest 2003; 33:1051–1069.

109. Eriksson JW, Buren J, Svensson M, Olivecrona T, Olivecrona G. Postprandial regulation of blood lipids and adipose tissue lipoprotein lipase in type 2 diabetes patients and healthy control subjects. Atherosclerosis 2003; 166:359–367.

110. Mero N, Syvanne M, Taskinen MR. Postprandial lipid metabolism in diabetes. Atherosclerosis 1998 (suppl 1):S53–S55.

111. Rashid S, Uffelman KD, Lewis GF. The mechanism of HDL lowering in hypertriglyceridemic, insulin-resistant states. J Diabetes Complications 2002; 16:24–28.

112. Feingold KR, Grunfeld C, Pang M, et al. LDL subclass phenotypes and triglyceride metabolism in non-insulin dependent diabetes. Arterioscler Thromb Vasc Biol 1992; 12:1496–1502.

113. Garvey WT, Kwon S, Zheng D, et al. Effects of insulin resistance and type 2 diabetes on lipoprotein subclass particle size and concentration determined by nuclear magnetic resonance. Diabetes 2003; 52:453–462.

114. Adams MR, Kinlay S, Blake GJ, Orford JL, Ganz P, Selwyn AP. Atherogenic lipids and endothelial dysfunction: mechanisms in the genesis of ischemic syndromes. Annu Rev Med 2000; 51:149–167.114.

115. Stemerman MB. Lipoprotein effects on the vessel wall. Circ Res 2000; 86:715–716.

116. Schwenke DC, D'Agostino RB Jr, Goff DC Jr, Karter AJ, Rewers MJ, Wagenknecht LE. Insulin resistance atherosclerosis study. Differences in LDL oxidizability by glycemic status: the insulin resistance atherosclerosis study. Diabetes Care 2003; 26:1449–1455.

117. Lamharzi N, Renard CB, Kramer F, et al. Hyperlipidemia in concert with hyperglycemia stimulates the proliferation of macrophages in atherosclerotic lesions: potential role of glucose-oxidized LDL. Diabetes 2004; 53:3217–3225.

118. De Graaf J, Hak-Lemmers HLM, Hectors MPC, et al. Enhanced susceptibility to in vitro oxidation of the dense low density lipoprotein subfraction in healthy subjects. Arterioscler Thromb 1991; 11:298–306.

119. Camejo G, Hurt-Camejo E, Bondjers G. Effect of proteoglycans on lipoprotein-cell interactions: possible contribution to atherogenesis. Curr Opin Lipidol 1990; 1:431–436.

120. Geleano NF, Milne R, Marcel YL, et al. Apoprotein B structure and receptor recognition of triglyceride-rich low density lipoprotein (LDL) is modified in small LDL but not in triglyceride-rich LDL of normal size. J Biol Chem 1994; 269:511–519.

121. Haraguchi G, Kobayashi Y, Brown ML, et al. PPAR(alpha) and PPAR(gamma) activators suppress the monocyte-macrophage apoB-48 receptor. J Lipid Res 2003; 44:1224–1231.

122. Tannock LR, Chait A. Lipoprotein-matrix interactions in macrovascular disease in diabetes. Front Biosci 2004; 9:1728–1742.

123. Rohrer L, Hersberger M, von Eckardstein A. High density lipoproteins in the intersection of diabetes mellitus, inflammation and cardiovascular disease. Curr Opin Lipidol 2004; 15:269–278.

124. Hedrick CC, Thorpe SR Fu MX, et al. Glycation impairs high-density lipoprotein function. Diabetologia 2000; 43:312–320.

125. Lopes-Virella MF, Virella G. The role of immune and inflammatory processes in the development of macrovascular disease in diabetes. Front Biosci 2003; 8:s750–s768.

126. Brown BE, Dean RT, Davies MJ. Glycation of low-density lipoproteins by methylglyoxal and glycolaldehyde gives rise to the in vitro formation of lipid-laden cells. Diabetologia 2005; 48:361–369.

127. Stamler J, Vacaro O, Neaton O, et al. Diabetes, other risk factors and 12 year cardiovascular mortality for men screened in the Multiple Risk Factors Intervention Trial. Diabetes Care 1993; 16:434–444.

128. Fontbonne A, Eschwege E, Cambien F, et al. Hypertriglyceridemia as a risk factor for coronary heart disease mortality in subjects with impaired glucose tolerance and diabetes: results from the 11 year follow-up of the Paris Prospective Study. Diabetologia 1989; 32:300–304.

129. Laakso M, Lehto S, Pentilla I, et al. Lipids and lipoprotein predicting coronary heart disease mortality and morbidity in patients with non-insulin-dependent diabetes. Circulation 1993; 88:1421–1430.

130. Turner RC, Millns H, Neil HA, et al. Risk factors for coronary artery disease in non-insulin dependent diabetes mellitus: United Kingdom Prospective Diabetes Study (UKPDS: 23). BMJ 1998; 316:823–828.

131. Liu J, Sempos C, Donahue RP, Dorn J, Trevisan M, Grundy SM. Joint distribution of non-HDL and LDL cholesterol and coronary heart disease risk prediction among individuals with and without diabetes. Diabetes Care 2005; 28:1916–1921.

132. Ratner R, Goldberg R, Haffner S, et al. Diabetes Prevention Program Research Group. Impact of intensive lifestyle and metformin therapy on cardiovascular disease risk factors in the diabetes prevention program. Diabetes Care 2005; 28:888–894.

133. Centers for Disease Control and Prevention (CDC). Data from the Behavioral Risk Factor Surveillance System. http://www.cdc.gov/diabetes/statistics/age/source.html.

134. Wong ND, Thakral G, Franklin SS, et al. Preventing heart disease by controlling hypertension: impact of hypertensive subtype, stage, age, and sex. Am Heart J 2003; 145:888–895.

135. Joffres MR, Hamet P, MacLean DR, L'italien GJ, Fodor G. Distribution of blood pressure and hypertension in Canada and the United States. Am J Hypertens 2001; 14:1099–1105.

136. Ko GT, Cockram CS, Chow CC, et al. Effects of body mass index, plasma glucose and cholesterol levels on isolated systolic hypertension. Int J Cardiol 2005; 101:429–433.

137. Feldt-Rasmussen B, Mathiesen ER, Deckert T, et al. Central role for sodium in the pathogenesis of blood pressure changes independent of angiotensin, aldosterone and catecholamines in type 1 (insulin-dependent) diabetes mellitus. Diabetologia 1987; 30:610–617.

138. Trujillo A, Eggena P, Barrett J, Tuck M. Renin regulation in type II diabetes mellitus: influence of dietary sodium. Hypertension 1989; 13:200–205.

139. Cooper ME. The role of the renin-angiotensin-aldosterone system in diabetes and its vascular complications. Am J Hypertens 2004; 17(11 Pt 2):16S–20S.

140. Candido KA, Jandeleit-Dahm Z, Cao SP, et al. Allen, Prevention of accelerated atherosclerosis by angiotensin-converting enzyme inhibition in diabetic apolipoprotein C-deficient mice. Circulation 2002; 106:246–253.

141. Candido TJ, Allen M, Lassila Z, et al. Irbesartan but not amlodipine suppresses diabetes-associated atherosclerosis. Circulation 2004; 109:1536–1542.

142. Brunner H, Cockcroft JR, Deanfield J, et al. Working group on endothelins and endothelial factors of the european society of hypertension. Endothelial function and dysfunction. Part II: association with cardiovascular risk factors and diseases. A statement by the Working Group on Endothelins and Endothelial Factors of the European Society of Hypertension. J Hypertens 2005; 23:233–246.

143. van Etten RW, de Koning EJ, Verhaar MC, Gaillard CA, Rabelink TJ. Impaired NO-dependent vasodilation in patients with type II (non-insulin-dependent) diabetes mellitus is restored by acute administration of folate. Diabetologia 2002; 45:1004–1010.

144. Schiffrin EL. State-of-the-art lecture. Role of endothelin-1 in hypertension. Hypertension 1999; 34:876–881.

145. McEniery CM, Qasem A, Schmitt M, Avolio AP, Cockcroft JR, Wilkinson IB. Endothelin-1 regulates arterial pulse wave velocity in vivo . J Am Coll Cardiol 2003; 42:1975–1981.

146. Wilkinson IB, Qasem A, McEniery CM, Webb DJ, Avolio AP, Cockcroft JR. Nitric oxide regulates local arterial distensibility in vivo . Circulation 2002; 105:213–217.
147. Wilkinson IB, McEniery CM. Arterial stiffness, endothelial function and novel pharmacological approaches. Clinical and Experimental Pharmacology and Physiology 2004; 31:795–799.
148. Miyata T, Sugiyama S, Suzuki D, Inagi R, Kurokawa K. Increased carbonyl modification by lipids and carbohydrates in diabetic nephropathy. Kidney Int Suppl 1999; 71:S54–S56.
149. Lehmann ED, Gosling RG, Sonksen PH. Arterial wall compliance in diabetes. Diabet Med 1992; 9:114–119.
150. Taylor AA. Pathophysiology of hypertension and endothelial dysfunction in patients with diabetes mellitus. Endocrinol Metab Clin North Am 2001; 30:983–997.
151. Salomaa V, Riley W, Kark JD, Nardo C, Folsom AR. Non-insulin-dependent diabetes mellitus and fasting glucose and insulin concentrations are associated with arterial stiffness indexes: the ARIC study. Atherosclerosis Risk in Communities Study. Circulation 1995; 91:1432–1443.
152. Franklin SS, Gustin W 4th, Wong ND, et al. Hemodynamic patterns of age-related changes in blood pressure: the framingham heart study. Circulation 1997; 96:308–315.
153. Lehmann ED, Hopkins KD, Rawesh A, et al. Relation between number of cardiovascular risk factors/events and noninvasive Doppler ultrasound assessments of aortic compliance. Hypertension 1998; 32:565–569.
154. Wilkinson IB, MacCallum H, Rooijmans DF, et al. Increased augmentation index and systolic stress in type 1 diabetes mellitus. Q J Med 2000; 93:441–448.
155. Natarajan R, Lanting L, Gonzales N, Nadler J. Formation of an F2-isoprostane in vascular smooth muscle cells by elevated glucose and growth factors. Am J Physiol 1996; 27 1(1 Pt 2):H159–H165.
156. Adler AI, Stratton IM, Neil HA, et al. Association of systolic blood pressure with macrovascular and microvascular complications of type 2 diabetes (UKPDS 36): prospective observational study. BMJ 2000; 12:412–419.
157. Viberti GC, Earle K. Predisposition to essential hypertension and the development of diabetic nephropathy. J Am Soc Nephrol 1992; 3(suppl 1):S27S33.
158. Colwell JA, Nesto RW. The platelet in diabetes: focus on prevention of ischemic events. Diabetes Care 2003; 267:2181–2188.
159. Ferroni P, Basili S, Falco A, Davi G. Platelet activation in type 2 diabetes mellitus. J Thromb Haemost 2004; 2:12821291.
160. Davi G, Catalano I, Averna M, et al. Thromboxane biosynthesis and platelet function in type II diabetes mellitus. N Engl J Med 1990; 322:17691974.
161. Leet H, Paton RC, Passa P, Caen JP. Fibrinogen binding and ADP-induced aggregation in platelets from diabetic subjects. Thromb Res 1981; 24:143150.
162. Vericel E, Januel C, Carreras M, Moulin P, Lagarde M. Diabetic patients without vascular complications display enhanced basal platelet activation and decreased antioxidant status. Diabetes 2004; 53:1046–1051.
163. Queen LR, Ji Y, Goubareva I, Ferro A. Nitric oxide generation mediated by beta-adrenoceptors is impaired in platelets from patients with Type 2 diabetes mellitus. Diabetologia 2003; 46:1474–1482.
164. Watala C, Boncer M, Golanski J, Koziolkiewcz W, Trojanowski Z, Walkowiak B. Platelet membrane lipid fluidity and intraplatelet calcium mobilization in type 2 diabetes. Eur J Haematol 1998; 61:319–326.
165. Eibl N, Krugluger W, Streit G, Schrattbauer K, Hopmeier P, Schernthaner G. Improved metabolic control decreases platelet activation markers in patients with type-2 diabetes. Eur J Clin Invest 2004; 34:205–209.
166. Sacco M, Pellegrini F, Roncaglioni MC, Avanzini F, Tognoni G, Nicolucci A. PPP Collaborative Group. Primary prevention of cardiovascular events with low-dose aspirin and vitamin E in type 2 diabetic patients: results of the Primary Prevention Project (PPP) trial. Diabetes Care 2003; 26:3264–3272.
167. Jones R.L. Fibrinopeptide-A in diabetes mellitus. Relation to levels of blood glucose, fibrinogen disappearance, and hemodynamic changes. Diabetes 1985; 34:836–843.
168. Horvath M, Pszota A, Rahoi K, Kugler Z, Evel S, Szigeti G. Fibrinopeptide A as thrombotic risk marker in diabetic and atherosclerotic coronary vasculopathy. J Med 1992; 23:93–100.
169. Morishita E, Asakura H, Jokaji H, Saito M, Uotani C, Kumabashiri I. Hypercoagulability and high lipoprotein (a) levels in patients with type II diabetes mellitus. Atherosclerosis 1996; 120:7–14.
170. Myrup B, Rossing P, Jensen T, Gram J, Kluft C, Jespersen J. Procoagulant activity and intimal dysfunction in IDDM. Diabetologia 1995; 38:73–78.
171. Kannel WB, D'Agostino RB, Wilson PW, Belanger AJ, Gagnon DR. Diabetes, fibrinogen, and risk of cardiovascular disease: the framingham experience. Am Heart J 1990; 120:672–676.
172. Lufkin EG, Fass DN, O'Fallon WM, Bowie EJW. Increased von Willebrand factor in diabetes mellitus. Metabolism 1979; 28:63–66.
173. Yarnell JW, Patterson CC, Sweetnam PM, Lowe GD. Haemostatic/inflammatory markers predict 10-year risk of IHD at least as well as lipids: the Caerphilly collaborative studies. Eur Heart J 2004; 25(12):1049–1056.
174. Bruno G, Merletti F, Biggeri A, et al. Casale monferrato study. Fibrinogen and AER are major independent predictors of 11-year cardiovascular mortality in type 2 diabetes: the casale monferrato study. Diabetologia 2005; 48:427–434.

175. Sobel BE, Schneider DJ. Platelet function, coagulopathy, and impaired fibrinolysis in diabetes. Cardiol Clin 2004; 22:511–526.
176. Brownlee M, Vlassara H, Cerami A. Inhibition of heparin-catalyzed human antithrombin III activity by nonenzymatic glycosylation. Diabetes 198; 33:532–535.
177. Ceriello A, Quatraro A, Dello Russo P, Marchi E, Barbanti M, Millani MR. Protein C deficiency in insulin dependent diabetes: a hyperglycemia-related phenomenon. Thromb Haemost 1990; 65:104–107.
178. Vague P, Juhan-Vague I, Aillaud MF, Badier C, Viard R, Alessi MC. Correlation between blood fibrinolytic activity, plasminogen activator inhibitor level, plasma insulin level and relative body weight in normal and obese subjects. Metabolism 1986; 35:250–253.
179. Schneider DJ, Hayes M, Wadsworth M, et al. Attenuation of neointimal vascular smooth muscle cellularity in atheroma by plasminogen activator inhibitor type 1 (PAI–1). J Histochem Cytochem 2004; 52:1091–1099.
180. Scarabin PY, Aillaud MF, Amouyel P, et al. Associations of fibrinogen, factor VII and PAI-1 with baseline findings among 10,500 male participants in a prospective study of myocardial infarction: the PRIME study. Thromb Haemost 1998; 80:749–756.
181. Johansson L, Jansson JH, Boman K, Nilsson TK, Stegmayr B, Hallmans G. Tissue plasminogen activator, plasminogen activator inhibitor-1, and tissue plasminogen activator/plasminogen activator inhibitor-1 complex as risk factors for the development of a first stroke. Stroke 2000; 31:26–32.
182. van Hoeven KH, Factor SM. A comparison of the pathological spectrum of hypertensive, diabetic and hypertensive-diabetic heart disease. Circulation 1990; 82:848–855.
183. Fang ZY, Prins JB, Marwick TH. Diabetic cardiomyopathy: evidence, mechanisms, and therapeutic implications. Endocr Rev 2004; 25:543–567.
184. Garcia MJ, McNamara PM, Gordon T, Kannel WB. Morbidity and mortality in diabetics in the Framingham population. Sixteen year follow-up study. Diabetes 1974; 23:105–111.
185. Karvounis HI, Papadopoulos CE, Zaglavara TA, et al. Evidence of left ventricular dysfunction in asymptomatic elderly patients with non-insulin-dependent diabetes mellitus. Angiology 2004; 55:549–555.
186. Diamant M, Lamb HJ, Smit JW, de Roos A, Heine RJ. Diabetic cardiomyopathy in uncomplicated type 2 diabetes is associated with the metabolic syndrome and systemic inflammation. Diabetologia 2005; 48:1669–1670.
187. Liao D, Cai J, Brancati FL, et al. Association of vagal tone with serum insulin, glucose, and diabetes mellitus – the ARIC study. Diabetes Res. Clin Prac 1995; 30:211–221.
188. Nesto R. Correlation between cardiovascular disease and diabetes mellitus: current concepts. Am J Med 2004; 8:116(suppl 5A):11S–22S.
189. Sajadieh A, Nielsen OW, Rasmussen V, Hein HO, Hansen JF. Prevalence and prognostic significance of daily-life silent myocardial ischaemia in middle-aged and elderly subjects with no apparent heart disease. Eur Heart J 2005; 26:1402–1409.
190. Takahashi N, Nakagawa M, Saikawa T, et al. Regulation of QT indices mediated by autonomic nervous function in patients with type 2 diabetes. Int J Cardiol 2004; 96:375–379.
191. Jokinen V, Ukkola O, Airaksinen KE, et al. Temporal changes in cardiovascular autonomic regulation in type II diabetic patients: association with coronary risk variables and progression of coronary artery disease. Ann Med 2003; 35:216–223.
192. Valensi P, Paries J, Attali JR. Cardiac autonomic neuropathy in diabetic patients: influence of diabetes duration, obesity, and microangiopathic complications the French multicenter study. Metabolism 2003; 52:815–820.
193. Atkins RC. The epidemiology of chronic kidney disease. Kidney Int Suppl 2005; 94:S14–S18.
194. US Renal Data System: USRDS 2003 Annual Data Report, Atlas of End-Stage Renal Disease in the United States, National Institutes of Health, National Institute of Diabetes and Digestive and Kidney Diseases. Bethesda: MD, 2003.
195. Pavkov ME, Bennett PH, Sievers ML, et al. Predominant effect of kidney disease on mortality in Pima Indians with or without type 2 diabetes. Kidney Int 2005; 68:1267–1274.
196. Dinneen SF, Gerstein HC. The association of microalbuminuria and mortality in non-insulin-dependent diabetes mellitus: a systematic overview of the literature. Arch Intern Med 1997; 15:1413–1418.
197. Stehouwer CD, Nauta JJ, Zeldenrust GC, Hackeng WH, Donker AJ, den Ottolander GJ. Urinary albumin excretion, cardiovascular disease, and endothelial dysfunction in non-insulin-dependent diabetes mellitus. Lancet 1992; 340:319–237.
198. Yudkin JS, Forrest RD, Jackson CA. Microalbuminuria as predictor of vascular disease in non-diabetic subjects. Lancet 1988; 2:530–533.
199. Standl E, Stiegler H. Microalbuminuria in a random cohort of recently diagnosed type 2 (non-insulin-dependent) diabetic patients living in the greater Munich area. Diabetologia 1993; 36:1017–1020.
200. Gerstein HC, Mann JF, Pogue J, et al. Yusuf for the HOPE study investigators. Prevalence and determinants of MA in high-risk diabetic and non-diabetic patients in the heart outcomes prevention evaluation study. Diabetes Care 2000; 23(suppl 2):B35–B39.
201. Gerstein HC, Mann JF, Yi Q, et al. HOPE study Investigators. Albuminuria and risk of cardiovascular events, death, and heart failure in diabetic and nondiabetic individuals. JAMA 2001; 286:421–426.
202. Asselbergs FW, Hillege HL, van Gilst WH. Framingham score and microalbuminuria: combined future targets for primary prevention? Kidney Int Suppl 2004; 92:S111–S114.

203. Go AS, Chertow GM, Fan D, McCulloch CE, Hsu CY. Chronic kidney disease and the risks of death, cardiovascular events, and hospitalization. N Engl J Med 2004; 351:1296–1306.
204. Attvall S, Fowelin J, Lager I, Von Schenck H, Smith U. Smoking induces insulin resistance—a potential link with the insulin resistance syndrome. J Intern Med 1993; 233:327–332.
205. Madsbad S, McNair P, Christensen MS, Christiansen C, Faber OK, Binder C, Transbol I. Influence of smoking on insulin requirement and metabolic status in diabetes mellitus. Diabetes Care 1980; 3:41–43.
206. Eliasson B. Cigarette smoking and diabetes. Prog Cardiovasc Dis 2003; 45:405–413.
207. Axelsen M, Eliasson B, Joheim E, Lenner RA, Taskinen MR, Smith U. Lipid intolerance in smokers. J Intern Med 1995; 237:449–455.
208. Mero N, Syvanne M, Eliasson B, Smith U, Taskinen MR. Postprandial elevation of ApoB-48-containing triglyceride-rich particles and retinyl esters in normolipemic males who smoke. Arterioscler Thromb Vasc Biol 1997; 17:2096–2102.
209. Eliasson M, Lundblad D, Hagg E. Cardiovascular risk factors in young snuff-users and cigarette smokers. J Intern Med 1991; 230:17–22.
210. Ambrose JA, Barua RS. The pathophysiology of cigarette smoking and cardiovascular disease: an update. J Am Coll Cardiol. 2004; 43:1731–1737.
211. Stevens RJ, Kothari V, Adler AI, Stratton IM. United kingdom prospective diabetes study (UKPDS) group. The UKPDS risk engine: a model for the risk of coronary heart disease in Type II diabetes (UKPDS 56). Clin Sci (Lond). 2001; 101:671–679.
212. Kothari V, Stevens RJ, Adler AI, et al. UKPDS 60: risk of stroke in type 2 diabetes estimated by the UK prospective diabetes study risk engine. Stroke 2002; 33:1776–1781.
213. Adler AI, Stevens RJ, Neil A, Stratton IM, Boulton AJ, Holman RR. UKPDS 59: Hyperglycemia and other potentially modifiable risk factors for peripheral vascular disease in type 2 diabetes. Diabetes Care 2002; 25:894–899.
214. D Al-Delaimy WK, Willett WC, Manson JE, Speizer FE, Hu FB. Smoking and mortality among women with type 2 diabetes: The Nurses' Health Study cohort. Diabetes Care 2001; 24:2043–2048.
215. Chaturvedi N, Stevens L, Fuller JH. Which features of smoking determine mortality risk in former cigarette smokers with diabetes? The world health organization multinational study group. Diabetes Care 1997; 20:1266–1272.
216. UK Prospective diabetes study group: intensive blood-glucose control with sulfonylureas or insulin compared with conventional treatment and risk of complications in patients with type 2 diabetes (UKPDS 33). Lancet 1998; 352:837–853.
217. DCCT research group. The effect of intensive treatment of diabetes on the development and progression of long-term complications insulin-dependent diabetes mellitus. N Engl Med 1993; 329:977–986.
218. Stratton IM, Adler AI, Neil HA, et al. Association of glycaemia with macrovascular and microvascular complications of type 2 diabetes (UKPDS 35): prospective observational study. BMJ 2000; 321:405–412.
219. Knatterud GL, Klimt CR, Levin ME, Jacobson ME, Goldner MG. Effects of hypoglycemic agents on vascular complications in patients with adult-onset diabetes. VII. Mortality and selected nonfatal events with insulin treatment. JAMA. 1978; 240:37–42.
220. Cleveland JC Jr, Meldrum DR, Cain BS, Banerjee A, Harken AH. Oral sulfonylurea hypoglycemic agents prevent ischemic preconditioning in human myocardium: two paradoxes revisited. Circulation 1997; 96:29–32.
221. Garratt KN, Brady PA, Hassinger NL, Grill DE, Terzic A, Holmes DR Jr. Sulfonylurea drugs increase early mortality in patients with diabetes mellitus after direct angioplasty for acute myocardial infarction. J Am Coll Cardiol 1999; 33:119–124.
222. Esposito K, Giugliano D, Nappo F, Marfella R; Campanian postprandial hyperglycemia study group. Regression of carotid atherosclerosis by control of postprandial hyperglycemia in type 2 diabetes mellitus. Circulation 2004; 110:214–219.
223. Abraira C, Duckworth W, McCarren M, et al. VA Cooperative study of glycemic control and complications in diabetes mellitus Type 2. Design of the cooperative study on glycemic control and complications in diabetes mellitus type 2: veterans affairs diabetes trial. J Diabetes Complications 2003; 17:314–322.
224. Nathan DM, Lachin J, Cleary P, et al. Diabetes control and complications trial; Epidemiology of diabetes interventions and complications research group. Intensive diabetes therapy and carotid intima-media thickness in type 1 diabetes mellitus. N Engl J Med. 2003; 348:2294–30.
225. Malmberg K, Ryden L, Efendic S, et al. Randomized trial of insulin-glucose infusion followed by subcutaneous insulin treatment in diabetic patients with acute myocardial infarction (DIGAMI study): effects on mortality at 1 year. J Am Coll Cardiol 1995; 26:57–65.
226. Malmberg K. Prospective randomised study of intensive insulin treatment on long term survival after acute myocardial infarction in patients with diabetes mellitus. DIGAMI (Diabetes mellitus, insulin glucose infusion in acute myocardial infarction) study group. BMJ. 1997; 314:1512–1515.
227. Malmberg K, Norhammar A, Wedel H, Ryden L. Glycometabolic state at admission: important risk marker of mortality in conventionally treated patients with diabetes mellitus and acute myocardial infarction: long-term results from the diabetes and insulin-glucose infusion in acute myocardial infarction (DIGAMI) study. Circulation 1999; 99:2626–2632.

228. Malmberg K, Ryden L, Wedel H, et al. DIGAMI 2 Investigators. Intense metabolic control by means of insulin in patients with diabetes mellitus and acute myocardial infarction (DIGAMI 2): effects on mortality and morbidity. Eur Heart J 2005; 26:650–661.

229. van den Berghe G, Wouters P, Weekers F, et al. Intensive insulin therapy in the critically ill patients. N Engl J Med 2001; 345:1359–1367. ICU

230. Carr JM, Sellke FW, Fey M, et al. Implementing tight glucose control after coronary artery bypass surgery. Ann Thorac Surg 2005; 80:902–909.

231. Langouche L, Vanhorebeek I, Vlasselaerxxs D, et al. Insulin therapy protects the central and peripheral nervous system of intensive care patients. Neurology 2005; 64:1348–1353.

232. DeFronzo RA, Barzilai N, Simonson DC. Mechanism of metformin action in obese and lean noninsulin-dependent diabetic subjects. J Clin Endocrinol Metab 1991; 73:1294–1301.

233. DeFronzo RA, Goodman AM. Efficacy of metformin in patients with non-insulin-dependent diabetes mellitus: the multicenter metformin study group. N Engl J Med 1995; 333:541–549.

234. Fontbonne A, Charles MA, Juhan-Vague I, et al. The effect of metformin on the metabolic abnormalities associated with upper-body fat distribution. BIGPRO Study Group Diabetes Care 1996; 19:920–926.

235. Mather KJ, Verma S, Anderson TJ. Improved endothelial function with metformin in type 2 diabetes mellitus. J Am Coll Cardiol 2001; 37:1344–1350.

236. Caballero AE, Delgado A, Aguilar-Salinas CA, et al. The differential effects of metformin on markers of endothelial activation and inflammation in subjects with impaired glucose tolerance: a placebo-controlled, randomized clinical trial. J Clin Endocrinol Metab 2004; 89:3943–3948.

237. UK prospective diabetes study group: effect of intensive blood-glucose control with metformin on complications in over-weight patients with type 2 diabetes (UK-PDS 34). Lancet 1998; 352:854–865.

238. Johnson JA, Majumdar SR, Simpson SH, Toth EL. Decreased mortality associated with the use of metformin compared with sulfonylurea monotherapy in type 2 diabetes. Diabetes Care 2002; 25:2244–2248.

239. Eurich DT, Majumdar SR, McAlister FA, Tsuyuki RT, Johnson JA. Improved clinical outcomes associated with metformin in patients with diabetes and heart failure. Johnson Diabetes Care 2005; 28:2345–2351.

240. Yki-Jarvinen H. Thiazolidinediones. New Engl J Med 2004; 351:1106–1118.

241. Reynolds K, Goldberg RB. Thiazolidinediones: beyond glycemic control. Trends in Endocrinol Metab 2005. In Press.

242. Spiegelman BM. PPAR-gamma: adipogenic regulator and thiazolidinedione receptor. Diabetes. 1998; 47:507–514.

243. Wellen KE, Uysal KT, Wiesbrock S, Yang Q, Chen H, Hotamisligil GS. Interaction of tumor necrosis factor-alpha- and thiazolidinedione-regulated pathways in obesity. Endocrinology 2004; 145:2214–2220.

244. Ouchi N, Kihara S, Funahashi T, Matsuzawa Y, Walsh K. Obesity, adiponectin and vascular inflammatory disease. Curr Opin Lipidol 2003; 14:561–566.

245. Da Ros R, Assaloni R, Ceriello A. The preventive anti-oxidant action of thiazolidinediones: a new therapeutic prospect in diabetes and insulin resistance. Diabet Med 2004; 21:1249–1252.

246. Caballero AE, Saouaf R, Lim SC, et al. The effects of troglitazone, an insulin-sensitizing agent, on the endothelial function in early and late type 2 diabetes: a placebo-controlled randomized clinical trial. Metabolism 2003; 52:173–180.

247. Li D, Chen K, Sinha N, et al. The effects of PPARγ ligand pioglitazone on platelet aggregation and arterial thrombus formation. Cardiovasc Research 2005; 65:907–912.

248. Zhang L, Chawla A. Role of PPARgamma in macrophage biology and atherosclerosis. Trends Endocrinol Metab 2004; 15:500–505.

249. Li AC, Brown KK, Silvestre MJ, Willson TM, Palinski W, Glass CK. Peroxisome proliferator-activated receptor gamma ligands inhibit development of atherosclerosis in LDL receptor-deficient mice. J Clin Invest 2000; 106:523–531.

250. Goldberg RB, Kendall DM, Deeg MA, et al. GLAI study investigators. A comparison of lipid and glycemic effects of pioglitazone and rosiglitazone in patients with type 2 diabetes and dyslipidemia. Diabetes Care 2005; 28:1547–1554.

251. Buse JB, Rubin CJ, Frederich R, et al. Muraglitazar, a dual (alpha/gamma) PPAR activator: a randomized, double-blind, placebo-controlled, 24-week monotherapy trial in adult patients with type 2 diabetes. Clin Ther 2005; 27:1181–1195.

252. Dormandy JA, Charbonnel B, Eckland DJ, et al. Secondary prevention of macrovascular events in patients with type 2 diabetes in the PROactive study (PROspective pioglitAzone clinical trial in macrovascular events): a randomised controlled trial. Lancet 2005; 366:1279–1289.

253. Yki-Jarvinen H. The PROactive study: some answers, many questions. Lancet. 2005; 366:1241–1242.

254. Masoudi FA, Inzucchi SE, Wang Y, Havranek EP, Foody JM, Krumholz HM. Thiazolidinediones, metformin, and outcomes in older patients with diabetes and heart failure: an observational study. Circulation 2005; 111:583–590.

255. Hartung DM, Touchette DR, Bultemeier NC, Haxby DG. Risk of hospitalization for heart failure associated with thiazolidinedione therapy: a medicaid claims-based case-control study. Pharmacotherapy 2005; 10:1329–1336.

256. Karter AJ, Ahmed AT, Liu J, Moffet HH, Parker MM. Pioglitazone initiation and subsequent hospitalization for congestive heart failure. Diabet Med 2005; 22:986–993.

257. Shah M, Kolandaivelu A, Fearon WF. Pioglitazone-induced heart failure despite normal left ventricular function. Am J Med 2004; 117:973–974.

258. Metformin and heart failure: innocent until proven guilty. Diabetes Care 2005; 28:2585–2587.

259. Guazzi M, Tumminello G, Matturri M, Guazzi MD. Insulin ameliorates exercise ventilatory efficiency and oxygen uptake in patients with heart failure-type 2 diabetes comorbidity. J Am Coll Cardiol 2003; 2:1044–1050.

260. Miyazaki Y, Mahankali A, Matsuda M, et al. Effect of pioglitazone on abdominal fat distribution and insulin sensitivity in type 2 diabetic patients. J Clin Endocrinol Metab 2002; 87:2784–2791.

261. Coutinho M, Gerstein HC, Wang Y, Yusuf S. The relationship between glucose and incident cardiovascular events: a metaregression analysis of published data from 20 studies of 95,783 individuals followed for 12.4 years. Diabetes Care 1999; 22:233–240.(80)

262. Haffner SM, Stern MP, Hazuda HP, Mitchell BD, Patterson K. Cardiovascular risk factors in confirmed prediabetic individuals. Does the clock for coronary heart disease start ticking before the onset of clinical diabetes? JAMA 1990; 263:2893–2898.(57)

263. 264. 264. _Hu FB, Stampfer MJ, Haffner SM, Solomon CG, Willett WC, Manson JE. Elevated risk of cardiovascular disease prior to clinical diagnosis of type 2 diabetes. Diabetes Care 2002; 25:1129–1134.

264. Orchard TJ, Temprosa M, Goldberg R, et al. Diabetes prevention program research group. The effect of metformin and intensive lifestyle intervention on the metabolic syndrome: the diabetes prevention program randomized trial. Ann Intern Med 2005; 142:611–619.

265. The diabetes prevention program research group. Lipid, lipoproteins, C-reactive protein and hemostatic factors at baseline in the diabetes prevention program. Diabetes Care 2005; 28:2472–2479.

266. Ratner R, Goldberg R, Haffner S, et al. Diabetes prevention program research group. Impact of intensive lifestyle and metformin therapy on cardiovascular disease risk factors in the diabetes prevention program. Diabetes Care 2005; 28:888–894.(132)

267. 269. _Chiasson JL, Josse RG, Gomis R, Hanefeld M, Karasik A, Laakso M. STOP–NIDDM trail research group. Acarbose for prevention of type 2 diabetes mellitus: the STOP–NIDDM randomised trial. Lancet 2002; 359:2072–2077.

268. Chiasson JL, Josse RG, Gomis R, Hanefeld M, Karasik A, Laakso M; STOP–NIDDM trial research group. Acarbose treatment and the risk of cardiovascular disease and hypertension in patients with impaired glucose tolerance: the STOP–NIDDM trial. JAMA 2003; 290:486–494.

269. Ohkubo Y, Kishikawa H, Araki E, et al. Intensive insulin therapy prevents the progression of diabetic microvascular complications in Japanese patients with non-insulin-dependent diabetes mellitus: a randomized prospective 6-year study. Diabetes Res Clin Pract 1995; 28:103–117.

270. American Diabetes Association: clinical practice recommendations 2003. Standards of medical care for patients with diabetes mellitus. Diabetes Care 2003; 26 (S1):S33–S50.

271. Meltzer S, Leiter L, Daneman D,et al. Clinical practice guidelines for the management of diabetes in Canada. Canadian Diabetes Association CMAJ 1998; 159(Suppl 8):S1–S29.

272. A desktop guide to type 2 diabetes mellitus: european diabetes policy group 1999. Diabet Med 1999; 16:716–730.

273. The American association of clinical endocrinologists medical guidelines for the management of diabetes mellitus: the AACE system of intensive diabetes self-management—2000 update. Endocr Pract 2000; 6:43–84.

274. European guidelines on cardiovascular prevention in clinical practice. Third joint task force of european and other societies on cardiovascular prevention in clinical practice. Executive summary. Eur Heart J 2003; 24:1601–1610.

275. Sheard NF, Clark NG, Brand-Miller JC, et al. Dietary carbohydrate (amount and type) in the prevention and management of diabetes (ADA statement). Diabetes Care 2004; 27:2266–2271.

276. Klein S, Sheard NF, Pi-Sunyer X, et al. Weight management through lifestyle modification for the prevention and management of type 2 diabetes: rationale and strategies: a statement of the american diabetes association, the north american association for the study of obesity, and the american society for clinical nutrition. Diabetes Care 2004; 27:2067–2073.

277. Knowler WC, Barrett-Connor E, Fowler SE, et al. Diabetes prevention program research group. Reduction in the incidence of type 2 diabetes with lifestyle intervention or metformin. N Engl J Med 2002; 346:393–403.

278. Samaha FF, Iqbal N, Seshadri P, et al. A low-carbohydrate as compared with a low-fat diet in severe obesity. N Engl J Med 2003; 348:2074–2081.

279. US Department of Health and Human Services: Physical Activity and Health: A Report of the Surgeon General: Centers for Disease Control and Prevention and National Center for Chronic Disease Prevention and Health Promotion. 1996. Washington, DC, U.S. Government Printing Office, 1996.

280. Vettor R, Serra R, Fabris R, Pagano C, Federspil G. Effect of sibutramine on weight management and metabolic control in type 2 diabetes: a meta-analysis of clinical studies. Diabetes Care 2005; 28:942–949.

281. O'Meara S, Riemsma R, Shirran L, Mather L, ter Riet G. A systematic review of the clinical effectiveness of orlistat used for the management of obesity. Obes Rev 2004; 5:51–68.

282. Pinkney J, Kerrigan D. Current status of bariatric surgery in the treatment of type 2 diabetes. Obes Rev 2004; 5:69–78.
283. Haffner SM, Alexander CM, Cook TJ, et al. Reduced coronary events in simvastatin treated patients with coronary heart disease and diabetes or impaired fasting glucose levels. Arch Intern Med 1999; 159:2661–2667.
284. Goldberg RB, Mellies MJ, Sacks FM, et al. Cardiovascular events and their reduction with pravastatin in diabetic and glucose-intolerant myocardial infarction survivors with average cholesterol levels. Subgroup analysis in the cholesterol and recurrent events (CARE) trial. Circulation 1998; 98:2513–2519.
285. Keech A, Colquhoun D, Best J, et al. LIPID study group. Secondary prevention of cardiovascular events with long-term pravastatin in patients with diabetes or impaired fasting glucose. Results from the LIPID trial. Diabetes Care 2003; 26:2713–2721.
286. Shepherd J, Cobbe SM, Ford I, et al. Prevention of coronary heart disease with pravastatin in men with hypercholesterolemia. West of scotland coronary prevention study group. N Engl J Med 1995; 333:1301–1307.
287. Downs JR, Clearfield M, Weis S, et al. Primary prevention of acute coronary events with lovastatin in men and women with average cholesterol levels: results of AFCAPS/TexCAPS. JAMA 1998; 279:1615–1622.
288. The ALLHAT officers and coordinators for the ALLHAT collaborative research group. Major outcomes in moderately hypercholesterolemic, hypertensive patients randomized to pravastatin vs. usual care: the antihypertensive and lipid-lowering treatment to prevet heart attack trial (ALLHAT–LLT). JAMA 2002; 288:2998–3007.
289. Sever PS, Poulter NR, Dahlof B, et al. Reduction in cardiovascular events with atorvastatin in 2,532 patients with type 2 diabetes: anglo-scandinavian cardiac outcomes trial—lipid-lowering arm (ascot-lla). Diabetes Care 2005; 28:1151–1157.
290. Heart protection study collaborative group. MCR/BHF heart protection study of cholesterol-lowering with simvastatin in 5963 people with diabetes: a randomized placebo-controlled trial. Lancet 2003; 361:2005–2016.
291. Heart protection study collaborative group. MCR/BHF heart protection study of cholesterol lowering with simvastatin in 20,536 high-risk individuals: a randomized placebo-controlled trial. Lancet 2002; 360:7–22.
292. Colhoun HM, Betteridge DJ, Durrington PN, et al. Primary prevention of cardiovascular disease with atorvastatin in type 2 diabetes in the collaborative atorvastatin diabetes study (CARDS): multicentre randomized placebo-controlled trial. Lancet 2004; 364:685–696.
293. Koskinen P, Manttari M, Manninen V, Huttunen JK, Heinonen OP, Frick MH. Coronary heart disease incidence in NIDDM patients in the helsinki heart study. Diabetes Care 1992; 15:820–825.
294. The bip study group. Secondary prevention by raising HDL cholesterol and reducing triglycerides in patients with coronary artery disease. The bezafibrate infarction prevention (BIP) study. Circulation 2000; 102:21–27.
295. Rubins HB, Robins SJ, Collins D, et al. Gemfibrozil for the secondary prevention of coronary heart disease in men with low levels of high-density lipoprotein cholesterol. N Engl J Med 1999; 341:410–418.
296. The field study investigators. Effects of long-term fenofibrate therapy on cardiovascular events in 9795 people with type 2 diabetes mellitus (the FIELD study): randomised controlled trial Lancet 2005; 366:1849–1861.
297. Rubins HB, Robins SJ, Collins D, et al. Diabetes, plasma insulin, and cardiovascular disease. Subgroup analysis from the department of veterans affairs high-density lipoprotein intervention trial (VA–HIT). Arch Intern Med 2002; 162:2597–2604.
298. Diabetes atherosclerosis intervention study investigators. Effect of fenofibrate on progression of coronary-artery disease in type 2 diabetes: the diabetes atherosclerosis intervention study, a randomized study. Lancet 2001; 357:905–910.
299. The coronary drug project research group. Clofibrate and niacin in coronary heart disease. JAMA 1975; 231:360–381.
300. Canner PL, Furberg CD, Terrin ML, McGovern ME. Benefits of niacin by glycemic status in patients with healed myocardial infarction (from the coronary drug project). Am J Cardiol 2005; 95:254–257.
301. Brown BG, Zhao XQ, Chait A, et al. Simvastatin and niacin, antioxidant vitamins, or the combination for prevent of coronary disease. N Eng J Med 2001; 345:1583–1592.
302. Grundy SM, Cleeman JI, Merz CN, et al. Coordinating committee of the national cholesterol education program. Coordinating committee of the national cholesterol education program: national heart, lung, and blood institute; american college of cardiology foundation; americam heart association. Implications of recent clinical trials for the national cholesterol education program adult treatment panel III guidelines. Circulation 2004; 110:227–239.
303. LaRosa JC, Grundy SM, Waters DD, et al. Treating to new targets (TNT) investigators. Treating to New Targets (TNT) Investigators. Intensive lipid lowering with atorvastatin in patients with stable coronary disease. N Engl J Med 2005; 352:1425–1435.
304. American diabetes association. Standards of medical care in diabetes. Diabetes Care 2005; 28(S1):S4–S36.

305. Genest J, Frohlich J, Fodor G, McPherson R; Working Group on hypercholesterolemia and other dyslipidemias. Recommendations for the management of dyslipidemia and the prevention of cardiovascular disease: summary of the 2003 update. CMAJ 2003; 169:921–924.

306. American diabetes association. Evidence-based nutrition principles and recommendations for the treatment and prevention of diabetes and related complications. Diabetes Care 2003; 26:S51–S61.

307. Yu-Poth S, Zhao G, Etherton T, Naglak M, Jonnalagadda S, Kris-Etherton PM. Effects of the national cholesterol education program's step I and II dietary intervention program on cardiovascular disease risk factors: a meta-analysis. Am J Clin Nutr 1999; 69:632–646.

308. Temme EH, Van Hoydonck PG, Schouten EG, Kesteloot H. Effects of a plant sterol-enriched spread on serum lipids and lipoproteins in mildly hypercholesterolemic subjects. Acta Cardiol 2002; 57:111–115.

309. Gylling H, Miettinen TA. Serum cholesterol and cholesterol and lipoprotein metabolism in hypercholesterolemic NIDDM patients before and during sitostanol ester-margarine treatment, Diabetologia 1994; 37:773–780.

310. Chandalia M, Garg A, Lutjohann D, von Bergmann K, Grundy SM, Brinkley LJ. Beneficial effects of high dietary fiber intake in patients with type 2 diabetes mellitus. N Eng J Med 2000; 342:1392–1398.

311. Anderson JW, Allgood LD, Turner J, Oeltgen PR, Daggy BP. Effects of psyllium on glucose and serum lipid responses in men with type 2 diabetes and hypercholesterolemia. Am J Clin Nutr 1999; 70:466–473.

312. Turley ML, Skeaff CM, Mann JI, Cox B. The effect of a low-fat, high-carbohydrate diet on serum high density lipoprotein cholesterol and triglyceride. Eur J Clin Nutr 1998; 52:728–732.

313. Garg A. High-monounsaturated-fat diets for patients with diabetes mellitus: a meta-analysis. Am J Clin Nutr 1998; 67:577S–582S.

314. Bravata DM, Sanders L, Huang J, et al. Efficacy and safety of low-carbohydrate diets. A systematic review. JAMA 2003; 289:1837–1850.

315. Emanuele N, Azad N, Abraira C, et al. Effect of intensive glycemic control on fibrinogen, lipids, and lipoproteins: veterans affairs coperative study in type II diabetes mellitus. Arch Intern Med 1998; 18:2485–2490.

316. Palumbo PJ. Metformin: effects on cardiovascular risk factors in patients with non-insulin-dependent diabetes mellitus. J Diabetes Complications 1998; 12:110–119.

317. Robins SJ, Collins D, Wittes JT, et al. VA-HIT study group. Veterans affairs high-density lipoprotein intervention trial. VA-HIT study group. Veterans affairs high-density lipoprotein intervention trial. Relation of gemfibrozil treatment and lipid levels with major coronary events: VA-HIT: a randomized controlled trial. JAMA 2001; 285:1585–1591.

318. Scharnagl H, Schinker R, Gierens H, Nauck M, Wieland H, Marz W. Effect of atorvastatin, simvastatin, and lovastatin on the metabolism of cholesterol and triacylglycerides in HepG2 cells. Biochemical Pharmacology 2001; 62:1545–1555.

319. Pontrelli L, Parris W, Adeli K, Cheung RC. Atorvastatin treatment beneficially alters the lipoprotein profile and increases low-density lipoprotein particle diameter in patients with combined dyslipidemia and impaired fasting glucose/type 2 diabetes. Metabolism 2002; 51:334–342.

320. Wagner AM, Perez A, Zapico E, Ordonez-Llanos J. Non-HDL cholesterol and apolipoprotein B in the dyslipidemic classification of type 2 diabetic patients. Diabetes Care 2003; 26:2048–2051.

321. Sniderman AD, Lamarche B, Tilley J, Seccombe D, Frohlich J. Hypertriglyceridemic hyperapoB in type 2 diabetes. Diabetes Care 2002; 25:579–582.

322. Friedberg CE, Janssen MJ, Heine RJ, Grobbee DE. Fish oil and glycemic control in diabetes. A meta-analysis. Diabetes Care 1998; 21:494–500.

323. Woodman RJ, Mori TA, Burke V, et al. Effects of purified eicosapentaenoic and docosahexaenoic acids on glycemic control, blood pressure, and serum lipids in type 2 diabetic patients with treated hypertension. Am J Clin Nutr 2002; 76:1007–1015.

324. Kris-Etherton P, Daniels SR, Eckel RH, et al. Summary of the scientific conference on dietary fatty acids and cardiovascular health: conference summary from the nutrition committee of the american heart association. Circulation 2001; 103:1034–1039.

325. Taylor AJ, Sullenberger LE, Lee HJ, Lee JK, Grace KA. Arterial Biology for the investigation of the treatment effects of reducing cholesterol (ARBITER) 2: a double-blind, placebo-controlled study of extended-release niacin on atherosclerosis progression in secondary prevention patients treated with statins. Circulation 2004; 110:3512–3517.

326. Gagne C, Bays HE, Weiss SR, et al. Ezetimibe study group. Efficacy and safety of ezetimibe added to ongoing statin therapy for treatment of patients with primary hypercholesterolemia. Am J Cardiol 2002; 90:1084–1091.

327. Crouse JR III. Hypertriglyceridemia: a contraindication to the use of bile acid binding resins. Am J Med 1987; 83:243–248.

328. Capuzzi DM, Morgan JM, Weiss RJ, Chitra RR, Hutchinson HG, Cressman MD. Beneficial effects of rosuvastatin alone and in combination with extended-release niacin in patients with a combined hyperlipidemia and low high-density lipoprotein cholesterol levels. Am J Cardiol 2003; 91:1304–1310.

329. Athyros VG, Papageorgiou AA, Athyrou VV, Demitriadis DS, Kontopoulos AG. Atorvastatin and micronized fenofibrate alone and in combination in type 2 diabetes with combined hyperlipidemia. Diabetes Care 2002; 1198–1202.

330. Shepherd J, Betteridge J, Van Gaal L, European consensus panel. Nicotinic acid in the management of dyslipidaemia associated with diabetes and metabolic syndrome: a position paper developed by a european consensus panel. Curr Med Res Opin 2005; 21:665–682.

331. Carlson LA, Hamsten A, AsplaundA. Pronounced lowering of serum levels of lipoprotein Lp(a) in hyperlipidemic subjects treated with nicotinic acid. J Intern Med 1989; 226:271–276.

332. Superko HR, Krauss RM. Differential effects of nicotinic acid in subjects with different LDL subclass patterns. Atherosclerosis 1992; 95:69–76.

333. Omar MA, Wilson JP, Cox TS. Rhabdomyolysis and HMG-CoA reductase inhibitors. Ann Pharmacother 2001; 35:1096–1107.

334. Elam MB, Hunninghake DB, Davis KB, et al. Effect of niacin on lipid and lipoprotein levels and glycemic control in patients with diabetes and peripheral arterial disease: the ADMIT study. A randomized trial. JAMA 2000; 284:1263–1270.

335. Grundy SM, Vega GL, McGovern ME, et al. Diabetes multicenter research group. Efficacy, safety, and tolerability of once-daily niacin for the treatment of dyslipidemia associated with type 2 diabetes. Arch Intern Med 2002; 162:1568–1576.

336. Shepherd J. Fibrates and statins in the treatment of hyperlipidemia: an appraisal of their efficacy and safety. Euro Heart J 1995; 16:5–13.

337. Athyros VG, Papageorgiou AA, Hatzikonstandinou HA, et al. Safety and efficacy of long-term statin-fibrate combinations in patients with refractory familial combined hyperlipidemia. Am J Cardiol 1997; 80:608–613.

338. Pierce LR, Wysowski DK, Gross TP. Myopathy and rhabdomyolysis associated with lovastatin-gemfibrozil combination therapy. JAMA 1990; 264:71–75.

339. Tal A, Rajeshawari M, Isley W. Rhabdomyolysis associated with simvastatin-gemfibrozil therapy. Southern Med J 1997; 90:546–547.

340. Pogson G, Kindred L, Carper B. Rhabdomyolysis and renal failure associated with cerivastatin-gemfibrozil combination therapy. Am J Card 1999; 83:1146.

341. Duell PB, Connor WE, Illingworth DR. Rhabdomyolysis after taking atorvastatin with gemfibrozil. Am J Cardiol 1998; 81:368–369.

342. Ellen RL, McPherson R. Long term efficacy and safety of fenofibrate and a statin in the treatment of combined hyperlipidemia. Am J Cardiol 1998; 81:60B–65B.

343. Iliadis EA, Rosenson RS. Long-term safety of pravastatin-gemfibrozil therapy in mixed hyperlipidemia. Clin Cardiol 1999; 22:25–28.

344. Murdock DK, Murdock AK, Murdock RW. Long-term safety and efficacy of combination gemfibrozil and HMG-CoA reductase inhibitors for the treatment of mixed lipid disorders. Am Heart J 1999; 138:151–155.

345. Vega GL, Ma PT, Cater NB, et al. Effects of adding fenofibrate (200mg/day) to simvastatin (10mg/day) in patients with combined hyperlipidemia and metabolic syndrome. Am J Cardiol 2003; 91:956–960.

346. Prueksaritanont T, Zhao JJ, Ma B, et al. Mechanistic studies on metabolic interactions between gemfibrozil and statins. Pharmacol Exp Ther 2002; 301:1042–1051.

347. Prueksaritanont T, Tang C, Qiu Y, Mu L, Subramanian R, Lin JH. Effects of fibrates on metabolism of statins in human hepatocytes. Drug Metabolism and Disposition 2002; 30:1280–1287.

348. Jones PH, Davidson MH. Reporting rate of rhabdomyolysis with fenofibrate + statin versus gemfibrozil + any statin. Am J Cardiol 2005; 95:120–122.

349. K/DOQI clinical practice guidelines for management of dyslipidemias in patients with kidney disease. Am J Kidney Dis 2003; 41:1–91.

350. Curb JD, Pressel SL, Cutler JA, et al. Effect of diuretic-based antihypertensive treatment on cardiovascular disease risk in older diabetic patients with isolated systolic hypertension. Systolic hypertension in the elderly program cooperative research group. JAMA 1996; 276:1886–1892.

351. Hansson L, Zanchetti A, Carruthers SG, et al. Effects of intensive blood-pressure lowering and low-dose aspirin in patients with hypertension: principal results of the hypertension optimal treatment (HOT) randomised trial. HOT study group. Lancet 1998; 351:1755–1762.

352. Tuomilehto J, Rastenyte D, Birkenhager WH, et al. Effects of calcium-channel blockade in older patients with diabetes and systolic hypertension. Systolic hypertension in europe trial investigators. N Engl J Med 1999; 340:677–684.

353. Effects of ramipril on cardiovascular and microvascular outcomes in people with diabetes mellitus: results of the HOPE study and MICRO-HOPE substudy. Heart outcomes prevention study investigators. Lancet 2000; 355:253–259.

354. Svensson P, de Faire U, Sleight P, Yusuf S, Ostergren J. Evaluation comparative effects of ramipril on ambulatory and office blood pressures: a HOPE substudy. Hypertension 2001; 38:E28–E32.

355. UK prospective diabetes study group tight blood pressure control and risk of macrovascular and microvascular complications in type 2 diabetes: UKPDS 38. BMJ 1998; 317:703–713.

356. UK prospective diabetes study group. Efficacy of atenolol and captopril in reducing risk of macrovascular and microvascular complications in type 2 diabetes: UKPDS 39. BMJ 1998; 317:713–720.

357. Lindholm LH, Hansson L, Ekbom T, Dahlof B, Lamke J, Linjer E, et al. Comparison of antihypertensive treatments in preventing cardiovascular events in elderly diabetic patients: results from the swedish trial in old patients with hypertension-2. STOP Hypertension–2 study group. J Hypertens 2000; 18:1671–1675.

358. Hansson L, Lindholm LH, Niskanen L, et al. Effect of angiotensin-converting-enzyme inhibition compared with conventional therapy on cardiovascular morbidity and mortality in hypertension: the captopril prevention project (CAPPP) randomised trial. Lancet 1999; 353:611–616.

359. Wing LM, Reid CM, Ryan P, et al. Second australian national blood pressure study group. A comparison of outcomes with angiotensin-converting—enzyme inhibitors and diuretics for hypertension in the elderly. N Engl J Med 2003; 348:583–592.

360. Whelton PK, Barzilay J, Cushman WC, et al. ALLHAT collaborative research group. Clinical outcomes in antihypertensive treatment of type 2 diabetes, impaired fasting glucose concentration, and normoglycemia: antihypertensive and lipid-lowering treatment to prevent heart attack trial (ALLHAT). Arch Intern Med 2005; 165:1401–1409.

361. Estacio RO, Jeffers BW, Hiatt WR, Biggerstaff SL, Gifford N, Schrier RW. The effect of nisoldipine as compared with enalapril on cardiovascular outcomes in patients with non-insulin-dependent diabetes and hypertension. N Engl J Med 1998; 338:645–652.

362. Tatti P, Pahor M, Byington RP, Di Mauro P, Guarisco R, Strollo G, Strollo F. Outcome results of the fosinopril versus amlodipine cardiovascular events randomized trial (FACET) in patients with hypertension and NIDDM. Diabetes Care 1998; 21:597–603.

363. Major cardiovascular events in hypertensive patients randomized to doxazosin vs chlorthalidone: the antihypertensive and lipid-lowering treatment to prevent heart attack trial (ALLHAT). ALLHAT collaborative research group. JAMA 2000; 283:1967–1975.

364. Lindholm LH, Ibsen H, Dahlof B, et al. LIFE study group. Cardiovascular morbidity and mortality in patients with diabetes in the losartan intervention for endpoint reduction in hypertension study (LIFE): a randomised trial against atenolol. Lancet 2002; 359:1004–1010.

365. Lindholm LH, Dahlof B, Edelman JM, et al. LIFE study group. Effect of losartan on sudden cardiac death in people with diabetes: data from the LIFE study. Lancet 2003; 362:619–620.

366. Dahlof B, Sever PS, Poulter NR, et al. ASCOT investigators. Prevention of cardiovascular events with an antihypertensive regimen of amlodipine adding perindopril as required versus atenolol adding bendroflumethiazide as required, in the anglo-scandinavian cardiac outcomes trial-blood pressure lowering arm (ASCOT-BPLA): a multicentre randomised controlled trial. Lancet 2005; 366:895–906.

367. Poulter NR, Wedel H, Dahlof B, et al. ASCOT investigators. Role of blood pressure and other variables in the differential cardiovascular event rates noted in the anglo-scandinavian cardiac outcomes trial-blood pressure lowering arm (ASCOT-BPLA). Lancet. 2005; 366:907–913.

368. Staessen JA, Birkenhager WH. Evidence that new antihypertensives are superior to older drugs. Lancet 2005; 366:869–871.

369. Chobanian AV, Bakris GL, Black HR, et al. National heart, lung, and blood institute joint national committee on prevention, detection, evaluation, and treatment of high blood pressure; national high blood pressure education program coordinating committee. The seventh report of the joint national committee on prevention, detection, evaluation, and treatment of high blood pressure: the JNC 7 report. JAMA 2003; 289:2560–2572.

370. 2003 European Society of Hypertension–European Society of Cardiology guidelines for the management of arterial hypertension Journal of Hypertension. 2003; 21:1011–1053.

371. Bakris GL, Williams M, Dworkin L, Elliott WJ, Epstein M, Toto R, et al. Preserving renal function in adults with hypertension and diabetes: a consensus approach. National kidney foundation hypertension and diabetes executive committees working group. Am J Kidney Dis 2000; 36:646–661.

372. Snow V, Weiss KB, Mottur-Pilson C, for the Clinical Efficacy Assessment Subcommittee of the American College of Physicians. The evidence base for tight blood pressure control in the management of type 2 diabetes mellitus. Ann Intern Med 2003; 138:587–602.

373. Turnbull F, Neal B, Algert C, et al. Blood pressure lowering treatment trialists' collaboration. Effects of different blood pressure-lowering regimens on major cardiovascular events in individuals with and without diabetes mellitus: results of prospectively designed overviews of randomized trials. Arch Intern Med 2005; 165:1410–1419.

374. Liebson PR, Grandits GA, Dianzumba S, Prineas RJ, Grimm RH, Neaton JD, et al. Comparison of five antihypertensive monotherapies and placebo for change in left-ventricular mass in patients receiving nutritional-hygienic therapy in the treatment of mild hypertension study (TOMHS). Circulation 1995; 91:698–706.

375. Brenner BM, Cooper ME, de Zeeuw D, Keane WF, Mitch WE, Parving HH, et al. Effects of losartan on renal and cardiovascular outcomes in patients with type 2 diabetes and nephropathy. N Engl J Med 2001; 345:861–869.

376. Bakris GL, Weir M. ACE inhibitors and protection against kidney disease progression in patients with type 2 diabetes: what's the evidence. J Clin Hypertens (Greenwich) 2002; 4:420–423.

377. Hamalainen H, Ronnemaa T, Virtanen A, et al. On behalf of the Finnish Diabetes Prevention Study Group. Improved fibrinolysis by an intensive lifestyle intervention in subjects with impaired glucose tolerance. The Finnish Diabetes Prevention Study. Diabetologia. 2005; 48:2248–2253.

378. Lyon CJ, Hsueh WA. Effect of plasminogen activator inhibitor–1 in diabetes mellitus and cardiovascular disease. Am J Med 2003; 115:Suppl 8A:62S–68S.

379. Chu NV, Kong AP, Kim DD, et al. Differential effects of metformin and troglitazone on cardiovascular risk factors in patients with type 2 diabetes. Diabetes Care 2002; 25:542–549.

380. Ceriello A. Fibrinogen and diabetes mellitus: is it time for intervention trials? Diabetologia 1997; 40:731–734.

381. Final report on the aspirin component of the ongoing physicians' health study research group. N Engl J Med 1989; 321:129–135.

382. The ETDRS investigators: Aspirin effects on mortality and morbidity in patients with diabetes mellitus: early treatment diabetic retinopathy study report 14. JAMA 1992; 268:1292–1300.

383. The antithrombotic trialists' collaboration, collaborative meta-analysis of randomized trials of antiplatelet therapy for prevention of death myocardial infarction and stroke in high risk patients. BMJ 2002; 324:71–86.

384. Colwell J. Aspirin for primary prevention of cardiovascular events in diabetes. Diabetes Care 2003; 26:3349–3350.

385. Roffi M, Chew DP, Mukherjee D, et al. Platelet glycoprotein IIb/IIIa inhibitors reduce mortality in diabetic patients with non-ST-segment-elevation acute coronary syndromes. Circulation 2001; 104:2767–2771.

386. American diabetes association: clinical practice recommendations 2003. Aspirin therapy in diabetes. Diabetes Care 2003; 26(S1):S87–S88.

387. Bhatt DL, Marso SP, Hirsch AT, Ringleb PA, Hacke W, Topol EJ. Amplified benefit of clopidogrel versus aspirin in patients with diabetes mellitus. Am J Cardiol 2002; 90(6):625–628.

388. The clopidogrel in unstable angina to prevent recurrent events trial investigators. Effects of clopidogrel in addition to aspirin in patients with acute coronary syndromes without ST-segment elevation. NEJM 2001; 345:494–502.

389. Bhatt DL, Topol EJ; CHARISMA executive committee: clopidogrel added to aspirin versus aspirin alone in secondary prevention and high-risk primary prevention: rationale and design of the clopidogrel for high atherothrombotic risk and ischemic stabilization, management, and avoidance (CHARISMA) trial. Am Heart J 2004; 148:263–268.

390. Angiolillo DJ, Fernandez-Ortiz A, Bernardo E, et al. Platelet function profiles in patients with type 2 diabetes and coronary artery disease on combined aspirin and clopidogrel treatment. Diabetes 2005; 54:2430–2435.

391. Neri Serneri GG, Coccheri S, Marubini E, Violi F. Drug evaluation in atherosclerotic vascular disease in diabetics (DAVID) study group. Picotamide, a combined inhibitor of thromboxane A2 synthase and receptor, reduces 2-year mortality in diabetics with peripheral arterial disease: the DAVID study. Eur Heart J 2004; 25:1845–1852.

392. Colwell JA. American diabetes association. Aspirin therapy in diabetes. Diabetes Care 2003; 26(Suppl 1):S87–S88.

393. American heart association: AHA scientific statement: AHA guidelines for primary prevention of cardiovascular disease and stroke:2002 update. Circulation 2002; 106:388–391.

394. Preventive services task force: aspirin for the primary prevention of cardiovascular events: recommendations and rationale. Ann Intern Med 2002; 136:157–160.

395. Ridker PM, Rifai N, Pfeffer MA, et al. Inflammation, pravastatin, and the risk of coronary events after myocardial infarction in patients with average cholesterol levels. Cholesterol and recurrent events (CARE) investigators. Circulation. 1998; 98:839–844.

396. Ridker PM, Cannon CP, Morrow D, et al. Pravastatin or atorvastatin evaluation and infection therapy-thrombolysis in myocardial infarction 22 (PROVE IT-TIMI 22) Investigators. C-reactive protein levels and outcomes after statin therapy. N Engl J Med 2005; 352:20–28.

397. Starkebaum G, Harlan JM. Endothelial cell injury due to copper-catalyzed hydrogen peroxide generation from homocysteine. J Clin Invest 1986; 77:1370–1376.

398. Meigs JB, Jacques PF, Selhub J, et al. Framingham offspring study: fasting plasma homocysteine levels in the insulin resistance syndrome: framingham offspring study. Diabetes Care 2001; 24:1403–1410.

399. Bonaa K. NORVIT: randomised trial of homocysteine-lowering with B-vitamins for secondary prevention of cardiovascular disease after acute myocardial infarction http://www.escardio.org/congresses/esc_congress_2005/

400. Danesh J, Collins, Peto R. Lipoprotein(a) and coronary heart disease : meta-analysis of prospective studies. Circulation 2000; 102:1082–1085.

401. Haffner SM, Moss SE, Klein BEK, Klein R. Lack of association between lipoprotein(a) concentrations and coronary heart disease mortality in diabetes: the wisconsin epidemiologic study of diabetic retinopathy. Metabolism 1992; 41:194–197.

402. Gazzaruso C, Garzaniti A, Falcone C, Geroldi D, Finardi G, Fratino P. Association of lipoprotein(a) levels and apolipoprotein(a) phenotypes with coronary artery disease in Type 2 diabetic patients and in non-diabetic subjects. Diabet Med 2001; 18:589–594.

403. Peripheral arterial disease in people with diabetes. Diabetes Care 2003; 26:3333–3341.

404. Leng GC, Price JF, Jepson RG: Lipid-lowering for lower limb atherosclerosis (cochrane review). Cochrane Database Syst Rev 2000; 2:CD000123.

405. Gæde P, Vedel P, Larsen N, Jensen GVH, Parving H-H, Pedersen O. Multifactorial intervention and cardiovascular disease in patients with type 2 diabetes. N Engl J Med 2003; 348:383–393.

406. Saydah SH, Fradkin J, Cowie CC. Poor control of risk factors for vascular disease among adults with previously diagnosed diabetes. J Am Med Assoc 2004; 291:335–342.

407. Eliasson B, Cederholm J, Nilsson P, Gudbjornsdottir S. Steering committee of the swedish national diabetes register. The gap between guidelines and reality: Type 2 diabetes in a national diabetes register 1996–2003. Diabet Med 2005; 22:1420–1426.

7 | Management of Elevated Low-Density Lipoprotein Cholesterol

Michael H. Davidson
Rush University Medical Center, Chicago, Illinois, U.S.A.

Jennifer G. Robinson
Departments of Epidemiology and Medicine, College of Public Health, University of Iowa, Iowa City, Iowa, U.S.A.

KEY POINTS

- LDL-C is a critical factor in all stages of atherogenesis and is an independent risk factor in all population studied.
- LDL-C magnifies cardiovascular when other risk factors are present.
- Cardiovascular risk reduction occurs in direct relation to the degree of LDL-C-lowering.
- Intensity of LDL-C-lowering therapy is guided by the level of risk.
- Lifestyle therapy is indicated for all patients with LDL-C above goal.
- Statins are the drugs of choice for reducing cardiovascular risk.
- Combination drug therapy may be considered for patients at high risk.

LOW-DENSITY LIPOPROTEIN AS A CARDIOVASCULAR RISK FACTOR
The Lipid Hypothesis

The lipid hypothesis was first proposed over 150 years ago when Virchow et al. described lipid accumulation as the hallmark of atherosclerotic plaque (1). Fifty years later, Ignatoski, Anitschkow and colleagues, in an experiment evaluating the effect of protein on the kidney, serendipitously found that rabbits developed atherosclerosis when fed a diet high in animal products (2). The biochemist Windhaus went on to elucidate the structure of cholesterol by the end of the second decade of the 20th century (3). As reviewed by Stamler (3), Keys (4), and others (5), as early as 1916, lower serum cholesterol levels and lower coronary heart disease (CHD) event rates were found in native Indonesian populations than in Dutch immigrants and familial hypercholesterolemia (FH) and its association with severe premature atherosclerosis had been described. Following World War I, between-country comparisons showed a "geographical" pathology for atherosclerotic disease. Countries with habitual diets high in cholesterol and fat were noted to have high levels of CHD, whereas atherosclerotic disease was rare in countries with diets high in vegetables and low in fat and cholesterol. As a result of famine and severe shortages of fat during both World Wars, regression of atherosclerosis as well as lower serum cholesterol levels and rates of CHD mortality were found in autopsy studies. When food consumption patterns returned to prewar levels, so did CHD mortality.

By 1941, cholesterol-laden foam cells were established as pivotal players in atherogenesis (6). Following the end of World War II, research into the pathogenesis of atherosclerosis greatly expanded. The multifactorial nature of atherosclerosis was demonstrated in a wide variety of animal models when animals fed cholesterol-supplemented diets developed accelerated atherosclerosis, especially when other risk factors, such as hypertension, were present. Plaque was also shown to regress after discontinuation of the atherogenic diet. These studies also found that circulating cholesterol-containing lipoproteins in plasma were the source of cholesterol in plaque. The Framingham Study, initiated in 1948, was the first prospective cohort study of men and women designed to study cardiovascular disease (CVD) (7). The Framingham researchers adopted the risk factor concept and over the next several decades went on to describe the relationship between risk factors and the lifetime risk of CVD. During the 1950s, metabolic ward studies by Keys, Hegsted, and others quantitated the response of blood cholesterol levels to changes in dietary saturated fat and cholesterol intake (8).

Autopsies of young U.S. soldiers killed in Korea found a high prevalence of coronary atherosclerosis, in contrast to its rarity in similarly aged Koreans (9). Migration studies established that environment, not genetics, was the crucial determinant of serum cholesterol levels and atherosclerotic disease. The best known of these studies, the Ni-Hon-San study, showed that Japanese men in Nipon, Japan, and the cities of Honolulu and San Francisco in the United States had progressively higher serum cholesterol levels accompanied by progressively higher risk of CHD resulting from an increasingly Westernized diet high in animal fat (10). Cross-country comparisons continued to yield similar findings. In the Seven Countries study, conducted between 1958 and 1964 and led by Keys, similar relationships between the mean serum cholesterol for a country and the rate of CHD were found (11). North Karelia, Finland, with a high intake of diary products, had the highest mean serum cholesterol level and the highest rate of CHD while Japan had the lowest levels of both. Comparisons of Bantu with Europeans in South Africa, and of rural and urban Guatelmalans, yielded similar findings (3).

During the late 1950s through the 1990s, more than 65 cohorts in 23 countries on four continents reported a remarkably consistent relationship between total serum cholesterol and CHD risk (3). The Multinational Monitoring of Trends and Determinants in Cardiovascular Disease (MONICA) study alone developed cohorts in 26 countries (12). Many of these studies have now followed participants for up to 30 years, clarifying the relationships between lifetime blood cholesterol levels, other cardiovascular risk factors, and the subsequent development of atherosclerotic coronary heart, cerebrovascular, and peripheral arterial disease. Low-density lipoprotein cholesterol (LDL-C) typically makes up 60% to 70% of total serum cholesterol. Although the earlier epidemiologic studies measured only total serum cholesterol, subsequent studies have found a similarly robust relationship between LDL-C and CVD risk, especially in those with preexisting CVD.

Despite the prodigious amount of data supporting the association between elevated cholesterol levels and CVD risk, final proof of the lipid hypothesis awaited the results of randomized controlled trials. In 1984, the Lipid Research Clinic trial was the first large trial to demonstrate a reduction in the risk of nonfatal and fatal CHD events using cholestyramine, a bile acid sequestering agent, to lower LDL-C (13). This primary-prevention trial enrolled over 3800 men with severe hypercholesterolemia. Those who received cholestyramine had a 13% reduction in LDL-C and a 19% reduction in CHD events after a mean 7.4 years of treatment. However, no reduction in overall mortality was observed, and in fact, a small number of excess deaths occurred in the cholestyramine group; although this did not reach clinical significance, leading major medical figures remained skeptical of the link between cholesterol and CHD risk (14). It was not until the Scandinavian Simavastatin Survival Study (4S) was published that the irrevocable clinical relevance of the lipid hypothesis was finally established (15). In a hypercholesterolemic population of 4444 patients with CHD, a 35% reduction in LDL-C with simvastatin 20 to 40 mg was shown to reduce overall mortality by 30%. In a meta-analysis of placebo-controlled statin trials, each 1% reduction in LDL-C correspondingly lowered the relative risk of nonfatal myocardial infarction (MI), CHD death, and stroke by 1%, regardless of the baseline risk of the population studied (16).

Magnitude of the Relationship

The largest of the prospective cohort studies, the Multiple Risk Factor Intervention Trial (MRFIT), included 361,662 men aged 35 to 57 who were screened in 18 U.S. cities between 1973 and 1975 (17). Prospective mortality data after 12 years of follow-up provide a very precise estimate of the risk associated with different levels of risk factors, which are comparable to other prospective cohort studies (3). In MRFIT, at every level of systolic blood pressure (BP), the risk of CHD death increased in a progressive and marked fashion with higher serum cholesterol levels (Fig. 1). For nonsmokers, whose absolute risk of CHD is two to three times lower than in smokers, elevated cholesterol levels contributed proportionately more to risk than in smokers. The relative risk of CHD death was three- to fourfold higher in the top quintile of cholesterol [245 mg/dL (6.33 mmol) or greater] than in the lowest [less than 180 mg/dL (4.7 mmol)] for nonsmokers. In smokers, relative risk was approximately two- to threefold fold higher in the highest compared to lowest cholesterol quintiles (3). In multivariate analysis, a cholesterol difference of 40 mg/dL (230 vs. 190 mg/dL) increased the risk of CHD death by 29%, a BP difference of 20 mmHg (118–138 mmHg) increased risk by 56%, smoking increased risk by 58%, and diabetes increased risk threefold. Each 1% increase in serum total cholesterol level was associated with an almost 2% higher CHD risk and it was estimated that 46% of excess CHD deaths were due to total cholesterol of 180 mg/dL (≥ 4.65 mmol) or greater (3) (17).

The relationship between serum total cholesterol and CHD mortality appears to be curvilinear in populations with high baseline absolute CHD risk (Fig. 2) (18). In lower-risk populations,

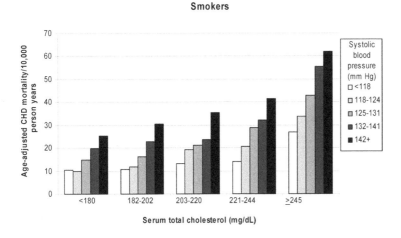

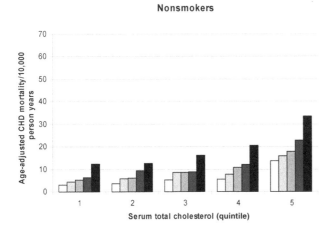

FIGURE 1   Age-adjusted coronary heart disease mortality per 10,000 person years in men aged 35 to 57 years at baseline without diabetes mellitus in the MRFIT over 12 years of follow-up. *Abbreviations*: MRFIT, Multiple Risk Factor Intervention Trial; CHD, coronary heart disease. *Source*: From Ref. 3.

the association between total cholesterol and CHD risk appears to be more linear. When epidemiologic data from populations with varying levels of baseline risk is considered, it appears an LDL-C level above 100 mg/dL (2.58 mmol) [or total cholesterol greater than 150 mg/dL (3.88 mmol)] appears to be atherogenic in both women and men (19,20). In animal models, atherosclerosis generally does not develop until LDL-C levels exceed 80 mg/dL (2.07 mmol). LDL-C levels as low as 25 to 60 mg/dL (0.65–1.55) appear to be sufficient for normal physiologic processes. Newborns have LDL-C levels of approximately 30 mg/dL (0.78 mmol). Although very low–density lipoproteins (VLDL-C) and high-density lipoprotein-cholesterol (HDL-C) also play important in atherogenesis, they have been less well studied. LDL-C has been identified as the primary target for clinical management in the major international guidelines (19,21).

Risk estimates from epidemiologic studies that used one measurement of baseline cholesterol level may "underestimate" the lifetime risk of CHD. Age is also a critical factor in determining the risk associated with LDL-C. In observational studies of primary prevention populations of men, adjustment for regression dilution bias (random fluctuation over time) and surrogate dilution effect (differences in LDL-C are smaller than differences in total cholesterol) showed that a 0.6 mmol (23 mg/dL or about 10%) lower serum cholesterol at age 40 was associated with a 54% lower risk of CHD over the next 15 to 20 years. A 10% lower LDL-C at age 50 was associated with 39% lower risk, 27% at age 60, and 20% after age 70 (22). However, the excess number of CHD deaths due to even modestly elevated cholesterol levels is actually greater with advancing age, simply because the absolute risk of CHD death increases, such that

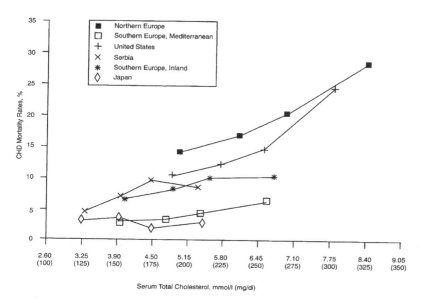

FIGURE 2   Twenty five-year coronary death and quartile of serum cholesterol concentration adjusted for age, cigarette smoking, and systolic blood pressure. *Abbreviation*: CHD, Coronary heart disease. *Source*: From Ref. 18.

the excess risk of CHD is three times greater in men aged 65 to 69 compared to those aged 45 to 49 (3). Although absolute risk of CHD is lower in women, much less attenuation in risk attributable to elevated cholesterol appears to occur in women with advancing age. Compared to women with total cholesterol levels ≥240 mg/dL, those with a 10% lower total cholesterol level have a lifetime risk 21% lower at age 40, 23% lower at age 50, 33% lower at age 60, 31% lower at age 70, and 14% lower at age 80 (23).

In trials of treatments that primarily lower LDL-C (statins, colestipol, diet, and ileal bypass surgery), performed primarily in populations with CHD (of which 75% were men), a 1 to 1 relationship between percent LDL-C reduction and percent relative risk reduction was apparent over two to six years (16,24). This is less than the 1 to 2 to 1 to 4 relationship between LDL-C and CHD risk seen in observational studies with follow-up of 15 to 20 years. At 10 years of follow-up, the risk reduction associated with lower cholesterol levels in the observational studies is more similar to the clinical trials. This may suggest either that the cumulative benefit from intervention early in the course of atherosclerosis is of greater benefit or simply that long-term treatment with statins (more than 5 years) results in greater relative risk reductions. These hypotheses are unlikely to be tested in clinical trials.

Women

Serum cholesterol concentrations increase steadily between the ages of 35 and 60 years in women and to a lesser degree in men (22). LDL-C levels are lower in women than in men prior to menopause. Although LDL-C concentration rises to higher levels in women than in men following menopause, LDL-C particle number remains lower in women (25). Similar associations between serum total cholesterol and the risk of CHD are seen in middle-aged and older women as in men, after adjustment for other risk factors (20,26,27). LDL-C continues to predict excess risk of CHD and stroke in women over the age of 65 in some cohorts (28) but not others (29,30). Non-HDL-C (total cholesterol minus HDL-C) may be a somewhat better predictor of CHD risk than LDL-C in women (31).

Advancing Age

Many studies have described a decline in serum cholesterol levels after age 65, more so in men than in women. Due at least in part to increasing comorbidity and weight loss, declining cholesterol synthesis may also play a role (28). Total cholesterol is inversely related to CHD mortality after age 80 (32).

Preexisting Cardiovascular Disease

In those with CVD, LDL-C more strongly predicts the risk of subsequent cardiovascular death than in those without evidence of disease at baseline. In middle-aged men with CVD, the risk of death from CVD over the next 10 years is threefold higher in those with a baseline untreated LDL-C level of 160 mg/dL or greater compared to those with an LDL-C lower than 100 mg/dL (33,34). The risk of cardiovascular death for those with CVD is two- to fivefold higher for a given level of LDL-C compared to those without CVD at baseline (33).

Region, Race, and Ethnicity

Although mean LDL-C levels and rates of CHD vary by region, estimates of the relative risk of death due to hypercholesterolemia in the MRFIT study are consistent with those from other cohort studies conducted in Australia and New Zealand, Belgium, Canada, Denmark, England, Finland, France, Germany, Israel, Italy, The Netherlands, Norway, Poland, Scotland, Spain, Switzerland, the United States and the USSR (3). Evidence of a curvilinear relationship between cholesterol and the risk of CHD death was found in the MRFIT study (35) but is less apparent in populations with lower absolute risk of CVD (Fig. 2) (18). Although CHD rates have fallen in industrialized countries over the last three decades, CHD rates continue to rise in industrializing countries as dietary consumption patterns become more "westernized" (36). A substantial proportion (more than 75%) of the 50% increase in CHD in men and 27% increase in women over the past 20 years has been attributed to rising total cholesterol levels (37). A recent international case–control study, INTERHEART, which included additional countries in central and eastern Europe, the Middle East, South Asia, China and Hong Kong, Southeast Asia and Japan, South America, Mexico, and Africa also found similar relationships between cholesterol and CHD risk (39,40). Some evidence, however, suggests that total cholesterol and LDL-C may be less strongly related to CHD risk in South Asians and related more to the high prevalence of diabetes and metabolic syndrome and lipoprotein(a) elevations (38).

In the United States, LDL-C levels tend to be lower in non-Hispanic black men and women than in non-Hispanic white and Mexican American men and women (41). Although mean LDL-C levels and rates of CHD and stroke differ among the various racial and ethnic groups in the United States, the association between total cholesterol and LDL-C and the relative risk of CHD and ischemic stroke risk are similar for blacks (42–44), Mexican Americans (45), men of Japanese ancestry (46), and Native Americans (47).

StrokePeripheral Vascular Disease, and Total Mortality

Stroke, lower extremity arterial disease, total CVD, and all-cause mortality also demonstrate a continuous, graded relationship to total cholesterol level, although the magnitude of the risk association is less than that for CHD events (48). Many epidemiologic studies have shown no relationship between total cholesterol level and stroke (49). However, when analyzed by stroke type, a 1 mmol/L (39 mg/dL, or about 28%) decrease in LDL-C was associated with a 15% reduction in ischemic stroke and a 19% increase in hemorrhagic stroke (50). In eastern Asian populations, stroke is more common than CHD and the risks of both types of stroke are less strongly associated with cholesterol and more strongly associated with BP levels (51).

As is stroke, lower extremity arterial disease, or peripheral vascular disease (PVD), is primarily a disease of those over age 60, with over 40% of those aged 75 years or more with evidence of lower extremity arterial occulsion (52,53). Risk factors for PVD are the same as those for CHD and stroke. LDL-C levels greater than 147 mg/dL (greater than 1.90 mmol) have been associated with an increased risk of developing either subclinical or clinical evidence of PVD (54).

Noncardiovascular Mortality

Some, but not all, studies have reported an inverse relationship between low serum cholesterol levels and all-cause mortality. In two cohorts of men ($n = 12,280$) aged 18 to 39 years at baseline, who were followed for 22 to 34 years, the lowest mortality rate occurred in those with total cholesterol levels lower than 160 mg/dL (4.14 mmol/L) at baseline (48). In a third cohort aged 35 to 39 at baseline, followed for 16 years, and another cohort of men and women aged 65 years or more, followed for 8 years, mortality rates were highest in those with baseline total cholesterol levels lower than 160 mg/dL (28,48).

Trends in Serum Cholesterol

In the final risk factor survey of the MONICA study performed between 1992 and 1998, the mean total cholesterol level of the 26 countries ranged from 213 to 244 mg/dL (5.5 to 6.3 mmol), with the lowest levels observed in China (Beijing) (12). Cholesterol rates had declined in most countries from the first surveys, which were performed approximately 10 years earlier. Cholesterol levels increased in the Poland, China, France, Italy, Yugoslavia, and the eastern part of Switzerland.

Data from the U.S. National Health and Nutrition Examination Surveys (NHANES) have shown consistent declines in cholesterol levels and in the percentage of individuals aged 20 years or more with serum total cholesterol levels of 240 mg/dL (≥ 6.22 mmol/L) since 1960 (41). Between the 1960–1962 survey and the 1999–2002 NHANES surveys, total serum cholesterol declined in women by 10% from 225 to 202 mg/dL (5.85 to 5.23 mmol/L) and in men by 8% from 220 to 203 mg/dL (5.70 to 5.23 mmol/L). Mean total cholesterol levels decreased for each age and sex group except for men and women aged 20 to 29 years. Most of the decline in serum cholesterol levels occurred prior to the 1988–1994 survey, with age-adjusted total cholesterol levels decreasing significantly only in women after this time period [207 to 204 mg/dL (5.36 to 5.287 mmol/L); men 204 to 202 mg/dL (5.36 to 5.28 mmol/L)]. Secular trends in obesity prevalence may have contributed to a slowing of the decline in cholesterol levels, with obesity prevalence increasing form 23% to 30% between these two surveys (55,56).

In large part, the decline in cholesterol levels occurred in men aged 60 years or more and women aged 50 years or more, who experienced at least 10 mg/dL (0.26 mmol/L) declines in both total and LDL-C. Non-Hispanic black men and women both experienced significant cholesterol declined during the period between 1988–1994 and 1999–2002 while cholesterol levels declined significantly only for Mexican American and non-Hispanic white women. A total serum cholesterol of 240 mg/dL (≥ 6.22 mmol/L) or greater defined the top quartile of the distribution in the 1960–1962 survey. However, by the 1988–1994 survey, 20% had total cholesterol levels of 240 mg/dL or more, and by 1999–2002 this had declined to 17% of the population. Mean LDL-C levels also declined during this time period from 131 to 126 mg/dL (3.39 to 3.26 mmol/L) in men and from 126 to 120 mg/dL (3.26 to 3.11 mmol/L) in women. Both non-Hispanic white and black men and women experienced significant declines. For Mexican American adults, a significant decline was observed only for women.

The decreases in total and LDL-C between 1976–1980 and 1988–1994 may have been influenced more by the increase in the use of cholesterol-lowering medication than secular dietary changes following the first set of recommendations from the National Cholesterol Education Program Adult Treatment Panel in 1988 (57). Although intake of saturated fat decreased by 11% during this time period, cholesterol intake actually increased in women. Significant increases in the use of cholesterol-lowering medication occurred, with the largest increase in those over age 60 (7% to 24% of men and 9% to 22% of women). Non-Hispanic white men were the most likely to be taking cholesterol-lowering medication in the 1999–2002 survey (11%) whereas 9% of non-Hispanic white women, 9% of black men, 6% of black women, 7% of Mexican American women, and 5% of Mexican American men were taking a cholesterol-lowering medication.

CRITICAL ROLE OF LDL-C IN ATHEROGENESIS

Plaque progresses through several pathologically distinct phases and the prevalence of advanced lesions varies widely depending on risk factor levels in a population (58). The earliest lesions, fatty streaks, can be seen as early as 2 years of age and are characterized by macrophage-derived foam cells containing lipid droplets. In countries with habitual atherogenic diets, fibrous plaques have begun to develop by the teenage years and are characterized by a thin fibrous cap overlying a lipid-rich core with smooth-muscle cell infiltration and extracellular matrix accumulation. By age 35, fibrous plaques constitute approximately half of coronary artery lesions in men and one-third of lesions in women (59). Advanced plaque develops as lesions become confluent with a large amount of extracellular lipid accumulation in the vessel intima. These lesions may be prone to rupture because of their high lipid content, increased inflammation, and an overlying thin fibrous cap. Complicated lesions arise as these plaques erode or rupture with overlying thrombosis. Usually thrombosis is nonocclusive and clinically silent. Reorganization occurs with further infiltration by smooth muscle and inflammatory cells and extracellular connective tissue matrix. Occlusive thrombus occurs about two-thirds of

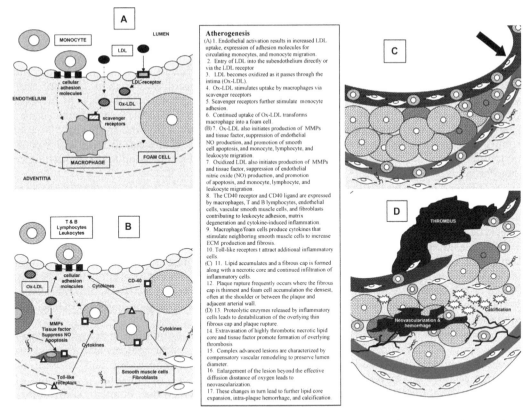

FIGURE 3 Initiation and progression of atherosclerotic plaque. *Abbreviations*: LDL-C, low-density lipoprotein, MMPs, matrix metalloproteinases; ECM, extracellular matrix; OX, oxidized; NO, nitric oxide.

the time on a nonstenotic lesion. By age 50, advanced plaque is present in 100% of individuals in Western populations (60). Even in relatively low-risk populations, one-half of individuals have atherosclerotic plaque by age 65 (8).

As described by Fuster, Libby, and others (58,61), LDL-C is a critical factor in all stages of atherogenesis, although other lipoproteins such as HDL-C and VLDL-C may play important roles as well (Fig. 3). Endothelial dysfunction, characterized by decreased nitric oxide synthesis, is the earliest manifestation of atherosclerosis. It may result from mechanical stress enhanced by hypertension, and other risk factors such as hypercholesterolemia, insulin resistance, tobacco use, and inflammation. Normal endothelial-dependent vasodilation becomes impaired after only 6 to 12 weeks in animals fed a high-cholesterol diet (62). A dysfunctional endothelium facilitates the entry of circulating lipoproteins, including LDL-C, into the intima. LDL-C molecules can infiltrate directly through the arterial endothelium or can be taken up by the LDL-C receptor. LDL-C becomes oxidized as it passes into the proteoglycan matrix of the intima although the precise mechanisms are unknown. Endothelial cells, fibroblasts, and leukocytes have all been shown to produce reactive oxygen species. Oxidation promotes LDL-C retention in the intima and stimulates uptake by macrophages via scavenger receptors SR-A and CD-36, thereby transforming the macrophage into a lipid-filled foam cell. Oxidized LDL-C also initiates a cascade of atherogenic processes, including transcription of proatherogenic genes, production of matrix metalloproteinases (MMPs) and tissue factor, suppression of endothelial nitric oxide production, and promotion of smooth muscle cell apoptosis.

Macrophages are derived from circulating monocytes recruited by the activated endothelial cells. Endothelial activation results in expression of cell adhesion molecules (CAMs) such as E- and P-selectins, which facilitate monocyte margination and adhesion. Other CAMs facilitate migration of the adhered monocytes into the arterial wall to become macrophages. Oxidized LDL-C also triggers monocyte, lymphocyte, and leukocyte migration, as well as macrophage transformation by activating nuclear factor-kappa B transcription factor, which in turn initiates a potent cascade of chemoattractants (monocyte chemoattractant protein-1, leukotriene B_4 (LTB_4), and monocyte-colony stimulating factor).

The CD40 receptor and CD40 ligand are expressed by macrophages, T and B lymphocytes, endothelial cells, vascular smooth muscle cells, and fibroblasts and are thought to contribute to leukocyte adhesion, matrix degeneration, and cytokine-induced inflammation. Macrophage/foam cells produce cytokines that stimulate neighboring smooth muscle cells to increase extracellular matrix production and fibrosis. Toll-like receptors in fibroblasts and macrophages in the adventitia and intima of coronary arteries may become activated by tissue injury to produce autoantigens and a variety of cytokines that attract additional inflammatory cells. The toll-like receptors have also been shown to be involved in progression and remodelling of atherothrombosis.

Continued exposure to the proatherogenic milieu promotes recruitment of inflammatory T and B monocytes, macrophages, and mast cells into the plaque, further lipid accumulation, formation of a necrotic lipid core, and fibrous cap formation. These inflammatory cells release proteolytic enzymes, including MMPs and plasminogen activators, which degrade extracellular matrix, leading to destabilization of the overlying thin fibrous cap and plaque rupture. Plaque rupture frequently occurs where the fibrous cap is thinnest and foam cell accumulation the densest, often at the shoulder or between the plaque and adjacent arterial wall. CD40 may also play a role in plaque rupture via effects on MMP production and increasing thrombogenicity. These cells also release cytokines that regulate macrophage uptake of modified LDL-C and other lipoproteins via the scavenger receptors.

In what appears to be a defense against lipoprotein accumulation, macrophages may undergo apoptosis in response to certain cytokines, including tumor necrosis factor and interleukins. Apoptosis appears to be an important link between inflammation and thrombosis. Lipid-rich plaques are extremely thrombogenic. Foam cell apoptosis results in exposure of intracellular membrane proteins and release of tissue factor, which may be major contributors to arterial thrombosis following plaque rupture.

Elevated blood LDL-C levels may also increase blood thrombogenicity and growth of thrombus. Lowering LDL-C levels with a statin has been shown to decrease thrombus growth by about 20%. The thrombogenicity of high LDL-C levels may share a common biological pathway with smoking and diabetes, which also increase thrombogenicity. These conditions all have higher levels of tissue factor and thrombin activation. Elevated levels of circulating monocytes in these conditions also appear to be a source of microparticles containing tissue factor. Higher levels of circulating tissue factor antigen have been associated with increased blood thrombogenicity in patients with CHD.

Complex advanced lesions are characterized by compensatory vascular remodeling to preserve lumen diameter. Enlargement of the lesion beyond the effective diffusion distance of oxygen leads to neovascularization. These changes, in turn, lead to further lipid core expansion, intraplaque hemorrhage, and calcification. Macrophages, attracted by oxidized LDL-C, produce cytokines, stimulating neovessel growth.

Importantly, plaque stabilization and regression may occur with aggressive lipid lowering. These fibrocalcific plaques are characterized by reduced lipid content and have the least inflammatory cell infiltration and microvessel content. Microvessels (vas vasora) may provide a pathway for reverse cholesterol transport and regress once the cholesterol core has been depleted.

NATIONAL CHOLESTEROL EDUCATION PROGRAM ADULT TREATMENT PANEL III GOALS FOR LDL-C
Identifying High-Risk Patients

The National Cholesterol Education Program Adult Treatment Panel III (NCEP ATP III) guidelines outline a nine-step approach to identifying high-risk patients and implementing the guidelines (Table 1). High-risk patients are identified by a fasting lipid profile (step 1). NCEP ATP III classifies an optimal LDL-C as less than 100 mg/dL and a desirable total cholesterol as less than 200 mg/dL. Along with assessing lipoprotein levels to determine high-risk status, the presence of clinical atherosclerosis, including peripheral arterial disease, abdominal aortic aneurysm, and symptomatic carotid artery disease, is then assessed (step 2). In NCEP ATP III, all clinical forms of atherosclerotic disease and diabetes represent a CHD risk equivalent. The

TABLE 1   Nine-Step Approach to Implementation of the National Cholesterol Education Program Adult Treatment Panel III Guidelines

1. Determine fasting lipoprotein levels.
2. Identify presence of clinical atherosclerosis.
3. Determine presence of major risk factors.
4. If 2+ risk factors present, calculate global risk score.
5. Determine risk category and establish LDL-C goal.
6. Initiate TLC diet if LDL-C is above goal.
7. Add drug therapy if LDL-C continues to exceed initiation levels.
8. Identify metabolic syndrome and treat if present after 3 mo of TLC.
9. Treat patients with elevated triglycerides to non-high-density lipoprotein goals.

Abbreviations: LDL-C, low-density lipoprotein cholesterol; TLC, therapeutic lifestyle change.
Source: From Ref. 63.

presence of major risk factors is then determined (step 3). According to ATP III, major risk factors (exclusive of LDL-C) that modify LDL-C goals include cigarette smoking, hypertension (BP greater than or equal to 140/90 mmHg or on antihypertensive medication), low HDL-C (less than 40 mg/dL), family history of premature CHD, and age (men, 45 years or older; women, 55 years or older). If two risk factors are present, the global risk score is calculated (step 4) (19).

CALCULATING THE GLOBAL RISK SCORE

The global risk score, which is calculated with the Framingham scoring, allows better targeting of intensive treatment to individuals who have multiple (2+) risk factors. The Framingham risk scoring system is used to estimate the 10-year CHD risk on the basis of age, total cholesterol, smoking status, and systolic BP. The total risk score sums the points for each risk factor, and the 10-year CHD risk is estimated from the total points. Individuals with multiple risk factors are divided into those with 10-year risk for CHD of greater than 20%, 10% to 20%, and less than 10% (19).

Once the risk category is determined, the LDL-C goal is established (step 5). For CHD and CHD risk equivalents, the LDL-C goal is less than 100 mg/dL; for individuals with multiple (2+) risk factors, the LDL-C goal is less than 130 mg/dL; and for individuals with 0 to 1 risk factors, the LDL-C goal is less than 160 mg/dL. The therapeutic lifestyle change (TLC) diet is then initiated (step 6) on the basis of risk category and LDL-C goal. For individuals with CHD or CHD risk equivalents (10-year risk greater than 20%), TLC is initiated for an LDL-C level greater than or equal to 100 mg/dL (19).

Drug therapy is added when the LDL-C continues to exceed initiation levels (step 7). For individuals with CHD or CHD risk equivalents, drug therapy is initiated for LDL-C levels greater than or equal to 100 mg/dL, with the goal of attaining an LDL-C level of less than 100 mg/dL and an optional goal of less than 70 mg/dL for very high–risk patients. When drugs are prescribed, attention to TLC should continue to be maintained and reinforced (Table 2) (19).

Individuals with metabolic syndrome should be identified and treated with drug therapy after three months of TLC (step 8). Factors characteristic of the metabolic syndrome include abdominal obesity, atherogenic dyslipidemia (elevated triglyceride (TG), small LDL-C particles, low HDL-C), raised BP, insulin resistance (with or without glucose intolerance), and prothrombotic and proinflammatory states. ATP III recognizes the metabolic syndrome as a secondary target of risk-reduction therapy (19).

As elevated TGs are also an independent risk factor for CHD, individuals with elevated TGs should be treated to achieve the target goal for LDL-C (step 9). In addition to weight reduction and increased physical activity, drug therapy can be considered in high-risk individuals with elevated TGs (greater than or equal to 200 mg/dL) to achieve the non–HDL-C goals. Achieving ATP III goals is a relatively complex, step-by-step process that requires a tape measure (to measure waist circumference) and a software device or score sheets to calculate the Framingham score to ensure that clinicians adhere closely to the guidelines (19).

The European guidelines also use a Systematic Coronary Risk Evaluation system to determine the eligibility of patients for therapeutic intervention. Patients with CHD, clinical noncoronary atherosclerosis, or a 5% or greater 10-year risk of fatal CVD (the NCEP ATP III utilizes an estimate of 10-year risk of total CHD events) should be treated with lipid-lowering

TABLE 2 Summary of Treatment Panel III (ATP III) Guidelines for dyslipidemia

	LDL-C Goal (mg/dL)	If TG >200 mg/dL, Non-HDL-C Goal (mg/dL)
Low Risk		
<2 risk factor	<160	<190
Moderate Risk		
(≥2 risk factors)	<130	<160
Moderately-to-High Risk		
(≥2 risk factors; and 10–20% 10-year risk)	<100	<130
Including those wth:	<100	<130
Advancing age		
Severe or poorly controlled risk factors		
TG≥200 mg/dL + non-HDL≥160 mg/dL		
HDL<40 mg/dL		
Metabolic syndrome		
Coronary calcium >75th percentile for age and sex		
High Risk	<70[b]	<100[d]
CHD, PAD, AAA, >50% carotid stenosis		
Diabetes[a]		
>20% 10-year CHD risk		
Creatinine >1.5 mg/dL[b]		
10–20% 10-year CHD risk plus hs-CRP >3.0[c]		
Very High Risk		
CVD plus:		
Diabetes		
Metabolic syndrome		
Multiple, severe or poorly controlled risk factors		
(including hs-CRP >3.0)		
Cigarette smoking		
Acute coronary syndrome		

[a]ADA recommends that all type 2 diabetics age >80 should lower LDL by at least 30% even if baseline LDL <100 mg/dL.
[b]High risk by National Kidney Foundation Guidelines.
[c]High risk by AHA/CDC Guidelines.
[d]ATP III optional goal.
Abbreviations: AAA: abdominal aortic aneurysm; CHD: coronary heart disease; CVD: cardiovascular disease; hs-CRP: highly sensitive assay for C-reactive protein; PAD, peripheral artery disease; TG: triglycerides
Source: From Refs. 63 and 64.

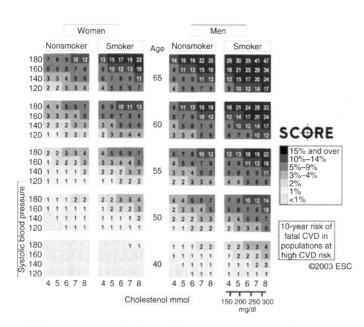

FIGURE 4 Ten-year risk of fatal CVD in high-risk regions of Europe by gender, age, systolic blood pressure, total cholesterol and smoking status. *Abbreviation*: CVD, cardiovascular disease.

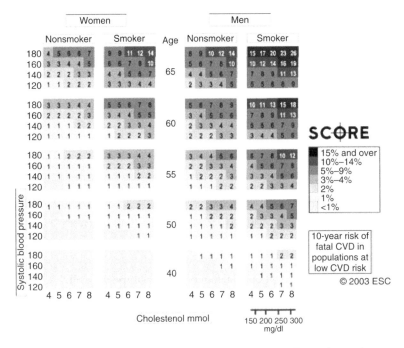

FIGURE 5 Ten-year risk of fatal CVD in low-risk regions of Europe by gender, age, systolic blood pressure, total cholesterol, and smoking status. *Abbreviation:* CVD, cardiovascular disease.

drugs, if dietary therapy fails achieve to an LDL-C goal of less than 2.5 mmol/L (100 mg/dL). The 5% 10-year risk calculation is determined by evaluating the risk factor or a color-coded chart (Figs. 4 and 5). Color charts allow for the easy determination of high-risk patients without the use of adding up point scales or the need for a risk calculator. To account somewhat for lifetime risk, the European guidelines recommend that for evaluating risk, the patient's age should be adjusted to 60 years. For patients with less than 5% 10-year risk of fatal CVD (after correction to age 60 years), the European guidelines recommend lifestyle changes only, and drug therapy is not indicated unless the patient has a very high serum cholesterol or FH (LDL ≥ 8 mmol/L or 240 mg/dL) (65).

Ratio Goals

A total cholesterol/HDL-C goal has been advocated by the Canadian guidelines (Table 3) (66). These guidelines are similar to the NCEP ATP III recommendation in that goals for LDL-C are more aggressive according to the risk classification. However, rather than non-HDL-C targets, the Canadian guidelines have a total cholesterol/HDL-C ratio less than 4. The advantage of this approach is that for patients with low HDL-C, more aggressive LDL-C lowering or HDL-C raising may be necessary to achieve both targets. As greater reduction in LDL-C is usually easier to achieve with the present therapies than significantly raising HDL-C, a ratio target of more than 4 may frequently require reducing LDL-C levels to less than 75 mg/dL in patients with low HDL-C. For example, a patient with an HDL-C of 30 mg/dL and TGs of 150 mg/dL would require a target total cholesterol of 120 mg/dL and an LDL-C of 60 mg/dL. For patients with higher HDL-C levels, an LDL-C lower than 100 mg/dL would most likely result in a ratio goal of less than 4. Therefore, by including a ratio target, the Canadian guidelines appropriately require more aggressive LDL-C-lowering in patients with low HDL-C based on clinical trials that have demonstrated that this subpopulation has a significantly higher residual risk of events on statin therapy. The ratio has been shown to be a better epidemiologic predictor of CV events than LDL-C and also appears to significantly improve event prediction on statin therapy. Thus, rather than having a more aggressive LDL-C goal for all patients, a ratio goal of less than 4 in conjunction with an LDL-C goal of less than 100 mg/dL (recently revised to an LDL-C goal of lower than 2.0 mmol/L or 80 mg/dL) may sufficiently identify the higher-risk patients who deserve more aggressive lipid-altering interventions.

TABLE 3 Canadian Dyslipidemia Guidelines

	Target level	
Risk category	**LDL-C level (mmol/L)**	**TC: HDL-C ratio**
High[a] (10-yr risk of CAD ≥20%, or history of diabetes mellitus[b] or any atherosclerotic disease)	<2.5	<4.0
Moderate (10-yr risk, 11–19%)	<3.5	<5.0
Low[c]	<4.5	<6.0

[a]Apolipoprotein B can be used as an alternative measurement, particularly for patients treated with statins. An optimal level of apolipoprotein B in a patient at high risk is <0.9 g/L, in a patient at moderate risk <1.05 gL, and in a patient at low risk <1.2 g/L.
[b]Includes patients with chronic kidney disease and those undergoing long-term dialysis.
[c]In the very low risk stratum, treatment may be deferred if the 10-year estimate of cardiovascular disease is <5% and the LDL-C level is <5.0 mmol/L.
Abbreviations: HDL-C, high-density lipoprotein cholesterol; LDL-C, low-density lipoprotein cholesterol; TC, total cholesterol; CAD, coronary artery disease.

The argument against a ratio target is based on a lack of evidence supporting HDL-C raising as a therapeutic target, and, thus, there is a concern that a ratio target would inappropriately emphasize the benefits of increasing HDL-C. However, because raising HDL-C by more than 25% with existing therapies is difficult, the most likely means to achieve a ratio goal of less than 4 would still require more aggressive LDL-C lowering.

Another ratio target that has been evaluated is the apolipoprotein (Apo) B/AI ratio. The ApoB/AI ratio is a better predictor of events in large population observational trials, such as the Apolipoprotein-Related Mortality Risk study (AMORIS) (67), and the best predictor of events on statin therapy, according to the Air Force/Texas Coronary Atherosclerosis Prevention Study (AFCAPS/TexCAPS) trial (68). ApoB measurements are most useful in patients with hypertriglyceridemia (HTG) because it incorporates all the atherogenic lipoproteins. Non-HDL-C correlates better with ApoB than LDL-C, especially in patients with HTG. The main reason the ApoB/AI ratio predicts better than the total cholesterol/HDL-C is that, in the hypertriglyceridemic population and in those with small dense LDL-C (ApoB/LDL-C greater than 1.0), the ApoB level is significantly more predictive of CV events than the total cholesterol level. Apo measurements are not universally available and are more expensive than a standard lipid profile to determine total cholesterol/HDL-C ratio and, therefore, the utilization of the ApoB/AI ratio as a therapeutic target will require additional justification based on a cost–benefit analysis. However, to define a therapeutic benefit of a lipid-altering treatment, putative changes in the ApoB/AI ratio may be useful for demonstrating an enhanced benefit of a therapy and may provide a helpful lipid surrogate end point for regulatory approval for novel therapies.

Adult Treatment Panel III Update

Since the publication of ATP III in 2001, seven major clinical trials of statin therapy with clinical endpoints have been published. These seven trials extended the benefits of statin therapy across a wide spectrum of at-risk populations and emphasized the importance of adhering to an LDL-C goal of less than 100 mg/dL in high-risk individuals. Four of these trials, the Heart Protection Study (HPS), the Pravastatin or Atorvastatin Evaluation and Infection Therapy (PROVE-IT) trial, Treating to New Targets (TNT), and Incremental Decrease in Endpoints through Aggressive Lipid Lowering (IDEAL) supported an even more aggressive LDL-C goal for patients at very high risk for CHD events. The ATP III revised the guidelines to recommend a therapeutic optional goal of LDL-C less than 70 mg/dL and non-HDL-C less than 100 mg/dL for patients at very high risk. The definition of "very high risk" was left deliberately up to clinical judgment. However, factors that favor the definition of very high risk include established CVD plus (a) multiple risk factors (especially diabetes); (b) several poorly controlled risk factors (especially continued cigarette smoking); (c) multiple risk factors of the metabolic syndrome [especially high TGs greater than or equal to 200 mg/dL plus non-HDL-C greater than or equal to 130 mg/dL with low HDL-C (less than 40 mg/dL)]; and (d), on the basis of PROVE-IT, patients with acute coronary syndromes. Although not specifically stated, the intent of the revised ATP III report suggests that CVD with recurrent events with an LDL-C less than 100 mg/dL should also be considered for the optional therapeutic goal of LDL-C less than 70 mg/dL (Table 2) (64).

The revised ATP III also encouraged continued focus on non-HDL-C for patients with elevated TGs and low HDL-C, thereby recommending niacin or fibrates in addition to statins for patients at their LDL-C goal but not yet at their non-HDL-C goals. When initiating LDL-C-lowering therapy in a person of high risk or modestly high risk, a reduction in LDL-C of at least 30% to 40% beyond dietary therapy should be achieved, if feasible.

In addition, for patients with a Framingham 10-year risk of 10% to 20%, therapeutic goals of LDL-C less than 100 mg/dL and non-HDL-C less than 130 mg/dL should be considered an option based on the results of the Anglo-Scandinavian Cardiac Outcomes Trial (ASCOT). Therefore, the revised ATP III report basically divides patients into five categories across the risk continuum: very high to high, modestly high, and moderate to low risk (64).

There were some noticeable differences between the revised ATP III recommendations from some of the professional organizations. In a divergence from the American Diabetes Association (ADA) guidelines, ATP III did not recommend a target goal of HDL-C greater than 40 mg/dL and TGs less than 150 mg/dL for diabetics. Also, for patients with diabetes without CVD, ATP III did not yet endorse the ADA concept of starting on LDL-C-lowering drugs when LDL-C is less than 100 mg/dL at baseline to lower LDL-C by at least 30% but, rather, left the decision to treat up to clinical judgment. ATP III also did not mention the National Kidney Foundation recommendation that patients with renal impairment (creatinine greater than 1.5 mg/dL) be classified as high risk.

The revised ATP III guidelines have formally endorsed the concept of "the lower, the better," especially for very high–risk patients. The panel also recognized the potential challenges of achieving the optional therapeutic target LDL-C of less than 70 mg/dL and non-HDL-C less than 100 mg/dL. The benefits of aggressive lipid control are well documented in clinical trials, but achieving improved outcomes in the at-risk population remains an elusive goal in many patients.

METABOLISM OF LDL-C

Almost all human cells have the capability of synthesizing cholesterol. The cellular cholesterol pool is regulated by nuclear receptors such as Liver X Receptor (LXR) and Farnesoid X Receptor, which protect the cells from cholesterol and bile acid toxicity, respectively. Oxysterols stimulate LXR, which regulates a large number of genes involved in cholesterol homeostasis. To protect the cells from free cholesterol toxicity, the ABC transporters such as ABCA1, ABCG1, ABCG5, and ABCG8 are upregulated to efflux cholesterol into HDL-C (ABCA1 and ABCG1) or bile (ABCG5 and ABCG8). As cellular cholesterol stores are depleted, sterol regulatory element-binding protein (SREBP)-2 stimulate the genes involved in cholesterol synthesis. Acetyl-CoA utilized for cholesterol biosynthesis derived from mitochondrial or cytoplasmic oxidation is transported to the cytoplasm where it is converted to 3-hydroxy-3-methylglutaryl-CoA (HMG-CoA). HMG-CoA is converted to mevalonate by the rate-limiting enzyme HMG-CoA reductase, which is bound to the endoplasmic reticulum. After a series of phosphorylations and other enzymatic changes, squalene is formed, which undergoes cyclization to yield lanosterol. Through a series of 19 additional reactions, lanosterol is converted to cholesterol.

The cellular supply of cholesterol is maintained at a steady level by three distinct mechanisms: (i) regulation of HMG-CoA reductase, (ii) regulation of excess free cholesterol through the activity of acyl-CoA:cholesterol acyltransferase (ACAT), and (iii) regulation of plasma cholesterol by LDL-C receptor–mediated uptake in hepatocytes and HDL-C-mediated reverse cholesterol transport.

HMG-CoA reductase, the rate-limiting enzyme for cholesterol biosynthesis, has a sterol-sensing domain that is downregulated by cholesterol. HMG-CoA reductase is most active in its unmodified dephosphorylated state. Phosphorylation, a modification reaction that deactivates the enzyme, is catalyzed by AMP-activated protein kinase (AMPK). AMPK is hormonally regulated, with glucagon and epinephrine inhibiting and insulin stimulating this enzyme. HMG-CoA reductase also undergoes proteolytic degradation when cellular cholesterol levels are elevated. When hepatic cellular cholesterol levels are low, SREBP and its cleavage-activating protein (SCAP) move to the Golgi apparatus where sterol synthesis is initiated. When sterol levels are high, the movement of SCAP is halted, preventing the activation of SREBP-2. Thereby, cellular cholesterol levels regulate cholesterol synthesis mediated by SREBP-2, and oxysterols activated by LXR enhance cholesterol efflux from cells.

Cholesterol is transported in the plasma predominantly as cholesteryl esters associated with lipoproteins. Cholesteryl esters are packaged into lipoproteins along with ApoB and TGs mediated by microsomal transfer protein into VLDL-C. The liver secretes VLDL-C and this TG-rich lipoprotein undergoes hydrolysis through the action of endothelial cell–associated lipoprotein lipase and hepatic lipases to form LDL-C, which are relatively TG depleted. LDL-C returns to the liver by LDL-C receptor–mediated uptake. The cholesterol in LDL-C is then excreted into bile as free cholesterol or as bile salts following conversion to bile acids in the liver.

The regulation of LDL-C levels are, therefore, controlled by the synthesis and secretion of VLDL-C by the liver, the rate of conversion of VLDL-C into LDL-C, and the clearance of VLDL-C by the LDL-C receptor on the surface of the hepatocyte. The hepatic LDL-C receptor gene is regulated by thyroxine and upregulated or downregulated in response to cellular cholesterol levels. Inhibition of HMG-CoA reductase or interrupting bile acid or biliary cholesterol reabsorption will result in decreased hepatic cholesterol stores and, subsequently, an upregulation of LDL-C receptors. The apo-B100 of LDL-C binds to the coiled binding domain of the LDL-C receptor, which is located inside coated pits on the cell surface. These pits facilitate the endocytosis of receptor-bound LDL-C, forming an endocytic vesicle. Within the endosome, the LDL-C receptor dissociates from LDL-C and recycles back to the cell surface where it can be reutilized to internalize LDL-C. The endosome then fuses with lysosomes to degrade the apoproteins into amino acids, and hydrolase splits the cholesteryl esters to produce free cholesterol. The free cholesterol suppresses HMG-CoA reductase, is converted back into cholesteryl esters by ACAT to form cytoplasmic lipid droplets, and turns off the synthesis of the LDL-C receptor in the endoplasmic reticulum (Fig. 6) (69).

GENETIC CAUSES OF ELEVATED LDL-C

The most common genetic cause of elevated LDL-C is familial combined hyperlipidemia (FCH) (70). In this disorder, ApoB is overproduced, resulting in the secretion of more VLDL-C particles

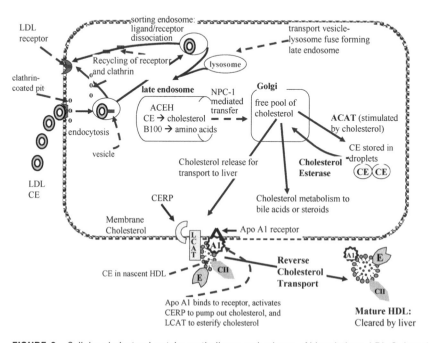

FIGURE 6 Cellular cholesterol uptake metbolisom and release. *Abbreviations*: LDL-C, low-density lipoprotein-cholesterol; HDL-C, high-density lipoprotein-cholesterol; ACAT, acyl-COA:cholesterol acyltransferase; CERP, cholesterol efflux regulatory protein; LCAT, lecithin:cholesterol acyltransferase.

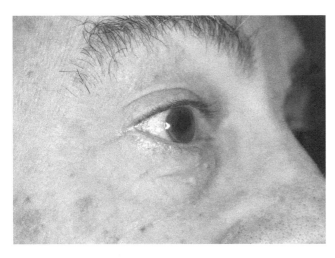

FIGURE 7 Xanthelasma.

rather than enlarged VLDL-C particles. There is also delayed clearance of postprandial TGs and an increased flux of free fatty acids. These abundant VLDL-C particles oversaturate the ability of lipoprotein lipase to break down all the TGs, resulting in TG-enriched LDL-C, which are further metabolized by hepatic lipase to form dense LDL-C particles. The more prevalent VLDL-C particles also exchange their TGs for cholesterol in HDL-C or LDL-C mediated by cholesteryl ester transfer protein, resulting in smaller HDL-C particles and small, dense LDL-C. The net result of this autosomal dominant disorder is a combined elevation of both TGs and LDL-C with low HDL-C and significantly increased risk of premature CHD. Because the serum TG is usually more than 200 mg/dL, non-HDL-C is a better target for treatment because this value includes all the TG-rich particles as well as LDL-C (71). In addition, because the LDL-C is small and dense, the total LDL-C level may not be significantly elevated and the ApoB/LDL-C ratio is frequently ≥ 1.0. This genetic disorder is important to diagnose because the risk of CHD is very high and family screening is advisable. Asian-Indians have a high incidence of FCH (72). Among family members, the lipid profile can vary from pure hypercholesterolemia to combined hyperlipidemia to isolated HTG. In patients with HTG, measuring ApoB can help confirm the diagnosis, because patients with familial HTG will usually have a normal ApoB level. Patients with FCH also may have a corneal arcus and xanthelasma (Fig. 7) but almost never have tendon xanthomas. The disorder may not be as evident in children or in premenopausal women. Weight gain, especially visceral fat increase, usually worsens the condition and patients are at much higher risk for the metabolic syndrome and Type 2 diabetes.

FH causes severe elevations of LDL-C levels due to the impairment or absence of the LDL-C receptor (73). The LDL-C receptor discovered by Drs. Brown and Goldstein is a complex protein that contains a binding domain to ApoB that is tightly coiled (Fig. 6) (74). Therefore, a mutation of even one amino-acid in the binding domain can unravel the coil and impair the ability of the receptor to bind ApoB. Most of the mutations are in the binding domain but many other mutations have been identified. Patients with FH have severe elevation of LDL-C and the disorder is present at birth. Homozygous FH (1 in 1,000,000) patients have no normal LDL-C receptors and the LDL-C levels often exceed 1000 mg/dL at birth, and these children develop severe atherosclerosis at an early age (75). The much more common heterozygous FH (1 in 500) (76) patients have half the number of normal LDL-C receptors and develop LDL-C levels between 200 and 400 mg/dL. On physical exam, the pathognomonic findings are tendonous xanthomas on the Achilles' heel and knuckles of the hands (Fig. 8). These patients also commonly develop a corneal arcus and xanthelasma, which are also present in patients with FCH. FH is more commonly found in French Canadians, Lebanese Christians, South African Afrikaners, and Jews of Lithuanian descent (17).

Familial defective ApoB is due to accumulation of LDL-C because of a defective ApoB rather than impaired LDL-C receptors. Familial defective ApoB patients have the ApoB mutation ApoB 3500. There is some evidence the LDL-C elevations are not as severe as FH, but often the clinical manifestations are identical (i.e., xanthomas with severe LDL-C elevations) (77). Other genetic causes of elevated LDL-C include autosomal dominant hypercholesterolemia (different from FH), which is due to mutations in proprotein convertase subtilisin/kexin type 9 (PCSK9). PCSK9 is

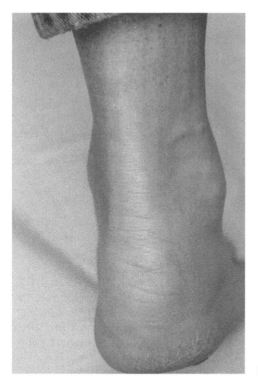

FIGURE 8 Achilles tendon xanthoma.

modified with the degradation of the LDL-C receptor but its molecular physiology is not fully understood (78).

SECONDARY CAUSES OF ELEVATED LDL-C

Any patient who presents with elevated LDL-C should be evaluated for secondary causes of hyperlipidemia. The major causes of secondary dyslipidemia include diabetes, hypothyroidism, chronic renal failure, nephritic syndrome, chronic liver disease, and certain drugs that raise LDL-C or TGs or lower HDL-C. A patient with newly diagnosed hypercholesterolemia should have a drug, diet, and family history performed and a physical exam. If secondary dyslipidemia is suspected, the workup should include a urinalysis to rule out significant proteinuria, a TSH to diagnose subclinical hypothyroidism, and chemistry profile to evaluate liver function, and alkaline phosphatase to detect obstructive biliary disease. Approximately 5% of women over the age of 40, with severe hypercholesterolemia (more than 300 mg/dL), were shown to have hypothyroidism. Hypothyroid individuals also appear to be more susceptible to statin-induced side effects, and hypothyroidism must be suspected in any patient who complains of statin intolerance. Other secondary causes of hyperlipidemia include anorexia nervosa, Cushing's syndrome, and porphyrias.

NONPHARMACOLOGICAL THERAPY

"Therapeutic lifestyle changes" is a term coined by the National Cholesterol Education Program Adult Treatment Panel III (NCEP ATP III) to incorporate a multifaceted nonpharmacologic approach to reducing the risk for CHD. The essential features of the therapeutic lifestyle changes are the following:

1. Reduction of saturated fat to less than 7% of total calories
2. Less than 200 mg/day of dietary cholesterol
3. Optional increases in plant sterols 2 g/day and viscous soluble fiber to enhance LDL-C lowering
4. Weight reduction
5. Increased physical activity

Dietary treatment should be targeted at saturated fat reduction to less than 7% of calories. Dietary studies have determined that reducing saturated fat to less than 7% of calories is necessary to have a significant reduction in LDL-C. The Seven Countries Study is the best evidence that saturated fat is the main culprit for inducing hypercholesterolemia around the world (4). Three intervention studies, the Boeing Fat Intervention Trial, Diet Alternative, and Dietary Effects on Lipoproteins and Thrombogenic Activity, demonstrated the benefits of lowering LDL-C by approximately 10% by decreasing saturated fat to less than 7% of calories (19).

The "Meats, Eggs, Dairy, Fried foods, In baked goods, Convenience foods, Table fats, Snacks" dietary assessment questionnaire is an easy-to-administer survey that can identify the source of overconsumption of saturated fat in most patients. Once the sources of saturated fat are identified, the challenge is to have the patient adhere to recommended dietary changes. One successful approach is to have the patient tell, or, ideally, write down for the physician or health professional the past one to two days of dietary intake. After reviewing the dietary intake, the patient can be informed of the various changes that will reduce his or her saturated fat intake (19).

For almost every high-saturated-fat food, there is an alternative low-fat food that will most likely be an acceptable alternative for patients. The benefits of a low dietary cholesterol intake on reducing serum cholesterol are less well established. Clinical studies with eggs have failed to demonstrate a significant increase in serum cholesterol with consuming up to two egg yolks/day (approximately 500 mg/day of dietary cholesterol).

There are three additional options to add to the diet to enhance LDL-C reduction: plant sterols, viscous soluble fiber, and soy protein. The cumulative benefits of all three dietary factors may lower LDL-C by approximately 20%, and, in conjunction with a low-saturated-fat diet, the total LDL-C reduction may approach 30%. A 20% to 30% reduction in LDL-C is sufficient for many patients to obviate the need for drug therapy. Plant sterols as either stanol esters (Benecol[TM]) or sterols (Take Control[TM]) are probably the most effective additional dietary ingredients to lower cholesterol. Several studies have demonstrated the benefits of both plant sterols and stanols in lowering LDL-C by 7% to 14% (79).

Soluble viscous fibers also lower LDL-C by approximately 5% to 10% depending on the daily amount consumed. There have been many studies to verify the LDL-C-lowering effects of both β-glucan in oat cereal and psyllium. Initially, the water solubility of the fiber was thought to cause the LDL-C-lowering effect, but nonviscous, water-soluble fibers, such as gum arabic, were shown not to lower LDL-C. To significantly lower LDL-C, a person should consume between 10 and 25 g/day of oat fiber or psyllium (80).

The benefits of soy protein on lowering LDL-C are less firmly established than those of viscous fiber and plant sterols, but, based on cumulative studies demonstrating a modest LDL-C reduction, the U.S. Food and Drug Administration (FDA) approved soy protein, at least 25 g/day (or four servings equal to 25 g/day noted on the food label), for the reduction of cardiovascular risk. In a meta-analysis of 38 soy protein studies, an overall mean of 9% LDL-C reduction was noted, with a range of 3.3% to 24% (81).

Soy protein contains isoflavones or phytoestrogens that may cause LDL-C reduction. However, other research suggests that the amino acid content of soy protein is responsible for hypocholesterolemia activity. Soy protein is mostly incorporated into low-fat foods, and there may be a substitution phenomenon in which hyperlipidemics who eat more soy protein will eat less fat-enriched foods. These theories regarding the hypocholesterolemic effects of soy protein are still being evaluated.

The most difficult challenge with increasing the amount of soy protein in the diet is the paucity of food products containing adequate soy amounts. A glass of soymilk contains approximately 7 to 8 g of soy protein. There are other products such as tofu, soybean curd, and vegetable burgers, which contain approximately 7 to 8 g of soy protein/serving. These food items are becoming more widely available, but for most Americans, they remain difficult food products to develop a taste for.

An alternative to reducing total fat in the diet, and usually saturated fat as well, is to increase the amount of monounsaturated and polyunsaturated fats. In fat-restrictive diets, many patients compensate by eating more calories from simple carbohydrates, which results in an increased glycemic load, leading to potential HTG and obesity. An attractive alternative to a low-fat diet is the Mediterranean diet. The Mediterranean diet is rich in complex carbohydrates and fiber, and the fat source is primarily monounsaturated fatty acids as found in olive oil. The Seven Countries Study, which was started in the early 1960s, demonstrated that Crete (an island

TABLE 4 Cholesterol Reduction with Approximately Equivalent Statin Doses

Dose (mg) of agent					Reduction (%)	
Atorvastatin	Simvastatin	Lovastatin	Pravastatin	Fluvastatin	Total cholesterol	Low-density lipoprotein cholesterol
—	10	20	20	40	22	27
10	20	40	40	80 XL	27	36
20	40	80			32	42
40	80				37	48
80					42	54

Note: Rosuvastatin 5, 10, 20, and 40 mg lowers LDL-C % by 42%, 46%, 52%, and 58%, respectively.

off of Greece) showed the lowest mortality from CHD and all causes (4). The Crete diet was not a low-fat diet; in fact, the fat intake was almost three times as much as that of the U.S. population. The major difference was the intake of olive oil. A more recent survey of CHD mortality also demonstrated a much lower CHD mortality among the Mediterranean populations compared to those in Northern Europe or the United States. In the Lyon Diet Study, 605 post-MI patients were randomly assigned to a Mediterranean-type diet versus an American Heart Association Step I diet. After a period of four years on the diet, although there were no differences in plasma lipids, the Mediterranean diet showed a 70% reduction in cardiac death and nonfatal MI. There is also evidence that olive oil reduces the risk of diabetes and obesity, which may relate to the lower glycemic load of the Mediterranean diet. Olive oil also inhibits the oxidation of LDL-C both in vitro and ex vivo. Olive oil contains phenolic compounds that, in addition to small amounts of vitamin E, provide the antioxidant effect. The phenolic content is most highly concentrated in extravirgin olive oils, but the content varies considerably because of climate and production techniques. The Mediterranean diet is also rich in wine, legumes, cereals, fruit, and vegetables that also provide antioxidant effects. Red wine, compared to white wine, contains many more flavonoids that are potent antioxidants. The net result of the Mediterranean diet is a diet rich in antioxidants, low in saturated fat, and with a low glycemic index. Therefore, many Americans may prefer a Mediterranean diet over a low-fat diet to reduce CHD risk.

PHARMACOLOGICAL THERAPY
Statins
Statins, HMG-CoA reductase inhibitors, are the most widely prescribed drugs to lower elevated LDL-C levels. By inhibiting HMG-CoA reductase, the rate-limiting enzyme for cholesterol

TABLE 5 HMG-CoA Reductase Inhibitor FDA-Approved Indications

Indication	HMG-CoA reductase inhibitors					
	Atorvastatin (Lipitor®)	Fluvastatin (Lescol®/XL)	Lovastatin (Altocor®/Mevacor®)	Pravastatin (Pravachol®)	Rosuvastatin (Crestor®)	Simvastatin (Zocor®)
Primary hypercholesterolemia	yes[a]	yes[a]	yes[a]	yes[a]	yes[a]	yes[a]
Mixed dyslipidemia	Yes[b]	Yes[b]	Yes[b]	Yes[b]	Yes[b]	Yes[b]
Hypertriglyceridemia	Yes[c]			Yes[c]	Yes[c]	Yes[c]
Primary dysbetalipoproteinemia	Yes[d]			Yes[d]		Yes[d]
Homozygous familial hyperlipidemia	Yes				Yes	Yes
Primary prevention coronary events			Yes	Yes		
Secondary prevention cardiovascular event(s)	Yes	Yes	Yes	Yes		Yes

[a]Includes heterozygous familial and nonfamilial hypercholesterolemia.
[b]Includes Fredrickson types IIa and IIb.
[c]Includes Fredrickson type IV.
[d]Includes Fredrickson type III.
Abbreviations: FDA, Food and Drug Administration; HMG-CoA, 3-hydroxy-3-methylglutaryl-CoA.

TABLE 6 Summary of the Comparative Pharmacokinetics of Statins in Healthy Volunteers

Variable	Atorvastatin	Fluvastatin	Lovastatin	Pravastatin	Rosuvastatin	Simvastatin
Prodrug	No	No	Yes	No	No	Yes
Lipophilicity (logP)	4.06	3.24	4.30	−0.23	−0.33	4.68
Affinity for Pgp transporter	Yes	No	Yes	Yes	No	Yes
t_{max} (h)	1.0–2.0	0.5–1.0	2.0–4.0	1.0–1.5	3.0–5.0	1.3–3.0
Absorption (%)	30	98	30–31	34	40–60	60–80
Hepatic first-pass metabolism (%)	20–30	40–70	40–70	50–70	50–70	50–80
Bioavailability (%)	12–14	29	<5	18	20	<5
Protein binding (%)	>98	>98	>95	43–54	88	95
Major metabolic enzyme	CYP3A4	CYP2C9	CYP3A4	Minimal CYP450	Minimal CYP4502C9	CYP3A4
Systemic active metabolites (No.)	Yes (2)	No	Yes (3)	No	Minimal	Yes (3)
Renal excretion (%)	≤2	<6	≥10	20	10	13
$t_{1/2}$ (h)	14–15	3.0	2.0	2.0	20	1.4–3.0

Abbreviations: CYP450, cytochrome P450; NA, not available; Pgp, P-glycoprotein; t_{max}, time of maximum circulating concentration; $t_{1/2}$, half-life.

synthesis, statins lower intracellular concentrations of cholesterol, thereby upregulating LDL-C receptors and enhancing clearance of LDL-C from the plasma. There are six statins on the market with varying degrees of LDL-C efficacy by dose (Table 4), different approved regulatory indications (Table 5), pharmacokinetic profiles (Table 6), and drug interactions (Table 7).

Clinically Relevant Differences Among the Statins
Table 5 lists the labeled indications for the statins and Table 8 summarizes the statin outcome trials. An objective synthesis of all the available statin data that includes efficacy, safety, pharmacokinetic interactions, and outcome trials can provide potential differentiating factors of each statin and the clinical relevance of these differences.

Lovastatin
Lovastatin is a short-half-life prodrug that is lipophilic and metabolized by the cytochrome P450 3A4 pathway. The immediate-release formulation should be administered with a meal, but the extended-release formulation (Altocor®) can be administered apart from food. Lovastatin has proven outcome benefits in primary prevention as demonstrated in the Air Force Texas (Coronary Atherosclerosis Prevention Study) (AFCAPS/TexCAPS) (68). Lovastatin is a generic statin and in the United States, therefore, if cost considerations are an overriding

TABLE 7 Clinically Relevant Statin Drug Interactions

Drug	Atorvastatin	Fluvastatin	Lovastatin	Pravastatin	Simvastatin	Rosuvastatin
Azole antifungals	+	−	+	−	?	−
CCBs	−	−	+	−	+	−
Cyclosporine	+	−	+	+	+	+
Erythromycin	+	−	+	−	+	−
Gemfibrozil	NA	−	+	+	+	+
Fenofibrate	−	−	NA	−	−	−
HIV PIs	+	−	+	−	+	−
Warfarin	+	+	+	+	+	+

Note: + indicates interaction reported; − indicates no interaction reported.
Abbreviations: CCB, calcium channel blocker (i.e., diltiazem, verapamil); PI, protease inhibitor; NA, not available.

TABLE 8 Outcomes Studies of Statin Medications

Study	Design	Patient characteristics	Treatment groups	Results
Primary Prevention				
Air Force/Texas Coronary Atherosclerosis Prevention Study	Multicenter, DB, PC, 5.6-yr follow-up	6,605 men and women; LDL-C 151 mg/dL; Age 58	Diet with placebo or lovastatin 20–40 mg/day	36% reduction in 1st major coronary event; 33% reduction in PTCA and CABG
Anglo-Scandinavian Cardiac Outcomes Trial–Lipid Lowering Arm	Multicenter, DB, PC, 3.36-yr follow-up	10,305 men and women; ≥3 additional CV risk factors, no h/o CHD; Median LDL-C 131 mg/dL; median age: 63	Diet with placebo or atorvastatin 10 mg/day	36% reduction in nonfatal myocardial infarction and fatal coronary heart disease; 27% reduction in fatal and nonfatal stroke; 21% reduction in total cardiovascular events; 29% reduction in total coronary events
Collaborative Atorvastatin Diabetes Study	Multicenter, DB, PC, 3.9-yr follow-up	2838 patients; Type II diabetes mellitus; ≥1 CHD risk factor(s)	Diet with placebo or atorvastatin 10 mg/day	37% reduction of major cardiovascular events; 27% of total mortality; 13.4% reduction of acute CVD events; 36% reduction of acute coronary events; 48% reduction of stroke
Prospective Study of Pravastatin in the Elderly at Risk	Multicenter, DB, PC, 3-yr follow-up	5,804 men ($n = 2804$) and women ($n = 3000$); Aged 70 to 82 yr	Diet with placebo or pravastatin 40 mg/day	15% reduction in combined endpoint (fatal/nonfatal MI or stroke); 19% reduction in total/nonfatal CHD; no effect on stroke (but 25% reduction in TIA)
West of Scotland Coronary Prevention Study	Multicenter, DB, PC, 5-yr follow-up	6,595 men; No history of MI; LDL-C 192 mg/dL; Age 55 yr	Diet with placebo or pravastatin 40 mg/day	30% reduction in nonfatal MI or CHD death; 22% reduction in death from any cause
Secondary Prevention				
Scandinavian Simvastatin Survival Study	Multicenter, DB, PC, 5.4-yr follow-up	4444 men and women; Angina or previous MI; Cholesterol 261 mg/dL; LDL-C 187 mg/dL; Age 60 yr	Diet with placebo or simvastatin 40 mg/day	Reduction in total mortality; 34% reduction in fatal/nonfatal MI and sudden cardiac death; 37% reduction in any coronary event
Cholesterol and Recurrent Events	Multicenter, DB, PC, 5-yr follow-up	4159 men and women; Previous MI; Mean LDL-C 139 mg/dL; Age 59 years	Diet with placebo or pravastatin 40 mg/day	24% reduction in CHD death or nonfatal MI; 37% reduction in fatal MI.
Heart Protection Study	Multicenter, DB, PC, 5-yr follow-up	20,536 adults; Coronary disease, other occlusive arterial disease, diabetes, or hypertension	Diet with placebo or simvastatin 40 mg/day	25% reduction in all-cause and coronary death and stroke; nonfatal MI reduced by 38%.
Long-term Intervention with Pravastatin in Ischaemic Disease	Multicenter, DB, PC, 6.1-yr follow-up	9014 men and women; Angina or previous MI; Median LDL-C 150 mg/dL; Age 62	Diet with placebo or pravastatin 40 mg/day	24% reduction in CHD death or nonfatal MI; 29% reduction in fatal or nonfatal MI.
Lescol Intervention Prevention Study	Multicenter, DB, PC, 3.9-yr follow-up	1667 men and women aged 18–80 yr post-angioplasty for CAD	Diet with placebo or fluvastatin 40 mg/day	22% lower rate of major coronary artery events (e.g., cardiac deaths, nonfatal MI, or reintervention procedure)

(Continued)

TABLE 8 *(Continued)*

Study	Design	Patient characteristics	Treatment groups	Results
Myocardial Ischemia Reduction with Aggressive Cholesterol Lowering	Multicenter, DB, PC, 16-week follow-up	3086 patients with ACS	Diet with placebo or atorvastatin 80 mg/day	Reduction in composite endpoint by 16%; ischemia reduced by 26%; stroke reduced by 50%
Pravastatin or Atorvastatin Evaluation and Infection Therapy	Multicenter, DB, PC, 1.5-yr follow-up	4162 patients with ACS	Atorvastatin 80 mg/day vs. pravastatin 40 mg/day	16% reduction of composite endpoint; 14% reduction in CHD death, MI, or revascularization; revascularizations reduced by 14%; unstable angina reduced by 29%
Treating to New Targets	Multicenter, DB, PC, 4.9-yr follow-up	10,001 men and women with CHD; Age 61; Median LDL-C 77 vs. 101 mg/dL	Atorvastatin 10 vs. 80 mg/day	22% reduction in composite CVD events

Abbreviations: DB, double blind; PC, placebo controlled; MI, myocardial infarction; CHD, coronary heart disease; CVD, cardiovascular disease; TIA, transient ischemic attack; LDL-C, low-density lipoprotein-cholesterol, PTCA, percutaneous transluminal coronary angioplasty; CABG, coronary artery bypass grafting; CAD, coronary artery disease.

issue for a patient, generic lovastatin would most likely provide the greatest LDL-C reduction (up to the limit of about a 40% decrease) for the cost.

Pravastatin

Pravastatin is a short-half-life hydrophilic statin that is not affected by food intake. Pravastatin is available at doses of 10 to 80 mg and provides LDL-C reductions of 25% to 40%. Pravastatin has shown cardiovascular benefits in patients with coronary disease (Cholesterol and Recurrent Events and Long-Term Intervention with Pravastatin in Ischaemic Disease), in high-risk primary prevention (West of Scotland Coronary Prevention Study), and in the elderly (Prospective Study of Pravastatin in the Elderly at Risk) (82–85).

Simvastatin

Simvastatin is a prodrug with a short half-life. It is lipophilic and metabolized by cytochrome P450 3A4. The drug may be administered without regard to food. Simvastatin, at doses of 5 to 80 mg, provides LDL-C reductions of 25% to 50%. For patients on potent 3A4 inhibitors, gemfibrozil or cyclosporine, the dose should not exceed 10 mg/day. For patients on verapamil or amiodarone (less potent 3A4 inhibitors), the dose of simvastatin should not exceed 20 mg/day (86). Simvastatin is the only statin to show a reduction in total mortality in both the 4S and HPS trials. Based on these outcome trials, simvastatin 40 mg is an approved starting dose for all high-risk patients (including diabetics) regardless of the baseline LDL-C level, and this is a unique indication among all the statins (86).

Fluvastatin

Fluvastatin is a synthetic, racemic mixture with a short half-life, metabolized by cytochrome 2C9. A new modified-release formulation of fluvastatin 80 mg, fluvastatin XL, provides enhanced efficacy and safety compared to the immediate-release dose. Because fluvastatin is metabolized by 2C9, there are significantly less drug interactions except for fluconazole (a 2C9 inhibitor) and warfarin. Fluvastatin 80 mg XL lowers LDL-C by approximately 35%. Fluvastatin is the only statin that has been shown not to be affected by gemfibrozil (87) and, therefore, is probably the statin of choice to combine with this fibrate. Although fluvastatin's pharmacokinetics are affected by concomitant cyclosporine, in the Assessment of Lescol in Renal Transplantation (ALERT) trial, post–renal transplant patients had a reduced incidence of cardiovascular events on fluvastatin and no patients developed rhabdomyolysis (88).

Therefore, the ALERT trial indicates that for patients post–renal transplant on cyclosporine, fluvastatin is probably the statin of choice.

Atorvastatin

Atorvastatin is a long-half-life, lipophilic statin metabolized by cytochrome P450 3A4. Atorvastatin at doses of 10 to 80 mg is the leading prescribed statin in the world, providing LDL-C reduction at 38% to 55%. Although the usual cautionary drug interactions exist for atorvastatin similar to other 3A4 metabolized statins, atorvastatin, in the clinical trial program, has an extremely low rate of myopathy (89). In almost 10,000 patients on atorvastatin in clinical trials, there have been no cases of drug-associated myopathy (CPK >10 × upper limit of normal (ULN) with symptoms). The atorvastatin 80 mg dose has an incidence of liver enzyme 3 × ULN of approximately 2.5%, which is the highest of all the statins, but a low incidence of 0.5% for all the other doses (90). The ASCOT trial showed the benefits of atorvastatin 10 mg in hypertensive patients (91), and the Collaborative Atorvastatin Diabetes Study demonstrated a benefit in diabetic patients (92). The TNT (93) and IDEAL (94) trials supported the improved clinical benefit of atorvastatin 80 mg over 10 mg of atorvastatin and 20 to 40 mg of simvastatin, respectively.

Rosuvastatin

Rosuvastatin is the most recent FDA-approved statin (doses 5–40 mg) for the treatment of dyslipidemia. Rosuvastatin, which has a structure similar to other synthetic statins, has a long half-life (20–24 hours) similar to atorvastatin and hydrophilicity comparable to pravastatin (95). Consequently, rosuvastatin is minimally metabolized and has no significant cytochrome P450 drug interactions. The efficacy of rosuvastatin is superior to that of other statins (96). Compared to atorvastatin, rosuvastatin provides approximately an 8% additional lowering of LDL-C on an equivalent dose level (96). This provides modestly more efficacy than a doubling of the dose of atorvastatin. Rosuvastatin also increases HDL-C slightly more than atorvastatin, especially at the highest doses (96).

The safety of rosuvastatin at doses of 5 to 10 mg is comparable to that of other statins in regard to liver function abnormalities and myopathy rates (97). The lack of cytochrome P450 metabolism for rosuvastatin allows this therapy to be used without precautions in patients who are on cytochrome P450 3A4–inhibiting drugs such as amiodarone, nefazodone, or ketoconazole. As compared to gemfibrozil, rosuvastatin has been shown not to have a pharmacokinetic interaction with fenofibrate. Therefore, the usual caution regarding the concomitant use of statin and fibrates may not apply with the combination of rosuvastatin and fenofibrate. Both gemfibrozil and cyclosporin significantly increase the area under the curve for rosuvastatin. In combination with these drugs, rosuvastatin should be initiated at the 5 mg dose and should not exceed 10 mg (98).

Safety Monitoring for Statin Therapy

Statin therapy is generally very safe, but patients should be warned about potential side effects such as myopathy or liver toxicity. Prior to initiating statin therapy, in addition to ruling out secondary causes of dyslipidemia, patients should have liver enzymes measured [alanine aminotransferase (ALT) and aspartate aminotransferase (AST)] and creatinine kinases (CK). Liver enzymes should be repeated after 6 to 12 weeks after initiating therapy and after each dose titration and then periodically thereafter. For patients on a statin dose, annual liver enzyme testing is appropriate. If ALT or AST increase to three times above the upper limit of normal, repeat enzymes should be conducted within the next week and if the elevations are persistent, the statin should be discontinued. If the liver enzymes are 1.5 to 3 times the ULN, the patient should undergo repeat measurements at more frequent intervals. After the baseline measurement of CK, repeat measurements are not necessary unless the patient develops muscle pain and weakness. Repeat CK measurements in asymptomatic patients are not necessary because sporadic CK elevation are common because of minor contusions or exercise and may inappropriately label the patient as statin intolerant. In a patient with muscle pain or weakness with a CK >10 × ULN, the statin should be discontinued. For patients with CK 5–10 × ULN, clinical judgment should be considered in regard to statin discontinuation. For patients with a normal or mildl-cy elevated CK elevation, the patient should continue the statin, unless the symptoms are intolerable or cause excessive concern regarding statin safety.

Rhabdomyolysis, which is defined as CK >10 × ULN with a creatinine elevation or CK > 10,000, is very rare (approximately 1 in 10,000 statin patients) and requires intravenous hydration after discontinuation of statin therapy. Statin myopathy is potentially due to the depletion of muscle ubiquinone (coenzyme Q10). The production of coenzyme Q10 is inhibited by statin therapy, but there is little clinical evidence as of yet whether oral coenzyme Q10 supplementation reduces the risk of myopathy.

Statin Intolerance

There are approximately 5% of hyperlipidemic patients who do not tolerate statins, usually because of myalgias or occasionally GI disturbance. Less than 1% discontinue statin use because of liver function abnormalities or myopathy (creatine phosphokinase greater than 10 × ULN with symptoms). Patients with liver function abnormalities or myopathy usually tolerate a lower dose of the statin, but patients with myalgias (muscle aches without creatine phosphokinase elevations) or GI complaints may continue to have symptoms on lower doses or different statins. The cause of myalgias is uncertain and in controlled trials, the incidence is far less than in clinical practice and similar to the placebo rate. Switching from one statin to another sometimes results in a statin the patient can tolerate. Although only anecdotal, some physicians have found success in preventing statin-induced myalgia by coadministering 50 to 100 mg of coenzyme Q10 (ubiquinone). Statins may decrease ubiquinone levels in skeletal muscles. Nonstatin therapy, such as the bile acid–binding polymer colesevelam, or the cholesterol absorption inhibitor ezetimibe, niacin, or fibrates, may also be used if statin intolerance is unavoidable. Many patients may tolerate an every-other-day dosing of a low dose statin alternating with an every-other-day dosing of ezetimibe.

Ezetimibe

Ezetimibe is the first of a new class of lipid-lowering drugs known as cholesterol absorption inhibitors (99). Ezetimibe localizes at the brush border of the small intestine and selectively inhibits the absorption of cholesterol from the intestinal lumen into enterocytes by binding to the Nieman Pick C1 like-1 sterol transporter (100). Further investigation is needed to determine the precise mechanism by which ezetimibe inhibits cholesterol absorption. Ezetimibe does not affect the absorption of TGs, fatty acids, bile acids, or fat-soluble vitamins, including vitamins A, D, and E, and alpha- and beta-carotenes (99,101). Following oral administration, ezetimibe is rapidly glucuronidated in the intestines, and once glucuronidated, it undergoes enterohepatic recirculation, thereby repeatedly delivering the drug to its site of action and minimizing systemic exposure (102). Notably, the glucuronide of ezetimibe is even more potent as a cholesterol absorption inhibitor than the parent compound, possibly because of its localization in the intestines (102). The enterohepatic recirculation may explain the long duration of action of ezetimibe; as such, its long elimination half-life permits once-daily dosing. Both ezetimibe and its glucuronide are recirculated enterohepatically and delivered back to the site of action in the intestine, resulting in multiple peaks of drug, accounting for a half-life of approximately 22 hours (103). The timing of dosing does not affect its activity (104), and food does not affect its bioavailability (105).

In animal models, ezetimibe decreased delivery of cholesterol from the intestine to the liver, reduced hepatic cholesterol stores, upregulated LDL-C receptors on liver cell membranes, and increased clearance of cholesterol from blood (99,106–109). In a two-week, double blind, placebo-controlled, crossover study of 18 hypercholesterolemic patients, ezetimibe 10 mg once daily inhibited intestinal cholesterol absorption by 54% as compared with placebo ($p < 0.001$) (110). Although hepatic cholesterol synthesis increased with ezetimibe, plasma LDL-C was reduced by 20% relative to placebo ($p < 0.001$).

Ezetimibe does not interact with drugs metabolized by cytochrome P450 (CYP) 1A2, 2D6, 2C8, 2C9, or 3A4, suggesting that it has low potential for participating in drug–drug interactions (111). Importantly, ezetimibe does not interact with statins, including atorvastatin, simvastatin, lovastatin, or fluvastatin (112–115). Accordingly, ezetimibe can be taken at the same time as the statin during coadministration therapy. Moreover, clinically significant interactions were not observed when ezetimibe was administered in conjunction with caffeine, dextromethorphan, midazolam, tolbutamide, antacid, cimetidine, oral contraceptives, warfarin, digoxin, or glipizide (111,116–122). Concomitant administration of fenofibrate (200 mg once daily) increased the mean maximum plasma concentration and area under the time versus plasma concentration curve for total ezetimibe by approximately 64% and 48%, respectively;

however, these effects were not clinically significant (83,120). The pharmacokinetics of fenofibrate were not significantly affected by ezetimibe (10 mg once daily) (83). Thus, its pharmacokinetic profile and novel mechanism of action make ezetimibe an ideal drug for use in combination therapy for hypercholesterolemia.

Efficacy of Ezetimibe

Ezetimibe Monotherapy

Monotherapy with ezetimibe has been shown to effectively reduce LDL-C in patients with hypercholesterolemia (123,124). In two randomized, placebo-controlled Phase III trials of 892 and 827 patients, 12 weeks of once-daily treatment with ezetimibe 10 mg decreased LDL-C by 17.7% and 18.2%, respectively, compared with increases of 1.1% and 1.4% with placebo ($p <$ 0.01). In both studies, ezetimibe also improved levels of total cholesterol (decreases of 12.5% and 12.4%, respectively, vs increases of 0.8% and 0.6%, respectively, with placebo), ApoB (decreases of 15.5% and 15.4%, respectively, vs decreases of 1.4% and 1.0%, respectively, with placebo), and HDL-C (increases of 1.3% and 1.0%, respectively, vs decreases of 1.6% and 1.3%, respectively, with placebo) (all $p < 0.01$) (123,124); in one study, ezetimibe improved levels of TGs (5.7% decrease) compared with placebo (5.7% increase; $p < 0.01$) (123).

Ezetimibe Plus Statin Coadministration Therapy

Ezetimibe was coadministered with a statin in four randomized, double blind, placebo-controlled, multicenter studies of patients with primary hypercholesterolemia (125–128). After patients were stabilized on the NCEP Step I diet (or stricter) and discontinued all previous lipid-lowering therapy; they entered a four-week, single blind placebo run-in period. Patients with baseline LDL-C levels between 145 mg/dL (3.35 mmol/L) and 250 mg/dL (6.48 mmol/L), and TGs ≤350 mg/dL (3.99 mmol/L) were then randomly assigned to daily treatment with ezetimibe alone, statin alone, ezetimibe plus statin, or placebo for 12 weeks. Ezetimibe was administered at a dosage of 10 mg once daily, whereas several statin dose levels were evaluated in monotherapy and in coadministration with ezetimibe (atorvastatin and simvastatin: 10 mg, 20 mg, 40 mg, or 80 mg; lovastatin and pravastatin: 10 mg, 20 mg, or 40 mg). In each study, ezetimibe plus statin coadministration was more effective in lowering LDL-C than statin alone. Notably, the greater efficacy of ezetimibe plus statin coadministration was seen at each statin dose level. Moreover, the coadministration of ezetimibe 10 mg daily with the lowest statin dose was as effective as statin monotherapy at the highest dose. For example, calculated LDL-C was equivalently reduced from baseline by ezetimibe 10 mg plus simvastatin 10 mg and by simvastatin 80 mg alone (46% vs. 45%) (125). Similarly, ezetimibe plus atorvastatin 10 mg was as effective as atorvastatin 80 mg alone (53% vs. 54%) (126); ezetimibe plus lovastatin 10 mg was as effective as lovastatin 40 mg alone (34% vs. 31%) (127); and ezetimibe plus pravastatin 10 mg was as effective at reducing LDL-C as pravastatin 40 mg (34% vs. 29%, $p < 0.05$) (128). Coadministration of ezetimibe plus statin (results pooled across doses) was also more effective than statin alone in raising HDL-C (except for ezetimibe plus pravastatin) and reducing TGs and ApoB. Notably, the efficacy of coadministration therapy was not influenced by age, race, gender, or level of CHD risk.

The overall safety profile of ezetimibe coadministration with statin therapy was generally similar to that of statin alone (125–128). There was no evidence that addition of ezetimibe to any dose of simvastatin, atorvastatin, lovastatin, or pravastatin increased the risk of any non-laboratory adverse event.

No cases of hepatitis, jaundice, or other clinical signs of liver dysfunction were reported with ezetimibe plus statin coadministration therapy. Incidence of elevations in ALT or AST ≥3 times ULN ranged from 0% to 0.8% with statin monotherapy, compared with 0% to 2.2% with ezetimibe plus statin coadministration. Clinically important elevations in CPK (≥10 times ULN) have been rarely observed with the ezetimibe plus statin therapy.

Bile Acid Sequestrants

Two of the most commonly prescribed bile acid sequestrants, cholestyramine and colestipol, have been in use since the 1980s. Bile acid sequestrants decrease intrahepatic cholesterol by interrupting enterohepatic circulation of bile acids, thereby increasing the synthesis of bile acids from cholesterol in the liver. This upregulates LDL-C receptor activity and increases clearance of LDL-C from the blood. Evidence of clinical benefit of bile acid sequestrants has been demonstrated in a number of clinical trials, including the Lipid Research Clinics-Coronary Primary Prevention trial (129) and the Familial Atherosclerosis Treatment study (FATS) (130).

Bile acid sequestrants are difficult to use in practice. Adherence to bile acid sequestrants is often an issue with their administration, in part because of the poor palatability of the drug, and the occurrence of gastrointestinal adverse effects, particularly constipation. Compliance with prescribed sequestrant therapy may be as low as 50%. Therefore, colesevelam, a novel bile acid sequestrant, has become the preferred drug of this class.

Colesevelam is a polyallylamine cross-linked with epichlorohydrin and alkylated with 1-bromodecane and 6-bromohexyltrimethylammonium bromide. Colesevelam did not inhibit the absorption of lovastatin when administered together.

Colesevelam is a novel, polymeric agent with bile-acid–binding activity. The ability of colesevelam to lower serum LDL-C levels has been demonstrated in several clinical trials in which approximately 1400 patients were evaluated. Compared to historical data with bile-acid sequestrants, colesevelam is four to six times more potent. Colesevelam is effective as monotherapy for patients with mild to moderate hypercholesterolemia and when coadministered with an HMG-CoA reductase inhibitor. In terms of its safety and tolerability, colesevelam is well accepted alone and in combination with statin therapy and lacks the constipating effect of typical bile acid sequestrants. There are three types of patients in whom colesevelam may be most appropriate. The first is a patient who has not achieved NCEP ATP III with maximal statin therapy (or maximally tolerated dose). Colesevelam may also be an option for the statin-intolerant patient or the patient who refuses to take a statin because of fear of side effects (131).

Niacin

Niacin or nicotinic acid is a soluble B vitamin that has favorable effects on all major lipid subfractions (Table 9) (132). The pharmacokinetics of niacin and its mechanism of action are not well understood, but niacin appears to reduce ApoB secretion, thereby lowering both VLDL-C and LDL-C, increasing ApoAI, and lowering Lp(a) (133). Niacin reduces the mobilization of free fatty acids from the periphery, probably by inhibiting hormone-sensitive lipase. Therefore, there is less TG substrate for VLDL-C synthesis and a reduced secretion of VLDL-C, which is the precursor of LDL-C (Fig. 9). Niacin may also inhibit diacylglycerol-2-acyltransferase, a key enzyme TG synthesis. On average, niacin lowers LDL-C by 10% to 20%, TGs by 20% to 40%, Lp(a) by 10% to 30%, and raises HDL-C by 15% to 30% (134). These effects are dose related and demonstrated in Figure 10 (135). Niacin is the only known approved lipid-altering drug (with the exception of estrogen) that lowers Lp(a) and is the most potent drug to raise HDL-C. Niacin appears to increase HDL-C by decreasing the hepatic uptake of Apo AI, thereby delaying catabolism (136). HDL-C can be taken up by hepatocytes by at least two cellular receptors. SRB1 binds HDL-C and cholesteryl ester is selectively taken up by hepatocytes. Once delipidated, the HDL-C particle is then released back into the circulation. This receptor is not affected by niacin. Niacin appears to inhibit another receptor that regulates holoparticle uptake and catabolism of HDL-C. This results in a longer circulating half-life for HDL-C and, theoretically, improved reverse cholesterol transport and increased potential for other antiatherogenic effects (137).

TABLE 9 Effects of Niacin

Niacin decreases	Niacin increases
Total cholesterol	HDL cholesterol
Total triglycerides	HDL_2 cholesterol
VLDL-C	HDL_3 cholesterol (less than HDL_2)
LDL-C	Apolipoproteins A-I, A-II
Small dense LDL-C	LP A-I
Lp(a)	LP A-I + A-II (less than LP A-I)
ApoB	LDL-C particle size
Total cholesterol/HDL-C	
LDL-C-C/HDL-C	
ApoB/A-I	

Abbreviations: LDL-C, low-density lipoprotein-cholesterol; HDL-C, high-density lipoprotein-cholesterol; VLDL, very-low-density lipoprotein; ApoB, Apo lipoprotein B; LP, lipoprotein.

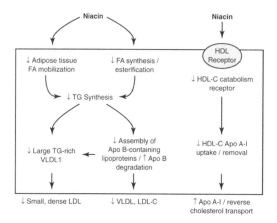

FIGURE 9   Pharmco-kinetics of niacin. *Abbreviations:* TG, triglyceride; LDL-C, low-density lipoprotein-choles-terol; VLDL-C, very-low-density lipoprotein; HDL-C, high-density lipoprotein-cholesterol;ApoA, Apolipoprotein-A; FA, fatty acid.

Niacin can cause significant hepatotoxicity and should be discontinued if liver enzymes (Serum glutamic-oxalocetic Transaminase and Serum glutamate-pyruvate transaminase) exceed three times the upper limit of normal. Patients who use over-the-counter niacin should be worried about the hazard of liver toxicity (138). Many over-the-counter niacin supplements may not be labeled as sustained release, but if niacin is combined with a fiber such as oat or rice bran, this can cause a sustained release and adversely affect the liver enzymes. Patients should generally be advised not to use over-the-counter niacin. Niacin can also increase uric acid levels, aggravating gout. Other side effects of niacin include a rash, gastrointestinal problems including worsening of esophageal reflux, or peptic ulcers, and headache. Rarely, skin lesions, usually in the axillary areas or elbows, known as acanthosis nigricans, can develop.

Niacin is often added to a statin in patients with combined hyperlipidemia, especially if the HDL-C is low or Lp(a) is high. There have been a number of studies that have evaluated the combination of a statin with niacin (139). The incidence of liver function abnormalities with the combination of a statin plus niacin is generally similar to niacin therapy alone at least when the combination of both drugs is at the starting doses (i.e., simvastatin 20 mg, pravastatin 40 mg, fluvastatin 40 mg plus niacin 1500–2000 mg/day). Myopathy has been reported with statins plus

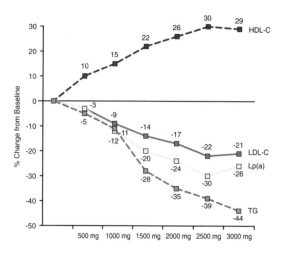

FIGURE 10   Dose–response of once-daily extended-release Niacin. *Abbreviations*: TG, Triglycleride; LDL-C, low-density lipoprotein-cholesterol; HDL-C, high-density lipoprotein cholesterol; Lp(a), lipoprotein(a). *Source*: From Ref. 140.

niacin, but the incidence appears to be less than expected with gemfibrozil (140). Myopathy has developed with the combination, after niacin-induced hepatotoxicity reduces the catabolism of the statin, resulting in markedly elevated statin levels. Therefore, unregulated sustained release niacins that have a higher incidence of hepatotoxicity should be avoided in combination therapy. The vast majority of combination trials have utilized either immediate-release niacin or Niaspan®. In one study, a single tablet containing both Niaspan® and lovastatin (Advicor®) was dose titrated from Niaspan® 500 mg plus lovastatin 10 mg to Niaspan® 2000 mg plus lovastatin 40 mg to target levels based on NCEP guidelines over a 16-week period (141). Once on a stable dose, the patients were followed further for 36 weeks. Over 600 patients were enrolled with LDL-C levels exceeding the NCEP ATP II levels for initiating drug therapy. At the 2000/40 mg dose, LDL-C was lowered by 47% and TG by 42%, and HDL-C increased by 30%. About 7% of patients withdrew as a result of flushing. There were no cases of drug-induced myopathy, and less than 1% had elevated liver enzymes more than $3 \times$ ULN.

Because of the safety data of Niaspan® in combination with a statin, recently, there has been a resurgence of interest in the utilization of combination therapy to maximize risk reduction in patients with dyslipidemia (135). Over the past several years, statins have established a large clinical trial base documenting both safety and outcome benefits. Niacin also has demonstrated CHD outcome benefits either as monotherapy or in combination with other lipid-lowering agents (Table 10) (130,142–146). The marked reductions in clinical events in the FATS and HDL-Atherosclerosis Treatment Study (HATS) trials, although relatively small trials, have provided intriguing data suggesting the importance of combining niacin with other lipid-lowering agents. Statins, in general, have demonstrated approximately a 30% reduction in CHD events, but in these small trials combining a statin with niacin, the reduction in CHD events was approximately 75%. This 75% reduction in clinical events with combining a statin with niacin is far more than what is expected with LDL-C reduction alone. This marked reduction in CHD events suggests that the other effects of niacin, such as raising HDL-C and lowering TG and Lp(a), contribute significantly to the benefits. Although the clinical benefits of changing the LDL-C particle size from small (pattern B) to large (pattern A) is not yet conclusively demonstrated, niacin is one of the most effective agents in modifying LDL-C particle size while statins are more effective in lowering the total LDL-C particle number (147,148).

The ATP III guidelines, by recommending non-HDL-C as well as LDL-C targets if the TG exceeds 200 mg/dL, have also enhanced the need for niacin therapy (63). Based on a recent evaluation of the safety and pharmacokinetics of statins in combination with fibrates or niacin, an algorithm was developed to utilize appropriate combination treatment if non-HDL-C goals have not been achieved (Fig. 11) (75).

TABLE 10 Niacin Coronary Heart Disease Endpoint Trials

Study	Population	Results
Coronary Drug Project	8341 post-MI men; Baseline TC 250 mg/dL—9.9% on trial; Baseline TG 177 mg/dL—26.1% on trial	27% reduction in definite nonfatal MI – 24% reduction in CVA. Total mortality decrease 10.6% at 15 yr.
Stockholm Ischemia Heart Study	555 consecutive MI survivors <70 yr old; open label clofibrate/niacin or placebo; Baseline TC 245 mg/dL—13% on trial; Baseline TG 208 mg/dL—19% on trial	36% reduction in CHD deaths
Familial Atherosclerosis Treatment Study	146 men with ApoB (125 mg/dL with CHD; Conventional therapy vs. niacin/colestipol or lovastatin/colestipol	73% reduction in CHD events in patients who received intensive lipid-lowering therapy
HDL Atherosclerosis Treatment Study	160 CHD patients with HDL <35 mg/dL, LDL-C <145 mg/dL; Treated 3 yr with niacin/simvastatin or placebo with or without antioxidants	Reduction of CHD events by 60% (on antioxidants) to 90% (off antioxidants)

Abbreviations: CHD, coronary heart disease; LDL-C, low-density lipoprotein; TG, triglyceride, MI, myocardial infarction; HDL-C, high-density lipoprotein-cholesterol; CVA, cerebrovascular disease.

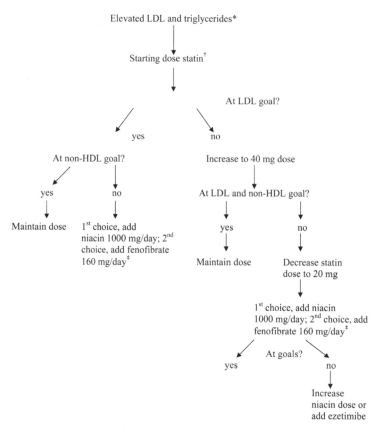

FIGURE 11   Algorithm to maximize safety of lipid-lowering therapy. *At baseline, check LFT, CK, thyroid profile; document presence of muscle soreness, tenderness, or pain. †FDA approved starting dose statins: lovastatin 20, 40mg; simvastatin 10, 20, 40mg; atorvastatin 10, 20, 40mg; fluvastatin 20, 40, 80mg XI; pravastatin 10, 20, 40mg. ‡or substitute niacin-ER/lovastatin combination tablet. Alternative options for patients at high risk for statin myopathy include ezetimibe plus niacin or fenofibrate. *Abbreviations*: LDL-C, low-density lipoprotein-cholesterol; HDL-C, high-density lipoprotein-cholesterol.

The utilization of niacin in diabetics has, in the past, been considered problematic because of the modest glucose-raising effects of niacin. A recent trial and a reevaluation of the Coronary Drug Project (CDP) (149,150) have provided helpful information in the utilization of niacin in patients with glucose elevations. A reevaluation of the CDP in the diabetic subpopulation demonstrated a similar reduction in clinical CHD events as the nondiabetic CHD population. This information provides support for the use of niacin to treat diabetic dyslipidemia and, although there may be a modest increase in serum glucose levels, the overall benefit is a marked reduction in cardiovascular events. In the Assessment of Diabetes Control and Evaluation of the Efficacy of Niaspan Trial (ADVENT) (151), 148 patients with Type 2 diabetes and dyslipidemia were randomized to 1000 mg/day, 1500 mg/day of Niaspan® or placebo; 47% of the patients were also taking statins.

In the ADVENT, extended-release niacin produced a significant effect on both TG and HDL-C levels. The increase in HDL-C was dose-dependent and was significantly greater at all time points for the niacin-treated groups than for the placebo group. In the 1000 mg niacin group, HDL-C increased up to 19% at 16 weeks. In the 1500 mg group, it increased up to 24%. The absolute increases in HDL-C at 16 weeks were 7.6 mg/dL in the 1000 mg group and 11 mg/dL in the 155 mg group, compared with 1.6 mg/dL among placebo-treated patients.

TG reductions were also dose-related. Reductions in the patients receiving lower-dose niacin were not significantly greater than those in placebo-treated patients. TG levels were reduced 28% in the 1500 mg niacin group at 16 weeks—a significant difference compared with placebo.

Changes in HbA1C levels were small in all treatment groups. HbA1C values in the 100 mg/day treatment group were not significantly different from the placebo group. Changes in HbA1C levels in the 1500 mg/day group reached marginal significance ($p = 0.048$) at 16 weeks. Increases in fasting blood glucose occurred between weeks 4 and 8 in the niacin-treated groups; levels returned to baseline by week 16.

ADVENT demonstrated that extended-release niacin, at the doses tested, is effective and well tolerated in patients who have Type 2 diabetes and atherogenic dyslipidemia—whether given alone or with a statin. Low doses of extended-release niacin are, therefore, an option for the treatment of dyslipidemia in patients who have glucose-controlled Type 2 diabetes.

Fibrates

There are five fibrates currently used in human therapy: clofibrate, gemfibrozil, fenofibrate, bezafibrate, and ciprofibrate. Only gemfibrozil and fenofibrate are available in the United States. Fibrates are peroxisome proliferator–activated receptor (PPAR)-alpha ligands. PPAR-alpha activated by fibrates form heterodimers with 9-*cis* retinoic acid receptor (RXR). The PPAR/RXR heterodimers bind to peroxisome proliferator response elements, upregulating the expression of these genes. PPAR-alpha activation by fibrates leads to increasing lipoprotein lipase expression and decreasing ApoCIII expression, which results in enhanced catabolism of TG-rich particles. Fibrates also increase expression of ApoAI and ApoAII (152). The net result of fibrate therapy is decreased HTG and an increase in HDL-C. LDL-C levels may also decrease, most likely because of a reduction of dense LDL-C, which is more atherogenic than buoyant LDL-C and has poor affinity for the LDL-C receptor. However, LDL-C may also increase in patients with HTG with fibrate therapy, but these are usually the less atherogenic buoyant LDL-C particles. Consequently, fibrates are used almost exclusively for patients with HTG and low HDL-C, but fibrates may lower LDL-C by 10% to 15% in patients without HTG.

There are several outcome trials that have used fibrates. In patients with HTG or low HDL-C, or both, these drugs reduce CHD events or the angiographic progression of atherosclerosis (Table 11). In patients with CHD and low HDL-C, the Veterans Affairs High-Density Lipoprotein Cholesterol Intervention Trial (VA-HIT) study (153) shows that gemfibrozil compares favorably to statin therapy, using a number needed to treat to prevent one-event analysis. The Bezafibrate Infarction Prevention (BIP) trial failed to demonstrate a significant overall benefit, but for patients with TGs greater than 200 mg/dL, there was a 40% CHD risk reduction ($p = 0.03$) (154). The mean LDL-C in the VA-HIT study was 111 mg/dL compared 148 mg/dL in the BIP trial. The lack of benefit for bezafibrate in the BIP trial compared to the significant benefit for gemfibrozil in the VA-HIT study suggests that fibrates need to be targeted at patients with high TGs or low HDL-C with a relatively low LDL-C.

The Fenofibrate Intervention and Event Lowering in Diabetes (FIELD) trial (155) did not reduce nonfatal and fatal myocardial interactions significantly (11% reduction, $p = 0.16$), but a secondary end point, which included fatal CVD events (nonfatal, fatal myocardial interactions, coronary revascularization, and stroke), was reduced significantly by 11% ($p = 0.035$). This study was compromised by a higher statin drop in rate-in the control group during the treatment period, which resulted in only minimal changes in the lipid profile between the two groups. The FIELD patients with preexisting CHD (approximately 20% of the study patients) had the highest statin drop-in during the study, and if the diabetics without CHD (approximately 80% of the study patients) are evaluated post hoc, there is a 25% CHD reduction, which is comparable to statin trials with diabetic patients. The greatest absolute reduction in CHD events (2.5%) was demonstrated in the patients with "dyslipidemia" (high TGs and low HDL-C). In the FIELD trial, fenofibrate was demonstrated to lower LDL-C by approximately 15% in this diabetic population without significant HTG. This significant decrease in LDL-C in the treatment group compared to placebo was abolished over time, probably because of the excessive statin drop-in rate in the placebo group.

While further LDL-C lowering may provide additional clinical benefits in patients with diabetes and/or metabolic syndrome, the post hoc analysis of clinical trials has demonstrated a very high residual risk even with low LDL-C levels. Surrogate endpoint trials also demonstrate significant atherosclerotic progression in diabetics on statins or a combination of statins and niacin. Because fibrates appear to have unique benefits in patients with insulin resistance, the combination of a statin and a fibrate is potentially most appropriate in this patient population. The Action to Control Cardiovascular Risk in Diabetes (156) trial will be testing this

TABLE 11 Fibrate Outcome Studies

Trial	Duration (yr)	n	Treatment	Primary endpoint	RRR	ARR	NNT
Primary Prevention							
HHS	5	4081	Gemfibrozil 600 mg b.i.d.	Fatal, nonfatal MI and cardiac death	34%	1.4%	71
FIELD	5	9795	Fenofibrate 200 mg	Fatal and nonfatal MI	11%	1.3%	77
FIELD Subgroup without CVD	5	7664	Fenofibrate 200 mg	Total MI cardiovascular events	19%	2.0%	50
Secondary Prevention							
BIP	6.2	3090	Bezafibrate 400 mg q.d.	Fatal, nonfatal MI, sudden death	9% (NS)	NA	NA
BIP subgroup TG >200	6.2	459	Bezafibrate 400 mg q.d.	Fatal, nonfatal MI, sudden death	39%	7.7%	13
VA-HIT	5.1	2531	Gemfibrozil 1200 mg q.d.	Nonfatal MI and CHD death	22%	4.4%	23

Abbreviations: N, number of participants; RRR, relative risk reduction; ARR, absolute risk reduction; NNT, number needed to treat; HHS, Helsinki Heart study; BIP, Bezafibrate Infarction Prevention Study; VA-HIT, Veterans Affairs High-Density Lipoprotein Intervention Trial; MI, Myocardial Infarction; FIELD, Fenofibrate Intervention and Event Lowering in Diabetes: TG, triglyceride; CHD, coronary heart disease.

hypothesis in approximately 10,000 diabetics on simvastatin randomized to fenofibrate or placebo to evaluate CHD outcomes.

The additive effects of simvastatin and fenofibrate on lipid parameters have been documented in the Simvastatin Plus Fenofibrate for Combined Hyperlipidemia trial (157). Simvastatin monotherapy (20 mg/day) was compared to combination therapy (simvastatin 20 mg/day plus fenofibrate 160 mg/day) in patients with combined hyperlipidemia (fasting TG levels 150 mg/dL or greater and 500 mg/dL or lower and LDL-C > 130 mg/dL). Mean LDL-C levels decreased significantly with combination therapy compared to monotherapy (31.2% and 25.8%, respectively, $p < 0.001$). In addition, mean HDL-C levels significantly increased with combination therapy compared to monotherapy (18.6% and 9.7%, respectively, $p < 0.001$) and no drug-related serious adverse events occurred (157).

In light of the residual risk of CHD events in statin trials within certain subgroups, combination therapy appears most appropriate in patients with high event rates despite optimal statin treatment. These subgroups include very high–risk patients with LDL-C levels greater than 70 mg/dL, diabetics, those with metabolic syndrome and elevated high-sensitivity C-reactive protein, and cigarette smokers. A recent survey demonstrated that 75% of patients with CVD met the definition of "very high risk" according to the NCEP ATP III update report (158). In this survey, only 18% of patients at "very high risk" had an LDL-C lower than 70 mg/dL and only 4% had an LDL-C lower than 70 mg/dL and a non-HDL-C lower than 100 mg/dL if TGs were greater than 200 mg/dL. These data support the utilization of more aggressive statin therapy and the implementation of combination therapy as necessary to achieve these optional targets in the very high–risk patient population.

DIFFICULT-TO-TREAT PATIENTS
Patient Profile #1: Hypercholesterolemia
Treatment Guidelines

High LDL-C, normal TG, and HDL-C. Patient example: 46-year-old man; nonsmoker; weight (Wt), 180; height (Ht), 5 ft 11 in.; BP, 130/88 Family history: Father died of myocardial infarction (MI) at age 74 years

Lipid Profile

Cholesterol: 250 mg/dL
TG: 100 mg/dL

HDL:	42 mg/dL
LDL-C:	188 mg/dL
Framingham 10-year risk:	10%
ATP III 10-year risk:	8%
LDL-C goal:	less than 130, optional goal less than 100 mg/dL

Therapy

Option 1: Starting Dose of Statin and Titrating the Dose to Goal

Table 4 depicts the efficacy of various statins throughout the dose range for percent LDL-C reduction. Many physicians prefer to start with the recommended starting dose of the statin, and, if the patient is not at the appropriate goal after 6 to 12 weeks of treatment, the dose is increased to the next level. After each titration, follow-up lipid profile and liver function tests are recommended at 6- to 12-week intervals.

Once the patient achieves the recommended goal with normal safety laboratory tests, follow-up is usually at 6- to 12-month intervals.

Option 2: Using a Flexible Start Dose

Some physicians prefer a higher start dose based on the percent LDL-C reduction required to achieve the goal. The advantage of this strategy is that a patient is more likely to achieve the recommended goal with fewer titration visits, and having more dramatic results over a shorter period may enhance patient satisfaction. If the patient has an exaggerated response to the higher statin dose, the dose can be downtitrated on the follow-up visit. This strategy is also best advocated for patients at high risk for cardiac events (e.g., patients with CHD or CHD risk equivalent).

Option 3: Starting Dose of Statin Plus Combination Therapy

Bile acid sequestrants (cholestyramine, colestipol, and colesevelam), niacin (Niaspan), and ezetimibe (a cholesterol absorption inhibitor) lower LDL-C, depending on the dose, by 15% to 20%. A 15% to 20% decrease in LDL-C is approximately equivalent to tripling the dose of the statin. For every doubling of the dose of the statin, there is a further decrease in LDL-C of approximately 6%. Therefore, adding one of the aforementioned nonstatin drugs to a starting dose results in LDL-C reductions equivalent to or greater than the highest available dose of the statin. This strategy is being used in patients who are intolerant to a high dose of a statin, in patients who do not achieve the recommended goals despite the use of a high dose of statin, or if more aggressive lipid-modifying therapy is necessary to achieve the desired treatment goals.

Option 4: Nonstatin Therapy for Patients with Mild Low-Density Lipoprotein Elevations

Some patients require an LDL-C reduction of less than 20% to achieve the recommended goals, and for these patients, nonstatin therapy is an option. Although statin therapy may result in LDL-C reduction far below the recommended goals, the proven benefits of statins in clinical trials and the ease of use lead to improved compliance, and, usually, cost issues still make statins the preferred option in most patients with mild LDL-C elevations. Nevertheless, some patients (and physicians) prefer nonsystemic therapies, such as the bile acid sequestrants or ezetimibe, for patients in whom modest LDL-C reduction achieves the recommended goals. For patients with significant cost constraints, over-the-counter immediate-release niacin may be a consideration; however, most pharmaceutical companies provide assistance programs and other options (although not U.S. FDA approved), which include pill cutting or alternate-day dosing of the statin to reduce cost.

Patient Profile #2: Hypercholesterolemia with Low High-Density Lipoprotein Cholesterol

High LDL-C, normal TG, low HDL-C

Patient example: 50-year-old man; smoker (two packs/day); Wt, 175 lb; Ht, 5′9″; body mass index (BMI), 25; BP, 130/80 mmHg

Family history: Mother died of MI at age 54

Lipid Profile

Cholesterol:	248 mg/dL
TG:	175 mg/dL
HDL-C:	38 mg/dL

Framingham 10-year risk: 21%
ATP III 10-year risk: 25%
LDL-C: 175 mg/dL
CV: age older than 74 year
LDL-C goal: less than 100 mg/dL
% LDL-C reduction to achieve goal: 43

Therapy

The treatment options for this patient are similar to those of Patient Profile #1 (high LDL-C, normal TG, and HDL-C); however, the low HDL-C and the cigarette smoking confer a much higher global risk for CHD. In addition to achieving the LDL-C treatment goal, special attention should be paid to attempting to raise the HDL-C. In patients such as this, smoking cessation would usually result in a significant increase in HDL-C. Therefore, smoking cessation should be strongly encouraged. Other causes of low HDL-C should also be considered, as in the following mnemonic:

L—Lack of exercise
O—Obesity
W—Postmenopausal status
H—Hypertriglyceridemia
D—Drugs such as anabolic steroids, testosterone, etc.
L—Lack of alcohol
C—Cigarette smoking

Because this patient is overweight, an exercise program should improve weight loss, lower TG values, and raise HDL-C. Physician advice to increase alcohol intake is generally not recommended because of other potentially adverse effects of alcohol. For patients who drink modestly, however, advice regarding the restriction of alcohol intake is not necessary.

In patients with high LDL-C and low HDL-C, the drug treatment options are similar to those of patients with isolated high LDL-C, with a potentially greater emphasis on combination drug therapy that may beneficially modify HDL-C levels. Statins remain the drugs of first choice. Based on the results of the large statin endpoint trials (West of Scotland Coronary Prevention Study, AFCAPS), patients with high LDL-C and low HDL have significant benefits for statin therapy. The percent reduction of events is even greater in the low HDL-C subjects. The main objective with this patient example is to achieve the LDL-C goal of less than 100 mg/dL. This requires a 46% reduction in LDL-C; therefore, beginning with a higher starting dose or a more potent statin, or both, is usually advisable. The Canadian guidelines recommend a total cholesterol HDL-C ratio goal of less than 4 for high-risk patients. A ratio goal may be achieved by more aggressive LDL-C lowering or by potentially increasing HDL-C. After initiating a statin, the next consideration involves whether to add a second drug (or use a combination of niacin plus lovastatin as a single tablet). Adding niacin to a statin is the most likely combination because niacin has the most significant effects on raising HDL-C. There have also been a number of trials that have demonstrated the safety of this combination and efficacy in inhibiting the development of atherosclerosis. Adding a fibrate is a less desirable combination for this patient profile because the TGs are not significantly elevated and, in the absence of insulin resistance, fibrates may be of limited clinical value.

Patient Profile #3: Combined Hyperlipidemia

High LDL-C ($\geq$130 mg/dL), moderate hypertriglyceridemia (200 to 500 mg/dL), and low HDL-C (lower than 40 mg/dL)

Patient example: 65-year-old woman; nonsmoker; Wt, 150 lb; Ht, 5'3''; BP, 140/88 mmHg; BMI, 26

Family history: Father died of MI at age 52 years

Lipid Profile

Cholesterol: 260 mg/dL
TG: 300 mg/dL

HDL-C:	33 mg/dL
LDL-C:	166 mg/dL
Non-HDL-C:	227 mg/dL
LDL-C goal:	less than 130 mg/dL
Non-HDL-C goal:	less than 160 mg/dL
10-year risk:	9%

Therapy

FCH is a relatively common genetic disorder associated with the overproduction of ApoB, which results in elevations of both LDL-C and TG. Family members may vary between pure hypercholesterolemia, combined hyperlipidemia, or isolated HTG. The disorder is dominantly inherited and is also associated with a family history of Type 2 diabetes. The ratio of ApoB/LDL-C is usually greater than or equal to 1.0; dense LDL-C or pattern B is present, and HDL-C is often low. On physical examination, premature corneal arcus or xanthelasma is occasionally present, but rarely are there tendon xanthomas. In patients with mixed dyslipidemia, other potential genetic causes include familial dysbetalipoproteinemia (type 3) or familial HTG. The treatments are usually similar; however, differentiating the potential genetic causes of HTG has prognostic implications, and, occasionally, the treatments may vary. In this patient profile, non-HDL-C becomes the primary target of therapy. Although ApoB may be a more accurate predictor of CHD risk and some physicians advocate direct measurements of LDL-C, the non-HDL, by incorporating LDL-C, intermediate-density lipoprotein, and VLDL-C, represents a target that contains all of the potentially atherogenic lipoproteins. ApoB, direct LDL-C, and lipoprotein subparticles are more expensive laboratory tests and not as widely available. If ApoB is measured, a goal of less than 90 mg/dL is the target for high-risk patients. Alternatively, an ApoB/AI ratio of less than 0.7 is an optimal target recommended by the Canadian guidelines.

Patients with combined hyperlipidemia often respond dramatically to weight loss, exercise, and lower-carbohydrate (lower-calorie) diets. Measurements of weight loss are usually a good guide to ascertain compliance to a prescribed diet and exercise program. Failure to lose weight usually means the patient is noncompliant or unable to adhere to the nonpharmacologic approaches. These are the types of patients in whom a referral to a dietitian or other experienced health professional in nonpharmacologic treatments is cost effective.

Drug therapy options are similar to those mentioned in Patient Profile #2. In this example, the patient requires a 22% reduction in LDL-C to achieve the ATP III goal of less than 130 mg/dL and a 30% reduction in non-HDL-C to achieve the goal of less than 160 mg/dL. These goals should be achieved with statin therapy alone; however, the use of more potent statins or a higher dose, or both, usually more effectively lowers TG levels. Combining a statin with niacin or a fibrate (preferably fenofibrate) is another possibility that may more effectively lower LDL-C and TG and raise HDL-C. Often, the preferred choice is a statin, starting with or titrating to a maximal dose, and if the goals are not achieved with monotherapy, titrating down the dose of the statin and adding niacin (or the combination pill of lovastatin plus Niaspan) or a fibrate (fenofibrate preferred). Another option is to add omega-3 fatty acid supplementation, 2 to 6 g/day (marine oil capsules), to a statin that is safe and usually well tolerated. Omega-3 fatty acids do not increase the HDL-C as much as niacin or a fibrate. After initiation of drug therapy, continued encouragement regarding diet, exercise, and weight loss are vital to the long-term success of the treatment of this patient population.

REFERENCES

1. Windhaus A. Uber den gehalt normaler and atheromatoser aorten an cholesterin und cholesterinester. Z Physiol Chem 1910; 67:174.
2. Anitschkow N. Experimental atherosclerosis in animals. In: Cowdry E, ed. Ateriosclerosis. New York: Macmillan, 1933:271–322.
3. Stamler J. Established major coronary risk factors. In: Marmot M, Elliott P, eds. Coronary Heart Disease Epidemiology: From Aetiology to Public Health. Oxford: Oxford University Press, 1992:35–66.
4. Keys A. From Naples to Seven Countries—a sentimental journey. Prog Biochem Pharmacol 1983; 19:1–30.
5. National Research Council (US) Food and Nutrition Board. Diet and Health Implications for Reducing Chronic Disease. Washington, DC: National Academy Press, 1989.

6. Leary T. The genesis of atherosclerosis. Arch Pathol 1941; 32:507–555.
7. Rothstein WG. A change of heart: how the Framingham Heart Study helped unravel the mysteries of cardiovascular disease. *JAMA* 2005; 293:1798–1799.
8. LaBarthe D. Epidemiology and Prevention of Cardiovascular Diseases. Gaithersberg, MD: Aspen Pub, 1998.
9. Enos W Jr, Holmes R, Beyer J. Coronary disease among United States soldiers killed in action in Korea. *JAMA* 1953; 152:1090–1093.
10. Worth R, Kato H, Rhoads G, Kagan K, Syme S. Epidemiologic studies of coronary heart disease and stroke in Japanese men living in Japan, Hawaii and California: mortality. Am J Epidemiol 1975; 102:481–490.
11. Keys A. Seven Countries : A Multivariate Analysis of Death and Coronary Heart Disease. Cambridge, Mass: Harvard University Press, 1980.
12. Tunstall-Pedoe H ed. For the WHO MONICA Project. MONICA Monograph and Multimedia Sourcebook 1979 to 2002. Geneva: World Health Organization, 2003.
13. Lipid Research Clinics Program. The Lipid Research Clinics Coronary Primary Prevention Trial results. II. The relationship of reduction in incidence of coronary heart disease to cholesterol lowering. *JAMA* 1984; 251:365–374.
14. McMichael J. Fats and atheroma. Br Med J 1979; 1(6167):890.
15. Scandinavism Simvastatin Survival Study Group. Randomised trial of cholesterol lowering in 4444 patients with coronary heart disease: the Scandinavism Simvastatin Survival Study. Lancet 1994; 344:1383–1389.
16. Robinson JG, Smith B, Maheshwari N, Schrott H. "Pleiotropic" effects of statins: Benefit beyond cholesterol reduction? A meta-regression analysis J Am Coll Cardiol 2005; 46:1855–1862.
17. Stamler J, Wentworth D, Neaton JD. Is relationship between serum cholesterol and risk of premature death from coronary heart disease continuous and graded? Findings in 356,222 primary screenees of the Multiple Risk Factor Intervention Trial (MRFIT). *JAMA* 1986; 256:2823–2828.
18. Verschuren WM, Jacobs DR, Bloemberg BP, et al. Serum total cholesterol and long-term coronary heart disease mortality in different cultures. Twenty-five-year follow-up of the seven countries study. JAMA 1995; 274:131–136.
19. National Cholesterol Education Panel. Third Report of the National Cholesterol Education Program (NCEP) Expert Panel on Detection, Evaluation, and Treatment of High Blood Cholesterol in Adults (Adult Treatment Panel III) Final Report. Circulation 2002; 106:3143–3421.
20. Sharrett AR, Ballantyne CM, Coady SA, et al. Coronary heart disease prediction from lipoprotein cholesterol levels, triglycerides, lipoprotein(a), apolipoproteins A-I and B, and HDL-C density subfractions: The Atherosclerosis Risk in Communities (ARIC) Study. Circulation 2001; 104:1108–1113.
21. European guidelines on cardiovascular disease prevention in clinical practice. Atherosclerosis 2003; 171:145–155.
22. Law MR, Wald NJ, Thompson SG. By how much and how quickly does reduction in serum cholesterol concentration lower risk of ischaemic heart disease? BMJ 1994; 308:367–372.
23. Lloyd-Jones DM, Wilson PWF, Larson MG, et al. Lifetime risk of coronary heart disease by cholesterol levels at selected ages. Arch Intern Med 2003; 163:1966–1972.
24. Cholesterol Treatment Trialists' (CTT) Collaborators. Efficacy and safety of cholesterol-lowering treatment: prospective meta-analysis of data from 90,056 participants in 14 randomised trials of statins. Lancet 2005; 366:1267–1278.
25. Bittner V. Perspectives on dyslipidemia and coronary heart disease in women. J Am Coll Cardiol 2005; 46:1628–1635.
26. Castelli WP, Garrison RJ, Wilson PW, Abbott RD, Kalousdian S, Kannel WB. Incidence of coronary heart disease and lipoprotein cholesterol levels. The Framingham Study. JAMA 1986; 256:2835–2838.
27. Dyer A, Stamler J, Shekelle R. Serum cholesterol and mortality from coronary heart disease in young, middle-aged, and older men and women from three Chicago epidemiologic studies. Ann Epidemiol 1992; 2:51–57.
28. Psaty BM, Anderson M, Kronmal RA, et al. The association between lipid levels and the risks of incident myocardial infarction, stroke, and total mortality: The Cardiovascular Health Study. J Am Geriatr Soc 2004; 52:1639–1647.
29. Eklund G, Carstensen J, Lindberg G, Gullberg B, L R, Tornberg S. Serum levels of cholesterol and ischemic heart disease mortality. The Varmland Study. Ann Epidemiol 1992; 2:121–128.
30. Higgins M, Keller J. Cholesterol, coronary heart disease, and total mortality in middle-aged and elderly men and women in Tecumseh. Ann Epidemiol 1992; 2:69–76.
31. Cui Y, Blumenthal RS, Flaws JA, et al. Non-high-density lipoprotein cholesterol level as a predictor of cardiovascular disease mortality. Arch Intern Med 2001; 161:1413–1419.
32. Anum EA, Adera T. Hypercholesterolemia and coronary heart disease in the elderly: a meta-analysis. Ann Epidemiol 2004; 14:705–721.
33. Pekkanen J, Linn S, Heiss G, et al. Ten-year mortality from cardiovascular disease in relation to cholesterol level among men with and without preexsiting cardiovascular disease. N Engl J Med 1990; 322:1700–1707.
34. Wong N, Wilson P, Kannel W. Serum cholesterol as a prognostic factor after myocardial infarction: The Framingham Study. Ann Intern Med 1991; 115:687–693.
35. Martin M, Hulley S, Browner W, Kuller L, et al. Serum cholesterol, blood pressure, and mortality: implications from a cohort of 361,622 men. Lancet 1986; 2:933–936.

36. Reddy KS. Cardiovascular disease in non-western countries. N Engl J Med 2004; 350:2438–2440.
37. Critchley J, Liu J, Zhao D, Wei W, Capewell S. Explaining the increase in coronary heart disease mortality in Beijing between 1984 and 1999. Circulation 2004; 110:1236–1244.
38. Reddy KS, Yusuf S. Emerging epidemic of cardiovascular disease in developing countries. Circulation 1998; 97:596–601.
39. Yusuf S, Hawken S, Ounpuu S, et al. Effect of potentially modifiable risk factors associated with myocardial infarction in 52 countries (the INTERHEART study): case-control study. Lancet 2004; 364:937–952.
40. Steyn K, Sliwa K, Hawken S, et al. Risk factors associated with myocardial infarction in Africa: The INTERHEART Africa Study. Circulation 2005; 112:3554–3561.
41. Carroll MD, Lacher DA, Sorlie PD, et al. Trends in serum lipids and lipoproteins of adults, 1960–2002. JAMA 2005; 294:1773–1781.
42. Jackson S, Burke G, Thach C, et al. Incidence and predictors of coronary heart disease among older African Americans—the Cardiovascular Health Study. J Natl Med Assoc 2001; 93:423–429.
43. Chambless LE, Heiss G, Shahar E, Earp MJ, Toole J. Prediction of ischemic stroke risk in the Atherosclerosis Risk in Communities Study. Am J Epidemiol 2004; 160:259–269.
44. Liao Y, McGee DL, Cooper RS. Prediction of coronary heart disease mortality in blacks and whites: pooled data from two national cohorts. Am J Cardiol 1999; 84:31–36.
45. Hunt KJ, Resendez RG, Williams K, Haffner SM, Stern MP, Hazuda HP. All-cause and cardiovascular mortality among Mexican American and Non-Hispanic white older participants in the San Antonio Heart Study-Evidence against the "Hispanic Paradox." Am. J. Epidemiol 2003; 158:1048–1057.
46. Stemmermann G, Chyou P-H, Kagan A, Nomura A, Yano K. Serum cholesterol and mortality among Japanese-American men. The Honolulu Heart Program. Arch Intern Med 1991; 151:969–972.
47. Howard BV, Lee ET, Cowan LD, et al. Rising tide of cardiovascular disease in American Indians: The Strong Heart Study. Circulation 1999; 99:2389–2395.
48. Stamler J, Daviglus ML, Garside DB, Dyer AR, Greenland P, Neaton JD. Relationship of baseline serum cholesterol levels in 3 large cohorts of younger men to long-term coronary, cardiovascular, and all-cause mortality and to longevity. JAMA 2000; 284:311–318.
49. Prospective Studies Collaboration. Cholesterol, diastolic blood pressure, and stroke: 13,000 strokes in 450,000 people in 45 prospective cohorts. Lancet 1995; 346:1647–1653.
50. Law M, Wald N, Rudinka A. Quantifying the effect of statins on low density lipoprotein cholesterol, ischaemic heart disease, and stroke: systematic review and meta-analysis. BMJ 2003; 326:1423–1427.
51. Eastern Stroke and Coronary Heart Disease Collaborative Research Group. Blood pressure, cholesterol, and stroke in eastern Asia. Lancet 1999; 352:1801–1807.
52. Paulose-Ram R, Gu Q, Eberhardt M, Gregg E, Geiss L, Engelgau M. Lower extremity disease among persons aged ≥40 years with and without diabetes - United States, 1999–2002. *MMWR* 2005; 54:1158–1160.
53. American Heart Association. Heart disease and stroke statistics—2005 update. http://american-heart.org/.
54. Kennedy M, Solomon C, Manolio TA, et al. Risk factors for declining ankle-brachial index in men and women 65 years or older: The Cardiovascular Health Study. Arch Intern Med 2005; 165:1896–1902.
55. Flegal KM, Carroll MD, Ogden CL, Johnson CL. Prevalence and trends in obesity among US adults, 1999–2000. JAMA 2002; 288:1723–1727.
56. Hedley AA, Ogden CL, Johnson CL, Carroll MD, Curtin LR, Flegal KM. Prevalence of overweight and obesity among US children, adolescents, and adults, 1999–2002. JAMA 2004; 291:2847–2850.
57. National Cholesterol Education Program. Report of the Expert Panel on Detection, Evaluation, and Treatment of High Blood Cholesterol in Adults. U.S. Dept Health and Human Services, 1989. NIH Pub No 89-2925.
58. Fuster V, Moreno PR, Fayad ZA, Corti R, Badimon JJ. Atherothrombosis and high-risk plaque: Part I: Evolving concepts. J Am Coll Cardiol 2005; 46:937–954.
59. Strong JP, Malcom GT, McMahan CA, et al. Prevalence and extent of atherosclerosis in adolescents and young adults: implications for prevention from the Pathobiological Determinants of Atherosclerosis in Youth Study. JAMA 1999; 281:727–735.
60. Report of a WHO Expert Committee. Prevention of Coronary Heart Disease. Geneva, Switzerland: World Health Organization, 1982.
61. Faxon DP, Fuster V, Libby P, et al. Atherosclerotic Vascular Disease Conference: Writing Group III: Pathophysiology. Circulation 2004; 109:2617–2625.
62. Herrmann J, Lerman L, Rodriguez-Porcel M, et al. Coronary vasa vasorum neovascularization precedes epicardial endothelial dysfunction in experimental hyperchoelsterolemia. Cardiovasc Res 2001; 51:762–766.
63. Executive Summary of the Third Report of the National Cholesterol Education Program (NCEP) Expert Panel on Detection, Evaluation, and Treatment of High Blood Cholesterol in Adults (Adult Treatment Panel III). JAMA 2001; 285:2486–2497.
64. Grundy SM, Cleeman JL, Merz CN, et al. Implications of recent clinical trials for the National Cholesterol Education Program Adult Treatment Panel III Guidelines. Circulation 2004; 110:227–239.
65. De Backer G, Ambrosioni E, Borch-Johnsen K, et al. European guidelines on cardiovascular disease prevention in clinical practice. Eur Heart J 2003; 24:1601–1610.

66. Genest J, Frohlich J, Fodor G, McPherson R, Working Group on Hypercholesterolemia and other dyslipidemias. Recommendations for the management of dyslipidemia and the prevention of cardiovascular disease: summary of the 2003 update. Can Med Assoc J 2003; 169:921–924.

67. Walldius G, Jungner I, Holme I, Aastveit AH, Kolar W, Steiner E. High apolipoprotein B, low apolipoprotein A-I, and improvement in the prediction of fatal myocardial infarction (AMORIS study): a prospective study. Lancet 2001; 358:2026–2033.

68. Downs JR, Clearfield M, Weiss S, et al. For the AFCAPS/TexCAPS Research Group. Primary prevention of acute coronary events with lovastatin in men and women with average cholesterol levels. JAMA 1998; 279:1615–1622.

69. Goldstein JL, Brown MS. Molecular medicine. The cholesterol quartet. Science 2001; 292:1394–1398.

70. Schaefer EJ, Genest JJ Jr, Ordovas JM, Salem DN, Wilson PWF. Familial lipoprotein disorders and premature coronary artery disease. Atherosclerosis 1994; 108(suppl):S41–S54.

71. Pischon T, Girman CJ, Sacks FM, et al. Non-high-density lipoprotein cholesterol and apolipoprotein B in the prediction of coronary heart disease in men. Circulation 2005; 112:3375–3383.

72. Enas EA, Yusuf S, Sharma S. Coronary artery disease in South Asians. Second meeting of the International Working Group. 16 March 1997, Anaheim, California. Indian Heart J 1998; 50:105–113.

73. Schneider WJ, Beisiegel U, Goldstein JL, Brown MS. Purification of the low density lipoprotein receptor, an acidic glycoprotein of 164,000 molecular weight. J Biol Chem 1982; 257:2664–2673.

74. Goldstein JL, Hobbs HH, Brown MS. Familial hypercholesterolemia. In: Scriver CR, Beaudet AL, Sly WS, Valle D, Stanbury JB, Wyngaarden JB, eds. The Metabolic and Molecular Bases of Inherited Disease. New York: McGraw-Hill, 1995:1981–2030.

75. Hoeg JM. Familial hypercholesterolemia: what the zebra can teach us about the horse. JAMA 1994; 271:543–546.

76. Goldstein JL, Schrott HG, Hazzard WR, Bierman EL, Motulsky AG. Hyperlipidemia in coronary heart disease, II. Genetic analysis of lipid levels in 176 families and delineation of a new inherited disorder, combined hyperlipidemia. J Clin Invest 1973; 52:1544–1568.

77. Innerarity TL, Weisgraber KH, Arnold KS, et al. Familial defective apolipoprotein B-100: low density lipoproteins with abnormal receptor binding. Proc Natl Acad Sci USA 1987; 84:6919–6923.

78. Timms KM, Wagner S, Samuels ME, et al. A mutation in PCSK9 causing autosomal-dominant hypercholesterolemia in a Utah pedigree. Hum Genet 2004; 114:349–353.

79. Davidson MH, Geohas CT. Efficacy of over-the-counter nutritional supplements. Curr Atheroscler Rep 2003; 5:15–21.

80. Davidson MH, Dugan LD, Burns JH, Bova J, Story K, Drennan KB. The hypocholesterolemic effects of beta-glucan in oatmeal and oat bran: a dose-controlled study. JAMA 1991; 265:1833–1839.

81. Anderson JW, Johnstone BM, Cook-Newell ME. Meta-analysis of the effects of soy protein intake on serum lipids. N Engl J Med 1995; 333:276–282.

82. Packard CJ, Shepherd J, Cobbe SM, et al. Influence of pravastatin and plasma lipids on clinical events in the West of Scotland Coronary Prevention Study (WOSCOPS). Circulation 1998; 97:1440–1445.

83. Sacks, FM, Pfeffer MA, Moye LA, et al. The effect of pravastatin on coronary events after myocardial infarction in patients with average cholesterol levels. N Engl J Med 1996; 335:1001–1009.

84. The Long-Term Intervention With Pravastatin in Ischemic Disease (LIPID) Study Group. Prevention of cardiovascular events and death with pravastatin in patients with coronary heart disease and a broad range of initial cholesterol levels. N Engl J Med 1998; 339:1349–1357.

85. Shepherd J, Blauw GJ, Murphy MB, et al. Pravastatin in elderly individuals at risk of vascular disease (PROSPER): a randomised controlled trial. Lancet 2002; 360:1623–1630.

86. Simvastatin. Physicians Desk Reference. MontVale, NJ: Medical Economics Company 2002.

87. Spence JD, Munoz CE, Hendricks L, et al. Pharmacokinetics of the combination of fluvastatin and gemfibrozil. Am. J. Cardiol 1995; 76:80A–83A.

88. Holdaas H, Fellstrom B, Jardine AG, et al. Effect of fluvastatin on cardiac outcomes in renal transplant recipients: a multicentre, randomised, placebo-controlled trial. Lancet 2003; 361:2024–2031.

89. Newman CB, Palmer G, Silbershatz H, Szarek M. Safety of atorvastatin derived from analysis of 44 completed trials in 9,416 patients. Am. J. Cardiol 2003; 92:670–676.

90. Atorvastatin. Physicians Desk Reference. MontVale, NJ: Medical Economics Company 2002.

91. Sever PS, Dahlof B, Poulter NR, et al. Prevention of coronary and stroke events with atorvastatin in hypertensive patients who have average or lower-than-average cholesterol concentrations, in the Anglo-Scandinavian Cardiac Outcomes Trial-Lipid Lowering Arm (ASCOT-LLA): a multicentre randomised controlled trial. Lancet 2003; 361:1149–1158.

92. Colhoun HM, Thomason MJ, Mackness MI, et al. Design of the Collaborative AtoRvastatin Diabetes Study (CARDS) in patients with type 2 diabetes. Diabet Med 2002; 19:201–211.

93. LaRosa JC, Grundy SM, Waters DD, et al, Treating to New Targets (TNT) Investigators. Intensive lipid lowering with atorvastatin in patients with stable coronary disease. N Engl J Med 2005; 352:1425–1435.

94. Pedersen TR, Faergeman O, Kastelein JJ, et al, Incremental Decrease in End Points Through Aggressive Lipid Lowering (IDEAL) Study Group. High-dose atorvastatin vs usual-dose simvastatin for secondary prevention after myocardial infarction: the IDEAL study: a randomized control trial. JAMA 2005; 294:2437–2445.

95. Davidson MH: Rosuvastatin: a highly efficacious statin for the treatment of dyslipidaemia. Expert Opin Invest Drugs 2002; 11:125–141.

96. Jones PH, Davidson MH, Stein EA, et al. Comparison of the efficacy and safety of rosuvastatin versus atorvastatin, simvastatin, and pravastatin across doses (STELLAR* Trial). Am. J. Cardiol 2003; 92:152–160.
97. Stein EA: Introduction: rosuvastatin—an efficacy assessment based on pooled trial data. Am J Cardiol 2003; 91:1C–2C.
98. Crestor; Rosuvastatin Calcium. IPR (trade) 630100, IPR (sample) 630200, API (sample) 23073–0. Package insert. Wilmington: AstraZeneca 2003.
99. Catapano AL. Ezetimibe: a selective inhibitor of cholesterol absorption. Eur Heart J 2001; (suppl E):E6–E10.
100. Davis HR, Compton DS, Hoos L, et al. Ezetimibe (SCH58235) localizes to the brush border of small intestinal enterocyte and inhibits enterocyte cholesterol uptake and absorption [abstr P3500]. Eur Heart J 2000; 21(suppl):636.
101. Knopp RH, Bays H, Manion CV, et al. Effect of ezetimibe on serum concentrations of lipid-soluble vitamins [abstr P175]. Atherosclerosis 2001; 2(suppl):90.
102. van Heek M, Farley C, Compton DS, et al. Comparison of the activity and disposition of the novel cholesterol absorption inhibitor, SCH58235, and its glucuronide, SCH60663. Br J Pharmacol 2000; 129:1748–1754.
103. Zetia [prescribing information]. North Wales, PA: Merck/Schering-Plough Pharmaceuticals; 2002.
104. Bays HE, Moore PB, Drehobl MA, et al. Effectiveness and tolerability of ezetimibe in patients with primary hypercholesterolemia: pooled analysis of two phase II studies. Clin Ther 2001; 23:1209–1230.
105. Punwani N, Pai S, Bach C, et al. Effect of food on oral bioavailability of SCH58235 in healthy male volunteers [abstr] [serial online]. AAPS Pharm Sci. 1(suppl):S486.
106. van Heek M, France CF, Compton DS, et al. In vivo metabolism-based discovery of a potent cholesterol absorption inhibitor, SCH58235, in the rat and rhesus monkey through the identification of the active metabolites of SCH48461. J Pharmacol Exp Ther 1997; 283:157–163.
107. Rosenblum SB, Huynh T, Alfonso A, et al. Discovery of 1-(4-fluorophenyl)-(3R)-[3-(4-fluorophenyl)-(3S)-hydroxypropyl]-(4S)-(4-hydroxyphenyl)-2-azetidinone (SCH58235): a designed, potent, orally active inhibitor of cholesterol absorption. J Med Chem 1998; 41:973–980.
108. van Heek M, Farley C, Compton DS, et al. Ezetimibe selectively inhibits intestinal cholesterol absorption in rodents in the presence and absence of exocrine pancreatic function. Br J Pharmacol 2001; 134:409–417.
109. van Heek M, Compton DS, Davis HR. The cholesterol absorption inhibitor, ezetimibe, decreases diet-induced hypercholesterolemia in monkeys. Eur J Pharmacol 2001; 415:79–84.
110. Sudhop T, Lutjohann D, Kodal A, et al. Inhibition of intestinal cholesterol absorption by ezetimibe in humans. Circulation 2002; 106:1943–1948.
111. Zhu Y, Statkevich P, Kosoglou T, et al. Effect of SCH 58235 on the activity of drug metabolizing enzymes in vivo [abstr PIII-43]. Clin Pharmacol Ther 2000; 67:152.
112. Zhu Y, Statkevich P, Kosoglou T, et al. Lack of a pharmacokinetic interaction between ezetimibe and atorvastatin [abstr PIII-15]. Clin Pharmacol Ther 2001; 69:68.
113. Kosoglou T, Meyer I, Veltri EP, Statkevich P, et al. Pharmacodynamic interaction between the new selective cholesterol absorption inhibitor ezetimibe and simvastatin. Br J Clin Pharmacol 2002; 54:309–319.
114. Reyderman L, Kosoglou T, Statkevich P, et al. No pharmacokinetic drug interaction between ezetimibe and lovastatin [abstr PIII-8]. Clin Pharmacol Ther 2001; 69:66.
115. Reyderman L, Statkevich P, Kosoglou T, et al. No pharmacokinetic drug interaction between ezetimibe and either cerivastatin or fluvastatin [abstr] [serial online]. AAPS Pharm Sci 2001; 3(suppl 3).
116. Statkevich P, Reyderman L, Kosoglou T, et al. Ezetimibe does not affect the pharmacokinetics and pharmacodynamics of glipizide [abstr PIII-12]. Clin Pharmacol Ther 2001; 69:67.
117. Kosoglou T, Statkevich P, Bauer KS, et al. Ezetimibe does not affect the pharmacokinetics and pharmacodynamics of digoxin [abstr] [serial online] AAPS Pharm Sci 2001; 3(suppl 3).
118. Keung AC, Kosoglou T, Statkevich P, et al. Ezetimibe does not affect the pharmacokinetics of oral contraceptives [abstr PII-89]. Clin Pharmacol Ther 2001; 69:55.
119. Bauer KS, Kosoglou T, Statkevich P, et al. Ezetimibe does not affect the pharmacokinetics or pharmacodynamics of warfarin [abstr PI-15]. Clin Pharmacol Ther 2001; 69:5.
120. Kosoglou T, Guillaume M, Sun S, et al. Pharmacodynamic interaction between fenofibrate and the cholesterol absorption inhibitor ezetimibe [abstr W6.1]. Atherosclerosis 2001; 2(suppl):38.
121. Krishna G, Kosoglou T, Ezzet F, et al. Effect of cimetidine on the pharmacokinetics of ezetimibe [abstr] [serial online]. AAPS Pharm Sci 2001; 3(suppl 3).
122. Courtney RD, Kosoglou T, Statkevich P, et al. Effect of antacid on the pharmacokinetics of ezetimibe. Clin Pharmacol Ther 2002; 71:80.
123. Dujovne CA, Ettinger MP, McNeer JF, et al. Efficacy and safety of a potent new selective cholesterol absorption inhibitor, ezetimibe, in patients with primary hypercholesterolemia. Am J Cardiol 2002; 90,1092–1097.
124. Knopp RH, Gitter H, Truitt T, et al. Effects of ezetimibe, a new cholesterol absorption inhibitor, on plasma lipids in patients with primary hypercholesterolemia. Eur Heart J. In press.
125. Davidson MH, McGarry T, Bettis R, et al. Ezetimibe coadministered with simvastatin in patients with primary. J Am Coll Cardiol 2002; 40:2125–2134.
126. Ballantyne C, Houri J, Notarbartolo A, et al. Effect of ezetimibe coadministered with atorvastatin in 628 patients with primary hypercholesterolemia: a prospective, randomized, double-blind trial. Circulation. In press.
127. Kerzner B, Corbelli J, Sharp S, et al. Efficacy and safety of ezetimibe coadministered with lovastatin in primary hypercholesterolemia. Am J Cardiol 2003; 91:418–424.

128. Melani L, Mills R, Hassman D, et al. Efficacy and safety of ezetimibe coadministered with pravastatin in patients with primary hypercholesterolemia: a prospective, randomized, double-blind trial. Eur Heart J. In press.

129. The Lipid research clinics coronary primary prevention trial results. I. Reduction in incidence of coronary heart disease. JAMA 1984; 251:351–364.

130. Brown G, Albers JJ, Fisher LD, et al. Regression of coronary artery disease as a result of intensive lipid-lowering therapy in men with high levels of apolipoprotein B. N Engl J Med 1990; 323:1289–1298.

131. Davidson MH, Dillon MA, Gordon B, et al. Colesevelam hydrochloride (cholestagel): a new, potent bile acid sequestrant associated with a low incidence of gastrointestinal side effects. Arch Intern Med 1999; 159:1893–1900.

132. Kreisberg RA. Niacin: a therapeutic dilemma. "One man's drink is another's poison." Am J Med 1994; 97:313–316.

133. Guyton JR. Effect of niacin on atherosclerotic cardiovascular disease. Am J Cardiol 1998; 82(12A):18U–23U.

134. Capuzzi DM, Guyton JR, Morgan JM, et al. Efficacy and safety of an extended-release niacin (Niaspan): a long-term study. Am J Cardiol 82(12A):74U–81U.

135. Guyton JR, Goldberg AC, Kreisberg RA, et al. Effectiveness of once-nightly dosing of extended-release niacin alone and in combination for hypercholesterolemia. Am J Cardiol 1998; 82:737–743.

136. Jin FY, Kamanna VS, Kashyap ML. Niacin decreases removal of high-density lipoprotein apolipoprotein A-I but not cholesterol ester by Hep G2 cells. Implication for reverse cholesterol transport. Arterioscler Thromb Vasc Biol 1997; 17:2020–2028.

137. Kamanna VS, Kashyap ML. Mechanism of action of niacin on lipoprotein metabolism. Curr Atheroscler Rep 2000; 2:36–46.

138. Gray DR, Morgan T, Chretien SD, et al. Efficacy and safety of controlled-release niacin in dyslipoproteinemic veterans. Ann Intern Med 1994; 121:252–258.

139. Bays H. Existing and investigational combination drug therapy for high-density lipoprotein cholesterol. Am J Cardiol 2002; 90(10B):30K–43K.

140. Davidson MH. Combination therapy for dyslipidemia: safety and regulatory considerations. Am J Cardiol 2002; 90(10B):50K–60K.

141. Kashyap ML, McGovern ME, Berra K, et al. Long-term safety and efficacy of a once-daily niacin/lovastatin formulation for patients with dyslipidemia. Am J Cardiol 2002; 89:672–678.

142. Blankenhorn DH, Nessim SA, Johnson RL, et al. Beneficial effects of combined colestipol-niacin therapy on coronary atherosclerosis and coronary venous bypass grafts. JAMA 1987; 257:3233–3240.

143. Coronary Drug Project Research Group. Clofibrate and niacin in coronary heart disease. JAMA 1975; 231:360–381.

144. Canner PL, Berge KG, Wenger NK, et al. Fifteen-year mortality in Coronary Drug Project patients: long-term benefit with niacin. J Am Coll Cardiol 1986; 8:1245–1255.

145. Brown BG, Zhao X-Q, Chait A, et al. Simvastatin and niacin, antioxidant vitamins, or the combination for the prevention of coronary disease. N Engl J Med 2001; 345:1583–1592.

146. Carlson LA, Rosenhamer G. Reduction of mortality in the Stockholm Ischaemic Heart Disease Secondary Prevention Study by combined treatment with clofibrate and nicotinic acid. Acta Med Scan 1988; 223:405–418.

147. Morgan JM, Baksh RI, Stanton M, et al. Beneficial effects of extended-release niacin on lipoprotein subclass distribution in patients with mixed dyslipidemia. Abstract presented at XIV Drugs Affecting Lipid Metabolism International Symposium. New York, New York, 2001.

148. Sakai T, Kamanna VS, Kashyap ML. Niacin, but not gemfibrozil, selectively increases Lp-AI, a cardioprotective subfraction of HDL-C, in patients with low HDL-C cholesterol. Arterioscler Thromb Vasc Biol 2001; 21:1783–1789.

149. Canner PL, Furberg CD, McGovern ME. Niacin decreases myocardial infarction and total mortality in patients with impaired fasting glucose or glucose intolerance: results from Coronary Drug Project [abstr]. Circulation 2002; 106:II-636.

150. Canner PL, Furberg CD, McGovern ME. Benefits of niacin in patients with versus without the metabolic syndrome and healed myocardial infarction (from the Coronary Drug Project). Am J Cardiol 2006; 97:477–479.

151. Grundy SM, Vega GL, McGovern ME, et al. Efficacy, safety, and tolerability of once-daily niacin for the treatment of dyslipidemia associated with type 2 diabetes: results of the assessment of diabetes control and evaluation of the efficacy of niaspan trial Arch Intern Med 2002; 162:1568–1576.

152. Fruchart JC, Staels B, Duriez P. The role of fibric acids in atherosclerosis. Curr Atheroscler Rep 2001; 3:83–92.

153. Rubins HB, Robins SJ, Collins D, et al. Diabetes, plasma insulin and cardiovascular disease. Subgroup analysis from the Department of Veterans Affairs High-density lipoprotein Intervention Trial (VA-HIT). Arch Intern Med 2002; 162:2597–2604.

154. Tenenbaum A, Motro M, Fisman EZ, Tanne D, Boyko V, Behar S. Bezafibrate for the secondary prevention of myocardial infarction in patients with metabolic syndrome. Arch Intern Med 2005; 165:1154–1160.

155. Keech A, Simes RJ, Barter P, et al. Field study investigators. Effects of long-term fenofibrate therapy on cardiovascular events in 9795 people with type 2 diabetes mellitus (the FIELD study): randomized controlled trial. Lancet 2005; 366:1849–1861.
156. Davidson MH, Maki KC, Pearson TA, et al. Results of the National Cholesterol Education (NCEP) Program Utilizing Novel E-Technology (NEPTUNE) II survey and implications for treatment under the recent NCEP writing group recommendations. Am J Cardiol 2005; 96:556–563.
157. Action to Control Cardiovascular Risk in Diabetes (ACCORD) http://www.accordtrial.org/public/index.cfm. Accessed 6-3-05.
158. Grundy SM, Vega LG, Yuan Z, Battisti WP, Brady WD, Palmisano J. Effectiveness and tolerability of simvastatin plus fenofibrate for combined hyperlipidemia (the SAFARI trial). Am J Cardiol 2005; 95:462–468.

8 | High-Density Lipoprotein Cholesterol

Peter P. Toth

Department of Preventive Cardiology, Sterling Rock Falls Clinic, Sterling, University of Illinois College of Medicine, Peoria, and Southern Illinois University School of Medicine, Springfield, Illinois, U.S.A.

Antonio M. Gotto, Jr.

Department of Medicine, Weill Medical College of Cornell University, New York, New York, U.S.A.

KEY POINTS

- There is significant residual risk for cardiovascular morbidity and mortality in clinical trials even with aggressive reductions in atherogenic lipoprotein burden (LDL-C and non–HDL-C).
- In epidemiologic studies (case-control and prospective cohort) conducted throughout the world, low serum levels of HDL-C are associated with increased risk for CHD, MI, stroke, and sudden death in both men and women. High levels of HDL-C are associated with reduced cardiovascular risk.
- Low serum levels of HDL-C are defined as less than 40 mg/dL (<1.03 mmol/L) in men, and <50 mg/dL (<1.29 mmol/L) in women. Although the NCEP has not defined targets for HDL-C therapy, some specialty groups have suggested targets.
- Low HDL-C is widely prevalent in the United States and Europe and is a characteristic feature of the metabolic syndrome, diabetes mellitus, and obesity. Low HDL-C is also highly prevalent among patients with CHD.
- Among elderly patients, HDL-C appears to be a better predictor of risk for CHD and stroke than LDL-C or TC.
- There is a large corpus of basic scientific investigation supporting the observation from epidemiologic studies that HDL exerts a broad range of antiatherogenic effects within the vasculature.
- It is likely that the most important antiatherogenic effect exerted by HDL is RCT, the process by which HDL extracts excess cholesterol from the periphery (e.g., macrophages) and delivers it to either steroidogenic organs or to the liver for elimination via the gastrointestinal tract.
- HDL is an important source and donor of apoproteins and also exerts potent anti-thrombotic, anti-inflammatory, and antioxidative effects. HDL also appears to foster normal endothelial cell function and viability.
- Conceptually, the process of RCT has been experimentally confirmed in both humans and in animal models. The functional characteristics of HDL and how best to apply these in the clinical setting will continue to be a focus of considerable investigation.
- Patients with low serum levels of HDL-C benefit from pharmacologic intervention with a variety of agents.
- The statins should be used as first-line agents in patients with CHD or a CHD risk equivalent and in those who have isolated low HDL-C or low HDL-C combined with elevated LDL-C (Fig. 11).
- Fibrate therapy reduces the risk for cardiovascular events in patients with hypertriglyceridemia and low HDL-C. However, the addition of a statin and/or other LDL-C–lowering agent may be necessary to maintain LDL-C at NCEP-defined target levels.
- Niacin is the most potent drug currently available for raising serum levels of HDL-C. It may be particularly efficacious when used in combination with a statin in patients with CHD and low HDL-C. Currently, there are no primary prevention trials evaluating the efficacy of niacin monotherapy.
- TZDs stimulate elevations in HDL-C in diabetics with insulin resistance.
- Judicious combinations of these drugs can give additive increases in serum HDL-C levels.
- Serum HDL-C lev els are responsive to numerous environmental and lifestyle influences.

- Cigarette smoking tends to decrease HDL-C, possibly by adversely affecting the activities of LCAT and CETP and by promoting insulin resistance.
- BMI is inversely correlated with serum HDL-C. Weight loss can relieve insulin resistance and is associated with varying degrees of HDL-C elevation once a stable weight is achieved.
- Weight loss promoted by sibutramine and rimonabant is associated with increased HDL-C. Orlistat therapy does not appear to induce significant elevations in HDL-C.
- There is some evidence that ω-3 polyunsaturated fatty acids (DHA, EPA) can beneficially affect HDL-C and its subfractions and possibly RCT.
- Alcohol stimulates hepatic apoA-I expression and alcohol consumption is associated with increased serum HDL-C. However, given the risks associated with alcohol consumption, recommending alcohol as a means to raising HDL-C is not advised.
- Physical activity is an important component of any strategy for reducing cardiovascular risk, but especially so for patients with low HDL-C. Exercise can relieve insulin resistance and stimulate elevations in HDL-C, though this rise, can in many cases, be modest. There does appear to be a dose-response relationship between exercise and serum HDL-C, but the magnitude of the response varies between individuals depending upon genetic and metabolic background.
- HRT is an important quality-of-life issue for many women, especially if they have menopausal symptoms. Although estrogen raises serum HDL-C, low HDL-C is not an indication for HRT in postmenopausal women.

INTRODUCTION

Recent clinical intervention trials have demonstrated that even with aggressive reductions in serum atherogenic lipoprotein burden achieved by statin therapy, there is still significant residual risk for cardiovascular morbidity and mortality (1,2). Clearly, when managing a patient's global cardiovascular risk, it is imperative that all modifiable risk factors such as hypertension, impaired glucose tolerance or diabetes, cigarette smoking, obesity, inactivity, and dyslipidemia be managed with appropriate lifestyle modification and pharmacologic intervention. The National Cholesterol Education Program (NCEP) has continued to place primary emphasis on the therapeutic reduction of serum low-density lipoprotein cholesterol (LDL-C) and nonhigh-density lipoprotein cholesterol (non–HDL-C) for decreasing the morbidity and mortality of atherosclerotic disease in all of its manifestations (3,4). However, much recent basic scientific and clinical investigation suggests that established and novel approaches to managing high-density lipoprotein (HDL) metabolism may also significantly affect the risk for atherosclerotic disease and its sequelae, including myocardial infarction (MI), stroke, sudden death, and claudication (5,6). HDLs are the structurally most complex and functionally most diverse lipoproteins. Low serum levels of HDL constitute a widely prevalent risk factor for atherosclerotic disease. This chapter will review the epidemiology, metabolism, and antiatherogenic effects of HDL, and will also provide a comprehensive overview of how to manage low levels of this lipoprotein through lifestyle modification and pharmacologic intervention.

EPIDEMIOLOGY

A considerable body of epidemiological data from many regions of the world has consistently demonstrated that low levels of HDL-C enhance the risk for developing atherosclerosis and coronary heart disease (CHD) independently of other coronary risk factors, while higher levels of HDL-C are associated with reduced risk for atherosclerotic diseases (Table 1) (7–13). In 1951, Barr and coworkers made two important early observations that suggested HDL may possess antiatherogenic potential: (*i*) young women tended to have higher concentrations of what were then known as α-lipoproteins, which correspond today with HDL; and (*ii*) individuals with atherosclerotic cardiovascular disease (CVD) had significantly lower concentrations of α-lipoprotein than healthy individuals. The Cooperative Lipoprotein Phenotyping Study, a case-control study across five US communities (Albany, New York; Evans County, Georgia; Framingham, Massachusetts; San Francisco, California; Honolulu, Hawaii), affirmed these findings: the inverse association of HDL-C with CHD persisted even after adjustment for LDL-C and triglycerides (8). A two-year case-control follow-up study of 6595 men aged 20 to 49 years living in the municipality of Tromso, Norway complemented

TABLE 1 Observational Studies That Demonstrated HDL-C as an Independent CHD Risk Factor

Study	Country (ethnicity)	*n* (% women)	Design	Finding
Cooperative Lipoprotein Phenotyping Study (8)	U.S. (multiethnic)	6859 (25)	Case-control	HDL-C was 3.81 mg/dL (0.1 mmol/L) lower in CHD cases vs. controls
Tromso Heart Study (16)	Norway	6595 (0)	2-year case-control	HDL-C three times more predictive than lower-density fractions
Israeli Ischemic Heart Disease Study (9)	Israel	8586 (0)	21-year longitudinal cohort	Men with isolated low HDL-C [<35 mg/dL (0.9 mmol/L)] at 36% greater risk for CHD death than men with higher HDL-C
Belgian Interuniversity Research on Nutrition and Health (14)	Belgium		10-year mortality follow-up	Found curvilinear relation between HDL-C and CVD mortality
Honolulu Heart Program (15)	U.S. (Japanese American)	8066 (0)	~20-year longitudinal cohort	HDL-C was protective for incident CHD, but the pattern was not consistent in the elderly
Monitoring of Trends and Determinants in Cardiovascular Disease (Augsburg) (10)	Germany	2087 (48)	8-year longitudinal cohort	HDL-C in the highest quartile associated with 70% lower hazard ratio for MI compared with the lowest quartile
Framingham Heart Study (11)	U.S.	5127	~50-year longitudinal cohort	50% reduction in CHD per . 5 mmol/L increase in HDL-C
Prospective Cardiovascular Muenster Study (18)	Germany	25502 (32)	8-year longitudinal cohort	Mean HDL-C 12 mg/dL (0.31 mmol/L) higher in women than men. Low HDL-C more common in subgroup with CHD than in subgroup without

these data (16). In the Tromso Heart Study, low serum levels of HDL-C made a three-fold greater contribution to the prediction of future CHD than did cholesterol from lower density fractions in this cohort.

The Framingham Heart Study also demonstrated that the risk for CHD varies continuously and inversely with HDL-C levels (17). The CHD risk decreased by half for each 20-mg/dL (0.5-mmol/L) increase in HDL-C (Fig. 1).

The Prospective Cardiovascular Münster Study supported the Framingham data: individuals with HDL-C levels <35 mg/dL were at three times greater risk for CHD compared with

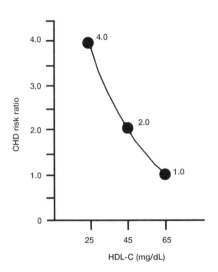

FIGURE 1 The relationship between serum HDL and risk for coronary heart disease in the Framingham Heart Study. CHD risk decreased by half for every 20 mg/dL (0.5 mmol/L) increment of high-density lipoprotein cholesterol (HDL-C). *Abbreviations*: CHD, coronary heart disease; HDL-C, high-density lipoprotein cholesterol. *Source*: From Ref. 17.

men who had HDL-C greater than or equal to 35 mg (18). In Japanese American men, aged 51 to 72 years, who had type 2 diabetes mellitus or abnormal glucose tolerance in the Honolulu Heart Program (HHP), low HDL-C was an independent predictor of CHD incidence (19). In the Physicians' Health Study, a low serum level of HDL-C is associated with an increased incidence of coronary artery disease (CAD) even in the presence of low total cholesterol (TC) (20). An analysis of four of the largest US epidemiologic studies (the Framingham Heart Study, the Lipid Research Clinics Prevalence Mortality Follow-up Study, the Lipid Research Clinics Primary Prevention Trial, and the Multiple Risk Factor Intervention Trial) indicated that, in general, each 1-mg/dL (0.03-mmol/L) increase in HDL-C confers a 2% decrease in CHD risk in men and a 3% decrease in women (Fig. 2) (21).

Among Japanese residents of Osaka, when comparing patients in the lowest to the highest quartile of serum HDL-C, the patients with the lowest HDL had a relative risk of 3.39 for MI and 4.17 for CAD. Among these patients, for every 1 mg/dL rise in HDL-C, the risk for MI and CAD decreased by 6.4% and 5.7%, respectively (22). In a recent analysis of data from the Nurses' Health Study, a 17 mg/dL elevation in HDL-C was associated with a 40% reduction in risk for developing CAD (23).

A population-based survey of US adults showed that 35.2% of men and 39.3% of women aged greater than or equal to 20 years had low HDL-C [<40 mg/dL (1.03 mmol/L) for men; <50 mg/dL (1.29 mmol/L) for women] (24). In a recent survey of 11 European countries, among 8545 patients with dyslipidemia, the prevalence of low HDL-C among women (<50 mg/dL or <1.29 mmol/L) was 40% and among men (<40 mg/dL or <1.03 mmol/L) was 33% (25). Low HDL-C is a defining feature of the metabolic syndrome and is common among patients with type 2 diabetes mellitus who have significant insulin resistance. Low HDL-C is also a common feature in men with CHD. Genest and colleagues, for example, found that the prevalence of HDL-C levels less than 35 mg/dL (<0.90 mmol/L) was threefold greater in patients with premature CHD than in healthy controls (57% vs. 19%, respectively) (26). In a study of 8500 men with CHD, 64% had HDL-C less than or equal to 40 mg/dL (1.03 mmol/L) (27). In the Quebec Cardiovascular Study, the prevalence of reduced HDL-C [<35 mg/dL (0.9 mmol/l)] was 50% in men with ischemic heart disease (IHD) compared with 30% in those not known to have IHD, and reduced HDL-C remained a significant predictor of IHD after adjustment for other risk factors (28).

The NCEP defines low HDL-C as less than 40 mg/dL (1.03 mmol/L) for all patients, although some authorities have also suggested a cut point <50 mg/dL (1.29 mmol/L) for women to account for their tendency to have higher concentrations of HDL-C compared with men (29). Although NCEP does not suggest a target to which HDL-C should be raised in

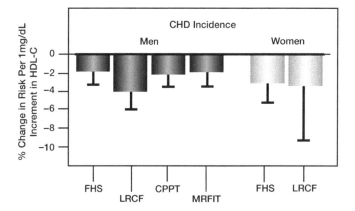

FIGURE 2   Effect of increasing HDL-C on CHD risk in four major studies. FHS, Framingham Heart Study; LRCF, Lipid Research Clinics Prevalence Mortality Follow-up Study; CPPT, Lipid Research Clinics Coronary Primary Prevention Trial; MRFIT, Multiple Risk Factor Intervention Trial. *Abbreviations*: HDL-C, high-density lipoprotein cholesterol; CHD, coronary heart disease; FHS, Framingham Heart Study; LRCF, Lipid Research Clinics Prevalence Mortality Follow-up Study; CPPT, Lipid Research Clinics Coronary Primary Prevention Trial; MRFIT, Multiple Risk Factor Intervention Trial. *Source*: From Ref. 21.

patients at risk, it does recommend that patients with low HDL-C be treated with lifestyle modification (weight loss, step I diet, smoking cessation, aerobic exercise) and pharmacologic intervention as indicated. When estimating 10-year Framingham risk scores, an HDL-C less than 40 mg/dL adds two points to the total score, while an HDL-C greater than or equal to 60 mg/dL allows for the substraction of one point since an HDL-C that exceeds this threshold is widely held to be protective. The Expert Group on HDL Cholesterol (30) and the European Consensus Panel on HDL-C (31) recommend that therapeutic effort be made to raise HDL to 40 mg/dL in patients with CAD and those at high risk for CAD (metabolic syndrome, diabetes mellitus, 10-year Framingham risk >20%). In a recent update to its management guidelines for diabetics, the American Diabetes Association recommends HDL-C targets of greater than or equal to 40 mg/dL in men, and greater than or equal to 50 mg/dL in women (32).

The Cardiovascular Health Study, a large, multicenter cohort study of elderly patients living in U.S. communities, assessed the relation between lipid parameters and risk for MI, stroke, and total mortality. Among 1954 men and 2931 women aged 65 and older who were at risk for MI or stroke, 436 subjects had a coronary event, 332 had an ischemic stroke, 104 a hemorrhagic stroke, and 1096 died during an average 7.5-year follow-up. For TC and LDL-C, the associations with MI and ischemic stroke were only marginally significant. On the other hand, HDL-C was inversely associated with MI risk [hazard ratio = 0.85 per standard deviation (SD) of 15.7 mg/dL (0.4 mmol/L), 95% confidence interval = 0.76–0.96]. For the outcome of ischemic stroke, high levels of HDL-C were associated with a decreased risk in men, but not women. Thus, in this population-based study of older adults, while most lipid measures were weakly associated with CHD events, the association between low HDL-C and increased MI risk was strong and consistent (33). In another study evaluating 3904 American men and women older than 71 years, low HDL-C was a better predictor for incident CHD morbidity and mortality than TC (34). Among patients 71 to 80 years of age, when comparing those with an HDL-C of less than 35 mg/dL to those with an HDL-C greater than 60 mg/dL, the relative risk for CHD mortality was 4.1. In the Northern Manhattan Stroke Study, HDL-C protected patients of all racial and ethnic groups studied older than 75 years from stroke according to a dose-response relation (35). Among Dutch patients greater than or equal to 85 years of age, risk for stroke or fatal CHD was independent of serum LDL-C. However, both of these outcomes were highly correlated with low HDL-C (36). In addition to being associated with increased risk for MI and stroke, low levels of HDL-C increase risk for restenosis after angioplasty (37) and severe premature atheromatous plaquing in the proximal left main coronary artery (38).

Concentrations of HDL-C have also been correlated with atherosclerotic disease progression. A recent imaging study included 1952 men and women aged 25 to 82 years who had at least one plaque present in the right carotid artery at baseline (39). All plaque images were computer-processed to yield a measure of plaque area in square millimeters and echogenicity, expressed as the gray-scale median. After seven years of follow-up, a new ultrasound screening assessed the changes in plaque area and echogenicity. In a multivariable adjusted model, HDL-C, age, systolic blood pressure, and current smoking were independent predictors of plaque growth. For a 1-SD (0.41 mmol/L) lower HDL-C level, mean (SE) plaque area increased by 0.93 mm^2 (0.44 mm^2; $P = 0.03$). Excluding users of lipid-lowering drugs from the analysis strengthened the HDL estimate (beta = 1.46 mm^2, $P = 0.002$). In a study of Japanese patients with CAD treated with pravastatin, elevations in serum HDL-C were associated with reductions in atheromatous plaque volume, whereas reductions in serum LDL-C and TC were not (40).

ANTIATHEROGENIC EFFECTS OF HIGH-DENSITY LIPOPROTEIN
Reverse Cholesterol Transport

HDL particles are a heterogeneous class of lipoproteins with diverse metabolic functions. Like other lipoproteins, the HDLs are organized macromolecular assemblies of lipids and proteins. The HDL surface is comprised of phospholipids, cholesterol, enzymes, and apoproteins. The hydrophobic core consists of triglycerides and cholesteryl esters. HDLs can bind to a variety of cell surface receptors and participate in the delivery of cholesteryl ester to steroidogenic organs and the hepatic parenchyma. In addition to carrying apoprotein (apo)

A-I and apo A-II, HDL is an important carrier and reservoir of a variety of apoproteins, including apo A-IV, CI, CII, CIII, D, E, and J, among others, and can transfer these moieties to other lipoproteins.

HDL plays a key role in the regulation of cholesterol balance in systemic tissues. Cholesterol is synthesized in all somatic cells and is driven from plasma into the subendothelial space and intima of the vasculature in response to a variety of thermodynamic, inflammatory, and histologic influences. Cholesterol is an important component of cell membranes, where it modulates fluidity of the hydrocarbon phase of phospholipid bilayers, regulates the activity of membrane-bound enzymes, and is a precursor to steroid hormone and bile salt biosynthesis. Peripheral cells are unable to catabolize cholesterol. Excess cholesterol must be transported back to the liver where the cholesterol can either be repackaged into apoprotein B100-containing lipoproteins, excreted into bile, or converted into bile salts via the activity of 7α-hydroxylase. HDLs transport excess cholesterol from the periphery back to the liver or to steroidogenic organs (adrenals, ovaries, testes, placenta) through a series of reactions that are collectively described as "reverse cholesterol transport" (RCT). If any individual step of RCT is defective, then there will be impaired capacity for the systemic clearance of cholesterol, cholesterol homeostasis is disturbed, and there is increased risk for developing atherosclerotic disease.

Apoprotein A-I

Apo A-I is the primary apoprotein constituent of HDL. ApoA-I is produced by both the intestine and the liver and can be secreted into plasma in its free form or as a surface coat constituent of chylomicrons and very low-density lipoproteins (VLDLs). ApoA-I can interact with macrophages (41) and hepatocytes (42,43) and stimulate the extracellular translocation of phospholipid and cholesterol (43). ApoA-I is thus an important means by which to deplete macrophages and foam cells of excess cholesterol, promoting HDL formation and "speciation" at the surface of the hepatocyte and within the subendothelial space. As the apoA-I undergoes progressively greater lipidation in the extracellular space, it forms pre-β-HDL and nascent discoidal HDL (ndHDL) (Fig. 3) (42).

Both apoA-I and ndHDL are efficient acceptors of cholesterol translocated out of hepatocytes and cholesterol-loaded peripheral cells (i.e., intimal macrophage foam cells). The overexpression of ApoA-I in a variety of animal models, including rabbits (45) and mice (46), significantly reduces atherosclerotic disease and can stimulate atheromatous plaque regression.

Multiple studies, including the European Concerted Action on Thrombosis and Disabilities Angina Pectoris Study (47), Apolipoprotein-related Mortality Risk Study (AMORIS) (Fig. 4) (48), and the Air Force/Texas Coronary Atherosclerosis Prevention Study (AFCAPS/TexCAPS) (49) trial all showed that as serum levels of apoA-I decrease, the risk for acute cardiovascular events increases.

A number of mutations in the gene for apo A-I have been documented and some are associated with increased risk for atherosclerosis in humans. In a detailed survey of apoA-I mutations, 23 have been found to predispose patients to some degree of hypoalphalipoproteinemia (i.e., decreased serum levels of HDL) (50). ApoA-I$_{Zavalla}$, which has an amino acid substitution of proline for leucine at position 159 (Leu$_{159}$→Pro), results in a 4-fold decrease in serum HDL and is associated with increased risk for CAD (51). ApoA-I$_{Nichinan}$ is characterized by the deletion of glutamic acid at position 235 (Glu$_{235}$); this significantly reduces the capacity of apoA-I to bind cells and promote cholesterol externalization (52). Patients with apoA-I(Lys$_{107}$→0), previously known as apoA-I Marburg or apoA-I Münster-2, have low HDL-C because of accelerated catabolism due to the deletion of lysine 107 (53,54). ApoA-I (L178P), in which a proline is substituted for the usual leucine residue at position 178, predisposes to endothelial cell dysfunction, increased arterial wall thickness, and premature CAD (55,56).

ATP-Binding Membrane Cassette Transport Protein A1

Cholesterol trafficking within cells is a complex and highly regulated process involving a variety of enzymes, membrane transport proteins, cell signaling molecules, and organelles. Maintaining intracellular cholesterol homeostasis and overall cellular integrity depends on the ability to balance cholesterol uptake with the capacity to mobilize and externalize excess cholesterol back into the extracellular milieu. The ATP-binding membrane cassette transport

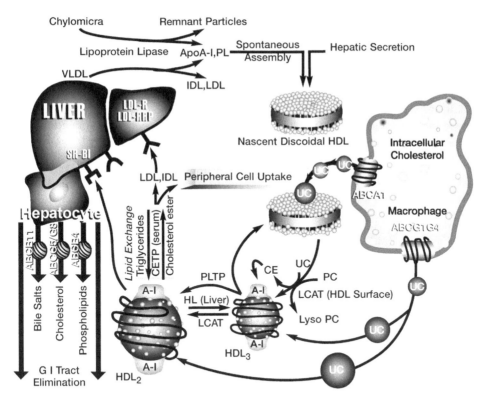

FIGURE 3 Metabolism of HDL and the flow of reverse cholesterol transport. In order to deliver peripheral cholesterol back to the liver or steroidogenic organs, apo A-I and nascent discoidal (pre-β) HDL interact with macrophages within the subendothelial space of blood vessel walls. HDL undergoes a series of cell receptor- and serum enzyme-dependent maturation reactions (i.e., "HDL speciation"). HDL can interact directly with a number of hepatocyte receptors. The cholesterol ester in HDL can also be delivered back to the liver via an "indirect pathway" for RCT, which depends upon CETP and the LDL and LDL-RRP receptors. *Abbreviations*: ABCA1 and G1/G4, ATP-binding membrane cassette transporters A1 and G1/G4; Apo A-I, apoprotein A-I; ApoE, apoprotein E; CE, cholesteryl ester; CETP, cholesterol ester transfer protein; HL, hepatic lipase; IDL, intermediate-density lipoprotein; LCAT, lecithin:cholesterol acyltransferase; LDL, low-density lipoprotein; LDL-R, low-density lipoprotein receptor; LDL-RRP, low-density lipoprotein receptor-related protein; lysoPC, lysophosphatidylcholine; PC, phosphatidylcholine; PGN, proteoglycans; PL, phospholipid; PLTP, phospholipid transfer protein; SR-BI, scavenger receptor BI; Trigly, triglyceride; UC, unesterified cholesterol; VLDL, very low-density lipoprotein. *Source*: From Ref. 44; with permission from Excerpta Media Inc.

protein A1 (ABCA1) regulates cholesterol exporting. This transporter is defective in the macrophages of patients with Tangier disease because of the deletion of nucleotides 3283 and 3284 in exon 22 of the ABCA1 gene (57). Tangier disease is a rare recessive disorder discovered on Tangier Island in the Chesapeake Bay. Patient's with Tangier disease have excessive tissue

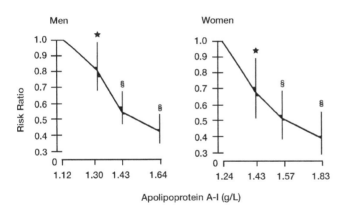

FIGURE 4 The Apolipoprotein-Related Mortality Risk Study demonstrated that decreased ApoA-I levels correlate with increased cardiovascular risk. *Source*: From Ref. 48; with permission from Elsevier.

cholesterol deposition and extremely low serum levels of apoA-I and HDL, resulting in hyperplastic orange tonsils, hepatosplenomegaly, and increased risk for atherosclerotic disease. The regulation of ABCA1 expression is complex. One important mechanism regulating ABCA1 activity involves increased intracellular oxysterol formation, resulting in the activation of liver X receptor-retinoid X receptor (LXR α-RXR) heterodimers and the induction of ABCA1 gene transcription so as to augment cholesterol externalization (58).

ABCA1 mediates the initial step in RCT. ABCA1 transports cholesterol and phospholipid into the extracellular spacej in an energy-dependent manner (59). ApoA-I in the subendothelial space functions as a reservoir for externalized cholesterol and phospholipid. As apoA-I acquires phospholipid, it binds cholesterol, leading to the formation of ndHDL. In the absence of adequate ABCA1 activity, apoA-I and ndHDL cannot mature and are rapidly catabolized and cleared from serum via renal elimination, resulting in hypoalphalipoproteinemia (Fig. 3). The exposure of macrophages to apoA-I increases the delivery of vesicles enriched with cholesterol from the Golgi apparatus to the plasma membrane, resulting in increased cholesterol efflux (60). Amino acid residues 220 to 231 in apoA-I facilitate specific binding to ABCA1 and are required for cellular lipid efflux and ndHDL formation (61). At least a portion of the cholesterol bound to ApoA-I may arise from passive diffusion down a concentration gradient into the extracellular space.

ABCA1 activity is an important determinant of serum levels of HDL, capacity for RCT, and risk for atherosclerotic disease. Transgenic mice overexpressing human ABCA1 demonstrate: (i) increased serum levels of HDL and apoA-I and augmented RCT as shown by increased biliary cholesterol excretion (62); and (ii) increased capacity to export cholesterol and phospholipid from macrophages and reduced risk for atherosclerotic disease (63). The overexpression of ABCA1 in mice homozygous for LDL receptor deficiency significantly retards rates of progression of atheromatous plaque progression (64). Dutch men who carry the R219K variant of ABCA1 (an arginine-to-lysine substitution at amino acid 219) in the Regression Growth Evaluation Statin Study (REGRESS) have higher HDL-C, lower triglycerides, slower progression of CAD, and lower risk for acute coronary events when compared with patients who do not have this mutation (65). Patients heterozygous for ABCA1 mutations that decrease the capacity for cholesterol efflux have reduced serum levels of HDL, increased triglyceride concentrations, and a threefold increased risk for CAD, with earlier onset compared with unaffected family members (66). In the latter investigation, each 8% change in ABCA1-mediated cholesterol efflux was associated with a 0.1 mmol/L change in serum HDL. ABCA1$_{Alabama}$ (C_{254}→T) is another example of a polymorphism that is associated with low HDL and increased risk for premature CAD (67). Heterozygotes for this mutation have a proline-to-leucine substitution (Pro85→Leu).

Lecithin:Cholesterol Acyltransferase

Lecithin:cholesterol acyltransferase (LCAT) catalyzes the esterification of cholesterol on the surface of ndHDL and HDL using the *sn*-2 fatty acid of phosphatidylcholine as an acyl chain donor. The esterified cholesterol partitions into the hydrophobic core of the HDL particle. This reaction creates a concentration gradient for unesterified cholesterol out of peripheral cells. As the HDL particle becomes more enriched with cholesteryl ester, it becomes progressively rounder and larger, leading to the successive formation of HDL$_3$ and then HDL$_2$. Another set of ATP binding membrane cassette transport proteins in the macrophage, ABCG1 and ABCG4, translocate intracellular cholesterol directly to HDL$_3$ and HDL$_2$ and provide additional molecular circuitry for driving RCT and facilitate the maturation of HDL (68,69).

Familial LCAT deficiency can be caused by mutations in the LCAT gene. For example, a substitution of proline for leucine (Leu$_{209}$→Pro) or isoleucine for methionine (Met$_{293}$→Ile), results in a complete or nearly complete loss of enzyme activity (70,71). The clinical features of complete (classic) LCAT deficiency include corneal opacities, anemia, proteinuria, and renal insufficiency (72). In contrast, patients with fish-eye disease develop massive corneal opacities (the basis for the name of the syndrome), but do not have anemia, proteinuria, or renal disease (73–76). A number of allelic variants in the LCAT gene can each cause fish-eye disease, a partial LCAT deficiency disorder in which the defective enzyme esterifies cholesterol in apoB-containing lipoproteins, but not in HDL (71,72,76,77). The LCAT mutation Pro$_{260}$→Stop results in a truncated enzyme with substantial reductions in serum HDL and apoA-I (70).

Patients with LCAT deficiency have a diminished capacity for cholesteryl ester formation and present with moderate to severe reductions in serum HDL. Kinetic studies have shown that complete or partial LCAT deficiency is associated with increased catabolic rates for serum apoA-I and apoA-II, although the catabolism of particles containing both apoproteins (LpA-I:A-II) appears to be greater than that of particles containing apoA-I without apoA-II (LpA-I) (73,78,79). Despite the hypoalphalipoproteinemia, no clear relationship between the severity of LCAT deficiency and the risk for atherosclerotic disease in humans has been identified. In part, this may be because of relatively efficient cholesterol efflux as a result of the higher proportion of LpA-I to LpA-I:A-II particles (73,78).

There are no known examples of LCAT overexpression in humans. In a transgenic rabbit model, however, human LCAT overexpression led to a dose-dependent increase in HDL-C levels (80). This was characterized by the presence of large HDL particles, with corresponding increases in apoA-I and plasma phospholipid concentrations. Plasma concentrations of apoB were markedly reduced. The results of this study suggest that the overexpression of human LCAT may lead to hyperalphalipoproteinemia and to reduced concentrations of apoB-containing atherogenic lipoproteins. Apo A-I is an activator of LCAT and depends on three strictly conserved arginine residues (positions 149, 153, and 160) within the α-helical repeat formed by amino acid residues 143-164 (81). ApoA-I$_{Mallorca}$ has reduced ability to activate LCAT and is associated with familial hypoalphalipoproteinemia (82).

Phospholipid Transfer Protein

Phospholipid transfer protein (PLTP) mediates the transfer of phospholipids from apoB100-containing lipoproteins (VLDL, LDL) to HDL (83). According to in vitro evidence, PLTP also facilitate, inducing "HDL conversion," a process whereby HDL$_3$ is remodeled into smaller and larger particles through a fusion reaction (84–86). The resulting conversion products include lipid-poor apoA-I, a precursor of pre-β-HDL (Fig. 3) (85). Because pre-β-HDL appears to be a key acceptor of cholesterol from macrophages, it has been suggested that PLTP might be antiatherogenic by promoting RCT (72,85,87). No human polymorphism resulting in PLTP overexpression has yet been identified.

Cholesteryl Ester Transfer Protein

Cholesteryl ester transfer protein (CETP) is a hepatically derived protein that binds to HDL. CETP mediates the equimolar exchange of cholesteryl esters from HDL for triglycerides in apoB-containing lipoproteins (chylomicrons, VLDL, and LDL). The cholesteryl ester transferred into apoB lipoproteins can subsequently enter multiple pathways for disposal. First, it can be delivered to the liver via the LDL receptor and the LDL receptor-related protein. Once taken up by the hepatocyte, the cholesterol can be: (i) secreted into bile via the activity of ABCBG5/G8; (ii) converted into bile acids by 7α-hydroxylase, with the resulting bile acids pumped into the biliary tree by ABCB11; or (iii) the cholesterol can be partitioned back into VLDL and resecreted into the circulation. Second, if the cholesteryl ester is not taken up by hepatocyte lipoprotein receptors, it can be delivered to peripheral tissues by VLDL remnants and LDL particles (Fig. 3).

A number of polymorphisms result in CETP deficiency states and hyperalphalipoproteinemia. CETP deficiency is best characterized in the Japanese, who have a relatively high prevalence of two polymorphisms: a G→A mutation in the 5′ splice donor site of intron 14 (Int14 G→A) and a substitution of glycine for aspartic acid (D$_{442}$→G) in exon 15 (88,89). The combined heterozygote frequency is approximately 9% (89). In subjects who are homozygous for CETP null mutations, HDL-C levels can be three to five times higher than normal. Heterozygosity results in partial CETP activity, with HDL-C elevations of 10% to 30% (90).

Although high HDL-C levels are generally considered antiatherogenic, some studies have shown a reduced capacity for RCT by the HDL of Japanese patients with inborn CETP deficiency states (90). This may be attributable to disruptions in key elements of RCT, including cholesterol efflux from macrophages, the esterification of cholesterol, and the transfer of cholesteryl esters to apo B100-containing lipoproteins (87). Such disruptions may hinder the transport of cholesterol to the liver for biliary excretion (87).

A crucial question regarding CETP deficiency is whether it influences atherosclerotic burden and coronary risk (75). Consequently, studies have been conducted to evaluate the association between CETP deficiency and the incidence or prevalence of CHD.

In the Omagari region of Japan, where there is a high prevalence of the intron 14 splicing defect, as well as a high rate of alcohol intake, HDL-C levels greater than 100 mg/dL occur in just over 1% of individuals (83). According to a population-based study in this rural area ($N = 104{,}505$), the frequency of ischemic ECG changes increased in subjects with HDL-C levels greater than or equal to 90 mg/dL. Moreover, subjects with CAD and genetic CETP deficiency had significantly higher HDL-C and apoA-I levels, accompanied by lower LDL-C and apoB levels, than their CAD counterparts who lacked the gene mutation. There was also a lower prevalence of marked hyperalphalipoproteinemia ($\geq$100 mg/dL) and of the intron 14 splicing defect (homozygous or heterozygous) in persons greater than or equal to 80 years of age compared with younger participants. Although these results indicate that the Int14 G$\rightarrow$A mutation may not be atheroprotective or confer longevity, they are inconclusive given the small sample size (88).

Initially, in a cross-sectional investigation, the HHP found that Japanese American men with heterozygous CETP deficiency and normal HDL-C levels (40–60 mg/dL) had an increased risk for CHD compared both with control subjects in the same HDL-C range and with heterozygotes whose HDL-C levels exceeded 60 mg/dL. This implies that heterozygous CETP deficiency may raise CHD risk if it is not accompanied by an elevation in HDL-C (75,91). The study also found that heterozygotes and controls with HDL-C levels greater than 60 mg/dL had a similarly low prevalence of CHD (91). More recently, however, a seven-year follow-up reported that HDL-C levels were significantly higher in CETP-deficient heterozygotes than in controls; furthermore, heterozygotes in each HDL-C stratum ($\leq$60 mg/dL and >60 mg/dL) were at lower risk for CHD compared with controls, although the trend was not statistically significant (92,93). The divergent results of the cross-sectional and longitudinal analyses may be partly explained by methodologic differences. It is also possible that the effects of CETP gene mutations may change with age (92).

Among Japanese men living in Kochi Prefecture, a cross-sectional study found that the $D_{442}\rightarrow$G and Int14G$\rightarrow$A mutations were each associated with HDL-C levels greater than or equal to 80 mg/dL. There was also an association between HDL-C levels greater than or equal to 80 mg/dL and a reduced prevalence of CHD (75). Based on this study, however, it is unclear whether genetic CETP deficiency is directly protective (93,94).

Other CETP gene polymorphisms have also been identified. In the Veterans Affairs HDL Intervention Trial (VA-HIT) men with the *Taq*I B2B2 genotype had reduced CETP activity, higher baseline HDL levels, and a 48% lower risk for CAD-related events compared with patients homozygous for the B1 allele (95). In contrast, the CETP polymorphism *EcoN*1 G/G is associated with reduced HDL-C levels and an increased risk for CAD (96).

The study of genetic CETP deficiency is important because it can help clarify the mechanisms of HDL metabolism. Although observational evidence does not consistently support the presence of an association between CETP deficiency and a reduction in coronary risk, pharmacologic agents for the inhibition of CETP are being developed (see "Emerging Therapies").

Hepatic Lipase

Hepatic lipase (HL) is synthesized by hepatocytes and is bound to heparan sulfate proteoglycans in the space of Disse and the endothelium lining hepatic sinusoids. HL has both phospholipase A1 and triglyceride lipase activities and plays an important role in HDL remodeling. HL hydrolyzes triglycerides and phospholipids during the conversion of larger, more buoyant HDL_2 to the smaller and denser HDL_3 (Fig. 3). HDLs enriched with triglyceride are particularly favorable targets for HL activity. As the HDL is catabolized to smaller species, it can become progressively unstable thermodynamically, resulting in the release of apo A-I from its surface coat. If the apo A-I is not rapidly relipidated by ABCA1, it is eliminated via the kidney. Consequently, increased HL activity can result in low serum levels of HDL.

A number of studies have evaluated the effect of HL mutations on serum HDL levels. Allelic variation in the gene for HL appears to regulate approximately 25% of the variation in HDL levels among humans (97). HL overexpression is at least partly etiologic for a high prevalence of low HDL among Turkish women (26%) and men (53%) (98). Among premenopausal normolipidemic women, the $C_{514}\rightarrow$T allele for the HL gene (LIPC) is associated with significantly lower HL activity, significantly higher levels of HDL_2, and significantly more buoyant LDL compared with the CC controls (99). Despite its association with decreased HL activity, the LIPC T-allele does not raise total HDL-C levels in all populations (100,101). Another mutation in the LIPC promoter region, $G_{250} \rightarrow A$, also gives rise to reduced enzyme activity (100). According to one study, the A genotype is associated with significantly higher HDL_2-C levels in white CAD patients, as well as with a trend toward increased HDL-C overall (100). Low HL activity is not necessarily associated with reduced risk for CAD. A number of studies show that when low HL activity is combined with CETP deficiency, risk for CAD increases (101). Given such findings, it is possible that for reduced HL activity to have a beneficial effect on the risk for atherogenesis, it may have to coexist with specific genetic and metabolic backgrounds. This will require additional basic scientific and clinical trial clarification.

Endothelial Lipase

Endothelial lipase (EL) is produced and secreted by endothelial cells and preferentially hydrolyzes acyl chains at the *sn*-1 position of phospholipids. When EL activity is decreased in mice either by polyclonal antibody inhibition (102) or inactivation by gene targeting (103), serum HDL levels increase substantially (25–60%). The role of EL in human RCT and HDL metabolism, the regulation of its activity, and the effects of gene polymorphisms on risk for CAD all require further characterization. One recent study among patients with metabolic syndrome showed that increased EL activity is highly correlated with significant reductions in serum HDL-C levels (104).

Hepatic High-Density Lipoprotein Receptors

The delivery of cholesteryl esters back to the liver for elimination in bile or conversion into bile salts is the final step in RCT. Scavenger receptor class B type I (SR-BI) is a high-affinity receptor for HDL, is located on the hepatocyte surface, and mediates selective cholesteryl ester uptake into hepatocytes (105–107). In the mouse, a deficiency of SR-BI reduces biliary cholesterol concentrations, increases cholesteryl ester content of HDL, and augments rates of atherogenesis (108). On the other hand, SR-BI overexpression in mice increases biliary cholesterol excretion, dramatically reduces serum HDL, and is antiatherogenic (109). The latter experiments illustrate the emerging concept that, it is not the absolute level of HDL that determines risk for atherosclerotic disease, but rather the RCT pathway's capacity to deliver excess cholesterol from the periphery back to the liver for disposal. The greater the capacitance for this centripetal flux of cholesterol back to the liver, the lower the likelihood for net accumulation of cholesterol in the periphery.

Selective cholesteryl ester uptake by SR-BI is dependent on interactions with multiple α-helical segments α in apoA-I (110), and targeted disruption of these sites impairs lipid transfer (111). Cholesteryl ester internalized by SR-BI is channeled to a membrane compartment where it is hydrolyzed to free cholesterol by a neutral cholesteryl ester hydrolase (112). Delipidated HDL is released back into the circulation where it can reinitiate another cycle of RCT. Other hepatic HDL receptors have also been identified. The α-chain of the mitochondrial F1-ATP synthetase is expressed on the surface of hepatocytes and functions as a high-affinity HDL receptor (113). After binding apoA-I, this receptor mediates HDL holoparticle endocytosis in a reaction that hydrolyzes ATP. Glycosylphosphatidylinositol-anchored HDL-binding protein 1 is a high-affinity HDL receptor that mediates selective lipid uptake in mice (114). Clearly, hepatic HDL delipidation and uptake is complex. The coordination and regulation of these uptake pathways are yet to be elucidated.

RCT is likely the most important antiatherogenic function of HDL. There is experimental support confirming the conceptual validity of RCT in both animals (115) and humans (116). Much basic scientific and clinical investigation is focused on identifying the means by which to increase the concentration and functionality of HDL in order to more specifically augment RCT for therapeutic purposes in patients at risk for CHD-related events (117).

In addition to driving RCT, HDL is likely atheroprotective secondary to its ability to mediate a broad range of antiatherogenic phenomena along the vessel wall. These are summarized in this section.

Effects on Endothelial Cell Function

Endothelial cell dysfunction is an important precursor to atherogenesis and is characterized by reduced nitric oxide production, increased production of reactive oxygen species such as superoxide anion and hydrogen peroxide, upregulation of adhesion molecule expression, and reduced tissue plasminogen activator (tPA) and increased plasminogen activator inhibitor-1 (PAI-1) production, among other changes. HDL stimulates endothelial cell nitric oxide production by stabilizing the mRNA transcripts for endothelial nitric oxide synthase (118). Consistent with this observation, as serum HDL-C increases, the degree of flow-mediated brachial artery vasodilatation increases (Fig. 5) (119), as does myocardial perfusion (120).

Activated dysfunctional endothelial cells express a variety of adhesion molecules along their surface that facilitate the binding and transmigration of inflammatory white cells (e.g., monocytes) into the subendothelial space. These adhesion molecules include vascular cell adhesion molecule-1 (VCAM-1) and intercellular adhesion molecule-1 (ICAM-1). Inhibiting the expression of adhesion molecules is associated with a reduced risk for the development of atherosclerosis in a variety of experimental models. Nuclear factor-(B (NF-κB) regulates a large number of inflammatory signaling pathways (121) including the expression of VCAM-1 and ICAM-1. HDL reduces NF-κB and adhesion molecule expression by inhibiting sphingosine kinase and sphingosine 1-phosphate production (Fig. 6) (122).

HDL stimulates endothelial cell proliferation (124) and migration (125) along denuded areas of vascular surfaces and inhibits endothelial apoptosis by transferring sphingosylphosphorylcholine and lysosulfatide, which reduce the activation of caspases 3 and 9 (126).

Antithrombotic Effects

Platelets are an important source of growth factors and inflammatory mediators capable of influencing atheromatous plaque stability and progression (127). Platelet-derived mediators include thrombospondin, platelet-derived growth factor, CD 40 ligand, and transforming growth factor-β, among others. Platelets also influence risk for such acute coronary syndromes as MI and unstable angina by forming acute thrombi along plaque fissure, ulcerations, and ruptures, ultimately leading to partial or total coronary luminal obstructions with myocardial ischemia (128,129).

HDL modulates the activity of platelets and a variety of thrombotic factors. A low serum HDL-C increases platelet aggregability in women taking oral contraceptives (130). HDL inhibits platelet thromboxane A2 production (131), decreases platelet reactivity in response to collagen or thrombin exposure (132), and enhances urokinase-mediated fibrinolysis (133). HDL potentiates the ability of proteins C and S to inactivate coagulation factor Va (134). HDL increases endothelial cell COX-2 expression (135), and functions as an arachidonic acid donor (136), thereby increasing biosynthesis of prostacyclin (PGI_2) (137), a vasodilator and inhibitor of platelet aggregation. HDL has also been shown to reduce thrombin-mediated platelet aggregation and fibrinogen binding by inhibiting formation of the intracellular messengers inositol 1,4,5-triphosphate and 1,2-diacylglycerol (138).

Antioxidative Activity

Oxidized LDL is highly inflammatory and proatherogenic (139). Transition metal cations and enzymes, such as NAD(P)H oxidase, lipoxygenase, and myeloperoxidase, promote the formation of reactive oxygen species that oxidize the fatty acids of phospholipids within LDL particles (140). Such oxidative processes yield highly reactive fatty acid free radicals, conjugated diene peroxy free radicals, and conjugated diene free radicals, among other injurious chemical

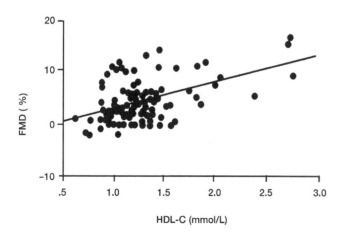

FIGURE 5 As serum HDL-C increases, the degree of flow-mediated brachial artery vasodilatation increases. To convert HDL-C values from mmol/L to mg/dL, multiply by 38.7. *Abbreviations*: HDL-C, high-density lipoprotein cholesterol. *Source*: From Ref. 119; with permission from Elsevier.

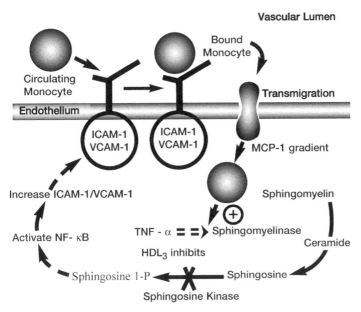

FIGURE 6 HDL reduces endothelial cell adhesion molecule expression. Endothelial cell adhesion molecules such as ICAM-1 and VCAM-1 promote the binding of circulating monocytes to activated, dysfunctional endothelium. Monocytes can then transmigrate into the subendothelial space in response to a monocyte chemoattract protein-1 (MCP-1) gradient, where they can establish an inflammatory nidus. Monocytes release TNF-α, a cytokine that activates sphingomyelinase. Sphingomyelinase catalyzes the conversion of sphingomyelin to ceramide. The ceramide can be converted into sphingosine. Sphingosine kinase phosphorylates sphingosine to sphingosine 1-phosphate. Sphingosine 1-phosphate is an activator of nuclear factor kappaB, which regulates the expression of adhesion molecules. HDL is an inhibitor of sphingosine kinase and can down-regulate the expression of endothelial ICAM-1 and VCAM-1. *Abbreviations*: MCP-1, monocyte chemoattract protein-1; TNF-α, tumor necrosis factor-alpha; NF-κB, nuclear factor kappaB;. *Source*: From Ref. 123; with permission from Elsevier.

species. Oxidized LDL induces endothelial dysfunction, facilitates the development of localized vasculitis secondary to autoantibody production, and stimulates monocyte/macrophage and T cell recruitment into the subendothelial space (141). Macrophages exposed to oxidized LDL upregulate the expression of scavenging receptors, such as CD36 and SR-A, which promote LDL binding and uptake. The continued internalization of oxidized LDL by macrophages leads to foam cell, fatty streak, and atheromatous plaque formation along the vessel wall (142,143).

HDL has significant antioxidative capacity and inhibits LDL oxidation (144). When evaluated in vitro, HDL inhibits LDL lipid peroxide generation by up to 90% in a concentration-dependent manner and significant inter-individual differences in the antioxidative capacity of HDL is observed (145). Young men (<40 years) with low HDL-C have greater endothelial dysfunction and higher in vivo levels of oxidized LDL compared with age-matched controls with normal HDL-C (146). HDL is a carrier for two important antioxidative enzymes: paraoxonase (PON; also known as aryldialkylphosphatase) and platelet-activating factor-acetylhydrolase (PAFA). PON is a glycoprotein synthesized by the liver and associates with HDL in serum. PON blocks LDL lipid peroxidation (147) and reduces cholesteryl ester hydroperoxides to less reactive hydroxides in atheromatous plaques (148). PON activity is decreased in patients with CAD and diabetes mellitus (149), chronic renal failure (150), MI (151), and smokers (152). PAFA also associates with HDL and hydrolyzes fatty acyl peroxides at the *sn*-2 position of phospholipids (153).

The apoprotein constituents of HDL also augment the antioxidative potential of HDL. Both apoA-I and apoA-II contain redox-sensitive methionine residues capable of reducing reactive cholesteryl ester hydroperoxides to relatively inert hydroxides (154). In human HDL, the Met(112) and Met(148) of apoA-1 and Met(26) of apoA-II are converted to methionine sulfoxide groups as lipid hydroperoxides are reduced to hydroxides (155). These methionine residues reduce the hydroperoxides of both cholesteryl esters and phospholipids and function independently of PON. CETP can render oxidized LDL less atherogenic by mediating the net transfer of lipid hydroperoxides from LDL to HDL (156). Once incorporated into HDL, the lipids are reduced and detoxified.

PHARMACOLOGIC MANAGEMENT OF LOW HIGH-DENSITY LIPOPROTEIN CHOLESTEROL
Statin Therapy

The publication of the first clinical event trials with statins in the mid-1990s yielded the most persuasive evidence that treatment of hypercholesterolemia produced coronary benefits with few safety concerns, especially in patients at high risk (157–159). In those trials, treatment predominantly induced reductions of TC and LDL-C; however, there were also modest (approximately 15%) decreases seen in triglyceride levels and increases of 5% to 8% in HDL-C. These other lipid changes may have contributed to the beneficial effects seen, although their potential contributions are difficult to quantify.

The statins induce elevations in HDL-C by two principal mechanisms. First, the statins inhibit factor Rho which leads to activation of peroxisome proliferator-activated receptor (PPAR)-α and hepatic expression of apoproteins A-I and A-II (160). Second, by decreasing serum VLDL and triglyceride levels, the statins reduce the amount of cholesteryl ester transferred out of HDL by CETP, thereby indirectly reducing its catabolism (161). In efficacy studies, the statins raise HDL-C by 5% to 13% (162,163), with rosuvastatin having a slightly better capacity than comparator statins to increase this lipoprotein (164).

AFCAPS/TexCAPS studied more than 6600 men ≥45 years) and women ≥55 years) who were free of CHD and whose mean baseline lipid levels were as follows: TC, 221 mg/dL (5.71 mmol/L); LDL-C, 150 mg/dL (3.89 mmol/L); HDL-C, 36 mg/dL (0.94 mmol/L) for men and 40 mg/dL (1.03 mmol/L) for women. Subjects were randomized to treatment with either lovastatin (20–40 mg/day) or matching placebo (165). A minority of this apparently healthy population had other cardiovascular risk factors such as hypertension (22%), smoking (12%), diabetes (2%) and family history of premature CHD (15%). Lovastatin reduced LDL-C by 25% and increased HDL-C by 6%. During an average follow-up of 5.2 years, lovastatin treatment was associated with a 37% reduction in the risk for an acute coronary event (fatal or nonfatal MI, sudden cardiac death or unstable angina). First heart attack was reduced by 40%, and the need for revascularization procedures was reduced by 33%. Across the tertiles of baseline HDL-C, the largest relative risk reduction associated with statin treatment versus placebo was observed in the patients in the lowest tertile (45% among patients in the lowest tertile vs. 15% in the highest tertile) (Fig. 7), although this trend was not statistically significant.

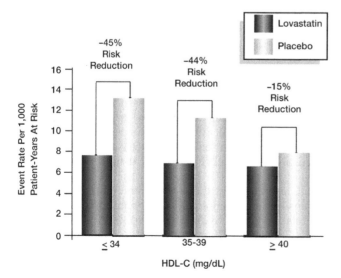

FIGURE 7 The Air Force/Texas Coronary Atherosclerosis Prevention Study (AFCAPS/TexCAPS). Across the tertiles of baseline HDL-C, the largest relative risk reduction associated with lovastatin treatment, 20 to 40 mg/day, versus placebo was observed in the patients in the lowest tertile (45% among patients in the lowest tertile vs. 15% in the highest tertile). *Abbreviation:* HDL-C, high-density lipoprotein cholesterol. *Source:* From Ref. 166.

A subsequent analysis assessed the relation between baseline and on-treatment lipid and apoprotein parameters and the risk for acute major coronary events (166). Baseline HDL-C, apoA-I, and apoB were among the significant predictors of acute major coronary events. However, only on-treatment apoA-I, apoB, and the ratio of apoB to apoA1 were predictive of subsequent risk; on-treatment LDL-C was not. On-treatment apoB, especially when combined with apoA1 to form the apoB/apoA-I ratio, may be more accurate than LDL-C in predicting the risk for a first acute major coronary event in the primary prevention setting.

In general, post hoc analyses of the other major statin trials suggest no heterogeneity of benefit across the range of HDL-C values in the study cohorts. One exception is the Prospective Study of Pravastatin in the Elderly at Risk (PROSPER) trial in which 5804 high-risk subjects, aged 70 to 82 years, were treated with pravastatin, 40 mg/day, versus placebo. The main study finding was a 19% to 23% reduction in CHD risk with treatment, but no reduction in the risk for stroke. A subsequent analysis examined the association of LDL-C and HDL-C with risk (167). Although risk reduction was not related to baseline LDL-C, there was a significant interaction when comparing the effects of treatment on those with lower baseline HDL-C and those with higher HDL-C ($P = 0.012$). Patients in the lowest two quintiles of HDL-C [<44 mg/dL (1.15 mmol/L)] had a 33% relative risk reduction with pravastatin treatment compared with placebo ($P < 0.0001$), but those with higher HDL-C showed no benefit. Therefore, in a high-risk elderly cohort, HDL-C less than 44 mg/dL (1.15 mmol/L) defined a subgroup that benefited from treatment.

In the Lipoprotein and Coronary Atherosclerosis Study (LCAS), patients with angiographic evidence of coronary disease were treated with fluvastatin, 20 mg twice daily, versus placebo (168). Of the 339 patients with biochemical and angiographic data, 68 who had baseline HDL-C less than 35 mg/dL (0.91 mmol/L) had mean HDL-C of 31.7 mg/dL (0.82 mmol/L), versus 47.4 mg/dL (1.23 mmol/L) in patients with baseline HDL-C greater than or equal to 35 mg/dL (0.91 mmol/L). Among patients on placebo, those with low HDL-C had significantly more angiographic progression than those with higher HDL-C. Fluvastatin significantly reduced progression among low–HDL-C patients, as measured by a decrease in the minimum lumen diameter (MLD): 0.065 ± 0.036 mm versus 0.274 ± 0.045 mm in placebo patients ($P = 0.0004$); respective decreases in MLD among higher–HDL-C patients were 0.036 ± 0.021 mm and 0.083 ± 0.019 mm ($P = 0.09$). The treatment effect of fluvastatin on MLD change was significantly greater among low–HDL-C patients than among higher–HDL-C patients ($P = 0.01$); among low–HDL-C patients, fluvastatin patients had improved event-free survival compared with placebo patients, although the study was not designed to assess clinical end points.

Statins are the drugs of choice for a wide range of patients with dyslipidemia in both the primary- and secondary-prevention settings. The statins also appear to disproportionately benefit patients with low HDL-C. In addition to modulating lipid metabolism, the statins exert a broad variety of pleiotropic effects that can also be induced by HDL, including the activation of endothelial nitric oxide synthase, down-regulation of adhesion molecule expression, and inhibition of LDL oxidation and platelet activation, among others (169). The statins should be first-line therapy in patients with isolated low HDL-C or low HDL-C combined with LDL-C levels that exceed NCEP-defined targets.

Fibrate Therapy

The fibrates are synthetic PPAR-α agonists that exert multiple direct and indirect effects on HDL metabolism. Fibrates, on average, raise serum HDL-C approximately 10% (4.1 mg/dL) (170). The fibrates stimulate hepatic HDL secretion by upregulating the expression of hepatic apoA-I and A-II. They also appear to potentiate RCT by stimulating macrophage expression of ABCA1 and hepatocyte SR-BI (171). The fibrates stimulate triglyceride and fatty acid catabolism by inducing the transcription of genes involved in lipoprotein lipase (LPL) expression and mitochondrial β-oxidation. As the triglycerides in large lipoproteins such as VLDL and chylomicrons undergo catabolism, surface coat mass (phospholipid and apoproteins) is released and can be used to assimilate HDL in serum. For this reason, low LPL activity is associated with hypertriglyceridemia and hypoalphalipoproteinemia. In patients with hypertriglyceridemia, HDL and LDL particles tend to become enriched with triglycerides because of increased rates of CETP exchange activity (Fig. 8). As these lipoproteins become progressively more enriched with triglycerides, they become better targets for HL, an enzyme that tends to catabolize HDL into its smaller isoforms. With continued catabolism,

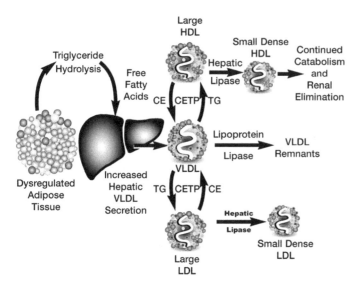

FIGURE 8 Effect of hypertriglyceridemia on lipoprotein metabolism. As adipose tissue metabolism becomes dysregulated in the milieu of insulin resistance, the rate of triglyceride hydrolysis increases. This results in increased: (i) flux of free fatty acids into the portal circulation and liver and (ii) hepatic production and secretion of VLDL. In an insulin resistant state, lipoprotein lipase activity is reduced. This results in elevated VLDL levels, high serum VLDL remnant levels, and hypertriglyceridemia. With excess triglyceride availability, CETP catalyzes the equimolar exchange of cholesterol ester in HDL for triglyceride. As the HDL becomes progressively more enriched with triglyceride it becomes a better target for lipolysis and catabolism by hepatic lipase. Large, buoyant LDL is converted into smaller, denser LDL via a similar mechanism. *Abbreviations*: HDL, high-density lipoprotein; CETP, Cholesteryl ester transfer protein; CE, cholesteryl ester; TG, triglyceride; VLDL, very low-density lipoprotein; LDL, low-density lipoproteins. *Source*: From Ref. 172.

the HDL particles can become unstable and may ultimately be eliminated via renal pathways. Consequently, controlling hypertriglyceridemia in patients with low HDL-C is an important therapeutic consideration.

LPL is bound to endothelial cells lining the vasculature within adipose tissue, myocardium, and skeletal muscle. Mutations in this enzyme can yield changes in both serum levels of HDL and risk for cardiovascular events. The substitution of glutamic acid for glycine at position 188 (Gly_{188}→Glu) in the LPL gene is associated with low HDL, hypertriglyceridemia, and increased risk for CHD (173). A substitution of serine for asparagine (Asn_{291}→Ser) predisposes both men and women to low HDL and increased risk for cardiovascular events (174,175). The Ser_{447}→Stop polymorphism, representing a premature truncation of the LPL molecule, increases HDL levels in Dutch men (172). In patients with mutations that lead to nonfunctional variants of LPL, hypertriglyceridemia tends to respond minimally to fibrate therapy.

The Helsinki Heart Study was a primary prevention trial evaluating the efficacy of gemfibrozil therapy (1200 mg/day) compared with placebo in 4081 men aged 40 to 55 years (177). Gemfibrozil therapy increased HDL-C by 11% and decreased LDL-C and triglycerides by 11% and 35%, respectively. It was also associated with a 34% reduction in the incidence of coronary mortality and MI compared with placebo. The investigators for this trial estimated that for every 1% increase in HDL-C induced by gemfibrozil therapy, the risk for CAD-related events decreased by 3% (178).

In VA-HIT, more than 2500 men with CHD were randomized to either gemfibrozil (1200 mg/day) or placebo (179). For entry into the trial, subjects had to have documented CAD, HDL-C levels of 40 mg/dL (1.03 mmol/L) or less, and LDL-C levels of no more than 140 mg/dL (3.62 mmol/L). The primary combined end-point was nonfatal MI or death from coronary causes. At the end of one year, HDL-C had increased by 6%, triglycerides were 31% lower, and there were no differences between the groups in LDL-C levels. After a median follow-up of 5.1 years, there was a 22% reduction in the risk for a primary end-point event and a 24% reduction in the combined endpoint of coronary death, nonfatal MI and stroke. In patients whose primary lipid abnormality is low HDL-C, raising HDL-C levels and lowering levels of triglycerides, without lowering LDL levels, may reduce the rate of coronary events. In follow-up, a multivariable Cox proportional hazards analysis showed that CHD events were reduced by 11% with gemfibrozil for every 5-mg/dL (0.13-mmol/L) increase in HDL-C ($P = 0.02$). Diabetic patients benefited most significantly with a 32% reduction in the combined primary end point, 41% reduction in CHD mortality, and 40% reduction in risk for stroke. During gemfibrozil treatment, only the increase in HDL-C significantly predicted a lower risk for CHD events, whereas neither triglyceride nor LDL-C levels at baseline or during the trial predicted CHD events by multivariable analysis. Thus, concentrations of HDL-C achieved with gemfibrozil treatment predicted a significant reduction in CHD events in patients with low HDL-C levels. However, the achieved HDL-C levels only partially explained the beneficial effect of gemfibrozil (180).

Multiple angiographic trials confirm the ability of fibrates to reduce rates of atheromatous plaque progression in coronary (181,182) and saphenous vein bypass grafts (183). Fibrates are a rational therapeutic choice for patients with low HDL-C, high triglycerides, and low-normal LDL-C. However, fibrate therapy can raise serum levels of LDL-C. Mechanistically this arises from the increased conversion of VLDL to LDL as LPL is activated. If LDL-C increases substantially, combination therapy with a statin may be necessary to help patients meet the overall lipoprotein goals recommended by the NCEP. If combination therapy is necessary, gemfibrozil should be avoided as this fibrate can block the glucuronidation of the statins, increasing the risk for adverse events (376). Fenofibrate is a safer choice since it has 1/15 times the risk for inducing adverse events when used in combination with statins compared with gemfibrozil (184,185).

Niacin Therapy

Niacin is the most potent drug currently available for raising serum levels of HDL-C, with elevations of up to 25% to 30%. For many years it was assumed that niacin raised HDL-C by blocking hepatic holoparticle uptake without impairing rates of RCT (186). A radically different view of the mechanisms of niacin has recently come into focus. Niacin does not appear to have a specific receptor in the liver. Niacin binds with high affinity to a receptor on both the adipocyte and the macrophage. The human and murine isoforms of this receptor are referred to as HM74 and PUMA-G (protein-upregulated in macrophages by interferon-γ) (187,188). The natural ligand for these receptors is, as yet, unknown. When niacin binds to this receptor in adipose tissue, hormone-sensitive triglyceride lipase is inhibited through a G-protein-mediated inhibition of adenylate cyclase. As lipolytic activity in adipose tissue decreases, less fatty acid is mobilized from triglyceride stores. This decreases the amount of fatty acid delivered to the liver, which reduces hepatic VLDL secretion and serum triglyceride levels. HDL-C levels will rise secondary to: (i) reduced triglyceride enrichment of this lipoprotein fraction by CETP; and (ii) reduced catabolism by HL. Niacin also upregulates the expression of ABCA1 along the macrophage membrane and this would be expected to increase rates of both ndHDL and HDL biosynthesis in the extravascular compartment, as well as the rate of RCT (189).

In the Coronary Drug Project, the efficacy of immediate-release niacin monotherapy (3 g of crystalline niacin daily) versus placebo was studied in a group of men with CAD (190). Although the effect on serum HDL-C levels was not specifically evaluated, niacin therapy reduced the risk of MI by 26%, stroke by 24%, and the need for coronary revascularization by 67% relative to placebo. There was no statistically significant effect on mortality after five years of follow-up. There was a high incidence of niacin discontinuation secondary to flushing. The flushing is most likely mediated by cyclooxygenase-generated prostaglandin D_2 (191).

In the three-year double-blind HDL-Atherosclerosis Treatment Study (HATS), 160 patients with coronary disease, low HDL-C levels [≤35 mg/dL (0.91 mmol/L) in men, and 40 mg/dL (1.03 mmol/L) in women], "normal" LDL-C levels ≤145 mg/dL (3.75 mmol/L), and triglyceride levels below 400 mg/dL (4.52 mmol/L) were randomly assigned to receive one of four regimens: simvastatin, 10 to 20 mg/day, plus 2–4 grams niacin per day; daily antioxidant vitamins (800 IU of vitamin E, 1000 mg of vitamin C, 25 mg of beta-carotene, and 100 μg of selenium); simvastatin-niacin plus antioxidants; or placebo (192). The mean levels of LDL-C and HDL-C cholesterol were unaltered in the antioxidant group and the placebo group; these levels changed substantially (by –42% and +26%, respectively) in the simvastatin-niacin group. The pre-specified primary angiographic end point was mean change per patient in percent coronary stenosis from the baseline to the final angiogram. The average stenosis progressed by 3.9% with placebo, 1.8% with antioxidants ($P = 0.16$ for the comparison with the placebo

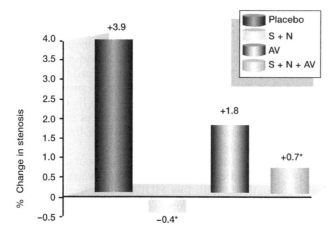

FIGURE 9 The high-density lipoprotein-Atherosclerosis Treatment Study: effect of Simvastatin plus Niacin, with or without Antioxidants, on coronary artery disease progression. *Source*: From Ref. 192.

group), and 0.7% with simvastatin-niacin plus antioxidants ($P < 0.01$), and regressed by 0.4% with simvastatin-niacin alone ($P < 0.001$) (Fig. 9).

The pre-specified clinical end point was the time to the first of the following events: coronary death, nonfatal MI, stroke, or revascularization. The frequency of the clinical end point was 24% with placebo; 3% with simvastatin-niacin alone; 21% in the antioxidant-therapy group; and 14% in the simvastatin-niacin-plus-antioxidants group. The risk for the composite primary end point was 90% lower in the simvastatin–niacin group than in the placebo group ($P = 0.03$) (Fig. 10).

An intriguing finding in HATS was that the protective increase in HDL_2 with simvastatin plus niacin was attenuated by concurrent therapy with antioxidants (193). Increases in HDL-C, especially HDL_2-C, were consistently higher in the simvastatin plus niacin group than in the simvastatin plus niacin and antioxidants group (25% vs. 18% and 42% vs. 0%, respectively). With simvastatin plus niacin, but not with simvastatin plus niacin and antioxidants, there were selective increases in apoA-I (64%) associated with LpA-I particles and in the proportion of large LpA-I particles relative to baseline. Thus, in CHD patients with low HDL-C, the combination of these lipid-modifying drugs substantially increased the amount of LpA-I and the relative proportion of large LpA-I particles, as well as the concentration of HDL_2-C.

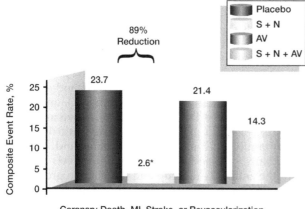

FIGURE 10 The high-density lipoprotein-Atherosclerosis Treatment Study: effect of Simvastatin plus Niacin, with or without Antioxidants, on cardiovascular events. *Abbreviation*: MI, myocardial infarction. *Source*: From Ref. 192.

However, the addition of antioxidants blunted these favorable effects, perhaps because of a selective effect on LpA-I. This unexpected adverse interaction between antioxidants and lipid therapy may have important implications for the management of CAD.

Carotid intima-media thickness (CIMT) measurements are a validated surrogate cardiovascular end point (194). In the Arterial Biology for the Investigation of the Treatment Effects of Reducing Cholesterol 2 (ARBITER 2) trial, patients with low HDL-C (<45 mg/dL) and established CAD already on statin therapy were randomized to the addition of either placebo or 1000 mg of sustained-release niacin (Niaspan; Kos Pharmaceuticals) (195). The primary endpoint for the trial was change in CIMT after one year. Compared with the group randomized to statin monotherapy, the patients receiving combination therapy experienced a 21% increase in HDL-C. There was a trend for serum HDL-C to rise for the full year of therapy. Statin monotherapy was associated with CIMT progression (mean increase 0.044 (0.10 mm; $P < 0.001$), whereas combination therapy was associated with CIMT stabilization (mean increase of 0.014 (0.104 mm; $P = 0.23$). Consistent with HATS, ARBITER 2 showed that combination of niacin with statin therapy decreases the rate of progression of atherosclerotic vascular disease.

Niacin is available in a number of formulations. Crystalline niacin (unmodified, or immediate-release) and Slo-Niacin (Upsher-Smith), a sustained-release compound, are available as over-the-counter preparations and are associated with significant hepatotoxicity when used at doses that exceed 2 g daily (196,197). Niaspan is an extended-release preparation that is formulated for slow absorption over approximately eight hours. Niaspan is probably the safest form of niacin currently available, with a low risk for hepatotoxicity and myopathy (198). Cutaneous flushing is a well-known side effect of niacin; although transient, it is bothersome and can lead to discontinuation of therapy (199,200). Because arachidonic acid, an essential fatty acid, is the precursor for prostaglandin biosynthesis by cyclooxygenase, fatty meals should be avoided for at least two hours before taking niacin. Alcohol and hot fluids exacerbate flushing and should also be avoided. In addition, patients can minimize cutaneous reactions by taking 325 mg of aspirin (a cyclooxygenase inhibitor) one hour before each niacin dose (199). Niacin can antagonize glycemic control, increase serum homocysteine levels, and promote proximal tubular reuptake of urate and increase risk for gouty flares, especially at high doses (201,202).

Thiazolidinedione Therapy

The thiazolidinediones (TZDs) are insulin-sensitizing agents that significantly affect lipoprotein metabolism and circulating levels of serum lipoproteins. The frequency of insulin resistance is demonstrated by the high prevalence of metabolic syndrome and the onset of adult type 2 diabetes mellitus in the United States of America and European countries. Low serum levels of HDL-C are a prominent feature of the insulin resistance syndrome. Reduced serum HDL-C is the result of three principal metabolic defects attributable to insulin resistance: (i) reduced transfer of surface coat mass from VLDL and chylomicrons to HDL secondary to inhibition of LPL activity; (ii) increased catabolism of triglyceride-enriched HDL by hepatic lipase; and (iii) decreased production of apoA-I, the major protein component of HDL, because apoA-I gene transcription is subject to regulation by insulin through an insulin response core element; therefore, expression of the gene may be altered in the presence of insulin resistance (203,204).

Pioglitazone (Actos; Takeda) and rosiglitazone (Avandia; GlaxoSmithKline) relieve insulin resistance and can stimulate elevations in HDL-C. The results of a meta-analysis suggesting that pioglitazone raises HDL-C significantly more than does rosiglitazone (205), were subsequently confirmed by a trial directly comparing pioglitazone at 45 mg daily with rosiglitazone at 4 mg twice daily in subjects with diabetes. The trial found that these drugs raised HDL-C by 5.2 ± 0.5 (14.9%) vs. 2.4 ± 0.5 (7.1%) mg/dL ($P < 0.001$) (26). Another recent trial of pioglitazone versus placebo reported that HDL-C levels rose by 19% from baseline with active therapy, while placebo-treated subjects experienced a 10% increase, a highly significant difference (207). In diabetic patients, the adjuvant use of a TZD with other therapies for the management of dyslipidemia can provide a valuable means of further raising HDL-C. The TZDs are not yet indicated for use in patients with metabolic syndrome without diabetes.

High-Density Lipoprotein Subfractions and Risk for Coronary Heart Disease

A relatively common misconception generated in recent years is that the smaller, denser HDL particles are "proatherogenic" while the larger, more buoyant HDL particles are "antiatherogenic."

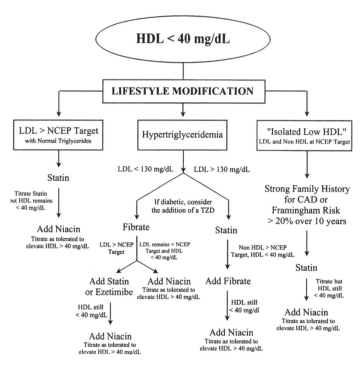

FIGURE 11   Algorithm for the management of low serum HDL-C. Treatment of isolated low HDL-C is generally reserved for high-risk patients. The use of an LDL-C lowering agent is a therapeutic option in moderately high-risk patients with an LDL-C level of 100 to 129 mg/dL (2.59–3.33 mmol/L) or in high-risk patients with an LDL-C level less than 100 mg/dL (2.59 mmol/L). *Abbreviations*: LDL, low-density lipoprotein; NCEP, National Cholesterol Education Program; HDL, high-density lipoprotein; TZD, thiazolidinedione; CAD, coronary artery disease. *Source*: From Refs. 3,6.

HDL particles of all sizes can exert antiatherogenic effects. A number of the antiatherogenic effects attributable to HDL, including the activation of prostacyclin expression and suppression of adhesion molecule expression, were elucidated with HDL_3, the smaller, denser isoform of HDL. As discussed above, all HDL subfractions participate in RCT, and it is the smaller HDL particles that have the highest affinity for cellular cholesterol because they are less saturated with cholesterol and cholesteryl ester than their larger lipid-laden counterparts. Although some studies have suggested that HDL_2 is more atheroprotective against CHD than HDL_3 (208,209), other studies such as the Physicians Health Study (20) and Caerphilly and Speedwell cohorts (210) demonstrate the opposite. In VA-HIT (180) and the Lopid Coronary Angiography Trial (211) trials, reductions in cardiovascular morbidity and mortality and rates of coronary and vein graft atheromatous plaque progression were driven by fibrate induced increases in serum HDL_3 levels. Consequently, it is the elevations in total HDL mass that are important when treating low HDL-C, and not necessarily the elevation of any one fraction over the other. Perhaps even more importantly, it is the functionality of the HDL produced in response to specific interventions that is likely the principal determinant of how any given change in serum HDL-C affects CAD development and progression.

THE EFFECTS OF LIFESTYLE FACTORS ON HIGH-DENSITY LIPOPROTEIN CHOLESTEROL

Blood lipid concentrations are determined by environmental factors (a physical, chemical, or biological exposure or a behavior pattern) and genetic factors, but the relative importance of the variables within these two categories, as well as their interaction effects, are unclear (212). An interaction effect is defined as "a different effect of an environmental exposure on a given parameter (e.g., HDL-C) in persons with different genotypes or, conversely, a different effect of a genotype on a given parameter in persons with different environmental exposures" (213). In the future, the study of gene-environment interactions may lead to a better understanding of interindividual variability in the HDL response to diet, exercise and other behaviors or exposures (214).

The following environmental factors are associated with HDL-C levels: cigarette smoking, body mass index, diet, alcohol consumption, physical exercise/energy expenditure, and use of hormone replacement therapy in women. Other factors that can affect HDL metabolism and function include vitamin supplementation (e.g., antioxidant vitamins as shown in the HATS trial), fasting, and weight loss. A variety of medications can also affect serum levels of HDL-C.

Almost 30 candidate genes have been identified for HDL metabolism and RCT (215). These genes encode apoproteins, enzymes and lipid transfer proteins, cellular receptors and transporters, and transcription factors (215,216). For each gene, there are a number of possible variations in the DNA sequence (217). Known as single nucleotide polymorphisms (SNPs), these variations can influence the level of expression or the structure and/or function of the protein (218). Although environmental factors may require a genetic predisposition in order to induce an observable effect, in this discussion, the term "environmental" will be used to designate factors whose assessment, unlike polymorphisms, is not DNA based (216).

Studies have reported that major environmental factors explain 14% to 28% of the variance in HDL-C levels, while selected candidate genes explain up to 4%, and gene-environment interactions account for 2%. The substantial role of environmental factors is consistent with the observed fluctuations in blood cholesterol levels worldwide over the past few decades, a phenomenon that is likely due to changes in diet, physical activity, smoking, and other behavioral patterns. However, the modest contribution of interaction effects implies that the genetic variants studied represent just a fraction of the polymorphisms operating in the population as a whole. Because the genetic and nongenetic predictors analyzed were identified before the study of gene-environment interactions became an established discipline, some determinants, which affect HDL-C levels only when interacting with other factors, may have been omitted (216,219–221).

CIGARETTE SMOKING

Cigarette smoking is associated with lower levels of total HDL-C (Fig. 12) (219,222–226) as well as decreased concentrations of both HDL_2-C and apoA-I (226–228). In one large epidemiologic study, individuals who smoked 15 to 24 cigarettes a day had significantly lower HDL-C levels compared with those smoking 1 to 14 cigarettes daily. Ex-smokers and nonsmokers had similar HDL-C levels, which were significantly higher than in smokers, indicating that HDL-C may increase in those who engage in smoking cessation (224).

The effect of smoking may vary by sex, lowering HDL-C levels more markedly in women than in men (219). In an analysis from the Framingham Offspring Study, the proportion of female smokers with HDL-C levels less than 35 mg/dL exceeded the proportion of male smokers with similarly low HDL-C levels by 18%, a significant difference (230).

Currently, drug treatment for smoking cessation involves either nicotine replacement therapy or bupropion. The latter is thought to reduce the urge to smoke by inhibiting the

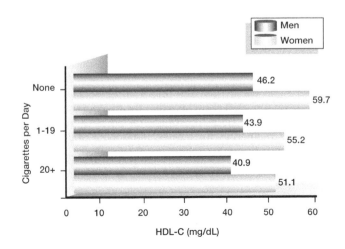

FIGURE 12 Cigarette smoking is associated with lower levels of total HDL-C in both men and women in the Framingham Offspring Study. *Abbreviation:* HDL-C, high-density lipoprotein cholesterol. *Source:* From Ref. 229.

uptake of norepinephrine and dopamine (231). Future therapies may include the investigational agent rimonabant, which is also discussed under "Weight Loss." Studies indicate that rimonabant is effective as a smoking cessation agent and that it raises HDL-C levels (232,233).

The mechanism underlying the association between smoking and low HDL-C is unclear, but a pattern of high triglycerides and low HDL-C observed in smokers may also be due to smoking-induced insulin resistance (224).

Gene-Environment Interactions

In addition, smoking is thought to inhibit the activity of LCAT, the enzyme that catalyzes the esterification of cholesterol within the HDL particle (226,228,234). ApoA-IV is an HDL-associated apoprotein that may act as a cofactor for LCAT (235–237). A substitution of histidine for glutamine at position 360 ($Gln_{360} \rightarrow His$) leads to a polymorphism that may diminish the ability of apoA-IV to activate LCAT, making carriers of this allele (i.e., apoA-IV-2) more susceptible to the LCAT-inhibiting effects of cigarette smoke (228,238).

One study conducted in Costa Rica, a country whose Mestizo population provides a relatively homogeneous genetic substrate for the investigation of gene-environment interactions, found that urban dwellers with the apoA-IV-2 allele had lower levels of HDL-C and apoA-I compared both with their rural counterparts and with apoA-IV-1 homozygotes, whether urban or rural (228). In part, this may be because of the effects of an urban lifestyle, which was characterized by increased cigarette smoking.

In another investigation, male CAD patients with the apoA-IV-2 allele had significantly higher LCAT levels than their apo A-IV-1 counterparts, while HDL-C levels were unchanged. In contrast, LCAT levels were similar in apoA-IV-2 versus apoA-IV-1 women, but HDL-C levels were lower, although the difference was not significant (237). This suggests that the inhibitory effect of apoA-IV-2 on LCAT activation may be sex-specific. Consequently, any interaction effect between apoA-IV-2 and smoking on HDL-C levels may be more adverse in women than in men.

It has also been reported that an interaction between smoking and the *Taq*IB polymorphism of the CETP gene significantly affects HDL-C levels in Turks, a population whose main lipid characteristic is low HDL-C (239). Men and women with the rare B2 allele, whether heterozygous or homozygous, had no decrease in HDL-C levels, even with greater than or equal to 20 cigarettes/day; in contrast, HDL-C levels declined significantly in B1B1 homozygotes who smoked greater than or equal to 20 cigarettes/day (239).

Body Mass Index

Body mass index (BMI) is calculated by dividing weight in kilograms by the square of height in meters (kg/m^2). In general, a BMI of 18.5 to 24.9 kg/m^2 is considered healthy. Individuals with a BMI of 25 kg/m^2 are about 10% over ideal bodyweight, and those with a BMI of 25 to less than 30 kg/m^2 are considered overweight. Obesity and extreme obesity are defined as a BMI of greater than or equal to 30 kg/m^2, and greater than or equal to 40 kg/m^2, respectively (240).

Inversely associated with levels of HDL-C (Fig. 13) and apoA-I in men and women, BMI accounts for 1% to 3% of the variability in each of these parameters (230,241,242), a pattern of association that appears to have a strong genetic component (243).

Body mass index represents adipose and lean tissue, and each of these components can have a distinct effect on lipid levels (245). An increase of 1 kg/m^2 in the fat mass index (FMI) lowered HDL-C levels by 1 mg/dL in middle-aged men and women after adjustment for multiple covariates. Similarly, an increase of 1 kg/m^2 in the fat-free mass index (FFMI) corresponded to an HDL decrease of 1 mg/dL in men, but there was no significant association in women. Although this and other research has found that fat mass and weight gain are significantly associated with decreasing levels of HDL-C (245–247), it has been reported elsewhere that the inverse association between BMI and HDL-C loses statistical significance after adjustment for adipose-free tissue mass. This implies that the association may be explained by the fat-free component of BMI, raising the question of whether BMI is an appropriate surrogate for body fat (248–250).

DIET

Macronutrients

To reduce LDL-C levels, NCEP guidelines recommend a diet low in saturated fat (<7% of total calories) and high in complex carbohydrates from fruits, vegetables and whole grains (50–60%

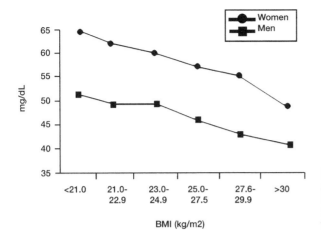

FIGURE 13 Body Mass Index (BMI) is inversely associated with HDL-C in the Framingham Offspring Study. *Abbreviation*: BMI, body mass index. *Source*: From Ref. 244; with permission from Elsevier.

of total calories) (3). However, this type of diet generally decreases or fails to increase HDL-C (251–253). In contrast, consumption of a diet high in saturated fat ($\geq$15% of calories) raises levels of HDL-C, HDL$_2$-C, and HDL$_3$-C (254,255).

Compared with saturated fat, hydrogenated fat (including *trans* fatty acids) appears to lower HDL-C without significantly affecting HDL$_2$-C and HDL$_3$-C level, although a decline in apoA-I levels has been observed. This may be because of an increase in apoA-I catabolism (256). Diets that emphasize the consumption of protein (25% of daily calories) or carbohydrates (58% of calories) also lower HDL-C (251).

The effects of macronutrients on HDL-C concentration and particle distribution are mediated by multiple mechanisms. According to one study, the decline in HDL-C levels due to a change from a high-fat to a low-fat diet correlates with a decrease in apoA-I production, whereas the variability in HDL-C levels among individuals on a fixed diet, whether high- or low-fat, correlates with an increase in apoA-I clearance (257). Because of this fundamental metabolic difference, it may be inappropriate to conclude that a low HDL-C level within a fixed diet carries the same risk for atherosclerosis as does a decrease in HDL-C level upon changing diets. This may help explain the reason as to why the inverse association between HDL-C levels and coronary risk seen in the U.S. and other western countries has not been observed in populations that traditionally consume a low-fat, high-complex-carbohydrate diet (257,258).

Unsaturated Fatty Acids

Eicosapentaenoic acid (EPA) and docosahexaenoic acid (DHA), the two principal ω-3 polyunsaturated fatty acids (PUFAs) are considered cardioprotective (259–261), with possible effects on lipoprotein metabolism, as well as on platelet and endothelial function, vascular reactivity, neutrophil and monocyte cytokine production, coagulation, fibrinolysis, and blood pressure (262). Both EPA and DHA are found in many popular fish, including salmon, lake trout, albacore tuna, sardines, herring, and mackerel. Since 2000, the American Heart Association has recommended at least two servings of fish per week for healthy adults. Alpha-linolenic acid, which is found in soybeans and in canola, walnut, and flaxseed oils, is a third and less potent type of ω-3 fatty acid (259). The NCEP advises that =10% of daily calories should come from polyunsaturated fat (3).

Studies of the effects of EPA and DHA on HDL-C concentrations have produced variable results, with a substantial number reporting either a nonsignificant change or a small percentage change that is considered physiologically insignificant (263,264). In the GISSI-Prevenzione trial, fish oil supplementation led to a 15% to 20% reduction in cardiovascular events, despite no difference in HDL-C levels between the intervention and the control groups (265). Similarly, in the Lyon Heart Study, which evaluated the effect of a Mediterranean-type diet emphasizing grains, vegetables, and fish, a 70% reduction in coronary risk was unrelated to serum concentrations of HDL-C (266,267).

The absence of an increase in plasma concentrations does not preclude the possibility of other antiatherogenic effects on HDL-C. Small studies have found that ω-3 supplementation can increase HDL_2-C levels, despite no change in HDL-C and a decline in HDL_3-C (262,268–270). There is also evidence that ω-3 fatty acids increase the plasma concentration of paraoxonase (269) as well as the amount of cellular cholesterol efflux, an early step in RCT (271).

The results of another small study involving recreationally active men suggest that exercise in combination with ω-3 fatty acids may be beneficial, particularly in augmenting a post-supplementation increase in HDL-C and in raising HDL_3-C levels (270). Possible reasons for the HDL-raising effect of physical activity are discussed in the section entitled "Physical Activity/Exercise."

Gene-Environment Interactions

The LIPC C_{514}→T polymorphism (see "Hepatic Lipase") may affect HL activity (272). One study has examined interaction effects between this polymorphism, dietary fat, and HDL-C measures in men and women from the Framingham Study. The investigators found that HDL-C and HDL_2-C levels increased significantly in heterozygotes (CT) or homozygotes (TT) of those who consumed <30% of energy from fat, an atypical response to reduced fat intake (214). Interestingly, TT homozygotes of those with a total fat intake greater than or equal to 30% had markedly lower levels of HDL-C and HDL_2-C compared with the CC and CT genotypes. When the model was adjusted for animal or vegetable fat, only the interactions between animal fat and the LIPC polymorphism were significant in determining HDL-C level, HDL particle size, large-HDL subfraction, and intermediate+small subfractions (214). These results suggest that the LIPC T-allele is associated with an altered response to animal fat intake.

Another study has shown a significant interaction between saturated fat intake and apoA-IV, the apoprotein that may also influence the effect of smoking on HDL-C (see "Cigarette Smoking," already dealt with earlier). Levels of HDL-C were 19% lower in carriers of the apoA-IV-2 allele who consumed a high- versus a low-saturated fat diet, but 6% higher in apoA-IV-1 homozygotes (228), a more characteristic response to increased fat intake (252). In this study, apoA-IV-2 carriers living in urban areas, where saturated fat intake was higher than in rural settings, had lower HDL-C levels compared both with their rural counterparts and with apoA-IV-1 homozygotes, whether urban or rural (228).

In women, a common G→A substitution in the −75 promoter region of the apoA-I gene appears to affect the HDL response to PUFAs. Higher PUFA consumption corresponded to an increase in HDL-C levels in women with the A allele, both heterozygous and homozygous, while those with the G/G genotype experienced a nonsignificant decrease in HDL-C (273). For men, there was no significant interaction between HDL-C levels and PUFA intake. The sex difference in the genotype-PUFA interaction suggests the presence of a hormonal effect, a hypothesis that seems plausible in part because estradiol enhances the activity of the apoA-I gene, whereas androgens decrease it.

The study of gene-nutrient interactions is termed "nutrigenomics." In the future, nutrigenomics may make it possible to develop personalized dietary recommendations for the reduction of cardiovascular risk (274).

Weight Loss

Obesity is a major health concern. In 2000, there were an estimated 300 million obese adults worldwide, an increase of 50% from the 200 million in 1995. The prevalence of obesity in the U.S. adult population has increased from 13% to 31% over the past four decades, while the prevalence of overweight has increased from 45% to 64% (275). Obesity is commonly considered to be a characteristic of industrialized societies, but evidence suggests that developing countries are also affected, with an estimated 115 million people suffering from obesity-related problems. Among these problems are cardiovascular risk factors, including low levels of HDL-C (276).

Despite the inverse association between BMI and HDL-C, weight reduction does not necessarily raise HDL-C levels (241,277,278). The HDL response to weight loss depends on several factors, including the modality used and the phase of the intervention period (acute weight loss or weight maintenance) (279–282). Increasingly, weight-loss interventions are being studied for their effects on the metabolic abnormalities and other cardiovascular risk factors associated with obesity. Research is also needed to identify the characteristics, both genetic and nongenetic, that can help predict an individual patient's response to a particular modality (283).

Dietary Interventions

In weight-loss diets, the percentage of daily calories from fat can range from 10% to 30%, with saturated fat content often not specified (284). Individual exceptions notwithstanding, the typical effect of a reduced-fat diet is to decrease HDL-C (252). According to a meta-analysis of five studies, each comparing a low-fat versus a low-carbohydrate ketogenic diet (with unrestricted fat intake), HDL-C levels with a low-carbohydrate regimen were approximately 5 mg/dL higher at six months, a significant between-group difference (284). It is not known, however, whether the improvement in HDL-C has an effect on the development of CVD (252,284,285). Furthermore, the HDL-C difference declined to a nonsignificant 3 mg/dL at one year (284). Similarly, after one year there was no significant between-group difference in weight loss, the primary end point (284–287).

Given the limited number of trials in the meta-analysis, as well as the moderate quality of their design (eg, none used blinded outcomes assessment), the use of self-reporting to measure dietary intake and adherence, and the substantial attrition rates (a problem common to most weight-loss studies, whether dealing with lifestyle or with pharmacology, and a potential source of bias), these results require corroboration in future trials.

Pharmacologic Interventions

Sibutramine and orlistat are the two main antiobesity drugs approved for use in the United Sates. These drugs have variable effects on HDL-C levels.

Sibutramine

Sibutramine, which acts centrally by inhibiting the reuptake of serotonin and norepinephrine, enhances the feeling of satiety (fullness); it may also affect the metabolic rate, increasing energy expenditure (288).

In a study of sibutramine 10 mg/day, HDL-C levels rose from 47 to 57 mg/dL after 24 months of treatment, accompanied by a weight loss of 8.9% versus 4.9% with placebo (289). The subjects, who qualified as obese, were also prescribed a low-fat, hypocaloric diet. Although sibutramine did not affect TC concentrations, the marked increase in HDL-C led to a reduction of 13.3% in the TC/HDL-C ratio, which is a significant predictor of cardiovascular risk (289,290). During the first six months, HDL-C levels increased similarly in the sibutramine and placebo groups. Once bodyweights stabilized, however, a between-group difference began to emerge, reaching significance in favor of sibutramine during the six-month to two-year maintenance phase (increases of 19.9% vs. 8.7% in men, and 20.9% vs. 12.4% in women) (289). In contrast, a one-year trial of sibutramine reported no change in HDL-C (280).

According to a retrospective analysis that included five randomized double-blind placebo-controlled trials of at least 12 months' duration, the HDL-raising effect of sibutramine may be independent of weight loss, particularly in patients with HDL-C levels of 40 to 50 mg/dL at baseline (291). These results, which have not yet been published in a peer-reviewed journal, must be considered preliminary. A meta-analysis of nine trials, each with a minimum duration of three months, reported that sibutramine significantly raises HDL-C by 20% in subjects with type 2 diabetes. Despite this overall effect, none of the individual trials showed a significant increase in HDL-C levels with sibutramine (292).

Orlistat

Orlistat is a peripherally acting drug that inhibits lipases in the gastrointestinal tract. This decreases energy intake by blocking the breakdown and subsequent absorption of nutrients (288,293).

In general, orlistat 120 mg t.i.d., together with a low fat hypocaloric diet, does not raise HDL-C levels in obese men and women, including those with type 2 diabetes, after one year of treatment (293–296). Although one study did report an increase of 11% from baseline at one year, a further increase during the second year of treatment was no longer significant (293). Moreover, one four-year placebo-controlled study found that orlistat blunts the effect of lifestyle measures on HDL-C levels in obese subjects, despite significant weight loss and a 37% decrease in progression to type 2 diabetes (297). While HDL-C rose in all participants, those who were randomized to placebo plus lifestyle interventions had significantly higher HDL-C levels than did those randomized to orlistat plus lifestyle measures (5% and 2.6% higher at one and four years, respectively).

Rimonabant

Currently, a novel endocannabinoid receptor antagonist, rimonabant, is being studied for the treatment of obesity (282). Rimonabant selectively blocks the CB_1 receptor, one of two cannabinoid receptor subtypes identified to date (282,288). The CB_1 receptor is located in the central nervous system (eg, the hypothalamus) and in a number of peripheral tissues, including adipocytes, the gastrointestinal tract, and muscle (283,298). In some animal models, obesity is associated with overactivation of the endocannabinoid system, resulting in hyperphagia, enhanced lipogenesis via hepatic and adipose tissue pathways, and decreased muscle (283,298–300). Blockade of the CB_1 receptor seems to modulate this overactivation, thereby preventing weight gain and associated metabolic abnormalities that increase cardiovascular risk.

A 12-month study involving overweight or obese subjects found that rimonabant at a dosage of 5 or 20 mg/day, together with a hypocaloric diet, significantly increased HDL-C levels from baseline by 14% and 19%, respectively. In all intervention groups, including placebo, HDL-C levels rose steadily and reached their peak at 36 weeks, after which there was a slight decline. Although rimonabant did not significantly affect TC level, the increase in HDL-C produced a significant reduction in the TC/HDL-C ratio with the 20-mg dose only (–15%) (281). Furthermore, the prevalence of the metabolic syndrome decreased from 53% to 26% in subjects receiving rimonabant 20 mg/day. This was significantly greater than the decline in the placebo group and was attributed primarily to the reduction in waist circumference and the increase in HDL-C levels. Weight loss was 3 kg in the 5-mg group and 7 kg in the 20-mg group, compared with 1.5 kg in placebo-treated subjects.

With rimonabant 20 mg/day, approximately 50% to 60% of the increase in HDL-C is accounted for by a reduction in bodyweight, indicating that the effect on HDL-C levels is partly independent of weight loss (282,298). Although the mechanisms responsible for the independent effect on HDL-C have not been identified, one possible explanation may involve adiponectin, a hormone secreted by adipocytes (282,301). Following weight loss, adiponectin levels increase (302). This change is positively and significantly correlated with an increase in HDL-C levels, an association shown to be independent of the degree of bodyweight reduction (302). Rimonabant has not yet been approved by the Food and Drug Administration for use in the United States.

Fasting

The Muslim holiday of Ramadan, which occurs during the ninth lunar month of the Islamic calendar, requires observant Muslims to eat and drink only twice each day: before dawn and after sunset (303). According to one study, healthy men and women had significantly higher HDL-C levels both mid-Ramadan and end-Ramadan compared with before Ramadan. In this study, the subjects' food intake was not analyzed, nor is it known whether a longer period of fasting would alter the effect on HDL-C.

Alcohol

According to observational evidence, moderate alcohol consumption is associated with a modestly reduced risk for CHD in a wide range of ethnic groups (304). Approximately half of this effect appears to be mediated by increases in HDL-C (305,306). Alcohol is also associated with increased concentrations of HDL_2 and, more notably, HDL_3 (306). The mechanism for the effect of alcohol on HDL-C may involve an increase in the transport rates of both apoA-I and apoA-II, with no significant change in the fractional catabolic rates (305). This increased production could help stimulate apoA-I-mediated cellular cholesterol efflux (305,307). Because of the risks involved in promoting alcohol consumption, however, it is generally considered an inadvisable HDL-raising strategy.

Physical Activity/Exercise

Physical inactivity contributes to low HDL-C levels (30), and exercise can raise HDL-C, with some evidence of a dose-response relationship in men and women (308–311). In addition, regular exercise can prevent the reduction in HDL-C levels associated with a low-fat diet (282,312,313).

Physical inactivity is also a risk factor for CHD, and exercise is linked to a reduction in coronary mortality (308,311,314,315). Although increased HDL-C may be one of several mechanisms for the cardioprotective effect of exercise (308,311), not all subjects experience improvements in the level of HDL-C or its subfractions (316–320). There may be several reasons for this, including the possibility that changes in HDL metabolism are more strongly associated with physical fitness than with physical activity (316,321) that individuals who start with a less favorable profile (ie, higher blood pressure, higher triglycerides, and lower HDL-C) experience greater change (318,322) that the HDL response is attenuated in women (318), and that factors such as intensity, frequency, and duration (308,316,320), as well as length of the training period (308), can influence the effect of exercise on HDL-C. In addition, genetic factors may play a role (discussed below).

Questions have also been raised about whether exercise directly increases HDL-C, or whether the increase results from an accompanying weight loss (323). A recent cross-sectional study in women found a stronger association between higher BMI levels and low HDL-C than between physical inactivity and low HDL-C. Within each category of BMI, however, physically active women had significantly higher HDL-C levels compared with those who were inactive (324).

The mechanism responsible for the exercise-induced modification of HDL is unclear. Exercise appears to interact with nutrients, adiposity, weight loss, and the activity of hormones and enzymes to modify the synthesis, transport, and clearance of lipids and lipoproteins (325). For example, aerobic exercise can increase the activity of LPL, which hydrolyzes triglycerides contained within lipoproteins (321,326). During hydrolysis, surface fragments are transferred from triglyceride-rich lipoproteins to HDL particles as part of a remodeling process. Evidence suggests that increased synthesis of HDL_3 and HDL_2 contributes to higher HDL levels in untrained and trained subjects, respectively (270,316). Exercise may also inhibit the CETP-mediated exchange of cholesteryl esters and triglycerides, thereby reducing the triglyceride enrichment of HDL and possibly decreasing its susceptibility to the lipolytic action of HL (327). In addition, it has been suggested that exercise improves insulin resistance (328). Because transcription of the apoA-I gene is subject to regulation by insulin through an insulin response core element, a lessening of insulin resistance may increase apoA-I gene expression (see "Thiazolidinedione Therapy").

Yet another effect of exercise may be to increase the resistance of LDL to oxidative modification (329). Although there appears to be no correlation between the lag phase of LDL, a measure of its susceptibility to oxidation, and HDL-C levels, this does not preclude the possibility that exercise may increase the antioxidant enzymatic activity of HDL.

Evidence-based guidelines issued by the Third Adult Treatment Panel (ATP III) of the NCEP recommend physical activity to reduce coronary risk and raise HDL-C levels (3). At the present time, however, the amount of exercise needed to produce an adequate HDL-C response, as well as the type, frequency, intensity, and duration, have not been determined and will vary individual to individual depending upon specific metabolic and genetic backgrounds.

Gene-Environment Interactions

Individual variability makes it difficult to identify an appropriate measure for the HDL response to exercise. In one study, physical training significantly raised mean HDL-C levels by 3.6 mg/dL, but the change in individual subjects ranged from a 66% increase to a 24% reduction compared with baseline (311). Among the factors that may influence the effect of exercise on HDL, there appears to be a genetic component. For example, endurance training has been shown to increase HDL-C levels in healthy men and women with either the CETP B1B1 or the B1B2 genotype, whereas HDL_2-C levels rose significantly from baseline in B1B1 individuals only (330).

The use of exercise for the modification of HDL-C raises several questions: (i) what are the causes of interindividual variability in the HDL response to exercise? (ii) what are the effects of exercise type, amount, intensity, frequency, and duration on HDL-C and its subfractions? (iii) what are the respective thresholds needed to produce a favorable HDL response? (iv) what are the mechanisms underlying the effect of physical exercise on HDL-C? (v) what is the relationship of weight loss to the association between exercise and HDL-C? and (vi) what is the most appropriate measure of an exercise-induced change in HDL-C (e.g., overall plasma level vs. the level of HDL_2-C or apoA-I)? Despite these unanswered questions, exercise is an important part of a healthy lifestyle. Exercise reduces coronary risk, and physicians are encouraged to prescribe regular exercise, particularly aerobic activity, for their patients (30,315,328,331).

Hormone Replacement Therapy

Postmenopausal HRT was once considered promising for the reduction of cardiovascular risk, but a series of trials with clinical end points have produced disappointing results. Although estrogen raises HDL-C levels (332–334), two placebo-controlled trials found that women assigned to active treatment had no change in the progression of atherosclerosis (332), no reduction in coronary risk (333), and an increased risk for endometrial hyperplasia (332). Moreover, in the Women's Health Initiative (WHI), which compared estrogen or estrogen plus a progestin versus placebo in approximately 26,000 women, there were increases in the relative risk for CHD (29%), stroke (40%), and embolic events (up to 100%), depending on the regimen used. A higher incidence of invasive breast cancer (26%) with estrogen plus progestin was also reported (335).

Evidence suggests that estrogen raises HDL-C levels by mechanisms that include an increase in the synthesis of apoA-I and a decrease in the activity of HL. By promoting cellular cholesterol efflux and reducing HDL catabolism, respectively, each of these mechanisms may be potentially antiatherogenic (336–338). The failure of estrogen to reduce coronary risk, despite this evidence, illustrates the complexity of the relationship between plasma HDL level and RCT, as well as the challenge of trying to associate any change in HDL-C levels with the underlying mechanisms involved in the development of CVD (339). It is possible, however, that a genetically determined subgroup of women could benefit from HRT (340). In the future, pharmacogenomic studies, including analyses of biological samples from the WHI, may identify genetic markers that predict variations in response to estrogen replacement, leading to the development of individualized therapeutic recommendations (341).

Secondary Effects of Drug Therapy

Several commonly prescribed drugs have secondary effects on HDL-C.

Antihypertensives

Beta-blockers, both selective (eg, propranolol) and nonselective (e.g., metoprolol and atenolol), lower HDL-C levels by 10% to 15%. However, beta-blockers with intrinsic sympathomimetic activity are more lipid neutral, although one study found a 12% decline in HDL-C levels with pindolol. The alpha-blockers (e.g., prazosin) either raise HDL-C or have no effect. As a rule, diuretics, calcium channel blockers, ACE inhibitors, and angiotensin II antagonists do not alter HDL-C levels (342).

Steroid Hormones

Steroid hormones include a range of drugs: androgenic-anabolic steroids, estrogens, progestins, estrogen receptor modulators, dehydroepiandrosterone (DHEA), and glucocorticoids. In hypogonadal men, testosterone replacement lowers HDL-C by 10% to 20%, whether administered sublingually, transdermally, or subcutaneously. The most harmful effect on HDL-C levels seems to come from oral testosterone formulations. In an observational study of athletes taking oral androgens, HDL-C decreased by 50% to 70%; moreover, comparisons of parenteral versus oral androgens have reported HDL reductions of 10% versus 40% to 50%, respectively (342). With progestins, the detrimental effect on HDL is proportional to their androgenicity. In the PEPI trial, for example, the HDL-raising effect of estrogen was blunted by the addition of medroxyprogesterone acetate, but not by micronized progesterone (308,314). Among oral contraceptives, only the progestin dl-norgestrel appears to lower HDL-C levels.

Unlike estrogen, which has been discussed elsewhere, tamoxifen and raloxifene, which are selective estrogen receptor modulators (SERMs), do not alter HDL-C levels, perhaps because of differential binding to the estrogen receptors. These drugs do appear to have an estrogen-like effect on LDL-C and possibly on triglycerides (342). DHEA, which is used as a nutritional supplement, acts as a weak androgen, lowering HDL levels by 10% to 20%. The effect of glucocorticoids on HDL-C is difficult to determine because they are often used to treat conditions that may also alter lipid metabolism. Nevertheless, prednisone is associated with

HDL increases of up to 67%, although a decrease was noted in patients with systemic lupus erythematosus, perhaps independent of the drug (342).

Antiretrovirals

Drugs used for the treatment of human immunodeficiency virus (HIV) appear to vary in their HDL-related effects (343). Nonnucleoside reverse transcriptase inhibitors (e.g., nevirapine) increase HDL-C levels by up to about 40% (344,345). However, the use of highly active antiretroviral therapy (HAART), which combines a protease inhibitor (eg, nelfinavir) with a nonnucleoside reverse transcriptase inhibitor and/or a reverse transcriptase inhibitor, has been associated with a neutral or an HDL-lowering effect (343,346). Antiretroviral therapy affects other lipid parameters as well, and a large observational study has reported that the risk for an MI in HIV-1–infected patients increases with longer exposure to combination antiretroviral therapy (347).

Anticonvulsants

Enzyme-inducing antiepileptic drugs (i.e., carbamazepine, phenobarbital, phenytoin), which are metabolized by hepatic P450 microsomes, tend to increase HDL-C levels, perhaps because of increased hepatic synthesis of apoA-I (348).

Immunosuppressants

Cyclosporine, a potent cyclic polypeptide immunosuppressant used in transplant patients, is associated with a range of adverse effects, including dyslipidemia. The effect of cyclosporine on HDL-C varies, but when levels are reduced, there is generally an accompanying increase in triglycerides.

EMERGING THERAPIES

Currently available drugs used to treat HDL-C also induce simultaneous changes in other lipid fractions. For this reason, it has been difficult to unequivocally prove the "HDL hypothesis," namely that raising HDL independent of reductions in atherogenic lipoprotein fractions reduces risk for cardiovascular morbidity and mortality. The development of multiple novel drug classes with more specific effects on HDL and the capacity for augmenting RCT independent of changes in apoB100-containing lipoproteins pose exciting new therapeutic possibilities for treating patients with low HDL in both the primary and secondary prevention settings.

LXRα Agonists

The liver X receptors (LXRs) are ligand-activated transcription factors that function as cholesterol sensors (349). LXRα is highly expressed in the liver, intestine, and in adipose tissue, as well as at lower levels in the adrenal glands, kidney, lung, and in macrophages, In contrast, LXRα has been found in almost every tissue tested (349,350). Acting as heterodimers with the retinoid X receptor (RXR), LXRα coordinately regulates the pathway for RCT, including the expression of ABCA1, ABCG1, CETP, and PLTP (90,349); LXRα also regulates the transcription of 7α-hydroxylase (351) and the excretion of biliary and intestinal cholesterol, the latter by modulating the expression of ABCG5 and ABCG8 in hepatocytes and enterocytes. The biological ligands for LXRα are oxysterols, such as 27-hydroxycholesterol and 24-(S),25-epoxycholesterol. Oxysterol binding leads to LXRα activation and heterodimerization with RXR. The LXRα-RXR heterodimer then binds to LXR response elements in the promoters of target genes, resulting in increased expression.

The treatment of mice with the synthetic LXRα agonist GW3965 reduces aortic atheromatous plaquing by approximately one-half (352). In contrast, when LXR expression by macrophages is knocked out, atherosclerosis is significantly exacerbated (353). One potential complication of LXRα-agonist therapy is the induction of hypertriglyceridemia and hepatic steatosis. LXRα induces sterol regulatory element-binding protein-1c, which in turn activates multiple enzymes responsible for triglyceride biosynthesis, including fatty acid synthase, acetyl coenzyme A carboxylase, and stearoyl coenzyme A desaturase-1. The recently developed LXRα agonist T0901317 raises HDL significantly without inducing triglyceride biosynthesis or steatosis (354). In addition, T0901317 therapy is associated with the regression and stabilization of atheromatous plaque and a reduction in plaque macrophage density (355). The LXRα agonists have not yet entered into human trials.

Apoprotein A-I Milano

Apo A-I$_{Milano}$ (Arg$_{173}$→Cys) and apo A-I$_{Paris}$ (Arg$_{151}$→Cys) are two important, rare cysteine variants of apoA-I that are associated with hypoalphalipoproteinemia but no apparent excess risk for CHD. These apoprotein variants are able to form homodimers and heterodimers with wild type apo A-I (356). Serum HDL levels in patients with these mutations are reduced because of impaired capacity to activate LCAT, reduced maturation of HDL, and increased catabolism and elimination. ApoA-I$_{Milano}$ was first identified in a family from Limone sul Garda, a small town in Northern Italy (357). Patients affected with this mutation are heterozygotes and have reduced atheromatous plaque burden and normal carotid IMT relative to age- and sex-matched controls (358). Despite having low serum levels of HDL-C, these patients can live well into their eighth and ninth decades.

ApoA-I$_{Milano}$ has become the subject of intensive investigation. ApoA-I$_{Milano}$ has a number of antiatherogenic properties, which include: (i) augmented capacity to induce cholesterol externalization by macrophages (359); (ii) blockade of ADP stimulated platelet aggregation and thrombus formation (360); (iii) and increased capacity to inhibit lipoxygenase-mediated phospholipid peroxidation relative to wild type apo A-I (361). A number of animal studies demonstrated that the intravenous infusion of recombinant apoA-I$_{Milano}$ could significantly reduce the magnitude of balloon injury-induced atherosclerosis relative to controls, could reverse atherosclerosis progression, and stimulate the depletion of lipids and macrophages from established atheromatous plaques (362–364). Sirtori and coworkers subsequently showed that a single 2 hour infusion of high-dose recombinant apoA-I$_{Milano}$ could induce a substantial reduction of lipid and atheromatous plaque volume within the carotid vessels of rabbits (365).

Given these data, recombinant apoA-I$_{Milano}$ has been incorporated into phospholipid vesicles comprised of 1-palmitoyl,2-oleoyl phosphatidylcholine for therapeutic use (ETC-216; Esperion Therapeutics, A Division of Pfizer Global Research & Development). In a small pilot study of 47 patients with a recent history of an acute coronary syndrome, five once weekly infusions of ETC-216 were shown to induce an average 4.3% regression in atheromatous plaque volume in target coronary lesions as measured by intravascular ultrasound relative to saline (377). This was a remarkable finding after such a short period of therapy, and highlights some important points. First, this was the first demonstration in humans that therapeutic HDL utilization independent of any other change in serum lipid (LDL or triglyceride) levels altered atheromatous plaque volume. Second, this study reinforced findings from animal studies that an intravenous HDL preparation could be used to induce atheromatous plaque resorption. Third, this study suggests that the intravenous infusion of bioengineered HDL may provide a means by which to acutely stabilize atheromatous plaque in patients at risk for acute coronary syndromes. Larger studies with ETC-216 are eagerly awaited.

Apoprotein A-I Mimetic Peptides

ApoA-I mimetic peptides are amphipathic helical peptides with antiatherogenic properties (366,367). A number of mimetic peptides have been developed and they have been shown to promote the externalization of intracellular cholesterol from macrophages (368). The one with the greatest potential for eventual clinical application is D4F. D4F is an edible, synthetic polypeptide comprised of the D-isomer of each of its constituent amino acids, making it resistant to hydrolysis by gastric peptidases. When ingested, D4F does not increase serum levels of apoA-I or HDL. Rather, it appears to augment the functionality of HDL. D4F supplementation has been shown to reduces LDL oxidation, monocyte chemotactic activity, and atherogenesis in mice fed high cholesterol diets (369). D4F has also been shown to reduce rates of atherosclerotic disease progression in the vein grafts of apo E-null mice (370).

CETP Inhibitors

Naturally occurring mutations that result in reduced CETP activity are associated with increased serum HDL-C. This has lead to the development of two inhibitors of CETP in an effort to therapeutically modulate protein activity and raise HDL-C. JTT-705 inhibits CETP, raises serum HDL-C, and decreases aortic atherosclerosis by 70% in rabbits (371). JTT-705 can raise HDL-C up to 37% in a dose-dependent fashion after one month of therapy in humans (372). Torcetrapib is another CETP inhibitor and can increase HDL in humans in a dose-dependent manner by up to 91% (373) and 106% (374). A variety of studies will be needed with these drugs in order to determine whether they produce sustained elevations in serum HDL, augment RCT, induce changes in plaque volume and stability, and decrease coronary morbidity and mortality (375).

■ Case Studies

Case One

The patient is a 39-year-old African American female who presents to clinic because she is concerned about her health. Both of her parents and four of seven siblings are diabetic. Both parents are also obese and have CAD, hyperlipidemia, and hypertension. Family members are urging her to undergo comprehensive evaluation for coronary risk and to be evaluated for diabetes.

The patient does not have any symptoms of myocardial ischemia. Her BMI is 35.2, she does not exercise, and she smokes one pack of cigarettes daily. She began smoking "socially" at age 15. Her blood pressure is 150/100 mmHg. Her fasting blood sugar measurements on two separate occasions spaced 10 days apart were 115 and 109 mg/dL. Her LDL-C is 165 mg/dL, triglycerides 275 mg/dL, and HDL-C is 30 mg/dL. C-reactive protein is 4.7. A 12-lead EKG reveals a normal sinus rhythm with no evidence of arrhythmia or ischemia. Serum TSH was 2.07. Apart from her obesity, her physical examination reveals no bruits, extra heart sounds, peripheral edema or other abnormalities. Surgical history is significant for tubal ligation at age 28 after her third child.

The patient was counseled to begin an exercise regimen, salt restriction, and weight loss diet to help reduce her insulin resistance and blood pressure. The patient meets NCEP criteria for the diagnosis of metabolic syndrome. Her risk factor profile, family history, and CRP greater than 3.0 place her at elevated risk for CHD. The patient was started on a baby aspirin daily, a combination ACE inhibitor with hydrochlorothiazide, and simvastatin 40 mg daily. After six weeks of therapy, her blood pressure decreased to 135/85 mmHg and her LDL-C decreased to 120 mg/dL, triglycerides decreased to 205 mg/dL, and her HDL-C increased to 37 mg/dL. Her hepatic transaminase levels remained normal. She was adamant about not starting additional medication. She wanted to be able to further optimize her risk factors through lifestyle modification. Over a six-month period of supervised lifestyle modification with a dietitian and exercise physiologist, she lost 40 pounds. Her fasting blood glucose was now routinely less than 100 mg/dL. She quit smoking "cold turkey" as a challenge to herself. On follow-up, her lipid profile showed LDL-C of 87 mg/dL, triglyceride 65 mg/dL, and HDL-C of 54 mg/dL.

Case Two

The patient is a 48-year-old Asian Indian male. The patient's father and paternal grandfather and great-grandfather all suffered MIs by their late 40s, died in their early to mid-50s. The patient is distressed by the possibility that history will repeat itself. He is a successful architect, married, and has three young children. The patient runs five miles three times per week and plays golf at least once a week. He is a strict vegetarian and his BMI is 22.5. He practices yoga. He does not smoke or consume alcohol. At present, he has no symptoms of CVD.

The patient's blood pressure is 100/50 mmHg, fasting blood sugar is 80, and his 12-lead EKG is normal. His fasting lipid profile reveals an LDL-C of 120 mg/dL, triglycerides 70 mg/dL, and HDL-C 21 mg/dL. The patient's past medical history and physical examination were normal. The patient was counseled about his low HDL-C against the background of a strong family history for premature CAD. Consistent with the findings of AFCAPS/TexCAPS, he was counseled to begin statin therapy in an effort to reduce his risk for CAD and raise his HDL. The patient was started on 40 mg of lovastatin therapy. After six weeks, his lipid profile showed LDL-C 83 mg/dL, triglyceride 50 mg/dL, and HDL-C 24 mg/dL. In an effort to further raise his HDL-C, he was gradually titrated up to 1500 mg of Niaspan daily. After six months of pharmacologic intervention, the patient's HDL-C rose to 38 mg/dL. He tolerated his combination therapy without complication. The patient himself insisted upon titration to the 2000-mg dose. After one year of combination therapy, his HDL-C rose to 41 mg/dL.

Case Three

The patient is a 57-year-old aeronautical engineer who underwent four-vessel coronary artery bypass graft (CABG) surgery two years ago following a posterior wall MI. He recently relocated to the area. After taking a statin for a few weeks, the patient discontinued treatment because of uncomfortable myalgias and resolved not to try another one. At the time of his first visit, he was taking a baby aspirin and was appropriately treated with a beta-blocker and an ACE inhibitor. He is happily married, and his job is going on well too. Recently promoted, he now supervises the development of a new satellite system, a position that stimulates far more excitement than stress. The patient works long hours, does not exercise, and admits that he frequently "eats on the run."

On physical examination, the patient is noted to have a BMI of 27 and his blood pressure is 120/75 mmHg. He is normoglycemic with a fasting blood sugar of 95 mg/dL. The patient's hsCRP level is 3.2, with LDL-C 215 mg/dL, triglycerides 390 mg/dL, and HDL 32 mg/dL. Renal indices and liver function tests are normal. Physical examination is unremarkable except for his well-healed median sternotomy incision site.

The patient was counseled about the importance of exercise and dietary modification in keeping with his dyslipidemia. He was also started on rosuvastatin 20 mg daily and advised about the warning signs of toxicity, including myalgias, proximal muscle weakness, right upper quadrant pain or nausea, or red or brown urine . A follow-up lipid profile revealed LDL-C 95 mg/dL, triglycerides 272 mg/dL, and HDL 37 mg/dL. Fenofibrate 160 mg daily was then added to the rosuvastatin. He. After six weeks of combination therapy, the patient's lipid profile improved further with LDL-C 85 mg/dL, triglycerides 165 mg/dL, and HDL 43 mg/dL. He was not manifesting any evidence of toxicity from combination therapy and had no difficulty tolerating his medications.

REFERENCES

1. Cannon CP, Braunwald E, McCabe CH, et al. Pravastatin or atorvastatin evaluation and infection therapy—thrombolysis in myocardial infarction 22 investigators. Comparison of intensive and moderate lipid lowering with statins after acute coronary syndromes. N Engl J Med 2004; 350:1495–1504.
2. LaRosa JC, Grundy SM, Waters DD, et al. Intensive lipid lowering with atorvastatin in patients with stable coronary disease. N Engl J Med. 2005; 352:1425–1435.
3. Expert Panel on Detection, Evaluation, and Treatment of High Blood Cholesterol in Adults. Executive summary of the third report of the National Cholesterol Education Program (NCEP) Expert Panel on Detection, Evaluation, and Treatment of High Blood Cholesterol in Adults (Adult Treatment Panel III). JAMA 2001; 285:2486–2497.
4. Grundy SM, Cleeman JI, Merz CN, et al. National Heart, Lung, and Blood Institute, American College of Cardiology Foundation, American Heart Association. Implications of recent clinical trials for the National Cholesterol Education Program Adult Treatment Panel III guidelines. Circulation 2004; 110 (2):227–239.
5. Gotto AM Jr, Brinton EA. Assessing low levels of high-density lipoprotein cholesterol as a risk factor in coronary heart disease, a working group report and update. J Am Coll Cardiol 2004; 43:717–724.
6. Toth PP. High-density lipoprotein and cardiovascular disease. Circulation 2004; 109:1809–1812.
7. Barr DP, Russ EM, Eder HA. Protein-lipid relationships in human plasma II. In atherosclerosis and related conditions. Am J Med 1951; 11:480–493.
8. Castelli WP, Doyle TG, Hames CG, et al. HDL and other lipids in coronary heart disease, the Cooperative Lipoprotein Phenotyping Study. Circulation 1977; 55:767–772.
9. Goldbourt U, Yaari S, Medalie JH. Isolated low HDL cholesterol as a risk factor for coronary heart disease mortality, a 21-year follow-up of 8000 men. Arterioscler Thromb Vasc Biol 1997; 17:107–113.
10. Keil U, Liese AD, Hense HW, et al. Classical risk factors and their impact on incident non-fatal and fatal myocardial infarction and all-cause mortality in southern Germany. Results from the MONICA Augsburg cohort study 1984–1992. Monitoring Trends and Determinants in Cardiovascular Diseases. Eur Heart J 1998; 19(8):1197–1207.
11. Castelli WP, Garrison RJ, Wilson PW, et al. Incidence of coronary heart disease and lipoprotein cholesterol level. JAMA 1986; 256:2835–2838.
12. Jacobs DR, Mebane IL, Bangdiwala SI, et al. High density lipoprotein cholesterol as a predictor of cardiovascular disease mortality in men and women, follow-up study of the Lipid Research Clinics Prevalence Study. Am J Epidemiol 1990; 131:32–47.
13. Kannel WB, Castelli WP, Gordon T. Cholesterol in the prediction of atherosclerotic diseases, new perspectives on the Framingham Study. Ann Intern Med 1979; 90:85–91.
14. de Backer G, de Bacquer D, Kornitzer M. Epidemiological aspects of high density lipoprotein cholesterol. Atherosclerosis. 1998 Apr; 137(suppl):S1–S6.
15. Reed D, Benfante R. Lipid and lipoprotein predictors of coronary heart disease in elderly men in the Honolulu Heart Program. Ann Epidemiol 1992 Jan–Mar; 2(1–2):29–34.
16. Miller NE, Thelle DS, Forde OH, Mjos OD. The Tromso heart-study. High-density lipoprotein and coronary heart-disease, a prospective case-control study. Lancet 1977; 1(8019):965–968.
17. Kannel WB. High-density lipoproteins, epidemiologic profile and risks of coronary artery disease. Am J Cardiol 1983; 52:9B–12B.
18. Assmann G, Cullen P, Schulte H. The Muenster Heart Study (PROCAM), results of follow-up at 8 years. Eur Heart J 1998; 19(Suppl A):A2–A11.
19. Laws A, Marcus EB, Grove JS, Curb JD. Lipids and lipoproteins as risk factors for coronary heart disease in men with abnormal glucose tolerance, the Honolulu Heart Program. J Intern Med 1993; 234:471–478.
20. Stampfer MJ, Sacks FM, Salvin S, et al. A prospective study of cholesterol, apolipoproteins, and the risk of myocardial infarction. N Engl J Med 1991; 325:373–381.
21. Gordon DJ, Probstfield JL, Garrison RJ, et al. High-density lipoprotein cholesterol and cardiovascular disease. Circulation 1989; 79:8–15.
22. Kitamura A, Iso H, Naito Y, et al. High-density lipoprotein cholesterol and premature coronary heart disease in urban Japanese men. Circulation 1994; 89:2533–2539.
23. Shai I, Rimm EB, Hankinson SE, et al. Multivariate assessment of lipid parameters as predictors of coronary heart disease among postmenopausal women. Potential implications for clinical guidelines. Circulation 2004; 110:2824–2830.
24. Ford ES, Giles WH, Dietz WH. Prevalence of the metabolic syndrome among US adults, Findings from the third National Health and Nutrition Examination Survey. JAMA 2002; 287(3):356–359.
25. Bruckert E, Baccara-Dinet M, McCoy F, Chapman J. High prevalence of low HDL-cholesterol in a pan-European survey of 8545 dyslipidaemic patients. Curr Med Res Opin 2005; 21:1927–1934.

26. Genest J Jr, McNamara JR, Ordovas JM, et al. Lipoprotein cholesterol, apolipoprotein A-I and B and lipoprotein (a) abnormalities in men with premature coronary artery disease. J Am Coll Cardiol 1992; 19:792–802.

27. Rubins HB, Robins SJ, Collins D, et al. Distribution of lipids in 8,500 men with coronary artery disease. Am J Cardiol 1995; 75:1196–1201.

28. Lamarche B, Despres JP, Moorjani S, et al. Triglycerides and HDL-cholesterol as risk factors for ischemic heart disease. Results from the Quebec cardiovascular study. Atherosclerosis 1996; 119(2):235–245.

29. Mosca L, Grundy SM, Judelson D, et al. Guide to preventive cardiology for women. AHA/ACC scientific statement, consensus panel statement. Circulation 1999; 99:2480–2484.

30. Sacks FM. The role of high-density lipoprotein (HDL) cholesterol in the prevention and treatment of coronary heart disease, expert group recommendations. Am J Cardiol 2002; 90:139–143.

31. Chapman MJ, Assmann G, Fruchart JC, et al. For the European Consensus Panel on HDL-C. Raising high-density lipoprotein cholesterol with reduction of cardiovascular risk, the role of nicotinic acid— a position paper developed by the European Consensus Panel on HDL-C. Curr Med Res Opin 2004; 20:1253–1268.

32. American Diabetes Association. Dyslipidemia management in adults with diabetes. Diabetes Care 2004; 27(suppl 1):S68–S71.

33. Psaty BM, Anderson M, Kronmal RA, et al. The association between lipid levels and the risks of incident myocardial infarction, stroke, and total mortality, The Cardiovascular Health Study. J Am Geriatr Soc 2004; 52(10):1639–1647.

34. Corti MC, Guralnik JM, Salive ME, et al. HDL-C predicts coronary heart disease mortality in older persons. JAMA 1995; 274:575–577.

35. Sacco RL, Benson RT, Kargman DE, et al. High-density lipoprotein cholesterol and ischemic stroke in the elderly. The Northern manhattan Stroke Study. JAMA 2001; 285:2729–2735.

36. Weverling-Rijnsburger AWE, Jonkers IJ, van Exel E, et al. High-density vs. low-density lipoprotein cholesterol as the risk factor for coronary artery disease and stroke in old age. Arch Intern Med 2003; 163:1549–1554.

37. Shah P, Amin J. Low high density lipoprotein level is associated with increased restenosis rate after coronary angioplasty. Circulation 1992; 85:1279–1285.

38. Pearson T, Bulkley B, Achuff S, et al. The association of low levels of HDL-C and arteriographically defined coronary artery disease. Am J Epidemiol 1979; 109:285–295.

39. Johnsen SH, Mathiesen EB, Fosse E, et al. Elevated high-density lipoprotein cholesterol levels are protective against plaque progression, a follow-up study of 1952 persons with carotid atherosclerosis the Tromso study. Circulation 2005; 112(4):498–504.

40. Ishikawa K, Tani S, Watanabe I, et al. Effect of pravastatin on coronary plaque volume. Am J Cardiol 2003; 92:975–977.

41. Aiello RJ, Brees, D, Francone OL. ABCA 1-deficient mice, insights into the role of monocyte lipid effluxin HDL formation and inflammation. Arterioscler Thromb Vasc Biol 2003; 23:972–980.

42. Basso F, Freeman L, Knapper CL, et al. Role of the hepatic ABCA1 transporter in modulating intrahepatic cholesterol and plasma HDL cholesterol concentrations. J Lipid Res 2003; 44:296–302.

43. Sahoo D, Trischuk TC, Chan T, et al. ABCA1-dependent lipid efflux to apolipoprotein A-I mediates HDL particle formation and decreases VLDL secretion from murine hepatocytes. J Lipid Res 2004; 45:1122–1131.

44. Toth PP. High-density lipoprotein as a therapeutic target-clinical evidence and treatment strategies. Am J Cardiol 2005; 96(suppl):50K–58K.

45. Miyazaki A, Sakuma S, Morikawa W, et al. Intravenous injection of rabbit apolipoprotein A-I inhibits the progression of atherosclerosis in cholesterol-fed rabbits. Arterioscler Thromb Vasc Biol 1995; 15:1882–1888.

46. Tangirala RK, Tsukamoto K, Chun SH, et al. Regression of atherosclerosis induced by liver-directed gene transfer of apolipoprotein A-1 in mice. Circulation 1999; 100:1816–1822.

47. Assmann G. Pro and con, high-density lipoprotein, triglycerides, and other lipid subfractions are the future of lipid management. Am J Cardiol 2000; 87(suppl):2B–7B.

48. Walldius G, Jungner I, Holme I, et al. High apolipoprotein B, low apolipoprotein A-I, and improvement in the prediction of fatal myocardial infarction (AMORIS study), a prospective study. Lancet 2001; 358:2026–2033.

49. Downs JR, Clearfield M, Weis S, et al. Primary prevention of acute coronary events with lovastatin in men and women with average cholesterol levels. Results of AFCAPS/TexCAPS. JAMA 1998; 279:1615–1622.

50. Sorci-Thomas MG, Thomas MJ. The effects of altered apolipoprotein A-I structure on plasma HDL concentration. Trends Cardiovasc Med 2002; 12:121–128.

51. Miller M, Aiello D, Pritchard H, et al. Apolipoprotein A-I Zavalla (Leu159?Pro), HDL cholesterol deficiency in a kindred associated with premature coronary artery disease. Arterioscler Thromb Vasc Biol 1998; 18:1242–1247.

52. Huang W, Sasaki J, Matsunaga A, et al. A single amino acid deletion in the carboxy terminal of apolipoprotein A-I impairs lipid binding and cellular interaction. Arterioscler Thromb Vasc Biol 2000; 20:210–216.

53. Tilly-Keisi M, Lichtenstein A, Ordovas J, et al. Subjects with ApoA-I (Lys107-0) exhibit enhanced fractional catabolic rate of Apo-A-I in Lp(AI) and ApoA-II in Lp(AI with AII). Arterioscler Thromb Vasc Biol 1997; 17:873–880.

54. Rall SC Jr, Weisgraber KH, Mahley RW, et al. Abnormal lecithin, cholesterol acyltransferase activation by a human apolipoprotein A-I variant in which a single lysine residue is deleted. J Biol Chem 1984; 259:10063–10070.

55. Hovingh GK, Brownlie A, Bisoendial RJ, et al. A novel apoA-I mutation (L178P) leads to endothelial dysfunction, increased arterial wall thickness, and premature coronary artery disease. J Am Coll Cardiol 2004; 44:1429–1435.

56. Ballantyne CM, Nambi V. Apolipoprotein A-I and high-density lipoprotein. J Am Coll Cardiol 2004; 44:1436–1438.

57. Brooks-Wilson A, Marcil M, Clee SM, et al. Mutations in ABCA1 in Tangier disease and familial high-density lipoprotein deficiency. Nat Genet 1999; 22, 336–345.

58. Venkateswaran A, Laffitte BA, Joseph SB, et al. Control of cellular cholesterol efflux by the nuclear oxysterol receptor LXRa. Proc Natl Acad Sci 2000; 97:12097–12102.

59. Attie AD, Kastelein JP, Hayden MR. Pivotal role of ABCA1 in reverse cholesterol transport influencing HDL levels and susceptibility to atherosclerosis. J Lipid Res 2001; 42:1717–1726.

60. Zha X, Gauthier A, Genest J, et al. Secretory vesicular transport from the Golgi is altered during ATP-binding cassette protein A1 (ABCA1) mediated cholesterol efflux. J Biol Chem 2003; 278:10002–10005.

61. Chroni A, Liu T, Gorshkova I, et al. The central helices of ApoA-I can promote ATP-binding cassette transporter A1 (ABCA1)-mediated lipid efflux. J Biol Chem 2003; 278(9):6719–6730.

62. Vaisman BL, Lambert G, Amar M, et al. ABCA1 overexpression leads to hyperalphalipoproteinemia and increased biliary cholesterol excretion in transgenic mice. J Clin Invest 2001; 108:303–309.

63. Singaraja RR, Fiever C, Castro G, et al. Increased ABCA1 activity protects against atherosclerosis. J Clin Invest 2002; 110:35–42.

64. Van Eck M, Singaraja RR, Ye D, Hildebrand RB, et al. Macrophage ATP-binding cassette transporter A1 overexpression inhibits atherosclerotic lesion progression in low-density lipoprotein receptor knockout mice. Arterioscler Thromb Vasc Biol 2006; 26:929–934.

65. Clee SM, Zwinderman AH, Engert JC, et al. Common genetic variation in ABCA1 is associated with altered lipoprotein levels and a modified risk for coronary artery disease. Circulation 2001; 103:1198–1205.

66. Clee SM, Kastelein JP, van Dam M, et al. Age and residual cholesterol efflux affect HDL cholesterol levels and coronary artery disease in ABCA1 heterozygotes. J Clin Invest 2000; 106:1263–1270.

67. Hong SH, Rhyne J, Zeller K, et al. ABCA1 (Alabama), a novel variant associated with HDL deficiency and premature coronary artery disease. Atherosclerosis 2002; 164:245–250.

68. Wang N, Lan D, Chen W, et al. ATP-binding cassette transporter G1 and G4 mediate cellular cholesterol efflux to high-density lipoproteins. Proc Natl Acad Sci USA 2004; 101:9774–9779.

69. Kennedy MA, Berrera GC, Nakamura K, et al. ABCG1 has a critical role in mediating cholesterol efflux to HDL and preventing cellular lipid accumulation. Cell Metabolism 2005; 1:121–131.

70. Kasid A, Rhyne J, Zeller K, et al. A novel TC deletion resulting in Pro260? Stop in the human LCAT gene is associated with a dominant effect on HDL-cholesterol. Atherosclerosis 2001; 156:127–132.

71. Online Mendelian Inheritance in Man. Johns Hopkins University. Available at, http://www.ncbi.nlm. nih.gov/entrez/query.fcgi?cmd = Retrieve&db = OMIM&dopt = Detailed&tmpl = dispomimTemplate&list_uids = 606967. Accessed March 20, 2006.

72. Rader DJ, Ikewaki K, Duverger N, et al. Markedly accelerated catabolism of apolipoprotein A-II (apoA-II) and high density lipoproteins containing apoA-II in classic lecithin, cholesterol acyltransferase deficiency and fish-eye disease. J Clin Invest 1994; 93:321–330.

73. Elkhalil L, Majd Z, Bakir R, et al. Fish-eye disease, structural and in vivo metabolic abnormalities of high-density lipoproteins. Metabolism 1997; 46:474–483.

74. Von Eckardstein A, Huang Y, Wu S, et al. Reverse cholesterol transport in plasma of patients with different forms of familial HDL deficiency. Arterioscler Thromb Vasc Biol 1995; 15:691–703.

75. Rader DJ. Inhibition of cholesteryl ester transfer protein activity, a new therapeutic approach to raising high-density lipoprotein. Curr Atheroscler Rep 2004; 6:398–405.

76. Klein H-G, Lohse P, Pritchard PH, et al. Two different allelic mutations in the lecithin-cholesterol acyltransferase gene associated with the fist eye syndrome. J Clin Invest 1992; 898:499–506.

77. K, Hill JS, Wang X, Pritchard PH. Recombinant lecithin, cholesterol acyltransferase containing a Thr123ÆIle mutation esterifies cholesterol in low density lipoprotein but not in high density lipoprotein. J Lipid Res 1993; 34:81–88.

78. Vaisman BL, Klein H-G, Rouis M, et al. Overexpression of human lecithin cholesterol acyltransferase leads to hyperalphalipoproteinemia in transgenic mice. J Biol Chem 1995; 20:12269–12275.

79. Cohen JC, Kiss RS, Pertsemlidis A, et al. Multiple rare alleles contribute to low plasma HDL cholesterol. Science 2004; 305(5685):869–872.

80. Hoeg JM, Vaisman BL, Demosky SJ Jr, et al. Lecithin, cholesterol acyltransferase overexpression generates hyperalphalipoproteinemia and a non-atherogenic lipoprotein pattern in transgenic rabbits. J Biol Chem 1996; 271:4396–4402.

81. Roosbeck S, Vanloo B, Duverger N, et al. Three arginine residues in apolipoprotein A-I are critical for activation of lecithin, cholesterol acyltransferase. J Lipid Res 2001; 42:31–40.

82. Martin-Campos JM, Julve J, Escola JJ, et al. ApoA-I (Mallorca) impairs LCAT activation and induces familial hypoalphalipoproteinemia. J Lipid Res 2002; 43:115–123.

83. Husskonen J, Olkkonen VM, Jauhiainen M, et al., The impact of phospholipid transfer protein (PLTP) on HDL metabolism. Atherosclerosis 2001; 155:269–281.

84. Cheung M, Wolfbauer G, Brown B, et al. Relationship between plasma phospholipid transfer protein activity and HDL subclasses among patients with low HDL and cardiovascular disease. Atherosclerosis 1999; 142:201–205.

85. Lusa S, Jauhiainen M, Metso J, et al. The mechanism of human plasma phospholipid transfer protein-induced enlargement of high-density lipoprotein particles, evidence for particle fusion. Biochem J 1996; 313:275–282.

86. Settasatian N, Duong M, Curtiss LK, et al. The mechanism of the remodeling of high density lipoproteins by phospholipid transfer protein. J Biol Chem 2001; 276:26898–26905.

87. Bruce C, Chouinard RA, Tall AR. Plasma lipid transfer proteins, high-density lipoproteins, and reverse cholesterol transport. Ann Rev Nutr 1998; 18:297–310.

88. Yamashita S, Maruyama T, Hirano K, et al. Molecular mechanisms, lipoprotein abnormalities and atherogenicity of hyperalphalipoproteinemia. Atherosclerosis 2000; 152:271–285.

89. Inazu A, Jiang X-C, Haraki T, et al. Genetic cholesteryl ester transfer protein deficiency caused y two prevalent mutations as a major determinant of increased levels of high density lipoprotein cholesterol. J Clin Invest 1994; 94:1872–1882.

90. Tall A, Jiang X, Silver D. George Lyman Duff memorial lecture, lipid transfer proteins, HDL metabolism, and atherogenesis. Arterioscler Thromb Vasc Biol 2000; 20:1185–1188.

91. Zhong S, Sharp DS, Grove JS, et al. Increased coronary heart disease in Japanese American men with mutation in the cholesteryl ester transfer protein gene despite increased HDL levels. J Clin Invest 1996; 97:2917–2923.

92. Curb JD, Abbott RD, Rodriguez BL, et al. A prospective study of HDL-C and cholesteryl ester transfer protein gene mutations and the risk of coronary heart disease in the elderly. J Lipid Res 2004; 45:948–953.

93. Wolfe ML, Rader DJ. Cholesteryl ester transfer protein and coronary artery disease. An observation with therapeutic implications. Circulation 2004; 110:1338–1340.

94. Moriyama Y, Okamura T, Inazu A, et al. A low prevalence of coronary heart disease among subjects with increased high-density lipoprotein cholesterol levels, including those with plasma cholesteryl ester transfer protein deficiency. Prev Med 1998; 27:659–667.

95. Brousseau ME, O'Connor JJ, Ordovas JM, et al. Cholesteryl ester transfer protein TaqI B2B2 genotype is associated with higher HDL cholesterol levels and lower risk of coronary heart disease endpoints in men with HDL deficiency. Veterans Affairs HDL Cholesterol Intervention Trial. Arterioscler Thromb Vasc Biol 2002; 22:1148–1154.

96. Wu JH, Lee YT, Hsu HC, et al. Influence of CETP gene variation on plasma lipid levels and coronary heart disease, a survey in Taiwan. Atherosclerosis 2001; 159:451–458.

97. Cohen J, Wand Z, Grundy S, et al. Variation at the hepatic lipase and apolipoprotein AI/CIII/AIV loci is a major cause of genetically determined variation in plasma HDL cholesterol levels. J Clin Invest 1994; 94:2377–2384.

98. Bersot TP, Vega GL, Grundy SM, et al. Elevated hepatic lipase activity and low levels of high-density lipoprotein in a normotriglyceridemic, nonobese Turkish population. J Lipid Res 1999; 40:432–438.

99. Carr MC, Ayobi AF, Murdoch SJ, et al. Contribution of hepatic lipase, lipoprotein lipase, and cholesteryl ester transfer protein to LDL and HDL heterogeneity in healthy women. Arterioscler Thromb Vasc Biol 2002; 22:667–673.

100. Zambon A, Deeb SS, Hokanson JE, et al. Common variants in the promoter of the hepatic lipasegene are associated with lower levels of hepatic lipase activity, buoyant LDL, and higher HDL2 cholesterol. Arterioscler Thromb Vasc Biol 1998; 18:1723–1729.

101. Jansen H, Verhoeven AJ, Sijbrands EJ. Hepatic lipase, a pro- or anti-atherogenic protein? J Lipid Res 2002; 43:1352–1362.

102. Jin W, Millar JS, Broedl U, et al. Inhibition of endothelial lipase causes increased HDL cholesterol levels in vivo. J Clin Invest 2003; 111:357–362.

103. Ishida T, Choi S, Kundu RK, et al. Endothelial lipase is a major determinant of HDL level. J Clin Invest 2003; 111:347–355.

104. Badellino KO, Wolfe ML, Reilly MP, Rader DJ. Endothelial lipase concentrations are increased in metabolic syndrome and associated with coronary atherosclerosis. PLOS Medicine 2006; 3(2):e22.

105. Trigatti BL, Rigotti A, Braun A. Cellular and physiological roles of SR-BI, a lipoprotein receptor which mediates selective lipid uptake. Biochim Biophys Acta 2000; 1529:276–286.

106. Krieger M. Scavenger receptor class B type I is a multiligand HDL receptor that influences diverse physiologic systems. J Clin Invest 2001; 108:793–797.

107. Van Eck M, Twisk J, Hoekstra M, et al. Differential effects of scavenger receptor BI deficiency on lipid metabolism in cells of the arterial wall and in the liver. J Biol Chem 2003; 278(26):23699–23705.

108. Kozarsky KF, Donahee MH, Glick JM, et al. Gene transfer and hepatic overexpression of the HDL receptor SR-BI reduces atherosclerosis in the cholesterol-fed LDL receptor-deficient mouse. Arterioscler Thromb Vasc Biol 2000; 20:721–727.

109. Williams DL, Llera-Moya M, Thuahnai ST, et al. Binding and cross-linking studies show that scavenger receptor BI interacts with multiple sites in apolipoprotein A-I and identifies the class A amphipathic α-helix as a recognition motif. J Biol Chem 2000; 275:18897–18904.

110. Liu T, Krieger M, Kan HY, et al. The effects of mutations in helices 4 and 6 of apoA-I on scavenger receptor class B type I (SR-BI)-mediated cholesterol efflux suggest that formation of a productive complex between reconstituted high density lipoprotein and SR-BI is required for efficient lipid transport. J Biol Chem 2002; 277:21576–21584.

111. Connelly MA, Kellner-Weibel G, Rothblat GH, Williams DL. SR-BI-directed HDL-cholesterol ester hydrolysis. J Lipid Res 2003; 44(2):331–341.

112. Martinez LO, Jacquet S, Esteve JP, et al. Ectopic β-chain of ATP synthase is an apolipoprotein A-I receptor in hepatic HDL endocytosis. Nature 2003; 421:75–79.

113. Ioka RX, Kang MJ, Kamiyama S, et al. Expression cloning and characterization of a novel glycosylphosphatidylinositol-anchored high density lipoprotein-binding protein, GPI-HBP-I. J Biol Chem 2003; 278:7344–7349.

114. Naik SU, Wang X, Da Silva JS, et al. Pharmacological activation of liver X receptors promotes reverse cholesterol transport in vivo. Circulation 2006; 113:90–97.

115. Eriksson M, Carlson LA, Miettinen TA, et al. Stimulation of fecal steroid excretion after infusion of recombinant proapolipoprotein A-I. Potential reverse cholesterol transport in humans. Circulation 1999; 100:594–598.

116. Toth PP, Davidson MH. Therapeutic interventions targeted at the augmentation of reverse cholesterol transport. Curr Opin Cardiol 2004; 19:374–379.

117. Nofer J, Kehrel B, Fobker M, et al. HDL and arteriosclerosis, beyond reverse cholesterol transport. Atherosclerosis 2002; 161:1–16.

118. Ramet ME, Ramet M, Lu, Q, et al. High-density lipoprotein increases the abundance of eNOS protein in human vascular endothelial cells by increasing its half-life. J Am Coll Cardiol 2003; 41(12):2288–2297.

119. Li X, Zhao S, Zhang S, et al. Protective effect of high-density lipoprotein on endothelium-dependent vasodilatation. Int J Cardiol 2000; 73:231–236.

120. Levkau B, Hermann S, Theilmeier G, et al. High-density lipoprotein stimulates myocardial perfusion in vivo. Circulation 2004; 110:3355–3359.

121. de Winther MPJ, Kanters E, Kraal G, Hofker MH. Nuclear factor κB signaling in atherogenesis. Arterioscler Thromb Vasc Biol 2005; 25:904–914.

122. Xia P, Vadas M, Rye K, et al. High-density lipoproteins (HDL) interrupt the sphingosine kinase signaling pathway. J Biol Chem 1999; 274:33143–33147.

123. Toth PP. Dis Mon 2001; 47:365–416.

124. Kimura T, Sato K, Malchinkhuu E, Tumora H, et al. High-density lipoprotein stimulates endothelial cell migration and survival through sphingosine 1-phosphate and its receptors. Arterioscler Thromb Vasc Biol 2003; 23:1283–1288.

125. Tamagaki T, Sawada S, Imamura H, et al. Effects of high-density lipoproteins on intracellular pH and proliferation of human vascular endothelial cells. Atherosclerosis 1996; 123:73–82.

126. Nofer JR, Levkau B, Wolinska I, et al. Suppression of endothelial cell apoptosis by high-density lipoproteins and HDL-associated lysosphingolipids. J Biol Chem 2001; 276:34480–34485.

127. Libby P. Current concepts of the pathogenesis of the acute coronary syndromes. Circulation 2001; 104:365–372.

128. Libby P. Molecular bases of the acute coronary syndromes. Circulation 1995; 91:2844–2850.

129. Fuster V. Elucidation of the role of plaque instability and rupture in acute coronary events. Am J Cardiol 1995; 76:24C–33C.

130. Bierenbaum ML, Fleischman AI, Stier A, et al. Increased platelet aggregation and decreased high density lipoprotein cholesterol in women on oral contraceptives. Am J Obstet Gynecol 1979; 134:638–641.

131. Beitz J, Mest HJ. Thromboxane A2 formation by washed platelets under the influence of low and high density lipoproteins. Prostaglandins Leukot Med 1986; 23:303–307.

132. Aviram M, Brook G. Characterization of the effect of plasma lipoproteins on platelet function in vitro. Haemostasis 1983; 13:344–350.

133. Saku K, Ahmad M, Glas-Greenwalt P, Kashyap ML. Activation of fibrinolysis by apolipoproteins of high density lipoproteins in man. Thromb Res 1985; 39 (1):1–80.

134. Griffin J, Kojima K, Banka C, et al. High-density lipoprotein enhancement of anticoagulant activities of plasma protein S and activated protein C. J Clin Invest 1999; 103:219–227.

135. Cockerill G, Saklatvala J, Ridley S, et al. High-density lipoproteins differentially modulate cytokine-induced expression of E-selectin and Cyclooxygenase-2. Arterioscler Thromb Vasc Biol 1999; 19:910–917.

136. Vinals M, Martinez-Gonzalez J, Badimon L. Regulatory effects of HDL on smooth muscle cell prostacyclin release. Arterioscler Thromb Vasc Biol 1999; 19:2405–2411.

137. Fleisher L, Tall A, Witte L, et al. Stimulation of arterial endothelial cell prostacyclin synthesis by high density lipoproteins. J Biol Chem 1982; 257:6653–6655.

138. Nofer J, Walter M, Kehrel B, et al. HDL3-mediated inhibition of thrombin-induced platelet aggregation and fibrinogen binding occurs via decreased production of phosphoinositide-derived second messengers 1,2-diacylglycerol and inositol 1,4,5-tris-phosphate. Arterioscler Thromb Vasc Biol 1998; 18:861–869.

139. Libby P, Ridker PM, Maseri A. Inflammation and atherosclerosis. Circulation 2002; 105:1135–1143.

140. Carr AC, McCall MR, Frei B. Oxidation of LDL by myeloperoxidase and reactive nitrogen species. Reaction pathways and antioxidant protection. Arterioscler Thromb Vasc Biol 2000; 20:1716–1723.

141. Hansson GK. Inflammation, atherosclerosis, and coronary artery disease. N Engl J Med 2005; 352:1685–1695.

142. Stary HC, Chandler AB, Glagov S, et al. A definition of initial, fatty streak, and intermediate lesions of atherosclerosis. Circulation 1994; 89:2462–2478.

143. Steinberg D, Gotto AM. Preventing coronary artery disease by lowering cholesterol levels. Fifty years from bench to bedside. JAMA 1999; 282:2043–2050.

144. Parthasarathy S, Barnett J, Fong L. High-density lipoprotein inhibits the oxidative modification of low-density lipoprotein. Biochim Biophys Acta 1990; 1044:275–283.

145. Mackness M, Abbott C, Arrol S, et al. The role of high-density lipoprotein and lipid-soluble antioxidant vitamins in inhibiting low-density lipoprotein oxidation. Biochemistry 1993; 294:829–834.

146. Toikka J, Ahotupa M, Viikari J, et al. Constantly low HDL-cholesterol concentration relates to endothelial dysfunction and increased in vivo LDL-oxidation in healthy young men. Atherosclerosis 1999; 147:133–138.

147. Heinecke J, Lusis A. Paraoxonase-gene polymorphisms associated with coronary heart disease, support for the oxidative damage hypothesis? Am J Hum Genet 1998; 62:20–24.

148. Aviram M, Hardak E, Vaya J, et al. Human serum paraoxonases (PON1) Q and R selectively decrease lipid peroxides in human coronary and carotid atherosclerotic lesions. Circulation 2000; 101:2510–2517.

149. Mackness MI, Harty D, Bhatnager D, et al. Serum paraoxonase activity in familial hypercholesterolemia and insulin-dependent diabetes mellitus. Atherosclerosis 1991; 86:193–199.

150. Dantioine T, Debord J, Charmes J, et al. Pathophysiology of renal disease. J Am Soc Nephrol 1998; 9:2082–2089.

151. Ayub A, Mackness M, Arrol S, et al. Serum paraoxonase after myocardial infarction. Arterioscler Thromb Vasc Biol 1999; 19:330–335.

152. James R, Leviev I, Righetti A. Smoking is associated with reduced serum paraoxonase activity and concentration in patients with coronary artery disease. Circulation 2000; 101:2252–2257.

153. Stremler KE, Stafforini DM, Prescott SM, et al. Human platelet-activating factor acetylhydrolase. Oxidatively fragmented phospholipids as substrates. J Biol Chem 1991; 266:11095–11103.

154. Garner B, Waldeck R, Witting P, et al. Oxidation of high density lipoproteins. II. J Biol Chem 1998; 273:6088–6095.

155. Garner B, Witting PK, Waldeck AR, et al. Oxidation of high density lipoproteins. I. J Biol Chem 1998; 273:6080–6087.

156. Christison JK, Rye KA, Stocker R. Exchange of oxidized cholesteryl linoleate between LDL and HDL mediated by cholesteryl ester transfer protein. J Lipid Res 1995; 36:1012–1021.

157. Scandinavian Simvastatin Survival Study Group. Randomized trial of cholesterol lowering in 4444 participants with coronary artery disease, the Scandinavian Simvastatin Survival Study (4S). Lancet 1994; 344:1383–1389.

158. Sacks FM, Pfeffer MA, Moye LA, et al. The effect of pravastatin on coronary events after myocardial infarction in patients with average cholesterol levels. N Engl J Med 1996; 335:1001–1009.

159. Shepherd J, Cobbe SM, Ford I, et al. For the West of Scotland Coronary Prevention Study Group. Prevention of coronary heart disease with pravastatin in men with hypercholesterolemia. N Engl J Med 1995; 333:1301–1307.

160. Martin G, Duez H, Blanquart C, et al. Statin-induced inhibition of the Rho-signaling pathway activates PPAR-α and induces HDL apoA-I. J Clin Invest 2001; 107:1423–1432.

161. Schaefer EJ, Asztalos BF. The effects of statins on high-density lipoproteins. Curr Atheroscler Rep 2006; 8:41–49.

162. Ballantyne CM, Blazing MA, Hunninghake DB, et al. Effect on high-density lipoprotein cholesterol of maximum doses of simvastatin and atorvastatin in patients with hypercholesterolemia, results of the comparative HDL efficacy and safety study (CHESS). Am Heart J 2003; 146:862–869.

163. Davidson MH, Ma P, Stein EA, et al. Comparison of effects on low-density lipoprotein cholesterol and high-density lipoprotein cholesterol with rosuvastatin versus atorvastatin in patients with type IIa or type IIb hypercholesterolemia. Am J Cardiol 2002; 89:268–275.

164. Jones PH, Davidson MH, Stein EA, et al. STELLAR Study Group. Comparison of the efficacy and safety of rosuvastatin versus atorvastatin, simvastatin, and pravastatin across doses (STELLAR* Trial). Am J Cardiol 2003; 92:152–160.

165. Downs JR, Clearfield M, Weis S, et al. For the AFCAPS/TexCAPS Research Group, Primary prevention of acute coronary events with lovastatin in men and women with average cholesterol levels. JAMA 1998; 279:1615–1622.

166. Gotto AM Jr, Whitney E, Stein EA, et al. Relation between baseline and on-treatment lipid parameters and first acute major coronary events in the Air Force/Texas Coronary Atherosclerosis Prevention Study (AFCAPS/TexCAPS). Circulation 2000; 101(5):477–484.

167. Packard CJ, Ford I, Robertson M, et al. For the PROSPER Study Group. Plasma lipoproteins and apolipoproteins as predictors of cardiovascular risk and treatment benefit in the PROspective Study of Pravastatin in the Elderly at Risk (PROSPER). Circulation 2005; 112(20):3058–3065.

168. Ballantyne CM, Herd JA, Ferlic LL, et al. Influence of low HDL on progression of coronary artery disease and response to fluvastatin therapy. Circulation 1999; 99(6):736–743.

169. Liao JK. Clinical implications for statin pleiotropy. Curr Opin Lipidol 2005; 6(6):624–629.

170. Birjmohun RS, Hutten BA, Kastelein JJP, Stroes ESG. Efficacy and safety of high-density lipoprotein cholesterol-increasing compounds. A meta-analysis of randomized controlled trials. J Am Coll Cardiol 2005; 45:185–197.

171. Fruchart JC. Peroxisome proliferator-activated receptor-a activation and high-density lipoprotein metabolism. Am J Cardiol 2001; 88 (suppl):24N–29N.

172. Bays H. Extended-release niacin/lovastatin: the first combination product for dyslipidemia. Expert Rev Cardiovasc Ther 2004; 2:89–105.

173. Nordestgaard B, Abildgaard S, Wittrup H, et al. Heterozygous lipoprotein lipase deficiency. Circulation 1997; 96:1737–1744.

174. Reymer P, Groenemeyer BE, Gagne E, et al. A lipoprotein lipase mutation (Asn291→Ser) is associated with reduced HDL cholesterol levels in premature atherosclerosis. Nature Genet 1995; 10:28–34.

175. Wittrup HH, Nordestgaard BG, Sillesen H, et al. A common mutation in lipoprotein lipase confers a 2-fold increase in risk of ischemic cerebrovascular disease in women but not in men. Circulation 2000; 101:2393–2397.

176. Kuivenhoven J, Groenemeyer B, Boer J, et al. Ser447 stop mutation in lipoprotein lipase is associated with elevated HDL cholesterol levels in normolipidemic males. Arterioscler Thromb Vasc Biol 1997; 17:595–599.

177. Frick MH, Elo O, Haapa K, et al. Helsinki Heart Study, primary-prevention trial with gemfibrozil in middle-aged men with dyslipidemia. Safety of treatment, changes in risk factors, and incidence of coronary heart disease. N Engl J Med 1987; 317:1237–1245.

178. Manninen V, Elo MO, Frick MH, et al. Lipid alterations and decline in the incidence of coronary heart disease in the Helsinki Heart Study. JAMA 1988; 260:641–651.

179. Rubins HB, Robins SJ, Collins D, et al. For the Veterans Affairs High-Density Lipoprotein Cholesterol Intervention Trial Study Group. Gemfibrozil for the secondary prevention of coronary heart disease in men with low levels of high-density lipoprotein cholesterol. N Engl J Med 1999; 341:410–418.

180. Robins SJ, Collins D, Wittes JT, et al. For the VA-HIT Study Group. Veterans Affairs High-Density Lipoprotein Intervention Trial. Relation of gemfibrozil treatment and lipid levels with major coronary events, VA-HIT, a randomized controlled trial. JAMA 2001; 285(12):1585–1591.

181. Ericsson CG, Hamsten A, Nilsson J, et al. Angiographic assessment of effects of bezafibrate on progression of coronary artery disease in young male postinfarction patients. Lancet 1996; 347:849–853.

182. Frick MH, Syvänne M, Nieminen MS, et al. Prevention of the angiographic progression of coronary and vein-graft atherosclerosis by gemfibrozil after coronary bypass surgery in men with low levels of HDL cholesterol. Circulation 1997; 96:2137–2143.

183. Karpe F, Taskinen MR, Nieminen MS, et al. Remnant-like lipoprotein particle cholesterol concentration and progression of coronary and vein-graft atherosclerosis in response to gemfibrozil treatment. Atherosclerosis 2001; 157(1):181–187.

184. Jones PH, Davidson MH. Reporting rate of rhabdomyolysis with fenofibrate + statin versus gemfibrozil + any statin. Am J Cardiol 2005; 95:120–122.

185. Bergman AJ, Murphy G, Burke J, et al. Simvastatin does not have a clinically significant pharmacokinetic interaction with fenofibrate in humans. J Clin Pharmacol 2004; 44:1054–1062.

186. Sakai T, Kamanna VS, Kashyap ML. Niacin, but not gemfibrozil, selectively increases LP-AI, a cardioprotective subfraction of HDL, in patients with low HDL cholesterol. Arterioscler Thromb Vasc Biol 2001; 21:1783–1789.

187. Tunaru S, Kero J, Schaub A, et al. PUMA-G and HM74 are receptors for nicotinic acid and mediate its anti-lipolytic effect. Nature Med 2003; 9:352–355.

188. Wise A, Foord SM, Fraser NJ, et al. Molecular identification of high and low affinity receptors for nicotinic acid. J Biol Chem 2003; 278:9869–9874.

189. Rubic T, Trottmann M, Lorenz RL. Stimulation of CD36 and the key effector of reverse cholesterol transport ATP binding cassette A1 in monocytoid cells by niacin. Biochem Pharmacol 2004; 67:411–419.

190. The Coronary Drug Project Research Group. Clofibrate and niacin in coronary heart disease. JAMA 1975; 231:360–381.

191. Carlson LA. Nicotinic acid, the broad-spectrum lipid drug. A 50th anniversary review. J Int Med 2005; 258:94–114.

192. Brown BG, Zhao XQ, Chait A, et al. Simvastatin and niacin, antioxidant vitamins, or the combination for the prevention of coronary disease. N Engl J Med 2001; 345(22):1583–1592.

193. Cheung MC, Zhao XQ, Chait A, et al. Antioxidant supplements block the response of HDL to simvastatin-niacin therapy in patients with coronary artery disease and low HDL. Arterioscler Thromb Vasc Biol 2001; 21(8):1320–1326.

194. Hodis HN, Mack WJ, LaBree L, et al. The role of carotid arterial intima-media thickness in predicting clinical coronary events. Ann Intern Med 1998; 128:262–269.

195. Taylor AJ, Sullenberger LE, Lee HJ, et al. Arterial Biology for the Investigation of the Treatment Effects of Reducing Cholesterol (ARBITER) 2, a double-blind, placebo-controlled study of extended-release niacin on atherosclerosis progression in secondary prevention patients treated with statins. Circulation 2004; 110(23):3512–3517.

196. Gray DR, Morgan T, Chretien SD, et al. Efficacy and safety of controlled-release niacin in dyslipoproteinemic veterans. Ann Intern Med 1994; 121:252–258.

197. McKenney JM, Proctor JD, Harris S, et al. A comparison of the efficacy and toxic effects of sustained-vs immediate release form of niacin in hypercholesterolemic patients. JAMA 1994; 271:672–677.
198. Goldberg A, Alagona P, Capuzzi DM, et al. Multiple-dose efficacy and safety of an extended-release form of niacin in the management of hyperlipidemia. Am J Cardiol 2000; 85:1100–1105.
199. Jungnickel PW, Maloley PA, Vander Tuin EL, et al. Effect of two aspirin pretreatment regimens on niacin-induced cutaneous reactions. J Gen Intern Med 1997; 12:591–596.
200. Mills E, Prousky J, Raskin G, et al. The safety of over-the-counter niacin. A randomized placebo-controlled trial [ISRCTNI8054903] BMC Clin Pharmacol 2003; 3:4.
201. Elam MB, Hunninghake DB, Davis KB, et al. Effect of niacin on lipid and lipoprotein levels and glycemic control in patients with diabetes and peripheral arterial disease. The ADMIT study, a randomized trial. JAMA 2000; 284:1263–1270.
202. Garg R, Malinow M, Pettinger M, et al. Niacin treatment increases plasma homocyst(e)ine levels. Am Heart J 1999; 138:1082–1087.
203. Lam JK, Matsubara S, Mihara K, et al. Insulin induction of apolipoprotein AI, role of Sp1. Biochemistry 2003; 42:2680–2690.
204. Moradian AD, Haas MJ, Wong NCW. Transcriptional control of apolipoprotein A-I gene expression in diabetes. Diabetes 2004; 53:513–520.
205. van Wijk JPH, de Koning EJP, Martens EP, Rabelink TJ. Thiazolidinediones and blood lipids in type 2 diabetes. Arterioscler Thromb Vasc Biol 2003; 23:1744–1748.
206. Goldberg RB, Kendall DM Deeg, MA, et al. A comparison of lipid and glycemic effects of pioglitazone and rosiglitazone in patients with type 2 diabetes and dyslipidemia. Diabetes care 2005; 28:1547–1554.
207. Dormandy JA, Charbonnel B, Eckland DJA, et al. On behalf of the PROactive investigators. Secondary prevention of macrovascular events in patients with type 2 diabetes in the PROactive Study (PROspective pioglitazone Clinical Trial In macroVascular Events), a randomised controlled trial. Lancet 2005; 366:1279-1289.
208. Salonen JT, Salonen R, Seppanen K, et al. HDL, HDL2, and HDL3 subfractions, and the risk of acute myocardial infarction. A prospective population study in eastern Finnish men. Circulation 1991; 84:129-139.
209. Lamarche B, Moorjani S, Cantin B, et al. Association of HDL2 and HDL3 subfractions with ischemic heart disease in men. Prospective results from the Quebec Cardiovascular Study. Arterioscler Thromb Vasc Biol 1997; 17:1098-1105.
210. Sweetnam PM, Bolton CH, Yarnell JW, et al. Associations of the HDL2 and HDL3 cholesterol subfractions with the development of ischemic heart disease in British men. The Caerphilly and Speedwell Collaborative Heart Disease Studies. Circulation 1994; 90:769-774.
211. Syvanne M, Nieminen MS, Frick MH, et al. For the Lopid Coronary Angiofraphy Trial Study group. Associations between lipoproteins and the progression of coronary and vein-graft atherosclerosis in a controlled trial with gemfibrozil in men with low baseline levels of HDL-C. Circulation 1998; 98:1993-1999.
212. Corella D, Ordovás JM. Single nucleotide polymorphisms that influence lipid metabolism, interaction with dietary factors. Annu Rev Nutr 2005; 25:341–390.
213. Ottman R. Gene-environment interaction, definitions and study designs. Prev Med 1996; 25:764–770.
214. Ordovas JM, Corella D, Demissie S, et al. Dietary fat intake determines the effect of a common polymorphism in the hepatic lipase gene promoter on high-density lipoprotein metabolism. Circulation 2002; 106:2315–2321.
215. Ordovas JM. HDL genetics, candidate genes, genome wide scans, and gene-environment interactions. Cardiovasc Drugs Ther 2002; 16:273–281.
216. Costanza MC, Cayanis E, Ross BM, et al. Relative contributions of genes, environment, and interactions to blood lipid concentrations in a general adult population. Am J Epidemiol 2005; 161:712–725.
217. National Human Genome Research Institute. National Institutes of Health. Talking glossary of genetic terms. Available at, http://www.genome.gov/glossary.cfm. Accessed January 3, 2006.
218. Smith GD, Ebrahim S. 'Mendelian randomization', can genetic epidemiology contribute to understanding environmental determinants of disease? Int J Epidemiol 2003; 32:1–22.
219. Ellison RC, Zhang Y, Qureshi MM, et al. For the investigators of the NHLBI Family Heart Study. Lifestyle determinants of high-density lipoprotein cholesterol, the National Heart, Lung, and Blood Institute Family Heart Study. Am Heart J 2004; 147:529–535.
220. Talmud PJ, Hawe E, Robertson K, et al. Genetic and environmental determinants of plasma high density lipoprotein cholesterol and apolipoprotein AI concentrations in healthy middle-aged men. Ann Hum Genet 2002; 66:111–124.
221. Gardner CD, Tribble DL, Yong DR, et al. Associations of HDL, HDL$_2$, and HDL$_3$ cholesterol and apolipoproteins A-I and B with lifestyle factors in healthy women and men, the Stanford Five City Project. Prev Med 2000; 31:346–356.
222. Craig WY, Palomaki GE, Haddow JE. Cigarette smoking and serum lipid and lipoprotein concentrations, an analysis of published data. Br Med J 1989; 298:784–788.
223. Imamura H, Tanaka K, Hirae C, et al. Relationship of cigarette smoking to blood pressure and serum lipids and lipoproteins in men. Clin Exp Pharmacol Physiol 1996; 23:397–402.
224. Cullen P, Schulte H, Assmann G. Smoking, lipoproteins and coronary heart disease risk. Data from the Münster Heart Study (PROCAM). Eur Heart J 1998; 19:1632–1641.

225. Wu D-M, Pai L, Sung P-K, Hsu L-L, Sun C-A. Joint effects of alcohol consumption and cigarette smoking on atherogenic lipid and lipoprotein profiles, results from a study of Chinese male population in Taiwan. Eur J Epidemiol 2001; 17:629–635.

226. Imamura H, Teshima K, Miyamoto N, Shirota T. Cigarette smoking, high-density lipoprotein cholesterol subfractions, and lecithin, cholesterol acyltransferase in young women. Metabolism 2002; 51:1313–1316.

227. Morgan J, Carey C, Lincoff A, Capuzzi D. High-density lipoprotein subfractions and risk of coronary artery disease. Curr Atheroscler Rep 2004; 6:359–365.

228. Campos H, López-Miranda J, Rodríguez C, et al. Urbanization elicits a more atherogenic lipoprotein profile in carriers of the apolipoprotein A-IV-2 allele than in A-IV-1 homozygotes. Arterioscler Thromb Vasc Biol 1997; 17:1074–1081.

229. Garrison R, Kannel WB, Fernleib M. Cigarette smoking and HDL cholesterol: the Framingham offspring study. Atherosclerosis 1978; 30:17–25.

230. Schaefer EJ, Lamon-Fava S, Ordovás JM, et al. Factors associated with low and elevated plasma high-density lipoprotein cholesterol and apolipoprotein A-I levels in the Framingham Offspring Study. J Lipid Res 1994; 35:871–882.

231. Mallin R. Smoking cessation, integration of behavioral and drug therapies. Am Fam Physician 2002; 65:1107–1114.

232. Reynolds J, Campbell RK. Emerging treatment for diabetes, obesity, and smoking. US Pharmacist 2005; 11:75–79.

233. Van Gaal LF, Rissanen AM, Scheen AJ, et al. For the RIO-Europe Study Group. Effects of the cannabinoid-1 receptor blocker rimonabant on weight reduction and cardiovascular risk factors in overweight patients, 1-year experience from the RIO-Europe study. Lancet 2005; 365:1389–1397.

234. McCall MR, van den Berg JJM, Kuypers FA, et al. Modification of LCAT activity and HDL structure. New links between cigarette smoke and coronary heart disease risk. Arterioscler Thromb 1994; 14:248–253.

235. Fisher RM, Burke H, Nicaud V, Ehnholm C, Humphries SE. On behalf of the EARS Group. Effect of variation in the apo A-IV gene on body mass index and fasting and postprandial lipids in the European Atherosclerosis Research Study II. J Lipid Res 1999; 40:287–294.

236. Gañán A, Corella D, Guillén M, et al. Frequencies of apolipoprotein A4 gene polymorphisms and association with serum lipid concentrations in two healthy Spanish populations. Hum Biol 2004; 76:253–266.

237. von Eckardstein A, Funke H, Chirazi A, et al. Sex-specific effects of the glutamine/histidine polymorphism in apo A-IV on HDL metabolism. Arterioscler Thromb 1994; 14:1114–1120.

238. Tenkanen H, Lukka M, Jauhiainen M, et al. The mutation causing the common apolipoprotein A-IV polymorphism is a glutamine to histidine substitution of amino acid 360. Arterioscler Thromb 1991; 11:851–856.

239. Hudoglugil U, Williamson DW, Huang Y, Mahley RW. An interaction between the TaqIB polymorphism of cholesterol ester transfer protein and smoking is associated with changes in plasma high-density lipoprotein cholesterol levels in Turks. Clin Genet 2005; 68:118–127.

240. American Heart Association. Body composition tests. Available at, http://www.americanheart.org/presenter.jhtml?identifier = 4489. Accessed January 19, 2006.

241. Eckel RH, Yost TJ. HDL subfractions and adipose tissue metabolism in the reduced-obese state. Am J Physiol 1989; 256(6 Pt 1):E740–E746.

242. Hu D, Hannah J, Gray RS, et al. Effects of obesity and body fat distribution on lipids and lipoproteins in nondiabetic American Indians, the Strong Heart Study. Obes Res 2000; 8:411–421.

243. Arya R, Lehman D, Hunt KJ, et al. Evidence for bivariate linkage of obesity and HDL-C levels in the Framingham Heart Study. BMC Genetics 2003; 4(suppl):S52.

244. Lamon-Fava S, Wilson PW, Scheaffer EJ, et al. Impact of body mass index on coronary heart disease risk factors in men and women: The Framingham offspring study. Arterioscler Thromb Vasc Biol 1996; 16:1509–1515.

245. Schubert CM, Rogers NL, Remsberg KE, et al. Lipids, lipoproteins, lifestyle, adiposity, and fat-free mass during middle age, the Fels Longitudinal Study. Int J Obes 2005. Available at, http://www.nature.com/ijo/journal/vaop/ncurrent/pdf/0803129a.pdf. Accessed January 20, 2006.

246. DeNino WF, Tchernof A, Dionne IJ, et al. Contribution of abdominal adiposity to age-related differences in insulin sensitivity and plasma lipids in healthy nonobese women. Diabetes Care 2001: 24:925–932.

247. Ferrara A, Barrett-Connor E, Shan J. Total, LDL, and HDL cholesterol decrease with age in older men and women. The Rancho Bernardo Study 1984–1994. Circulation 1997; 96:37–43.

248. Williams PT. Health effects resulting from exercise versus those from body fat loss. Med Sci Sports Exerc 2001; 33(6 suppl):S611–S621.

249. Pietrobelli A, Lee RC, Capristo E, et al. An independent, inverse association of high-density-lipoprotein-cholesterol concentration with nonadipose body mass. Am J Clin Nutr 1999; 69:614–620.

250. Daniels SR, Khoury PR, Morrison JA. The utility of body mass index as a measure of body fatness in children and adolescents, differences by race and gender. Pediatrics 1997; 99:804–807.

251. Appel LJ, Sacks FM, Carey VJ, et al. For the OmniHeart Collaborative Research Group. Effects of protein, monounsaturated fat, and carbohydrate intake on blood pressure and serum lipids. Results of the OmniHeart randomized trial. JAMA 2005; 294:2455–2464.

252. Dansinger ML, Gleason JA, Griffith JL, et al. Comparison of the Atkins, Ornish, Weight Watchers, and Zone diets for weight loss and heart disease risk reduction. JAMA 2005; 293:43–53.

253. Walden CE, Retzlaff BM, Buck BL, et al. Differential effect of National Cholesterol Education Program (NCEP) Step II Diet on HDL cholesterol, its subfractions, and apoprotein A-I levels in hypercholesterolemic women and men after 1 year. The beFIT Study. Arterioscler Thromb Vasc Biol 2000; 20:1580–1587.

254. Hodson L, Skeaff CM, Chisholm W-AH. The effect of replacing dietary saturated fat with polyunsaturated or monounsaturated fat on plasma lipids in free-living young adults. Eur J Clin Nutr 2001; 55:908–915.

255. Berglund L, Oliver EH, Fontanez N, et al. For the DELTA investigators. HDL-subpopulation patterns in response to reductions in dietary total and saturated fat intakes in healthy subjects. Am J Clin Nutr 1999; 70:992–1000.

256. Matthan NR, Welty FK, Barrett HR, et al. Dietary hydrogenated fat increases high-density lipoprotein apo A-I catabolism and decreases low-density lipoprotein apoV-100 catabolism in hypercholesterolemic women. Arterioscler Thromb Vasc Biol 2004; 24:1092–1097.

257. Brinton EA, Eisenberg S, Breslow JL. A low-fat diet decreases high density lipoprotein (HDL) cholesterol levels by decreasing HDL apolipoprotein transport rates. J Clin Invest 1990; 85:144–151.

258. Beard CM, Barnard J, Robbins DC, et al. Effects of diet and exercise on qualitative and quantitative measures of LDL and its susceptibility to oxidation. Arterioscler Thromb Vasc Biol 1996; 16:201–207.

259. American Heart Association. New guidelines focus on fish, fish oil, omega-3 fatty acids. Available at, http://www.americanheart.org/presenter/jhtml?identifier = 3006624. Accessed February 9, 2006.

260. Kris-Etherton P, Daniels SR, Eckel RH, et al. For the Conference Planning and Writing Committee. Summary of the Scientific Conference on Dietary Fatty Acids and Cardiovascular Health. Conference summary from the Nutrition Committee of the American Heart Association. Circulation 2001; 103:1034–1039.

261. Mattson FH, Grundy SM. Comparison of effects of dietary saturated, monounsaturated, and polyunsaturated fatty acids on plasma lipids and lipoproteins in man. J Lipid Res 1985; 26:194–202.

262. Mori TA, Burke V, Puddy IB, et al. Purified eicosapentaenoic and docosahexaenoic acids have differential effects on serum lipids and lipoproteins, LDL particle size, glucose, and insulin in mildly hyperlipidemia men. Am J Clin Nutr 2000; 71:1085–1094.

263. Effects of omega-3 fatty acids on cardiovascular risk factors and intermediate markers of cardiovascular disease. Evidence Report/Technology Assessment No. 93. Agency for Healthcare Research and Quality. Public Health Service. U.S. Department of Health and Human Services. Available at, http://www.ncbi.nlm.nih./gov/books/bs.fcgi?rid = hstatia.chapter.35161. Accessed February 9, 2006.

264. Harris WS. n-3 Fatty acids and serum lipoproteins, human studies. Am J Clin Nutr 1997; 65(suppl):1645S–1654S.

265. Marchioli R, Barzi F, Bomba E, et al. On behalf of the GISSI-Prevenzione investigators. Early protection against sudden death by n-3 polyunsaturated fatty acids after myocardial infarction. Time-course analysis of the results of the Gruppo Italiano per lo Studio delle Sopravvivenza nell'Infaarto Miocardico (GISSI)-Prevenzione. Circulation 2002; 150:1897–1903.

266. Renaud S, de Lorgeril M, Delaye J, et al. Cretan Mediterranean diet for prevention of coronary heart disease. Am J Clin Nutr 1995; 61(6 suppl):1360S–1367S.

267. de Lorgeril M, Salen P, Martin J-L, et al. Mediterranean diet, traditional risk factors, and the rate of cardiovascular complications after myocardial infarction. Final report of the Lyon Diet Heart Study. Circulation 1999; 99:779–785.

268. Woodman RJ, Mori TA, Burke V, et al. Effects of purified eicosapentaenoic and docosahexaenoic acids on glycemic control, blood pressure, and serum lipids in type 2 diabetic patients with treated hypertension. Am J Clin Nutr 2002; 76:1007–1015.

269. Calabresi L, Villa B, Canavesi M, et al. An w-3 polyunsaturated fatty acid concentrate increases plasma high-density lipoprotein 2 cholesterol and paraoxonase levels in patients with familial combined hyperlipidemia. Metabolism 2004; 53:153–158.

270. Thomas TR, Smith B, Donahue OM, et al. Effects of omega-3 fatty acid supplementation and exercise on low-density lipoprotein and high-density lipoprotein subfractions. Metabolism 2004; 53:749–754.

271. Montoya MT, Porres A, Serrano S, et al. Fatty acid saturation of the diet and plasma lipid concentrations, lipoprotein particle, concentrations, and cholesterol efflux capacity. Am J Clin Nutr 2002; 75:484–491.

272. Carr MC, Hokanson JE, Zambon A, et al. The contribution of intraabdominal fat to gender differences in hepatic lipase activity and low/high density lipoprotein heterogeneity. J Clin Endocrinol Metab 2001; 86:2831–2837.

273. Ordovas JM, Corella D, Cupples LA, et al. Polyunsaturated fatty acids modulate the effects of the APOA1 G-A polymorphism on HDL-cholesterol in a sex-specific manner, the Framingham Study. Am J Clin Nutr 2002; 75:340–346.

274. Ordovas JM. Gene–diet interaction and plasma lipid responses to dietary intervention. Biochem Soc Interact 2002; 30(Pt2):68–73.

275. Overweight, obesity, and healthy weight among persons 20 years of age and over, according to sex, age, race, and Hispanic Origin, United States, 1960–62, 1971–74, 1976–80, 1988–94, and 1999–2000. Centers for Disease Control and Prevention. Department of Health and Human Services. Available at, http://www.cdc.gov/nchs/data/hus/tables/2003/03hus/068.pdf. Accessed March 1, 2006.

276. Han TS, van Leer EM, Seidell JC, Lean MEJ. Waist circumference action levels in the identification of cardiovascular risk factors, prevalence study in a random sample. Br Med J 1995; 311:1401–1405.
277. Katzel LI, Coon PJ, Rogus E, Krauss RM, Goldberg AP. Persistence of low HDL-C levels after weight reduction in older men with small LDL particles. Arterioscler Thromb Vasc Biol 1995; 15:299–305.
278. Dattilo AM, Kris-Etherton PM. Effects of weight reduction on blood lipids and lipoproteins: a meta-analysis. Am J Clin Nutr 1992; 56:320–328.
279. Davidson MH, Hauptman J, DiGirolamo M, et al. Weight control and risk factor reduction in obese subjects treated for 2 years with orlistat. A randomized controlled trial. JAMA 1999; 281:235–242.
280. Wadden TA, Berkowitz RI, Womble LG, et al. Randomized trial of lifestyle modification and pharmacotherapy for obesity. N Engl J Med 2005; 353:2111–2120.
281. Després J-P, Golay A, Sjöström L. For the Rimonabant in Obesity—Lipids Study Group. Effects of rimonabant on metabolic risk factors in overweight patients with dyslipidemia. N Engl J Med 2005; 252:2121–2134.
282. Van Gaal LF, Mertens IL, Ballaux D. What is the relationship between risk factor reduction and degree of weight loss. Eur Heart J 2005; 7(suppl L):L21–L26.
283. Pagotto U, Pasquali R. Fighting obesity and associated risk factors by antagonizing cannabinoid type 1 receptors. [Comment] Lancet 2005; 365:1363–1364.
284. Nordmann AJ, Nordmann A, Briel M, et al. Effects of low-carbohydrate vs low-fat diets on weight loss and cardiovascular risk factors Arch Intern Med 2006; 166:285–293.
285. Stern L, Iqbal N, Seshadri P, et al. The effects of low-carbohydrate versus conventional weight loss diets in severely obese adults, one-year follow-up of a randomized trial. Ann Intern Med 2004; 140:778–785.
286. Samaha FF, Iqbal N, Seshadri P, et al. A low-carbohydrate as compared with a low-fat diet in severe obesity. N Engl J Med 2003; 348:2074–2081.
287. Yancy WS Jr, Olsen MK, Guyton JR, et al. A low-carbohydrate, ketogenic diet versus a low-fat diet to treat obesity and hyperlipidemia. Ann Intern Med 2004; 140:769–777.
288. Finer N. Does pharmacologically induced weight loss improve cardiovascular outcome? Impact of anti-obesity agents on cardiovascular risk factors. Eur Heart J Suppl 2005; 7(suppl L):L32–L38.
289. James WPT, Astrup A, Finer N, et al. For the STORM Study Group. Effect of sibutramine on weight maintenance after weight loss, a randomised trial. Lancet 2000; 356:2119–2125.
290. Lemieux I, Lamarche B, Couillard C, et al. Total cholesterol/HDL ratio vs LDL cholesterol/HDL ratio as indices of ischemic heart disease risk in men. The Quebec Cardiovascular Study. Arch Intern Med 2001; 161:2685–2692.
291. James WPT, Van Gaal L, Hewkin A, Blakesley V. Weight-loss independent effects of sibutramine on HDL cholesterol, results of a retrospective analysis. [Abstract] Presented at the 14th European Congress on Obesity, Athens, Greece, 1–4 June 2005 [Abstr No. P502]. Obes Rev 2005; 6(S1):145.
292. Vettor R, Serra R, Fabris R, et al. Effect of sibutramine on weight management and metabolic control in type 2 diabetes. A meta-analysis of clinical studies. Diabetes Care 2005; 28:942–949.
293. Rössner S, Sjöström L, Noack R, et al. On behalf of the European Orlistat Obesity Study Group. Obes Res 2000; 8:49–61.
294. Sjöström L, Rissanen A, Andersen T, et al. For the European Multicentre Orlistat Study Group. Randomised placebo-controlled trial of orlistat for weight loss and prevention of weight regain in obese patients. Lancet 1998; 352:167–173.
295. Kelley DE, Bray GA, Pi-Sunyer FX, et al. Clinical efficacy of orlistat therapy in overweight and obese patients with insulin-treated type 2 diabetes. Diabetes Care 2002; 25:1033–1041.
296. Lucas CP, Boldrin MN, Reaven GM. Effect of orlistat added to diet (30% of calories from fat) on plasma lipids, glucose, and insulin in obese patients with hypercholesterolemia. Am J Cardiol 2003; 91:961–964.
297. Torgerson JS, Hauptman J, Boldrin MN, Sjöström L. XENical in the Prevention of Diabetes in Obese Subjects (XENDOS) study. A randomized study of orlistat as an adjunct to lifestyle changes for the prevention of type 2 diabetes in obese patients. Diabetes Care 2004; 27:155–161.
298. Pi-Sunyer FX, Aronne LJ, Heshmati HM, et al. For the RIO-North America Study Group. Effect of rimonabant, a cannabinoid-1 receptor blocker, on weight and cardiometabolic risk factors in overweight or obese patients. RIO-North America, a randomized controlled trial. JAMA 2006; 295:761–775.
299. Di Marzo V, Bifulco M, De Petrocellis L. The endocannabinoid system and its therapeutic exploitation. Nat Rev Drug Discov 2004; 3:771–784.
300. Cota D, Marsicano G, Tschop M, et al. The endogenous cannabinoid system affects energy balance via central orexigenic drive and peripheral lipogenesis. J Clin Invest 2003; 112:423–431.
301. Lawlor DA, Davey Smith G, Ebrahim S, et al. Plasma adiponectin levels are associated with insulin resistance, but do not predict future risk of coronary heart disease in women. J Clin Endocrinol Metab 2005; 90:5677–5683.
302. Baratta R, Amato S, Degano C, et al. Adiponectin relationship with lipid metabolism is independent of body fat mass, evidence from both cross-sectional and intervention studies. J Clin Endocrinol Metab 2004; 89:2665–2671.
303. Qujeq D, Bijani K, Kalavi K, et al. Effects of Ramadan fasting on serum low-density and high-density lipoprotein-cholesterol concentrations. Ann Saudi Med 2002; 22:297–299.
304. Yusuf S, Ounpuu S, Dans T, et al. On behalf of the INTERHEART Study investigators. Effect of potentially modifiable risk factors associated with myocardial infarction in 52 countries (the INTERHEART study): case-control study. Lancet 2004; 364:937–952.

305. De Oliveira e Silva ER, Foster D, Harper MM, et al. Alcohol consumption raises HDL cholesterol levels by increasing the transport rate of apolipoproteins A-I and A-II. Circulation 2000; 102:2347–2352.
306. McConnell MV, Vavouranakis I, Wu LL, et al. Effects of a single, daily alcoholic beverage on lipid and hemostatic markers of cardiovascular risk. Am J Cardiol 1997; 80:1226–1228.
307. van der Gaag MS, van Tol A, Vermunt SH, et al. Alcohol consumption stimulates early steps in reverse cholesterol transport. J Lipid Res 2001; 42:2077–2083.
308. Kokkinos PF, Fernhall B. Physical activity and high density lipoprotein cholesterol levels. What is the relationship? Sports Med 1999; 28:307–314.
309. Williams PT. High-density lipoprotein cholesterol and other risk factors for coronary heart disease in female runners. N Engl J Med 1996; 334:1298–1301.
310. Skoumas J, Pitsavos C, Panagiotakos DB, et al. Physical activity, high-density lipoprotein cholesterol and other lipid levels, in men and women from the ATTICA study. Lipids Health Dis 2003, 2, 3. Available at http://www.Lipidworld.com/content/2/1/3. Accessed February 3, 2006.
311. Leon AS, Gaskill SE, Rice T, et al. Variability in the response of HDL cholesterol to exercise training in the HERITAGE Family Study. Int J Sports Med 2002; 23:1–9.
312. Welty FK, Stuart E, O'Meara M, Huddleston J. Effect of addition of exercise to therapeutic lifestyle changes diet in enabling women and men with coronary heart disease to reach Adult Treatment Panel III low-density lipoprotein goal without lowering high-density lipoprotein cholesterol. Am J Cardiol 2002; 89:1201–1204.
313. Wood PD, Stefanick ML, Williams PT, Haskell WL. The effects on plasma lipoproteins of a prudent weight-reducing diet, with or without exercise, in overweight men and women. N Engl J Med 1991; 325:461–466.
314. Berlin JA, Colditz GA. A meta-analysis of physical activity in the prevention of coronary heart disease. Am J Epidemiol 1990; 132:612–628.
315. Grundy SM, Pasternak R, Greenland P, et al. Assessment of cardiovascular risk by use of multiple-risk-factor assessment equations. A statement for healthcare professionals from the American Heart Association and the American College of Cardiology. J Am Coll Cardiol 1999; 34:1348–1359.
316. Kantor MA, Cullinane EM, Sady SP, et al. Exercise acutely increases lipoprotein-cholesterol and lipoprotein lipase activity in trained and untrained men. Metabolism 1987; 36:188–192.
317. Kraus WE, Houmard JA, Duscha BD, et al. Effects of the amount and intensity of exercise on plasma lipoproteins. N Engl J Med 2002; 347:1483–1492.
318. Wilmore JH. Dose-response, variation with age, sex, and health status. Med Sci Sports Exerc 2001; 33(6 suppl):S622–S634.
319. Eisenmann JC, Womack CJ, Reeves MJ, et al. Blood lipids of young distance runners, distribution and inter-relationships among training volume, peak oxygen consumption, and body fatness. Eur J Appl Physiol 2001; 85:104–112.
320. Duncan GE, Anton SD, Sydeman SJ, et al. Prescribing exercise at varied levels of intensity and frequency. A randomized trial. Arch Intern Med 2005; 165:2362–2369.
321. Zhang JQ, Smith B, Langdon MM, et al. Changes in LPLA and reverse cholesterol transport variables during 24-h postexercise period. Am J Physiol Endocrinol Metab 2002; 283:E267–E274.
322. Couillard C, Després J-P, Lamarche B, et al. Effects of endurance exercise training on plasma HDL cholesterol levels depend on levels of triglycerides. Evidence from men of the Health, Risk Factors, Exercise Training and Genetics (HERITAGE) Family Study. Arterioscler Thromb Vasc Biol 2001; 21:1226–1232.
323. Health effects resulting from exercise versus those from body fat loss. Med Sci Sports Exerc 2001; 33(6 suppl):S611–S621.
324. Mora S, Lee I-M, Buring JE, Ridker PM. Association of physical activity and body mass index with novel and traditional cardiovascular biomarkers in women. JAMA 2006; 295:1412–1419.
325. Durstine JL, Haskell WL. Effects of exercise training on plasma lipids and lipoproteins. Exerc Sport Sci Rev 1994; 22:477–521.
326. Borggreve SE, de Vries R, Dullaart RPF. Alterations in high-density lipoprotein metabolism and reverse cholesterol transport in insulin resistance and type 2 diabetes mellitus, role of lipolytic enzymes, lecithin, cholesterol acyltransferase and lipid transfer protein. Eur J Clin Investig 2003; 33:1051–1069.
327. Gill JMR, Al-Mamari A, Ferrell WR, et al. Effects of a moderate exercise session on postprandial lipoproteins, apolipoproteins and lipoprotein remnants in middle-aged men. Atherosclerosis 2006; 185:87–96.
328. Thompson PD, Buchner D, Piña IL, et al. Exercise and physical activity in the prevention and treatment of atherosclerotic cardiovascular disease. A statement from the Council on Clinical Cardiology (Subcommittee on Exercise, Rehabilitation, and Prevention) and the Council on Nutrition, Physical Activity, and Metabolism (Subcommittee on Physical Activity). Circulation 2003; 107:3109–3116.
329. Sánchez-Quesada JL, Ortega H, Payés-Romero A, et al. LDL from aerobically-trained subjects shows higher resistance to oxidative modification than LDL from sedentary subjects. Atherosclerosis 1997; 132:207–213.
330. Wilund KR, Ferrell RE, Phares DA, et al. Changes in high-density lipoprotein-cholesterol subfractions with exercise training may be dependent on cholesteryl ester transfer protein (CETP) genotype. Metabolism 2002; 51:774–778.

331. Thompson PD, Rader DJ. Does exercise increase HDL cholesterol in those who need it the most? [Editorial] Arterioscler Thromb Vasc Biol 2001; 21:1097–1098.

332. Herrington DM, Reboussin DM, Brosnihan B, et al. Effects of estrogen replacement on the progression of coronary-artery atherosclerosis. N Engl J Med 2000; 343:522–529.

333. Hulley S, Grady D, Bush T, et al. For the Heart and Estrogen/progestin Replacement Study (HERS) Research Group. Randomized trial of estrogen plus progestin for secondary prevention of coronary heart disease in postmenopausal women. JAMA 1998; 280:605–613.

334. Effects of estrogen or estrogen/progestin regimens on heart disease risk factors in postmenopausal women. The Postmenopausal Estrogen/Progestin Interventions (PEPI) trial. The Writing Group for the PEPI trial. JAMA 1995; 273:199–203.

335. Effects of conjugated equine estrogen in postmenopausal women with hysterectomy. The Women's Health Initiative randomized controlled trial. JAMA 2004; 291:1701–1712.

336. Krauss RM. Individualized hormone-replacement therapy? [Editorial] N Engl J Med 2002; 346:1017–1018.

337. Jin F-Y, Kamanna VS, Kashyap ML. Estradiol stimulates apolipoprotein A-I–but not A-II–containing particle synthesis and secretion by stimulating mRNA transcription rate in HepG2 cells. Arterioscler Thromb Vasc Biol 1998; 18:999–1006.

338. Tikkanen MHJ, Nikkila EA, Juusi T, Sipinen SU. High density lipoprotein-2 and hepatic lipase, reciprocal changes produced by estrogen and norgestrel. J Clin Endocrinol Metab 1982; 54:1113–1117.

339. Tall AR, Wang N, Mucksavage P. Is it time to modify the reverse cholesterol transport model? [Commentary] J Clin Invest 2001; 108:1273–1275.

340. Fan Y-M, Dastidar P, Jokela H, et al. Review, hepatic lipase C-480T genotype-dependent benefit from long-term hormone replacement therapy for atherosclerosis in postmenopausal women. J Clin Endocrinol Metab 2005; 90:3786–3792.

341. Louth K. WHI Broad Agency Announcement (BAA) Solicitation in Federal Business Opportunities. Request for Proposals No. NHLBI-WH-06–09. January 6, 2006. National Institutes of Health. National Heart, Lung, and Blood Institute. Available at, http://www.nhlbi.nih.gov/whi/index.html. Accessed March 20, 2006.

342. Donahoo WT, Kosmiski LA, Eckel RH. Drugs causing dyslipoproteinemia. Endocrinol Metab Clin North Am 1998; 27:677–697.

343. Behrens G, Dejam A, Schmidt H, et al. Impaired glucose tolerance, beta cell function and lipid metabolism in HIV patients under treatment with protease inhibitors. AIDS 1999; 13:F63–F70.

344. van Leth F, Phanuphak P, Stroes E, et al. Nevirapine and efavirenz elicit different changes in lipid profiles in antiretroviral-therapy-naïve patients infected with HIV-1. PloS Medicine 2004, 1, 064–074. Available at, http://www.plosmedicine.org.

345. Fisac C, Virgili N, Ferrer E, et al. A comparison of the effects of nevirapine and nelfinavir on metabolism and body habitus in antiretroviral-naïve human immunodeficiency virus-infected patients, a randomized controlled study. J Clin Endocrinol Metab 2003; 88:5186–5192.

346. Riddler SA, Smit E, Cole SR, et al. Impact of HIV infection and HAART on serum lipids in men. JAMA 2003; 289:2978–2982.

347. Combination antiretroviral therapy and the risk of myocardial infarction. The Data Collection on Adverse Events of Anti-HIV Drugs (DAD) Study Group. N Engl J Med 2003; 349:1993–2003.

348. Aynaci FM, Orhan F, Örem A, et al. Effect of antiepileptic drugs on plasma lipoprotein (a) and other lipid levels in childhood. Child Neurol 2001; 16;364–385.

349. Zelcer N, Tontonoz P. Liver X receptors as integrators of metabolic and inflammatory signaling. J Clin Invest 2006; 116:607–614.

350. Repa JJ, Mangelsdorf DJ. The role of orphan nuclear receptors in the regulation of cholesterol homeostasis. Annu Rev Cell Dev Biol 2000; 16:459–481.

351. Chiang JYL, Kimmel R, Stroup D. Regulation of cholesterol 7a-hydroxylase gene (CYP7A1) transcription by the liver orphan receptor (LXRa). Gene 2001; 626:257–265.

352. Joseph SB, McKilligan E, Pei L, et al. Synthetic LXR ligand inhibits the development of atherosclerosis in mice. Proc Natl Acad Sci USA 2002; 99:7604–7609.

353. Tangirala RK, Bischoff ED, Joseph SB, et al. Identification of macrophage liver X receptors as inhibitors of atherosclerosis. Proc Natl Acad Sci USA 2002; 99:11896–11901.

354. Miao B, Zondlo S, Gibbs S, et al. Raising HDL-C without inducing hepatic steatosis and hypertriglyceridemia by a selective LXR modulator. J Lipid Res 2004; 45:1410–1417.

355. Levin N, Bischoff ED, Daige CL, et al. Macrophage liver X receptor is required for antiatherogenic activity of LXR agonists. Arterioslcer Thromb Vasc Biol 2005; 25:135–142.

356. Franceschini G, Calabresi L, Tosi C, et al. Apolipoprotein AIMilano, disulfide-linked dimers increase high density lipoprotein stability and hinder particle interconversion in carrier plasma. J Biol Chem 1990; 265:12224–12231.

357. Franceschini G, Sirtori CR, Capurso A, et al. A-I Milano apoprotein, decreased high density lipoprotein cholesterol levels with significant lipoprotein modifications and without atherosclerosis in an Italian family. J Clin Invest 1980; 66:892–900.

358. Sirtori CR, Calabresi L, Franceschini G, et al. Cardiovascular status of the carriers of the apolipoprotein AI Milano mutant. The Limone sul Garda Study. Circulation 2001; 103:1949–1954.

359. Franceschini G, Calabresi L, Chiesa G, et al. Increased cholesterol efflux potential of sera from ApoA-I Milano carriers and transgenic mice. Arterioscler Thromb Vasc Biol 1999; 19:1257–1262.

360. Li D, Weng S, Yang B, et al. Inhibition of arterial thrombus formation by ApoA1 Milano. Arterioscler Thromb Vasc Biol 1999; 19:378–383.

361. Bielicki JK, Oda MN. Apolipoprotein A-IMilano and apolipoprotein A-IParis exhibit an antioxidant activity distinct from that of wild-type apolipoprotein A-I. Biochemistry 2002; 41:2089–2096.

362. Ameli S, Hultgardh-Nilsson A, Regnstrom J, et al. Effect of immunization with homologous LDL and oxidized LDL on early atherosclerosis in hypercholesterolemic rabbits. Arterioscler Thromb Vasc Biol 1996; 16:1074–1079.

363. Shah PK, Nilsson J, Laul S, et al. Effects of recombinant apolipoprotein A-I(Milano) on aortic athero-sclerosis in apolipoprotein E-deficient mice. Circulation 1998; 97:780–785.

364. Shah PK, Yano J, Teyes O, et al. High-dose recombinant apolipoprotein A-I(Milano) mobilizes tissue cholesterol and rapidly reduces plaque lipid and macrophage content in apolipoprotein E-deficient mice. Potential implications for acute plaque stabilization. Circulation 2001; 103:3047–3050.

365. Chiesa G, Monteggia E, Marchesi M, et al. Recombinant apolipoprotein A-I(Milano) infusion into rab-bit carotid artery rapidly removes lipid from fatty streaks. Circ Res 2002; 90:974–980.

366. Navab M, Anantharamaiah GM, Reddy ST, et al. Apolipoprotein A-I mimetic peptides. Arterioscler Thromb Vasc Biol 2005; 25:1325–1331.

367. Garber DW, Datta G, Chaddha M, et al. A new synthetic class A amphipathic peptide analogue pro-tects mice from diet-induced atherosclerosis. J Lipid Res 2001; 42:545–552.

368. Mendez A, Anantharamaiah GM, Segrest JP, Oram JF. Synthetic amphipathic helical peptides that mimic apolipoprotein A-I in clearing cellular cholesterol. J Clin Invest 1994; 94:1698–1705.

369. Navab M, Anantharamaiah GM, Hama S, et al. Oral administration of an apoA-I mimetic peptide synthesized from D-amino acids dramatically reduces atherosclerosis in mice independent of plasma cholesterol. Circulation 2002; 105:290–292.

370. Li X, Chyu K, Neto JR, et al. Differential effects of apolipoprotein A-I-mimetic peptide on evolving and established atherosclerosis in apolipoprotein E-null mice. Circulation 2004; 110:1701–1705.

371. Okamoto H, Yonemori F, Wakitani K, et al. A cholesteryl ester transfer protein inhibitor attenuates atherosclerosis in rabbits. Nature 2000; 406:203–207.

372. de Grooth GJ, Kuivenhoven JA, Stalenhoef AF, et al. Efficacy and safety of novel cholesteryl ester transfer protein inhibitor, JTT-705, in humans, a randomised phase II dose-response study. Circulation 2002; 105:2159–2165.

373. Clark RW, Sutfin TA, Ruggeri RB, et al. Raising high-density lipoprotein in humans through inhibi-tion of cholesteryl ester transfer protein, an initial multidose study of torcetrapib. Arterioscler Thromb Vasc Biol 2004; 24:490–497.

374. Brousseau ME, Schaefer EJ, Wolfe ML, et al. Effects of an inhibitor of cholesteryl ester transfer pro-tein on HDL cholesterol. N Engl J Med 2004; 350:1505–1515.

375. Barter PJ, Brewer HB, Chapman MJ, et al. Cholesteryl ester transfer protein. A novel target for rais-ing HDL and inhibiting atherosclerosis. Arterioscler Thromb Vasc Biol 2003; 23:160–167.

376. Prueksaritanont T, Zhao JJ, Ma B, et al. Mechanistic studies on metabolic interactions between gem-fibrozil and statins. J Pharmacol Exp Ther 2002; 301:1042–1051.

377. Nissen SE, Tsunoda T, Tuzcu EM, et al. Effect of recombinant apoA-I Milano on coronary atherosclerosis in patients with acute coronary syndromes, a randomized controlled trial. JAMA 2003; 290:2292–2300.

9 | Triglycerides and Risk for Atherosclerotic Disease

Gérald Luc, Patrick Duriez, and Jean-Charles Fruchart
Department of Atherosclerosis, INSERM U545, University of Lille 2, Institut Pasteur de Lille, Lille, France

KEY POINTS

- Plasma triglyceride levels are the results of an interaction between genetic and environmental factors. Among known genetic factors are apoE, lipoprotein lipase, apoCIII, and apoAV gene polymorphisms. The environmental factors are drugs (retinoids, antiproteases, corticoids, antihypertensive agents...) and alcohol consumption, but in a majority of subjects, overweight which induces the metabolic syndrome.
- Triglycerides are considered an independent risk factor for atherosclerosis, but the risk associated with triglycerides is more pronounced in the presence of a high low-density lipoprotein (LDL) and/or low high-density lipoprotein (HDL) level.
- No clinical trial was specifically published in hypertriglyceridemic subjects with metabolic syndrome, but fibrates (gemfibrozil and bezafibrate) appear to prevent coronary and cerebrovascular events in subjects with hypertriglyceridemia-low HDL levels.
- The therapeutic strategy in hypertriglyceridemic patients is firstly to initiate lifestyle changes or stop hypertriglyceridemic drug if possible, secondly to decrease non-HDL-cholesterol (total cholesterol-HDL-cholesterol) levels below the initially defined objective regards the atherosclerotic risk of the patient using statins or a combination of statins with other hypocholesterolemic drugs such as ezetimibe, and thirdly to prescribe fibrate treatment (with the exception of gemfibrozil) in the presence of the association hypertriglyceridemia–low HDL-cholesterol.

INTRODUCTION

Hypertriglyceridemia, which can be defined as fasting triglyceride levels greater than 150 mg/dL, is a prevalent form of dyslipoproteinemia in all populations. The underlying pathophysiological mechanisms that result in elevations of plasma triglycerides are heterogeneous and, in most cases, incompletely understood. This heterogeneity leads to difficulty in the diagnosis and prediction of a future ischemic attack, as coronary heart disease (CHD) risk is likely to differ according to the type of biological mechanisms causing the hyperlipoproteinemia.

HYPERTRIGLYCERIDEMIA AND CARDIOVASCULAR RISK

Multivariate analyses performed in most prospective cohort studies have shown an absence of association between triglycerides and CHD risk, whereas this association is significant with univariate analysis. The absence of any significant association in multivariate analysis is mainly due to adjustment for HDL-cholesterol (HDL-C). Indeed, triglycerides and HDL-C are negatively and highly correlated, and low HDL-C has always been a powerful risk factor in all cohort studies. Furthermore, hypertriglyceridemia is frequently associated with a set of other complex abnormalities such as small dense LDL, hyperinsulinemia, and noninsulin-dependent diabetes, each having a role in atherogenesis. Finally, the intra- and inter-individual variability of serum triglycerides is likely to weaken the strength of the relationship between triglycerides and CHD.

However, despite factors that tend to diminish the relationship between triglycerides and CHD risk, a meta-analysis including more than 46,000 men and nearly 11,000 women in prospective cohort studies in the United States and in different European countries has shown that the univariate relative risk estimates for cardiovascular disease (CVD) associated with a 1 mmol/L (87 mg/dL) increase in triglycerides are significantly high, on an average of 1.32 ($p < 0.05$) and 1.76 ($p < 0.05$) in men and women, respectively. These relative risks were attenuated after adjustment for HDL-C but remained significant: 1.14 and 1.37 in men and women, respectively. Thus, even after adjustment for HDL-C (and other usual risks factors), a statistically significant increase in the risk of incident CVD was associated with triglycerides; the relative risk, however, being higher in women than in men. Strong evidence has therefore emerged that triglyceride-rich particle levels [principally very-low-density lipoprotein (VLDL)] are at least partly a risk factor, independent of variations in HDL-C.

Triglycerides independently predict CHD in cohorts, and combinations of adverse levels of the three major lipid risk factors—total cholesterol (TC), triglycerides, and HDL-C—have no greater impact on CHD than that expected from their individual contribution (1). Geographic comparisons also show differences between countries. In men, the relative risk was clearly higher in Scandinavia (2.49 for 1 mmol/L increase in triglycerides) than in other European countries (1.25) and the United States (1.34). A similar difference was observed for women in Scandinavia (2.02) and the United States (1.71) (2).

NON-HIGH-DENSITY LIPOPROTEIN CHOLESTEROL AS A RISK FACTOR

The measurement of non-HDL-C (total serum cholesterol minus HDL-C) is useful for identifying dyslipoproteinemia, characterizing risk for CHD, and assessing response to hypolipidemic therapy, as suggested by the following:

(i)   VLDLs are heterogeneous. A fraction of these particles, which are richer in cholesterol and poorer in triglycerides than VLDLs as a whole may constitute a particularly atherogenic group of lipoproteins (3).
(ii) An increase in large VLDL, particularly present in hypertriglyceridemic patients, possesses a high atherogenic potential because the particles can be taken up by macrophages and cause the formation of foam cells, a hallmark of early atherosclerotic lesions, and these are associated with procoagulant and prothrombotic factors in plasma (4).
(iii) The Friedewald formula used to calculate LDL cholesterol (LDL-C) from TC, triglyceride, and HDL-C plasma levels is progressively less accurate as plasma triglyceride concentrations increase and the formula is generally considered inapplicable when triglyceride levels exceed 400 mg/dL (5) or in diabetic patients because of the altered composition of VLDL or in the presence of high levels of remnants in the intermediate-density lipoprotein (IDL) density range.

The use of non-HDL-C as a tool to assess risk has the advantage of including all of the cholesterol considered atherogenic in lipoprotein particles [VLDL, IDL, LDL, and lipoprotein(a)]. Non-HDL-C is a therapeutic target in subjects with triglycerides above 200 mg/dL. This is particularly true in diabetic subjects, with CHD risk increasing along with increasing non-HDL-C, but not with increasing LDL cholesterol (6).

ETIOLOGY AND PATHOPHYSIOLOGY

Hypertriglyceridemia is the consequence of genetic and environmental factors. Most hypertriglyceridemic patients probably have two or more such disorders even if it is difficult to establish them in each individual. Mechanistically, hypertriglyceridemia is due to a decreased catabolism of plasma triglyceride-rich lipoproteins (chylomicrons and VLDL) and their remnants or an increased hepatic secretion of VLDL, or both.

Genetic Factors

The metabolism of triglyceride-rich lipoproteins depends on a number of protein activities. The genes coding for these proteins have, therefore, been analyzed by analyzing the relationship between their polymorphisms and serum triglyceride levels (Table 1).

Lipoprotein Lipase

Lipoprotein lipase (LPL) plays a major role in the catabolism of triglyceride-rich lipoproteins by hydrolyzing triglycerides from the core of these particles. Mutations in the LPL gene leading to LPL deficiency have been found in severe hypertriglyceridemic patients suffering from hyperchylomicronemia (type-I hyperlipoproteinemia).

TABLE 1 Genetic Factors Promoting Hypertriglyceridemia

Gene/protein	Function or pathophysiology	Mutations/ polymorphisms	CHD risk
Lipoprotein lipase	Hydrolysis of triglycerides	>200 mutations Homozygosity (hyperchylomicronemia—type I) Chylomicrons VLDL LDL HDL	Pancreatitis
		Heterozygosity VLDL LDL HDL	CHD risk x 2–5
ApoCII	Cofactor of lipoprotein lipase	Homozygosity (hyperchylomicronemia—type I)	Pancreatitis
		Heterozygosity TG or	?
Hepatic lipase	Catabolism of triglyceride-rich and cholesterol-rich lipoproteins	~10 common and rare mutations	
		Homozygosity	Hypertriglyceridemia, accumulation of β VLDL and HDL
		Heterozygosity	Hypertriglyceridemia, accumulation of β VLDL and HDL observed in a few mutations
ApoCIII	Inhibitor of apo CII activated lipoprotein lipase	Mutations in the insulin response element of the promoter	
	Uptake of TG-rich lipoproteins	TG (interaction with smoking ?)	
ApoAV	Stimulus of lipolysis ?	Polymorphisms - 1131T/C S19W TG	?
ApoE	Uptake of remnants	Allele e2: TG /remnants Allele e4: TG LDL e2/e2 genotype + other genetic or environmental factor: dyslipoproteinemia (type III)	CHD and peripheral vascular risk
PPAR γ	Transcription factor regulating several genes involved in lipid and glucose metabolism	P12 A of PPARg2 12A - interaction with dietary fat: if >37% energy, a supplementation with *n*-3 fatty acids decrease TG	?
PPAR α	Transcription factor regulating several genes involved in lipid metabolism	L162V TG (possible interaction with dietary polyunsaturated fatty acids) 7G>C:G/G genotype associated with a higher response to fibrate	?
FCHL	Overproduction of VLDL-apoB Increase in apoB levels	Metabolic syndrome + genetic factors (LPL; apoAI/CIII/AIV/AV genecluster; ASP; USF1)	1.7–5
Familial hypertriglyceridemia	Overproduction of triglycerides into VLDL		

Abbreviations: ASP, acylation stimulation protein; CHD coronary heart disease; FCHL, familial combined hyperlipoproteinemia; HDL, high-density lipoprotein; LDL, low-density lipoprotein; LPL, lipoprotein lipase; PPAR, peroxisome proliferator activated receptor; TG, triglycerides; USF, upstream transcription factor; VLDL, very-low-density-lipoprotein.

Hyperchylomicronemia is a rare disorder (frequency 1/1,000,000) characterized by severe hypertriglyceridemia, as triglyceride levels are often above 2000 mg/dL. Most patients are detected in infancy, but diagnosis is not noted before the fourth decade in some subjects. Triglyceride plasma levels are checked because of clinical manifestations such as abdominal pain sometimes due to acute pancreatitis, which can be fatal. In half of the patients, papuloeruptive xanthomas have appeared on the skin at one time or another.

Plasma triglycerides are essentially carried in chylomicrons. The VLDL fraction level is often moderately increased whereas LDL-C and HDL-C are low. No premature atherosclerosis seems to result from this hyperlipoproteinemia, even if peripheral or coronary atherosclerosis or both have sometimes been observed before the age of 55 (7). The occurrence of atherosclerosis could be due to the presence of other usual risk factors and/or the appearance of diabetes favored by the recurrence of bouts of acute pancreatitis.

The deficit in LPL activity, which leads to hyperchylomicronemia, can be due to mutations in the LPL gene inducing a loss of LPL activity, or in the apolipoprotein (apo) CII gene, the obligatory cofactor of LPL. For both types of mutations, a homozygous or double heterozygous state needs to be present to induce hyperchylomicronemia. More than 200 mutations in the LPL gene associated with LPL deficiency have been reported, these mutations being mainly (75% of them) in exons 5 and 6 of the gene, which correspond to the sequence for the catalytic site of the enzyme. The presence of heterozygosity for LPL deficiency leads to moderate hypertriglyceridemia associated with low HDL-C levels as early as under the age of 40 (8). In a meta-analysis, the effect of the four most frequent LPL mutations was assessed. For three of these mutations (G188E, D9N, and N291S) that were associated with a decrease in LPL activity, plasma triglycerides increased by 20% to 78% and HDL-C decreased by 3 to 10 mg/dL in heterozygous carriers (9,10). Two of these mutations (G188E and D9N) were associated with a risk of CVD, five times and two times more, respectively, than in noncarriers (10). Conversely, subjects with S447X mutation had lower triglyceride levels and trend toward a decrease in the incidence of vascular disease (11).

Apolipoprotein CII

ApoCII is an obligatory positive cofactor of LPL. A deficit in apoCII due to the presence of apo CII mutations in the homozygous state is a rare disorder. The patients carrying these abnormalities are severely hypertriglyceridemic (type-I hyperlipoproteinemia) because of a deficiency in LPL activity, and heterozygotes can be hypertriglyceridemic (12).

Hepatic Lipase

Hepatic lipase participates in the catabolism of triglyceride-rich and cholesterol-rich remnant particles as well as in that of HDL. The effects of hepatic lipase deficiency are hypertriglyceridemia and a rise in HDL-C levels. The presence of V73M and L334P mutations in the heterozygote state are found more frequently in subjects with combined hypertriglyceridemia and hyperalphalipoproteinemia than in normolipidemic controls (13).

Apolipoprotein CIII

ApoCIII has been proposed as an inhibitor of apoCII-activated LPL, acting either by direct LPL inhibition or by displacement of apoCII from triglyceride-rich lipoproteins. ApoCIII lowers the cellular uptake of apoB-containing lipoproteins mediated through the LDL receptor (14) and plays a role in their hepatic uptake. Two potential variants of apoCIII (−482C>T and −455T>C), due to mutations in the promoter region mediating the expression of the gene to insulin, have been described and appear particularly interesting. The presence of the less frequent allele has been associated with higher triglyceride levels than in subjects carrying the other alleles for both polymorphisms. Interaction between the presence of polymorphism −482C>T and smoking is interesting as no difference in triglycerides was displayed in nonsmokers, whereas smoking carriers of the rare allele had higher triglycerides than the noncarriers with a dose allele-effect (15). Furthermore, subjects carrying the −455C variant had higher triglyceride levels and higher CHD risk than noncarriers, this effect being accentuated in subjects with metabolic syndrome (16,17).

Apolipoprotein AV

ApoAV was recently identified when an orthologous sequence spanning the apoAI/CIII/AIV gene cluster was compared in humans and in mice (18). Mice with targeted inactivation of the apoAV gene have a marked rise in serum triglycerides compared to controls because of an accumulation of VLDL, while mice overexpressing this gene have reduced triglyceride levels (18). Sequence analysis of the apoAV gene revealed mutations in apoAV (Q145X; Q139X), which predicted the generation of a truncated apoAV in severe hypertriglyceridemic subjects (triglycerides >1200 mg/dL) presenting no mutations in LPL and apoCII genes. Hypertriglyceridemic subjects were heterozygous or homozygous carriers of these mutations, the former being closely associated with the presence of a second allele of one or two previously described triglyceride-raising minor apoAV haplotypes (see below) (19,20).

A number of polymorphisms have been described in the apoAV gene and the respective effect of each polymorphism on triglyceride levels assessed. Globally, two single nucleotide polymorphisms (−1131T/C and S19W) were associated with higher triglyceride levels compared to noncarriers. However, comparisons between populations suggest that the influence of the apoAV gene on lipid metabolism, which is not yet clearly established, may be dependent on both race and gender (21). The apoAV S19W polymorphism is a functional polymorphism and in a population of healthy middle-aged men, homozygosity for this allelic variant is associated with the highest plasma triglycerides among all polymorphic variants described in the apoA1/C3/A4/A5 gene cluster (22).

Apolipoprotein E

Three common alleles (ε2, 3, and 4) acting at a single gene locus code for three major isoforms of the protein, E2, E3, and E4 in plasma, determine six apoE phenotypes. The various isoforms interact differently with specific lipoprotein receptors and ultimately alter the circulating levels of cholesterol and triglycerides. A number of studies have identified the impact of a specific allele on plasma lipid levels. They have shown that subjects carrying the allele ε2 or ε4 have higher triglyceride levels than subjects with the more frequent E3/E3 phenotype (23–25), but only allele ε4 leads to an elevated CHD relative risk (24,26).

The apoE genotype has been studied in disorders associated with hyperlipoproteinemia. Type-III hyperlipoproteinemia or dysbetalipoproteinemia results from factors that directly overload remnant lipoprotein production or disrupt removal pathways. An association between apoE2/2 and type-III hyperlipoproteinemia has been known for decades (27). This disorder is characterized by increased cholesterol and triglycerides (with a ratio between these levels expressed in mg/dL frequently around 1), the presence of β-VLDL, which are cholesterol-rich remnants of triglyceride-rich lipoproteins, specific xanthomas and premature vascular disease, and both CHD and peripheral arterial disease (28). Although the frequency of the apoε2/2 genotype is 0.5% to 1.0% in Caucasian populations, type-III hyperlipoproteinemia occurs with a frequency of 1.5 per 5000 (29). Thus, the ε2/2 genotype contributes to type-III hyperlipoproteinemia without being its sole cause. Subjects carrying the ε2/2 genotype without hyperlipoproteinemia have rather lower cholesterol and triglyceride levels than subjects with the wild genotype (E3/3). Genetic (30) or environmental factors could shift a normolipidemia toward type-III hyperlipoproteinemia in an ε2/2 subject.

■ Case Study for Type-III Hyperlipoproteinemia

E.D. is a 36-year-old man in whom hyperlipoproteinemia was discovered during familial screening, his father having a high cholesterol level. The patient was clinically well, but his weight had increased over the two previous years after stopping intensive physical activity, his body mass index (BMI) increasing from 27.0 to 32.1 kg/m². With the exception of abdominal obesity (waist circumference: 104 cm), the clinical examination showed nothing remarkable. The ultrasound examination of carotid and peripheral arteries was normal. No extravascular deposit was noted.

The two first lipid measurements (without any treatment) showed cholesterol at 469 and 404 mg/dL and triglycerides at 508 and 433 mg/dL. HDL-C was 68 and 59 mg/dL. Thyroid-stimulating hormone (TSH) was normal and no diabetes was noted. ApoE phenotype was determined from plasma and was defined as apo E2/2, and type-III hyperlipoproteinemia was diagnosed.

A diet was prescribed, the patient lost 6 kg and thereafter his weight remained stable. The weight loss had no influence on lipid levels. Fenofibrate therapy was initiated and the results on lipid levels were as follows after two and six months of therapy: cholesterol: 181 and 166 mg/dL; triglycerides: 113 and 84 mg/dL. Fenofibrate was well tolerated and the treatment was continued.

Remarks

(i) Type-III hyperlipoproteinemia was suspected because of elevated concentrations (expressed in mg/dL) of cholesterol and triglycerides.

(ii) The clinical examination showed no extravascular lipid deposits, particularly no tuberoeruptive xanthomas or xanthoma striata palmaris. These cholesterol deposits are not constant (and rather rare in the authors' experience) in type-III hyperlipoproteinemia.

(iii) The diagnosis was confirmed because of the association of mixed hyperlipoproteinemia with the apoE2/2 phenotype. Determination of the apoE2/2 phenotype requires a specialized laboratory. A lipoprotein electrophoresis could be carried out to find a broad-beta band (a large band between pre-beta and beta lipoproteins), but this analysis is no longer performed in clinical laboratories.

(iv) Type-III hyperlipoproteinemia appeared in this patient because of the association of apoE2 homozygosity and one or several other factors. These factors could be genetic factors such as those determining the hypercholesterolemia in his father or environmental factors such as obesity. These factors often induce an overproduction of VLDL and then remnants that $\varepsilon 2/2$ subjects have difficulty clearing because of poor binding of apoE2 to hepatic receptors.

(v) Hypolipidemic treatment is justified because of the high risk of CHD and peripheral arterial disease in subjects with type-III hyperlipoproteinemia, even if clinical trials to verify the clinical efficacy of treatment have not been performed because of the relatively small number of subjects with this pathology. Fibrates are usually very effective in this disease, as in the patient described above, but nicotinic acid or statins could also be used (31).

Peroxisome Proliferator Activated Receptor

Peroxisome Proliferator Activated Receptor Gamma

Peroxisome proliferator–activated receptor gamma (PPARγ) controls adipocyte differentiation, and regulates lipid and glucose homeostasis. Therefore, the PPARγ gene may affect insulin sensitivity and, by a sequence of steps, the synthesis of triglycerides and their plasma levels.

The association of triglycerides and the presence of PPAR polymorphisms have been analyzed in different populations, diabetic or not, obese or not, in both women and men. The results of analyses of the association between the Pro12Ala polymorphism of the PPARγ2 gene and lipids are divergent, showing either no association (32,33), higher triglycerides in subjects with Ala12 (34), or lower triglyceride levels in Ala12 subjects compared with those carrying Pro12Pro allele (35). These differences were perhaps due to an inter action between this polymorphism and environmental factors, particularly dietary fatty acids (FA). Indeed, in subjects carrying the 12Ala allele, supplementation with *n*-3 fatty acid decreased triglyceride levels in those fed with a dietary fat intake below 37% of total energy intake whereas the PPARγ2 polymorphism had no effect on subjects eating above 37% fat (32).

Peroxisome Proliferator–Activated Receptor Alpha

Peroxisome proliferator–activated receptor alpha (PPARα) is a nuclear transcription factor regulating a number of genes involved in lipoprotein metabolism. Several variants were found in the gene. The association of these variants with serum lipids showed that only L162V and intron 7G>C polymorphisms appeared to be associated with triglyceride levels. Triglyceride levels were 20% to 30% lower in subjects carrying the L162V variant, especially women (36,37). A few studies suggest a gene-nutrient and gene-hypolipidemic treatment interaction in relation to serum triglycerides. A variation in polyunsaturated fatty acid (PUFA) intake leads to a large modification in serum triglycerides in 162V carriers compared to that observed in 162L homozygotes. Triglycerides were then 28% higher in 162V than in 162L/L subjects with low PUFA intake (<4%) whereas triglycerides were 4% lower when PUFA was above 8% (38). Furthermore, the intron 7 G/G genotype was associated with a higher fenofibrate response in type 2 diabetes (Fig. 1) (39).

Alterations in Bile Acid Metabolism

A positive correlation between bile acid turnover and plasma VLDL triglyceride levels has been recognized. Interruption of the enterohepatic circulation of bile acids with cholestyramine transiently increased plasma triglyceride levels, whereas the increase in biliary acid pool after the administration of chenodeoxycholic acid decreased them. It is therefore assumed that a primary

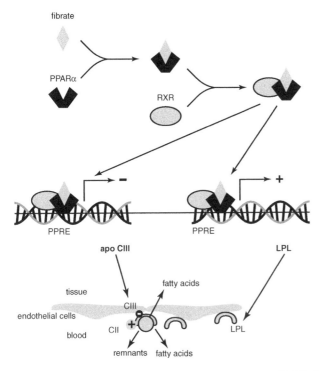

FIGURE 1 Peroxisome proliferator–activated receptor (PPAR) alpha induces transcription of lipoprotein lipase (LPL) gene and negative regulation of apolipoprotein (apo) CIII gene: Peroxisome proliferator response element (PPRE), consisting of imperfect direct repeats of the sequence TGACCT spaced by a single base pair, have been identified in the upstream regulatory sequences of several PPAR-targeted genes. The retinoic X receptor (RXR) ligand, 9 cis-retinoic acid, enhances PPAR action by activating the RXR, which forms a heterodimer with PPAR that binds to the PPRE to induce gene transcription. Upon activation by fibrates, PPAR could (a) increase the expression of LPL gene by binding of the heterodimer PPARα/RXR to the PPRE (b) repress apoCIII promoter by two modes of action. In a direct mechanism, nonproductive binding of PPAR–RXR heterodimers displaces hepatocyte nuclear factor-4 from the element CIIIB and thereby inhibits transactivation by transforming growth factor–signal transduction. Alternatively, in a multistep process, PPAR–RXR could bind a Rev-DR2 element in Rev-erb gene promoter (B), and increase its expression. Then monomers of Rev-erb antagonize activation by ROR1 and repress the activity of human apoCIII promoter (C). Moreover, upon activation of PPAR, the negative autoregulation of Rev-erb could be diminished because of a competition between PPAR–RXR and homodimers of Rev-erb. *Source*: From Refs. 39, 40.

defect in bile acid metabolism stimulates VLDL triglyceride production. Mutations and polymorphisms have been checked in genes involved in bile acid metabolism. With the exception of a rare mutation in the gene coding ileal bile acid transporter gene, no mutation or polymorphism was in a higher proportion in familial hypertriglyceridemic subjects than in controls (42). However, many other genes, which play a role in bile acid or salt metabolism, have not yet been explored.

Familial Hypertriglyceridemia

Several inherited hypertriglyceridemic disorders other than hyperchylomicronemia have been delineated from the analysis of lipid levels in families. Among these, familial combined hyperlipoproteinemia (FCHL) and familial hypertriglyceridemia (FHTG) were defined many years ago (43,44).

FCHL is the most common inherited hyperlipoproteinemia with a frequency of approximately 1% in all populations examined and is found in 1% to 20% of the patients with premature myocardial infarction before the age of 60. Affected individuals have elevated VLDL or LDL concentrations or both, and the lipid phenotype frequently modifies with time, these changes being probably related to modifications in environmental factors such as diet or weight. Patients with FCHL can, therefore, present a variable phenotype, hypertriglyceridemia, hypercholesterolemia, or mixed hyperlipoproteinemia. FCHL is a disorder that is not fully expressed until the third decade of life because it is associated with the accumulation of central abdominal fat, which appears progressively with age. Several other syndromes appear to exhibit overlapping biological markers with FCHL, namely hyperapobetalipoproteinemia and LDL subclass pattern B (corresponding to a predominance of small dense LDL). FHTG appears as an inherited disease in which all affected relatives have hypertriglyceridemia.

The underlying process in FCHL appears to be overproduction of apoB in lipoproteins (VLDL, IDL, and LDL) with a proportional increase in VLDL triglyceride secretion (45), whereas an overproduction of triglycerides into VLDL is observed in FHTG (46,47). The two disorders are often associated with a decrease in the catabolism of VLDL particles. Disparity in the turnover rates of apoB and triglycerides between these two disorders is accompanied by a higher VLDL triglycerides/apoB ratio in FCHL than in FHTG and in normolipidemic subjects.

The CHD risk of subjects afflicted with FCHL is elevated 1.7 to 5 times compared to spouse-control subjects (48–50) as well as subjects with FHTG (48,50). Because of the absence of a specific clinical or biological FCHL feature, the diagnosis requires familial screening, which is not a simple matter. The diagnosis is only established by family studies and cannot, therefore, be confirmed in a single patient. Family studies showed that about 50% of the subjects were hyperlipidemic. However, the demonstration of an elevated apoB concentration in plasma (>90th percentile adjusted for age and gender) was a strong indicator of this dyslipoproteinemia in individuals. The presence of small dense LDL (pattern B) is also a consistent feature of the disease whatever the lipid phenotype, and even persists despite a sporadic normolipidemic pattern (51) or a reduction in triglycerides with gemfibrozil (52).

Resistance to the normal action of insulin as observed in the metabolic syndrome is related to alterations in lipid metabolism. Subjects with insulin resistance develop excessive postprandial release of free fatty acids (FFAs) from adipocytes. The high flux of FFA into the liver leads to an overproduction of triglycerides and apoB, thereby contributing to an elevation in the concentration of VLDL. Furthermore, insulin resistance contributes to decreased LPL activity, resulting in reduced clearance of triglyceride-rich lipoproteins. Triglyceride enrichment of lipoproteins leads to an increase in the serum concentrations of small dense LDL and a decrease in HDL-C levels due to hepatic lipase activity. Insulin resistance is associated with alterations in lipid metabolism such as hypertriglyceridemia, increased apoB levels, low HDL-C levels, and a predominance of small dense LDL particles. All these features of the metabolic syndrome are very similar to those of FCHL.

As in the metabolic syndrome, FCHL subjects often present with an excess of abdominal fat with impaired insulin action both on the suppression of the decrease in serum FFA and on stimulation of glucose disposal during a euglycemic clamp. Resistance to normal insulin action is related to excessive postprandial release of FFA from fat cells. All consequent metabolic disorders such as hepatic overproduction of VLDL, decreased LPL activity, presence of high levels of small dense LDL, and decrease in HDL-C concentration are characteristics of FCHL. FCHL subjects were shown to be more insulin-resistant than controls and a change in insulin resistance is associated with a change in lipid phenotype expression. FCHL subjects with hypertriglyceridemia or combined hyperlipoproteinemia tend to be more insulin-resistant than hypercholesterolemic FCHL subjects (53).

An overlap obviously exists between FCHL and the metabolic syndrome. But even if insulin resistance and overweight were modulators of the FCHL phenotype, insulin resistance would not be fully explained by the increase in BMI. Insulin resistance therefore appears as a characteristic feature of FCHL, but visceral obesity and insulin resistance do not fully account for the elevated levels of apoB and small dense LDL in this disorder (50,53,54). FCHL, therefore, appears as a subtype of the metabolic syndrome with higher apoB and smaller dense LDL levels than most insulin-resistant subjects. These FCHL subjects are at high CHD risk because apoB is a better predictor of future cardiovascular events than LDL-C levels (55–57) and are, therefore, candidates for aggressive lipid-lowering interventions. A number of genetic studies have been preformed to find genetic traits at the origin of the particular lipid phenotype observed in FCHL patients. It is likely that FCHL is heterogenous and that the presence of one or several mutations and/or functional polymorphisms transforms a metabolic syndrome into an FCHL phenotype.

A deficit of LPL activity was noted in about one-third of the families with FCHL (58). However, mutations in these LPL genes, such as those found in obligatory heterozygous parents of children with LPL deficiency, were infrequent (59), and it was concluded that LPL mutations are one of the predisposing genetic factors for FCHL (60). The absence of LPL mutations, despite decreased LPL activity, may be due to other abnormalities. Increased apoCIII expression is associated with impaired clearance of triglyceride-rich lipoproteins due to direct inhibition of LPL by apoCIII. A linkage between FCHL and the apoAI/CIII/AIV gene cluster has been reported but not verified in other populations (61,62). More recently, the discovery of apoAV has established the importance of two distinct alleles of the apoAI/CIII/AIV/AV multigene cluster in the transmission of FCHL (63).

FCHL is characterized by overexpression of VLDL by the liver. An abnormality in fatty acid metabolism could induce both an increase in the hepatic synthesis of triglycerides by the liver and an adaptation in LPL activity corresponding to findings discussed above.

Adipose tissue is the body's major site for storage and mobilization of FFA. Hormone-sensitive lipase (HSL) plays a major role in the release of FFA from adipocytes. HSL does not seem to have a primary role in the pathogenesis of FCHL, its gene expression (mRNA) remaining unmodified in the adipose tissue of FCHL patients compared to controls (64), and there is no evidence of linkage between HSL intragenic markers and FCHL (65). This does not exclude an intra-adipocyte lipolytic defect, as marked resistance to the lipolytic effect of catecholamine has already been demonstrated (66).

The uptake and intracellular esterification of FA by adipocytes is mediated by the action of the acylation stimulation protein (ASP) (67). Because impaired ASP activity has been reported in hyperapobetalipoproteinemia, a condition apparently related to FCHL, a reduced rate of fatty acid uptake into adipocytes may result in an increased flux of FFA to the liver and consequently in increased hepatic VLDL synthesis, which is characteristic of FCHL. However, no molecular mechanism or genetic traits of genes involved in the ASP activity system constituted by a protein cascade and the ASP receptor have been found. In Finnish FCHL families, a common haplotype of upstream transcription factor 1 (USF1) gene was associated with FCHL. USF1 could be a factor for the major gene determining the appearance of FCHL because USF1 encodes a transcription factor expressed mainly in adipose tissue known to regulate several glucose and lipid metabolism genes (68).

■ **Case Study for FCHL**

A 45-year-old patient was referred to the Metabolic Department in 2002 after bouts of angina pectoris in 2000. The examination in the Department of Cardiology noted evidence of a silent myocardial infarction on electrocardiogram. A therapeutic regimen for CHD was prescribed and the coronary insufficiency was stabilized.

Clinically, the patient appeared well. His weight was 90 kg and height 179 cm with a BMI of 28.1 kg/m^2. His waist circumference was 103 cm. The patient had never smoked, his blood pressure (BP) was normal (120/72 mmHg), and no history of high BP was found. The patient had nine brothers and sisters, two of whom had myocardial infarction before the age of 40.

Several hypolipidemic drugs had been prescribed since 2000, but the patient stopped all drugs eight weeks earlier because of the apparent lack of efficacy on blood lipids. Serum lipids were 277, 453, and 38 mg/dL for TC, triglycerides, and HDL-C, respectively. Blood glucose was 97 mg/dL, plasma creatinine and TSH were normal. Transaminases were 31 [upper limit of normal (ULN) < 40] and 63 (<40) for SGOT and SGPT, respectively.

The patient's physical activity was moderate both during and outside his professional activity. The patient was seen by a dietician who advised a decrease in saturated fat intake to obtain a hypocaloric diet.

Remarks

(i) FCHL was probably the diagnosis for this patient. Indeed, hypertriglyceridemia and premature CHD in the patient as well as in two first-degree relatives support this diagnosis. This patient also had metabolic syndrome diagnosed by a high waist circumference [>94 (or 102) cm in a European Caucasian man], hypertriglyceridemia (>150 mg/dL) and low HDL-C (<40 mg/dL).

(ii) The increase in SGPT was moderate and probably related to a hepatic steatosis frequently noted in the metabolic syndrome. The prescription of a hypolipidemic drug is not contraindicated by this moderate abnormality.

The first objective in treating this patient with CHD is to decrease LDL cholesterol to below 100 mg/dL and non-HDL-C below 130 mg/dL. The initial LDL-C level could not be calculated by the Friedewald formula because of the hypertriglyceridemia (>400 mg/dL).

Non-HDL-C was therefore calculated (239 mg/dL) and clearly elevated. Non-HDL-C is a therapeutic target when triglycerides are above 200 mg/dL.

Dietary measures were instituted and simvastatin 20 mg/day was prescribed and progressively titrated. Non-HDL-C decreased to 173 mg/dL (average of two measurements) (−28%) with simvastatin 80 mg/day. Because the patient was unable to reach his non-HDL-C goal, he was switched to atorvastatin at 80 mg/day and the non-HDL-C decreased to 154 mg/dL (average of three measurements).

Fenofibrate 200 mg (micronized form) was prescribed along with atorvastatin. With this combination, serum lipids decreased to 199, 188, 39, and 122 mg/dL for TC, triglycerides, HDL-C, and LDL-C, respectively.

Remarks
(i) The patient had suffered a myocardial infarction and was, therefore, in a high-risk category. The goal of treatment was to decrease LDL-C below 100 mg/dL. No formal clinical trials have addressed the question "does altering risk factors in a population of FCHL patients alter the risk?" However, different drugs (statins and fibrates) have shown their clinical efficacy in subjects with hyperlipoproteinemia such as those observed with FCHL and metabolic syndrome.
(ii) When a statin is moderately effective, two strategies can be used: either a change of statin, or combining it with another hypolipidemic drug. A fibrate was indicated in this patient because of the presence of hypertriglyceridemia and low HDL-C. Fibrates (gemfibrozil, bezafibrate) have indeed shown particular clinical efficacy in this group of patients. Bezafibrate would have been preferred to fenofibrate but gemfibrozil was not prescribed because of its ability to inhibit the glucuronidation of statins, an important elimination pathway for these drugs. Fenofibrate has been shown to reduce the rate of progression of atherosclerotic lesions in diabetic patients (The Diabetes Atherosclerosis Intervention Study) (69).

Although adherence to the pharmacologic regimen was excellent, LDL cholesterol remained higher than the National Cholesterol Education Program (NCEP) goal. Consequently, ezetimibe was added. Lipid levels normalized with triple combination therapy—TC: 163 mg/dL, triglycerides: 174 mg/dL, HDL-C: 40 mg/dL, and LDL-C: 88 mg/dL.

Remarks
Nicotinic acid should have been prescribed instead of ezetimibe because nicotinic acid has demonstrated its CHD protective effect in secondary prevention, as well as its hypotriglyceridemic and increased HDL-C effects. Conversely, ezetimibe has not yet demonstrated a capacity to reduce cardiovascular morbidity and mortality, but its hypocholesterolemic strength is greater than that of nicotinic acid and it is better tolerated.

Pathological and Environmental Factors Contributing to Increased Triglycerides
Drugs
A number of drugs affect lipoprotein metabolism and could affect CHD risk in patients. Diuretics and beta-blockers have a strong tendency to affect serum lipids adversely, whereas the peripherally acting alpha-blocking agents consistently result in beneficial effects. Most of the other antihypertensive agents [calcium channel blockers, angiotensin-converting enzyme (ACE) inhibitors, angiotensin II receptor antagonists, and drugs that act centrally] are lipid-neutral. The effect of steroid hormones varies with the drug, dose, and route of administration. In general, androgens lower HDL-C and have a variable effect on LDL-C. The effects of progestins vary greatly depending on their androgenicity, and estrogens are beneficial except when hypertriglyceridemia occurs with oral estrogens. Glucocorticoids raise HDL-C and may also increase triglycerides and LDL-C. Retinoids increase triglycerides and LDL-C and also reduce HDL-C. Interferons can cause hypertriglyceridemia. Following organ transplantation, a dyslipoproteinemia often ensues. This is partly caused by the medications used to prevent rejection (glucocorticoids, cyclosporine, and FK-506) and requires close attention and, in some patients, drug therapy to prevent coronary artery disease (70).

Antihypertensives
Thiazide diuretics such as chlorthalidone and hydrochlorothiazide have long been known to increase TC and triglyceride. HDL-C remains unaltered but VLDL and LDL-C both increase.

These changes probably reflect the adverse effects of these drugs on glucose tolerance and tend to be accompanied by an increase in uric acid. The effects, which are most marked in obese males and postmenopausal females, can be minimized by weight reduction and adherence to a modified fat diet Spironolactone, indapamide, ACE inhibitors and calcium antagonists appear to have no adverse effects on serum lipids. Long-term administration of beta-blockers without intrinsic sympathomimetic activity (ISA) to patients with hypertension or CHD is associated with 15% to 30% increase in serum triglyceride and 6% to 8% decrease in HDL-C levels. There appears to be little or no difference between nonselective drugs such as propranolol and cardioselective drugs such as atenolol in this respect. However, beta-blockers with ISA have a much less marked influence on serum lipids, and alpha-blockers cause an increase in HDL-C.

The mechanism of the lowering effects of beta-blockers on hypertriglyceridemia and HDL-C is unclear but may involve a decrease in LPL due to inhibition of adenyl cyclase in adipocytes. There is evidence that removal of triglycerides from plasma is impaired during beta blockade and this can lead to marked increases in serum triglycerides in individuals with a genetic predisposition to hypertriglyceridemia.

Oral Contraceptives

Arterial thromboses occurring with oral contraceptive (OC) use do not seem to be atheromatous in nature. A study by the Lipid Research Clinics of 2000 of OC users and nonusers found that users had higher levels of TC, triglycerides, and LDL and VLDL cholesterol, while the elevation of HDL-C was minimal. The effects of combinations of hormones in OCs depend on their composition. OCs with high or medium doses of estrogen cause a rise in TC, triglycerides, and LDL and VLDL cholesterol. HDL-C rises slightly with 19-norsteroids and declines with norgestrel. The ratio of total to HDL-C is, on the whole, increased. OCs with low estrogen doses induce a decline in HDL-C while the levels of TC and triglycerides remain unchanged. A high dose progestin-only pill induces increase in LDL-C and decrease in HDL-C. TC tends to increase with 19-norsteroids and decline with norgestrel, while triglycerides vary slightly. With smaller doses of progestin, less-intense effects are noted. The theoretic atherogenic risk determined by the levels and ratio of total and HDL-C is thus increased with some hormonal combinations. OCs can be prescribed for women with normal lipid balance after a pretreatment lipid profile determination. Lipid balance should be reassessed regularly. OCs are contraindicated in cases of moderate or severe hypercholesterolemia and primary hypoHDLemia. Combined OCs may be used in cases of mild hyperlipoproteinemia in which other contraceptive methods are not possible if regular monitoring is provided (71).

Menopause, Hormonal Replacement Therapy

The relationship between menopause and cardiovascular risk factors was analyzed in samples of French women. Three thousand four hundred and forty women between 45 and 65 years of age who received a systematic check-up between January 1991 and April 1993 were enrolled in this study. Women were classified as premenopausal ($n = 1233$), postmenopausal ($n = 1774$) if they had not menstruated in the 12 months before the examination, and perimenopausal ($n = 433$) if they met at least two of the following criteria: elevated serum levels of follicle-stimulating hormone, irregular menses, amenorrhea for less than 12 months, hot flushes. The effect of menopause on cardiovascular risk factors was determined in 2167 women between 45 and 65 years of age (premenopausal $n = 790$, postmenopausal $n = 1377$), none of whom were at the time treated with hormonal replacement therapy (HRT). In addition, the effect of progestin was assessed in a group or 397 perimenopausal women, and the effect of combined estrogen and progestin replacement therapy in another group of 1746 postmenopausal women. Menopause was associated with higher levels of serum cholesterol (248 mg/dL vs. 228 mg/dL), triglycerides (105 mg/dL vs. 87 mg/dL), apoB (130 mg/dL vs. 110 mg/dL), apoAI (190 mg/dL vs. 180 mg/dL), as well as with elevated diastolic BP (79.7 mmHg vs. 77.0 mmHg). Multivariate analysis indicated that these effects were independent of age, BMI, blood glucose, smoking, alcohol intake, exercise, and parity.

Perimenopausal women treated with progestin alone ($n = 95$) were compared to perimenopausal women not using HRT ($n = 302$). There were no statistically significant differences in the levels of cholesterol, triglycerides, apoB, apoAI, blood glucose, and BP between the two groups. Postmenopausal women using a combination of estrogen and progestin ($n = 369$) had significantly lower levels of serum cholesterol (236 mg/dL vs. 248 mg/dL), triglycerides

(87 mg/dL vs. 105 mg/dL), apoB (120 mg/dL vs. 130 mg/dL), systolic (131.9 mmHg vs. 137.9 mmHg) and diastolic (76.9 mmHg vs. 79.7 mmHg) BP than postmenopausal women without hormonal therapy ($n = 1377$), taking into account confounding variables. In contrast, serum apoAI levels were not altered by the combined hormonal therapy. It was concluded that menopause is associated with the aggravation of multiple cardiovascular risk factors and that the deleterious factors are affected by combination hormone replacement therapy (72).

Another recent study assessed the benefits and risks of HRT in preventing cardiovascular events by conducting a meta-analysis of all randomized trials of HRT. All relevant randomized clinical trials were identified in MEDLINE (1966–2001), HealthSTAR (1975–2001), and Cochrane Library databases. The search terms were hormone replacement or HRT, estrogen, progesterone, women, and heart disease. Meta-analysis of the randomized clinical trials involving 21,066 patients revealed that HRT did not reduce mortality compared to control group [1.9% vs. 1.9%, odds ratio (OR) 1.05, 95% CI 0.86–1.30, $p = 0.58$] or the incidence of myocardial infarction (3.7% vs. 3.7%, OR 1.04, 95% CI 0.90–1.21, $p = 0.58$) or the revascularization rate (6.4% vs. 6.8%, OR 0.95, 95% CI 0.85–1.08, $p = 0.50$). The acute coronary syndrome rate was 9.1% in the HRT group versus 9.3% with OR 1.00, 95% CI 0.90 to 1.12, $p = 0.98$. Therefore, HRT use is not associated with reduced death, myocardial infarction, or revascularization rate (73).

In direct contrast to the observational studies, both primary and secondary prevention trials on female reproductive hormones have found no benefit for CHD. It is likely that uncorrected biases in the observational studies lead to an overestimation of any benefits of hormone use. Hormones are not indicated for the prevention of CHD, particularly in the light of the increased risk of stroke and venous thrombosis. Their use for other indications (menopausal symptoms, osteoporosis) needs to be tempered by the risk of CVD (74).

All-Trans-Retinoic Acid and 13-cis Retinoic Acid

Hypertriglyceridemia is a metabolic complication of retinoid therapy (74). A phase-I trial of all-trans-retinoic acid (ATRA) was conducted to establish the maximum tolerable dose (MTD) of ATRA given once daily to patients with solid tumors. Cancer patients, for whom no standard therapy was available, were treated with ATRA once daily. The pharmacokinetics of ATRA was assessed on day one and weekly in 31 patients who received doses of 110 mg/m^2 or above per day. Patients were followed for toxicity and response. Correlations of toxicity frequency and doses were sought using pharmacokinetic parameters. An assessment was also made between the correlation of changes in ATRA pharmacokinetics, and the concentration of ATRA metabolites in plasma were sought. A total of 49 patients received ATRA at doses ranging from 45 to 309 mg/m^2/day. Hypertriglyceridemia was dose limiting at 269 mg/m^2 day. Other frequent toxicities included mucocutaneous dryness and headache. The recommended once-daily ATRA dose is 215 mg/m^2, although significant interindividual variability is observed in toxicity and plasma retinoid concentrations (75). It has been demonstrated that retinoids increase human apoCIII expression at the transcriptional level via the retinoid X receptor. This increase in apoCIII expression contributes to the hypertriglyceridemic action of retinoids (74).

Administration of 13-cis -retinoic acid (isotretinoin) for acne is occasionally accompanied by hyperlipoproteinemia. It is not known why some patients develop this side effect. The goal of a recent study was to determine whether isotretinoin triggers a familial susceptibility to hyperlipoproteinemia and the metabolic syndrome. Tests were carried out on 102 persons whose triglyceride levels increased at least 89 mg/dL (hyperresponders) and 100 patients whose triglyceride levels changed less than 9 mg/dL or less (nonresponders) during isotretinoin therapy for acne. Parents of 71 hyperresponders and 60 nonresponders were also evaluated. Hyperresponders and nonresponders had similar pretreatment body weight and plasma lipid levels. When evaluated again approximately four years after completion of isotretinoin therapy, hyperresponders were more likely to have hypertriglyceridemia [triglyceride level >177 mg/dL; OR, 4.8 (95% CI, 1.6–13.8)], hypercholesterolemia [cholesterol level >252 mg/dL; OR, 9.1 (95% CI, 1.9–43)], truncal obesity [waist-to-hip ratio (WHR) >0.90; OR, 11.0 (95% CI, 2.0–59)], and hyperinsulinemia [insulin–glucose ratio >7.2; OR, 3.0 (95% CI, 1.6–5.7)]. In addition, more hyperresponders had at least one parent with hypertriglyceridemia [OR, 2.6 (95% CI, 1.2–5.7)] or a ratio of TC to HDL-C that exceeded 4.0 [OR, 3.5 (95% CI, 1.5–8.0)]. Lipid response to isotretinoin was closely associated with the apoE gene. Therefore, people who develop hypertriglyceridemia during isotretinoin therapy for acne are at increased risk for future hyperlipoproteinemia and the metabolic syndrome as are their parents (76).

Whole body and adipose tissue insulin sensitivity were assessed in 15 healthy male volunteers before and after five days of administration of isotretinoin (1 mg/kg/day), which increased plasma triglyceride from 0.85 ± 0.13 to 114 ± 19 mg/dL ($p < 0.02$), but did not change whole body insulin-mediated glucose disposal and lipolysis. These observations are consistent with isotretinoin-induced inhibition of VLDL-triglyceride clearance. The suppression of endogenous glucose production and the reduction in subcutaneous adipose glycerol concentrations by insulin remained equally unaffected after isotretinoin administration. It was concluded that the impaired clearance of triglyceride-rich particles secondary to a five-day isotretinoin administration does not impair insulin-mediated antilipolysis or glucose disposal (77).

Atypical and Typical Antipsychotics
Individuals with psychiatric disorders tend to have excessive morbidity. Typically, they have high rates of respiratory illnesses, infectious diseases, substance abuse (including smoking), obesity, diabetes mellitus, and CVD. Persons with schizophrenia and affective disorders also have a high prevalence of risk factors for CVD such as diabetes and obesity, which are about 1.5 to 2.0 times higher than in the general population; this translates into increased mortality rates due to CVD. The use of certain psychotropics results in metabolic abnormalities such as obesity, dyslipoproteinemia, glucose dysregulation, and the metabolic syndrome, which exacerbate the already elevated risk of CVD and diabetes in this group of people. Therefore, the use of psychotropic agents that result in, for example, excessive weight gain not only add another complication for physicians managing a patient with schizophrenia but may also have serious prognostic and cost implications with respect to treatment-related diabetes and coronary disease incidence. The recent American Diabetes Association Consensus Panel concluded that some agents are associated with greater diabetes risk than others (78).

There is a four-fold risk of metabolic syndrome in patients with schizophrenia. In The Northern Finland 1966 Birth Cohort study, the high prevalence of metabolic syndrome in schizophrenia appeared even at a relatively young age and underscores the need to select antipsychotic medications with no or little capacity to induce metabolic side effects. It is also essential to develop comprehensive efforts directed at controlling weight and diet and improving physical activity (79). Individual antipsychotic medications are associated with different degrees of treatment-induced increases in body weight and adiposity, ranging from modest effects (<2 kg) with amisulpride, ziprasidone, and aripiprazole to clinically significant increases with olanzapine (4–10 kg) (80). Both nonobese clozapine- and olanzapine-treated groups displayed significant insulin resistance and impairment of glucose effectiveness compared to risperidone-treated subjects. Patients taking clozapine and olanzapine must be examined for insulin resistance and its consequences (81). Changes in fasting plasma levels of TC, HDL-C, and triglycerides were significantly different in the two treatment groups with worsening of the lipid profile among patients treated with olanzapine in comparison with aripiprazol. The observed effects on weight and lipids indicate a potentially lower metabolic and cardiovascular risk in patients treated with aripiprazole compared to those treated with olanzapine (82). A retrospective cohort chart review was performed of 191 randomly selected patients who were being treated with ziprasidone or olanzapine in an integrated health care system. A significant weight gain was observed in olanzapine-treated patients ($p < 0.001$) but not in the ziprasidone-treated cohort ($p > 0.05$). Furthermore, adverse metabolic changes associated with olanzapine administration were significant with respect to effects on TC ($p = 0.01$), triglycerides ($p = 0.05$) and hemoglobin A1C (HbA1C) ($p < 0.05$), whereas significant favorable metabolic effects were observed in ziprasidone-treated patients as regards TC ($p < 0.05$), LDL-C ($p < 0.01$), HDL-C ($p < 0.05$) and HbA1C ($p < 0.05$). Olanzapine-treated patients exhibited significant weight increase, whereas ziprasidone-treated patients exhibited weight loss. Olanzapine treatment was also associated with significant adverse effect on patients' lipid profile and HbA1C. These adverse metabolic effects were not observed in ziprasidone-treated patients though favorable effects were observed on TC, LDL-C, HDL-C, and HbA1C (83).

Despite concerns about the adverse effects of second-generation antipsychotics on weight regulation, glucose, and lipid metabolism, little is known about the relationship between these agents and the metabolic syndrome. In a recent study the relationship between second-generation antipsychotics and the metabolic syndrome has been explored. Twenty-six (29.2%) of the 89 patients fulfilled criteria for the metabolic syndrome. Presence of the syndrome was associated with older age, higher BMI, and higher values for each individual criterion of the metabolic syndrome but not with specific diagnoses or antipsychotic treatment regimens. Presence of abdominal obesity was most sensitive (92.0%), while fasting glucose above 110 mg/dL was most specific (95.2%) in correctly identifying the presence of metabolic syndrome. Sensitivity was 100% when combining abdominal obesity and elevated fasting blood glucose (84).

A recent two-year evaluation has suggested that clinically or statistically significant BMI increases as well as high blood glucose and lipid levels were not unavoidably correlated with the use of the atypical antipsychotic agents olanzapine and risperidone, and could be minimized by careful monitoring, a regimen of dietary control, and a moderate activity level in a residential population of individuals with mental retardation (85).

Chronic Glucocorticoid Therapy

Glucocorticoids continue to be a potent therapeutic tool for various medical conditions; however, their side effects pose challenges. Steroid diabetes is treated primarily with prandial insulin, either regular or rapid (lispro or aspart). Intermediate insulin is prescribed less frequently for fasting hyperglycemia. Osteoporosis is the most debilitating of potential glucocorticoid side effects, with bisphosphonates the mainstay in prevention and treatment (86). Elevations of total plasma cholesterol, triglycerides, LDL-C, and HDL-C are often reported. Dyslipoproteinemia can range from mild to significant. The elevation of various lipid subfractions is probably mediated by increased plasma insulin levels, impaired lipid catabolism, and increased lipid production in the liver. The major adverse effects of glucocorticoids on the cardiovascular system include dyslipoproteinemia and hypertension. These effects may predispose treated patients to coronary artery disease if high doses and prolonged courses are used. Accordingly, corticosteroids should be used judiciously in patients with other risk factors for CVD, and attention should be paid to risk modification. Low dose and alternate day therapy may reduce the incidence of complications in corticosteroid therapy. The mechanisms of these adverse effects are complex and have not yet been fully explained (87). Dyslipoproteinemia responds to therapy similar to that of nonglucocorticoid-induced lipid disorders.

Immunosuppressants

Cardiovascular morbidity including coronary artery disease, left ventricular hypertrophy, and mortality are high in patients following renal transplantation. CVD is thought to be due to traditional (hypertension, hyperlipoproteinemia, diabetes mellitus, and smoking) as well as nontraditional (microinflammation) cardiovascular risk factors. Furthermore, immunosuppressive drugs, namely, calcineurin inhibitors, sirolimus, and steroids, have been reported to adversely affect cardiovascular risk factors (e.g., hypertension, hyperlipoproteinemia, and hyperglycemia). Experimental studies suggest that a steroid-induced increase in VLDL synthesis is one of the mechanisms involved. Similar changes can occur spontaneously in patients with Cushing's syndrome. Studies in renal transplant patients on cyclosporin show that this drug causes an increase in serum cholesterol, reflecting an increase in LDL-C. Similar abnormalities occur in patients receiving steroids and cyclosporin after renal or cardiac transplantation, especially those with a background of CHD. Evidence from comparative trials and from conversion studies suggests that BP, hyperlipoproteinemia, and hyperglycemia after renal transplantation may be differentially affected by the calcineurin inhibitors, cyclosporine, and tacrolimus. In the European Tacrolimus versus Cyclosporin A Microemulsion Renal Transplantation Study, 557 patients were randomly allocated to therapy with tacrolimus versus cyclosporine. Tacrolimus resulted in a significantly lower time-weighted average of serum cholesterol and mean arterial BP but a higher time-weighted average of blood glucose than cyclosporine. A mean 10-year coronary artery disease risk estimate was significantly lower in men treated with tacrolimus (10.0% vs. 13.2%; $p < 0.01$) but was unchanged in women (4.7% vs. 7.0%). Tacrolimus and cyclosporine microemulsion have compound-specific effects on cardiovascular risk factors that differentially affect the predicted rate of coronary artery disease (88). Conversion from cyclosporine to tacrolimus is recommended for kidney transplant patients in whom there has been a progressive fall in renal function. It leads to stabilization or even improvement of transplant function and a reduction in cardiovascular risk factors (89).

Steroid-induced adverse effects after transplantation include cosmetic, metabolic, and cardiovascular complications. Steroid withdrawal or avoidance with cyclosporine-based regimens have been hampered by an unacceptably high rate of acute rejections and increased rates of graft loss. Recently the results of several large, randomized trials of steroid withdrawal/avoidance with tacrolimus-based immunosuppression in renal transplant recipients have become available. Data from the THOMAS trial clearly indicate that steroid withdrawal three months after transplantation from a initial regimen of tacrolimus, mycophenolate mofetil (MMF), and steroids, is safe as far as acute rejection rate and graft survival are concerned. If an induction therapy with daclizumab is used in combination with tacrolimus and MMF (CARMEN trial), even steroid avoidance is safe as far as acute rejection rate and graft survival are concerned. Finally, in the ATLAS trial, steroid avoidance with basiliximab in combination with tacrolimus (resulting in tacrolimus monotherapy) or alternatively with tacrolimus and MMF, both resulted in similar graft survival, but higher rates of acute rejection. To conclude, steroid use may be completely avoided three months after transplantation when the tacrolimus and MMF are combined with daclizumab induction. Tacrolimus monotherapy may be used with basiliximab induction at the price of higher rates of acute rejection, but with unaffected graft survival. Thus tacrolimus-based immunosuppression with or without interleukin-2 receptor antagonist induction has made steroid withdrawal or avoidance a realistic option in renal transplantation (90).

Highly Active Antiretroviral Therapy

Dyslipoproteinemia, characterized by elevated serum levels of triglycerides and reduced levels of TC, LDL-C, and HDL-C, has been recognized in patients with human immunodeficiency virus (HIV) infection. It is thought that elevated levels of circulating cytokines such as tumor necrosis factor-alpha and interferon-alpha may alter lipid metabolism in patients with HIV infection. Both HIV and demographic characteristics were found to influence lipid values and glucose homeostasis in the absence of antiretroviral treatment. More advanced HIV is associated with less favorable lipid and glucose homeostatic profiles. The independent association between HIV RNA levels and various lipid parameters suggests that viral replication has a direct effect on lipid levels. Interpretation of the effects of various regimens and drugs in HIV treatment on metabolic parameters must take into account the stage of HIV infection and the demographic characteristics of the population studied (91).

Protease inhibitors (PIs) [highly active antiretroviral therapy (HAART)] have been associated with a syndrome of fat redistribution, insulin resistance, and hyperlipoproteinemia. In a cohort of HIV-infected patients, the prevalence of diabetes was 12% among those who were taking PIs compared to 0% among those who were not. The incidence of newly diagnosed diabetes during a three-year period was 7.2%. Diabetes occurred only in the group taking PIs. Diabetic subjects were older than their nondiabetic counterparts. This study suggests that PIs increase the likelihood of diabetes developing with increasing age in patients infected with HIV (92). Twelve months after treatment initiation with PIs, statistically significant increases in TC and triglyceride levels were observed in HIV-infected patients under conditions of standard treatment (93). It has been estimated that hypercholesterolemia and hypertriglyceridemia occur in more than 50% of PI recipients after two years of therapy, and that the risk of developing hyperlipoproteinemia increases with the duration of treatment with PIs (94). Postprandial clearance of triglyceride-rich lipoproteins is delayed in HIV-positive individuals receiving antiretroviral therapy. Compared with HIV-positive individuals not on PIs, those taking PIs do not have increased postprandial triglyceride-rich lipoproteins but do have increased postprandial atherogenic IDLs and LDLs (95). Patients with elevated lipid values at baseline have the greatest risk of developing hypercholesterolemia and hypertriglyceridemia after starting lopinavir/ritonavir, whereas antiretroviral-naive patients coinfected with hepatitis C have a low risk (96).

The mechanism of action of PIs on lipoprotein metabolism is largely unknown. Using cultured human and rat hepatoma cells and primary hepatocytes from transgenic mice, it has been demonstrated that PI treatment inhibits proteasomal degradation of nascent apoB, the principal protein component of triglyceride and cholesterol-rich plasma lipoproteins. Unexpectedly, PIs also inhibit the secretion of apoB. This is associated with the inhibition of cholesteryl-ester synthesis and microsomal triglyceride transfer-protein activity. However, in the presence of oleic acid, which stimulates neutral-lipid biosynthesis, protease-inhibitor treatment increased secretion of apoB-lipoproteins above controls. These findings suggest a molecular basis for protease-inhibitor-associated hyperlipoproteinemia (97).

In general, the treatment of hyperlipoproteinemia should follow only NCEP guidelines. Efforts should be made to modify/control CHD risk factors (i.e., smoking, hypertension, and diabetes mellitus) and maximize lifestyle modifications, primarily dietary intervention and exercise, in these patients. Where indicated, treatment usually consists of rosuvastatin, pravastatin, or atorvastatin for patients with elevated serum levels of LDL-C. Simvastatin and lovastatin are significantly metabolized by cytochrome P450 enzymes (CYP3A4) and are therefore not recommended for coadministration with PIs.

A fibric acid derivative (gemfibrozil or fenofibrate) should be used in patients with primary hypertriglyceridemia. However, it must be kept in mind that PIs, such as nelfinavir and ritonavir, induce enzymes involved in the metabolism of fibric acid derivatives and may, therefore, reduce the lipid-lowering activity of coadministered gemfibrozil or fenofibrate. In certain patients, 3-hydroxy-3-methylglutaryl coenzyme A (HMG-CoA) reductase inhibitors may be used in combination with fibric acid derivatives, but patients should be carefully monitored for liver and skeletal muscle toxicity. Select patients may experience improvements in serum lipid levels when their offending PI(s) is/are exchanged for efavirenz, nevirapine, or abacavir; however each patient's virological and immunological status must be taken into close consideration (88).

The majority of the studies examining the incidence of CVD events demonstrated an increase in CV event rate with HAART in the HIV-infected population. Overall, CHD risk appears to be greater in the HIV-infected population than in the general population, and increased CV risk is associated with HAART, particularly with PI use. Despite the relative risk of CHD being significantly high (the hazard ratio for myocardial infarction ranging between 1.3 and 7.1), the absolute risk for CHD remains low, with the CV event rates ranging between 1 and 7 per 1000 person-years. Although there is a general consensus that the benefits of HAART far outweigh toxicity-related risks of the treatment, prolonged survival among HIV-infected patients will probably favor the use of different antiretroviral regimens with potentially less CV toxicity in the future (98).

Atazanavir (ATV) is a once-daily PI that has not been associated with clinically relevant increases in TC, fasting LDL-C, or fasting triglyceride concentrations, and may limit the need for lipid-lowering strategies to reduce the risk of CVD (99). In hyperlipidemic, antiretroviral-experienced patients with HIV-1 RNA levels below 50 copies/mL and CD4+ cell counts above 500 cells/mm^3, the substitution of abacavir for hyperlipoproteinemia-associated PIs in combination antiretroviral regimens improves lipid profiles, maintains virological suppression over a 28-week period, and simplifies treatment (100). Replacing PI with efavirenz, nevirapine, or abacavir improved the lipid profile, with more marked results in nonlipodystrophic patients. Significant decrease in the levels of triglycerides occurred over the first year in all treatments; however, at 24 months, most of the initial loss had been regained. Several insulin resistance markers show a trend toward improvement. Conversely, no improvements in morphological abnormalities were observed (101). Current evidence suggests that simplified maintenance therapy (SMT) with abacavir rather than continued PI, increases the risk of virological failure, although this increased risk may be confined to patients with prior mono or dual therapy with reverse transcriptase inhibitors. There is not enough evidence to prove whether SMT, along with efavirenz and nevirapine, influences the risk of virological failure. SMT with any of the three drugs reduces the risk of therapy discontinuation, and SMT with abacavir reduces plasma cholesterol (102).

Environmental Factors

Excess Alcohol Consumption

Alcohol is a common cause of secondary hypertriglyceridemia, especially in males, and usually results in an increase in VLDL and sometimes chylomicron levels. Even moderate consumption of alcohol on a regular basis results in significantly higher serum triglycerides than those found in total abstainers. The hypertriglyceridemic effect of alcohol is most marked in subjects with preexisting primary hypertriglyceridemia, and is enhanced by concomitant consumption of fat. One postulated mechanism is that alcohol is preferentially oxidized in the liver, which results in an economy of FFA and its increased availability for triglyceride synthesis. Withdrawal of alcohol results in a rapid decrease in triglyceride levels.

An increased level of HDL-C is a common consequence of regular heavy alcohol consumption as is hypertriglyceridemia; however, concomitant elevation of both lipids together with a raised gamma-glutamyl transpeptidase is pathognomonic. The increase in HDL-C reflects increase in both HDL$_2$ and HDL$_3$, the former being due to the increase in LPL activity that accompanies regular drinking.

Effects of Physical Activity on Triglycerides

Effect of Training on Blood Lipids. The association between changes in fat mass (FM), abdominal visceral fat (AVF), and abdominal subcutaneous fat (ASF) on blood lipid changes subsequent to aerobic exercise training has been explored. The sample included 613 participants (428 white and 185 black, 46% men) from the HERITAGE Family Study. Total FM was determined by densitometry, whereas AVF and ASF cross-sectional areas were determined by computed tomography at the L4 to L5 level. Blood lipid measurements included TC, HDL-C, LDL-C, triglycerides, and the TC/HDL-C ratio, which were obtained before and after 20 weeks of supervised aerobic exercise. Body fat accounted for 26% to 36% of the variance in baseline blood lipids, and changes in body fat accounted for 7% to 21% of the variation in changes in blood lipids with exercise training. The pattern of loadings indicated similar relationships between body fat and blood lipids at baseline, and their respective changes with exercise training. Greater fat loss, characterized by loss of FM, AVF, and ASF, was associated with a greater blood lipid response characterized by an increase in HDL-C and decrease in LDL-C, triglycerides, and TC/HDL-C ratio (103).

Effect of Detraining on Body Composition and Insulin Sensitivity in Young Healthy Subjects. Two months after discontinuing regular training, female dancers experience significant elevations in basal and postprandial insulin, triglyceride, and FFA levels. This result appears to be partly related to increased central fatness but not body mass, indicating that the early development of obesity due to reduced physical activity may not necessarily depend on weight alone (104).

Health Exercise for Early Postmenopausal Women. After menopause, women face many changes that may lead to loss of health-related fitness (HRF), especially if sedentary. Many exercise recommendations are therefore relevant for early postmenopausal women, but may not meet their specific needs because they are based mainly on studies in men. A systematic review for randomized, controlled exercise trials was conducted on postmenopausal women (aged 50–65 years) on components of HRF. In total, nine reported on lipids, two on glucose and one on insulin. Based on these studies, early postmenopausal women could benefit from 30 minutes of daily moderate walking in one to three sessions combined with a resistance-training program twice a week. For a sedentary person, walking is feasible and can be incorporated into everyday life. A feasible way to start resistance training is to perform 8 to 10 repetitions of 8 to 10 exercises for major muscle groups starting with 40% of one repetition, maximum. Based on limited evidence, such exercise might also improve flexibility, balance and coordination, decrease hypertension, and improve dyslipoproteinemia (105).

Training in Elderly Subjects. Previous studies have demonstrated that frail octogenarians have reduced capacity for cardiovascular adaptations to endure exercise training. A recent study determined the magnitude of cardiovascular and metabolic adaptations to high-intensity endurance exercise training in healthy, nonfrail elderly subjects. Ten subjects [eight men, two women, 80.3 years (SD 2.5)] completed 10 to 12 months (108 exercise sessions) of a supervised endurance exercise-training program consisting of 2.5 sessions/week (SD 0.2), 58 min/session (SD 6), at an intensity of 83% (SD 5) of peak heart rate. Primary outcomes were maximal attainable aerobic power [peak aerobic capacity (VO_2 peak)]; serum lipids, oral glucose tolerance, and insulin action during a hyperglycemic clamp; body composition by dual-energy X-ray absorptiometry, and energy expenditure using doubly labeled water and indirect calorimetry. The training program resulted in a 15% (SD 7) increase in VO_2 peak [22.9 (SD 3.3) to 26.2 mL/kg/min (SD 4.0); $p < 0.0001$]. Favorable lipid changes included reductions in TC (−8%; $p = 0.002$) and LDL-C (−10%; $p = 0.003$), with no significant change in HDL-C or triglycerides. Insulin action improved, as shown by a 29% increase in glucose disposal rate relative to insulin concentration during the hyperglycemic clamp. Fat mass decreased by 1.8 kg (SD 1.4) ($p = 0003$); lean mass did not change. Total energy expenditure increased by 400 kcal/day because of an increase in physical activity. No change occurred in resting metabolism. In summary, healthy nonfrail octogenarians can adapt to high-intensity endurance exercise training with improvements in aerobic power, insulin action, and serum lipid and lipoprotein risk factors for CHD; however, adaptations in aerobic power and insulin action are attenuated compared with middle-aged individuals (106).

Effects of Aerobic Exercise Programs in Type 2 Diabetes. Under insulin-resistant conditions, regular aerobic exercise can increase insulin sensitivity, thereby improving the lipid profile. Although patients are advised to exercise as part of their therapy, this is usually unsuccessful unless it is part of a supervised exercise program. Because current therapeutic strategies are often ineffective in reducing insulin resistance and improving the adverse lipid profile, the use of a supervised exercise program may have a role in the treatment of these patients. In a recent study, patients were studied before and after a six-month exercise program. All patients were given an initial training session and an individualized exercise program based on the American College of Sports Medicine guidelines and were asked to exercise for 20 to 40 minutes at 60% to 85% of maximal oxygen uptake (VO_{2max}) four times per week in the mode of aerobic activity of their choice. Patients were then randomized into a supervised or unsupervised group. Supervised patients saw the exercise trainer once every week for an exercise session and an account of the previous week's activity. A plan for the activity for the following week was agreed. The exercise trainer did not see patients in the unsupervised group after their initial contact. In the supervised and unsupervised groups at baseline, there was no difference in age, BMI, or percent HbA1c. In the supervised group, after six months of exercise, there was a significant decrease in BMI (30.6 ± 2.0 to 29.6 ± 2.7, $p < 0.03$), body weight, total body fat, and trunk fat ($p < 0.03$, < 0.004, and < 0.005). The decrease in body weight was due to a decrease in body fat. Patients in this group increased their VO_2 and power, which are measures of aerobic fitness and muscle strength, respectively ($p < 0.001$ and $p < 0.003$). There was no significant change in these measurements in the unsupervised group. The change in these measurements from zero to six months between groups was significant for body fat, trunk fat, VO_{2max}, and power ($p < 0.004$, < 0.002, < 0.05, and < 0.006). There was no difference in fasting lipid profile before the exercise program in the two groups, although HDL-C tended to be lower in the unsupervised group. After six months of exercise, there was a significant decrease in fasting plasma triglyceride ($p < 0.05$) and nonesterified fatty acids (NEFA) concentrations ($p < 0.04$) in the supervised group but not in the unsupervised group. Plasma TC and LDL-C levels were no different in the two groups at baseline and showed no significant change after six months. HDL-C increased significantly in both groups after six months ($p < 0.001$). In the supervised group, there was a significant decrease in VLDL triglyceride concentration ($p < 0.01$), VLDL cholesterol concentration ($p < 0.007$) and VLDL apoB concentration ($p < 0.01$), but there was no change in the VLDL triglyceride/apoB, VLDL triglyceride/cholesterol, or VLDL cholesterol/apoB ratio. The change in these measurements from zero to six months between groups was significant for VLDL apoB concentration ($p < 0.002$) (107).

In this study, a within-group analysis demonstrated that a supervised exercise program in type 2 diabetic patients resulted in a decrease in triglyceride concentrations and a decrease in VLDL apoB secretion rate with no change in VLDL apoB catabolism. Insulin resistance improved, NEFA concentrations decreased, and HDL-C levels increased after the program. However, the change in VLDL apoB secretion rate between the supervised and the unsupervised exercise group was not significantly different, perhaps because of large between-subject variation in VLDL apoB secretion rate and modified activity levels of some subjects in the unsupervised group. There is considerable evidence that dyslipoproteinemia and insulin resistance are associated with increased body fat and, in particular, with visceral adiposity. In obesity, an association has been demonstrated between VLDL apoB secretion and body fat and also with visceral fat. In the current study, the supervised exercise program resulted in a significant decrease in body and trunk fat. At six months, the change in VLDL apoB was significantly related to the change in body fat but not to the change in trunk FM. This may be because of the small sample size in the current study. Because abdominal adipocytes have a high lipolytic capacity, it is possible that an increased flux of NEFAs in the portal vein to the liver may stimulate hepatic secretion of VLDL apoB or may contribute to increased triacylglycerol accumulation in the liver, which is associated with hepatic insulin resistance. Increased levels of circulating NEFAs, as found in the patients in this study, have also been shown to be associated with insulin resistance. Although both NEFAs and insulin resistance decreased with exercise, it was impossible to demonstrate a relationship between the change in NEFAs and insulin resistance. Decreased NEFA concentrations in the presence of reduced insulin levels after supervised exercise suggest an improvement in insulin sensitivity in adipose tissue. This has also been demonstrated in a study of obese nondiabetic subjects, in whom aerobic exercise training for three months decreased basal lipolysis and HSL activity. VLDL particles are removed from the vascular compartment either by complete hydrolysis to IDL and subsequently LDL particles or by direct removal of the partially delipidated particle via the LDL, LDL-related receptor protein, or VLDL receptor in the liver. LPL activity will determine the rate of VLDL hydrolysis to IDL.

There is evidence that the ability of insulin to increase LPL activity is impaired in type 2 diabetes and that increased physical exercise in the patients with the condition, increases LPL activity. However, in the current study, the improvement in insulin sensitivity with the supervised exercise program had no impact on VLDL catabolism. In conclusion, the within-group analysis suggested that an exercise program reduced VLDL apoB pool size by decreasing VLDL apoB secretion rate. The failure to find a significant difference in the change of VLDL apoB secretion rate between the supervised and the unsupervised exercise groups may be due to the large between-subject variation in VLDL apoB secretion rate and the increase in activity levels in some subjects in the unsupervised group. We hypothesize that a decrease in VLDL apoB secretion rate may be due to an increase in hepatic insulin sensitivity. A decrease in NEFA flux from adipose tissue to the liver may indirectly improve hepatic insulin resistance and decrease intrahepatic lipid availability, thereby contributing to the decrease in VLDL apoB secretion rate. This study suggests that the decrease in triglycerides with regular exercise in type 2 diabetes may be due to a decrease in VLDL apoB secretion rate (107).

Post hoc analysis of long-term effects of different amounts of increased energy expenditure [metabolic equivalents (METS) per hour per week] through voluntary aerobic physical activity was performed on 179 type 2 diabetic subjects [age 62 ± 1 years (mean $\pm$ SE)] randomized in a physical activity counseling intervention. Subjects were followed for two years and divided into six groups based on their increments in METs per hour per week: group 0 (no activity, $n = 28$), group 1 to 10 (6.8 ± 0.3, $n = 27$), group 11 to 20 (17.1 ± 0.4, $n = 31$), group 21 to 30 (27.0 ± 0.5, $n = 27$), group 31 to 40 (37.5 ± 0.5, $n = 32$), and group over 40 (58.3 ± 1.8, $n = 34$). At baseline, the six groups did not differ as to energy expenditure, age, sex, diabetes duration, and all parameters measured. After two years, in group 0 and in group 1 to 10, no parameter changed; in groups 11 to 20, 21 to 30, 31 to 40, and over 40, HbA1C, BP, total serum cholesterol, triglycerides, and estimated percent of 10-year CHD risk improved ($p < 0.05$). In group 21 to 30, 31 to 40, and over 40, body weight, waist circumference, heart rate, fasting plasma glucose, serum LDL and HDL-C also improved ($p < 0.05$). METs per hour per week correlated positively with changes of HDL-C and negatively with those of other parameters ($p < 0.001$). After two years, per capita yearly costs of medications increased ($p = 0.008$) by US \$393 in group 0, did not significantly change in group 1 to 10 (US \$206, $p = 0.09$), and decreased in group 11 to 20 (US \$196, $p = 0.01$), group 21 to 30 (US \$593, $p = 0.009$), group 31 to 40 (US \$660, $p = 0.003$), and group over 40 (US \$579, $p = 0.001$). Energy expenditure over 10 METs/hr/wk obtained through aerobic leisure time physical activity is sufficient to achieve health and financial advantages, but full benefits are achieved with energy expenditure over 20 METs/hr/wk (108).

Pathology Associated with Hypertriglyceridemia
Obesity, Insulin Resistance
The abnormalities most closely associated with insulin resistance and/or compensatory hyperinsulinemia involve changes in lipoprotein metabolism. Indeed, the relationship between insulin resistance, compensatory hyperinsulinemia, and hypertriglyceridemia has been known for more than 30 years. It is now apparent that the link between insulin resistance and dyslipoproteinemia is much greater, and consists of more than an increase in plasma triglyceride concentrations.

Obesity is associated with increased storage of lipids in nonadipose tissues such as skeletal muscle, liver, and pancreatic beta cells. These lipids constitute a continuous source of long-chain fatty acyl CoA (LC-CoA) and derived metabolites such as diacylglycerol and ceramide, acting as signalling molecules on protein kinases activities [in particular, the protein kinase C (PKC) family], ion channel, gene expression, and protein acylation. In skeletal muscle, the increase in LC-CoA and diacylglycerol translocates and activates specific PKC isoforms, which will phosphorylate serine residues on insulin receptor substrate-1, thereby preventing its phosphorylation on tyrosine and association with phosphatidylinositol triphosphokinase. This interrupts the insulin-signalling pathway leading to the stimulation of glucose transport and induces insulin resistance. In pancreatic beta cells, short-term excess of FA or LC-CoA activates PKC and also directly stimulates insulin exocytosis. Long-term exposure to FFA leads to increased basal and blunted glucose-stimulated insulin secretion by affecting gene expression, an increase in K(ATP) channel activity, and uncoupling of the mitochondria (109).

The interplay of insulin resistance at the level of the muscle and adipose tissue and normal hepatic insulin sensitivity leads to the atherogenic lipoprotein profile that is characteristic of insulin-resistant individuals (110). The disordered crosstalk between adipose tissue and the liver, results in an imbalance of the machinery that orchestrates the regulation of VLDL production. A number of studies indicate that adipocytokines, in particular adiponectin, are seminal players in the regulation of fat metabolism in the liver (111). Insulin resistance is associated with excessive flux of substrates for VLDL assembly to the liver as well as the upregulation of the machinery generating large VLDL particles in excess (Fig. 2) (111). Studies in individuals with either normal or elevated plasma triglyceride concentrations have defined highly significant direct relationships between insulin resistance, compensatory hyperinsulinemia, hepatic VLDL-triglyceride secretion, and plasma triglyceride concentrations. Based upon these data, it has been suggested that the major cause of elevated plasma triglyceride concentrations in nondiabetic individuals is an increase in hepatic VLDL-triglyceride secretion rate, secondary to insulin resistance and the resultant hyperinsulinemia (112–115).

Although there is widespread agreement that the four variables in question are highly correlated, there is controversy concerning the causal relationship between them. One view is that resistance to insulin regulation of muscle and adipose tissue leads to higher ambient levels of both insulin and FFA, and these two changes stimulate hepatic VLDL triglyceride secretion, leading to an increase in plasma triglyceride concentration in insulin-resistant individuals (116,117). This formulation postulates that higher ambient insulin concentrations present in insulin-resistant individuals act on the liver to increase the rate at which incoming FFA are converted to VLDL triglycerides; the higher the plasma FFA concentrations, the greater the increase in VLDL triglyceride secretion (117). Alternatively, evidence has recently been put forward that hypertriglyceridemia occurs in insulin-resistant, nondiabetic individuals because of resistance to the normal ability of insulin to inhibit hepatic VLDL triglyceride secretion (118).

In the absence of this postulated effect of insulin to inhibit hepatic VLDL triglyceride secretion, it is suggested that the increase in plasma FFA concentrations in insulin-resistant

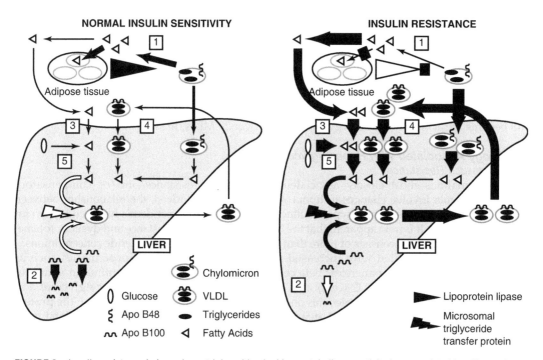

FIGURE 2   Insulin resistance induces hypertriglyceridemia: Lipoprotein lipase activity is upregulated in adipose tissue and may become insulin resistant (1). Furthermore, the uptake of fatty acids by adipose tissue could be reduced in insulin resistance increasing their uptake by the liver (2). Secretion of very-low-density lipoprotein (VLDL) by the liver results from the complex, posttranscriptional regulation of apolipoprotein B (apoB) metabolism in the liver. In the presence of low levels of hepatic triglycerides and cholesterol, much of the constitutively synthesized apoB is degraded by both proteasomal and nonproteasomal pathways (3). When excess triglycerides, and to a lesser extent, cholesterol, are present, and in the presence of active microsomal triglyceride transfer protein, apoB is targeted for secretion (4). The major sources of triglycerides in the liver: uptake of fatty acids (FA) released by lipolysis of adipose tissue triglycerides (2), uptake of triglycerides in VLDL (5) and chylomicrons remnants (6), and hepatic de novo lipogenesis (the synthesis of FA from glucose) (7) are all abnormally increased in insulin resistance.

individuals will be sufficient to overcome hepatic insulin resistance and stimulate hepatic VLDL triglyceride synthesis and secretion (119). Evidence in support of this hypothesis is derived entirely from discerning experiments. For example, insulin rapidly inhibits VLDL triglyceride secretion from cultured rat and human hepatocytes and HepG2 cells (120), and the rapid infusion of insulin inhibits VLDL triglyceride secretion in humans, associated with a substantial decrease in plasma FFA concentration (119).

An obvious explanation for this observation is that an acute insulin infusion will profoundly decrease adipose tissue lipolysis, dramatically lowering FFA concentrations (121–123). The increased flux of FA from adipose tissue can be expanded beyond fatty acid release. Since the enzyme LPL in adipose tissue is upregulated by insulin (124), adipose tissue is an important site for the disposal of dietary triacylglycerol in the postprandial period (125). The process of triglyceride-fatty acid uptake by adipose tissue, may also become insulin-resistant in obesity. This process comprises two steps (126). The first step is the action of LPL on the chylomicron-triglyceride. There are many demonstrations that acute insulin activation of adipose tissue LPL becomes "insulin resistant" in obesity (125). The second step involves the uptake of the FA released by LPL into the adipocyte. The evidence here is less clear-cut, with some evidence for a reduction in this process in obesity, but other evidence against such a reduction (125).

Increased assembly and secretion of VLDL by the liver results from the complex, post-transcriptional regulation of apo B metabolism in the liver. In the presence of low levels of hepatic triglycerides and cholesterol, much of the constitutively synthesized apo B is degraded by both proteasomal and nonproteasomal pathways. When excess triglycerides, and to a lesser extent, cholesterol, are present, and in the presence of active microsomal triglyceride transfer protein, apoB is targeted for secretion. The major sources of triglycerides in the liver include: uptake of FA released by lipolysis of adipose tissue triglycerides, uptake of FA in VLDL and chylomicron remnants, and hepatic de novo lipogenesis (the synthesis of FA from glucose). All these sources are abnormally increased in the setting of insulin resistance (127).

Increased plasma levels of triglycerides in VLDL not only are common characteristics of the dyslipoproteinemia associated with insulin resistance and type 2 diabetes mellitus, but are the central pathophysiological feature of the abnormal lipid profile. Overproduction of VLDL leads to increased plasma levels of triglycerides which, via an exchange process mediated by cholesteryl ester transfer protein, results in the enrichment of HDL and LDL particles with triglycerides. This makes these particles better substrates for hepatic lipase, an enzyme that can catabolize HDL and convert large, buoyant LDL to its smaller, denser, and more atherogenic form (127).

Type 2 Diabetes (Noninsulin-Dependent Diabetes)

Hyperglycemia develops when insulin secretion is inadequate for the degree of insulin resistance. The transition from normal to impaired glucose tolerance and type 2 diabetes is mainly dependent on the progressive deterioration of beta-cell function. The total amount of insulin secreted may be normal or even increased, but temporal insulin secretion may be disturbed. This particularly concerns the early phase of insulin secretion, resulting in postprandial hyperglycemia. Where insulin sensitivity decreases by only about 40%, insulin secretion decreases five-fold in the transition from normal to diabetic glucose tolerance. Importantly, type 2 diabetes begins years, possibly decades, before diagnosis.

Dyslipoproteinemia is common in patients with type 2 diabetes. Patients with type 2 diabetes are at high risk for complications associated with atherosclerosis and should therefore receive preventive lifestyle and pharmacologic interventions.

At the level of the adipocyte, impaired insulin action leads to increased rates of intracellular hydrolysis of triglycerides with the release of NEFA. The rise in NEFA provides substrate for the liver, which, in the presence of impaired insulin action and relative insulin deficiency, is associated with complex alterations in plasma lipids:

1. Plasma VLDL levels are raised.
   - (*i*) Increased VLDL levels are associated with postprandial hyperlipoproteinemia that is compounded by impaired LPL activity. The latter may be independently associated with coronary artery disease (CAD).
   - (*ii*) Remnant particles can deliver more cholesterol to macrophages than LDL particles.
   - (a) Thrombogenic alterations in the coagulation system also ensue from hypertriglyceridemia.

2. Plasma HDL-C levels are reduced.
   (*i*)   The reduction in cardioprotective HDL-C means a reduction in cholesterol efflux from systemic tissues such as the vasculature—the first step in reverse cholesterol transport to the liver (see also the chapter on High-Density Lipoprotein Cholesterol).
   (*ii*) The antioxidant and antiatherogenic activities of HDLs are reduced when circulating levels are low.
3. LDL particles become small and dense. Small, dense LDL particles are held to be more atherogenic than their larger, buoyant counterparts because they
   (a)   are more liable to oxidation
   (b)   may more readily adhere to and subsequently invade the arterial wall
   (c)   have reduced clearance from serum because of decreased affinity for the LDL receptor.

Metabolic and lipid abnormalities can often be improved with lifestyle changes, including dietary modification, weight loss, smoking cessation and increased exercise. Although attainment of better glycemic control may improve diabetic dyslipoproteinemia, pharmacological intervention is usually required.

The Metabolic Syndrome
The metabolic syndrome is a constellation of interrelated risk factors of metabolic origin—metabolic risk factors—that appear to directly promote the development of atherosclerotic CVD. The metabolic syndrome has received increased attention in the past few years. A recent statement from the American Heart Association (AHA) and the National Heart, Lung, and Blood Institute (NHLBI) intends to provide up-to-date guidance for professionals on the diagnosis and management of the metabolic syndrome in adults (128). In accordance with this proposal of the AHA and the NHLBI, a person with any three of the five following categorical cutpoints has the metabolic syndrome:

1. Elevated waist circumference[a,b]
   102 cm and above ($\geq$ 40 in.) in men, 88 cm and above ($\geq$ 35 in.) in women
2. Elevated triglycerides
   150 mg/dL or above or on drug treatment for elevated triglycerides[c]
3. Reduced HDL-C below 40 mg/dL in men, below 50 mg/dL in women or on drug treatment for reduced HDL-C[c]
4. Elevated BP 130 mmHg or above of systolic BP or 85 mmHg or above of diastolic BP or on antihypertensive drug treatment in a patient with a history of hypertension
5. Elevated fasting glucose 100 mg/dL or above or on drug treatment for elevated glucose

Type 1 Diabetes (Insulin-Dependent Diabetes Mellitus)
A recent study has reported that total and lipoprotein cholesterol levels were similar, but triglycerides in IDL and LDL were higher in type 1 diabetics than in control subjects. Most of the marker sterols were transported by LDL and HDL in both groups. The percentage of cholesteryl esters was lower in triglyceride-rich lipoproteins of diabetic patients than control subjects (129).

It has been shown that intensive treatment of type 1 diabetes results in greater weight gain than conventional treatment. The changes in lipid levels and BP that occur with excessive weight gain are similar to those seen in the insulin resistance syndrome and may, over time,

---

[a]To measure waist circumference, locate the top of the right iliac crest. Place a measuring tape in a horizontal plane around the abdomen at the level of the iliac crest. Before reading the tape measure, ensure that the tape is snug but does not compress the skin and is parallel to the floor. Measurement is made at the end of a normal expiration.
[b]Some U.S. adults of non-Asian origin (e.g., white, black, and Hispanic) with marginally increased waist circumference [e.g., 94–102 cm (37–39 in.) in men and 80–88 cm (31–35 in.) in women] may have inherited contribution to insulin resistance and should benefit from changes in lifestyle habits, similar to men with categorical increases in waist circumference. A lower waist circumference cutpoint [e.g., =90 cm (35 in.) in men and =80 cm (31 in.) in women] appears to be appropriate for Asian-Americans.
[c]Fibrates and nicotinic acid are the most commonly used drugs for elevated triglycerides and reduced HDL-C. Patients taking one of these drugs are presumed to have high triglycerides and low HDL-C.

increase the risk of coronary artery disease in this subset of subjects (130). Nevertheless, it has recently been reported that without sufficient insulin treatment, it is difficult to obtain an acceptable level of glycoregulation, avoidance of dyslipoproteinemia, and maintenance of body mass in patients with type 1 diabetes mellitus. On the other hand, it is sometimes difficult to prevent weight gain, endogenous hyperlipoproteinemia, and iatrogenic insulin resistance. A sample of 52 patients with type 1 diabetes with no late complications or long duration of disease was selected. Among them 19 (36.5%) were treated with insulin in four or five doses, and 33 (63.5%) conventionally, in two doses. In the group treated conventionally, a significantly higher mean value of BMI was found compared to those on intensified insulin treatment $(23.2 \pm 2.0 \text{ kg/m}^2$, and $21.2 \pm 1.2 \text{ kg/m}^2$, respectively, $p < 0.01$) and the proportion of those overweight was also significantly higher (27.3% vs. 0%, $p = 0.012$). Higher mean values of systolic (134.2 ± 17.6 mmHg vs. 123.4 ± 12.7, $p < 0.05$) and diastolic (83.2 ± 10.1 vs. 74.0 ± 9.7, $p < 0.01$) BP were noted. Biochemical indicators of glycoregulation were significantly worse with a higher total dose of applied insulin (55.9 ± 8.5 IU vs. 46.3 ± 10.0 IU, $p < 0.01$), and insulin units per kg of body weight (0.84 ± 0.11 IU/kg vs. 0.77 ± 0.15 IU/kg, $p < 0.05$). These results indicate that intensified insulin treatment is a more favorable variant at the level of insulin resistance, which might be present in patients treated with two higher insulin doses, and is probably reduced. It therefore improves metabolic outputs, BP values, and BMI (131).

There has been controversy over the hypothesis that serum lipids affect the development and progression of microvascular complications in patients with type 1 diabetes. Nevertheless, it is now recognized that high triglyceride levels are an independent predictive factor of both renal and retinal complications in patients with type 1 diabetes (132). The EURODIAB Prospective Complications Study examined risk factors in the prediction of CHD and differences in men and women. Baseline risk factors and CHD at follow-up were assessed in 2329 type 1 diabetic patients without prior CHD. CHD was defined as physician-diagnosed myocardial infarction, angina pectoris, coronary artery bypass graft surgery, and/or Minnesota-coded ischemic electrocardiograms or fatal CHD. One hundred and fifty-one patients developed CHD, and the seven-year incidence rate was 8.0 (per 1000 person-years) in men and 10.2 in women. Multivariate standardized Cox proportional hazard models showed that age (hazard ratio 1.5), albumin excretion rate (1.3 in men and 1.6 in women), WHR (1.3 in men), smoking (1.5 in men), fasting triglycerides (1.3 in women) or HDL-C (0.74 in women), and systolic BP (1.3 in women) were predictors of CHD (133).

Thyroid

Thyroid hormones influence all major metabolic pathways. Their most obvious known action is an increase in basal energy expenditure by increasing protein, carbohydrate, and lipid metabolism. With specific regard to lipid metabolism, thyroid hormones affect the synthesis, mobilization, and degradation of lipids, although degradation is influenced more than synthesis. The main and best-known effects on lipid metabolism include: (i) enhanced utilization of lipid substrates; (ii) an increase in the synthesis and mobilization of triglycerides stored in adipose tissue; (iii) an increase in the concentration of NEFA; and (iv) an increase in lipoprotein-lipase activity. While severe hypothyroidism is usually associated with an increased serum concentration of TC, LDL-C, apoB, Lp(a) levels, and possibly triglyceride levels, the occurrence of acute myocardial infarction in hypothyroid patients is not frequent. However, hypothyroid patients appear to have an increased incidence of residual myocardial ischemia following myocardial infarction. Even in subclinical hypothyroidism characterized by raised serum TSH levels with normal serum thyroid hormone concentrations, the preponderance of evidence suggests that TC, LDL-C, and possibly triglycerides are increased, whereas HDL-C and Lp(a) remain unchanged. Mild hyperlipoproteinemia is present and may contribute to an increased risk of atherogenesis. Prudent substitution therapy with L-thyroxine is indicated in patients with both overt and subclinical hypothyroidism, with or without angina, to counteract the cardiovascular risk resulting from dyslipoproteinemia (134).

Subclinical and overt hypothyroidism is a relatively common disorder in the general population. Most lipid abnormalities in patients with overt hypothyroidism are resolved with thyroid hormone replacement therapy (135). In subclinical hypothyroidism, thyroxine replacement reduces TC and LDL-C, with no effect on triglycerides. Effects on HDL-C, Lp(a), and apoA1 and apoB require further study. Clinical trials to date have not shown any beneficial effect of thyroid hormone treatment on serum lipid levels in patients with subclinical hypothyroidism. More extensive prospective studies are needed to clarify many issues (136). The lipid-altering effects of the thyroid hormone make it an appealing target for drug development. The development of specifically targeted thyroid hormone analogues that could potentially treat hyperlipoproteinemia without causing systemic thyrotoxicosis is currently ongoing (135).

Obstructive Liver Disease

Prolonged cholestasis due to primary biliary cirrhosis or other causes is accompanied by marked hyperlipoproteinemia due to the presence of high concentrations of lipoprotein X (Lp-X). The latter is also found in familial lecithin:cholesterol acyltransferase (LCAT) deficiency, but in biliary obstruction its presence reflects substrate excess rather than enzyme deficiency, due to the reflux of biliary lecithin into plasma. This interacts with free cholesterol, albumin, and apoC in plasma and, if these events occur at a rate that exceeds the cholesterol-esterifying capacity of LCAT, Lp-X is formed. Demonstration of the presence of Lp-X in jaundiced plasma on agar gel electrophoresis is diagnostic.

Lipoprotein X (Lp-X) is an abnormal lipoprotein that appears in the sera of patients with obstructive jaundice and is thus a marker for cholestasis. It is a spherical particle that aggregates strongly. Phospholipids and unesterified cholesterol make up the bulk of Lp-X, which is an LDL. Proteins, cholesteryl esters, and triglycerides together make up 12% of the composition of Lp-X. Lithocholic acid is the major bile acid in Lp-X. Three species of Lp-X have been isolated (Lp-X1, Lp-X2, and Lp-X3). Because of its aggregating properties, Lp-X complexes with enzymes such as alkaline phosphatase. Electrophoretic and immunochemical methods are available for assay of Lp-X. The fact that bile lipoprotein can be converted to Lp-X by addition of albumin, and Lp-X can be converted to bile lipoprotein by the addition of bile salts, may suggest that the integrity of the Lp-X molecule depends on a certain critical bile salts to albumin ratio. Phospholipase in plasma is implicated in the catabolism of Lp-X. The role of Lp-X in cholestasis is apparently related to the removal of free cholesterol from the circulation as a consequence of its aggregating properties. The presence of Lp-X in serum does not allow discrimination between intra- and extra-hepatic cholestasis. In addition, Lp-X is present in the plasma of patients with familial plasma LCAT deficiency (137).

Cutaneous xanthomata occur if hyperlipoproteinemia is marked, sometimes accompanied by xanthomatous neuropathy, but without accelerated atherosclerosis, as was first pointed out by Ahrens and colleagues 40 years ago. Effective control of hyperlipoproteinemia may require extreme measures such as plasma exchange. Fibrates can aggravate hypercholesterolemia whereas anion-exchange resins are ineffective. HMG-CoA reductase inhibitors may cause myopathy in patients with cholestasis due to decreased biliary excretion.

Gout

Hypertriglyceridemia is a common accompaniment of gout. In one series, 8 out of 33 patients with primary hyperuricemia and normal renal function had a fasting triglyceride level of over 175 mg/dL, two of whom had values over 1225 mg/dL. One of these had high levels of VLDL and chylomicrons, the remainder only VLDL. There appears to be no direct metabolic link between hyperuricemia and hypertriglyceridemia in that treatment with allopurinol has no effect on triglyceride levels, and the relationship may simply reflect the fact that obesity, alcohol, and thiazides are common causes of both abnormalities. However, patients with primary hypertriglyceridemia often have raised uric acid levels and it has been reported that some fibrates, notably fenofibrate, reduce both triglyceride and uric acid levels in such individuals. On the other hand, nicotinic acid compounds can reduce triglycerides but aggravate hyperuricemia.

Progressive Partial Lipodystrophy

This rare disorder, which is sometimes familial, usually affects females and is characterized by the progressive loss of subcutaneous fat from the upper half of the body. Sometimes, this is associated with apparent redistribution of fat, resulting in gross obesity of the lower limbs. Other features are glucose intolerance, which may progress to frank diabetes, hepatic dysfunction, severe hypertriglyceridemia, and glomerulonephritis. The cause of the disorder is unknown.

Storage Disorders

Hypertriglyceridemia is a feature of both Gaucher's disease and glycogen storage disease and has been shown to remit following the creation of a porto-caval shunt.

Renal Dysfunction

Nephrotic Syndrome. Often, severe hyperlipoproteinemia is common in the nephrotic syndrome. Hypoalbuminemia appears to play a central role probably by diverting increased amounts of FFA to the liver and thus stimulating lipoprotein synthesis. Other causes of hypoalbuminemia can have the same effect. The most common phenotypes are types na and nb although type IV and V phenotypes can also occur. Serum cholesterol is inversely correlated with serum albumin and falls temporarily after albumin infusions. Accelerated vascular disease can be a major consequence of persistent hyperlipoproteinemia and used to be difficult to treat, since fibrates frequently precipitated myositis. However, the advent of HMG-CoA reductase inhibitors may offer new hope to these patients.

Chronic Renal Failure on Dialysis or Posttransplant Hyperlipoproteinemia. It is common in patients with chronic renal failure, including those on hemodialysis, but in contrast to the nephrotic syndrome, hypertriglyceridemia is much more frequent than hypercholesterolemia. CVD is a major cause of mortality and morbidity in patients with chronic kidney disease (CKD) and yet the prevalence of hyperlipoproteinemia is much higher in them than the general population (138). Although LDL-Cl levels in patients who undergo hemodialysis are normal or near normal, increased oxidized LDL, triglycerides, and Lp(a) and decreased HDL-C have been noted. Patients who receive peritoneal dialysis have a more atherogenic lipid profile with the same abnormalities. Furthermore, the LDL particles of peritoneal dialysis patients are small and dense (139). As the majority of patients with CKD die of cardiovascular causes, the Kidney Disease Outcomes Quality Initiative guidelines on dyslipoproteinemias in CKD suggest that all patients should be evaluated for dyslipoproteinemias. Generally, the treatment approach parallels that suggested by the NCEP Adult Treatment Panel III guidelines in which the main focus of treatment is the level of LDL-C. Patients with CKD should be considered in the high-risk category and aggressive therapeutic intervention initiated to reduce the risk of cardiovascular events (138). The emerging consensus is that dialysis patients should be treated aggressively with an LDL-C goal below 100 mg/dL (139).

Conclusion. To conclude this part, genetic and environmental factors interact to determine triglyceride levels. With the exception of rare patients suffering a characterized form of hyperlipoproteinemia (i.e., type-I and type-III hyperlipoproteinemia) because of the presence of mutations in a homozygous or double heterozygous state in a particular gene and in whom this genetic factor has a high penetrance, it would not be possible, in current practice, to precisely determine genetic factors responsible for hypertriglyceridemia in most patients. Conversely, environmental factors such as alcohol intake or overweight are easier to evaluate.

EFFECTS OF HYPOLIPIDEMIC DRUGS ON SERUM TRIGLYCERIDES
Statins

Inhibitors of HMG-CoA reductase (statins) act by decreasing the intracellular synthesis of cholesterol. This results is an increase in hepatocyte LDL-receptor expression and increased serum clearance of LDL-C. Another metabolic consequence is the reduced entry of LDL into the circulation (140). The main effect of statins is then a considerable decrease in LDL-C, the maximal reduction in plasma cholesterol concentrations being induced by treatment with a statin ranging from 24% to 64% (Table 2). Globally, all statins lower plasma triglyceride concentrations but atorvastatin, simvastatin, and rosuvastatin have the greatest effect with a decrease of 17% observed in clinical trials, all doses combined (141). However, the effect of statins on triglycerides depends on their baseline serum levels (Table 3). In subjects with normal triglyceride levels, the effect of statins is small while the magnitude of triglyceride reduction achieved as baseline triglycerides increase ranges from −30% to −40% in subjects with triglycerides above 250 mg/dL (152,153). Furthermore, the hypotriglyceridemic effect of statins is parallel to the decrease in LDL-C in hypertriglyceridemic subjects (142,154). Statins simultaneously

TABLE 2   Effects of Hypolipidemic Drugs on Plasma Lipid Concentrations Expressed as Percentage Changes

	Triglycerides	LDL cholesterol	HDL cholesterol	References
Statins				
Atorvastatin	−17	−36	7	(141,144,217)
Fluvastatin	−10	−30	7	(141,144,217)
Lovastatin	−15	−30	7	(141,144,217)
Pravastatin	−12	−27	12	(141,144,217)
Rosuvastatin	−18	−46	9	(141,218,219)
Simvastatin	−17	−34	6	(141,144,217)
Fibrates				
Bezafibrate	−38		10	(220)
Ciprofibrate	−24	−22	12	(152,221)
Fenofibrate	−21	−17	6	(152)
Gemfibrozil	−36	−5	10	(222)
Nicotinic acid	−30	−15	25	(156,157)
n-3 fatty acids	−55	−5	−2	

Abbreviations: LDL, low-density lipoprotein; HDL, high-density lipoprotein.

reduce the concentrations of remnant lipoprotein particle (155,156) and postprandial triglyceridemia (157). The mechanism behind the decrease in triglyceride levels is essentially an increase in VLDL and VLDL remnant catabolism (158,159) probably through the increased uptake of these particles by LDL receptors.

Fibrates

The prototypical fibric acid, clofibrate, is no longer used. The related drugs partly resemble short-chain FA and act by activating the nuclear transcription factor, peroxisome proliferator–activated receptor alpha (PPARα), upregulating a large number of genes such as those coding for apoAI, apoAII, LPL, and some involved in reverse cholesterol transport as well in the fatty oxidation of the liver. Fibrates downregulate genes such as apoCIII and a few involved in the inflammatory process in the artery wall. However, fibrates are not entirely specific for PPARα and a few of them also weakly activate PPARγ, but this is not known to have a clinical role (39).

Four fibrates (bezafibrate, ciprofibrate, fenofibrate, gemfibrozil) are available, but not in all countries. These drugs are the most effective hypotriglyceridemic ones (Table 2), because of an increase in the catabolism of triglyceride-rich lipoproteins by a rise in LPL activity (due to an increase in LPL gene expression and a decrease in apoCIII gene expression) (39,147). LDL-C concentrations increase during fibrate treatment in a small percentage of subjects (the so-called "Beta effect"), and the LDL-C lowering effect of fibrates partly depends on the drug used and the initial LDL-C level. Fibrates are also effective in raising HDL-C due to a large increase in apoAI synthesis not completely counterbalanced by an increase in catabolism (159) (personal results). Fibrates increase the buoyancy of LDL particles, a potentially favorable effect (160).

Nicotinic Acid

Nicotinic acid (niacin) is effective in decreasing triglycerides, TC, and LDL-C cholesterol, and increasing HDL-C (Table 2). The major limitations to the use of plain niacin are cutaneous flush and itching, mucous membrane irritation including diarrhea and metabolic disturbances

TABLE 3   Hypotriglyceridemic Effects of Statins Expressed as the Percentage of Triglyceride Decrease According to Triglyceride Baseline

Baseline triglycerides (mg/dl)	Simvastatin (40 mg)	Lovastatin (40 mg)	Pravastatin (40 mg)	Rosuvastatin (10 mg)
<150	−7	4	−4	
150–250	−22	−14	−15	
>250	−29	−30	−35	
<200	−	−	−	−16
≥200	−	−	−	−29

Note: −, data not reported.

(increases in glucose, uric acid, and hepatic enzymes). Time-released nicotinic acid has been developed in an attempt to overcome these side effects, but the available formulations have been less effective and/or more hepatotoxic than plain niacin.

A recent intermediate-time release niacin formulation (Niaspan®) given once daily at the dose of up to 2 g/day at bedtime appears efficacious and better tolerated than plain niacin and less hepatotoxic than extended release niacin. About 50% to 80% of the patients taking Niaspan experience flushing, but this side effect becomes infrequent or resolves after a few weeks of treatment (161). Niaspan has no or only mild side effects on the liver and minimally modifies glycosylated hemoglobin in type 2 diabetes (162).

The effect of Niaspan on lipid and lipoprotein levels is dose-dependent. The main effects at the dose of 2000 mg/day are a decrease in triglycerides (−30%) and a large increase in HDL-C (+25%). Niaspan moderately decreases LDL-C (−15%) and is particularly effective in decreasing Lp(a) levels (−25%) (150,151,163).

The biological mechanism explaining the modulation of lipid and lipoprotein levels through niacin is only partly known. Niacin tends to diminish lipolysis in adipocytes (164), possibly by inhibiting hormone sensitive lipase (165). As a result, a smaller quantity of FFA is transported to the liver and in turn, the liver esterifies fewer of these FFA into triglycerides. Reduced triglyceride production results in decreased hepatic VLDL secretion, which can in turn lead to a decreased generation of LDL particles. In addition, niacin reduces hepatic HDL catabolism by blocking holoparticle uptake of this lipoprotein (166).

Omega-3 Fatty Acids

Omega-3 FA used as hypolipidemic drugs are essentially of marine origin, i.e., eicosapentaenoic acid (EPA) and docosahexaenoic acid (DHA). This treatment decreases triglycerides by 25% to 50%, while LDL-C tends to rise by 5% to 25% and HDL-C by 7% to 13% (Table 2). Omega-3 fatty acid from plants (alpha-linolenic acid) has a similar effect on lipids to that of omega-6 fatty acid enriched oils and so is not equivalent to marine omega-3 FA. Fish oils were moderately concentrated in omega-3 FA in old preparations (35%), but more recent ones such as Omacor® have a higher quantity of omega-3 FA (85%). The hypotriglyceridemic effect is higher for the concentrated formulation than for the former (167,168). The mechanisms by which marine *n*-3 FA modulate serum lipids are primarily a decrease in VLDL synthesis (169). Omacor is effective in decreasing serum triglyceride levels (−45%) in severe hypertriglyceridemic patients (170).

Thiazolidinediones

Thiazolidinediones are oral antihyperglycemic agents that reduce insulin resistance in peripheral tissues and decrease hepatic glucose production (171). They are potent, synthetic ligands for PPARγ activation, which mediate the physiological response by altering the transcription of genes that regulate glucose and lipid metabolism (172). Currently, there are two thiazolidinediones available: rosiglitazone and pioglitazone. However, at usual clinical doses, pioglitazone also activates PPARα while rosiglitazone seems to be an almost pure PPARγ agonist (173). The differential effect could explain the findings that pioglitazone tends to reduce triglyceride concentration (approximately −20%) with no or little effect on LDL-C whereas rosiglitazone has a variable effect on triglycerides and increases LDL-C levels (+8 to +16%). Both drugs increase HDL-C (+5 to +13%) (174–176).

Antiobesity Drugs

Orlistat acts as an inhibitor of gastric, pancreatic, and carboxylester lipase, which consequently results in both a decreased absorption of fat and the excretion of unabsorbed cholesterol and triglycerides. This effect should facilitate weight loss in obese subjects because the intake of excess dietary fat is one of the leading causes of obesity. Weight loss is also known to be associated with an improvement in the serum lipid profile.

In obese subjects, orlistat had a significant but modest and favorable effect on TC and LDL-C, –17 and –13 mg/dL, respectively, no effect on HDL-C, and a small one on triglycerides (–7 mg/dL). It is difficult to determine whether these effects were due to weight loss induced by the drug or the consequence of a direct effect of the drug through inhibition of intestinal lipid absorption, but it was probably due to weight loss because similar weight loss obtained by other means had a similar effect on lipids (52). Orlistat can be used to treat severe hyperchylomicronemia due to excess absorption of dietary triglyceride.

Sibutramine is a pharmacological agent for weight loss. Sibutramine acts by blocking the neuronal reuptake of serotonine and norepinephrine and enhancing postprandial satiety. After six months of treatment, weight decreases by five kilograms, on an average. Triglycerides decrease and HDL-C increases in obese subjects taking sibutramine, these changes being proportional to the magnitude of weight loss (177).

Rimonabant is a recently developed drug prescribed to obese patients. Rimonabant acts by blocking the endocannabinoid-1 receptor present in the hypothalamus but also in other tissues such as the adidpocyte. Subjects taking rimonabant had a decrease in triglycerides and an increase in HDL-C levels associated with weight loss, but these lipid changes appear to be greater than those presumed to be due to weight loss alone. These specific lipid effects are perhaps due to the effect of rimonabant on adipocytes (178).

Combination of Hypolipidemic Drugs

Hypertriglyceridemic subjects frequently have lipid abnormalities other than high triglyceride levels such as low HDL-C and high LDL-C. All these abnormalities are rarely normalized by only one hypolipidemic drug. A combination of two or more drugs yields significantly better results than monotherapy. Statins have largely shown their efficacy in lowering LDL-C, leading to a reduction in cardiovascular risk. Fibrates, such as gemfibrozil and bezafibrate, have proven their favorable clinical effects, particularly in individuals with insulin resistance or high triglycerides/low HDL-C levels. Niacin reduces CHD risk, but its LDL-C lowering effect is considerably less than that of statins. Each of these hypolipidemic drugs decreases CHD risk by changing plasma lipids in different ways. Even if no clinical trial using a combination of hypolipidemic drugs has really proved a reduction in CHD risk, it is likely that the simultaneous effects of lowering LDL-C and decreasing triglycerides/raising HDL-C are cumulative in reducing the cardiovascular risk.

Statin/Fibrate Combination Therapy

The use of combined fibrate/statin has been limited because of earlier reports suggesting a 3% to 5% risk of myopathy occasionally associated with severe complications, including rhabdomyolysis and renal failure. However, it seems that this high frequency of severe myopathy was due to the use of gemfibrozil, which particularly interacts with statin metabolism (179). The frequency of side effects of other statin/fibrates besides statin/gemfibrozil combination has been rare. Between 1989 and 2000, there were 29 published case reports of rhabdomyolysis with acute renal failure sometimes secondary to the combination of fibrates and statins. In each case, gemfibrozil was the fibrate incriminated (180). The number of cases of rhabdomyolysis reported per million prescription of fibrate/statin therapy was 0.58 and 8.6 when fenofibrate and gemfibrozil were used in association with statin (cerivastatin excluded) (181). Adding fibrate to statin improved the lipoprotein profile compared to statin monotherapy with a greater decrease in triglycerides and increase in HDL-C and to a lesser extent a more marked lowering of LDL-C (182–186).

Nevertheless, combination therapy with statins and fibrates requires careful selection and monitoring of patients. First, the benefit/risk ratio has to be carefully evaluated in patients presenting risk factors that may predispose to severe myopathy. These factors include increased age, female gender, renal or liver disease, hypothyroidism, excessive alcohol intake, surgery, and vigorous exercise. Patients with abnormal renal or liver functions, or elderly patients have to be excluded unless the benefit/risk ratio is favorable. Second, if a fibrate has already been begun (the dose of a fibrate is usually fixed), the statin should usually be started at a low dose and gradually titrated after checking clinical and serum parameters. Patients should be counseled with regard to the risks and warning signs of myopathy (e.g., muscle pain, weakness, and dark urine) and therapy discontinued if they develop any of these warning signs. Renal function as well serum creatine phosphokinase and transaminases are regularly checked. Statin/fibrate therapy can be continued even if transaminases rise to three times ULN or creatine phosphokinase to five times ULN without symptoms. Repeat measurements should be made regularly every three months. A rise in enzymes above these limits needs repeat measurement and discontinuation of one of the two drugs if the abnormality persists.

Statin/Niacin Combination Therapy

The combination of a statin with niacin is an attractive option in patients with mixed hyper-lipoproteinemia because both have excellent safety histories for improving cardiovascular outcomes. In a recent randomized angiographic trial, the frequency of the clinical end point was reduced by 89% in patients taking simvastatin–niacin combination therapy compared to placebo, e.g., 24% with placebo and 3% with simvastatin-niacin. Moreover, simvastatin plus niacin reduced cardiovascular events by 40% in patients with metabolic syndrome (187). A number of clinical trials compared niacin and the combined use of niacin and statins. Adding a statin to niacin enhances the LDL-C and triglyceride lowering effects from –20% to −35% and –28% to −33%, respectively. The increase in HDL-C observed with niacin was not really modified during the statin-niacin combination (188). The combination of statin with niacin is safe.

Statin-Omega-3 Combination Therapy

High doses (3–5 g/day) of omega-3 FA (corresponding to 1–1.5 g EPA-DHA per day) have been shown to reduce triglycerides by 20% to 30%. Combining omega-3 FA with statins is an attractive option in patients suffering from mixed hyperlipoproteinemia. There have been few studies on the combination of statins and omega-3 FA. The supplementation of pravastatin or simvastatin (20 mg/day) with 3 to 3.6 g/day of omega-3 FA significantly lowers cholesterol and triglyceride concentrations by 7% and 9%, respectively, when subjects taking the combination were compared with those taking only statins (189,190). In contrast, the addition of omega-3 FA (1.68 g/day) was not effective in decreasing triglycerides in subjects already taking atorva-statin of 10 mg/day. However, the addition of omega-3 FA did increase HDL-C and decreased postprandial hypertriglyceridemia effectively (191). Interestingly, the concentration of small dense atherogenic LDL decreases in the plasma of subjects treated with statin-omega-3 combination therapy (190,191).

CLINICAL TRIALS
Clinical Trials Using Fibrates

Among the four fibrates used in clinical practice, only two, gemfibrozil and bezafibrate, were studied for their efficacy in decreasing the incidence of CVD in humans. Fenofibrate was evaluated in diabetes [the Fenofibrate Intervention and Event Lowering in Diabetes (FIELD) Study] (Table 4) (192).

Primary Prevention

The Helsinki Heart Study

Gemfibrozil (1200 mg/day) was tested in the Helsinki Heart Study, a randomized, double-blind five-year trial that included 4081 dyslipidemic and CHD-free men aged 40 to 55 years (193). To be included, subjects had to have non-HDL-C of 200 mg/dL or above. The means of age and BMI in randomized subjects were 47.3 years and 26.6 kg/m^2, respectively. At baseline, means of TC, LDL-C, HDL-C, and triglycerides were 289, 189, 47, and 242 mg/dL, respectively. Gemfibrozil effectively decreased triglycerides (-35%), TC (-9%) and LDL-C (-9%), while HDL-C increased by 9%.

The rates of major cardiac endpoints (nonfatal and fatal myocardial infarction or sudden cardiac death) were 4.1% and 2.7% in the placebo and treated groups, respectively. This 34% reduction in the incidence of CHD was significant ($p < 0.002$) (193). The changes in serum HDL-C and LDL-C levels were both statistically and significantly associated with the decline in CHD incidence within the gemfibrozil-treated group whereas the large decrease in triglyc-eride levels had relatively little effect on CHD incidence (194).

In this study, serum triglyceride concentration in association with an LDL-C/HDL-C ratio is a strong predictor of cardiac events. The relative risk in the group of subjects with triglycerides above 201 mg/dL and an LDL-C/HDL-C ratio above 5 was 3.8 times higher that the risk for subjects with triglycerides below 201 mg/dL and cholesterol ratio of 5 and above. Moreover, subjects with high risk profited most from treatment with gemfibrozil with a 71% lower incidence of CHD events than the corresponding placebo subgroup. Another subgroup classification showed that gemfibrozil was also very efficient in subjects with hypertriglyc-eridemia (>200 mg/dL) and low HDL-C (<42 mg/dL) (195).

TABLE 4 Characteristics and Results of Clinical Trials Using Fibrates

		Placebo event rate (%)	Treatment event rate (%)	RRR	NNT to prevent one event	Triglycerides (mg/dL)	Baseline LDL cholesterol (mg/dL)	HDL cholesterol (mg/dL)
Primary prevention								
HHS							Criteria of inclusion non-HDL-C $\geq$200 mg/dl	
Gemfibrozil	All cohort (CHD)	4.1	2.7	−34	71	242	189	47
	Tg > 200 (mg/dL) and HDL-C (<42 mg/dL)	8	2.7	−66	19			
Secondary prevention								
VA-HIT						Criteria of inclusion		
						≤300	≤140	≤40
Gemfibrozil	All cohort (CHD + stroke)	26.1	20.4	−22	18	161	111	32
	All cohort (CHD)	21.7	17.3	−20	23			
	Insulin-resistant (CHD + stroke)	31.7	23.2	−28	12	179	109	31
	Non-insulin-resistant (CHD + stroke)	20.7	17.1	−20	28	153	113	32
BIP						Criteria of inclusion		
						≤300	≤180	≤45
Bezafibrate	All cohort (CHD)	15	13.6	−9.4 (ns)	71	145	148	35
	Metabolic syndrome	18.4	14.1	−23	23	170	146	33
	Tg >200 mg/dl and HDL-C <35 mg/dl	22.3	13	−42	11			
Prevention in diabetes								
FIELD						Criteria of inclusion		
						116–250	87–438	OR cholesterol /HDL-C = 4
Fenofibrate	All cohort (CHD)	5.9	5.2	−11 (ns)	143	151	119	43
	All cohort (MI)	4.2	3.2	−24	100			
	All cohort (CVD)	13.9	12.5	−11	69			
	Metabolic syndrome	14.5	13.1	−9.7 (ns)	71			
	Tg > 150 mg/dL and HDL-C < 40 (men) and 50 (women) mg/dL	16.3	14.0	−14 (ns)	43			

Abbreviations: CHD, coronary death + nonfatal myocardial infarction; MI, myocardial infarction; CVD, cardiovascular disease = CVD death, MI, stroke, coronary or carotid revascularisation; ns, non significant–; otherwise $p < 0.05$; HDL, high-density lipoprotein; VA-HII, Veterans Affairs High-Density Lipoprotein Cholesterol Intervention Trial; HHS, Helsinki Heart Study; BIP, Bezafibrate Infarction Prevention; LDL, low-density lipoprotein; FIELD, Fenofibrate Intervention and Event Lowering in Diabetes; Tg, triglyceride.

A post hoc analysis showed that the favorable preventive effect of gemfibrozil was mainly concentrated in overweight subjects (BMI > 26 kg/m^2) with low HDL-C (<42 mg/dL) and high triglyceride levels (>204 mg/dL). Indeed, among these subjects, the placebo group had a CHD incidence 2.6 times that found in the group of subjects with normal HDL-C and triglyceride levels and the reduction in CHD risk was 78%. Furthermore, the treatment effect was consistently favorable in overweight subjects with high blood glucose and/or hypertension and/or smoking and/or sedentary lifestyle (196).

Secondary Prevention

Veterans Affairs High-Density Lipoprotein Cholesterol Intervention Trial
The Veterans Affairs High-Density Lipoprotein Cholesterol Intervention Trial (VA-HIT) was a randomized clinical trial including subjects in secondary prevention whose major lipid abnormality

was a low level of HDL-C. The patients were eligible for this trial if they were men with documented CHD, an HDL-C 40 mg/dL or below and LDL cholesterol of 140 mg/dL or below. Two thousand five hundred and thirty-one subjects were randomized to either gemfibrozil (1200 mg/day) or placebo, and were followed for an average of five years. Their mean age was 64 and their mean BMI was 29 kg/m^2. The average lipids at baseline were cholesterol, 175 mg/dL, HDL-C, 32 mg/dL, LDL-C, 111 mg/dL, and triglycerides, 160 mg/dL (197).

The CHD (first nonfatal myocardial infarction or CHD death) event rates were 21.7% and 17.3% in patients receiving placebo and gemfibrozil, respectively. The 22% (95% CI 7–35%) lower relative reduction in CHD incidence was significant ($p = 0.006$) (197). There was also a significant reduction in cerebrovascular events (198).

A post hoc analysis used the measurements of plasma fasting glucose and insulin levels at baseline to divide subjects into subgroups relative to the presence of diabetes mellitus (defined by plasma glucose value ≥126 mg/dL or history of diabetes) and insulin resistance determined according to the homeostasis model assessment of insulin resistance (HOMA-IR) index. Higher waist circumference (109 cm) and BMI (31.5 kg/m^2) were measured in subjects with insulin resistance whether diabetic or not, and compared to those without insulin resistance (100 cm and 27.6 kg/m^2 respectively). The rate of cardiovascular events in subjects with insulin resistance was associated with hypertriglyceridemia (~170 mg/dL) compared to those without insulin resistance (triglycerides ~140 mg/dL) while HDL-C was globally similar in all subgroups. Gemfibrozil appeared more efficacious in the group of subjects with insulin resistance, reducing CHD events by 28% ($p = 0.02$) compared to the group with lower HOMA-IR, CHD incidence decreasing by 20% ($p = 0.06$) in this last subgroup. Gemfibrozil, moreover, tends to be essentially cardioprotective in subjects with low HDL-C (<29 mg/dL) and/or triglycerides (>180 mg/dL) and without insulin resistance, whereas the efficacy of gemfibrozil was similar in subjects with insulin resistance whatever the HDL-C and triglyceride levels (199). The most favorable effect of gemfibrozil in subjects with insulin resistance was concordant with the results of another post hoc analysis of VA-HIT. In subjects without diabetes, gemfibrozil indeed appeared more efficacious among those with the highest level of fasting plasma insulin (200). Finally, if on-trial HDL-C is a good predictor of CHD outcomes, no more than 23% of the decrease in CHD incidence could be explained by lipid level changes. This is probably because of other effects of gemfibrozil such as a direct anti-inflammatory effect in the artery wall.

The Bezafibrate Infarction Prevention Study. In the Bezafibrate Infarction Prevention study, 3122 patients who were mainly men (>90%) aged 45 to 74 years, with a recent history of myocardial infarction (≥6 months <5 years) or stable angina pectoris, were randomized to receive either 400 mg of bezafibate or placebo. To be eligible for randomization, patients were required to have TC between 180 and 250 mg/dL, LDL-C of 180 mg/dL or below (≤160 for patients <50 years), HDL-C 45 mg/dL or below, and triglycerides 300 mg/dL or below.

The mean age of enrolled subjects was 60 and BMI 27.7 kg/m^2. They were followed for an average of 6.2 years. Baseline lipids were TC 212 mg/dL, HDL-C 34.6 mg/dL, LDL-C 148 mg/dL, and triglycerides 145 mg/dL. Bezafibrate increased HDL-C by 18% and decreased triglycerides by 21%, while TC and LDL-C slightly decreased in patients treated with bezafibrate. Among these patients, the rate of the primary endpoint (nonfatal and fatal myocardial infarction or sudden death) was 13.6% versus 15.0% in the placebo group, i.e., a nonsignificant reduction of 9.4% ($p = 0.26$). No difference in the incidence of ischemic stroke was noted (201).

A post hoc analysis of CHD incidence dividing subjects according to baseline triglycerides and HDL-C showed that bezafibrate reduced the primary endpoint rate in the group of patients with triglycerides 200 mg/dL or above and HDL-C below 35 mg/dL, whereas no benefit was observed in patients with triglycerides below 200 mg/dL or triglycerides 200 mg/dL or below and HDL-C 35 mg/dL or below (202).

Another post hoc analysis was performed to evaluate the efficacy of bezafibrate in patients with metabolic syndrome. Almost half (47%) of the patients randomized in the trial met a definition near that of ATP III (i.e., at least three out of five factors, a high waist circumference from ATP III's criteria being replaced by a high BMI ≥28 kg/m^2). No difference between the placebo and bezafibrate groups appeared at baseline in terms of clinical and laboratory characteristics. Baseline TC and LDL-C were similar in patients with metabolic syndrome compared to the whole cohort whereas HDL-C was slightly lower (33 mg/dL) and triglycerides higher (170 g/dL) than those measured in the whole cohort. Bezafibrate effectively increased HDL-C (+14%; $p < 0.001$) and decreased triglyceride levels (-26%; $p < 0.001$) in patients with metabolic syndrome. The CHD rate was 18.4% in subjects randomized to placebo and 14.1% in subjects randomized to bezafibrate, for risk reduction of 25% ($p = 0.03$) (201).

Prevention in Diabetes
The Fenofibrate Intervention and Event Lowering in Diabetes Study
The FIELD study was the single clinical event study using fibrate specifically only on diabetic patients. Nine thousand seven hundred and ninety-five people aged 50 to 75 years (63% males) were included in the FIELD study, a randomized controlled trial. The patients had a diagnosis of type 2 diabetes mellitus not taking statin therapy, TC of 116 to 250 mg/dL and a TC/HDL-C ratio 4 and above, or plasma triglycerides of 87 to 438 mg/dL. Four thousand eight hundred and ninety-five and 4900 patients took fenofibrate and placebo, respectively, in a double-blind pattern over a five-year duration. Twenty-two percent of the patients had a history of CVD at entry. About 5.9% of the patients on placebo and 5.2% of those receiving fenofibrate had a major coronary event (coronary death or nonfatal myocardial infarction), i.e., a nonsignificant 11% relative reduction. There was no benefit from fenofibrate concerning coronary death whereas the incidence of nonfatal myocardial infarction significantly decreased by 24%. Considering all CVD events including CHD death, myocardial infarction, stroke, and coronary and carotid revascularization, fenofibrate significantly decreased their incidence by 11% (12.5% vs. 13.9%, $p = 0.035$). Fenofibrate therapy significantly reduced microvascular disease as evidenced by lesser progression of albuminuria (11% vs. 10%, $p < 0.002$) and reduced need of laser treatment for retinopathy (5.2% vs. 3.6%, $p < 0.001$). The data suggest that 69 diabetic patients need to be treated for five years to prevent one CVD related event (203).

The FIELD study showed that fenofibrate did not reduce the incidence of major CHD events (coronary death and nonfatal myocardial infarction) in diabetic patients in a statistically significant fashion. This absence of significant results is due either to fenofibrate itself or to the design of this trial. Indeed, as prevention clinical trials in diabetes [heart protection study (HPS), collaborative atorvastatin diabetic study (CARDS)] were published after the beginning of the FIELD study and primary-care doctors or specialist physicians were free to adapt hypolipidemic treatment, a number of patients took statins during the study, the rate being lower in the fenofibrate-allocated patients than in the placebo group. After adjustment for new lipid-lowering therapy, fenofibrate reduced the risk of CHD events by 19% ($p = 0.01$) and total CVD events by 15% ($p = 0.004$). Finally, fenofibrate was generally well tolerated in patients taking both fenofibrate and statin.

Nicotinic Acid
Several clinical trials evaluated the effect of nicotinic acid on the rate of cardiovascular outcomes. The Coronary Drug Project was the only one to have used nicotinic acid as monotherapy. This six-year randomized, placebo-controlled trial included subjects with previous myocardial infarction. Subjects were treated with various drugs (conjugated estrogens, dextrothyroxin, clofibrate, nicotinic acid) or placebo in parallel groups. Mean baseline TC was 250 mg/dL and triglycerides, 177 mg/dL.

Nicotinic acid was given at a dosage of 1 g three times daily and decreased cholesterol by 10% and triglycerides by 26% compared to placebo. LDL-C and HDL-C were not determined in this study because measurements were not available at the time of this trial (1966–1975). However, more recent data indicate that immediate-release nicotinic acid decreases LDL-C and triglycerides by about 15% and 26%, respectively, and this was the most powerful drug on the market to increase HDL-C ($\sim$22+%) (204).

Nicotinic acid decreased nonfatal myocardial infarction by 26% (13.8% in the placebo group; 10.2% in the treatment group) ($p < 0.005$) and major CHD events (coronary death and nonfatal myocardial infarction) by 15% (30.1% vs. 25.6%) ($p < 0.01$). The stroke rate also decreased (-24%; $p < 0.05$) (205). Even if the trial was discontinued in 1975 and the drug no longer recommended because of the absence of a significant difference in the incidence of cardiovascular death between nicotinic acid and placebo groups, subjects were followed up for an additional nine years. This posttrial follow-up study showed a 10.6% relative reduction in total mortality ($p < 0.0001$) among men originally assigned to the nicotinic acid group indicating a beneficial effect on fatal CVD long after withdrawal of the study drug, which makes understanding the mechanism more complicated (206).

Another clinical trial using nicotinic acid was the Stockholm Ischemic Heart Disease study. This trial was a five-year randomized open-label trial, which included 555 survivors of myocardial infarction below 70 years of age. Subjects were treated with a combination of nicotinic acid and clofibrate or placebo. Cholesterol and triglycerides were 245 and 208 mg/dL at baseline and decreased by 13% and 19%, respectively, in the treated patients compared to placebo. A significant reduction in ischemic heart disease mortality was observed. Moreover, total mortality decreased by 26% ($p < 0.05$). An analysis by subgroup showed that the benefit of combined treatment was essentially observed in subjects with high triglycerides (>136 mg/dL) whereas those with the lower triglyceride levels at baseline had little or no benefit, a finding similar to those from clinical trials using fibrates (207).

Several other trials used nicotinic acid, but in combination with one or two other hypolipidemic drugs (clofibrate, gemfibrozil, cholestyramine, lovastatin, simvastatin). Most of them were angiographic studies aimed at assessing the effect of the drug regimen on coronary atherosclerotic lesions. With the exception of one study, the Harvard Atherosclerosis Reversibility Project (HARP) Study, which showed no significant differences in lesion modification (208), five other studies showed a favorable effect with either a lesser progression or even an average angiographic regression in the treated group compared to placebo. Even if a difference in clinical endpoints between treatment and placebo groups was not the main objective of these studies, most of them analyzed the incidence of cardiovascular events and, with the exception of the HARP Study, showed a significant decrease in combined cardiovascular events (cardiovascular death, nonfatal myocardial infarction, revascularization procedure) in treated patients compared to those taking placebo (187,209–213).

Statins

The favorable effect of HMG-CoA reductase inhibitors (statins) on clinical event endpoints has been largely demonstrated across a broad range of patient cohorts. Among the six statins prescribed, four—lovastatin, simvastatin, pravastatin, and atorvastatin—have provided evidence of a decrease in the incidence of CHD and stroke events. The clinical effect of statins is largely considered as a consequence of a reduction in LDL-C (214). Statins also decrease triglyceride levels, but to a moderate extent. Initial and post hoc analyses of these trials have evaluated the clinical effect of statins in patients with hypertriglyceridemia or conditions associated with high triglyceride levels such as metabolic syndrome (Table 5).

The 4S was the first trial to demonstrate that statin therapy could reduce CHD rates in a secondary-prevention population (215). A subsequent subgroup analysis showed, in subjects with high LDL-C, a greater effect of simvastatin in the quartile where subjects had the lowest HDL-C (<39 mg/dL) and highest triglycerides (>159 mg/dL) compared to the quartile where patients had the highest HDL-C (>52 mg/dL) and lowest triglycerides (<98 mg/dL). The incidence of major coronary events was 35.9% and 19% in the former and 20.8% and 18.0% in the latter in placebo and treated groups, respectively (216). Excluding patients with diabetes did not alter these results.

In other clinical trials using statins, the analysis evaluated the effect of baseline triglyceride levels on clinical event rates. The population was divided into thirds or in two groups according to medians. Globally, no difference in the effect of the different statins appeared in the incidence of major CHD events according to triglyceride levels. A few studies [HPS, cholesterol and recurrent events (CARE)] tend to show a decrease in the efficacy of statins when triglyceride levels are elevated whereas others [long-term intervention with pravastatin in inchemic disease (LIPID), air force coronary atherosclerosis prevention study/texas coronary atherosclerosis prevention study (AFCAPS/TexCAPS)] show no heterogeneity in the effects of treatment related to triglycerides, unlike the results of the 4S. Taken together, the results of clinical trials using statins suggest that the clinical effect of these drugs is mediated through a decrease in LDL cholesterol whatever the baseline serum triglycerides.

Omega-3 Fatty Acids

Fish oils moderately concentrated in marine omega-3 FA (EPA and DHA) decrease triglyceride levels. Although a large number of randomized controlled trials comparing omega-3 FA and placebo on the incidence of cardiovascular events have been carried out, no decrease in

TABLE 5 Results of Clinical Trials of Statins in Primary and Secondary Prevention in Groups of Subjects Defined by Triglyceride Subgroups

Trial (I: primary; II: secondary)	Triglycerides (mg/dL)	Placebo event rate (%)	Statin event rate (%)	RRR	p	NNT to prevent one event	Baseline LDL cholesterol
WOSCOPS (I)	<148	6.3	4.4	−29	0.024	53	192
	≥148	9.4	6.6	−32	0.003	36	
AFCAPS/TexCAPS (I)					ns	50	150
4S (II)	<98	20.8	18.0	−13	ns		178
	>159	35.9	19.0	−47	0.001	6	192
CARE (II)	<144	27	19	−32	<0.001	13	139
	≥144	26	22	−15	0.07	25	
LIPID (II)	<133	15	12	−25	<0.05	25	150
	133-230	15	12	−24	<0.05	33	
	>230	16	14	−24	<0.05	25	
HPS (II or high risk)	<175	23.7	18.3	−23	<0.05	19	131
	≥175-350	27.3	21.6	−21	<0.05	18	
	≥350	27.1	23.2	−26	<0.05	26	

Note: Nonfatal MI or CHD death in WOSCOPS, LIPID; nonfatal MI, CHD death, coronary-artery bypass grafting or percutaneous transluminal coronary angioplasty in CARE, major vascular events (total CHD, total stroke, revascularizations) in HPS; nonfatal or fatal MI, unstable angina, or sudden cardiac death in AFCAPS.
Abbreviations: LDL, low-density lipoprotein, HDL, high-density lipoprotein.

combined cardiovascular events or fatal or nonfatal myocardial infarction, whatever the fish or vegetable source or the dose, was noted in a meta-analysis. While triglycerides globally decreased by 35 mg/dL, HDL-C was not modified, and LDL-C increased by 5 mg/dL (217). The GISSI prevention trial showed a significant decrease in CHD outcomes (combined death, myocardial infarction, stroke) in patients surviving myocardial infarction and taking omega-3 FA (1g/day), but the dose was not sufficient to decrease triglyceride levels. So, the favorable effect of omega-3 fatty acid intake in this trial was probably due to effects other than the hypotriglyceridemic one (218).

Comparison Between Treatments

The incidence of CHD and stroke is reduced by statins. This effect appears to be related to a decrease in LDL-C and is proportional to the duration of treatment (214). Furthermore, the effect of statins on the reduction of CHD incidence seems independent of the presence of hypertriglyceridemia/low HDL-C or the metabolic syndrome. In contrast, fibrates are essentially effective in CHD and stroke prevention in patients with insulin resistance or hyperlipoproteinemia often associated with the metabolic syndrome, i.e., hypertriglyceridemia/low HDL-C.

Table 6 shows the results of different trials using statins and fibrates in secondary prevention in subjects with hypertriglyceridemia or metabolic syndrome, expressed in absolute terms. The number of patients to be treated needed to prevent a new major CHD event [number needed to treat (NNT)] is an excellent parameter to assess the absolute efficacy of a treatment. Therapy with simvastatin in 4S, where patients had high values of LDL-C resulted in the lowest NNT. In contrast, fibrate (gemfibrozil or bezafibrate) therapy provided the next lowest NNT compared with statin trials where patients had moderately elevated LDL-C. Converse to gemfibrozil and bezafibrate, fenofibrate did not seem to be more efficient in the prevention of CVD in diabetic patients with metabolic syndrome or hypertriglyceridemia/low HDL-C than in those not having these abnormalities (203).

Comparison with other hypolipidemic drugs is not possible yet because of the absence of clinical trials in hypertriglyceridemic patients. Niacin is theoretically a useful drug in patients with hypertriglyceridemia/low HDL-C, but no data are available to specifically evaluate this drug in hypertriglyceridemic or insulin-resistant subjects. Other trials using a combination of niacin with one or two other hypolipidemic drugs are angiographic studies including small numbers of patients, making interpretation of clinical results awkward. There has, however, been a clear tendency toward clinical efficacy of combined therapy with niacin compared to

TABLE 6 Trials Using Statins and Fibrates in Secondary Prevention, in Subjects with Hypertriglyceridemia or Metabolic Syndrome

	Triglycerides	NNT to prevent one event	Baseline LDL cholesterol
4S (simvastatin)	>159	6	192
CARE (pravastatin)	≥144	25	139
LIPID (pravastatin)	>230	25	150
HPS (simvastatin)	>350	26	131
VA-HIT (gemfibrozil)	Insulin-resistant	12	109
BIP (bezafibrate)	Metabolic syndrome	23	146
	Tg >200 mg/dL and HDL-C <35 mg/dL	11	
FIELD (fenofibrate)	Metabolic syndrome Tg > 150 mg/dL and	71	119
	HDL-C < 40 (men) and 50 (women) mg/dL	43	

Abbreviations: VA-HIT, Veterans Affairs High-Density Lipoprotein Cholesterol Intervention Trail; FIELD, Fenofibrate Intervention and Event Lowering in Diabetes; BIP, Bezafibrate Infarclion Prevention; LDL, low-density lipoprotein; HDL-C, high-density lipoprotein–cholesterol; Tg, triglyceride.

placebo in two recent angiographic trials, which include subjects with moderate hypertriglyceridemia and low HDL-C levels (187,213).

EVALUATION AND MANAGEMENT IN A HYPERTRIGLYCERIDEMIC PATIENT

The diagnosis of hypertriglyceridemia has to be confirmed by two or more measurements performed in a one-to-two-week interval. Blood has to be drawn after a 12-hour fast and in a subject in a stable metabolic state (two to three months after a transitory pathology such as an infectious episode or surgery) (Table 7).

Inter-day triglyceride plasma concentrations vary in a subject, this variation being larger when concentrations are elevated. It is consequently necessary to have a few measurements to evaluate the right metabolic state and to take a few measurements during the treatment phase

TABLE 7 Diagnostic Strategy in a Patient with Hypertriglyceridemia

Hypertriglyceridemia confirmed by two to three lipid screenings (total cholesterol, triglycerides, HDL cholesterol) after a 12-hour fast and in a stable metabolic state.
Check for factors inducing hypertriglyceridemia:
1. Drugs
    contraceptive pill
    retinoids
    antipsychotics
    corticoids
    immunosuppressants
    antiretroviral therapy
2. Environmental factor
    excessive alcohol intake
3. Genetic factors
    hyperchylomicronemia (LPL deficiency)
    type III hyperlipoproteinemia
    familial hypertriglyceridemia
    familial combined hyperlipidemia
4. Pathology
    obesity - insulin resistance - type 2 diabetes mellitus - metabolic syndrome
    type 1 diabetes
    hypothyroidism
    obstructive liver disease
    progressive partial lipodystrophy
    renal dysfunction: nephrotic syndrome, chronic renal failure

Abbreviations: LPL, lipoprotein lipase; HDL, high-density lipoprotein.

for the same reason. Simultaneous with triglyceride measurements, TC and HDL-C have to be determined. LDL-C can be calculated by the Friedewald formula only if triglyceride levels are below 400 mg/dL. LDL-C could be measured using direct methods but it has been suggested that this kind of method should be avoided when triglycerides are above 800 mg/dL or in the presence of type-III hyperlipoproteinemia or monoclonal gammapathy. Ignorance of LDL-C is however initially not clinically important for therapy in severe hypertriglyceridemia. Non-HDL-C can easily be calculated when triglycerides are above 200 mg/dL.

The second diagnostic step is to find the presence of factors responsible for the development of hypertriglyceridemia.

- The prescription of drugs such as anti-AIDS drugs, contraceptive pills, retinoids, or corticoids is usually made after asking the patient questions or consulting his history.

Pathologies inducing hypertriglyceridemia are often already known before the first measurement of triglyceride levels. However, they must be systematically checked:

- Renal pathology by measuring plasma creatinine and screening albuminuria with urine sticks.
- Hypothyroidism by TSH dosage.
- Insulin-dependent diabetes with severe insulinopenia can induce a severe hypertriglyceridemia. Hypertriglyceridemia then appears when diabetes is discovered or when patients stop insulin injections.
- Susceptibility to alcohol has to be systematically assessed.

Comments

1. The evaluation of alcohol intake has to be performed during the evaluation of diet. Abrupt questions about alcohol consumption often lead to an underestimation, or less frequently, an overestimation of alcohol consumption. A complete evaluation of diet including alcohol intake is the first step toward treatment and is, therefore, almost always obligatory.
2. Considerable interindividual variability exists concerning alcohol intake and elevated triglycerides. A few subjects drinking a moderate quantity of alcohol can present an elevated level of triglycerides, whereas others display hyperlipoproteinemia after high intake only.
3. If hypertriglyceridemia were partially or totally dependent on alcohol intake, a short test, stopping alcohol consumption (replaced by drink without sugar such as mineral water to avoid an abrupt increase in dietary carbohydrates, which could induce hypertriglyceridemia) for five to seven days, would make an assessment possible. A sharp drop in fasting triglycerides would prove the alcohol effect.

■ Case Study for Hypertriglyceridemia in a Subject Having Sensitivity to Alcohol Intake

A 32-year-old man was referred to the Lipid Clinic for hypertriglyceridemia. Hypertriglyceridemia was discovered as an incidental finding because of asthenia. The subject appeared healthy. His weight was 72 kg and height, 180 cm or BMI, 22.2 kg/m². The clinical examination was normal and the medical history revealed no disease in the past. No history of abdominal pain or diabetes was found. The patient took no medication with the exception of a benzodiazepine for the last two weeks. The first lipid screening showed TC of 175 mg/dL, triglycerides of 1235 mg/dL and HDL-C of 63 mg/dL. Blood glucose, plasma creatinine, and TSH were normal. Second lipid measurements confirmed the first ones: TC, 183 mg/dL, triglycerides, 1050 mg/dL, and HDL-C, 59 mg/dL; hepatic enzymes, SGOT, SGPT, and GGT were 58 (ULN 40), 39 (ULN 40), and 283 (ULN 30), respectively. Dietary analysis showed a moderate excess in saturated fat and alcohol intake evaluated at about 45 g/day (two beers and three drinks of wine per day).

Comments

1. Susceptibility of a patient to hypertriglyceridemia related to alcohol intake was immediately evoked in relation to:
    - The absence of overweight, diabetes, or other pathologies and drugs potentially leading to hypertriglyceridemia
    - A high HDL-C level
2. An increase in GGT is not a strong argument because an elevation of this hepatic enzyme due to steatosis is frequently noted in patients with hypertriglyceridemia, whatever its cause.

3. The association between triglyceride levels and alcohol intake showed a large interindividual variation, probably corresponding to genetic factors modulating alcohol and lipid metabolism. The alcohol quantity inducing hypertriglyceridemia is quite variable from one individual to another.
4. The only tool to prove the cause and effect relationship between alcohol intake and hypertriglyceridemia is an abstinence test. The patient is asked to replace alcoholic drinks with mineral water (without adding sugar) for five to seven days. If alcohol is the cause of hypertriglyceridemia, triglyceride levels drop sharply.

The situation was explained and the subject asked to replace beer and wine by still or gaseous mineral water. A week later, the subject was able to stop alcohol completely and fasting triglycerides were 160 mg/dL, TC, 220 mg/dL HDL-C, 56 mg/dL, and GGT, 152.

Comments
1. A decrease in GGT argues in favor of the subject stopping alcohol consumption for a week.
2. The large decrease in triglycerides between the first measurement and the one after stopping alcohol intake supports a causative effect of alcohol in hypertriglyceridemia.
3. The therapeutic consequence is the decrease in or suppression of alcohol intake. It is likely that each individual has a threshold alcohol intake, above which hypertriglyceridemia appears, but the determination of this threshold is, of course, very difficult.
4. The case shows a subject with a large increase in hypertriglyceridemia entirely due to alcohol consumption, but alcohol can be only partially causative in moderate hypertriglyceridemia.

The third diagnostic step is to check for a genetic factor. In usual clinical activity, it is not possible to check all known genetic factors. A few can, however, be evaluated by laboratory tests or familial screening:

1. Hyperchylomicronemia. The patient has to be referred to a specialized clinical center to evaluate LPL activity and determine the treatment.
2. Type-III hyperlipoproteinemia (see above).
3. Familial hypertriglyceridemia or FCHL.

The diagnosis for FHTG and FCHL is dependent on familial screening. Sometimes, the presence of premature CHD in family members noted by asking the hypertriglyceridemic propositus is a strong element in diagnosing FHTG or FCHL. High plasma apoB can also be an indication in determining the diagnosis of FCHL.

The final step in diagnosis is to determine a pathology prone to induce hypertriglyceridemia: insulin resistance including type 2 diabetes and/or metabolic syndrome, type 1 diabetes, thyroid, liver, or renal dysfunction.

Globally, all information needed to determine the factors causing hypertriglyceridemia precisely are easily obtained by asking the patient or through standard biochemical parameters. The most difficult is probably to diagnose FCHL, but this pathology can be included in the framework of the metabolic syndrome and treated like it.

Therapeutic Strategies
Therapeutic strategy obviously depends on the findings during the diagnostic phase. Drugs that are not obligatory can be stopped (retinoids, contraceptive pills) and replaced by other therapeutic tools. Other drugs such as antipsychotics and antiretroviral therapy are often essential, and the prescribed drug should be chosen for the smallest effect on lipid metabolism, although the major aim would be to treat the initial disease.

Evidence of a relationship between alcohol consumption and hypertriglyceridemia (see above) means eliminating intake. Moderate consumption could be acceptable, but the threshold beyond which hypertriglyceridemia appears is difficult to appreciate.

Treatments for pathologies inducing hypertriglyceridemia must be improved. Insulin injection often helps normalize triglyceride levels in insulin-dependent diabetes. An improvement in renal pathology is likely to reduce hyperlipoproteinemia.

The first step is to evaluate the sensitivity of triglyceride plasma levels to dietary fats. Most patients with severe hypertriglyceridemia (>1000 mg/dL) not due to alcohol intake present with such sensitivity. The therapeutic aim is to lower triglycerides below 1000 mg/dL, the risk of pancreatitis increasing significantly when triglycerides are above this threshold. Patients are prescribed an isocaloric diet restricted in total fat (10–20 g/day). In general, compliance with this extreme diet is usually poor. A possibility is to adapt a diet containing about 20 g fat/day comprised of medium-chain triglycerides. Medium-chain triglycerides exist as oils used for dressing or margarines for cooking. Another approach for reducing severe hypertriglyceridemia is to couple restrictions in dietary fat with combination drug therapy comprised of a fibrate, nicotinic acid, and omega-3 FA, which frequently decrease triglyceride levels. These drugs have no effect on type-I hyperchylomicronemic patients. Tetrahydrolipstatin (Orlistat) is a selective inhibitor of gastric and pancreatic lipase, and can reduce exogenous triglyceride absorption. Orlistat 120 mg t.i.d. with meals reduced triglyceride levels by 35% in hyperchylomicronemic (219) and type-V hyperlipoproteinemic patients (220), alone, with diet, and with usual hypertriglyceridemic drugs.

■ Case Study for Hyperchylomicronemia

JG, a 15-year-old girl, was referred to the lipid clinic because of marked hypertriglyceridemia (2540 mg/dL). The patient was admitted to the Emergency Department for abdominal pain. Milky serum was observed and triglycerides measured. Moderately elevated plasma and urine levels of lipase were noted. An edematous aspect of the pancreas was observed on computed tomography scan. Taken together, these findings suggested edematous pancreatitis. Fasting and gastric aspiration lead to a rapid disappearance of pain and the serum lipase level returned to normal. The patient was seen at the lipid clinic four days later and questioned. She was found to have had a few bouts of abdominal pain in the past. No secondary cause of hypertriglyceridemia was found. Her BMI was normal at 21.4 kg/m². Her father displayed hypertriglyceridemia (353 mg/dL) while her mother and brother were normolipidemic. Fasting hypertriglyceridemia was again found (1455 mg/dL). Cholesterol was normal at 175 mg/dL and HDL-C low at 32 mg/dL. LPL activity measured in plasma after intravenous injection of heparin was very low. A diet low in fat was explained: 20 g/day instead about 80 g/day before hospitalization. A telephone follow-up with a dietician was proposed. Two months later, the patient was seen again. She felt no abdominal pain. Triglycerides were 1753 mg/dL and diet evaluation showed a fat intake around 40 g/day. A low-fat diet (20 g/day) was proposed, combined with medium-chain triglycerides (20 g/day). Two months later, this diet seemed to be better tolerated and followed, but triglycerides remained elevated at 1050 g/day. Orlistat was prescribed (120 mg t.i.d.) in combination with diet and two months later, triglycerides decreased to 628 mg/dL. The treatment was continued.

Comments

1. Type-I hyperlipoproteinemia is frequently detected and diagnosed in a patient suffering from abdominal pain, occasionally corresponding to pancreatitis.

2. LPL deficiency was evident in this patient, but the presence of severe hypertriglyceridemia in a young patient in the absence of any secondary cause (for example, retinoid, which would have been prescribed for acne at this age) seems a reasonable diagnosis even if LPL activity could not be measured. First-degree relatives frequently have moderate hypertriglyceridemia.

3. The aim of the treatment is to decrease the transport of triglycerides by chylomicrons. A low-fat diet is then prescribed to decrease the exogenous influx of triglycerides in chylomicrons, as well as medium-chain triglycerides, which are absorbed by the gut and pass into the blood to reach the liver directly without being incorporated into chylomicrons. Orlistat decreases the absorption of FA by the intestine and also the triglyceride flux toward chylomicrons. Combined treatment probably improves compliance, which is often poor: a single meal rich in fat can increase triglyceride levels significantly and can lead to pancreatitis.

Metabolic syndrome accompanied or not accompanied by type 2 diabetes is certainly the most frequent situation. Risk assessment is essential to determine therapeutic strategies. Cigarette smoking, BP, age, and lipid levels are key factors in this evaluation. Smoking cessation and the normalization of BP are part of the CHD prevention strategy. Weight reduction through lifestyle changes such as a reduction in calorie intake and an increase in physical activity is a major aim in treating this high-risk situation. Weight loss and physical activity have a strong impact on preventing the onset of diabetes in nondiabetic patients with metabolic syndrome.

What hypolipidemic drug is appropriate for patients with hypertriglyceridemia and metabolic syndrome?

No clinical trial has directly evaluated the clinical effect of a drug in patients with metabolic syndrome. Only subgroup analyses are available to determine the advantage of different drugs in this clinical situation. An international consensus has emerged along with guidelines developed in the United States, Canada, Europe, Australia, and New Zealand. The first step is to determine LDL-C or non-HDL-C goal. Non-HDL-C could be used as soon as triglyceride levels are above 200 mg/dL. For that, a patient's risk category has to be determined, whether clinical CVD is present or not, as well as the major risk factors other than LDL or non-HDL-C. These risk factors are:

- Cigarette smoking (current or ex-smoker for less than three years)
- Hypertension (BP ≥ 140/90 mmHg or on antihypertensive medication)
- Low HDL-C (<40 mg/dL)
- Family history of premature CHD (CHD in male first-degree relative <55 years; CHD in female first-degree relative <65 years)
- Age (men ≥ 45 or 50 years in men; ≥ 55 or 60 years in women)
- HDL-C of 60 mg/dL or above counts as a negative risk factor; its presence removes one risk factor from the total count.

The highest risk category is defined by CHD or CHD equivalents. Three types of patients are included in this category:

1. Patients with CHD, peripheral arterial disease, abdominal aortic aneurysm and symptomatic carotid artery disease.
2. Patients with diabetes: American and Canadian guidelines include all diabetic patients in this category, but all diabetic patients do not appear to be at high risk. Recent French guidelines consider diabetic patients in this category only if they have two other risk factors (smoking, high BP, low HDL-C, familial history of premature CHD, age >50 years for men, >60 for women, creatinine clearance <60 mL/min, microalbuminuria >30 mg/24 hours).
3. Patients with a 10-year risk of CHD above 20% as estimated by the Framingham risk score: it should however be noted that this estimation cannot be easily applied by General Physicians in clinical practice. Patients with a 10-year risk over 10% have essentially two or more risk factors, but a number of patients with two risk factors have a risk below the threshold.

In these patients, the aim is to decrease LDL-C below 100 mg/dL or non-HDL-C below 130 mg/dL.

The second category consists of patients in primary prevention with two or more risk factors in whom a 10-year risk is 20% or below. Their LDL-C or non-HDL-C goals are below 130 or 160 mg/dL, respectively.

The third category consists of patients in primary prevention having zero to one risk factor. Their LDL-C or non-HDL-C goals are below 160 or 190 mg/dL, respectively.

Another more detailed classification is used in France for patients in primary prevention: the LDL-C goal is to decrease this parameter below 220, 190, 160, and 130 mg/dL in patients with 0, 1, 2 or +2 risk factors, respectively.

Therapeutic lifestyle change is frontline therapy for lowering LDL-C. If LDL-C or non-HDL-C goals are not reached after a few months of dietary and lifestyle changes, drugs have to be considered. Drugs used in patients with high LDL-C or non-HDL-C are primarily the statins. The strategy for the use of statins or other hypocholesterolemic drugs such as ezetimibe and for their combination is not in the scope of this chapter and will not be described here. Statin treatment moderately reduces triglyceride levels and has little effect on HDL-C. The persistence of low HDL-C and high triglyceride levels tends to suggest a combination of drugs. Niacin or a fibrate (with the exception of gemfibrozil and rather bezafibrate than fenofibrate) can be prescribed. Fibrates seem particularly efficient clinically in patients with insulin resistance or with the association of hypertriglyceridemia/low HDL-C. In patients with a metabolic syndrome and LDL-C below

110 mg/dL (or non-HDL-C <140 mg/dL), gemfibrozil is effective in decreasing cardiovascular risk.

■ Case Study

A 53-year-old subject was referred to the Lipid Clinic because of mixed hyperlipoproteinemia. This patient suffered thoracic pain on effort; the cardiac examination showed a positive stress ECG. Angiography revealed a 70% stenosis of the left anterior descending coronary artery. Angioplasty and stenting were performed and the patient's anginal symptoms resolved.

Six months later, the subject was clinically well. No familial history of premature atherosclerosis and hyperlipoproteinemia was reported, but the patient had lost contact with several family members. The cardiologist reported his weight as 87 kg and height as 176 cm, i.e., a BMI of 28.1 kg/m^2, waist circumference of 103 cm and BP of 145/88 mmHg. Lifestyle changes (diet and physical activity) were advised during hospitalization in the Cardiology Department and a three-week cardiac rehabilitation period was initiated.

In the Lipid Clinic, the patient took simvastatin 20 mg qd, Plavix, and a beta-blocker. All drugs were tolerated and compliance appeared excellent. His weight was 86 kg and BP 132/82 mmHg. The patient was an ex-smoker, having stopped tobacco for two years.

Initial biochemical profile (before the prescription of simvastatin) was—TC: 195 mg/dL, triglycerides: 415 mg/dL, HDL-C: 33 mg/dL, glucose: 112 mg/dL, TSH: 2.1 (normal values: 0.3–3.6). Transaminases were moderately elevated, SGOT and SGPT at 1.2 and 2.1 ULN, respectively.

After eight weeks of treatment with simvastatin, cholesterol was 153 mg/dL, triglycerides, 373 mg/dL, HDL-C, 35 mg/dL. SGOT and SGPT were stable at 1.4 and 2.3 ULN, respectively.

Remarks

1. LDL-C could not be calculated because of high triglyceride levels (>400 mg/dL). So, non-HDL-C was used.
2. This case study can be examined from two angles:
   - First, the patient presented with CHD and was classified in the high-risk category. Therefore the goal was to obtain non-HDL-C below 130 mg/dL. Statin therapy was effective in reaching this goal (non-HDL-C with simvastatin 20 mg qd: 118 mg/dL).
   - Secondly, the patient suffered from metabolic syndrome because of the presence of all these diagnostic criteria:

■ Waist circumference above 102 cm.

■ HDL-C below 40 mg/dL.

■ Triglycerides above 150 mg/dL

■ BP above 130/85 mmHg

■ Fasting blood glucose above 100 mg/dL

The patient was prescribed simvastatin 20 mg and bezafibrate 400 mg qd. The patient was seen eight weeks later. The combination was clinically well tolerated. SGOT and SGPT were 1.6 and 1.5 ULN, respectively. The lipid profile improved—cholesterol: 156 mg/dL, triglycerides: 229 mg/dL, HDL-C: 40 mg/dL, i.e., non-HDL-C: 116 mg/dL.

Comments

■ As the patient has a metabolic syndrome and glucose intolerance, lifestyle changes were of major importance to prevent future diabetes and a new CHD event. Unfortunately, the patient was not able to decrease his weight.

■ As hypertriglyceridemia/low HDL-C and insulin resistance are high-risk CHD factors and fibrates are demonstrated to decrease CHD risk in this scenario, a statin/fibrate combination should be considered. Another solution is to use a statin/niacin combination. However, these combinations have not been evaluated by clinical trials at this time.

■ The addition of bezafibrate was efficacious in this patient.

■ Triglyceride and HDL-C are rarely normalized by fibrates alone. However, statistical analyses have shown that the effect of fibrate on CHD incidence is probably larger than that obtained by the effect on lipids alone, as a direct anti-inflammatory effect on the artery wall is probably important (221).

■ The high levels of SGOT and SGPT in the initial biochemical analysis probably reflect hepatic steatosis in the patient, a common pathology observed in insulin resistance. Paradoxical decreases in transaminases during treatment with bezafibrate were probably due to an improvement in the hepatic metabolism of triglycerides and a regression in steatosis.

REFERENCES

1. Yarnell JW, Patterson CC, Sweetnam PM, et al. Do total and high density lipoprotein cholesterol and triglycerides act independently in the prediction of ischemic heart disease? Ten-year follow-up of Caerphilly and Speedwell Cohorts. Arterioscler Thromb Vasc Biol 2001; 21:1340–1345.
2. Austin MA, Hokanson JE, Edwards KL. Hypertriglyceridemia as a cardiovascular risk factor. Am J Cardiol 1998; 81:B7–B12.
3. Havel RJ. Postprandial hyperlipidemia and remnant lipoproteins. Curr Opin Lipidol 1994; 5:102–109.
4. Havel R. McCollum Award Lecture, 1993: triglyceride-rich lipoproteins and atherosclerosis-new perspectives. Am J Clin Nutr 1994; 59:795–796.
5. Senti M, Pedro Botet J, Nogues X, et al. Influence of intermediate-density lipoproteins on the accuracy of the Friedewald formula. Clin Chem 1991; 37:1394–1397.
6. Liu J, Sempos C, Donahue RP, et al. Joint distribution of non-HDL and LDL cholesterol and coronary heart disease risk prediction among individuals with and without diabetes. Diabetes Care 2005; 28:1916–1921.
7. Benlian P, Degennes JL, Foubert L, et al. Premature atherosclerosis in patients with familial chylomicronemia caused by mutations in the lipoprotein lipase gene. N Engl J Med 1996; 335:848–854.
8. Bijvoet S, Gagne SE, Moorjani S, et al. Alterations in plasma lipoproteins and apolipoproteins before the age of 40 in heterozygotes for lipoprotein lipase deficiency. J Lipid Res 1996; 37:640–650.
9. Wittrup HH, Tybjaerg-Hansen A, Nordestgaard BG. Lipoprotein lipase mutations, plasma lipids and lipoproteins, and risk of ischemic heart disease. A meta-analysis. Circulation 1999; 99:2901–2907.
10. Hokanson JE. Functional variants in the lipoprotein lipase gene and risk cardiovascular disease. Curr Opin Lipidol 1999; 10:393–399.
11. Clee S, Loubser O, Collins J, et al. The LPL S447X cSNP is associated with decreased blood pressure and plasma triglycerides, and reduced risk of coronary artery disease. Clin Genet 2001; 60:293–300.
12. Hegele RA, Breckenridge WC, Cox DW, Maguire GF, Little JA, Connelly PW. Elevated LDL triglyceride concentrations in subjects heterozygous for the hepatic lipase S267F variant. Arterioscler Thromb Vasc Biol 1998; 18:1212–1216.
13. Gehrisch S, Kostka H, Tiebel M, et al. Mutations of the human hepatic lipase gene in patients with combined hypertriglyceridemia/hyperalphalipoproteinemia and in patients with familial combined hyperlipidemia. J Mol Med 1999; 77:728–734.
14. Clavey V, Lestavel-Delattre S, Copin C, et al. Modulation of lipoprotein B binding to the LDL receptor by exogenous lipids and apolipoproteins CI, CII, CIII, and E. Arterioscler Thromb Vasc Biol 1995; 15:963–971.
15. Waterworth DM, Talmud PJ, Bujac SR, et al. Contribution of apolipoprotein C-III gene variants to determination of triglyceride levels and interaction with smoking in middle-aged men. Arterioscler Thromb Vasc Biol 2000; 20:2663–2669.
16. Sturm R. Increases in clinically severe obesity in the United States, 1986–2000. Arch Intern Med 2003; 163:2146–2148.
17. Olivieri O, Bassi A, Stranieri C, et al. Apolipoprotein C-III, metabolic syndrome, and risk of coronary artery disease. J Lipid Res 2003; 44:2374–2381.
18. Pennacchio LA, Olivier M, Hubacek JA, et al. An apolipoprotein influencing triglycerides in humans and mice revealed by comparative sequencing. Science 2001; 294:169–173.
19. Oliva CP, Pisciotta L, Li VG, et al. Inherited apolipoprotein A-V deficiency in severe hypertriglyceridemia. Arterioscler Thromb Vasc Biol 2005; 25:411–417.
20. Marcais C, Verges B, Charriere S, et al. Apoa5 Q139X truncation predisposes to late-onset hyperchylomicronemia due to lipoprotein lipase impairment. J Clin Invest 2005; 115:2862–2869.
21. Klos KL, Hamon S, Clark AG, et al. APOA5 polymorphisms influence plasma triglycerides in young, healthy African Americans and whites of the CARDIA Study. J Lipid Res 2005; 46:564–571.
22. Talmud PJ, Hawe E, Martin S, et al. Relative contribution of variation within the APOC3/A4/A5 gene cluster in determining plasma triglycerides. Hum Mol Genet 2002; 11:3039–3046.
23. Robins SJ, Collins D, Wittes JT, et al. Relation of gemfibrozil treatment and lipid levels with major coronary events: VA-HIT: a randomized controlled trial. JAMA 2001; 285:1585–1591.
24. Luc G, Bard JM, Arveiler D, et al. Impact of apolipoprotein E polymorphism on lipoproteins and risk of myocardial infarction. The ECTIM Study. Arterioscler Thromb 1994; 14:1412–1419.
25. Dallongeville J, Lussier Cacan S, Davignon J. Modulation of plasma triglyceride levels by apoE phenotype: a meta-analysis. J Lipid Res 1992; 33:447–454.
26. Eichner JE, Kuller LH, Orchard TJ, et al. Relation of apolipoprotein E phenotype to myocardial infarction and mortality from coronary artery disease. Am J Cardiol 1993; 71:160–165.
27. Utermann G, Hees M, Steinmetz A. Polymorphism of apolipoprotein E and occurrence of dysbetalipoproteinaemia in man. Nature 1977; 269:604–607.
28. Mahley RW, Rall SCJ. Type III hyperlipoproteinemia (dysbetalipoproteinemia), the role of apolipoprotein E in normal and abnormal lipoprotein metabolism. In: Scriver CR, Beaudet AL, Sly WS, Valle D, eds. The Metabolic Basis of Inherited Disease. New York: Mc Graw Hill, 1989:1195–1213.
29. Davignon J, Gregg RE, Sing CF. Apolipoprotein E polymorphism and atherosclerosis. Arteriosclerosis 1988; 8:1–21.
30. Feussner G, Piesch S, Dobmeyer J, et al. Genetics of type III hyperlipoproteinemia. Genet Epidemiol 1997; 14:283–297.

31. van Dam M, Zwart M, de Beer F, et al. Long term efficacy and safety of atorvastatin in the treatment of severe type III and combined dyslipidaemia. Heart 2002; 88:234–238.

32. Lindi V, Schwab U, Louheranta A, et al. Impact of the Pro12Ala polymorphism of the PPAR-gamma2 gene on serum triacylglycerol response to n-3 fatty acid supplementation. Mol Genet Metab 2003; 79:52–60.

33. Vaccaro O, Mancini FP, Ruffa G, et al. Fasting plasma free fatty acid concentrations and Pro12Ala polymorphism of the peroxisome proliferator-activated receptor (PPAR) gamma2 gene in healthy individuals. Clin Endocrinol (Oxf) 2002; 57:481–486.

34. Swarbrick MM, Chapman CM, McQuillan BM, et al. A Pro12Ala polymorphism in the human peroxisome proliferator-activated receptor-gamma 2 is associated with combined hyperlipidaemia in obesity. Eur J Endocrinol 2001; 144:277–282.

35. Pihlajamaki J, Miettinen R, Valve R, et al. The Pro12A1a substitution in the peroxisome proliferator activated receptor gamma 2 is associated with an insulin-sensitive phenotype in families with familial combined hyperlipidemia and in nondiabetic elderly subjects with dyslipidemia. Atherosclerosis 2000; 151:567–574.

36. Khan QH, Pontefract DE, Iyengar S, et al. Evidence of differing genotypic effects of PPARalpha in women and men. J Med Genet 2004; 41:79.

37. Nielsen EM, Hansen L, Echwald SM, et al. Evidence for an association between the Leu162Val polymorphism of the PPARalpha gene and decreased fasting serum triglyceride levels in glucose tolerant subjects. Pharmacogenetics 2003; 13:417–423.

38. Tai ES, Corella D, Demissie S, et al. Polyunsaturated fatty acids interact with the PPARA-L162V polymorphism to affect plasma triglyceride and apolipoprotein C-III concentrations in the Framingham Heart Study. J Nutr 2005; 135:397–403.

39. Fruchart JC, Duriez P, Staels B. Peroxisome proliferator-activated receptor-alpha activators regulate genes governing lipoprotein metabolism, vascular inflammation and atherosclerosis. Curr Opin Lipidol 1999; 10: 245–257.

40. Coste H, Rodriguez JC. Orphan nuclear hormone receptor Rev-erb alpha regulates the human apolipoprotein CIII promoter. J Biol Chem 2002; 277:27120–27129.

41. Foucher C, Rattier S, Flavell DM, et al. Response to micronized fenofibrate treatment is associated with the peroxisome-proliferator-activated receptors alpha G/C intron7 polymorphism in subjects with type 2 diabetes. Pharmacogenetics 2004; 14:823–829.

42. Love MW, Craddock AL, Angelin B, et al. Analysis of the Iieal bile acid transporter gene, SLC10A2, in subjects with familial hypertriglyceridemia. Arterioscler Thromb Vasc Biol 2001; 21:2039–2045.

43. Goldstein JL, Schrott HG, Hazzard WR, et al. Hyperlipidemia in coronary heart disease. II Genetics analysis of lipid levels in 176 families and delineation of a new inherited disorder, combined hyperlipidemia. J Clin Invest 1973; 52:1544–1568.

44. Nikkila EA, Aro A. Family study of serum lipids and lipoproteins in coronary heart-disease. Lancet 1973; 1:954–959.

45. Venkatesan S, Cullen P, Pacy P, et al. Stable isotopes show a direct relation between VLDL apoB overproduction and serum triglyceride levels and indicate a metabolically and biochemically coherent basis for familial combined hyperlipidemia. Arterioscler Thromb 1993; 13:1110–1118.

46. Kissebah AH, Alfarsi S, Adams PW. Integrated regulation of very low density lipoprotein triglyceride and apolipoprotein-B kinetics in man: normolipemic subjects, familial hypertriglyceridemia and familial combined hyperlipidemia. Metab 1981; 30:856–868.

47. Chait A, Albers JJ, Brunzell JD. Very low density lipoprotein overproduction in genetic forms of hypertriglyceridaemia. Eur J Clin Invest 1980; 10:17–22.

48. Austin MA, McKnight B, Edwards KL, et al. Cardiovascular disease mortality in familial forms of hypertriglyceridemia: A 20-year prospective study. Circulation 2000; 101:2777–2782.

49. Voors-Pette C, de Bruin TW. Excess coronary heart disease in familial combined hyperlipidemia, in relation to genetic factors and central obesity. Atherosclerosis 2001; 157:481–489.

50. Hopkins PN, Heiss G, Ellison RC et al. Coronary artery disease risk in familial combined hyperlipidemia and familial hypertriglyceridemia: a case-control comparison from the National Heart, Lung, and Blood Institute Family Heart Study. Circulation 2003; 108:519–523.

51. Veerkamp MJ, de Graaf J, Bredie SJ, et al. Diagnosis of familial combined hyperlipidemia based on lipid phenotype expression in 32 families: results of a 5-year follow-up study. Arterioscler Thromb Vasc Biol 2002; 22:274–282.

52. Pi-Sunyer FX. A review of long-term studies evaluating the efficacy of weight loss in ameliorating disorders associated with obesity. Clin Ther 1996; 18:1006–1035.

53. Veerkamp MJ, de Graaf J, Stalenhoef AF. Role of insulin resistance in familial combined hyperlipidemia. Arterioscler Thromb Vasc Biol 2005; 25:1026–1031.

54. Purnell JQ, Kahn SE, Schwartz RS, et al. Relationship of insulin sensitivity and ApoB levels to intra-abdominal fat in subjects with familial combined hyperlipidemia. Arterioscler Thromb Vasc Biol 2001; 21:567–572.

55. Lamarche B, Moorjani S, Lupien PJ, et al. Apolipoprotein A-I and B levels and the risk of ischemic heart disease during a five-year follow-up of men in the Quebec cardiovascular study. Circulation 1996; 94:273–278.

56. Moss AJ, Goldstein RE, Marder VJ, et al. Thrombogenic factors and recurrent coronary events. Circulation 1999; 99:2517–2522.

57. Talmud PJ, Hawe E, Miller GJ, et al. Nonfasting apolipoprotein B and triglyceride levels as a useful predictor of coronary heart disease risk in middle-aged UK men. Arterioscler Thromb Vasc Biol 2002; 22:1918–1923.

58. Babirak SP, Brown BG, Brunzell JD. Familial combined hyperlipidemia and abnormal lipoprotein lipase. Arterioscler Thromb 1992; 12:1176–1183.

59. Nevin DN, Brunzell JD, Deeb SS. The LPL gene in individuals with familial combined hyperlipidemia and decreased LPL activity. Arterioscler Thromb 1994; 14:869–873.

60. de Bruin TW, Mailly F, van Barlingen HH, et al. Lipoprotein lipase gene mutations D9N and N291S in four pedigrees with familial combined hyperlipidaemia. Eur J Clin Invest 1996; 26:631–639.

61. Tahvanainen E, Pajukanta P, Porkka K, et al. Haplotypes of the ApoA-I/C-III/A-IV gene cluster and familial combined hyperlipidemia. Arterioscler Thromb Vasc Biol 1998; 18:1810–1817.

62. Dallingathie GM, Trip MV, Rotter JI, et al. Complex genetic contribution of the apo AI-CIII-AIV gene cluster to familial combined hyperlipidemia–identification of different susceptibility haplotypes. J Clin Invest 1997; 99:953–961.

63. Eichenbaum-Voline S, Olivier M, Jones EL, et al. Linkage and association between distinct variants of the APOA1/C3/A4/A5 gene cluster and familial combined hyperlipidemia. Arterioscler Thromb Vasc Biol 2004; 24:167–174.

64. Ylitalo K, Nuotio I, Viikari J, et al. C3, hormone-sensitive lipase, and peroxisome proliferator-activated receptor gamma expression in adipose tissue of familial combined hyperlipidemia patients. Metab 2002; 51:664–670.

65. Pajukanta P, Porkka KV, Antikainen M, et al. No evidence of linkage between familial combined hyperlipidemia and genes encoding lipolytic enzymes in Finnish families. Arterioscler Thromb Vasc Biol 1997; 17:841–850.

66. Reynisdottir S, Eriksson M, Angelin B, et al. Impaired activation of adipocyte lipolysis in familial combined hyperlipidemia. J Clin Invest 1995; 95:2161–2169.

67. Cianflone K, Maslowska M, Sniderman A. The acylation stimulating protein-adipsin system. Int J Obes Relat Metab Disord 1995; 19(Suppl 1):S34–S38.

68. Pajukanta P, Lilja HE, Sinsheimer JS, et al. Familial combined hyperlipidemia is associated with upstream transcription factor 1 (USF1). Nat Genets 2004; 36:371–376.

69. Effect of fenofibrate on progression of coronary-artery disease in type 2 diabetes: the Diabetes Atherosclerosis Intervention Study, a randomised study. Lancet 2001; 357:905–910.

70. Donahoo WT, Kosmiski LA, Eckel RH. Drugs causing dyslipoproteinemia. Endocrinol Metab Clin North Am 1998; 27:677–697.

71. Bakir R, Hilliquin P. Lipids, lipoproteins, arterial accidents and oral contraceptives. Contracept Fertil Sex (Paris) 1986; 14:81–87.

72. Dallongeville J, Marecaux N, Isorez D, et al. Multiple coronary heart disease risk factors are associated with menopause and influenced by substitutive hormonal therapy in a cohort of French women. Atherosclerosis 1995; 118:123–133.

73. Cho L, Mukherjee D. Hormone replacement therapy and secondary cardiovascular prevention: a meta-analysis of randomized trials. Cardiology 2005; 104:143–147.

74. Rossouw JE. Coronary heart disease in menopausal women: implications of primary and secondary prevention trials of hormones. Maturitas 2005; 51:51–63.

75. Conley BA, Egorin MJ, Sridhara R, et al. Phase I clinical trial of all-trans-retinoic acid with correlation of its pharmacokinetics and pharmacodynamics. Cancer Chemother Pharmacol 1997; 39:291–299.

76. Rodondi N, Darioli R, Ramelet AA, et al. High risk for hyperlipidemia and the metabolic syndrome after an episode of hypertriglyceridemia during 13-cis retinoic acid therapy for acne: a pharmacogenetic study. Ann Intern Med 2002; 136:582–589.

77. Stoll D, Binnert C, Mooser V, et al. Short-term administration of isotretinoin elevates plasma triglyceride concentrations without affecting insulin sensitivity in healthy humans. Metab 2004; 53:4–10.

78. Casey DE. Metabolic issues and cardiovascular disease in patients with psychiatric disorders. Am J Med 2005; 118(Suppl 2):15S–22S.

79. Saari KM, Lindeman SM, Viilo KM, et al. A 4-fold risk of metabolic syndrome in patients with schizophrenia: the Northern Finland 1966 Birth Cohort study. J Clin Psychiatry 2005; 66:559–563.

80. Newcomer JW. Metabolic risk during antipsychotic treatment. Clin Ther 2004; 26:1936–1946.

81. Henderson DC, Cagliero E, Copeland PM, et al. Glucose metabolism in patients with schizophrenia treated with atypical antipsychotic agents: a frequently sampled intravenous glucose tolerance test and minimal model analysis. Arch Gen Psychiatry 2005; 62:19–28.

82. McQuade RD, Stock E, Marcus R, et al. A comparison of weight change during treatment with olanzapine or aripiprazole: results from a randomized, double-blind study. J Clin Psychiatry 2004; 65(Suppl 18):47–56.

83. Brown RR, Estoup MW. Comparison of the metabolic effects observed in patients treated with ziprasidone versus olanzapine. Int Clin Psychopharmacol 2005; 20:105–112.

84. Straker D, Correll CU, Kramer-Ginsberg E, et al. Cost-effective screening for the metabolic syndrome in patients treated with second-generation antipsychotic medications. Am J Psychiatry 2005; 162:1217–1221.

85. McKee JR, Bodfish JW, Mahorney SL, et al. Metabolic effects associated with atypical antipsychotic treatment in the developmentally disabled. J Clin Psychiatry 2005; 66:1161–1168.

86. Trence DL. Management of patients on chronic glucocorticoid therapy: an endocrine perspective. Prim Care 2003; 30:593–605.

87. Sholter DE, Armstrong PW. Adverse effects of corticosteroids on the cardiovascular system. Can J Cardiol 2000; 16:505–511.
88. Kramer BK, Boger C, Kruger B, et al. Cardiovascular risk estimates and risk factors in renal transplant recipients. Transplant Proc 2005; 37:1868–1870.
89. Hohage H, Hillebrandt U, Welling U, et al. Cyclosporine and tacrolimus: influence on cardiovascular risk factors. Transplant Proc 2005; 37:1036–1038.
90. Kramer BK, Kruger B, Mack M, et al. Steroid withdrawal or steroid avoidance in renal transplant recipients: focus on tacrolimus-based immunosuppressive regimens. Transplant Proc 2005; 37:1789–1791.
91. El Sadr WM, Mullin CM, Carr A, et al. Effects of HIV disease on lipid, glucose and insulin levels: results from a large antiretroviral-naive cohort. HIV Med 2005; 6:114–121.
92. Salehian B, Bilas J, Bazargan M, et al. Prevalence and incidence of diabetes in HIV-infected minority patients on protease inhibitors. J Natl Med Assoc 2005; 97:1088–1092.
93. Levy AR, McCandless L, Harrigan PR, et al. Changes in lipids over twelve months after initiating protease inhibitor therapy among persons treated for HIV/AIDS. Lipids Health Dis 2005; 4:4.
94. Penzak SR, Chuck SK. Management of protease inhibitor-associated hyperlipidemia. Am J Cardiovasc Drugs 2002; 2:91–106.
95. Stein JH, Merwood MA, Bellehumeur JB, et al. Postprandial lipoprotein changes in patients taking antiretroviral therapy for HIV infection. Arterioscler Thromb Vasc Biol 2005; 25:399–405.
96. Montes ML, Pulido F, Barros C, et al. Lipid disorders in antiretroviral-naive patients treated with lopinavir/ritonavir-based HAART: frequency, characterization and risk factors. J Antimicrob Chemother 2005; 55:800–804.
97. Liang JS, Distler O, Cooper DA, et al. HIV protease inhibitors protect apolipoprotein B from degradation by the proteasome: a potential mechanism for protease inhibitor-induced hyperlipidemia. Nat Med 2001; 7:1327–1331.
98. Bozkurt B. Cardiovascular toxicity with highly active antiretroviral therapy: review of clinical studies. Cardiovasc Toxicol 2004; 4:243–260.
99. Cahn PE, Gatell JM, Squires K, et al. Atazanavir-a once-daily HIV protease inhibitor that does not cause dyslipidemia in newly treated patients: results from two randomized clinical trials. J Int Assoc Physicians AIDS Care (Chic Ill) 2004; 3:92–98.
100. Keiser PH, Sension MG, DeJesus E, et al. Substituting abacavir for hyperlipidemia-associated protease inhibitors in HAART regimens improves fasting lipid profiles, maintains virologic suppression, and simplifies treatment. BMC Infect Dis 2005; 5:2.
101. Fisac C, Fumero E, Crespo M, et al. Metabolic benefits 24 months after replacing a protease inhibitor with abacavir, efavirenz or nevirapine. AIDS 2005; 19:917–925.
102. Bucher HC, Kofler A, Nuesch R, et al. Meta-analysis of randomized controlled trials of simplified versus continued protease inhibitor-based antiretroviral therapy in HIV-1-infected patients. AIDS 2003; 17:2451–2459.
103. Ardern CI, Katzmarzyk PT, Janssen I, et al. Race and sex similarities in exercise-induced changes in blood lipids and fatness. Med Sci Sports Exerc 2004; 36:1610–1615.
104. Chen SY, Chen SM, Chang WH, et al. Effect of 2-month detraining on body composition and insulin sensitivity in young female dancers. Int J Obes (Lond) 2005.
105. Asikainen TM, Kukkonen-Harjula K, Miilunpalo S. Exercise for health for early postmenopausal women: a systematic review of randomised controlled trials. Sports Med 2004; 34:753–778.
106. Evans EM, Racette SB, Peterson LR, et al. Aerobic power and insulin action improve in response to endurance exercise training in healthy 77-87 yr olds. J Appl Physiol 2005; 98:40–45.
107. Alam S, Stolinski M, Pentecost C, et al. The effect of a six-month exercise program on very low-density lipoprotein apolipoprotein B secretion in type 2 diabetes. J Clin Endocrinol Metab 2004; 89:688–694.
108. Di Loreto C, Fanelli C, Lucidi P, et al. Make your diabetic patients walk: long-term impact of different amounts of physical activity on type 2 diabetes. Diabetes Care 2005; 28:1295–1302.
109. Assimacopoulos-Jeannet F. Fat storage in pancreas and in insulin-sensitive tissues in pathogenesis of type 2 diabetes. Int J Obes Relat Metab Disord 2004; 28(Suppl 4):S53–S57.
110. Reaven GM. Compensatory hyperinsulinemia and the development of an atherogenic lipoprotein profile: the price paid to maintain glucose homeostasis in insulin-resistant individuals. Endocrinol Metab Clin North Am 2005; 34:49–62.
111. Taskinen MR. Type 2 diabetes as a lipid disorder. Curr Mol Med 2005; 5:297–308.
112. Shumak SL, Zinman B, Zuniga-Guarjardo S, et al. Triglyceride-rich lipoprotein metabolism during acute hyperinsulinemia in hypertriglyceridemic humans. Metab 1988; 37:461–466.
113. Lewis GF, Uffelman KD, Szeto LW, et al. Effects of acute hyperinsulinemia on VLDL triglyceride and VLDL apoB production in normal weight and obese individuals. Diabetes 1993; 42:833–842.
114. Malmstrom R, Packard CJ, Watson TD, et al. Metabolic basis of hypotriglyceridemic effects of insulin in normal men. Arterioscler Thromb Vasc Biol 1997; 17:1454–1464.
115. Annuzzi G, Iovine C, Mandarino B, et al. Effect of acute exogenous hyperinsulinaemia on very low density lipoprotein subfraction composition in normal subjects. Eur J Clin Invest 2001; 31:118–124.
116. Lewis GF, Uffelman KD, Szeto LW, et al. Interaction between free fatty acids and insulin in the acute control of very low-density lipoprotein production in humans. J Clin Invest 1995; 95:158–166.
117. Julius U. Influence of plasma free fatty acids on lipoprotein synthesis and diabetic dyslipidemia. Exp Clin Endocrinol Diabetes 2003; 111:246–250.

118. Annuzzi G, De Natale C, Iovine C, et al. Insulin resistance is independently associated with postprandial alterations of triglyceride-rich lipoproteins in type 2 diabetes mellitus. Arterioscler Thromb Vasc Biol 2004; 24:2397–2402.
119. Lewis GF, Steiner G. Acute effects of insulin in the control of VLDL production in humans. Implications for the insulin-resistant state. Diabetes Care 1996; 19:390–393.
120. Au CS, Wagner A, Chong T, et al. Insulin regulates hepatic apolipoprotein B production independent of the mass or activity of Akt1/PKBalpha. Metab 2004; 53:228–235.
121. Mook S, Halkes CC, Bilecen S, et al. In vivo regulation of plasma free fatty acids in insulin resistance. Metab 2004; 53:1197–1201.
122. Carpentier AC, Frisch F, Cyr D, et al. On the suppression of plasma nonesterified fatty acids by insulin during enhanced intravascular lipolysis in humans. Am J Physiol Endocrinol Metab 2005; 289:E849–E856.
123. Watt MJ, Carey AL, Wolsk-Petersen E, et al. Hormone-sensitive lipase is reduced in the adipose tissue of patients with type 2 diabetes mellitus: influence of IL-6 infusion. Diabetologia 2005; 48:105–112.
124. Sadur CN, Eckel RH. Insulin stimulation of adipose tissue lipoprotein lipase. Use of the euglycemic clamp technique. J Clin Invest 1982; 69:1119–1125.
125. Coppack SW, Fisher RM, Gibbons GF, et al. Postprandial substrate deposition in human forearm and adipose tissues in vivo. Clin Sci (Lond) 1990; 79:339–348.
126. Sniderman AD, Cianflone K, Summers L, et al. The acylation-stimulating protein pathway and regulation of postprandial metabolism. Proc Nutr Soc 1997; 56:703–712.
127. Ginsberg HN, Zhang YL, Hernandez-Ono A. Regulation of plasma triglycerides in insulin resistance and diabetes. Arch Med Res 2005; 36:232–240.
128. Grundy SM, et al. Circulation 2005.
129. Gylling H, Tuominen JA, Koivisto VA, et al. Cholesterol metabolism in type 1 diabetes. Diabetes 2004; 53:2217–2222.
130. Purnell JQ, Hokanson JE, Marcovina SM, et al. Effect of excessive weight gain with intensive therapy of type 1 diabetes on lipid levels and blood pressure: results from the DCCT. Diabetes Control and Complications Trial. JAMA 1998; 280:140–146.
131. Kulenovic I, Rasic S, Grujic M. Metabolic control and body mass index in patients with type 1 diabetes on different insulin regimens. Bosn J Basic Med Sci 2004; 4:23–28.
132. Hadjadj S, Duly-Bouhanick B, Bekherraz A, et al. Serum triglycerides are a predictive factor for the development and the progression of renal and retinal complications in patients with type 1 diabetes. Diabetes Metab 2004; 30:43–51.
133. Soedamah-Muthu SS, Chaturvedi N, Toeller M, et al. Risk factors for coronary heart disease in type 1 diabetic patients in Europe: the EURODIAB Prospective Complications Study. Diabetes Care 2004; 27:530–537.
134. Pucci E, Chiovato L, Pinchera A. Thyroid and lipid metabolism. Int J Obes Relat Metab Disord 2000; 24(Suppl 2):S109–S112.
135. Pearce EN. Hypothyroidism and dyslipidemia: modern concepts and approaches. Curr Cardiol Rep 2004; 6:451–456.
136. Ineck BA, Ng TM. Effects of subclinical hypothyroidism and its treatment on serum lipids. Ann Pharmacother 2003; 37:725–730.
137. Narayanan S. Biochemistry and clinical relevance of lipoprotein X. Ann Clin Lab Sci 1984; 14:371–374.
138. Chan CM. Hyperlipidaemia in chronic kidney disease. Ann Acad Med Singapore 2005; 34:31–35.
139. Prichard SS. Impact of dyslipidemia in end-stage renal disease. J Am Soc Nephrol 2003; 14:S315–S320.
140. Bilheimer DW, Grundy SM, Brown MS, et al. Mevinolin and colestipol stimulate receptor-mediated clearance of low density lipoprotein from plasma in familial hypercholesterolemia heterozygotes. Proc Natl Acad Sci USA 1983; 80:4124–4128.
141. Edwards JE, Moore RA. Statins in hypercholesterolaemia: A dose-specific meta-analysis of lipid changes in randomised, double blind trials. BMC Fam Pract 2003; 4:18.
142. Stein EA, Lane M, Laskarzewski P. Comparison of statins in hypertriglyceridemia. Am J Cardiol 1998; 81:66B–69B.
143. Schaefer EJ, Mcnamara JR, Tayler T, et al. Comparisons of effects of statins (atorvastatin, fluvastatin, lovastatin, pravastatin, and simvastatin) on fasting and postprandial lipoproteins in patients with coronary heart disease versus control subjects. Am J Cardiol 2004; 93:31–39.
144. Cheng JW. Rosuvastatin in the management of hyperlipidemia. Clin Ther 2004; 26:1368–1387.
145. Schuster H. Rosuvastatin—a highly effective new 3-hydroxy-3-methylglutaryl coenzyme A reductase inhibitor: review of clinical trial data at 10–40 mg doses in dyslipidemic patients. Cardiology. 2003; 99:126–139.
146. Schaefer EJ, Lamonfava S, Cole T, et al. Effects of regular and extended-release gemfibrozil on plasma lipoproteins and apolipoproteins in hypercholesterolemic patients with decreased HDL cholesterol levels. Atherosclerosis 1996; 127:113–122.
147. Desager JP, Horsmans Y, Vandenplas C, et al. Pharmacodynamic activity of lipoprotein lipase and hepatic lipase, and pharmacokinetic parameters measured in normolipidaemic subjects receiving ciprofibrate (100 or 200 mg/day) or micronised fenofibrate (200 mg/day) therapy for 23 days. Atherosclerosis 1996; 124:S65–S73.

148. Betteridge DJ. Ciprofibrate—a profile. Postgrad Med J 1993; 69 (Suppl 1): S42–S47.
149. Durrington PN, Mackness MI, Bhatnagar D, et al. Effects of two different fibric acid derivatives on lipoproteins, cholesteryl ester transfer, fibrinogen, plasminogen activator inhibitor and paraoxonase activity in type IIb hyperlipoproteinaemia. Atherosclerosis 1998; 138:217–225.
150. Goldberg A, Alagona P Jr., Capuzzi DM, et al. Multiple-dose efficacy and safety of an extended-release form of niacin in the management of hyperlipidemia. Am J Cardiol 2000; 85:1100–1105.
151. Morgan JM, Capuzzi DM, Guyton JR. A new extended-release niacin (Niaspan): efficacy, tolerability, and safety in hypercholesterolemic patients. Am J Cardiol 1998; 82:29U–34U.
152. Drmanac S, Heilbron DC, Pullinger CR et al. Elevated baseline triglyceride levels modulate effects of HMGCoA reductase inhibitors on plasma lipoproteins. J Cardiovasc Pharmacol Ther 2001; 6:47–56.
153. Ordovas JM. The quest for cardiovascular health in the genomic era: nutrigenetics and plasma lipoproteins. Proc Nutr Soc 2004; 63:145–152.
154. Branchi A, Fiorenza AM, Rovellini A, et al. Lowering effects of four different statins on serum triglyceride level. Eur J Clin Pharmacol 1999; 55:499–502.
155. Sauvage Nolting PR, Twickler MB, Dallinga-Thie GM, et al. Elevated remnant-like particles in heterozygous familial hypercholesterolemia and response to statin therapy. Circulation 2002; 106:788–792.
156. Stein DT, Devaraj S, Balis D, et al. Effect of statin therapy on remnant lipoprotein cholesterol levels in patients with combined hyperlipidemia. Arterioscler Thromb Vasc Biol 2001; 21:2026–2031.
157. Boquist S, Karpe F, Danell-Toverud K, et al. Effects of atorvastatin on postprandial plasma lipoproteins in postinfarction patients with combined hyperlipidaemia. Atherosclerosis 2002; 162:163–170.
158. Chan DC, Watts GF, Barrett PH, et al. Regulatory effects of HMG CoA reductase inhibitor and fish oils on apolipoprotein B-100 kinetics in insulin-resistant obese male subjects with dyslipidemia. Diabetes 2002; 51:2377–2386.
159. Watts GF, Barrett PH, Ji J, et al. Differential regulation of lipoprotein kinetics by atorvastatin and fenofibrate in subjects with the metabolic syndrome. Diabetes 2003; 52:803–811.
160. de Graaf J, Hendriks JC, Demacker PN, et al. Identification of multiple dense LDL subfractions with enhanced susceptibility to in vitro oxidation among hypertriglyceridemic subjects. Normalization after clofibrate treatment. Arterioscler Thromb 1993; 13:712–719.
161. Capuzzi DM, Guyton JR, Morgan JM, et al. Efficacy and safety of an extended-release niacin (Niaspan): a long-term study. Am J Cardiol 1998; 82:74U–81U.
162. Grundy SM, Vega GL, Mcgovern ME, et al. Efficacy, safety, and tolerability of once-daily niacin for the treatment of dyslipidemia associated with type 2 diabetes: results of the assessment of diabetes control and evaluation of the efficacy of niaspan trial. Arch Intern Med 2002; 162:1568–1576.
163. Goldberg AC. A meta-analysis of randomized controlled studies on the effects of extended-release niacin in women. Am J Cardiol 2004; 94:121–124.
164. Carlson LA. Nicotinic acid and inhibition of fat mobilizing lipolysis. Present status of effects on lipid metabolism. Adv Exp Med Biol 1978; 109:225–238.
165. Tunaru S, Kero J, Schaub A, et al. PUMA-G and HM74 are receptors for nicotinic acid and mediate its anti-lipolytic effect. Nat Med 2003; 9:352–355.
166. Jin FY, Kamanna VS, Kashyap ML. Niacin decreases removal of high-density lipoprotein apolipoprotein A-I but not cholesterol ester by Hep G2 cells—Implication for reverse cholesterol transport. Arterioscler Thromb Vasc Biol 1997; 17:2020–2028.
167. Harris WS. Fish oils and plasma lipid and lipoprotein metabolism in humans: a critical review. J Lipid Res 1989; 30:785–807.
168. Calabresi L, Villa B, Canavesi M, et al. An omega-3 polyunsaturated fatty acid concentrate increases plasma high-density lipoprotein 2 cholesterol and paraoxonase levels in patients with familial combined hyperlipidemia. Metab 2004; 53:153–158.
169. Harris WS, Connor WE, Illingworth DR, et al. Effects of fish oil on VLDL triglyceride kinetics in humans. J Lipid Res 1990; 31:1549–1558.
170. Harris WS, Ginsberg HN, Arunakul N, et al. Safety and efficacy of Omacor in severe hypertriglyceridemia. J Cardiovasc Risk 1997; 4:385–391.
171. Saltiel AR, Olefsky JM. Thiazolidinediones in the treatment of insulin resistance and type II diabetes. Diabetes 1996; 45:1661–1669.
172. Lehmann JM, Moore LB, Smith-Oliver TA, et al. An antidiabetic thiazolidinedione is a high affinity ligand for peroxisome proliferator-activated receptor gamma (PPAR gamma). J Biol Chem 1995; 270:12953–12956.
173. Sakamoto J, Kimura H, Moriyama S, et al. Activation of human peroxisome proliferator-activated receptor (PPAR) subtypes by pioglitazone. Biochem Biophys Res Commun 2000; 278:704–711.
174. van Wijk JP, de Koning EJ, Martens EP, et al. Thiazolidinediones and blood lipids in type 2 diabetes. Arterioscler Thromb Vasc Biol 2003; 23:1744–1749.
175. Yki-Jarvinen H. Thiazolidinediones. N Engl J Med 2004; 351:1106–1118.
176. Goldberg RB, Kendall DM, Deeg MA, et al. A comparison of lipid and glycemic effects of pioglitazone and rosiglitazone in patients with type 2 diabetes and dyslipidemia. Diabetes Care 2005; 28:1547–1554.
177. Dujovne CA, Zavoral JH, Rowe E, et al. Effects of sibutramine on body weight and serum lipids: a double-blind, randomized, placebo-controlled study in 322 overweight and obese patients with dyslipidemia. Am Heart J 2001; 142:489–497.

178. Van Gaal LF, Rissanen AM, Scheen AJ, et al. Effects of the cannabinoid-1 receptor blocker rimonabant on weight reduction and cardiovascular risk factors in overweight patients: 1-year experience from the RIO-Europe study. Lancet 2005; 365:1389–1397.
179. Prueksaritanont T, Zhao JJ, Ma B, et al. Mechanistic studies on metabolic interactions between gemfibrozil and statins. J Pharmacol Exp Ther 2002; 301:1042–1051.
180. Shek A, Ferrill MJ. Statin-fibrate combination therapy. Ann Pharmacother 2001; 35:908–917.
181. Jones PH, Davidson MH. Reporting rate of rhabdomyolysis with fenofibrate + statin versus gemfibrozil + any statin. Am J Cardiol 2005; 95:120–122.
182. Shepherd J. Fibrates and statins in the treatment of hyperlipidaemia: an appraisal of their efficacy and safety. Eur Heart J 1995; 16:5–13.
183. Athyros VG, Papageorgiou AA, Hatzikonstandinou HA, et al. Safety and efficacy of long-term statin-fibrate combinations in patients with refractory familial combined hyperlipidemia. Am J Cardiol 1997; 80:608–613.
184. Pauciullo P, Borgnino C, Paoletti R, et al. Efficacy and safety of a combination of fluvastatin and bezafibrate in patients with mixed hyperlipidaemia (FACT study). Atherosclerosis 2000; 150:429–436.
185. Taher TH, Dzavik V, Reteff EM, et al. Tolerability of statin-fibrate and statin-niacin combination therapy in dyslipidemic patients at high risk for cardiovascular events. Am J Cardiol 2002; 89:390–394.
186. Grundy SM, Vega GL, Yuan Z, et al. Effectiveness and tolerability of simvastatin plus fenofibrate for combined hyperlipidemia (the SAFARI trial). Am J Cardiol 2005; 95:462–468.
187. Brown BG, Zhao XQ, Chait A et al. Simvastatin and niacin, antioxidant vitamins, or the combination for the prevention of coronary disease. N Engl J Med 2001; 345:1583–1592.
188. Guyton JR, Capuzzi DM. Treatment of hyperlipidemia with combined niacin-statin regimens. Am J Cardiol 1998; 82:82U–84U.
189. Nordoy, Bonaa, Nilsen, et al. Effects of Simvastatin and omega-3 fatty acids on plasma lipoproteins and lipid peroxidation in patients with combined hyperlipidaemia. J of Internal Med 1998; 243:163–170.
190. Contacos C, Barter PJ, Sullivan DR. Effect of pravastatin and omega-3 fatty acids on plasma lipids and lipoproteins in patients with combined hyperlipidemia. Arterioscler Thromb 1993; 13:1755–1762.
191. Nordoy A, Hansen JB, Brox J, et al. Effects of atorvastatin and omega-3 fatty acids on LDL subfractions and postprandial hyperlipemia in patients with combined hyperlipemia. Nutr Metab Cardiovasc Dis 2001; 11:7–16.
192. Keech A. Fenofibrate Intervention and Event Lowering in Diabetes (FIELD) study, a randomized, placebo-controlled trial: baseline characteristics and short-term effects of fenofibrate. Cardiovasc Diabetol 2005; 4:13.
193. Frick MH, Elo O, Haapa K, et al. Helsinki Heart Study: primary-prevention trial with gemfibrozil in middle-aged men with dyslipidemia. Safety of treatment, changes in risk factors, and incidence of coronary heart disease. N Engl J Med 1987; 317:1237–1245.
194. Manninen V, Elo MO, Frick MH, et al. Lipid alterations and decline in the incidence of coronary heart disease in the Helsinki Heart Study. JAMA 1988; 260:641–651.
195. Manninen V, Tenkanen L, Koskinen P, et al. Joint effects of serum triglycerides and LDL cholesterol and HDL cholesterol concentrations on coronary heart disease risk in the Helsinki Heart Study. Circulation 1992; 85:37–45.
196. Tenkanen L, Manttari M, Manninen V. Some coronary risk factors related to the insulin resistance syndrome and treatment with gemfibrozil: Experience from the Helsinki Heart Study. Circulation 1995; 92:1779–1785.
197. Rubins HB, Robins SJ, Collins D, et al. Gemfibrozil for the secondary prevention of coronary heart disease in men with low levels of high-density lipoprotein cholesterol. Veterans Affairs High-Density Lipoprotein Cholesterol Intervention Trial Study Group. N Engl J Med 1999; 341:410–418.
198. Bloomfield RH, Davenport J, Babikian V, et al. Reduction in stroke with gemfibrozil in men with coronary heart disease and low HDL cholesterol: The Veterans Affairs HDL Intervention Trial (VA-HIT). Circulation 2001; 103:2828–2833.
199. Robins SJ, Rubins HB, Faas FH, et al. Insulin resistance and cardiovascular events with low HDL cholesterol: the Veterans Affairs HDL Intervention Trial (VA-HIT). Diabetes Care 2003; 26:1513–1517.
200. Rubins HB, Robins SJ, Collins D, et al. Diabetes, plasma insulin, and cardiovascular disease: subgroup analysis from the Department of Veterans Affairs high-density lipoprotein intervention trial (VA-HIT). Arch Intern Med 2002; 162:2597–2604.
201. Tenenbaum A, Motro M, Fisman EZ, et al. Bezafibrate for the secondary prevention of myocardial infarction in patients with metabolic syndrome. Arch Intern Med 2005; 165:1154–1160.
202. Secondary prevention by raising HDL cholesterol and reducing triglycerides in patients with coronary artery disease: the Bezafibrate Infarction Prevention (BIP) study. Circulation 2000; 102:21–27.
203. The FIELD study i. Effects of long-term fenofibrate therapy on cardiovascular events in 9795 people with type 2 diabetes mellitus (the FIELD study): randomised controlled trial. Lancet 366:1849–1861.
204. Birjmohun RS, Hutten BA, Kastelein JJ, et al. Efficacy and safety of high-density lipoprotein cholesterol-increasing compounds: a meta-analysis of randomized controlled trials. J Am Coll Cardiol 2005; 45:185–197.
205. Clofibrate and niacin in coronary heart disease. JAMA 1975; 231:360–381.
206. Canner PL, Berge KG, Wenger NK, et al. Fifteen year mortality in Coronary Drug Project patients: long-term benefit with niacin. J Am Coll Cardiol 1986; 8:1245–1255.

207. Carlson LA, Rosenhamer G. Reduction of mortality in the Stockholm Ischaemic Heart Disease Secondary Prevention Study by combined treatment with clofibrate and nicotinic acid. Acta Med Scand 1988; 223:405–418.
208. Sacks FM, Pasternak RC, Gibson CM, et al. Effect on coronary atherosclerosis of decrease in plasma cholesterol concentrations in normocholesterolaemic patients. Harvard Atherosclerosis Reversibility Project (HARP) Group Lancet 1994; 344:1182–1186.
209. Blankenhorn DH, Nessim SA, Johnson RL, et al. Beneficial effects of combined colestipol-niacin therapy on coronary atherosclerosis and coronary venous bypass grafts. JAMA 1987; 257:3233–3240.
210. Cashin Hemphill L, Mack WJ, Pogoda JM, et al. Beneficial effects of colestipol-niacin on coronary atherosclerosis. A 4-year follow-up [see comments]. JAMA 1990; 264:3013–3017.
211. Brown G, Albers JJ, Fisher LD, et al. Regression of coronary artery disease as a result of intensive lipid-lowering therapy in men with high levels of apolipoprotein B [see comments]. N Engl J Med 1990; 323:1289–1298.
212. Kane JP, Malloy MJ, Ports TA, et al. Regression of coronary atherosclerosis during treatment of familial hypercholesterolemia with combined drug regimens. JAMA 1990; 264:3007–3012.
213. Whitney EJ, Krasuski RA, Personius BE, et al. A randomized trial of a strategy for increasing high-density lipoprotein cholesterol levels: effects on progression of coronary heart disease and clinical events. Ann Intern Med 2005; 142:95–104.
214. Law MR, Wald NJ, Rudnicka AR. Quantifying effect of statins on low density lipoprotein cholesterol, ischaemic heart disease, and stroke: systematic review and meta-analysis. Br Med J 2003; 326:1423.
215. Pedersen TR, Kjekshus J, Berg K, et al. Randomised trial of cholesterol lowering in 4444 patients with coronary heart disease: The Scandinavian Simvastatin Survival Study (4S). Lancet 1994; 344:1383–1389.
216. Ballantyne CM, Olsson AG, Cook TJ, et al. Influence of low high-density lipoprotein cholesterol and elevated triglyceride on coronary heart disease events and response to simvastatin therapy in 4S. Circulation 2001; 104:3046–3051.
217. Hooper L, Thompson RL, Harrison RA, et al. Omega 3 fatty acids for prevention and treatment of cardiovascular disease. Cochrane Database Syst Rev 2004; CD003177.
218. Dietary supplementation with n-3 polyunsaturated fatty acids and vitamin E after myocardial infarction: results of the GISSI-Prevenzione trial. Gruppo Italiano per lo Studio della Sopravvivenza nell'Infarto miocardico. Lancet 1999; 354:447–455.
219. Wierzbicki AS, Reynolds TM, Crook MA. Usefulness of Orlistat in the treatment of severe hypertriglyceridemia. Am J Cardiol 2002; 89:229–231.
220. Tzotzas T, Krassas GE, Bruckert E. Administration of orlistat in a patient with familial hyperchylomicronemia. Atherosclerosis 2002; 165:185–186.
221. Pineda TI, Gervois P, Staels B. Peroxisome proliferator-activated receptor alpha in metabolic disease, inflammation, atherosclerosis and aging. Curr Opin Lipidol 1999; 10:151–159.

10 | Safety of Dyslipidemic Agents

Stefano Bellosta, Rodolfo Paoletti, and Alberto Corsini

Department of Pharmacological Sciences, University of Milan, Milan, Italy

KEY POINTS

- Lipid-lowering monotherapy is well tolerated and is associated with a low frequency of adverse events.
- However, many patients with lipid-lowering therapy do not reach the current treatment goals on the lipid profile. Therefore, a combination therapy between classes of lipid-lowering agents is strongly recommended by the current guidelines.
- Since lipid-lowering drugs are prescribed on a long-term basis, interactions with other drugs deserve attention as many patients will typically receive drugs for concomitant conditions during the course of therapy.
- Knowledge of the metabolic pathways responsible for the metabolism of lipid-lowering agents allows the prediction and prevention of possible drug interaction among these agents and other drugs, thus improving the benefit of lipid-lowering therapy in terms of both efficacy and safety.

INTRODUCTION

Despite the continuous decline in the incidence of atherosclerosis-related deaths in the past two to three decades, coronary heart disease (CHD), cerebrovascular disease, and peripheral vascular disease are still the leading cause of mortality in Western nations (1). For patients with elevated levels of total cholesterol, low-density lipoprotein cholestrol (LDL-C), or triglycerides (TGs), or reduced high-density lipoprotein cholesterol (HDL-C) values, pharmacological treatment is based on the patient's risk factor status and LDL-C levels (2). Currently, several classes of hypolipidemic drugs are available, including the 3-hydroxy-3-methylglutaryl coenzyme A (HMG-CoA) reductase inhibitors (statins), fibrates, nicotinic acid, resins, and ezetimibe (1,3).

The issue of safety and tolerance of these drugs is particularly important in the primary and secondary prevention of cardiovascular disease (CVD), where the risk of long-term therapy must be considered in the context of achievable benefits (4). In general, lipid-lowering monotherapy is well tolerated and has a low frequency of adverse events. The statins are a well-established class of drugs in the treatment of hypercholesterolemia, and members of this class have been shown to reduce the risk of cardiovascular morbidity and mortality in patients with or at risk for CHD in several clinical trials (1,2,5). Statins are the most powerful agents for lowering LDL-C, with reductions in the range of 20% to 60%. However, several large surveys have shown that many patients do not reach the current treatment goals for the lipid profile after statin therapy. Therefore, combinations of therapy between statins and other classes of lipid-lowering agents (e.g., ezetimibe, fibrates, resins, and nicotinic acid) are recommended for some patients by the current guidelines. Moreover, since lipid-lowering drugs are prescribed on a long-term basis, possible interactions with other drugs deserve attention as many patients will typically receive drugs for concomitant conditions during the course of therapy (4). This chapter will cover the issue of safety of the hypolipidemic agents both in monotherapy and in combination with other drugs.

STATINS

The statins are a well-established class of drugs in the treatment of hypercholesterolemia, and members of this class have been shown to reduce the risk of cardiovascular morbidity and mortality in patients with or at risk for CHD in several clinical trials, even in those with normal LDL-C levels (1,3,6,7).

TABLE 1   Clinical Pharmacokinetics of HMG-CoA Reductase Inhibitors

Parameter	Atorvastatin	Fluvastatin	Fluvastatin XL	Lovastatin	Pravastatin	Rosuvastatin	Simvastatin
T_{max} (hr)	2–3	0.5–1	4	2–4	0.9–1.6	3	1.3–2.4
C_{max} (ng/mL)	27–66	448	55	10–20	45–55	37	10–34
Bioavail-ability (%)	12	19–29	6	5	18	20	5
Lipo-philicity	Yes	Yes	Yes	Yes	No	No	Yes
Protein binding (%)	80–90	>99	>99	>95	43–55	88	94–98
Meta-bolism	CYP3A4	CYP2C9	CYP2C9	CYP3A4	Sulfation	CYP2C9, 2C19 (minor)	CYP3A4
Meta-bolites	Active	Inactive	Inactive	Active	Inactive	Active (minor)	Active
Trans-porter proteins substrate	Yes	Yes	Yes	Yes	Yes/No	Yes	Yes
$T1/2$ (hr)	15–30	0.5–2.3	4.7	2.9	1.3–2.8	20.8	2–3
Urinary excretion (%)	2	6	6	10	20	10	13
Fecal excretion (%)	70	90	90	83	71	90	58

Note: Based on a 40 mg oral dose, with the exception of fluvastatin XL (80 mg).
Abbreviation: CYP, cytochrome P.
Source: Adapted from Refs. 8 and 9.

Pharmacokinetics

Statins are very selective inhibitors of HMG-CoA reductase, and usually do not show any relevant affinity toward other enzymes or receptor systems (8). This suggests that, at the pharmacodynamic level (i.e., at their site of action), statins are not prone to interfering with other drugs. However, at the pharmacokinetic level (i.e., absorption, distribution, metabolism, and excretion of a given drug), the available statins have important differences, including half-life, systemic exposure, maximum plasma concentration (C_{max}), bioavailability, protein binding, lipophilicity, metabolism, presence of active metabolites, and excretion routes (Table 1).

The liver biotransforms all statins, which accounts for their overall low systemic bioavailability. The apparent total body clearance is very high because of an important hepatic first-pass effect. All statins undergo extensive microsomal metabolism by the cytochrome P (CYP)450 isoenzyme systems, with the exceptions of pravastatin, which is transformed enzymatically in the liver cytosol, and rosuvastatin, which is only partly metabolized by the CYP2C9 (Tables 1 and 2).

About one-third of all drugs currently available in clinical practice are biotransformed in the liver primarily by the CYP450 3A4 system (Table 2) (10).

The CYP3A4 isoenzyme is responsible for the metabolism of lovastatin, simvastatin, and atorvastatin. Fluvastatin is metabolized primarily by the CYP2C9 enzyme, with CYP3A4 and CYP2C8 contributing to a lesser extent (8).

Adverse Effects

Several clinical trials have largely dispelled doubts about the safety and tolerability of statins. In fact, the common adverse effects associated with statin therapy are relatively mild and often transient (gastrointestinal symptoms, headache, nausea, rash, loss of concentration, sleep disturbance) (Table 3) (1–3). The most important adverse effects associated with statins are asymptomatic increases in liver transaminases and myopathy. Moreover, the incidence of side effects might be higher in clinical situations where patients are not monitored as closely as they are in clinical trials, as pointed out in a Food and Drug Administration (FDA) adverse event

TABLE 2   Human Cytochrome P (CYP)450 Isoenzymes Known to Oxidize Clinically Used Drugs

CYP1A2	CYP2C9	CYP2C19	CYP2D6	CYP2E1	CYP3A4
Acetaminophen	Alprenolol	Diazepam	Amitriptyline	Acetaminophen	Amiodarone
Caffeine	Diclofenac	Ibuprofen	Codeine	Etanol	Atorvastatin
Theophylline	Fluvastatin	Mephenytoin	Debrisoquine	Halothane	Clarithromycin
	Hexobarbital	Methylphenobarbital	Flecainide		Cyclosporine
	Phenytoin	Omeprazole	Imipramine		Diltiazem
	Rosuvastatin	Proguanyl	Metoprolol		Erythromycin
	Tolbutamide	Phenytoin	Mibefradil		Ketoconazole
	Warfarin		Nortriptyline		Itraconazole
			Pherexiline		Lacidipine
			Propafenone		Lovastatin
			Propranolol		Mibefradil
			Sparteine		Midazolam
			Thioridazine		Nefazodone
			Timolol		Nifedipine
					Protease inhibitors
					Quinidine
					Sildenafil
					Simvastatin
					Terbinafine
					Verapamil
					Warfarin

report (AER) (11). The worldwide withdrawal of cerivastatin in August 2001 because of its association with fatal rhabdomyolysis further underscores the importance of considering the safety profile of the available statins (12).

LIVER TRANSAMINASE ELEVATIONS

During initial postmarketing surveillance of the available statins, elevations in hepatic transaminases were reported at incidences of up to 1% (1,13); the elevations were dose related and comparable among statins, although not significantly increased compared to placebo (13). The majority of liver abnormalities occur within the first three months of therapy and require monitoring. The symptoms of hepatitis induced by statins (fatigue, sluggishness, anorexia, and weight loss) resemble those of an influenza-like syndrome. Serum alanine aminotransferase (ALT) concentrations are usually only moderately elevated (e.g., two to three times the upper limit of the normal range). The symptoms subside almost overnight after the drug is discontinued, but serum ALT concentrations may not return to normal levels for several weeks, depending on the degree of the elevation. On the other hand, minor, isolated elevations in serum ALT concentrations (such as increases to 1.5 times the upper limit of the normal range) can be ignored in the absence of symptoms. It is reasonable to measure ALT at baseline and three to six months after therapy is initiated or 6 to 12 weeks after a statin is titrated. As part of routine toxicity surveillance, it is reasonable to monitor liver function tests twice yearly while patients are on statin therapy (1).

TABLE 3   Adverse Effects of Statins

Location	Effect
Gastrointestinal tract	Abdominal pain, nausea, diarrhea
Immune system	Lupus-like syndrome
Liver	Hepatitis, loss of appetite, weight loss, increased serum aminotransferases
Muscles	Muscle pain or weakness, myositis, rhabdomyolysis with renal failure
Nervous system	Loss of concentration, sleep disturbance, headache, peripheral neuropathy
Protein binding	Diminished binding of warfarin
Skin	Rash

TABLE 4   Factors Contributing to Myopathy/Rhabdomyolysis Exacerbation

Age
Diabetes
Excessive alcohol intake
Female gender
Heavy physical activity
Hypothyroidism
Liver disease
Metabolic rate
Renal disease
Surgery
Trauma

MYOPATHY

The term "myopathy" designates any acquired or inherited disorder of skeletal muscle that causes proximal muscle weakness, with difficulty in arising from a chair or raising arms above the head (4,14). Duration of statin therapy before the onset of myopathy varies from a few weeks to more than two years. Statin-associated myopathy represents a broad clinical spectrum of disorders (14), from myalgia [muscle complaints without serum creatine kinase (CK) elevations], myositis (muscle symptoms with CK elevations), and rhabdomyolysis (markedly elevated CK levels, usually >10 times upper the normal limit and creatine elevation). However, patients have been also described who developed myositis and rhabdomyolysis while receiving statin therapy despite normal serum CK levels, thus pointing out the inadequacy of CK testing for statin-associated myopathy (4,10,14).

The epidemiology of statin-associated myopathy is poorly described and mainly focused on rhabdomyolysis. The occurrence of both myopathy and rhabdomyolysis during statin clinical trials is rare; the incidence of severe myopathy is 0.1% to 0.5%, while the incidence of rhabdomyolysis is 0.02% to 0.04% (15,16). Myopathy with statins is dose dependent, however, and the risk of its development increases when drugs that slow statin metabolism are administered concurrently (4). The symptoms progress toward rhabdomyolysis as long as patients continue to take the drug. It should be noted that the development of myopathy is induced by a complex interaction between drugs, disease, genetics, and concomitant therapy. Several risk factors that predispose patients to myopathy/rhabdomyolysis include increased age, female gender, renal or liver disease, diabetes mellitus, hypothyroidism, debilitated status, surgery, trauma, excessive alcohol intake, and heavy exercise (Table 4) (4). The mechanism by which statins cause myopathy is not completely understood (4,15). However, the clinical association appears to be dose dependent, and the risk is known to increase when statins are prescribed in combination with agents that are also myotoxic when used as monotherapy or increase the serum concentration of the statin (8,17). For example, one study reported a 0.15% incidence of myopathy with lovastatin monotherapy, which increased to 2%, 5%, and 28%, respectively, in patients receiving concomitant niacin, gemfibrozil, or cyclosporine plus gemfibrozil (18).

RHABDOMYOLYSIS

Rhabdomyolysis is a syndrome that results from severe skeletal muscle injury and myocyte lysis, causing the widespread release of myoglobin with production of dark brown urine secondary to myoglobinuria (1,19). Rhabdomyolysis is often characterized by marked elevations of CK levels to >100 times the upper limit of normal (ULN), and is accompanied by myoglobinuria, myoglobinemia, and evidence of target organ damage such as decreased renal function or acute renal failure (16). Importantly, the progression from myopathy to rhabdomyolysis can usually be reversed by an early diagnosis, hydration, and the withdrawal of the interacting agents (16,17). An analysis of data from the Adverse Event Reporting System of the U.S. FDA shows that as of June 2001, fatal rhabdomyolysis was reported at rates of less than one death per one million prescriptions for all statins, except cerivastatin which had an incidence of more than three deaths per one million prescriptions (12). The incidence of fatal rhabdomyolysis has been estimated using databases from the FDA and is low, resulting in 0.15 deaths per one million prescriptions. This figure uses as the denominator the number of prescriptions, not the number of individuals using the medication (10). Clinical trials results support a low incidence of severe muscle problems with statin therapy.

A compilation of randomized, placebo controlled statin trials revealed that among 83,858 patients randomly assigned to receive either statin treatment or placebo, there were only 49 cases of myositis and seven cases of rhabdomyolysis in the statin groups, compared with 44 cases of myositis and five cases of rhabdomyolysis in the placebo groups (10). However, these results in volunteer study participants who were followed by lipid researchers may underestimate the incidence when statins are used in unselected populations followed with less precision (10). Thus, although there are significant limitations to the interpretation of the reported adverse events, this information has valuable implications for clinical practice.

A recent meta-analysis of data from 79,701 participants in 13 randomized trials of statins has reported nine cases of rhabdomyolysis in the statin group and six in the placebo group (20). Important caveats in reviewing safety data from clinical trials, however, are that many of the patients excluded from trials receive these agents in clinical practice and that patients in clinical trials differ from those seen in general practice in that the former are generally better informed and monitored and perhaps more compliant (17). For example, clinical trials protocols often exclude patients who may be more prone to myopathy, such as the elderly or who may have abnormal liver test results at baseline, and assumptions about safety may be overestimated (4,8,15,17,21). Therefore, the results in volunteer study participants who were monitored by lipid researchers may underestimate the incidence of myopathy when statins are used in unselected populations monitored with less precision. Nevertheless, a recent study, which was conducted to estimate the incidence of hospitalized rhabdomyolysis in statin-treated patients in the ambulatory setting, reported a risk rate for rhabdomyolysis similar to that observed in clinical trials (22).

Muscular Symptoms

If the frequency of severe myopathy associated with lipid-lowering drugs is well evaluated, the frequency of milder symptoms remains largely unknown. It must be kept in mind that mild musculoskeletal symptoms with hypolipidemic drugs are far more frequent then severe myopathy. Moreover, mild muscular symptoms are often overlooked by doctors and their frequency is probably underestimated. This is particularly important when patients are treated with high dosages of statins, as the incidence of myopathy increases with dosage. Statins are more frequently associated with a variety of skeletal muscle complaints including myalgia, with or without serum CK elevations, cramps, and weakness. These mild symptoms are poorly assessed and only few data are available regarding the frequency, which may affect patients (15,16). While cramps and stiffness are the most frequent symptoms, tendonitis-associated pain is surprisingly common, being reported in almost half the cases. Pain is often diffused, and a majority of patients reported pain during rest and in the lying position. The impact of these mild symptoms on daily activities might not be negligible in a subset of patients, and the genetic background might play a role in predisposing to low-grade myopathy.

Review of two databases (19,23) showed that myalgia contributed to 6% to 25% of all adverse events associated with statins although its real incidence may be lower. In contrast, myalgia was rarely reported in clinical trials with an incidence (1–5%), which was not different from placebo and considered unrelated to statin therapy (10). Consequently, there is no consensus that statins are responsible for these myalgic complaints although many clinicians believe that statins can induce myalgia without CK elevations. In contrast to severe myopathy, no risk factors have been identified for mild muscle symptoms with the exception of some rare cases of preexisting myopathy. A recent observational study focused on the muscle side effects of statins with a specific focus on mild muscle symptoms (24). In this study, Franc et al. used a questionnaire to identify patients (16% of the total) who experienced muscle symptoms related to lipid-lowering therapy (LLT), mainly statins, including cramps, stiffness, and tendonitis-associated pain. Interestingly, a clear chronological link between symptoms and the LLT was revealed either because symptoms appeared soon after drug initiation or because of an improvement after drug withdrawal. There is a clear need, therefore, to better estimate the relevance, and to characterize the risk factors for this statin-associated muscular symptoms.

EFFECT OF STATINS ON COENZYME Q10 LEVELS

Coenzyme Q10 (ubiquinone), a component of the mitochondrial respiratory chain, is a derivative of mevalonate, and its levels might be affected by statin treatment. Ubiquinone is very lipophilic and it is carried by both the LDL and the HDL in plasma. Nevertheless, ubiquinone is taken up from the diet to only a very limited extent, and redistribution of this lipid via the circulation does not occur to any appreciable extent (25,26). For this reason, the relevance of serum levels of ubiquinone is questionable. Indeed, conflicting results have been reported on the effect of statin treatment on Q10 plasma levels (25,27). Most recently described mitochondrial myopathies are due to defects in nuclear DNA, including coenzyme Q10 deficiency, and mutations in genes that control mitochondrial DNA abundance. However, an open label study of Q10 concentration in muscle from statin-treated patients with increased CK showed that statin drug-related myopathy is associated with a mild decrease in muscle CoQ10 concentration, which does not cause histochemical or biochemical evidence of mitochondrial myopathy in most patients (28).

PROTEINURIA

Rosuvastatin and pravastatin are the only two statins with a significant (10–30%) renal clearance, including active tubular secretion (4). Phase III trials have shown a dose-dependent increase in stick-positive proteinuria in patients receiving 5, 10, 20 or 40 mg/day of rosuvastatin (0.2, 0.6, 0.7, and 1.2%, respectively). With 80 mg the proteinuria was significantly higher (>10%) (29). It is interesting to note that proteinuria was detectable also with other statins without any dose-dependent relationship (29,30). Experimental data indicate a predominance of lower molecular weight proteins, suggesting decreased reabsorption of normally filtered proteins (i.e., tubular proteinuria) rather than increased glomerular leakage of proteins as the primary etiology of the proteinuria seen in patients treated with statins (31). Nevertheless, only the postmarketing data will give the final answer to this matter.

NEUROPATHY

The diagnosis of peripheral neuropathy secondary to statin use poses a challenge for clinicians, because many of these patients have concomitant disease states such as diabetes or renal failure that predispose them to neuropathy (32,33). Moreover, confirmation that the neuropathy is associated with statin therapy requires prolonged follow-up, as symptom resolution may take weeks to months. The epidemiologic evidence suggests that a link between statins and neuropathy may exist; however, the incidence is low, affecting approximately 1 person per 14,000 person-years of treatment (34,35), and that the cardioprotective benefit of statin therapy far outweighs the risk of developing peripheral neuropathy (32). The current evidence for a possible link between statins and peripheral neuropathy is based entirely on observational data and, as such, it has many limitations, including possible bias and unknown confounders (32). Further studies are needed to determine the incidence of peripheral neuropathy with long-term use, assess patient-specific risk factors, and investigate potential mechanisms. In the interim, physicians should be aware of this potential toxicity and monitor patients appropriately; that is, statins should be considered the cause of peripheral neuropathy when other etiologies have been excluded (35).

HIGH-DOSE STATIN THERAPY

Finally, it is important to mention that the more recent trials addressing the benefit of high dosages of statins in CHD patients raise concerns on the safety of this therapy. All the trials, indeed, have shown an increased incidence of liver transaminases elevations (36,37), myopathy (37,38), and in noncardiovascular deaths (39). Nevertheless, it is worthwhile to mention that, in the aforementioned trials, intensive LLT was associated with a greater reduction in CVD incidence. Therefore, these observations from one side raise concerns on the use of high doses of statins, but at the same time suggest the potential benefit obtainable from lipid-lowering drugs.

Combination Therapy

The National Cholesterol Education Program adenosine triphosphate (ATP) III report (2) extended the use of lipid-lowering treatments to a larger number of high-risk CHD patients who often receive more than one medication. Therefore, the potential of drug–drug interactions emerges as a relevant factor in determining the safety profile of statins. An extensive FDA search on statin-associated rhabdomyolysis, covering the period from January 1990 through March 2002, showed that among 3339 reports of rhabdomyolysis, about 58% of the cases were associated with concomitant medications affecting statin metabolism including mibefradil, fibrates, cyclosporine, macrolides, warfarin, digoxin, and azole antifungal agents (10).

Pharmacological differences are evident among the statins, and these may affect their safety and potential for drug interactions (8). These differences can affect the potential for drug interactions with statins (8). These interactions can result in markedly increased or decreased plasma concentrations of some drugs within this class. Concomitant use of certain drugs such as fibrates, erythromycin, itraconazole, and immunosuppressive drugs such as cyclosporine can increase blood levels of statins and, consequently, the risk for myopathy (40). The relationship between altered plasma concentrations and adverse effects or toxicity might not be linear (41,42). Other variables affect this concentration–effect relationship including rapid changes in the concentrations, concomitant LLT, or host genetic factors that code for different forms or amounts of metabolizing enzymes and drug receptors. Special populations at high risk of cardiovascular disease, such as patients with CHD, dyslipidemia, diabetes, hypertension, nephrotic disease, HIV, organ transplant patients and the elderly, deserve particular attention to avoid clinically relevant interactions. Nevertheless, the incidence of both myopathy and rhabdomyolysis is very low despite coprescription of statins with competing substrates or inhibitors of their metabolism being commonplace (43). Indeed, up to one-third of prescriptions issued for statins were in combination with drugs that could potentially interact with them, although side effects occurred in only 3% of these patients (16).

STATIN INTERACTIONS WITH CYTOCHROME P450 INHIBITORS

Induction or inhibition of CYP450 isoenzymes is an important cause of drug interactions (8). Competitive inhibition between drugs at the enzymatic level is common and may serve to alter the disposition of statins, leading to increased plasma levels and greater risk of adverse events (Table 5).

Pharmacokinetic interactions (e.g., increased bioavailability) resulting in myositis and rhabdomyolysis have been reported following concurrent use of statins and different classes of drugs (Table 6) (4).

Fluvastatin, which is primarily metabolized by CYP2C9, and rosuvastatin and pravastatin, which are eliminated by other metabolic routes, are less subject to this interaction than other available statins. Nevertheless, a 5- to 23-fold increase in pravastatin bioavailability has been reported in the presence of cyclosporine A (4). This suggests that cyclosporine may interact with statins via mechanisms not limited to CYP3A4 inhibition. It has been postulated that competition for carrier-mediated transport across the bile canalicular membrane between rosuvastatin, pravastatin, and cyclosporine leads to a reduced clearance of these statins (8). A cyclosporine–pravastatin interaction may occur also at the level of *p*-glycoprotein, another transport protein (8). FDA AERs on statin-associated rhabdomyolysis (11) and postmarketing surveillance (44) have confirmed an increased risk of myopathy when pravastatin is combined with cyclosporine. On the other hand, fluvastatin shows a far milder interaction with cyclosporine, most likely because fluvastatin is primarily recognized by CYP2C9 rather than CYP3A4 (8). These findings supported the assessment of lescol in renal transplantation (ALERT) trial in renal transplantation patients with hypercholesterolemia treated with cyclosporine with or without fluvastatin (45). Adverse event rates were similar in both treatment groups, as were the rates of discontinuation because of adverse events. The incidence of ALT elevations ($\geq$3x ULN) or CK elevations ($\geq$5x ULN) was similar in fluvastatin- and placebo-treated patients, and no elevations were accompanied by musculoskeletal symptoms. The safety profile is perhaps the most remarkable aspect of this trial, as all the renal transplant patients enrolled were on cyclosporine, 80% were on prednisone, and 95% received concomitant cardiovascular medications (45). However, caution should be exercised when fluvastatin is combined with substrates for CYP2C9. For example, potentiation of the anticoagulant effects of warfarin (8), and increased bioavailability, peak plasma concentrations, and plasma half-life of fluvastatin have been reported when fluvastatin is coadministered with diclofenac and fluconazole (46,47).

TABLE 5 Inhibitors and Inducers of the Cytochrome P450 Enzymatic Pathway

CYP substrates (statins)	Inhibitors	Inducers
CYP3A4 Atorvastatin, lovastatin, simvastatin	Ketoconazole, itraconazole, fluconazole, erythromycin, clarithromycin, tricyclic anti- depressants, nefazodone, venlafaxine, fluvoxamine, fluoxetine, sertraline, cyclosporine A, tacrolimus, mibefradil, diltiazem, verapamil, protease inhibitors, midazolam, corticosteroids, grapefruit juice, tamoxifene, amiodarone	Phenytoin, phenobarbital, barbitu- rates, rifampin, dexamethasone, cyclophosphamide, carba- mazepine, troglitazone, omeprazole
CYP2C9 Fluvastatin, rosuvastatin (2C19-minor)	Ketoconazole, fluconazole, sulfaphenazole	Rifampin, phenobarbital, phenytoin, troglitazone

Source: Adapted from Ref. 4.

Dyslipidemia, one of the major metabolic abnormalities associated with HIV infection, appears to be related to the use of protease inhibitors (PIs), because of increased hepatic TG synthesis (48). Statins are being used increasingly in HIV-infected patients. However, cases of myalgia, rhabdomyolysis, and transaminases elevations have been reported with statins (49,50) due to the fact that PIs are inhibitors of the CYP3A4/5 isoenzymes (Table 3). The PI ritonavir has the most pronounced inhibiting effects on CYP3A4 of all the PIs, and rhabdomyolysis has been reported when it was coadministered with simvastatin. In addition, the pharmacokinetics of both simvastatin and atorvastatin were altered by the PI nelfinavir.

Finally, inhibitors of CYP3A4 isoenzyme activity, such as cimetidine and grapefruit juice, increase the oral availability and pharmacokinetic parameters of statins, thus potentially increasing their systemic exposure and side effects. In particular, the administration of 200 mL of double-strength grapefruit juice three times a day for two days, followed on day 3 by the administration of lovastatin together with 200 mL of juice, and additional doses of 200 mL 30 minutes and 90 minutes after statin intake, increased the lovastatin concentration–time curve (AUC) and C_{max} 15-fold and 12-fold, respectively (51). The same experiment was carried out with simvastatin, and the AUC and C_{max} increased 16-fold and 9-fold, respectively (52). However, despite the high concentrations of simvastatin and simvastatin acid when coadminis-tered with grapefruit juice, the HMG-CoA reductase inhibitory activity AUC and C_{max} increased only from threefold to fivefold (52). Under the same experimental conditions, grapefruit juice significantly increased up to 3.3-fold the AUC of atorvastatin, while no changes were observed in the pharmacokinetics of pravastatin. The interaction potential of even high amounts of grape-fruit juice with CYP3A4 substrates dissipates within three to seven days after ingestion of the last dose of juice (53). Both in vitro and in vivo studies have shown that furanocoumarin deriv-atives with geranyloxy side chains contained in the juice play a role in this effect. In vitro exper-iments confirmed that furanocoumarins from grapefruit juice are both competitive and

TABLE 6 Selected Drugs That May Increase Risk of Myopathy and Rhabdomyolysis When Used Concomitantly with Statins

CYP3A4 inhibitors/substrates
  Cyclosporine, tacrolimus
  Macrolides (azithromycin, clarithromycin, erythromycin)
  Azole antifungals (itraconazole, ketoconazole)
  Calcium antagonists (mibefradil, diltiazem, verapamil)
  Nefazodone
  Protease inhibitors (amprenavir, indinavir, nelfinavir, ritonavir,
    saquinavir)
  Sildenafil
  Warfarin
Others
  Digoxin
  Fibrates (gemfibrozil)
  Niacin

Source: Adapted from Refs. 8 and 16.

mechanism-based inhibitors of CYP3A4, and all contribute comprehensively to the grapefruit juice–drug interaction (54). However, other juice components might participate (55). More recent data show that daily consumption of a glass of regular-strength grapefruit has a minimal effect on plasma concentrations of statin (approximately 30–40% increase) after a 40 mg evening dose of lovastatin (56). It may be concluded that the interaction between grapefruit juice and statins does not represent a great concern, unless doses >1 qt/day of juice are consumed (53).

STATINS AND CALCIUM ANTAGONISTS

Many hypercholesterolemic patients are also hypertensive and may be receiving antihypertensive therapy with calcium channel antagonists. Of particular note is the interaction of statins with mibefradil, which was withdrawn from the global market because of a range of serious drug–drug interactions (8). Several cases of statin-associated rhabdomyolysis were reported in patients receiving mibefradil (57).

Verapamil and diltiazem, which are weak inhibitors of CYP3A4 (44), both increase the plasma concentration of simvastatin up to fourfold, and diltiazem increases the plasma concentration of lovastatin to the same magnitude (58,59). Cases of rhabdomyolysis have also been reported with the association of diltiazem with atorvastatin or simvastatin (60,61), suggesting a need for some caution in using these agents simultaneously.

STATIN INTERACTIONS WITH CYTOCHROME P450 INDUCERS

CYP450 inducers (Table 5) may reduce statin plasma levels. This seems to be the case with troglitazone (now withdrawn from the U.S. market), a thiazolidinedione antidiabetic agent that induces the CYP3A4 enzyme (62). Analogously, it has been shown that rifampicin, another inducer, greatly decreases the plasma concentrations of simvastatin (63).

Phenytoin, another inducer of CYP3A4, can alter the lipid-lowering efficacy of both atorvastatin and simvastatin (64). It has also been reported that the herbal supplement St. John's wort decreases plasma concentrations of simvastatin but not of pravastatin (65), this interaction most likely being caused by the enhancement of the CYP3A4-mediated first-pass metabolism of simvastatin in the small intestine and liver by this herbal supplement.

INTERACTIONS BETWEEN STATINS AND FIBRIC ACID DERIVATIVES

The interaction of statins with fibrates deserves particular attention because myopathy can occur with either drug alone, and the effects may be additive (8). Reports of statin-associated myopathies, based in part on the U.S. FDA information, outlined that the risk of rhabdomyolysis and other adverse effects with statin use can be compounded by other factors including altered renal and hepatic functioning, hypothyroidism and concomitant medications (2). Many (58%) of the 3399 cases of statin-associated myopathy that were reported were linked to combination with some class of drugs (2). The main classes of drugs responsible for interaction with statins were fibrates (gemfibrozil), cyclosporine, erythromycin, clarithromycin, warfarin, digoxin, and some antifungals (Table 6). The reason of potential interaction with statins can be attributed on a pharmacokinetic level and many of them are related to the cytochrome 3A4 that is responsible for the metabolism of many of these classes of drugs. Differences in biotransformation can affect the potential for drug interactions with statins. As reported above, all statins (except pravastatin) undergo extensive microsomal metabolism by the CYP450 isoenzyme systems. As a result of these, a number of drugs may increase the risk of myopathy and rhabdomyolysis when used concomitantly with statins (Table 6). The rate of fatal rhabdomyolysis was 16 to 80 times higher with the recently withdrawn statin, cerivastatin, than with the other five clinically used statins, a difference that appears to be related to the marked interaction (relative to that of other statins) between cerivastatin and gemfibrozil (12). (For a detailed overview of statin–fibrate interaction please see the section on fibrates.)

OTHER STATIN INTERACTIONS

The efficacy of drug therapy results from the complex interplay of multiple processes that govern drug disposition and response. Most studies to date have focused on the contribution of drug-metabolizing enzymes to the drug disposition process. However, over the past decade, it has become increasingly apparent that carrier-mediated processes, or protein transporters, also play critical roles in the overall disposition of numerous drugs in clinical use. In addition to their roles in xenobiotic transport, drug transporters often mediate important physiologic functions via transport of endogenous substrates such as amino acids, bile acids, and hormones that are critical for maintenance of normal homeostasis (66). Two major superfamilies, ATP-binding cassette and solute carrier transporters are involved in drug disposition (67). Table 7 shows some of the different drugs that are recognized by protein transporters at the level of the liver.

Changes in the absorption and excretion of drugs independent of CYP metabolism can alter drug disposition and may contribute to the interaction potential of statins. Transport proteins are, at least in part, responsible for the low and variable disposition of all statins (Table 2) (68). Indeed, interactions with other drugs at the *p*-glycoprotein level could potentially be responsible for the rhabdomyolysis observed after statin–digoxin combination therapy. Digoxin is a *p*-glycoprotein substrate/inhibitor, and its narrow therapeutic range makes any drug–drug interaction important, warranting the monitoring of digoxin levels. In fact, acute interactions have been observed with simvastatin (69), and coadministration of atorvastatin 80 mg/day and digoxin 0.25 mg/day for 20 days increased systemic exposure to digoxin by inhibition of *p*-glycoprotein (70). However, administration of atorvastatin 10 mg/day with digoxin did not affect mean steady-state concentrations of digoxin (70).

Polymorphisms in the protein transporters may also impact statin activity and are another factor to be considered in addressing the role of these transporters in terms of lipid-lowering activity and drug safety. Indeed, it has been shown that a variant of the organic anion transport protein in Japanese patients is involved in cases of myopathy following pravastatin treatment (71).

Clinical trials in which patients have received niacin in combination with fluvastatin, pravastatin, or simvastatin have also not reported myopathy (4), although the number of patients in these trials was low. However, in case reports, niacin has been associated with rhabdomyolysis in combination with lovastatin, pravastatin, or simvastatin, but not with atorvastatin or fluvastatin (4). A new lovastatin and prolonged-release niacin combination product has recently become available, and no cases of myopathy have been reported in a recent open-label study with this combination (72). Clinically important interactions have not been observed between statins and other drugs used in cardiovascular diseases, such as propranolol, angiotensin-converting enzyme inhibitors, angiotensin receptor blockers (the "sartans"), and thiazide diuretics (8).

Another interesting interaction occurs between statins and antithrombotic agents. The administration of statins to patients receiving warfarin caused a small potentiation of the

TABLE 7 Summary of the Major Human Liver Sinusoidal Canalicular Membrane Transporters Involved in Transport of Therapeutic Drugs

Common name of transporter	Gene family name	Subcellular location	Known drug substrates
OATP-A	SLC21A3	S	Fexofenadine, rosuvastatin, UK-191,005
OATP-C/2	SLC21A6	S	Atorvastatin, cerivastatin, simvastatin, rosuvastatin, pravastatin, pitavastatin, fluvastatin, gemfibrozil, lovastatin, ezetimibe, BSP, eicosanoids, conjugated steroids, cyclosporine
OATP-8	SLC21A8	S	BSP, rosuvastatin
OATP-B	SLC21A9	S	Fexofenadine, UK-191,005
OAT3	SLC22A8	S?	Fluvastatin, pravastatin, cimetidine
MDR1	ABCB1	C	Atorvastatin, simvastatin, lovastatin, pravastatin, cyclosporine, taxol, vinblastine, doxorubicin, digoxin, talinolol, loperamide, erythromycin
MRP2	ABCC2	C	Pravastatin, atorvastatin, methotrexate, grepafloxacin, cefodizime, irinotecan, conjugates of a variety of drugs
MRP1	ABCC1	L	Anticancer agents, anionic conjugates with glutathione, sulfate or glucuronide
BCRP	ABCP	L	Cerivastatin, pitavastatin, fluvastatin, pravastatin, rosuvastatin

Abbreviations: S, sinusoidal; C, canalicular; L, lateral membranes; ND, not determined; ATP-binding cassette; BSP, bromosulphophthalein.

TABLE 8 Comparison of Pharmacokinetic Properties of Fibric Acid Derivatives

	Bezafibrate	Ciprofibrate	Clofibrate	Fenofibrate	Gemfibrozil
Oral bioavailability (%)	100		100	60	100
Volume of distribution	17 L		14.5 L	0.89 L/kg	
$t_{1/2}$ in healthy volunteers (hr)	1.5–3.0	81	15	19–27	1.3
$t_{1/2}$ in patients with renal failure (hr)	9.2	172	30–110	143	
Protein binding (%)	95	99	96	>99	98
Route of elimination	Renal (unchanged)	Renal	Renal (metabolites)	Renal (glucuronide)	Renal (glucuronide)

Abbreviation: $t_{1/2}$, half-life.

anticoagulant effect, requiring a warfarin dosage reduction, and a recent FDA report has documented cases of rhabdomyolysis when all statins were given in combination with warfarin (11). The mechanism underlying the interaction between statins and warfarin is due to a competition at the cytochrome level. Conflicting data have been reported on the effect of statin on clopidogrel-inhibited platelet aggregation in patients undergoing coronary stenting; at the moment there are no clear reasons to exclude the potential association of these classes of drugs in patients at high risk for coronary disease (4).

Pharmacogenomics

Finally, evidence suggests that genetic polymorphisms may play a potentially key role in the efficacy, safety, and tolerability of all medications. Under clinical trials conditions, interindividual variations in response to statin therapy are clearly apparent, and seem to be largely independent of the dose and drug used (16). These variations in response to statins may be due to differences in receptor-mediated LDL catabolism as they occur to a similar extent in patients with both heterozygous familial hypercholesterolemia (FH) and non-FH, including a group of FH patients with the same mutation.

The cholesterol-lowering effect and tolerability of simvastatin is affected by CYP2D6 polymorphism and CYP2C9, which is responsible for the metabolism of fluvastatin, is also polymorphic (16).

FIBRATES
Pharmacokinetics

The fibrates are largely excreted by the kidney and therefore accumulate in the serum of patients with renal failure (Table 8).Renal failure is a relative contraindication to the use of fibrates, as is hepatic dysfunction. Combined statin-fibrate therapy should be avoided in patients with compromised renal function (1,3).

Adverse Effects

Fibric acid derivatives (fibrates) usually are well tolerated. Side effects may occur in 5% to 10% of patients, but most often are not sufficient to cause discontinuation of the drug. Gastrointestinal side effects occur in up to 5% of patients. Other side effects are reported infrequently and include rash, urticaria, hair loss, myalgias, fatigue, headache, impotence, and anemia (Table 9).

TABLE 9 Adverse Effects of Fibrates

Location	Effect
Gastrointestinal tract	Stomach upset, abdominal pain, cholesterol-saturated bile, increase in gallstone incidence (1–2%)
Genitourinary tract	Erectile dysfunction
Liver	Increased of serum aminotransferases
Muscles	Myositis with impaired renal function
Plasma proteins	Interference with binding of warfarin, with reduction of dosage by 30%
Skin	Rash

Minor increases in liver transaminases and decreases in alkaline phosphatase have been reported (1,3). All fibrates increase biliary cholesterol concentrations and can increase the lithogenicity of bile causing gallstones (1).

Combination Therapy
Anticoagulants
Clofibrate, bezafibrate, and fenofibrate have been reported to potentiate the action of oral anticoagulants, in part by displacing them from their binding sites on albumin. Careful monitoring of the prothrombin time and reduction in dosage of the anticoagulant may be appropriate when treatment with a fibrate is begun.

COMBINATION FIBRATES–STATINS

Concomitant use of a fibrate and a statin may offer a therapeutic advantage to patients with dyslipidemia, especially in those patients whose LDL-C is controlled by statin, but whose HDL-C and/or TG levels are not within goal (1,2). However, there is often reluctance to prescribe statins and fibrates concomitantly because of the concern that drug–drug interactions will increase the risk of myopathy and rhabdomyolysis.

As monotherapy, both statins and fibrates have been reported to cause myopathy. An enhanced risk of myopathy with the combined use of a statin and a fibrate is therefore not unexpected. There have been numerous reports in the medical literature of gemfibrozil/ statin-associated rhabdomyolysis. However, cases of fenofibrate-associated myopathy, either as monotherapy or in combination, appear to be exceedingly rare (73). There are also reports documenting cases of myopathy when patients were switched from a combination of a statin with fibrate to a statin with gemfibrozil or bezafibrate (74,75). Evaluations of the pharmacoepidemiological reports of rhabdomyolysis have also demonstrated a notable difference in the reporting rates for gemfibrozil as compared to fenofibrate. FDA AER database evaluations have demonstrated a substantially lower rate of rhabdomyolysis for fenofibrate compared to gemfibrozil, even when greater use of gemfibrozil in clinical practice was taken into consideration (76,77). Until recently, the mechanism by which fibrates may increase the risk of myopathy has not been fully understood. The interaction between statins and fibrates was considered a class effect for fibrates until recent pharmacokinetic and mechanistic studies demonstrated the pharmacological differences between gemfibrozil and fenofibrate. When used in combination with any statin medication, fenofibrate resulted in fewer reports of rhabdomyolysis than did gemfibrozil. Only 2.3% (14 of 606) of the total number of reports of rhabdomyolysis for fenofibrate and statin therapies were associated with fenofibrate/cerivastatin combination therapy, compared to 88% (533 of 606) that were associated with gemfibrozil/ cerivastatin therapy. Likewise, the number of reports of rhabdomyolysis per million prescriptions dispensed was approximately 33 times lower for fenofibrate than for gemfibrozil when used in combination with cerivastatin (76).

Additionally, the number of reports of rhabdomyolysis per million prescriptions dispensed was approximately 15 times lower for fenofibrate than for gemfibrozil with 0.58 reports per million prescriptions dispensed for fenofibrate versus 8.6 reports for gemfibrozil (76).

Both fenofibrate and gemfibrozil are similar with regard to metabolism via glucuronidation and renal excretion; however, they differ significantly in that they utilize different families of the hepatic glucuronidation enzymes [uridine diphosphate-glucuromosyl-transferases (UGT) 1A1, 1A3, 1A9 and 2B7 for fenofibrate; all the isoforms but UGT 1A10 for gemfibrozil] (78). These differences have significant clinical implications in that most statins are glucuronidated by the same family of enzymes as gemfibrozil, thereby competing for conversion of statins from the open form to the lactone form that undergoes hepatic metabolism catalyzed by CYP450 (Fig. 1). In addition, while fenofibrate is only a mild inhibitor of CYP2C9, gemfibrozil is a potent inhibitor of both CYP2C9 and CYP2C8, thus leading to potential interaction with fluvastatin and rosuvastatin. Finally, fibrates, like many other drugs, are recognized by protein transporters involved in drug disposition present in different tissues (79). The organic anion transporting polypeptides in the liver mediate the uptake of many organic anions, including the statins (Table 7) (79). Interaction between gemfibrozil and statins may result from interaction with transporters at the level of the liver, due to either the reduced uptake into hepatocytes by transporters or by reduced biliary secretion (79). In summary, many pharmacokinetic mechanisms are responsible for the interaction between gemfibrozil and the statins.

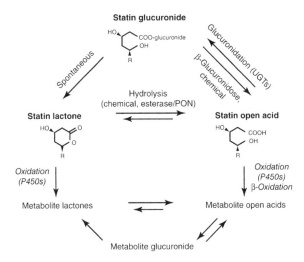

FIGURE 1 Metabolic pathways of statins.

Based on these considerations, in patients that may benefit from a combination of a statin and a fibrate, fenofibrate should be the preferred option to provide the patient with the maximal benefit to risk ratio.

EZETIMIBE

Ezetimibe is the first of a new class of drugs that specifically reduces the intestinal absorption of cholesterol (80,81).

Pharmacokinetics

Following oral administration, the drug is rapidly adsorbed and extensively metabolized (>80%) in the intestinal cell to the pharmacologically active glucuronide derivative before secretion into the blood (82). Ezetimibe is avidly taken up by the liver from the portal blood and excreted into the bile, resulting in low peripheral blood concentrations. The glucuronide conjugate is hydrolyzed and absorbed and is equally effective in inhibiting sterol absorption. Total ezetimibe (sum of "parent" ezetimibe plus ezetimibe-glucuronide) concentrations reach a maximum one to two hours postadministration, followed by the enterohepatic recycling and slow elimination. This enterohepatic recycling is responsible for a half-life in the body of approximately 22 hours (82). Because of the rapid glucuronidation, approximately 90% of total ezetimibe concentrations measured at 30 minutes and nearly 100% of those measured at 24 hours represent the glucuronide compound. Ezetimibe and its conjugate are >90% bound to plasma proteins. Eighty percent of an ezetimibe dose is eliminated fecally, predominantly as ezetimibe, with 10% eliminated renally, mainly as ezetimibe-glucuronide. Patients with compromised renal function (creatinine clearance 10–30 mL/min/1.73 m^2) exhibit greater AUCs (about 50% increase) of total ezetimibe without any alteration in C_{max} compared with patients having normal kidney function (82).

No significant difference in pharmacokinetics has been observed between sexes, races, ages, or with food intake. No dosage adjustment is necessary in patients with mild impairment or mild-to-severe renal insufficiency. Because of the prominent role of the liver in excretion, the drug is contraindicated in severe liver disease (82).

Adverse Effects

Current data suggest that ezetimibe is well tolerated by patients (82). No serious complications directly attributable to ezetimibe use have been reported. Chest pain, arthralgia, diarrhea, dizziness, and headache occur slightly more frequently with ezetimibe than with placebo. Hives, rash, flatulence, loose stools, abdominal discomfort, fatigue, and myalgia occur at an incidence similar to that in patients receiving placebo (Table 10). Liver or skeletal muscle

TABLE 10 Adverse Effects of Ezetimibe

Location	Effect
Thorax	Chest pain
Gastrointestinal tract	Abdominal discomfort, flatulence, diarrhea, loose stools
Muscles	Myalgia, fatigue, arthralgia
Nervous system	Dizziness, headache
Respiratory apparatus	Sinusitis, pharyngitis, and upper respiratory tract infection
Skin	Hives, rash

dysfunction has not been associated with ezetimibe when used alone or in combination with other agents. Laboratory analyses during the phase II and III trials involving over 2000 patients found that less than 1% of patients experienced a rise in alanine aminotransferase or aspartate aminotransferase greater than or equal to three times the upper reference limit, with no difference in incidence between placebo and ezetimibe groups. Similarly, less than 1% of patients had an increase in their CK activity greater than or equal to 10 times the upper limit of normal and this was not different from the placebo control group.

Sinusitis, pharyngitis, and upper respiratory tract infection occur more commonly in patients receiving ezetimibe than placebo. Viral infections also occurred more frequently among patients receiving ezetimibe compared with placebo. It remains to be determined whether a true relationship exists between acquiring infections and using ezetimibe.

Combination Therapy

Overall, ezetimibe has a favorable drug–drug interaction profile, as evidenced by the lack of clinically relevant interactions between ezetimibe and a variety of drugs commonly used in patients with hypercholesterolemia (83,84). Ezetimibe does not have significant effects on plasma levels of statins, fibrates, digoxin, glipizide, warfarin, and triphasic oral contraceptives. Concomitant administration of food, antacids, cimetidine, or statins had no significant effect of ezetimibe bioavailability. Although coadministration with gemfibrozil and fenofibrate increased the bioavailability of ezetimibe, the clinical significance of this interaction still remains to be fully elucidated. Nonetheless, the coadministration with fibrate is not recommended at this time owing to the lack of clinical trial data demonstrating the long-term efficacy and safety of this treatment. In contrast, coadministration with the resin cholestyramine significantly decreased ezetimibe oral bioavailability. Hence, ezetimibe and cholestyramine should be administered several hours apart to avoid attenuating the efficacy of ezetimibe. Finally, higher ezetimibe exposures were observed in patients receiving concomitant cyclosporine, and ezetimibe caused a small, but statistically significant, effect on plasma levels of cyclosporine. Because treatment experience in patients receiving cyclosporine is limited, physicians are advised to exercise caution when initiating ezetimibe in the setting of cyclosporine coadministration, and to carefully monitor cyclosporine levels (83).

BILE ACID SEQUESTRANTS

The bile acid sequestrants (resins) are highly positively charged and bind negatively charged bile acids. Colestipol and cholestyramine are useful in hyperlipoproteinemias involving isolated increases in LDL. In patients who have hypertriglyceridemia as well as elevated LDL levels, very low-density lipoprotein levels may be further increased during treatment with the resins (1,3).

Pharmacokinetics

Because of their large size, resins are not absorbed, and the bound bile acids are excreted in the stool. Because over 95% of bile acids are normally reabsorbed, interruption of this process depletes the liver's pool of bile acids, and hepatic bile acid synthesis increases. As a result, hepatic cholesterol content declines, stimulating the production of LDL receptors, an effect similar to that of statins (1,3). Hence, the resins are without effect in patients with homozygous FH who have no functioning receptors, but they may be useful in patients with receptor-defective combined heterozygous states (1).

TABLE 11 Adverse Effects of Bile Acid Sequestrants (Resins)

Location	Effect
Drug interactions	Binding of warfarin, digoxin, digitalis glycosides, tetracycline, iron salts, ascorbic acid, thyroxine, thiazide diuretics, folic acid, and statins
Electrolytes	Hyperchloremic acidosis in children and patients with renal failure
Gastrointestinal tract	Abdominal fullness, nausea, gas, constipation, hemorroids, anal fissure, activation of diverticulitis, diminished absorption of vitamin D in children
Liver	Mild serum aminotransferases elevation, exacerbated by cotreatment with statins
Metabolic system	Increased serum triglycerides (10%)

Adverse Effects

The resins are quite safe, as they are not systemically absorbed. Because they are administered as a chloride salt, rare instances of hyperchloremic acidosis have been reported in children or patients with renal failure because of chlorine ions released in exchange for bile acid (1,3). Severe hypertriglyceridemia is a contraindication to the use of cholestyramine and colestipol because these resins increase TG levels.

The main objections of patients taking resins are bloating and dyspepsia (Table 11) (1,3). However, these symptoms can be substantially reduced if the drug is completely suspended in liquid several hours before ingestion. Otherwise, the dosage can be adjusted to minimize these symptoms. Constipation can be prevented by adequate daily water or fiber (psyllium) intake if necessary. Resins may bind and interfere with the absorption of vitamin D, and other fat-soluble vitamins, but this effect is negligible, except possibly in children. Malabsorption of vitamin K may occur rarely, leading to hypoprothrombinemia. Prothrombin time should be measured frequently in patients who are taking resins and anticoagulants. Resins can also bind polar compounds, including warfarin, digoxin, digitalis glycosides, tetracycline, iron salts, ascorbic acid, thyroxine, thiazide diuretics, folic acid, and statins. To avoid such an effect, these substances should be given two hours before or four hours after the resins (1,3).

NICOTINIC ACID (NIACIN)

Nicotinic acid (niacin) is one of the oldest drugs used to treat dyslipidemia and is the most versatile in that it favorably affects virtually all lipid parameters (1,3).

Pharmacokinetics

The pharmacological doses of regular (crystalline) niacin used to treat dyslipidemia are almost completely absorbed, and peak plasma concentrations are achieved within 30 to 60 minutes. The half-life is about 60 minutes, which accounts for the necessity of twice- or thrice-daily dosing. At lower doses, most niacin is taken up by the liver; only the major metabolite, nicotinuric acid, is found in the urine. At higher doses, a greater proportion of the drug is excreted in the urine as unchanged nicotinic acid (1).

Adverse Effects

Two of niacin's side effects, flushing and dyspepsia, limit patients compliance (1,3). The cutaneous effects include flushing (warmth, redness, itching, and/or tingling of the skin) and pruritus of the face and upper trunk, skin rashes, and acanthosis nigricans. Flushing and associated pruritus occur in up to 70% to 80% of patients. This effect is attributable to the metabolism of nicotinic acid via the conjugation pathway, resulting in nicotinuric acid, which is associated with prostaglandin-mediated vasodilation. Taking an aspirin each day alleviates the flushing in many patients. Flushing is worse when therapy is initiated or the dosage is increased, it recurs if only one or two doses are missed, and it is more likely to occur when niacin is consumed with hot beverages or with ethanol-containing beverages or spicy food. Flushing is minimized if therapy is initiated with low doses (100–250 mg twice daily) and if the drug is taken after breakfast or at bedtime. As the immediate-release formulation of nicotinic acid is predominantly metabolized via the conjugation pathway, this treatment is associated with a high rate of flushing. The most common, medically serious side effects are hepatotoxicity, manifested as elevated serum transaminases and hyperglycemia (1,3).

The availability of a once-daily prolonged-release formulation of nicotinic acid (Niaspan), in which nicotinic acid is absorbed over an 8- to 12-hour period leading to more balanced metabolism, offers safety and tolerability advantages over earlier nicotinic acid formulations. While flushing is still the major side effect of treatment, data from head-to-head comparison of prolonged-release and immediate-release nicotinic acid showed that there were significantly fewer flushing episodes per patient with the prolonged-release preparation compared with the immediate-release preparation. Considerable elevation of liver function enzymes is also avoided with prolonged-release nicotinic acid (1,3).

Dry skin, a frequent complain, can be dealt with by using skin moisturizers, and acanthosis nigricans can be dealt with by using lotions or creams containing salicylic acid. Patients with a history of peptic ulcer disease should not take niacin because it reactivated ulcer disease. In patients with diabetes mellitus, niacin-induced insulin resistance can exacerbate hyperglycemia, and the dosages of antiglycemic medications may have to be adjusted in these patients. Niacin also may elevate uric acid levels and precipitate gout. As a precaution, uric acid levels should be monitored at regular intervals in patients treated with prolonged-release nicotinic acid, particularly in those with gout (1,3).

An overview of data from clinical trials, as well as postmarketing experience, indicate a very low incidence of elevated liver function enzymes with prolonged-release nicotinic acid, either alone or in combination with a statin (<1%), and no increase in the incidence of myopathy (when used in combination with a statin) compared with statin therapy alone. Nevertheless, clinicians are advised to monitor for evidence of skeletal muscle myopathy, as well as for changes in liver function, measuring liver transaminases and alkaline phosphatase at initiation, after six weeks of therapy and every four to six months thereafter (1,3).

CONCLUSIONS

The issue of safety and drug tolerance is particularly important in primary and secondary prevention of cardiovascular disease, where the risk of long-term therapy must be considered in the context of achievable benefits. Currently, several classes of hypolipidemic drugs are available, including statins, fibrates, nicotinic acid, resins, and ezetimibe. In general, lipid-lowering monotherapy is well tolerated and has a low frequency of adverse events. However, several large surveys have shown that many patients with LLT do not reach the current treatment goals for the lipid profile. Therefore, a potential combination therapy between statins and other classes of lipid-lowering agents (e.g., ezetimibe, fibrates and nicotinic acid) is strongly recommended by the current guidelines. Moreover, because lipid-lowering drugs are prescribed on a long-term basis, possible interactions with other drugs deserve attention, as many patients will typically receive drugs for concomitant conditions during the course of therapy. A knowledge of the metabolic pathways responsible for the metabolism of lipid-lowering agents allows the prediction and prevention of possible drug interaction among these agents and other drugs, thus improving the benefit of LLT in terms of both efficacy and safety.

REFERENCES

1. Mahley RW, Bersot TP. Drug therapy for hypercholesterolemia and dyslipidemia. In: Brunton LL, ed. Goodman and Gilman's the Pharmacological Basis of Therapeutics. New York: McGraw Hill, 2005:933–966.
2. Third Report of the National Cholesterol Education Program Expert Panel on detection, evaluation, and treatment of high blood cholesterol in adults (Adult Treatment Panel III) final report. Circulation 2002; 106(25):3143–3421.
3. Knopp RH. Drug treatment of lipid disorders. N Engl J Med 1999; 341(7):498–511.
4. Bellosta S, Paoletti R, Corsini A. Safety of statins: focus on clinical pharmacokinetics and drug interactions. Circulation 2004; 109(23 suppl 1):III50–III57.
5. Grundy SM, Cleeman JI, Merz CN, et al. Implications of recent clinical trials for the National Cholesterol Education Program Adult Treatment Panel III guidelines. Circulation 2004; 110(2):227–239.
6. Grundy SM, Vega GL, Yuan Z, et al. Effectiveness and tolerability of simvastatin plus fenofibrate for combined hyperlipidemia (the SAFARI trial). Am J Cardiol 2005; 95(4):462–468.
7. MRC/BHF Heart Protection Study of cholesterol lowering with simvastatin in 20,536 high-risk individuals: a randomised placebo-controlled trial. Lancet 2002; 360(9326):7–22.

8. Corsini A, Bellosta S, Baetta R, et al. New insights into the pharmacodynamic and pharmacokinetic properties of statins. Pharmacol Ther 1999; 84(3):413–428.
9. White CM. A review of the pharmacologic and pharmacokinetic aspects of rosuvastatin. J Clin Pharmacol 2002; 42(9):963–970.
10. Thompson PD, Clarkson P, Karas RH. Statin-associated myopathy. JAMA 2003; 289(13):1681–1690.
11. Omar MA, Wilson JP. FDA adverse event reports on statin-associated rhabdomyolysis. Ann Pharmacother 2002; 36(2):288–295.
12. Staffa JA, Chang J, Green L. Cerivastatin and reports of fatal rhabdomyolysis. N Engl J Med 2002; 346(7):539–540.
13. Farmer JA, Torre-Amione G. Comparative tolerability of the HMG-CoA reductase inhibitors. Drug Saf 2000; 23(3):197–213.
14. Pasternak RC, Smith SC Jr., Bairey-Merz CN, et al. ACC/AHA/NHLBI clinical advisory on the use and safety of statins. J Am Coll Cardiol 2002; 40(3):567–572.
15. Rosenson RS. Current overview of statin-induced myopathy. Am J Med 2004; 116(6):408–416.
16. Corsini A. The safety of HMG-CoA reductase inhibitors in special populations at high cardiovascular risk. Cardiovasc Drugs Ther 2003; 17(3):265–285.
17. Ballantyne CM, Corsini A, Davidson MH, et al. Risk for myopathy with statin therapy in high-risk patients. Arch Intern Med 2003; 163(5):553–564.
18. Tobert JA. Efficacy and long-term adverse effect pattern of lovastatin. Am J Cardiol 1988; 62(15): 28J–34J.
19. Hamilton-Craig I. Statin-associated myopathy. Med J Aust 2001; 175(9):486–489.
20. Baigent C, Keech A, Kearney PM, et al. Efficacy and safety of cholesterol-lowering treatment: prospective meta-analysis of data from 90,056 participants in 14 randomised trials of statins. Lancet 2005; 366(9493):1267–1278.
21. Mukhtar RY, Reckless JP. Statin-induced myositis: a commonly encountered or rare side effect? Curr Opin Lipidol 2005; 16(6):640–647.
22. Graham DJ, Staffa JA, Shatin D, et al. Incidence of hospitalized rhabdomyolysis in patients treated with lipid-lowering drugs. JAMA 2004; 292(21):2585–2590.
23. Ucar M, Mjorndal T, Dahlqvist R. HMG-CoA reductase inhibitors and myotoxicity. Drug Saf 2000; 22(6):441–457.
24. Franc S, Dejager S, Bruckert E, et al. A comprehensive description of muscle symptoms associated with lipid-lowering drugs. Cardiovasc Drugs Ther 2003; 17(5–6):459–465.
25. Elmberger PG, Kalen A, Lund E, et al. Effects of pravastatin and cholestyramine on products of the mevalonate pathway in familial hypercholesterolemia. J Lipid Res 1991; 32(6):935–940.
26. Chojnacki T, Dallner G. The uptake of dietary polyprenols and their modification to active dolichols by the rat liver. J Biol Chem 1983; 258(2):916–922.
27. Silver MA, Langsjoen PH, Szabo S, et al. Effect of atorvastatin on left ventricular diastolic function and ability of coenzyme Q10 to reverse that dysfunction. Am J Cardiol 2004; 94(10):1306–1310.
28. Lamperti C, Naini AB, Lucchini V, et al. Muscle coenzyme Q10 level in statin-related myopathy. Arch Neurol 2005; 62(11):1709–1712.
29. FDA. FDA document 2004 P-0113/CP1. Federal Drug Administration, 2004.
30. Vidt DG, Cressman MD, Harris S, et al. Rosuvastatin-induced arrest in progression of renal disease. Cardiology 2004; 102(1):52–60.
31. Shepherd J, Hunninghake DB, Stein EA, et al. Safety of rosuvastatin. Am J Cardiol 2004; 94(7):882–888.
32. Backes JM, Howard PA. Association of HMG-CoA reductase inhibitors with neuropathy. Ann Pharmacother 2003; 37(2):274–278.
33. Executive Summary of The Third Report of The National Cholesterol Education Program Expert Panel on detection, evaluation, and treatment of high blood cholesterol in adults (Adult Treatment Panel III). JAMA 2001; 285(19):2486–2497.
34. Gaist D, Garcia Rodriguez LA, Huerta C, et al. Are users of lipid-lowering drugs at increased risk of peripheral neuropathy? Eur J Clin Pharmacol 2001; 56(12):931–933.
35. Chong PH, Boskovich A, Stevkovic N, et al. Statin-associated peripheral neuropathy: review of the literature. Pharmacotherapy 2004; 24(9):1194–1203.
36. Cannon CP, Braunwald E, McCabe CH, et al. Intensive versus moderate lipid lowering with statins after acute coronary syndromes. N Engl J Med 2004; 350(15):1495–1504.
37. Pedersen TR, Faergeman O, Kastelein JJ, et al. High-dose atorvastatin vs. usual-dose simvastatin for secondary prevention after myocardial infarction: the IDEAL study: a randomized controlled trial. JAMA 2005; 294(19):2437–2445.
38. de Lemos JA, Blazing MA, Wiviott SD, et al. Early intensive vs. a delayed conservative simvastatin strategy in patients with acute coronary syndromes: phase Z of the A to Z trial. JAMA 2004; 292(11):1307–1316.
39. LaRosa JC, Grundy SM, Waters DD, et al. Intensive lipid lowering with atorvastatin in patients with stable coronary disease. N Engl J Med 2005; 352(14):1425–1435.
40. Gotto AM Jr. Safety and statin therapy: reconsidering the risks and benefits. Arch Intern Med 2003; 163(6):657–659.
41. Martin J, Krum H. Cytochrome P450 drug interactions within the HMG-CoA reductase inhibitor class: are they clinically relevant? Drug Saf 2003; 26(1):13–21.

42. Phillips PS, Haas RH, Bannykh S, et al. Statin-associated myopathy with normal creatine kinase levels. Ann Intern Med 2002; 137(7):581–585.
43. Bottorff M. "Fire and forget?"—pharmacological considerations in coronary care. Atherosclerosis 1999; 147(suppl 1):S23–S30.
44. Gruer PJ, Vega JM, Mercuri MF, et al. Concomitant use of cytochrome P450 3A4 inhibitors and simvastatin. Am J Cardiol 1999; 84(7):811–815.
45. Holdaas H, Fellstrom B, Jardine AG, et al. Effect of fluvastatin on cardiac outcomes in renal transplant recipients: a multicentre, randomised, placebo-controlled trial. Lancet 2003; 361(9374):2024–2031.
46. Kantola T, Backman JT, Niemi M, et al. Effect of fluconazole on plasma fluvastatin and pravastatin concentrations. Eur J Clin Pharmacol 2000; 56(3):225–229.
47. Transon C, Leemann T, Vogt N, et al. In vivo inhibition profile of cytochrome P450TB (CYP2C9) by (+/−)-fluvastatin. Clin Pharmacol Ther 1995; 58(4):412–417.
48. Lenhard JM, Croom DK, Weiel JE, et al. HIV protease inhibitors stimulate hepatic triglyceride synthesis. Arterioscler Thromb Vasc Biol 2000; 20(12):2625–2629.
49. Penzak SR, Chuck SK, Stajich GV. Safety and efficacy of HMG-CoA reductase inhibitors for treatment of hyperlipidemia in patients with HIV infection. Pharmacotherapy 2000; 20(9):1066–1071.
50. Cheng CH, Miller C, Lowe C, et al. Rhabdomyolysis due to probable interaction between simvastatin and ritonavir. Am J Health Syst Pharm 2002; 59(8):728–730.
51. Kantola T, Kivisto KT, Neuvonen PJ. Grapefruit juice greatly increases serum concentrations of lovastatin and lovastatin acid. Clin Pharmacol Ther 1998; 63(4):397–402.
52. Lilja JJ, Kivisto KT, Neuvonen PJ. Grapefruit juice-simvastatin interaction: effect on serum concentrations of simvastatin, simvastatin acid, and HMG-CoA reductase inhibitors. Clin Pharmacol Ther 1998; 64(5):477–483.
53. Lilja JJ, Kivisto KT, Neuvonen PJ. Duration of effect of grapefruit juice on the pharmacokinetics of the CYP3A4 substrate simvastatin. Clin Pharmacol Ther 2000; 68(4):384–390.
54. Guo LQ, Yamazoe Y. Inhibition of cytochrome P450 by furanocoumarins in grapefruit juice and herbal medicines. Acta Pharmacol Sin 2004; 25(2):129–136.
55. Honda Y, Ushigome F, Koyabu N, et al. Effects of grapefruit juice and orange juice components on P-glycoprotein- and MRP2-mediated drug efflux. Br J Pharmacol 2004; 143(7):856–864.
56. Rogers JD, Zhao J, Liu L, et al. Grapefruit juice has minimal effects on plasma concentrations of lovastatin-derived 3-hydroxy-3-methylglutaryl coenzyme A reductase inhibitors. Clin Pharmacol Ther 1999; 66(4):358–366.
57. Schmassmann-Suhijar D, Bullingham R, Gasser R, et al. Rhabdomyolysis due to interaction of simvastatin with mibefradil. Lancet 1998; 351(9120):1929–1930.
58. Azie NE, Brater DC, Becker PA, et al. The interaction of diltiazem with lovastatin and pravastatin. Clin Pharmacol Ther 1998; 64(4):369–377.
59. Mousa O, Brater DC, Sunblad KJ, et al. The interaction of diltiazem with simvastatin. Clin Pharmacol Ther 2000; 67(3):267–274.
60. Peces R, Pobes A. Rhabdomyolysis associated with concurrent use of simvastatin and diltiazem. Nephron 2001; 89(1):117–118.
61. Lewin JJ III, Nappi JM, Taylor MH. Rhabdomyolysis with concurrent atorvastatin and diltiazem. Ann Pharmacother 2002; 36(10):1546–1549.
62. Lin JC, Ito MK. A drug interaction between troglitazone and simvastatin. Diabetes Care 1999; 22(12):2104–2106.
63. Kyrklund C, Backman JT, Kivisto KT, et al. Rifampin greatly reduces plasma simvastatin and simvastatin acid concentrations. Clin Pharmacol Ther 2000; 68(6):592–597.
64. Murphy MJ, Dominiczak MH. Efficacy of statin therapy: possible effect of phenytoin. Postgrad Med J 1999; 75(884); 359–360.
65. Sugimoto K, Ohmori M, Tsuruoka S, et al. Different effects of St John's wort on the pharmacokinetics of simvastatin and pravastatin. Clin Pharmacol Ther 2001; 70(6):518–524.
66. Ho RH, Kim RB. Transporters and drug therapy: implications for drug disposition and disease. Clin Pharmacol Ther 2005; 78(3):260–277.
67. Ayrton A, Morgan P. Role of transport proteins in drug absorption, distribution, and excretion. Xenobiotica 2001; 31(8–9):469–497.
68. Wang E, Casciano CN, Clement RP, et al. HMG-CoA reductase inhibitors (statins) characterized as direct inhibitors of P-glycoprotein. Pharm Res 2001; 18(6):800–806.
69. Bizzaro N, Bagolin E, Milani L, et al. Massive rhabdomyolysis and simvastatin. Clin Chem 1992; 38(8 Pt 1):1504.
70. Boyd RA, Stern RH, Stewart BH, et al. Atorvastatin coadministration may increase digoxin concentrations by inhibition of intestinal P-glycoprotein-mediated secretion. J Clin Pharmacol 2000; 40(1):91–98.
71. Morimoto K, Oishi T, Ueda S, et al. A novel variant allele of OATP-C (SLCO1B1) found in a Japanese patient with pravastatin-induced myopathy. Drug Metab Pharmacokinet 2004; 19(6):453–455.
72. Kashyap ML, McGovern ME, Berra K, et al. Long-term safety and efficacy of a once-daily niacin/lovastatin formulation for patients with dyslipidemia. Am J Cardiol 2002; 89(6):672–678.
73. Corsini A, Bellosta S, Davidson MH. Pharmacokinetic interactions between statins and fibrates. Am J Cardiol 2005; 96(9A):44–49.

74. Oldemeyer JB, Lund RJ, Koch M, et al. Rhabdomyolysis and acute renal failure after changing statin-fibrate combinations. Cardiology 2000; 94(2):127–128.

75. Kamaliah MD, Sanjay LD. Rhabdomyolysis and acute renal failure following a switchover of therapy between two fibric acid derivatives. Singapore Med J 2001; 42(8):368–372.

76. Jones PH, Davidson MH. Reporting rate of rhabdomyolysis with fenofibrate + statin versus gemfibrozil + any statin. Am J Cardiol 2005; 95(1):120–122.

77. Alsheikh-Ali AA, Kuvin JT, Karas RH. Risk of adverse events with fibrates. Am J Cardiol 2004; 94(7):935–938.

78. Prueksaritanont T, Tang C, Qiu Y, et al. Effects of fibrates on metabolism of statins in human hepatocytes. Drug Metab Dispos 2002; 30(11):1280–1287.

79. Shitara Y, Sato H, Sugiyama Y. Evaluation of drug-drug interaction in the hepatobiliary and renal transport of drugs. Annu Rev Pharmacol Toxicol 2005; 45:689–723.

80. Mauro VF, Tuckerman CE. Ezetimibe for management of hypercholesterolemia. Ann Pharmacother 2003; 37(6):839–848.

81. Flores NA. Ezetimibe + simvastatin (Merck/Schering-Plough). Curr Opin Investig Drugs 2004; 5(9): 984–992.

82. Kosoglou T, Statkevich P, Johnson-Levonas AO, et al. Ezetimibe: a review of its metabolism, pharmacokinetics and drug interactions. Clin Pharmacokinet 2005; 44(5):467–494.

83. Davidson MH, Toth PP. Combination therapy in the management of complex dyslipidemias. Curr Opin Lipidol 2004; 15(4):423–431.

84. Bays H, Stein EA. Pharmacotherapy for dyslipidaemia-current therapies and future agents. Expert Opin Pharmacother 2003; 4(11):1901–1938.

11 | The Metabolic Syndrome: Identification and Management of the Patient at High Risk for Cardiovascular Disease

Charles Reasner
University of Texas Health Science Center and Texas Diabetes Institute, Zarzamora, San Antonio, Texas, U.S.A.

KEY POINTS

- The metabolic syndrome is a clustering of cardiovascular risk factors associated with central obesity and insulin resistance.
- The IDF definition requires the presence of central obesity and provides ethnic specific cut points for diagnosis.
- The prevalence of diabetes is the highest in developed countries and will increase as populations become more obese.
- In children, central obesity is associated with a threefold increase in insulin levels, a doubling of fasting TG levels, a decrease in the HDL-C of 20 mg/dL, and an increase in the systolic blood pressure of 15 to 20 mmHg.
- Fasting hyperglycemia is due to the failure of insulin to suppress glucose production by the liver.
- Postprandial hyperglycemia is caused by decreased uptake of glucose by muscle and a failure of insulin to suppress hepatic glucose production.
- Abdominal obesity leads to insulin resistance through a variety of mechanisms including: overproduction of FFA, overproduction of cytokines causing insulin resistance, and decreased production of adiponectin.
- Visceral fat cells are larger and more metabolically active than subcutaneous fat cells.

DEFINITION

The association of insulin resistance with a clustering of cardiovascular risk factors including central obesity, hypertension, dyslipidemia, and abnormal glucose tolerance was referred to as the "insulin resistance syndrome" by Reaven in 1988 (1). Over the last several years, the term "metabolic syndrome" has come to be preferred to "the insulin resistance syndrome" to describe individuals with these metabolic abnormalities, which put them at increased risk of developing both cardiovascular complications and diabetes. Several expert groups have developed criteria to define the metabolic syndrome. The most widely cited definitions are from the World Health Organization (2) and the National Cholesterol Education Program (NCEP) Adult Treatment Panel (ATP) III (3). The core components for each group include: obesity, impaired glucose regulation, dyslipidemia, and hypertension (Tables 1 and 2). The definition used in this chapter is the International Diabetes Federation (IDF) criteria adopted in 2005 (Table 3) (4).

In September 2005, the American Diabetes Association (ADA) and the European Association for the Study of Diabetes (EASD) issued a joint statement calling for a critical reappraisal of the metabolic syndrome (5). They questioned the pathogenic link between the individual risk factors, the validity of the cut points for each risk factor, and the evidence that treating the "syndrome" was more effective than treating the components. The IDF definition of the metabolic syndrome (Table 3) addresses some of these issues. First, in the IDF definition of the metabolic syndrome, central obesity is recognized as an important causative factor and is a prerequisite component for the diagnosis. The causal link between central obesity and the components of the metabolic syndrome will be discussed in the pathogenesis section of this chapter. Central obesity can be easily assessed using waist circumference. Second, the IDF has made a "first attempt" to provide ethnic group specific cut points for some risk factors such as waist circumference. Table 4 lists the Ethnic Specific values

TABLE 1 World Health Organization Clinical Criteria for the Metabolic Syndrome

Hypertension
Triglyceride
Central obesity
Microalbuminuria

Note: In order to make a diagnosis of the metabolic syndrome a patient must present with (*i*) glucose intolerance, impaired glucose tolerance of diabetes and/or (*ii*) insulin resistance, together with two or more of the components mentioned in the Table.
Source: From Ref. 2.

for waist circumference. However, several of the objections made in the joint ADA and EASD statements are valid.

My view, and that of the American Heart Association and the National Heart, Lung and Blood Institute, is that the metabolic syndrome identifies patients at risk for cardiovascular disease and encourages early lifestyle changes (6). Because each risk factor confers a continuous risk for cardiovascular disease, assigning any single cut point may falsely imply that above a certain number you are at high risk, while just below it the risk is low. At the present time these cut points are pragmatic estimates taken from various data sources. As more robust data sets become available, ethnic specific cut points will be warranted. Additionally, in future definitions risk factors themselves may be modified. For example, physical inactivity and markers of inflammation are associated with obesity, insulin resistance, and heart disease and are not presently part of the syndrome. Certainly, additional research to better understand the link between obesity, insulin resistance, and risk factors for heart disease is needed. For now, our recognition of the metabolic syndrome provides earlier identification of patients at risk for heart disease and encourages appropriate lifestyle and pharmacologic interventions of modifiable risk factors for heart disease.

PREVALENCE

Regardless of the definition used, large numbers of U.S. adults have the metabolic syndrome. The National Health and Nutrition Examination Survey (NHANES) 1999 to 2002, is the most scientifically rigorous sample of the U.S. population (7). A total of 3601 men and women aged more than 20 years were included in the survey. Using the NCEP definition the prevalence of metabolic syndrome was 33.7% of men and 35.4% of women. In comparison, the prevalence using the IDF definition was 39.9% of men and 38.1% of women. The largest difference in prevalence was found in Mexican-American men among whom the age-adjusted prevalence was 40.3% using the NCEP definition and 50.6% using the IDF definition. The percent agreement between the two definitions was 89.8% among men and 96% among women.

In a sample of 4060 predominantly European adults from South Australia, the metabolic syndrome was present in 19.4% of men and 14.4% of women using the ATP III definition (8). Using the IDF definition, the metabolic syndrome was identified in 26.4% of men and 15.7% of

TABLE 2 Adult Treatment Panel III Clinical Identification of the Metabolic Syndrome Three or More of the Following Risk Factors

Risk factor	Defining level
Central obesity	Waist circumference
Men	>102 cm (>40 in.)
Women	>88 cm (>35 in.)
Triglycerides	>150 mg/dL (1.7 mmol/L)
High-density lipoprotein cholesterol	
Men	<40 mg/dL (1.03 mmol/L)
Women	<50 mg/dL (1.29 mmol/L)
Blood pressure	>130/>85 mmHg
Fasting glucose	>110 mg/dL (6.1 mmol/L)

Source: From Ref. 3.

TABLE 3 The 2005 International Diabetes Federation Definition of Metabolic Syndrome

Raised TG level: >150 mg/dL (1.7 mmol/L), or specific treatment for this lipid abnormality
Reduced high-density lipoprotein cholesterol: <40 mg/dL (1.03 mmol/L) in males and <50 mg/dL (1.29 mmol/L) in females, or specific treatment for this lipid abnormality
Raised blood pressure: systolic BP >130 or diastolic BP >85 mmHg, or treatment of previously diagnosed hypertension
Raised fasting plasma glucose: >100 mg/dL (5.6 mmol/L), or previously diagnosed type 2 diabetes

Note: For a person to be defined as having the metabolic syndrome they must have the following:
Central obesity (defined as waist circumference >94cm for Europid men and >80cm for Europid women, with ethnicity specific values for other groups) (Table 4) and any two of four factors mentioned in the Table.
Source: From Ref. 4.

women. In this population, the IDF using a smaller waist circumference categorized 15% to 20% more individuals as having the metabolic syndrome. While the prevalence of the metabolic syndrome in these surveys is staggering, the data are now over eight years old and the prevalence has almost certainly increased. Because the IDF definition of metabolic syndrome requires the presence of central obesity, as the populations of the world become more obese, we will see the prevalence of the metabolic syndrome increase. Figure 1 shows the prevalence of obesity in countries throughout the world. While 20% to 30% of men and women in the Americas and many European countries are obese, being overweight is still unusual in Asia, India, and Africa. It is likely that the greatest explosion in the metabolic syndrome will be seen in developing countries as their populations become obese.

In the United States, among the segments of the population that are growing fatter, the fastest is children and teenagers. Data derived from the NHANES III between 1988 to 1994 and 1999 to 2000 showed that the prevalence of overweight (more than or equal to 95% of BMI for age) among adolescents aged 12 to 19 years of age increased from 11% to 16% (Fig. 2). Among adolescent boys, prevalence increased from 12% to 13% in non-Hispanic whites, 11% to 21% in non-Hispanic African Americans, and from 14% to 28% in Mexican Americans. Among adolescent girls, overweight prevalence increased from 9% to 12% in non-Hispanic whites, 16% to 27% in non-Hispanic African Americans, and 15% to 19% in Mexican-Americans (Fig. 2) (10).

The role of obesity in childhood and the development of the metabolic syndrome were highlighted by a study done by Weiss and colleagues (Fig. 3) (11). The effect of varying degrees of obesity on the prevalence of metabolic syndrome and its relation to insulin resistance in a large, multiethnic, multiracial cohort of children and adolescents was examined. A standard glucose tolerance test was administered to 439 obese, 31 overweight, and 20 nonobese children and adolescents. Baseline measurements included blood pressure and plasma lipids, C-reactive protein (CRP), and adiponectin levels. Levels of triglyceride (TG), high-density lipoprotein cholesterol (HDL-C), and blood pressure were adjusted for age and sex. Because the body mass index (BMI) varies according to age, the value for age and sex was standardized with the use of conversion to a Z-score (Fig. 3). The prevalence of the metabolic syndrome increased with the severity of obesity and reached 50% in severely obese youngsters. The prevalence of metabolic syndrome increased significantly with

TABLE 4 Ethnic Specific Values for Waist Circumference

Country/ethnic group	Waist circumference
Europids	
Men	>94 cm
Women	>80 cm
South Asians, Chinese	
Men	>90 cm
Women	>80 cm
Japanese	
Men	>85 cm
Women	>90 cm

Note: In the United States, the Adult Treatment Panel III values (102 cm male, 88 cm female) are still being used. European cut points are recommended for Sub-Saharan Africans and Eastern Mediterranean and Middle East (Arab) populations. South Asian values are recommended for South and Central Americans.
Source: From Ref. 4.

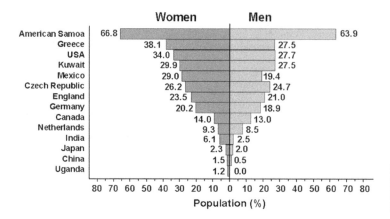

FIGURE 1 Prevalence of obesity defined as a body mass index $\geq 30 \, kg/m^2$ by country. *Source*: From Ref. 9.

increasing insulin resistance and the degree of obesity. Compared to their normal-weight siblings, obese children saw a doubling of their fasting TG levels, an increase in systolic blood pressure of 20 mmHg, and a decrease of 20 mg/dL in their level of HDL-C. The fasting glucose was essentially unchanged because of a compensatory three- to fourfold rise in fasting plasma insulin levels (Fig. 3). This study represents one of the clearest examples of the metabolic consequences of obesity, because the 12- and 13-year-old children in this study had no medical problems other than obesity. It also should provide a clear signal that as the population develops greater degrees of obesity at younger ages, the prevalence of the metabolic syndrome will only increase.

PATHOGENESIS
Normal Insulin Action

In order to better understand the insulin-resistant state we should first review insulin action under normal conditions. In the fasting state, approximately 85% of glucose production is derived from the liver, with the remainder produced by the kidney (12–14). The liver of healthy subjects produces glucose at the rate of approximately 2.0 mg/kg/min (12,15–17). Over half of this glucose production is essential to meet the needs of the brain and other neural tissues, which utilize glucose at a constant rate of 1 to 1.2 mg/kg/min (18). Because neural glucose metabolism does not require insulin, brain glucose uptake occurs at the same rate in the fasting and fed state and is not altered by insulin resistance. Most of the remaining glucose is metabolized by muscle, which requires insulin (15,19). In the fed state, carbohydrate ingestion leads to an increase in plasma glucose concentration and stimulates insulin release from the pancreatic beta cells. The resultant elevation in plasma insulin (*i*)

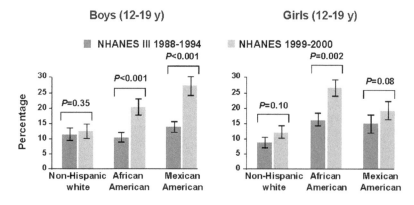

FIGURE 2 Prevalence and trends in overweight among U.S. children and adolescents. Overweight is defined as body mass index $\geq 95\%$ for age. *Abbreviation*: NHANES, National Health and Nutrition Examination Survey. *Source*: From Ref. 10.

Parameter*	Nonobese (n=20)	Overweight (n=31)	Moderately Obese (n=244)	Severely Obese (n=195)
Weight, kg	42	57	86	100
BMI	18	24	33	41
TG,[†] mg/dL	48	83	105	97
HDL-C,[†] mg/dL	59	47	41	40
SBP,[†] mm Hg	106	116	121	124
Glucose,[‡]	87	87	91	90
Insulin,[†] µU/mL	10	15	31	39
Metabolic syndrome prevalence, %	0	0	39	50

Mean age of study participants ~12 years.

* Mean baseline values; [†]$p<0.001$; [‡]$p=0.04$ for trend across all weight groups adjusted for sex, pubertal stage, and race and ethnic groups.

FIGURE 3 Relationship between changes in weight in children and components of the metabolic syndrome. *Abbreviations*: BMI, body mass index; TG, triglyceride; HDL-C, high-density lipoprotein cholesterol. *Source*: From Ref. 11.

suppresses hepatic glucose production and (*ii*) stimulates glucose uptake by peripheral tissues (12,15,19–24). The majority (~80–85%) of glucose that is taken up by peripheral tissues is disposed of in muscle (12,15,19,21–25), with only a small amount (~4–5%) being metabolized by adipocytes (25).

Although fat tissue is responsible for only a small amount of total body glucose disposal, it plays a very important role in the maintenance of total body glucose homeostasis through the release of free fatty acids (FFA). Small increments in the plasma insulin exert a potent antilipolytic effect, leading to a marked reduction in the plasma-free fatty acid level (26). The decline in plasma-free fatty acids concentration results in increased glucose uptake in muscle (27) and reduces hepatic glucose production (28–30).

Insulin Action in Resistant Individuals
Liver
Insulin resistance results in the failure of insulin to suppress hepatic glucose production, following carbohydrate ingestion. Postprandial hyperglycemia then, is the sum of two inputs of glucose following a meal, one from the liver and another from the diet. The glucose released by the liver can be derived from either glycogenolysis or gluconeogenesis (31). Radioisotope turnover studies, using lactate, alanine, and glycerol, have shown that ~90% of the increase in hepatic glucose production above baseline can be accounted for by accelerated gluconeogenesis (32,33).

Muscle
Studies employing the euglycemic insulin clamp in combination with femoral artery/vein catheterization have examined the effect of insulin on leg glucose uptake in type 2 diabetic and control subjects. Because bone is metabolically inert and adipose tissue takes up less than 5% of an infused glucose load (25,34,35), muscle represents the major tissue responsible for leg glucose uptake. In response to a physiologic increase in plasma insulin concentration (~80–100 (µU/mL), leg (muscle) glucose uptake increases linearly, reaching a plateau value of 10 mg/kg leg weights per minute (36). In contrast, in lean type 2 diabetic subjects, the onset of insulin action is delayed for ~40 minutes and the ability of the insulin to stimulate leg glucose uptake is markedly blunted (36). During the last hour of the insulin clamp study, when the effect of insulin was at its peak, the rate of glucose uptake in muscle was reduced by 50% in the insulin-resistant diabetic group (36).

Thus, insulin resistance involving both muscle and liver leads to abnormal glucose metabolism. In the basal state, the liver represents a major site of insulin resistance, and this is reflected by the overproduction of glucose. This accelerated rate of hepatic glucose output is the primary determinant of the elevated fasting plasma glucose concentration in type 2 diabetic individuals. In the fed state, the defects in insulin-mediated glucose uptake by muscle and the lack of suppression of hepatic glucose production by insulin contribute approximately equally to the disturbance in whole body glucose homeostasis in type 2 diabetes.

Fat Cell

Obesity is the most common acquired cause of insulin resistance. Interestingly, a similar degree of insulin resistance is seen in obese nondiabetic and lean type 2 diabetic individuals (37–39). However, lean diabetic subjects manifest marked glucose intolerance, whereas the obese non-diabetic individuals have normal plasma glucose (12). This difference is explained by the plasma insulin response to a glucose challenge. Obese nondiabetic individuals secrete more than twice as much as insulin as lean nondiabetic controls and compensate for the insulin resistance. In contrast, normal-weight diabetic subjects are unable to augment the secretion of insulin sufficiently to compensate for the insulin resistance. When obesity and diabetes coexist in the same individual, the severity of insulin resistance is only slightly greater than that in either the normal-weight diabetic or obese nondiabetic individuals (12).

Obese, insulin-resistant individuals have increased FFA levels in their blood (40–44). FFA are stored as TGs in adipocytes and serve as an important energy source during conditions of fasting. Utilizing the hyperinsulinemic, euglycemic clamp in 1146 nondiabetic, normotensive individuals, Ferrannini showed a progressive loss of insulin sensitivity when the BMI increased from 18 kg/m^2 to 38 kg/m^2 (45). The increase in insulin resistance with weight gain is directly related to the amount of visceral adipose tissue (VAT) (46,47). The VAT refers to fat cells located within the abdominal cavity and includes omental, mesenteric, retroperitoneal, and perinephric adipose tissue. In lean individuals, VAT represents 20% of fat in men and 6% of fat in women. Obese individuals have an expanded fat cell mass characterized by visceral adiposity.

Visceral fat cells have a high lipolytic rate, which is especially refractory to insulin (48,49). Increased lipolysis of fat results in elevations of plasma FFAs and causes insulin resistance in muscle and liver (12,15,27,29,30,42,50,51) and impairs insulin secretion (29,52,53). In addition to FFAs that circulate in plasma in increased amounts, type 2 diabetic and obese nondiabetic individuals have increased stores of TGs in muscle (54,55) and liver (26,56) and the increased fat content correlates closely with the presence of insulin resistance in these tissues. Finally, FFAs released into the portal circulation drain into the liver, where they stimulate production of very low-density lipoproteins (VLDL) particles (46).

Visceral fat cells are active endocrine cells producing many cytokines including leptin, tumor necrosis factor alpha, and interleukin 6 (Fig. 4). These factors drain into the portal circulation and reduce insulin sensitivity in peripheral tissues (58). VAT is also the site of pro-duction of adiponectin—a hormone associated with increased insulin sensitivity. Obesity is associated with decreased levels of adiponectin. Chromosomal locus 3q27 codes for adiponectin and is associated with insulin resistance and type 2 diabetes. Adiponectin has a number of antiatherosclerotic properties including: suppression of endothelial inflammatory response, decreasing vascular smooth muscle proliferation, decreasing vascular cell adhesion molecule-1 expression, and suppressing conversion of macrophages to foam cells. In humans, higher levels of adiponectin are associated with a lower risk of myocardial infarction (59).

Increased VAT may also lead to elevated levels of cortisol, which would increase insulin resistance. Intraabdominal fat has a high activity of the enzyme 11 beta-hydroxysteroid

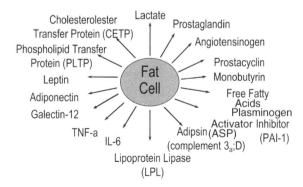

FIGURE 4 Depiction of adipose tissue derived proteohormones (adipocytokines). Overproduction in obesity promotes the development of the metabolic syndrome. *Source*: From Ref. 57.

All Fat Cells Are Not Created Equal

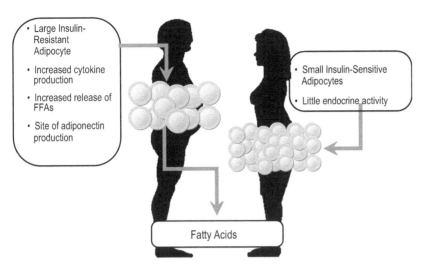

FIGURE 5 Differential activity of central versus peripheral fat cells. *Abbreviation*: FFAS, Free fatty acids. *Source*: From Ref. 57.

dehydrogenase. This enzyme converts inactive cortisone to active cortisol. In a weight-loss intervention trial carried out in obese, nondiabetic individuals, the best predictor of improvement in insulin sensitivity was a decrease in visceral adiposity (60).

Fat cell size is an important predictor of the development of diabetes (61) (Fig. 5). Small, newly differentiated adipocytes are more insulin sensitive than large, lipid-laden fat cells. The smaller cells are able to take up glucose and store lipid. In contrast, the larger cells have low rates of insulin stimulated glucose uptake, less suppression of lipolysis, and a higher rate of cytokine production. Visceral fat cells tend to be larger and more metabolically active than subcutaneous fat cells (62,63).

CELLULAR MECHANISMS OF INSULIN RESISTANCE

The stimulation of glucose metabolism by insulin requires that the hormone must first bind to specific receptors that are present on the cell surface (Fig. 6) (12,64–67). After insulin has bound to and activated its receptor, "second messengers" initiate a series of events involving a cascade of phosphorylation-dephosphorylation reactions (12,64–67) that result in the stimulation of intracellular glucose metabolism. The initial step in glucose metabolism involves activation of the glucose transport system, leading to the influx of glucose into insulin target tissues, primarily muscle (12,68,69). The free glucose is metabolized by a series of enzymatic steps that are under the control of insulin. Insulin resistance and the resulting increase in FFAs block every step in the glycogen synthesis pathway (Fig. 7).

The insulin receptor is a glycoprotein consisting of two α-subunits and two β-subunits linked by disulfide bonds (Fig. 6) (12,64–67). The α-subunit of the insulin receptor is entirely extracellular and contains the insulin-binding domain. The β-subunit has an extracellular domain, a transmembrane domain, and an intracellular domain that expresses insulin stimulated kinase activity directed toward its own tyrosine residues. Insulin receptor phosphorylation of the β-subunit, with subsequent activation of insulin receptor tyrosine kinase, represents the first step in the action of insulin on glucose metabolism (64–67).

The binding of insulin to tyrosine kinase stimulates two distinct pathways: the glycogen synthesis pathway and the mitogenic pathway (Fig. 6). Once activated, tyrosine kinase phosphorylates specific intracellular proteins, of which at least nine have been identified (69). Four of these belong to the family of insulin receptor substrate proteins: IRS-1, IRS-2, IRS-3, IRS-4 (the others include Shc, Cbl, Gab-1, p60 (dok), and APS). In muscle, IRS-1 serves as the major docking protein that interacts with the insulin receptor tyrosine kinase and undergoes tyrosine

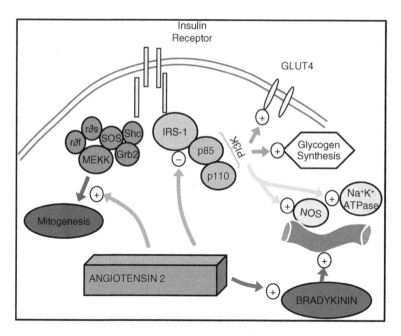

FIGURE 6   The mitogenic pathway and glycogen synthesis pathway. Insulin resistance and the resulting hyperinsulinemia leads to increased stimulation of both pathways.

phosphorylation. This leads to the activation of the enzyme PI-3 kinase (64–67). PI-3 kinase activation stimulates glucose transport (64–67) and glycogen synthesis 64,65). Inhibitors of PI-3 kinase impair glucose transport (70) by interfering with the translocation of GLUT-4 transporters from their intracellular location (68,69) and block the activation of glycogen synthase (70). The action of insulin to increase protein synthesis and inhibit protein degradation also is mediated by PI-3 kinase (72,73). Insulin also promotes hepatic TG synthesis and this lipogenic

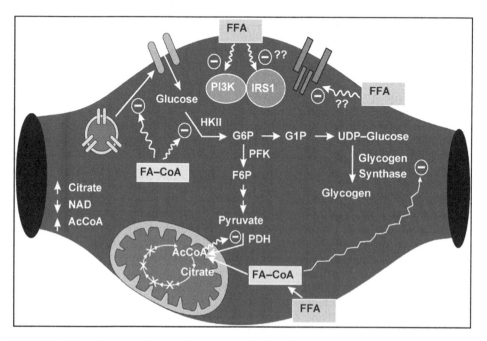

FIGURE 7   The mitogenic pathway and glycogen synthesis pathway in muscle. Overstimulation of the mitogenic pathway by insulin promotes cell growth and proliferation. *Abbreviation*: FFA, free fatty acid.

effect of insulin also appears to be mediated via the PI-3 kinase pathway (64). Thus all of the anabolic effects of insulin are mediated through the IRS/P13K pathway. In liver, IRS-2 serves as the primary docking protein that undergoes tyrosine phosphorylation and mediates the effect of insulin on hepatic glucose production, gluconeogenesis, and glycogen formation (74). In adipocytes, Cbl represents another substrate which is phosphorylated following its interaction with the insulin receptor tyrosine kinase, and which is required for stimulation of GLUT-4 translocation (75).

In muscle, insulin stimulates a second pathway, the mitogen-activated protein (MAP) signaling pathway (Fig. 7). Activation of this pathway plays an important role in the production of mitogens, which promote cell growth, proliferation, and differentiation. Blockade of the MAP kinase pathway prevents the stimulation of cell growth by insulin but has no effect on the anabolic actions of the hormone (76–78).

INSULIN SIGNAL TRANSDUCTION DEFECTS IN INSULIN RESISTANCE
Insulin Receptor Number and Affinity

Muscle and liver represent the major tissues responsible for the regulation of glucose homeostasis in vivo, and insulin binding to solubilized receptors obtained from skeletal muscle and liver biopsies has been shown to be normal in both obese and lean diabetic individuals (79–83). The insulin receptor gene has been sequenced in a large number of type 2 diabetic patients from diverse ethnic populations using denaturing-gradient gel electrophoresis or single-stranded conformational polymorphism analysis, and, with very rare exceptions (84), physiologically significant mutations in the insulin receptor gene have not been observed (85,86). Therefore, a structural gene abnormality in the insulin receptor is unlikely to be a common cause of insulin resistance.

Insulin Receptor Tyrosine Kinase Activity

Insulin receptor tyrosine kinase activity has been examined in skeletal muscle and hepatocytes from normal weight and obese diabetic subjects. Most investigators (79,80,87–90) have found reduced tyrosine kinase activity. Interestingly, weight loss with normalization of blood glucose levels has been shown to correct the defect in insulin receptor tyrosine kinase activity (91). This observation suggests that the defect in tyrosine kinase may be acquired and results from some combination of hyperglycemia and/or insulin resistance, which are reversed with weight loss.

Insulin Signaling (IRS-1 and PI-3 Kinase) Defects

A physiologic increase in the plasma insulin concentration stimulates tyrosine phosphorylation of the insulin receptor and IRS-1 in lean healthy subjects to 150% to 200% of basal values (90,92–94). In obese nondiabetic subjects, the ability of insulin to activate these two early insulin receptor signaling events in muscle is reduced, while in type 2 diabetics insulin has no significant stimulatory effect on either insulin receptor or IRS-1 tyrosine phosphorylation. The association of p85 protein and PI-3 kinase activity with IRS-1 also is greatly reduced in obese nondiabetic and type 2 diabetic subjects compared to lean healthy subjects (90–95). In the insulin-resistant, normal glucose-tolerant offspring of two type 2 diabetic parents, IRS-1 tyrosine phosphorylation and the association of p85 protein/PI-3 kinase activity with IRS-1 are also markedly decreased (93). These insulin-signaling defects are correlated closely with the severity of insulin resistance (93). In summary, a defect in the association of PI-3 kinase with IRS-1 and its subsequent activation appears to be a characteristic abnormality in type 2 diabetics and is closely correlated with *in vivo* muscle insulin resistance.

The profound defect of the PI-3-kinase signaling pathway in insulin-resistant individuals contrasts markedly with the ability of insulin to stimulate MAP kinase pathway activity (Fig. 6) (90). Hyperinsulinemia increases MEK1 activity and ERK1/2 phosphorylation activity to the same extent, in lean healthy as in insulin-resistant obese nondiabetic and type 2 diabetic patients (90). Maintenance of insulin stimulation of the MAP kinase pathway in the presence of insulin resistance in the PI-3 kinase pathway may be important in the development of atherosclerosis (Fig. 7). Insulin resistance in the anabolic (IRS/PI-3 kinase) pathway, with its compensatory hyperinsulinemia, would lead to excessive stimulation of the MAP kinase pathway in vascular tissue. This would result in the proliferation of vascular smooth muscle cells, increased collagen formation, and increased production of growth factors and inflammatory cytokines, possibly explaining the accelerated rate of atherosclerosis in type 2 diabetic individuals.

CLINICAL MANIFESTATIONS OF THE METABOLIC SYNDROME

The clinical manifestations of the metabolic syndrome are classified as the "risk factors" in the IDF guidelines (Fig. 3). I will discuss my approach to these risk factors in the context of three commonly seen patient types.

■ Case: A Patient with the Metabolic Syndrome and Atherogenic Dyslipidemia

A 56-year-old Mexican-American female presents for routine follow-up. Her past medical history is unremarkable. She shares a family history of diabetes with her mother, maternal grandmother, and two of four older sisters diagnosed with type 2 diabetes. Her mother had a myocardial infarction at age 51 and one of her sisters has had a three-vessel coronary artery bypass graft. The patient is on no medications. The patient has no scheduled exercise program but says she is "on her feet all day" at work.

Physical examination is remarkable for a well-developed woman with a blood pressure of 110/78 mmHg. Her BMI is 29 with a waist circumference of 88 cm. Acanthosis nigricans is present on the back of the neck. The remainder of the physical examination is unremarkable.

Lab findings show a fasting blood glucose of 112 mg/dL. The two-hour glucose value following a 75 g glucose load was 180 mg/dL. Fasting lipid profile revealed an LDL-C of 114 mg/dL, HDL-C of 41 mg/dL and TGs of 160 mg/dL. A CBC, UA, SMA20, and thyroid function tests were normal. A baseline electrocardiogram (ECG) was unremarkable.

ATHEROGENIC DYSLIPIDEMIA

The lipoprotein profile characteristic of the metabolic syndrome is termed "atherogenic dyslipidemia." Atherogenic dyslipidemia is defined by the triad of high TG levels, low levels HDL-C, and the presence of small, dense low-density lipoprotein (LDL) particles. The atherogenic lipid profile is strongly associated with insulin resistance and typically precedes the diagnosis of type 2 diabetes (96,97). The pathogenesis of "atherogenic dyslipidemia" is outlined in Figure 8.

ELEVATED TRIGLYCERIDE LEVELS

Insulin resistance or an extensive mass of VAT results in an enhancement of lipolysis and increased fatty acid flux to the liver. In the liver, fatty acids are re-esterified into TGs and incorporated into VLDL (99). The result is an increase in VLDL production and hypertriglyceridemia

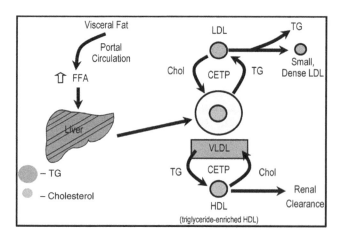

FIGURE 8 Relationship between visceral fat and the development of "atherogenic dyslipidemia" characterized by (i) an increase in small, dense LDL partices, (ii) elevated levels of VLDL triglycerides, and (iii) low levels of HDL-cholesterol. *Abbreviations*: FFA, free fatty acid; LDL, low-density lipoproteins; CETP, cholesterol ester Transfer protein; VLDL, very low-density lipoproteins; HDL, high density lipoproteins; TG, triglyceride; chol, cholesterol *Source*: From Ref. 98.

(100,101). Elevated FFA levels can also act to enhance insulin resistance (102), which exacerbates the problem. VLDL particles are removed from the circulation by several high-affinity receptors that recognize its surface apoproteins (apo) B, C, and E. Glycosylation of these proteins may reduce their affinity for hepatic receptor-mediated clearance and increase their uptake by vascular macrophages (103,104). Therefore, when a patient develops diabetes elevated TG levels result from both an overproduction and reduced catabolism of TG-rich VLDL.

LOW LEVELS OF HIGH-DENSITY LIPOPROTEIN CHOLESTEROL

HDL promotes the primary mechanism of lipid efflux from peripheral tissues, "reverse cholesterol transport," has anti-inflammatory properties and blocks LDL uptake by macrophages (105,106). HDL-C levels are lowered in patients with the metabolic syndrome as a result of elevated cholesteryl ester transfer protein (CETP) activity, which enriches HDL particles with TG and apoE (Fig. 8). More apoE molecules per particle may promote greater HDL catabolism through receptor-mediated clearance. In addition, removal of cholesterol from the HDL particle results in an increase in small, lipid-poor HDL particles. ApoA-I, the primary apoprotein of HDL, appears to dissociate more easily from the smaller HDL species; free apoA-I is then filtered in the kidney (100). ApoA-I deficiency subsequently leads to a decrease in the new HDL production.

SMALL, DENSE LOW-DENSITY LIPOPROTEIN PARTICLES

LDL particles are an end product of VLDL metabolism. While the LDL concentration is not elevated in individuals with the metabolic syndrome, there is a qualitative difference seen related to the particle size and density. Elevated VLDL and TG levels stimulate CETP activity, transferring TG from VLDL to LDL (Fig. 8). Subsequent exposure to lipases further depletes LDL-TG, leaving a population of the smaller, denser, and cholesterol-rich particles. This LDL subclass has a reduced affinity for the normal apoB clearance receptor. If the patient develops diabetes, glycosylation of apoB protein may also diminish the apoB receptor affinity (107). This leads to a greater opportunity for LDL oxidation by free radicals, preferential uptake by the scavenger receptors on tissue macrophages, and an increased foam cell formation. The atherogenic potential of small, dense LDL particles may also derive from their greater ease of penetration into the vascular tissues.

ASSOCIATED RISK FACTORS

The atherogenic triad has also been associated with a prothrombotic state (108). The lipid abnormalities, together with hyperinsulinemia, are thought to induce plasminogen activator inhibitor expression, inhibit platelet aggregation, elevate serum levels of factor VII, and increase blood and plasma viscosity (109,110). In a similar manner, a proinflammatory state, as identified by the inflammatory marker CRP, has been linked with an increase in the number of coronary heart disease (CHD) events in men and women (111–113). Patients with newly diagnosed diabetes have a 1.84-fold increased risk of having elevated CRP levels, compared with patients without diabetes (114). The frequent concurrence of many suspected individual cardiovascular risk factors makes it more difficult to identify any one of them as a truly independent predictor of CHD. However, it is clear that a particular cluster of these features increases the risk for CHD at any level of LDL-C (115).

LIPID GOALS FOR PATIENTS WITH THE METABOLIC SYNDROME

Since 1988, the NCEP has issued several consensus reports addressing clinical management of high blood cholesterol based on the emergence of scientific information (116). Each successive report has recommended progressively stricter lipid goals and indications for treatment that are directly related to an individual's degree of CHD risk (115). The highest risk is assigned to patients with clinically established CHD or other evidence of atherosclerosis. The guidelines recommend treating all components of the atherogenic lipid profile. High LDL-C is the primary therapeutic target because of the significant cardiovascular benefits associated with LDL-C lowering demonstrated in primary and secondary prevention trials with statins (115).

For patients in the high-risk category, the treatment goal for LDL-C lowering is lesser than 100 mg/dL (115). However, once the LDL-C goal is achieved, many patients will still have persistent abnormalities of TG and HDL-C.

Elevated TG and low HDL-C levels are most often found together but may occur by themselves. Hypertriglyceridemia is a secondary target for lipid management. Serum TG values of more than 200 mg/dL may increase an individual's risk for CHD events substantially above that predicted by LDL-C values alone (96). Some recommend lipid-lowering therapy targeted at correcting the serum level of non–HDL-C (total serum cholesterol minus HDL-C), representing the cholesterol carried by VLDL, intermediate-density lipoprotein, LDL, and Lp(a). All of these particles contain apoB and are atherogenic. Target non–HDL-C levels are 30 mg/dL above the LDL-C value goal (115).

Low HDL-C is the most consistent predictor of CHD events in type 2 diabetics (117). ATP III increased the threshold for low HDL-C from the previous level of less than 35 mg/dL to less than 40 mg/dL (115). In addition, the most recent American Heart Association guidelines for cardiovascular disease prevention in women have raised this threshold to less than 50 mg/dL (118). In patients with the metabolic syndrome, a low HDL-C level, as part of an atherogenic profile or as a single factor, should be targeted, with goals of more than or equal to 40 mg/dL in men and more than or equal to 50 mg/dL in women.

Our patient meets the IDF definition of the metabolic syndrome. Her strong family history of both diabetes and heart disease along with her abnormal lipid profile put her at a very high risk of developing both diabetes and cardiovascular disease.

Because obesity and physical inactivity enhance CHD risk, we recommended lifestyle modifications. Weight loss and exercise can decrease TG levels and increase HDL-C. In addition, LDL-C levels may be lowered by 15 to 25 mg/dL (117). Patients with atherogenic dyslipidemia, however, will usually require drug therapy to achieve lipid goals. Pharmacologic therapeutic options were discussed with the patient.

PHARMACOLOGIC THERAPY

The various classes of drugs used in the treatment of adult dyslipidemia provide a range of lipid alterations (Table 5) (115). Clinical trials have established the value of these agents as monotherapy and in combination.

STATINS

LDL-C is the initial target of therapy in a patient with the metabolic syndrome and atherogenic dyslipidemia. Statins (3-hydroxy-3-methylglutaryl co-enzyme A reductase inhibitors), the most powerful LDL-C–lowering class, should be the initial treatment option. In both primary and

TABLE 5   Drugs for the Treatment of Adult Dyslipidemia

Drug class	Lipid/lipoprotein	Effects
HMG CoA reductase	LDL-C	−18–55%
Inhibitors (statins)	HDL-C	+5–15%
	TG	−7–30%
Bile acid sequestrants	LDL-C	−15–30%
	HDL-C	+3–5%
	TG	No change, or increase
Niacin	LDL-C	−5–25%
	HDL-C	+15–35%
	TG	−20–50%
Fibric acids	LDL-C	−5–20%[a]
	HDL-C	+10–20%
	TG	−20–50%

[a]Levels may rise in patients with hypertriglyceridemia.
Abbreviations: LDL-C, low-density lipoprotein cholesterol; HDL-C, high-density lipoprotein cholesterol TG, triglyceride; HMG CoA, 3-hydroxy-3-methylglutaryl coenzyme A.
Source: From Ref. 112.

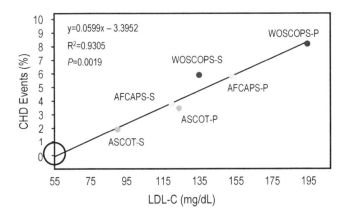

FIGURE 9 Clinical trials demonstrating a reduction in cardiovascular events as cholesterol is lowered with "statin" therapy. Patients in these trials were free of known cardiovascular disease. *Abbreviations*: CHD, coronary heart disease; LDL-C; low density lipoproteins-cholesterol. *Source*: From Ref. 119.

secondary prevention trials, statin therapy has shown consistent reductions in cardiovascular events between LDL-C levels of 100 and 200 mg/dL (Figs. 9 and 10).

The Heart Protection Study randomized over 20,000 patients, considered to be at clinical risk of experiencing a new CHD event by virtue of prior CHD, other atherosclerotic disease, or diabetes (120). This high-risk population included 5963 men and women with diabetes, including 2912 with no prior evidence of vascular disease (121). After an average follow-up of five years, there was a 24% relative risk reduction in major vascular events (CHD death, myocardial infarction, stroke, or revascularization) with simvastatin treatment ($p < 0.0001$) in the total population. Notably, individuals with baseline LDL-C levels less than 100 mg/dL derived the same 24% reduction in major vascular events as patients with baseline LDL-C levels greater than 130 mg/dL. Based on the consistent reduction in CHD risk and the safety of statins demonstrated in these randomized clinical trials, it is recommended that all patients at high risk for cardiovascular disease be placed on statin therapy independent of LDL-C level. While Statin therapy is universally accepted, the LDL-C treatment target is more controversial.

The European Diabetes Policy Group and the IDF recommend an LDL-C less than 115 mg/dL for high-risk patients (122). The initial NCEP ATP III guidelines suggest a primary target of LDL-C less than 100 mg/dL in high-risk patients; however, an update to these guidelines (123) suggested that very high-risk patients may have an optional lower target of 70 mg/dL. The Treating to New Targets (TNT) study and the Incremental Decrease In End points through Aggressive Lipid Lowering (IDEAL) trial were designed to answer this question.

The TNT study (124) compared the effect of atorvastatin 80 mg daily to atorvastatin 10 mg daily in over 10,000 individuals with known cardiovascular disease. Baseline LDL-C in both groups was about 155 mg/dL. The mean on treatment LDL-C was 77 mg/dL in the atorvastatin 80 mg group compared to 101 mg/dL in the atorvastatin 10 mg/dL group (Fig. 11)

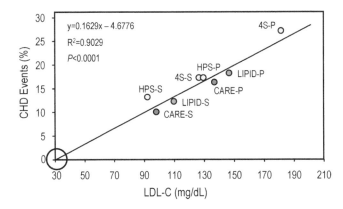

FIGURE 10 Clinical trials demonstrating a reduction in cardiovascular events as cholesterol is lowered with "statin" therapy. Patients in these trials had known cardiovascular disease. *Abbreviations*: CHD, coronary heart disease; LDL-C; low density lipoproteins-cholesterol. *Source*: From Ref. 119.

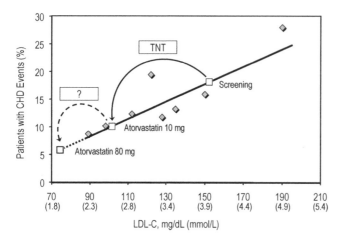

FIGURE 11 Study design of the Treating to New Targets Study. Patients with known heart disease were randomized to low dose versus high dose atorvastatin treatment to determine if greater cholesterol lowering would result in greater reductions in cardiovascular events. *Abbreviation*: CHD, coronary heart disease. *Source*: From Ref. 125.

The reduction in LDL-C in this study had no impact on total mortality (Table 6). The 22% reduction in cardiovascular events seen with the high-dose statin therapy was offset by a similar increase in noncardiovascular deaths. In addition, high-dose statin therapy was associated with more drug-related adverse events (8.1% vs. 5.8%). Of most concern, were the 60 cases of transaminase elevations above three times the upper limit of normal with atorvastatin 80 mg daily compared to the nine cases seen with atorvastatin 10 mg daily.

The IDEAL trial (126) compared therapy with simvastatin 20–40 mg daily to atorvastatin 80 mg daily in 8882 patients with known coronary artery disease (Table 7). As was the case in the TNT trial, there was no difference in total mortality between patients treated to an LDL-C target below 100 mg/dL. Surprisingly, there was no reduction in cardiovascular events with more aggressive LDL-C lowering in this large, well-designed clinical trial.

In addition to lifestyle changes, our patient was started on 10 mg of atorvastatin. After three months of therapy her repeat lipid profile showed an LDL-C of 82 mg/dL with an HDL-C of 42 mg/dL and serum TG levels of 134 mg/dL.

COMBINATION THERAPY

Statins primarily target LDL-C abnormalities. The reduction in major coronary events in landmark statin trials has varied between 25% and 38% (Fig. 12). Because our patient presented with abnormal TG and HDL-C levels, it may be beneficial to add an agent to address these lipid abnormalities. Fibric acid derivatives and niacin preparations address these abnormalities characteristic of "atherogenic dyslipidemia."

FIBRATES

The fibric acid derivatives include gemfibrozil, fenofibrate, and bezafibrate. Fibrates effectively reduce TG levels (128) and have modest effects on LDL-C and HDL-C levels. The Helsinki Heart

TABLE 6 Treating to New Targets Mortality

	Number of patients (%)	
	Atorvastatin 10 mg/d ($n = 5006$)	Atorvastatin 80 mg/d ($n = 4995$)
All-cause mortality	282 (5.6)	284 (5.7)
Cardiovascular	155	126
CHD	127	101
Stroke death	8	7
Noncardiovascular death	127	158
Cancer	75	85
Other	52	73

Note: A 22% reduction in cardiovascular events was offset by a 22% increase in noncardiovascular events.

TABLE 7 Incremental Decrease in End Points Through Aggressive Lipid Lowering Study: Effect of Treatment

	Number of patients (%)	
	Simvastatin 20 mg/d ($n = 4449$)	Atorvastatin 80 mg/d ($n = 4439$)
All-cause mortality	374 (8.4)	366 (8.2)
Cardiovascular mortality	218 (4.9)	223 (5.0)
CHD mortality	178 (4.0)	175 (3.9)
Total stroke (fatal/nonfatal)	174 (3.9)	151 (3.4)
Noncardiovascular mortality	156 (3.5)	143 (3.2)
Cancer	112 (2.5)	99 (2.2)
Suicide/violence/accidental	9 (0.2)	5 (0.1)
Other	30 (0.7)	32 (0.7)

Note: $p > .05$ versus placebo for all comparisons (not significant).
Source: From Ref. 126.

Study evaluated the effect of gemfibrozil in 4081 hyperlipidemic men without prior evidence of CHD (129). Treatment with gemfibrozil reduced TG levels by 26% and LDL-C levels by 10%, and raised HDL-C levels by 6% from baseline. After five years, the rate of nonfatal myocardial infarction or CHD-related death was significantly reduced by gemfibrozil treatment.

The Veterans Affairs High-Density Lipoprotein Intervention Trial (VA-HIT) enrolled 2531 men with known CHD, low HDL-C levels, and normal LDL-C levels, including 1092 with diabetes or impaired fasting glucose (130). Treatment with gemfibrozil reduced TG levels by 31% and LDL-C levels by 2%, and raised HDL-C levels by 6% from baseline. In the total population, major coronary events were reduced 22% more with gemfibrozil treatment than with placebo over a five-year period (131). The benefit tended to be greater in patients with diabetes than in those without diabetes (35% vs. 18%; $p = 0.07$).

The Diabetes Atherosclerosis Intervention Study evaluated the coronary angiographic effects of fenofibrate treatment in 418 patients with type 2 diabetes and documented CHD. Mean values for lipids at baseline were typical of diabetes, with LDL-C levels of 130 mg/dL, HDL-C levels of 39 mg/dL, and TG levels of 229 mg/dL. Treatment with fenofibrate reduced

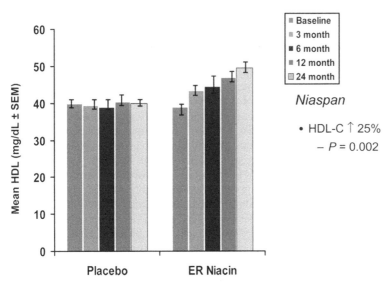

FIGURE 12 Changes in HDL-C with 1000 g of Niaspan over 2 years. A progressive increase in HDL-C was seen with no change in Niaspan dose. *Abbreviations*: HDL-C, high-density lipoprotein cholesterol. *Source*: From Ref. 127.

TG levels by 28% and LDL-C levels by 6%, and raised HDL-C levels by 7% from baseline. After three years, the rate of atherosclerotic stenoses progression was less with fenofibrate than placebo (2.10% vs. 3.65%; $p = 0.02$). Although the trial was not powered to assess clinical outcomes, there were fewer coronary events in the fenofibrate group than in the placebo group (38 vs. 50) (132).

The Fenofibrate Intervention and Event Lowering in Diabetes (FIELD) study (133) was designed to assess the effect of fenofibrate on cardiovascular disease in patients with diabetes both with and without known heart disease. Patients with type 2 diabetes between 50 and 75 years of age were randomized to treatment with fenofibrate 200 mg daily versus placebo. Nine thousand seven hundred and ninety five patients from 63 centers in Australia, New Zealand, and Finland were studied for five years making this by far the largest study ever completed in a diabetic population. The baseline lipid levels on no lipid altering medication included a mean LDL-C of 118 mg/dL (5.03 mmol/L), an HDL-C of 42.6 mg/dL (1.1 mmol/L), and a TG level was 153.3 mg/dL (1.7 mmol/L) in both groups. The primary endpoint was the first occurrence of either a nonfatal myocardial infarction or death from CHD.

At the end of the trial, a nonsignificant 11% reduction ($p = 0.16$) in the primary outcome of first myocardial infarction or coronary heart death was seen in the treatment group. This corresponded to a 24% reduction in nonfatal myocardial infarction in fenofibrate-treated patients ($p = 0.01$) and a 19% increase in coronary disease mortality ($p = 0.22$) A post hoc sub-group analysis showed a significant reduction in events in patients without previous cardio-vascular events but no benefit in patients with known preexisting cardiovascular disease.

The nonsignificant 11% decrease in the primary endpoint of coronary events in diabetics treated with fenofibrate was surprising and the nonsignificant 11% increase in overall mortal-ity is disturbing. Prior to the FIELD study, the VA-HIT provided the largest sample of diabetic patients treated with a fibric acid derivative. In VA-HIT, 769 diabetics with known heart disease were randomized either placebo or gemfibrozil 1200 mg daily for five years. Baseline LDL-C and TG levels were similar to those seen in the FIELD trial, while HDL-C levels were significantly lower at 31 mg/dL. In the VA-HIT diabetics treated with gemfibrozil had a 32% reduction in cardiovascular events ($p = .004$). The event reduction was due to a 22% reduction in myocardial infarction and a 41% reduction in cardiovascular death.

The reason(s) for the disappointing effect seen with fenofibrate in the FIELD study are unknown. The authors point out a greater use of statin therapy in patients allocated to the placebo group than in those on fenofibrate. While no patients were on statin therapy at the start of the study, statin therapy could be added during the study at the discretion of the patient's physician. In patients with known heart disease, 23% of placebo-allocated and 14% of fenofibrate-allocated patients received statins. In the primary-prevention patients, the corre-sponding numbers are 16% placebo-treated and 7% fenofibrate-treated. Because the vast major-ity of patients in this study did not receive statins, the "drop-in" statin effect can only be a partial explanation. If patients were censored at the time of starting lipid-lowering therapy, the benefit of fenofibrate was a nonsignificant 14% reduction in primary events ($p = 0.10$).

In my view, the most likely explanation for the disappointing effect of fenofibrate on cardiovascular event reduction in the FIELD trial was the lack of treatment effect on HDL-C lev-els. After four months of treatment, HDL-C levels had increased 5% in patients randomized to therapy with fenofibrate. The initial increase in HDL-C seen in this study is similar to that seen in the VA-HIT trial (130). In the VA-HIT, diabetic patients' HDL-C levels increased to 5% com-pared to the 8% increase in nondiabetic individuals and the 5% increase in HDL-C was main-tained throughout the entire five-year study. However, in the FIELD trial the initial increase in HDL-C was not sustained. By close study, the increase in HDL-C was only 1%. In the FIELD study, the LDL-C level was reduced by 12% and TG levels were 29% lower after four months of treatment. The reductions in LDL-C and TGs were maintained throughout the study. Thus, the attenuation of effect on HDL-C–raising with fenofibrate is not likely due to a decrease in com-pliance with taking the medication as the lipid effects on LDL-C and TGs were maintained.

Analysis of the lipid values from the VA-HIT demonstrated that baseline HDL-C and TG levels were significant predictors of cardiovascular events, whereas, during the trial, only con-centrations of HDL-C significantly predicted a reduction in cardiovascular endpoints (134). Change in TG levels was not predictive of a reduction in cardiovascular risk with gemfibrozil therapy. Similarly, the 29% reduction in TG levels with fenofibrate therapy did not result in a significant reduction in the primary endpoint of nonfatal myocardial infarction or coronary death in the FIELD trial.

Although no clinical outcome trials of statin-fibrate treatment have been reported, combination therapy has been shown to be very effective in lowering TG and LDL-C levels in diabetic patients in small clinical studies. After six months, the combination of atorvastatin 20 mg and fenofibrate 200 mg/day reduced TG levels by 50% and LDL-C levels by 46% from baseline (135). After one year, treatment with simvastatin 20 mg and bezafibrate 400 mg/day reduced TG levels by 42% and LDL-C levels by 29% (136). HDL-C levels were increased by 21% with atorvastatin and fenofibrate and by 25% with simvastatin and benzofibrate (135,136).

Fibrate therapy is generally safe and well tolerated (137). Gastrointestinal symptoms are the most frequent adverse events reported. Fibrates are also associated with a small risk of myopathy (less than 0.1%) (138). Use of statin-fibrate therapy has raised concern following reports in the literature of fatal rhabdomyolysis, especially with cerivastatin and gemfibrozil (139,140). More recent analyses show that statin-fibrate use is generally safe; in controlled clinical trials, including nearly 600 patients treated with this combination, only 1% of patients were withdrawn because of myalgias (115). Fenofibrate appears to be associated with a lower risk of myopathy than gemfibrozil, when used in combination with a statin.

NIACIN

Niacin is the most effective pharmacologic agent currently available for increasing HDL-C levels (115). In the ARBITER 3 trial (141), 1000 mg of Niaspan daily increased HDL-C by 25% after 24 months of therapy. The maximal effect of Niaspan to raise HDL-C may not be seen for 18 months (Fig. 13).

Clinically, niacin's ability to decrease cardiovascular events was shown in the Coronary Drug Project, where CHD patients with hypercholesterolemia experienced a 27% relative reduction in nonfatal myocardial infarction rates and an 11% reduction in long-term mortality (145,146). Recently, these results were analyzed by baseline fasting and one-hour blood glucose levels (147). In this post-hoc analysis, niacin reduced nonfatal myocardial infarction and total mortality to a similar extent across all baseline glucose levels, even in patients with fasting blood glucose greater than or equal to 126 mg/dL. Other trials of niacin in combination with LDL-C–lowering drugs have demonstrated significant regression of coronary stenoses and reductions in clinical events in patients with hypercholesterolemia (148–150).

Statins and niacin have complementary actions on the atherogenic lipid profile. The HDL-Atherosclerosis Treatment Study (HATS), which enrolled 160 patients with CHD, included 34 patients with diabetes or impaired fasting glucose levels (151,152). Substantial improvements were seen in this subgroup; simvastatin-niacin treatment was associated with a 31% decrease in LDL-C levels, a 40% decrease in TG levels, and a 30% increase in HDL-C levels, while placebo or antioxidant treatments alone had little effect (152). After three years, average coronary stenosis progressed by 1.1% in these patients taking simvastatin-niacin

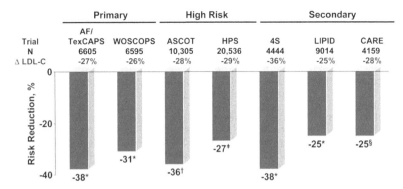

Major coronary events defined as: fatal or nonfatal myocardial infarction (MI), unstable angina, sudden cardiac death in AF/TexCAPS; nonfatal MI or coronary death in WOSCOPS, ASCOT, HPS, LIPID, CARE; coronary death, nonfatal MI, silent MI, resuscitated cardiac arrest in 4S.
* $p<0.001$; † $p=0.0005$; ‡ $p<0.0001$; § $p=0.002$.
LaRosa J et al. *JAMA.* 1999;282:2340-2346; HPS Collaborative Group. *Lancet.* 2002;360:7-22; Sever PS et al. *Lancet.* 2003;361:1149-1158.

FIGURE 13 Relationship between change in LDL-C and reduction in cardiovascular disease with "statin" therapy. Trials are stratified by level of patient risk from lowest (*left*) to highest (*right*). *Abbreviation*: LDL-C; low density lipoproteins-cholesterol. *Source*: From Refs. 142–144.

versus 4.8% in those not taking this combination ($p < 0.05$). The composite cardiovascular end-point (CHD death, myocardial infarction, stroke, or revascularization) occurred in 11% of sim-vastatin-niacin–treated patients compared with 21% of those not taking simvastatin-niacin (RRR = 48%; p = NS), suggesting that substantial reductions in risk may be achieved with combination therapy. Smaller studies have shown that statin-niacin combinations also increase LDL particle size and the antiatherogenic HDL_2 subclass to a greater extent than statin monotherapy in patients with diabetes (153,154). The first combination tablet for dys-lipidemia, containing lovastatin and niacin ER (Advicor®, Kos Pharmaceuticals, Inc., Miami, Florida, U.S.A.), was shown to provide similar alterations in lipids to those seen in HATS in a one-year study (155).

In the past, niacin has been considered to be relatively contraindicated in individuals with the metabolic syndrome because of concern that the modest hyperglycemic response to niacin may cause the individual to become diabetic. The hyperglycemic response to niacin is felt to be due to a secondary rebound in circulating oxidized FFAs, leading to reduced insulin-stimulated glucose uptake and increased hepatic glucose output (102). The Arterial Disease Multiple Interventions Trial evaluated niacin therapy in 125 participants with diabetes and vas-cular disease for a period of one year. Niacin (average dose, 2.5 g/day) increased glucose lev-els by 8.1 mg/dL in the diabetic patients compared with an increase of 6.3 mg/dL in the nondiabetic patients, and A1C concentrations were not significantly changed from baseline (156). Similarly, the Assessment of Diabetes Control and Evaluation of the Efficacy of Niaspan Trial randomized 148 type 2 diabetic patients to placebo or extended-release niacin (niacin ER). Dose-dependent increases in HDL-C and decreases in TG occurred with niacin ER 1000 and 1500 mg, and these changes were accompanied by negligible increases in A1C (157). In HATS, the combination of simvastatin and niacin was associated with small increases in fasting blood glucose during the first few months, which subsequently returned to baseline levels for the remainder of the study in the subgroup of patients with diabetes (158).

Based on this accumulating evidence, the ADA recommends that niacin less than or equal to 2 g/day can be used safely in diabetic patients with frequent glucose monitoring and adjust-ment of antidiabetic medication as necessary (159). Other potentially serious adverse events associated with statin-niacin combination therapy include hepatotoxicity and myopathy (137). At moderate doses, however, these events are rare. In the one-year study of lovastatin/niacin ER (40/2000 mg/day), the incidence of elevated liver transaminases was less than 0.5%, simi-lar to the rates reported with statin monotherapy (154).

Our patient was started on 500 mg of Niaspan daily. She was given a 325 mg aspirin tablet to reduce the potential flushing. After one month at this dose, the Niaspan was increased to 1000 mg daily. After three months of combined atorvastatin and Niaspan, the patient's LDL-C was 84 mg/dL, her TG levels were 98 mg/dL, and her HDL-C was 46 mg/dL.

■ Case: A Patient with the Metabolic Syndrome and Impaired Fasting Glucose

A 56-year-old African American female presents for evaluation of abnormal glucose tolerance. She denies polyuria, polydipsia, or recent weight change. Her 51-year-old sister has been recently diag-nosed with diabetes, which also afflicts her mother and maternal grandmother. Present medications include a diuretic, ACE-inhibitor, and beta-blocker for hypertension. Physical examination is significant for central obesity and well-controlled hypertension. A fasting lipid panel is normal with an LDL-C of 85 mg/dL, HDL-C of 60 mg/dL, and TGs of 130 mg/dL. Her fasting glucose is 112 mg/dL. The patient requests therapy to prevent diabetes.

A mismatch between the patterns of nutrient intake and physical activity is responsible for the epidemic of obesity and diabetes seen in modern industrialized societies (160). The major component of physical fitness that has been related to the primary prevention of diabetes is aerobic exercise. "Cardiorespiratory fitness" is largely determined by habitual physical activity and is often used as an objective measure of the pattern of recent physical activity.

PHYSICAL ACTIVITY AND FITNESS IN THE PRIMARY PREVENTION OF DIABETES

Observational studies. Five thousand nine hundred and ninety males, University of Pennsylvania alumni, aged 39 to 68 years at baseline were followed on an average of 14 years (161). Two hundred and two cases of diabetes occurred during 98,524 man-years of observation. After adjustment for age, BMI, hypertension, and parental history of diabetes, the investigators observed a 6% lower risk of diabetes for each 500 kcal/wk of self-reported leisure-time physical activity ($p = 0.01$).

As part of the Nurses' Health Study, 87,253 U.S. female nurses aged 34 to 59 were followed for an average of eight years, during which time 1303 were diagnosed with diabetes (162). Women who reported vigorous exercise at least once per week had a 33% lower age-adjusted risk of developing diabetes compared with women reporting no exercise ($p = 0.0001$). Similarly, an inverse relationship was seen between self-reported physical exercise and diabetes risk in 21,271 U.S. male physicians aged 40 to 84 years who were followed through 105,141 man-years, during which 285 developed diabetes (163).

Significant graded inverse associations were consistently observed between levels of self-reported physical activity and incident diabetes over long follow-up periods in established cohorts of men in the British Regional Heart Study (164), men and women in the Study of Eastern Finns (165), and women in the Iowa Women's Health Study (166), Nurses' Health Study (167,168), Women's Health Study (169), and Women's Health Initiative Observational Study (170). Each of the existing prospective studies of baseline fitness exposures and incident diabetes has shown that higher levels of fitness protect against the development of diabetes in women and men (171–174).

CARDIORESPIRATORY FITNESS AND THE DEVELOPMENT OF DIABETES

Lynch et al. (172) followed 897 Finnish men aged 42 to 60 for four years, during which time 46 cases of diabetes were identified with a two-hour postchallenge glucose level. Cardiorespiratory fitness was measured at baseline with ventilatory gas analysis during a maximal bicycle ergometry test. After adjusting for several confounders including age, BMI, and baseline glucose levels, odds ratios (95% confidence interval) for incident diabetes were 1.0 (referent), 0.77 (0.32–1.85), 0.26 (0.08–0.82), and 0.15 (0.03–0.79) in men in the first, second, third, and fourth quartile of fitness, respectively. Aerobics Center Longitudinal Study (174) followed 7442 men aged 30 to 79 years with normal glucose metabolism who had two clinical examinations an average of six years apart. An inverse relationship between cardiovascular fitness and the development of both impaired fasting glucose and diabetes was demonstrated.

Interventional Trials

The rate of progression to diabetes over a six-year period was assessed in four groups of Chinese patients with impaired glucose tolerance (175). The interventions were control, diet, exercise, or diet plus exercise. Diet alone reduced risk by 31%. Exercise alone was even more effective, reducing risk 46%. The combination of diet plus exercise (42% reduction) was no better than exercise alone.

Two large randomized controlled studies conducted in Finland and the United States examined the effect of a comprehensive lifestyle intervention on the progression to diabetes in high-risk women and men with impaired glycemic control (176,177). In both studies, the lifestyle intervention included regular physical activity (greater than or equal to 150 min/wk of moderate to vigorous intensity activities), modest weight loss (greater than or equal to 7% of baseline weight was targeted), reduction in fat intake, and increase in whole grains, fruits, and vegetables. Results of the studies were remarkably similar. During a mean follow-up of three to four years, the risk of developing diabetes was greater than or equal to 60% lower for those in the lifestyle intervention compared with those in the control group. In the Finnish trial, study participants who met the intervention target of greater than or equal to four hours of moderate intensity activity per week, but who did not meet the weight-loss goal, had a 70% lower risk of developing diabetes than those in the control arm ($p \geq 5$) (177,178). Therefore, regular exercise is able to prevent diabetes in the absence of weight loss.

Weight loss in the absence of exercise is also effective at preventing diabetes. The Xenical in the prevention of Diabetes in Obese Subjects (179) study randomized 3304 obese subjects to lifestyle changes alone versus orlistat: 120 mg/daily plus lifestyle changes. After an average follow-up of four years, individuals in the lifestyle only group had lost an average of 4.1 kg while orlistat-treated individuals lost an average of 6.9 kg. A 50% reduction in the development of diabetes in orlistat-treated patients (18% vs. 9%) was observed in patients with impaired fasting glucose at baseline.

Our patient was informed that she had impaired glucose tolerance and the metabolic syndrome. She was told that this information in addition to her strong family history of diabetes puts her at great risk of developing diabetes in the future. She was started on a diet and exercise regimen as implemented in the Diabetes Prevention Program.

PHARMACOLOGIC INTERVENTIONS FOR DIABETES PREVENTION

The Study to Prevent Non-Insulin–Dependent Diabetes Mellitus trial evaluated the effect of the glucosidase inhibitor acarbose to prevent the development of diabetes in subjects with impaired glucose tolerance (180). Individuals taking acarbose were 25% less likely to develop diabetes than placebo treated subjects. The Diabetes Prevention Program compared the effect of metformin versus lifestyle changes in the prevention of diabetes (Fig. 14) (181). After an average follow-up of 2.8 years, lifestyle changes were about twice as effective at preventing diabetes, as metformin. The Troglitazone in the Prevention of Diabetes Study compared the effect of troglitazone: 400 mg daily to placebo to prevent the development of diabetes in young women with a history of gestational diabetes (182). Therapy with troglitazone reduced the risk of developing diabetes over a four-year period about 60%. Thus, pharmacologic therapy with weight-loss agents, antidiabetic agents, and insulin sensitizers has been shown to delay the onset of diabetes. To date, no pharmacologic agent has been shown to be superior to diet and exercise, in the prevention of diabetes. Our patient was not started on pharmacologic therapy.

▓ Case: A Patient with Polycystic Ovary Syndrome

A 23-year-old female presents with a chief complaint of hirsutism and weight gain. She has noted excessive facial hair growth on her face, chest, and abdomen over the last two years. She has a documented weight gain of 20 kg between age 17 and 18. She had pubarche at age nine but has never had regular menses. She has never had more than five periods in a year. She has had unprotected intercourse with her husband for the past two years and has not become pregnant.

Family history is significant for early onset of pubarche, irregular menses, and hirsutism in her mother and two older sisters. Her 50-year-old mother had diabetes since age 40. The patient denies breast discharge, change in ring or shoe size, use of steroids, and deepening of voice.

Physical examination is pertinent for the presence of acanthosis nigricans and hyperpigmentation on the neck and groin. Terminal hair is present on the upper lip, chest, and abdomen. Blood pressure is 130/80 mmHg, BMI is 31, and waist circumference is 38 inches.

Laboratory assessment shows free testosterone levels are 1.5 times the upper limit of normal. The Luteinizing hormone (LH): Follicle-stimulating hormone (FSH) ratio was greater than 2.0 on two determinations. Serum prolactin, dehydroepiandrosterone sulfate (DHEA-S), 17-OH progesterone, and a 24-hour urine-free cortisol were normal. A fasting lipid profile showed a LDL-C of 110 mg/dL, TGs of 160 mg/dL, and HDL-C of 52 mg/dL. Fasting glucose is 106 mg/dL. Abdominal/pelvic ultrasound is significant for multiple cysts of the ovary.

A diagnosis of polycystic ovary syndrome (PCOS) is made based on the combination of oligomenorrhea, elevated levels of ovarian androgens, positive family history, multiple ovarian cysts, and exclusion of other hormonal disorders.

It is quite clear that PCOS has a variety of causes and may be inherited (183–187). Disorders, which affect the hypothalamic-pituitary-ovarian axis as well as genetic causes of insulin resistance, may lead to a similar clinical picture. Dunaif and colleagues have shown defects in the insulin-signaling pathways in both fat and skeletal muscle in patients with the PCOS (188–190). Because insulin resistance

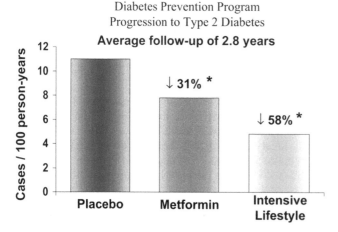

Diabetes Prevention Program
Progression to Type 2 Diabetes

Average follow-up of 2.8 years

↓ **31%** *

↓ **58%** *

Cases / 100 person-years

Placebo   Metformin   Intensive Lifestyle

FIGURE 14 The Diabetes prevention program compared the effect of metformin to lifestyle changes in the prevention of diabetes. *Source*: From Ref. 182.

and hyperinsulinemia play a central role in the development of the metabolic syndrome, the term "syndrome XX" has been suggested to describe this sex-specific metabolic syndrome (190,192). Obesity may cause or exacerbate PCOS. Up to 75% of women with PCOS in some series are obese (193). Not surprisingly, women in the United States with PCOS have a higher body weight than European women with the same diagnosis (193–196).

PCOS is present in 10% of reproductive age females making it the most common metabolic abnormality in young women (197–199). A clinical diagnosis of PCOS can be made in a woman who has oligomenorrhea (fewer than nine menstrual cycles per year) or amenorrhea and elevated levels of ovarian androgens (200). Patients will often present with cutaneous manifestations of androgen excess such as hirsutism, male pattern hair loss, or acne. Before a diagnosis of PCOS is made, other causes of androgen excess such as congenital adrenal hyperplasia, adrenal or ovarian tumors producing androgens, and hyperprolactinemia or Cushing's syndrome should be ruled out.

The symptoms of PCOS usually begin around menarche (201) but may present several years after puberty, usually as a result of significant weight gain. Premature pubarche may predict future PCOS. About half of young girls with premature pubarche will develop ovarian hyperandrogenism (202).

Women with PCOS are more efficient at making ovarian androgens than estrogen (203,204). Ovarian theca cells synthesize androstenedione, which can be converted by 17 beta-hydroxysteroid dehydrogenase (17b-HSD) to testosterone in the theca cell or aromatized by the aromatase enzyme in the granulosa cell to form estrone (Fig. 15) LH produced in pulsatile fashion by the anterior pituitary gland is responsible for theca cell androgen production while FSH stimulates aromatase activity within the granulose cell and regulates the production of estrone. An increase in the production of LH in relation to FSH will result in preferential production of adrenal androgen.

The pulse frequency of the hypothalamic hormone gonadotropin-releasing hormone (GnRH) determines the relative proportion of LH and FSH release from the anterior pituitary (Fig. 15). Increasing the pulse frequency of GnRH favors the production of LH, while a slower frequency favors FSH production (205). Because women with PCOS have an increased LH:FSH ratio, one of the causes of PCOS may be an increased pulse frequency of GnRH. This may be a primary defect or a result of low levels of progesterone in a woman with oligomenorrhea (206).

Hyperinsulinemia, which results from insulin resistance can cause or exacerbate PCOS. Insulin enhances the action of LH to stimulate the production of androgen by the theca cells. Insulin also inhibits the production of sex hormone–binding globulin (SHBG), the main protein, which binds testosterone. Because only unbound or "free" testosterone is active, a decrease in SHBG will increase the proportion of active testosterone.

CARDIOVASCULAR DISEASE IN POLYCYSTIC OVARY SYNDROME

A risk factor model analysis of 1462 women in Sweden who underwent an assessment in a prospective population study estimated a four- to sevenfold increased risk of myocardial infarction in women with PCOS compared with age-matched controls (207). In this study, women with PCOS were more likely to be diabetic (15% vs. 2.3%), and with a threefold increased incidence of hypertension, an increased waist-hip ratio, and higher levels of insulin. In a study from the Czech Republic (208), 28 women with PCOS were compared with 752 control women matched for BMI, waist-hip ratio, hypertension, dyslipidemia, and smoking.

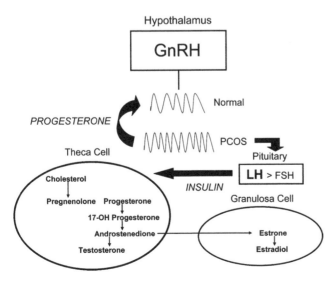

FIGURE 15 Pathway of ovarian androgen and estrogen production. In PCOS an increase in the pulse frequent of GnRH increases LH production which stimulats androgen production by Theca cells. *Abbreviations*: LH, Luteinizing hormone; PCOS, polycystic ovary syndrome; FSH, follicle-stimulating hormone; GnRH, gonadotropine-releasing hormone. *Source*: From Ref. 205.

Women with PCOS were more likely to be diabetic (32% vs. 8%), and have diagnosed coronary artery disease (21% vs. 5%) than control subjects.

In Holland, 346 lean (BMI: 24.4 kg/m^2) women with PCOS had an increased prevalence of hypertension, diabetes mellitus, and cardiac symptoms (209). Echocardiographic evidence of cardiac dysfunction was seen in women under age 30 with PCOS independent of weight (210). A Mayo clinic study of 36 nondiabetic women aged 30 to 45 with PCOS revealed a threefold higher level of coronary artery calcification compared to control women (211). Women with PCOS had twofold higher coronary artery calcification than a group of control obese women. In a study of 102 women aged 40 to 61 with PCOS compared to 118 control subjects, the mean coronary calcification score was 25.2 versus 4.1, respectively (212). PCOS, BMI, smoking, increased levels of insulin, and low levels of HDL-C were all associated with an increase in coronary calcification.

The Nurses' Health Study is a prospective study of 101,000 female nurses. Oligomenorrhea was associated with a 2- to 2.5-fold increased risk of developing diabetes (213). A 14 year prospective surveillance of 82,439 nurses aged 20 to 35 in this study showed a history of oligomenorrhea was associated with a 100% increase in fatal and a 50% increase in nonfatal coronary artery disease (214). While androgen status was not measured in this study, it is likely that the majority of women in this study with oligomenorrhea would have met the criteria for PCOS.

Obesity is associated with reduced fertility. In the Nurses' Health Study, infertility increases above a BMI 26 mg/m^2 (215). In addition, fat distribution is even more important than BMI in determining fertility. Comparing women with a waist:hip ratio less than 0.8 and more than 0.8 who had artificial insemination, women with central obesity were less likely to become pregnant (216). Eighty-seven Australian women with PCOS who desired fertility were placed on a gradual weight-loss program emphasizing sensible eating and exercise. Twenty of the women dropped out but 90% of those who stayed in the study ovulated and 78% became pregnant (217). A subsequent randomized controlled trial of 84 women meeting weekly with 87 control subjects showed a six-month weight loss of 4.7 versus 1.3 kg with 61 versus 21% becoming pregnant by 18 months (218). No distinct benefit of diets limiting fat versus carbohydrates has been found in this condition (219).

Our patient was placed on a hypocaloric diet designed to lead to a weight loss of one pound per week. She was advised to do aerobic exercise for 30 to 45 minutes five days per week and participate in resistance training for 30 to 45 minutes twice weekly.

PHARMACOLOGIC TREATMENT OF PCOS

A reduction in insulin levels will lower the production of ovarian androgens. Both metformin and the thiazolidinediones (TZDs) (pioglitazone and rosiglitazone) have been used to treat PCOS. Metformin directly inhibits the production of ovarian androgens (220,221) and decreases the amount of insulin necessary to control glucose by inhibiting hepatic glucose production. A meta-analysis of 13 studies in which metformin was administered to 543 women (222) showed women treated with metformin were 3.9 times more likely to ovulate compared with placebo-treated patients. Similarly, women treated with a combination of metformin and clomiphene were 4.4 times more likely to ovulate compared to women given clomiphene alone. Women who conceive while taking metformin have a lower rate of miscarriage and gestational diabetes (223–226). Metformin is a category B drug for pregnancy.

The TZDs directly reduce ovarian steroid synthesis (227) and indirectly lower ovarian androgen synthesis by reducing levels of insulin. The TZDs are the most potent insulin sensitizers available and have a major impact on fat and muscle and improve insulin sensitivity at the liver to a lesser degree. In a double-blind, randomized, placebo-controlled trial-ovulation was significantly more frequent in women given troglitazone (192). Levels of free testosterone decreased and SHBG increased in a dose-dependent manner. Similar findings were seen with rosiglitazone (228,229) and pioglitazone (230). TZDs are category C drugs for pregnancy.

In a study of normal weight, women with PCOS (BMI: 24 kg/m^2) (231) treated for six months with 850 mg of metformin twice-daily versus 4 mg of rosiglitazone twice-daily, versus both or neither, ovulatory cycles were more frequent with metformin. Testosterone improved with both therapies and there was no evidence of synergistic effect. When metformin therapy was compared to laparoscopic ovarian drilling, ovulation occurred in 55% of metformin treated patients and 53% of women treated surgically (232). Live birth rates were higher in metformin-treated women (82% of pregnancies vs. 65%). Metformin has been shown to reduce first trimester pregnancy loss in two additional studies (233,234). Because metformin is a category B drug for pregnancy it is not contraindicated during pregnancy, although it cannot be stated to be safe. Most experts recommend it be discontinued when the patient becomes pregnant. Some have advocated using metformin during the first 12 weeks of pregnancy in women who have a history of early pregnancy loss (235).

After three months of diet therapy, the patient expressed a desire to become pregnant. Metformin was given as an initial dose of 500 mg po daily and titrated to 1000 mg twice daily over one month. After four months of combined diet and metformin treatment, the patient became pregnant.

REFERENCES

1. Reaven GM. Role of insulin resistance in human disease. Diabetes 1988; 37:1595–1607.
2. World Health Organization. Definition, diagnosis and classification of diabetes mellitus and its complications. Report of a WHO consultation, 1999.
3. Executive summary of the Third Report of the National Cholesterol Eduction Program (NCEP) Expert Panel on detection, evaluations, and treatment of high blood cholesterol in Adults (Adult Treatment Panel III). JAMA 2001; 285:2486–2497.
4. International Diabetes Federation: The IDF consensus worldwide definition of the metabolic syndrome. Available from http://www.idf.org/webdata/docs/Metabolic_ syndrome_definition.pdf. Accessed 2 September 2005.
5. Kahn R, Buse J, Ferrannini E, Stern M. The metabolic syndrome: time for a critical appraisal: Joint statement from the American Diabetes Association and the European Association for the Study of Diabetes. DiabetesCare 2005; 28:2289–2304.
6. Circulation AHA 1051649.
7. Ford ES. Prevalence of the metabolic syndrome defined by the International Diabetes Federation Among Adults in the U.S. Diabetes Care 2005; 28:2745–2749.
8. Adams RJ, Appleton S, Wilson DH, et al. Population Comparison of Two Clinical Approaches to the Metabolic Syndrome: Implications of the new International Diabetes Federation consensus definition. Diabetes Care 2005; 28:2777–2779.
9. International obesity Task Force, 2003.
10. Ogden CL, Flegal KM, Carroll MD, Johnson CL. Prevalence and trends in overweight among US children and adolescents, 1999–2000. JAMA 2002; 288:1728–1732.
11. Weiss R, Dziura J, Burgert TS, et al. Obesity and the metabolic syndrome in children and adolescents. N Engl J Med 2004; 350:2362–2374.
12. DeFronzo RA. Pathogenesis of type 2 diabetes mellitus: metabolic and molecular implications for identifying diabetes genes. Diabetes 1997; 5:117–269.
13. Gerich JE, Meyer C, Woerle HJ, Stumvoll M. Renal gluconeogenesis. Its importance in human glucose homeostasis. Diabetes Care 2001; 24:382–391.
14. Ekberg K, Landau BR, Wajngot A, et al. Contributions by kidney and liver to glucose production in the postabsorptive state and after 60 h of fasting. Diabetes 1999; 48:292–298.
15. DeFronzo RA. Lilly Lecture. The triumvirate: beta cell, muscle, liver. A collusion responsible for NIDDM. Diabetes 1988; 37:667–687.
16. Groop LC, Bonadonna RC, Del Prato S, et al. Glucose and free fatty acid metabolism in non-insulin dependent diabetes mellitus. Evidence for multiple sites of insulin resistance. J Clin Invest 1989; 84:205–215.
17. DeFronzo RA, Ferrannini E, Simonson DC. Fasting hyperglycemia in non-insulin-dependent diabetes mellitus: contributions of excessive hepatic glucose production and impaired tissue glucose uptake. Metabolism 1989; 38:387–395.
18. Huang SC, Phelps ME, Hoffman EJ, Sideris K, Selin CJ, Kuhl DE. Non-invasive determination of local cerebral metabolic rate of glucose in man. Am J Physiol 1980; 238:E69–E82.
19. DeFronzo RA, Jacot E, Jequier E, Maeder E, Wahren J, Felber JP. The effect of insulin on the disposal of intravenous glucose: results from indirect calorimetry. Diabetes 1981; 30:1000–1007.
20. DeFronzo RA. Pathogenesis of type 2 (non-insulin dependent) diabetes mellitus: a balanced overview. Diabetologia 1992; 35:389–397.
21. Katz LD, Glickman MG, Rapoport S, Ferrannini E, DeFronzo RA. Splanchnic and peripheral disposal of oral glucose in man. Diabetes 1983; 32:675–679.
22. Ferrannini E, Bjorkman O, Reichard GA Jr., et al. The disposal of an oral glucose load in healthy subjects. Diabetes 1985; 34:580–588.
23. Mitrakou A, Kelley D, Veneman T, et al. Contribution of abnormal muscle and liver glucose metabolism to postprandial hyperglycemia in NIDDM. Diabetes 1990; 39:1381–1390.
24. Mandarino L, Bonadonna R, McGuinness O, Wasserman D. Regulation of muscle glucose uptake in vivo. Handbook of physiology, section 7. The endocrine system. In: Jefferson LS. AD Cherrington, eds. The Endocrine Pancreas and Regulation of Metab. Oxford University Press, 2001:2 803–848.
25. Jansson P-A, Larsson A, Smith U, Lonroth P. Lactate release from the subcutaneous tissue in lean and obese men. J Clin Invest 1994; 93:240–246.

26. Ryysy L, Hakkinen AM, Goto T, et al. Hepatic fat content and insulin action on free fatty acids and glucose metabolism rather than insulin absorption are associated with insulin requirements during insulin therapy in type 2 diabetic patients. Diabetes 2000; 49:749–758.

27. Santomauro A, Boden G, Silva M, et al. Overnight lowering of free fatty acids with acipimox improves insulin resistance and glucose tolerance in obese diabetic and non-diabetic subjects. Diabetes 1999; 48:1836–1841.

28. Bergman RN. Non-esterified fatty acids and the liver: why is insulin secreted into the portal vein? Diabetologia 2000; 43:946–952.

29. Boden G. Role of fatty acids in the pathogenesis of insulin resistance and NIDDM. Diabetes 1997; 46:3–10.

30. McGarry JD. Banting lecture 2001: dysregulation of fatty acid metabolism in the etiology of type 2 diabetes. Diabetes 2002; 51:7–18.

31. Cherrington AD, Stevenson RW, Steiner KE, et al. Insulin, glucagon, and glucose as regulators of hepatic glucose uptake and production in vivo. Diabetes Metab Rev 1987; 3:307–332.

32. Consoli A, Nurjahn N, Capani F, Gerich J. Predominant role of gluconeogenesis in increased hepatic glucose production in NIDDM. Diabetes 1989; 38:550–556.

33. Nurjhan N, Consoli A, Gerich J. Increased lipolysis and its consequences on gluconeogenesis in noninsulin-dependent diabetes mellitus. J Clin Invest 1992; 89:169–175.

34. Bjorntorp P, Berchtold P, Holm J. The glucose uptake of human adipose tissue in obesity. Eur J Clin Invest 1971; 1:480–485.

35. Frayn KN, Coppack SW, Humphreys SM, Whyte PL. Metabolic characteristics of human adipose tissue in vivo. Clin Sci 1989; 76:509–516.

36. DeFronzo RA, Gunnarsson R, Bjorkman O, Olsson M, Wahren J. Effects of insulin on peripheral and splanchnic glucose metabolism in non-insulin-dependent (type II) diabetes mellitus. J Clin Invest 1985; 76:149–155.

37. Bonadonna RC, Bonora E. Glucose and free fatty acid metabolism in human obesity: relationships to insulin resistance. Diabetes Rev 1997; 5:21–51.

38. Reaven GM, Chen Y-DI, Donner CC, Fraze E, Hollenbeck CB. How insulin resistant are patients with non-insulin-dependent diabetes mellitus? J Clin Endocrinol Metab 1985; 61:32–36.

39. Lillioja A, Mott DM, Zawadzki JK, Young AA, Abbott WG, Bogardus C. Glucose storage is a major determinant of in vivo 'insulin resistance' in subjects with normal glucose tolerance. J Clin Endocrinol Metab 1986; 62:922–927.

40. Jallut D, Golay A, Munger R, et al. Impaired glucose tolerance and diabetes in obesity: a 6 year follow-up study of glucose metabolism. Metabolism 1990; 39:1068–1075.

41. Golay A, DeFronzo RA, Ferrannini E, et al. Oxidative and non-oxidative glucose metabolism in non-obese Type 2 (non-insulin dependent) diabetic patients. Diabetologia 1988; 31:585–1591.

42. Golay A, Felber JP, Jequier E, DeFronzo RA, Ferrannini E. Metabolic basis of obesity and noninsulin-dependent diabetes mellitus. Diabetes Metab Rev 1988; 4:727–747.

43. Hales CN. The pathogenesis of NIDDM. Diabetologia 1994; 37:S162–S168.

44. Reaven GM, Hollenbeck C, Jeng C-Y, Wu MS, Chen Y-DI. Measurement of plasma glucose, free fatty acid, lactate, and insulin for 24 hours in patients with NIDDM. Diabetes 1988; 37:1020–1104.

45. Ferrannini E, Natali A, Bell P, Cavallo-Perin P, Lalic N, Mingrone G. On behalf of the European Group for the Study of Insulin Resistance (EGIR). Insulin resistance and hypersecretion in obesity. J Clin Invest 1997; 100:1166–1173.

46. Montague CT, O'Rahilly S. The Perils of Portliness: causes and consequences of visceral adiposity. Diabetes 2000; 49:883–888.

47. Kelley DE, Williams KV, Price JC, McKolanis TM, Goodpaster BH, Thaete FL. Plasma fatty acids, adiposity and variance of skeletal muscle insulin resistance in type 2 diabetes mellitus. J Clin Endocrinol Metab 2001; 86:5412–5419.

48. Bjorntorp P. Metabolic implications of body fat distribution. Diabetes Care 1991; 14:1132–1143.

49. Arner P. Regional adiposity in man. J Endocrinol 1997; 155:191–192.

50. Thiebaud D, DeFronzo RA, Jacot E, et al. Effect of long-chain triglyceride infusion on glucose metabolism in man. Metab 1982; 31:1128–1136.

51. Kelley De, Mandarino LJ. Fuel selection in human skeletal muscle in insulin resistance. A reexamination. Diabetes 2000; 49:677–683.

52. Kashyap S, Belfort R, Pratipanawatr T, et al. Chronic elevation in plasma free fatty acids impairs insulin secretion in non-diabetic offspring with a strong family history of T2DM. Diabetes 2002; 51(Suppl 2):A12.

53. Carpentier A, Mittelman SD, Bergman RN, Giacca A, Lewis GF. Prolonged elevation of plasma free fatty acids impairs pancreatic beta-cell function in obese nondiabetic humans but not in individuals with type 2 diabetes. Diabetes 2000; 49:399–408.

54. Goodpaster BH, Thaete FL, Kelley BE. Thigh adipose tissue distribution is associated with insulin resistance in obesity and in type 2 diabetes mellitus. Am J Clin Nutr 2000; 71:885–892.

55. Greco AV, Mingrone G, Giancaterini A, et al. Insulin resistance in morbid obesity. Reversal with intramyocellular fat depletion. Diabetes 2002; 51:144–151.

56. Miyazaki Y, Mahankali A, Matsuda M, et al. Effect of pioglitazone on abdominal fat distribution and insulin sensitivity in type 2 diabetic patients. J Clin Endocrinol Metab 2002; 87:2784–2791.

57. Staiger H, Haring HU. Adipocytokines: fat-derived humoral mediators of metabolic homeostasis. Exp clin Endocrin & Diab 2005; 113:67–79.

58. Kelley, DE. The Impact of Obesitgy, Regional Adiposity and Ectopic Fat on the Pathophysiology of Type 2 Diabetes; Council on Obesity Diabetes Education—2003; 12–20.
59. Pischon T, Girman CJ, Hotamisligil GS, et al. Plasm adiponectin levels and risk of myocardial infarction in men. JAMA 2004; 291:1730–1737.
60. Goodpaster BH, Kelley DE, Wing RR, Meier A, Thaete FL. Effects of weight loss on insulin sensitivity in obesity: influence of regional adiposity. Diabetes 1999; 48:839–847.
61. Weyer C, Foley JE, Bogardus C, Tataranni PA, Pratley RE. Enlarged subcutaneous abdominal adipocyte size, but not obesity itself, predicts type 2 diabetes independent of insulin resistance. Diabetologia 2000; 43:1498–1506.
62. Hotamisligil GS, Arner S, Caro P, Atkinson JF, Spiegelman RL, Bruce M. Increased adipose tissue expression of tumor necrosis factor-alpha in human obesity and insulin resistance. J Clin Invest 1995; 95:2409–2415.
63. Kern PA, Saghizadeh, M, Ong JM, Bosch RJ, Deem R, Simsolo RB. The expression of tumor necrosis factor in human adipose tissue: regulation by obesity, weight loss, and relationship to lipoprotein lipase. J Clin Invest 1995; 95:2111–2119.
64. Saltiel AR, Kahn CR. Insulin signaling and the regulation of glucose and lipid metabolism. Nature 2001; 414:799–806.
65. Virkamaki A, Ueki K, Kahn CR. Protein-protein interaction in insulin signaling and the molecular mechanisms of insulin resistance. J Clin Invest 1999; 103:931–943.
66. Pessin JE, Saltiel AR. Signaling pathways in insulin action: molecular targets of insulin resistance. J Clin Invest 2000; 106:165–169.
67. Whitehead JP, Clark SF, Urso B, James DE. Signalling through the insulin receptor. CurOpin Cell Biol 2000; 12:222–1228.
68. Shepherd PR, Kahn BB. Glucose transporters and insulin action. Implications for insulin resistance and diabetes mellitus. N Engl J Med 1999; 341:248–2457.
69. Garvey WT. Insulin action and insulin resistance: diseases involving defects in insulin receptors, signal transduction, and the glucose transport effector system. Am J Med 1998; 105:331–345.
70. Okada T, Sakuma L, Fukui Y, Hazeki O, Ui M. Essential role of phosphatidylinositol 3-kinase in insulin-induced glucose transport and antilipolysis in rat adipocytes. J Biol Chem 1994; 269:3568–3573.
71. Cross D, Alessi D, Vandenheed J, McDowell H, Hundal H, Cohen P. The inhibition of glycogen synthase kinase-3 by insulin-like growth factor 1 in the rat skeletal muscle cell line L6 is blocked by wortmannin but not rapamycin. Biochem J 1994; 303:21–26.
72. Thomas G, Hall MN. TOR signalling and control of cell growth. Cur Opin Cell Biol 1997; 9:782–787.
73. Nave BT, Ouwens M, Withers DJ, Alessi DR, Shepherd PR. Mammalian target of rapamycin is a direct target for protein kinase B: identification of a convergence point for opposing effects of insulin and amino-acid deficiency on protein translation. Biochem J 1999; 344(Pt 2):427–431.
74. Kerouz NJ, Horsch D, Pons S, Kahn CR. Differential regulation of insulin receptor substrates-1 and -2 (IRS-1 and IRS-2) and phosphatidylinositol 3-kinase isoforms in liver and muscle of the obese diabetic (ob/ob) mouse. J Clin Invest 1997; 100:3164–3172.
75. Chiang SH, Baumann CA, Kanzaki M, et al. Insulin-stimulated GLUT4 translocation requires the CAP-dependent activation of TC10. Nature 2001; 410:944–948.
76. Boulton TG, Nye SH, Robbins DJ, et al. ERKs: a family of protein-serine/threonine kinases that are activated and tyrosine phosphorylated in response to insulin and NGF. Cell 1991; 65:663–675.
77. Lazar DF, Wiese RJ, Brady MJ, et al. Mitogen-activated protein kinase kinase inhibition does not block the stimulation of glucose utilization by insulin. J Biol Chem 1995; 270:20801–20807.
78. Dorrestijn J, Ouwens DM, Van den Berghe N, Box JL, Maassen JA. Expression of dominant-negative Ras mutant does not affect stimulation of glucose uptake and glycogen synthesis by insulin. Diabetologia 1996; 39:558–563.
79. Caro JF, Sinha MK, Raju SM, et al. Insulin receptor kinase in human skeletal muscle from obese subjects with and without non-insulin dependent diabetes. J Clin Invest 1987; 79:1330–1337.
80. Caro JF, Ittoop O, Pories WJ, et al. Studies on the mechanism of insulin resistance in the liver from humans with non-insulin-dependent diabetes. Insulin action and binding in isolated hepatocytes, insulin receptor structure, and kinase activity. J Clin Invest 1986; 78:249–258.
81. Comi RJ, Grunberger G, Gorden P. Relationship of insulin binding and insulin-stimulated tyrosine kinase activity is altered in type II diabetes. J Clin Invest 1987; 79:453–462.
82. Klein HH, Vestergaard H, Kotzke G, Pedersen O. Elevation of serum insulin concentration during euglycemic hyperinsulinemic clamp studies leads to similar activation of insulin receptor kinase in skeletal muscle of subjects with and without NIDDM. Diabetes 1995; 344:1310–1317.
83. Obermaier-Kusser B, White MF, Pongratz DE, et al. A defective intramolecular autoactivation cascade may cause the reduced kinase activity of the skeletal muscle insulin receptor from patients with non-insulin-dependent diabetes mellitus. J Biol Chem 1989; 264:9497–9503.
84. Cocozza S, Procellini A, Riccardi G, et al. NIDDM associated with mutation in tyrosine kinase domain of insulin receptor gene. Diabetes 1992; 41:521–526.
85. Moller DE, Yakota A, Flier JS. Normal insulin receptor cDNA sequence in Pima Indians with non-insulin-dependent diabetes mellitus. Diabetes 1989; 38:1496–1500.

86. Kusari J, Verma US, Buse JB, Henry RR, Olefsky JM. Analysis of the gene sequences of the insulin receptor and the insulin-sensitive glucose transporter (GLUT4) in patients with common-type non-insulin-dependent diabetes mellitus. J Clin Invest 1991; 88:1323–1330.

87. Wilden PA, Kahn CR. The level of insulin receptor tyrosine kinase activity modulates the activities of phosphatidylinositol 3-kinase, microtubule-associated protein, and S6 kinases. Mol Endo 1994; 8:558–567.

88. Nyomba BL, Ossowski VM, Bogardus C, Mott DM. Insulin-sensitive tyrosine kinase relationship with in vivo insulin action in humans. Am J Physiol 1990; 258:E964–E974.

89. Nolan JJ, Friedenberg G, Henry R, Reichart D, Olefsky JM. Role of human skeletal muscle insulin receptor kinase in the in vivo insulin resistance of noninsulin-dependent diabetes and obesity. J Clin Endocrinol Metab 1994; 78:471–477.

90. Krook A, Bjornholm M, Galuska D, et al. Characterization of signal transduction and glucose transport in skeletal muscle from type 2 diabetic patients. Diabetes 2000; 49:284–292.

91. Freidenberg GR, Reichart D, Olefsky JM, Henry RR. Reversibility of defective adipocyte insulin receptor kinase activity in non-insulin dependent diabetes mellitus. Effect of weight loss. J Clin Invest 1988; 82:1398–1406.

92. Wajtaszewski JFP, Hansen BF, Kiens B, Richter EA. Insulin signaling in human skeletal muscle. Time course and effect of exercise. Diabetes 1997; 46:1775–1781.

93. Pratipanawatr W, Pratipanawatr T, Cusi K, et al. Skeletal muscle insulin resistance in normoglycemic subjects with a strong family history of type 2 diabetes is associated with decreased insulin-stimulated insulin receptor substrate-1 tyrosine phosphorylation. Diabetes 2001; 50:2572–2578.

94. Laville M, Auboeuf D, Khalfallah Y, Vega N, Riou JP, Vidal H. Acute regulation by insulin of phosphatidylinositol-3-kinase, Rad, Glut 4, and lipoprotein lipase in mRNA levels in human muscle. J Clin Invest 1996; 98:43–49.

95. Kim Y-B, Nikoulina S, Ciaraldi TP, Henry RR, Kahn BB. Normal insulin-dependent activation of Akt/protein kinase B, with diminished activation of phosphoinositide 3-kinase, in muscle in type 2 diabetes. J Clin Invest 1999; 104:733–741.

96. Haffner SM. Management of dyslipidemia in adults with diabetes. Diabetes Care 1998; 21:160–178.

97. Austin MA, King MC, Vranizan KM, Krauss RM. Atherogenic lipoprotein phenotype. A proposed genetic marker for coronary heart disease risk. Circulation 1990; 82:495–506.

98. Http://www.lipidsonline

99. Sztalryd C, Kraemer FB. Regulation of hormone-sensitive lipase in streptozotocin-induced diabetic rats. Metabolism 1995; 44:1391–1396.

100. Ginsberg HN. Diabetic dyslipidemia: basic mechanisms underlying the common hypertriglyceridemia and low HDL cholesterol levels. Diabetes 1996; 45(suppl 3):S27–S30.

101. Brown MS, Kovanen PT, Goldstein JL. Regulation of plasma cholesterol by lipoprotein receptors. Science 1981; 212:628–635.

102. Boden G, Chen X, Ruiz J, White JV, Rossetti L. Mechanisms of fatty acid-induced inhibition of glucose uptake. J Clin Invest 1994; 93:2438–2446.

103. Bucala R, Makita Z, Vega G, et al. Modification of low density lipoprotein by advanced glycation end products contributes to the dyslipidemia of diabetes and renal insufficiency. Proc Natl Acad Sci USA. 1994; 91:9441–9445.

104. Verges BL. Dyslipidaemia in diabetes mellitus. Review of the main lipoprotein abnormalities and their consequences on the development of atherogenesis. Diabetes Metab 1999; 25(suppl 3):32–40.

105. Tall AR. An overview of reverse cholesterol transport. Eur Heart J 1998; 19(suppl A):A31–A35.

106. Rohrer L, Hersberger M, von Eckardstein A. High density lipoproteins in the intersection of diabetes mellitus, inflammation and cardiovascular disease. Curr Opin Lipidol 2004; 15:269–278.

107. Howard BV. Insulin resistance and lipid metabolism. Am J Cardiol 1999; 84(suppl 1):28–32.

108. Calles-Escandon J, Garcia-Rubi E, Mirza S, Mortensen A. Type 2 diabetes: one disease, multiple cardiovascular risk factors. Coron Artery Dis 1999; 10:23–30.

109. Rosenson RS, Lowe GDO. Effects of lipids and lipoproteins on thrombosis and rheology. Atherosclerosis 1998; 140:271–280.

110. Reaven GM. Multiple CHD risk factors in type 2 diabetes: beyond hyperglycaemia. Diabetes Obes Metab 2002; 4(suppl 1):S13–S18.

111. Ridker PM, Hennekens CH, Buring JE, Rifai N. C-reactive protein and other markers of inflammation in the prediction of cardiovascular disease in women. N Engl J Med 2000; 342:836–843.

112. Koenig W, Sund M, Fröhlich M, et al. C-Reactive protein, a sensitive marker of inflammation, predicts future risk of coronary heart disease in initially healthy middle-aged men: results from the MONICA (Monitoring Trends and Determinants in Cardiovascular Disease) Augsburg Cohort Study, 1984 to 1992. Circulation 1999; 99:237–242.

113. Danesh J, Collins R, Appleby P, Peto R. Association of fibrinogen, C-reactive protein, albumin, or leukocyte count with coronary heart disease: meta-analyses of prospective studies. JAMA 1998; 279:1477–1482.

114. Ford ES. Body mass index, diabetes, and C-reactive protein among U.S. adults. Diabetes Care 1999; 22:1971–1977.

115. Expert Panel on Detection, Evaluation, and Treatment of High Blood Cholesterol in Adults. National Cholesterol Education Program (Adult Treatment Panel III): full report. NIH Publication No. 02-5215. September 2002. Bethesda, MD: NIH National Heart, Lung, and Blood Institute; 2002.

116. Expert Panel on Detection, Evaluation, and Treatment of High Blood Cholesterol in Adults. Report of the National Cholesterol Education Program Expert Panel on Detection, Evaluation, and Treatment of High Blood Cholesterol in Adults. Arch Intern Med 1988; 148:36–69.

117. American Diabetes Association. Management of dyslipidemia in adults with diabetes. Diabetes Care 2002; 25(suppl 1):S74–S77.

118. Mosca L, Appel LJ, Benjamin EJ, et al. Evidence-based guidelines for cardiovascular disease prevention in women. Circulation 2004; 109:672–693.

119. O' Keefe JH, Cordain L, Harris WH, Moe Rm, Vogal R. Optimal low-density lipoprotein is 50 to 70 mg/dl lower is better and physiologically normal. J Am Coll Cardiol 2004; 43:2142–2146.

120. Heart Protection Study Collaborative Group. MRC/BHF Heart Protection Study of cholesterol lowering with simvastatin in 20 536 high-risk individuals: a randomised placebo-controlled trial. Lancet 2002; 360:7–22.

121. Heart Protection Study Collaborative Group. MRC/BHF Heart Protection Study of cholesterol-lowering with simvastatin in 5963 people with diabetes: a randomised placebo-controlled trial. Lancet 2003; 361:2005–2016.

122. A desktop guide to type 2 diabetes mellitus: European Diabetes Policy Group 1999, Diabet Med 1999; 16:716–730.

123. Grundy SM, Cleeman JI, Merz CN, et al. Coordinating Committee of the National Cholesterol Education Program. Implications of recent clinical trials for the National Cholesterol Education Program Adult Treatment Panel III guidelines. Circulation 2004; 110:227–239.

124. LaRosa JC, Grundy SM, Waters DD, et al. Treating to New Targets (TNT) Investigators. Treating to New Targets (TNT) Investigators. Intensive lipid lowering with atorvastatin in patients with stable coronary disease. N Engl J Med 2005; 352:1425–1435.

125. Kastelein JJP. The future of best practice. Atherosclerosis 1999; 143 (Suppl): S17–S21.

126. Pederson TR, Faergeman O, Kastelein JJP, et al. For the Incremental Decrease in End Points Through Aggressive Lipid Lowering (IDEAL) Study Group. High-dose atorvastatin vs usual-dose simvastatin for secondary prevention after myocardial infarction. The IDEAL Study: A Randomized Controlled Trial. JAMA 2005; 294:2437–2445.

127. Taylor AJ, et al. ARBITER 2: Adouble-blind placebo-controlled study of extended release niacin on athero sclerosis progression in secondary prevention patients treated with statins. Circulation 2004; epub ahead of print ARBITER 3: AHA November 2005, Dallas TX.

128. Expert Panel on Detection, Evaluation, and Treatment of High Blood Cholesterol in Adults. Executive Summary of the Third Report of the National Cholesterol Education Program (NCEP) Expert Panel on Detection, Evaluation, and Treatment of High Blood Cholesterol in Adults (Adult Treatment Panel III). JAMA 2001; 285:2486–2497.

129. Koskinen P, Mänttäri M, Manninen V, Huttunen JK, Heinonen OP, Frick MH. Coronary heart disease incidence in NIDDM patients in the Helsinki Heart Study. Diabetes Care 1992; 15:820–825.

130. Rubins HB, Robins SJ, Collins D, et al. Diabetes, plasma insulin, and cardiovascular disease: subgroup analysis from the Department of Veterans Affairs high-density lipoprotein intervention trial (VA-HIT). Arch Intern Med 2002; 162:2597–2604.

131. Rubins HB, Robins SJ, Collins D, et al, for the Veterans Affairs High-Density Lipoprotein Cholesterol Intervention Trial Study Group. Gemfibrozil for the secondary prevention of coronary heart disease in men with low levels of high-density lipoprotein cholesterol. N Engl J Med 1999; 341:410–418.

132. Diabetes Atherosclerosis Intervention Study Investigators. Effect of fenofibrate on progression of coronary-artery disease in type 2 diabetes: the Diabetes Atherosclerosis Intervention Study, a randomised study. Lancet 2001; 357:905–910.

133. The FIELD Study investigators. www.thelancet.com published online Nov 14, 2005.

134. Robins SJ, Collins D, Wittes JT, et al. For the VA-HIT Study Group. Relation of gemfibrozil treatment and lipid levels with major coronary events: VA-HIT: A randomized controlled tiral. JAMA 2001; 285:1585–1591.

135. Athyros VG, Papageorgiou AA, Athyrou VV, Demitriadis DS, Kontopoulos AG. Atorvastatin and micronized fenofibrate alone and in combination in type 2 diabetes with combined hyperlipidemia. Diabetes Care 2002; 25:1198–1202.

136. Gavish D, Leibovitz E, Shapira I, Rubinstein A. Bezafibrate and simvastatin combination therapy for diabetic dyslipidaemia: efficacy and safety. J Intern Med 2000; 247:563–569.

137. Expert Panel on Detection, Evaluation, and Treatment of High Blood Cholesterol in Adults (Adult Treatment Panel III). Third Report of the National Cholesterol Education Program (NCEP) Expert Panel on Detection, Evaluation, and Treatment of High Blood Cholesterol in Adults (Adult Treatment Panel III) final report. Circulation 2002; 106:3143–3421.

138. Pasternak RC, Smith SC, Jr., Bairey-Merz CN, Grundy SM, Cleeman JI, Lenfant C. ACC/AHA/NHLBI clinical advisory on the use and safety of statins. J Am Coll Cardiol 2002; 40:567–572.

139. Omar MA, Wilson JP. FDA adverse event reports on statin-associated rhabdomyolysis. Ann Pharmacother 2002; 36:288–295.

140. Ballantyne CM, Corsini A, Davidson MH, et al. Risk for myopathy with statin therapy in high-risk patients. Arch Intern Med 2003; 163:553–564.

141. American Heart Association, Dallas, Texas, November, 2005.

142. LaRosa JC, He J, Vupputuri S. Effect of Statins on risk of coronary disease. A meta-analysis of randomized controlled trials. JAMA 1999; 282:2340–2436.

143. Heart Protection Study Collaborative Group. MRC/BHF Heart Protection Study of cholesterol lowering with simvastatin in 20536 high-risk individuals: A randomized placebo-controlled trial. Lancet 2002; 360:7–22.

144. Sever PS, Dahlöf B, Poulter NR, Wedel H, Beevers G, Caulfield M, Collins R, Kjeldsen SE, Kristinsson A, Mcinnes GT, Mehlsen J, Nieminen M, O'Brien E, Ostergren J, for the ASCOT investigators. Prevention of coronary and stroke events with atorvastatin in hypertensive patients who have average or lower-than-average cholesterol concentrations, in the Anglo-Scandinavian Cardiac Outcomes Trial – Lipid Lowering Arm (ASCOT-LLA): A multicentre randomized controlled trial. Lancet 2003; 361: 1149–1167.

145. The Coronary Drug Project Research Group. Clofibrate and niacin in coronary heart disease. JAMA 1975; 231:360–381.

146. Canner PL, Berge KG, Wenger NK, et al. for the Coronary Drug Project Research Group. Fifteen year mortality in Coronary Drug Project patients: long-term benefit with niacin. J Am Coll Cardiol 1986; 8:1245–1255.

147. Canner PL, Furberg CD, McGovern ME. Niacin decreases myocardial infarction and total mortality in patients with impaired fasting glucose or glucose intolerance: results from the Coronary Drug Project [abstract 3138]. Circulation 2002; 106(suppl II):II-636.

148. Kane JP, Malloy MJ, Ports TA, Phillips NR, Diehl JC, Havel RJ. Regression of coronary atherosclerosis during treatment of familial hypercholesterolemia with combined drug regimens. JAMA 1990; 264:3007–3012.

149. Blankenhorn DH, Nessim SA, Johnson RL, Sanmarco ME, Azen SP, Cashin-Hemphill L. Beneficial effects of combined colestipol-niacin therapy on coronary atherosclerosis and coronary venous bypass grafts. JAMA 1987; 257:3233–3240.

150. Brown G, Albers JJ, Fisher LD, et al. Regression of coronary artery disease as a result of intensive lipid-lowering therapy in men with high levels of apolipoprotein B. N Engl J Med 1990; 323:1289–1298.

151. Brown BG, Zhao XQ, Chait A, et al. Simvastatin and niacin, antioxidant vitamins, or the combination for the prevention of coronary disease. N Engl J Med 2001; 345:1583–1592.

152. Morse JS, Brown BG, Zhao X-Q, et al. Niacin plus simvastatin protect against atherosclerosis progression and clinical events in CAD patients with low HDLc and diabetes mellitus or impaired fasting glucose [abstract 842-3]. J Am Coll Cardiol 2001; 37(suppl A):262A.

153. Van JT, Pan J, Wasty T, Chan E, Wu X, Charles MA. Comparison of extended-release niacin and atorvastatin monotherapies and combination treatment of the atherogenic lipid profile in diabetes mellitus. Am J Cardiol 2002; 89:1306–1308.

154. Pan J, Lin M, Kesala R, Van J, Charles M. Niacin treatment of the atherogenic lipid profile and Lp(a) in diabetes. Diabetes Obes Metab 2002; 4:255–261.

155. Kashyap ML, McGovern ME, Berra K, et al. Long-term safety and efficacy of a once-daily niacin/lovastatin formulation in patients with dyslipidemia. Am J Cardiol 2002; 89:672–678.

156. Elam MB, Hunninghake DB, Davis KB, et al, for the ADMIT Investigators. Effect of niacin on lipid and lipoprotein levels and glycemic control in patients with diabetes and peripheral arterial disease. The ADMIT study: a randomized trial. JAMA 2000; 284:1263–1270.

157. Grundy SM, Vega GL, McGovern ME, et al, for the Diabetes Multicenter Research Group. Efficacy, safety, and tolerability of once-daily niacin for the treatment of dyslipidemia associated with type 2 diabetes: results of the Assessment of Diabetes Control and Evaluation of the Efficacy of Niaspan Trial. Arch Intern Med 2002; 162:1568–1576.

158. Zhao X-Q, Morse JS, Dowdy AA, et al. Safety and tolerability of simvastatin plus niacin in patients with coronary artery disease and low high-density lipoprotein cholesterol (The HDL Atherosclerosis Treatment Study). Am J Cardiol 2004; 93:307–312.

159. American Diabetes Association. Dyslipidemia management in adults with diabetes. Diabetes Care 2004; 27(suppl 1):S68–S71.

160. Eaton SB, Konner M, Shostak M. Stone agers in the fast lane: chronic degenerative diseases in evolutionary perspective. Am J Med 1988; 84:739–749.

161. Helmrich SP, Ragland DR, Leung RW, Paffenbarger RS Jr. Physical activity and reduced occurrence of non-insulin-dependent diabetes mellitus. N Engl J Med 1991; 325:147–152.

162. Manson JE, Rimm EB, Stampfer MJ, et al. Physical activity and incidence of non-insulin-dependent diabetes mellitus in women. Lancet 1991; 338:774–778.

163. Manson JE, Nathan DM, Krolewski AS, Stampfer MJ, Willett WC, Hennekens CH. A prospective study of exercise and incidence of diabetes among US male physicians. JAMA 1992; 268:63–67.

164. Wannamethee SG, Shaper AG, Alberti KG. Physical activity, metabolic factors, and the incidence of coronary heart disease and type 2 diabetes. Arch Intern Med 2000; 160:2108–2116.

165. Hu G, Lindstrom J, Valle TT, et al. Physical activity, body mass index, and risk of type 2 diabetes in patients with normal or impaired glucose regulation. Arch Intern Med 2004; 164:892–896.

166. Folsom AR, Kushi LH, Hong CP. Physical activity and incident diabetes mellitus in postmenopausal women. Am J Public Health 2000; 90:134–138.

167. Hu FB, Manson JE, Stampfer MJ, et al. Diet, lifestyle, and the risk of type 2 diabetes mellitus in women. N Engl J Med 2001; 345:790–797.

168 Hu FB, Sigal RJ, Rich-Edwards JW, et al. Walking compared with vigorous physical activity and risk of type 2 diabetes in women: a prospective study. JAMA 1999; 282:1433–1439.

169. Weinstein AR, Sesso HD, Lee IM, et al. Relationship of physical activity vs body mass index with type 2 diabetes in women. JAMA 2004; 292:1188–1194.

170. Hsia J, Wu L, Allen C, et al. Physical activity and diabetes risk in postmenopausal women. Am J Prev Med 2005; 28:19–25.

171. Carnethon MR, Gidding SS, Nehgme R, Sidney S, Jacobs DR Jr., Liu K. Cardiorespiratory fitness in young adulthood and the development of cardiovascular disease risk factors. JAMA 2003; 290:3092–3100.

172. Lynch J, Helmrich SP, Lakka TA, et al. Moderately intense physical activities and high levels of cardiorespiratory fitness reduce the risk of non-insulin-dependent diabetes mellitus in middle-aged men. Arch Intern Med 1996; 156:1307–1314.

173. Sawada SS, Lee IM, Muto T, Matuszaki K, Blair SN. Cardiorespiratory fitness and the incidence of type 2 diabetes: prospective study of Japanese men. Diabetes Care 2003; 26:2918–2922.

174. Wei M, Gibbons LW, Mitchell TL, Kampert JB, Lee CD, Blair SN. The association between cardiorespiratory fitness and impaired fasting glucose and type 2 diabetes mellitus in men. Ann Intern Med 1999; 130:89–96.

175. Pan XR, Li GW, Hu YH, et al. Effects of diet and exercise in preventing NIDDM in people with impaired glucose tolerance. The Da Qing IGT and Diabetes Study. Diabetes Care 1997; 20:537–544.

176. Knowler WC, Barrett-Connor E, Fowler SE, et al. Reduction in the incidence of type 2 diabetes with lifestyle intervention or metformin. N Engl J Med 2002; 346:393–403.

177. Tuomilehto J, Lindstrom J, Eriksson JG, et al. Prevention of type 2 diabetes mellitus by changes in lifestyle among subjects with impaired glucose tolerance. N Engl J Med 2001; 344:1343–1350.

178. Laaksonen DE, Lindstrom J, Lakka TA, et al. Physical activity in the prevention of type 2 diabetes: the Finnish Diabetes Prevention Study. Diabetes 2005; 54:158–165.

179. 9th International Congress on Obesity. Sao Paulo: Brazil, 2002.

180. Chiasson JL, Josse RG, Gomis R, Hanefeld M, Karasik A, Laakso M. STOP-NIDDM Trial Research Group. Acarbose for prevention of type 2 diabetes mellitus: the STOP-NIDDM randomized trial. Lancet 2002; 359:2072–2077.

181. Diabetes Prevention Program Research Group: Knowler WC, Barrett-Connor E, Fowler SE, et al. Reduction in the incidence of type 2 diabetes with lifestyle intervention or metformin. New Engl J Med 2002; 346:393–403.

182. Buchannan T, Xiang AH, Peters RK, et al. Preservation of pancreatic [beta]-cell function and prevention of type 2 diabetes by pharmacological treatment of insulin resistance in high-risk Hispanic women. Diabetes 2002; 51:2796–2803.

183. Azziz R, Kashar-Miller MD. Family history as a risk factor for the polycystic ovary syndrome. J Pediatr Endocrinol Metab 2000; 13:1303–1306.

184. Urbanek M, Legro R, Driscoll DA, et al. Thirty-seven candidate genes for polycystic ovary syndrome: strongest evidence for linkage is with follistatin. Proc Natl Acad Sci USA 1999; 86:8573–8578.

185. Ehrmann DA, Sturis J, Byrne MM, Karrison T, Rosenfield RL, Polonsky KS. Insulin secretory defects in polycystic ovary syndrome: relationship to insulin sensitivity and family history of non-insulin-dependent diabetes mellitus. J Clin Invest 1995; 96:520–527.

186. Legro RS, Driscoll D, Strauss JF III, Fox J, Dunaif A. Evidnece for a genetic basis for hyperandrogenemia in polycystic ovary syndrome. Proc Natl Acad Sci USA 1998; 95:14956–14960.

187. Kahsar-Miller MD, Nixon C, Boots LR, Go RC, Azziz R. Prevalence of polycystic ovary syndrome (PCOS) in first-degree relatives of patients with PCOS. Fertil Seril 2001; 75:53–58.

188. Dunaif A, Segal KR, Futterweit W, Dobrjansky A. Profound peripheral insulin resistance, independent of obesity, in polycystic ovary syndrome. Diabetes 1989; 38:1165–1174.

189. Dunaif A. Insulin resistance and the polycystic ovary syndrome: mechanism and implications for pathogenesis. Endocr Rev 1997; 18:774–800.

190. Dunaif A, Wu X, Lee A, Diamanti-Kandarakis E. Defects in insulin receptor signaling in vivo in the polycystic ovary syndrome (PCOS). Am J Physiol Endocrinol Metab 2001; 281:E392–E399.

191. National Cholesterol Education Program (NCEP) Expert Panel on Detection, Evaluation, and Treatment of High Blood Cholesterol in Adults (Adult Treatment Panel III). The Third Report of the National Cholesterol Education Program (NCEP) Expert Panel on Detection, Evaluation, and Treatment of High Blood Cholesterol in Adults (Adult Treatment Panel III): Final report. Circulation 2002; 105:3143–31421.

192. Sam S, Dunaif A. Polycystic ovary syndrome: Syndrome XX? Trends Endocrinol Metab 2003; 14:365–370.

193. Azziz R, Ehrmann D, Legro RS, et al. Troglitazone improves ovulation and hirsutism in the polycystic ovary syndrome: a multicenter, double blind, placebo-controlled trial. J Clin Endocrinol Metab 2001; 86:1626–1632.

194. Franks S. Polycystic ovary syndrome: a changing perspective. Clin Endocrinol (Oxf) 1989; 31:87–120.

195. Conway GS, Honour JW, Jacobs HS. Heterogeneity of the polycystic ovary syndrome: clinical, endocrine and ultrasound features in 556 patients. Clin Endocrinol (Oxf) 1989; 30:459–470.

196. Carmina E, Legro RS, Stamets K, Lowell J, Lobo RA. Difference in body weight between American and Italian women with polycystic ovary syndrome: Influence of the diet. Hum Reprod 2003; 18:2289–2293.

197. Knochenhauer E, Key TJ, Kahsar-Miller M, Waggoner W, Boots LR, Assiz R. Prevalence of the polycystic ovary syndrome in unselected black and white women of the southeastern United States: A Prospective study. J Clin Endocrinol Metab 1998; 83:3078–3082.

198. Diamanti-Kandarakis E, Kouli CR, Bergiele AT, et al. A survey of the polycystic ovary syndrome in the Greek island of Lesbos: hormonal and metabolic profile. J Clin Endocrinol Metab 1999; 84:4006–4011.

199. Asuncion M, Calvo RM, San Millan JL, Sancho J, Avila S, Escobar-Morreale HE. A prospective study of the prevalence of the polycystic ovary syndrome in unselected Caucasian women from Spain. J Clin Endocrinol Metab 2000; 85:2434–2438.

200. Ayala C, Steinberger E, Smith KD, Rodriguez-Rigau L, Petak SM. Serum testosterone levels and reference ranges in reproductive-age women. Endocr Pract. 1999; 5:322–329.

201. Franks S. Adult polycystic ovary syndrome begins in childhood. Best Pract Res Clin Endocrinol Metab 2002; 16:263–272.

202. Ibanez L, Valls C, Marcos MV, Ong K, Dunger DB, De Zegher F. Insulin sensitization for girls with precocious pubarche and with risk for polycystic ovary syndrome: effects of prepubertal initiation and postpubertal discontinuation of metformin treatment. J Clin Endocrinol Meta 2004; 89:4331–4337.

203. Nelson VL, Legro RS, Strauss JF III, McAllister JM. Augmented androgen production is a stable steroidogenic phenotype of propagated theca cells from polycystic ovaries. Mol Endocrinol 1999; 13:946–947.

204. Nelson VL, Qin KN, Rosenfield RL, et al. The biochemical basis for increased testosterone production in theca cells propagated from patients with polycystic ovary syndrome. J Clin Endocrinol Metab 2001; 85:5925–5933.

205. Haisenleder DJ, Dalkin AC, Ortolano GA, Marshall JC, Shupnik MA. A pulsatile gonadotropin-releasing hormone stimulus is required to increase transcription of the gonadotropin subunit genes: evidence for differential regulation of transcription by pulse frequency in vivo. Endocrinology 1991; 128:509–517.

206. Eagleson CA, Gingrich MB, Pastor CL, et al. Polycystic ovarian syndrome: evidence that flutamide restores sensitivity of the gonadotropin-releasing hormone pulse generator to inhibition by estradiol and progesterone. J Clin Endocrinol Metab 2000; 85:4047–4052.

207. Dahlgren E, Janson PO, Johansson S, Lapidus L, Oden A. Polycystic ovary syndrome and risk for myocardial infarction: evaluated from a risk factor model based on a prospective population study of women. Acta Obstet Gynecol Scand 1992; 71:599–604.

208. Cibula D, Cifkova R, Fanta M, Poledne R, Zivny J, Skibova J. Increased risk of non-insulin dependent diabetes mellitus, arterial hypertension and coronary heart disease in perimenopausal women with a history of the polycystic ovary syndrome. Hum Reprod 2000; 15:785–789.

209. Elting MW, Korsen TJ, Bezemer PD, Schoemaker J. Prevalence of diabetes mellitus, hypertension and cardiac complaints in a follow-up study of a Dutch PCOS population. Hum Reprod 2001; 16:556–560.

210. Orio F Jr., Palomba S, Cascella T, et al. Early impairment of endothelial structure and function in young normal-weight women with polycystic ovary syndrome. J Clin Endocrinol Metab 2004; 89:4588–4593.

211. Christian RC, Dumesic DA, Behrenbeck T, Oberg AL, Sheedy PF II, Fitzpatrick LA. Prevalence and predictors of coronary artery calcification in women with polycystic ovary syndrome. J Clin Endocrinol Metab 2003; 88:2562–2568.

212. Talbott E, Zborowski JV, McHugh-Pemu K, et al. Metabolic cardiovascular syndrome and its relationship to coronary calcification in women with polycystic ovarian syndrome. Presented at: 3rd International Workshop on Insulin Resistance, February 17–19, 2003, New Orleans, LA.

213. Solomon CG, Hu FB, Dunaif A, et al. Long or highly irregular menstrual cycles as a marker for risk of type 2 diabetes mellitus. JAMA 2001; 286:2421–2426.

214. Solomon CG, Hu FB, Dunaif A, et al. Menstural cycle irregularity and risk for future cardiovascular disease. J Clin Endocrinol Metab 2002; 87:2013–2017.

215. Rich-Edwards JW, Goldman MB, Willett WC, Hunter DJ, Stampfer MJ, Colditz GA, Manson JE. Adolescent body mass index and infertility caused by ovulatory disorder. Am J Obstet Gynecol 1771; 171–177.

216. Zaadstra BM, Seidell JC, Van Noord PA, et al. Fat and female fecundity: prospective study of effect of body fat distribution on conception rates. BMJ 1993; 306:484–487.

217. Clark AM, Thornley B, Tomlinson L, Galletley C, Norman RJ. Weight loss in obese infertile women results in improvement in reproductive outcome for all forms of fertility treatment. Hum Reprod 1998; 13:1502–1505.

218. Moran LJ, Noakes M, Clifton PM, Tomlinson L, Galletly C, Norman RJ. Dietary composition in restoring reproductive and metabolic physiology in overweight women with polycystic ovary syndrome. J Clin Endocrinol Metab 2003; 88:812–819.

219. Stamets K, Taylor DS, Kunselman A, Demers LM, Pelkman CL, Legro RS. A randomized trial of the effects of two types of short-term hypocaloric diets on weight loss in women with polycystic ovary syndrome. Fertil Steril 2004; 81:630–637.

220. Mansfield R, Galea R, Brincat M, Hole D, Mason H. Metformin has direct effects on human ovarian steroidogenesis. Fertil Steril 2003; 79:956–962.

221. Attia GR, Rainey WE, Carr BR. Metformin directly inhibits androgen production in human thecal cells. Fertil Steril 2001; 76:517–524.

222. Lord JM, Flight IHK, Nroman RJ. Insulin-sensitising drugs (metformin, troglitazone, rosiglitazone, pioglitazone, D-chi-ro-inositol) for polycystic ovary syndrome. Cochrone Database Syst Rev 2003; 3:CD003053.

223. Glueck CJ, Goldenberg N, Pranikoff J, Loftspring M, Sieve L, Wang P. Height, weight, and motor-social development during the first 18 months of life in 126 infants born to 109 mothers with polycystic

ovary syndrome who conceived on and continued metformin through pregnancy. Hum Reprod 2004; 19:1323–1330.

224. Glueck CJ, Wang P, Kobayashi S, Phillips H, Sieve-Smith L. Metformin therapy throughout pregnancy reduces the development of gestational diabetes in women with polycystic ovary syndrome. Fertil Steril 2002; 77:520–525.

225. Glueck CJ, Wang P, Goldenberg N, Sieve-Smith L. Pregnancy outcomes among women with polycystic ovary syndrome treated with metformin. Hum Reprod 2002; 17:2858–2864.

226. Gluck CJ, Phillips H, Cameron D, Sieve-Smith L, Wang P. Continuing metformin throughout pregnancy in women with polycystic ovary syndrome appears to safely reduce first-trimester spontaneous abortion: a pilot study. Fertil Steril 2001; 75:46–52.

227. Mitwally MF, Witchel SF, Casper RF. Troglitazone: a possible modulator of ovarian steroidogenesis. J Soc Gynecol Investig 2002; 9:163–167.

228. Ghazeeri G, Kutteh WH, Bryer-Ash M, Haas D, Ke RW. Effect of rosiglitazone on spontaneous and clomiphene citrate-induced ovulation in women with polycystic ovary syndrome. Fertil Steril 2003; 79:562–566.

229. Belli SH, Graffigna MN, Oneto A, Otero P, Schurman L, Levalle OA. Effect of rosiglitazone on insulin resistance, growth factors, and reproductive disturbances in women with polycystic ovary syndrome. Fertil Steril 2004; 81:624–629.

230. Romualdi D, Guido M, Ciampelli M, et al. Selective effects of pioglitazone on insulin and androgen abnormalities in normo- and hyperinsulinaemic obese patients with polycystic ovary syndrome. Hum Reprod 2003; 18:1210–1218.

231. Baillargeon JP, Jakubowicz DJ, Iuorno MJ, Jakubowicz S, Nestler JE. Effects of metformin and rosiglitazone, alone and in combination, in nonobese women with polycystic ovary syndrome and normal indices of insulin sensitivity. Fertil Steril 2004; 82:893–890.

232. Palomba S, Orio F JR, Nardo LG, et al. Metformin administration versus laparoscopic ovarian diathermy in clomiphene citrate-resistant womenw with polycystic ovary syndrome: a prospective parallel randomized double-blind placebo-controlled trial. J Clin Endocrinol Metab 2004; 89:4801–4809.

233. Jakubowicz DJ, Iuorno MJ, Jakubowicz S, Roberts KA, Nestler JE. Effects of metformin on early pregnancy loss in the polycystic ovary syndrome. J Clin Endocrinol Metab 2002; 87:524–529.

234. Gluck CJ, Wang P, Goldenberg N, Sieve-Smith L. Pregnancy outcomes among women with polycystic ovary syndrome treated with metformin. Hum Reprod 2002; 17:2858–2864.

235. Bloomgarden ZT. Definitions of the insulin resistance syndrome: The 1st World Congress on the Insulin Resistance Syndrome. Diabetes Care 2004; 27:824–830.

12 | Inflammatory Mediators and C-Reactive Protein

John A. Farmer
Baylor College of Medicine, Houston, Texas, U.S.A.

KEY POINTS

- The pathogenesis of atherosclerosis is best regarded as a syndrome with a variety of predisposing factors. Inflammation has been implicated by epidemiologic, pathologic, and clinical studies as a major pathogenetic factor in the initiation and progression of atherosclerosis.
- Multiple inflammatory markers had been validated as prognostic indicators of cardiac risk in clinical trials. However, C-reactive protein has been determined to be the most clinically useful and may represent a target for therapy in addition to the well-documented role and risk stratification.
- C-reactive protein determination is most useful in subjects classified as being of moderate risk in primary prevention.
- The measurement of C-reactive protein has been validated in a variety of populations and clinical trials.
- C-reactive protein may provide prognostic information even in subjects with relatively normal lipid levels.

INTRODUCTION

Age-adjusted cardiovascular mortality has been steadily declining for the past several decades in the United States (1). The longevity is the consequence of a better ability to detect subclinical atherosclerotic vascular disease using new technologies, coupled with significant advances in both medical therapy and interventional techniques, such as angioplasty and coronary artery bypass surgery. While a unified hypothesis of atherosclerosis remains elusive, the concept of risk factor identification and modification has gained credence in the prevention of coronary heart disease (CHD). Basic science, clinical, and epidemiologic studies provide a theoretical framework for atherosclerosis as a syndrome with multiple factors' playing a potential role in its initiation and progression. The major modifiable risk factors for atherosclerosis include hypertension, dyslipidemia, diabetes mellitus, obesity, and the use of tobacco products. While seemingly distinct, these risk factors may share common pathways that are involved in atherogenesis. A growing number of investigators have explored chronic, low-grade inflammation as an important pathologic feature of plaque formation, with a potential impact on cardiovascular risk assessment and treatment.

Reliable, reproducible, and easily measurable risk factors that can predict the presence and severity of atherosclerosis with a relatively high degree of sensitivity and specificity are necessary to establish risk stratification guidelines and shape algorithms to guide the intensity of therapeutic interventions. The risk score derived from the Framingham Heart Study database estimates 10-year coronary risk based on six easily measurable variables: age, sex, smoking, blood pressure, total cholesterol, and high-density lipoprotein cholesterol (HDL-C) (2). Low risk is defined as the probability of developing a cardiac event of less than 10% in the next decade (<1% per year). High risk in asymptomatic patients is defined as a 20% risk or higher over 10 years and is considered to be equivalent to having a history of previous CHD.

The Framingham risk prediction model accurately predicts short-term risk in several trials (2). However, in certain clinical situations, the calculation may not reflect a patient's risk accurately. For example, a young man with familial hypercholesterolemia has a relatively low short-term risk using the Framingham algorithm because of the impact of age on the total point score, but a high lifetime probability of developing symptomatic atherosclerosis because of his long-term exposure to dyslipidemia. The Framingham risk score has also been criticized because it is based on data from a predominantly middle-class, Caucasian-American cohort and thus might not extrapolate to other populations or socioeconomic groups. A study of women categorized at low risk by the algorithm reported that 32% of these women nevertheless had evidence of subclinical atherosclerosis (3). In a Scottish study, the Framingham risk score underestimated coronary risk by 48% in manual laborers versus 31% in nonmanual laborers (4). While the Framingham Risk Score has definite merit, consideration of other traditional risk factors (such as body mass index, family history of early CHD, level of physical activity) and emerging risk factors, such as inflammatory markers, may help improve the utility of risk prediction in clinical practice.

THE USE OF INFLAMMATORY MARKERS IN THE PREDICTION OF CARDIOVASCULAR RISK

Before any marker can be recommended for inclusion in screening for atherosclerosis, strict criteria should be met and verified. The ideal marker for risk assessment should be relatively inexpensive, standardized, and have broadly reproducible data in support of its potential to predict the clinical probability of developing a subsequent cardiac event. Also, if the marker is directly involved in the pathogenic process—as opposed to being a pure statistical risk predictor without demonstrable, direct pro-atherosclerotic activity—prospective clinical trial evidence should demonstrate that alteration of the clinical marker by treatment would decrease the incidence of cardiovascular events. Hypertension and dyslipidemia clearly fulfill these criteria and are routinely employed in risk stratification.

Emerging risk factors include homocysteine, fibrinolytic parameters, and a variety of inflammatory mediators [e.g., serum amyloid A (SAA), myeloperoxidase, cellular adhesion molecules (CAMs), and lipoprotein-associated phospholipase A_2 (Lp-PLA$_2$)]. However, based on a large body of clinical, epidemiologic, and experimental evidence that has related the circulating levels of C-reactive protein (CRP) to the presence and severity of atherosclerosis, CRP has emerged at the forefront of inflammatory markers of CHD and may have therapeutic implications.

Characteristics and Measurement of CRP

CRP is an acute phase reactant that was initially utilized in clinical situations as an indirect marker of infection or to monitor the degree of disease activity in a variety of collagen vascular diseases such as rheumatoid arthritis or systemic lupus erythematosus. The range of normal values of CRP employing the early clinical assays was quite wide and additionally demonstrated considerable inter- and intraindividual variability. The wide range of normal values and poor reproducibility of the results of the assay limited the role of CRP as a clinically useful measurement for the assessment of acute or chronic inflammation. However, high-sensitivity clinical assays have subsequently been developed that have improved the determination of CRP greatly (5). Serial measurement of high-sensitivity CRP (hsCRP) demonstrates a significant improvement in degree of reproducibility in clinically stable subjects. The development of hsCRP thus allowed for the evaluation of the degree of inflammation as a potential diagnostic marker for the primary assessment of patients' clinical risk status for CHD in a variety of epidemiological trials (Table 1).

MECHANISMS OF INFLAMMATION IN THE PATHOGENESIS OF ATHEROSCLEROSIS

Before discussing the role of CRP in cardiovascular risk assessment further, a brief discussion of the improved understanding of the effect of inflammation in atherogenesis is necessary. The *common soil hypothesis* centers on the observation that the major modifiable CHD risk factors have features of both inflammation and oxidative stress, which alter the normal structure and function of the vascular endothelium in a number of ways that promote plaque formation (Fig. 1) (8). Oxidative stress and inflammation cause the endothelium to shift to a prothrombotic state that is also characterized by a preponderance of vasoconstrictive stimuli. In addition, the barrier to the movement of atherogenic lipoproteins [e.g., low-density lipoprotein (LDL)] across the endothelium is altered, and apolipoprotein-B containing particles migrate more easily into the subendothelial space, where they are oxidized and scavenged by the monocyte-macrophage system. The uptake of oxidized LDL by the monocyte-macrophage system results in the subsequent conversion of these cells into the lipid-laden foam cell that are the earliest identifiable histologic substrate for atherosclerosis.

Studies of inflammation have improved understanding of the biologic properties of the atherosclerotic lesion and subsequent degree of plaque vulnerability (12). The concept of the *vulnerable plaque* has taken hold as an important pathological principle in CHD, based on

TABLE 1   Studies of the Relation of C-Reactive Protein to Coronary Risk

Study	N (% Female)	Median CRP in Pts w/CVD (mg/L)	Median CRP in Pts w/o CVD (mg/L)	RR for CHD[a]
In patients without preexisting CHD				
PHS (6)	543 cases (0), 543 controls	1.40	1.13	2.9
WHS (7)	122 cases (100), 244 controls	6.45	3.75	4.8
RPS (8)	2459 cases (28), 3969 controls (31)	1.75[b]	1.28[b]	1.45
HHP (9)	369 cases (0), 1348 controls (0)	0.74	0.54	1.6
ARIC (10)	608 cases (32), 740 controls (59)	4.05[b]	3.04[b]	2.53

Study	N (% Female)	CRP in Pts w/ Recurrent CHD	CRP in Pts w/o Recurrent CHD	Major finding
In patients with preexisting CHD				
Tommasi et al. (11)	64 post-MI pts (14) followed for 13 months	3.61	2.07	Only elevated CRP independently associated with CHD events

[a]Of highest quartile versus lower quartile (PHS, WHS, HHP, ARIC), or highest third versus lowest third (RPS).
[b]Geometric mean (RPS) or weighted mean (ARIC).
Abbreviations: PHS, Physicians' Health Study; WHS, Women's Health Study; RPS, Reykjavik Prospective Study; HHP, Honolulu Heart Program; ARIC, Atherosclerosis Risk in Communities; CHD, coronary heart disease; CRP, C-reactive protein; MI, myocardial infarction; RR, relative risk.

autopsy studies that demonstrated the majority of heart attacks were associated with only mildly-to-moderately stenotic lesions. Rupture of these culprit lesions appeared to initiate a thrombogenic cascade that would cause acute, ischemic episodes. This observation spawned a significant body of research that has shifted interest away from the quantitative burden of atherosclerotic vascular disease to its qualitative features. Vulnerable plaques are now well characterized (Table 2).

Inflammatory Cellular Elements of Atherosclerosis
Monocytes
The monocyte cell line serves a variety of host defense mechanisms because of the inherent ability of these cells to scavenge cellular breakdown products and remove them from the involved area. Mononuclear macrophages are thus a major cellular constituent of both the chronic inflammatory process and as a defense mechanism against infection (12). However, the role of monocytes in the pathogenesis of atherosclerosis involves more than simple scavenging functions.

Reduction of the number of monocytes or a reduction in the rate of their migration into areas of atherosclerosis is associated with a decrease in the extent of the degree of

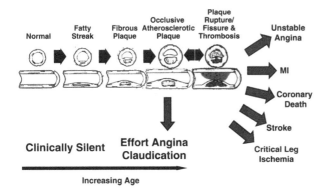

FIGURE 1   Atherosclerosis: a progressive process. *Abbreviation*: MI, myocardial infarction. *Source*: Courtesy of Ganz.

TABLE 2 Pathologic Features of the Vulnerable Atherosclerotic Plaque

Thin, friable fibrous cap
High macrophage content
Lipid-rich core
Moderate stenosis (<50% blockage)
Few smooth muscle cells

atherosclerosis (13). The monocytes that migrate into areas prone to the development of atherosclerosis are not fully differentiated and retain the ability to both proliferate at an increased rate and alter their inherent functional capabilities (14). Monocytes demonstrate the ability to transform functionally into tissue scavenger cells (macrophages). The transformation is mediated by a variety of stimuli, including a number of colony-stimulating factors (e.g., granulocyte-monocyte colony-stimulating factor, or GM-CSF) (15). The ability of the monocyte to function as a scavenger cell plays a pivotal role in the development and progression of atherosclerosis.

The transformation of monocytes into macrophages results in the capacity to synthesize and secrete multiple active mediators that also may play a role in atherosclerosis in addition to the ability to perform the scavenger function (16). The monocyte-macrophage cell line has the innate capacity to proliferate within the area of atherosclerosis and is the major source of the characteristic cellular component of the inflammatory process. Macrophages phagocytize not only necrotic cellular debris, but also native and modified lipoproteins. The term *"foam cell"* was derived from the pathologic appearance of the macrophage following lipid ingestion (17).

The recognition, binding, and internalization of lipoproteins by the macrophage are receptor mediated. The classic LDL receptor is predominantly localized in the liver and recognizes both apolipoproteins B and E (18). In contrast, the primary receptor on the macrophage is called the scavenger receptor because it recognizes both native and modified LDL. An important observation was that macrophage uptake of native LDL is quantitatively minimal compared with the relatively rapid uptake of LDL that has been oxidized, glycated, or acetylated (19). Modification of LDL appears to be a key step in facilitating foam cell formation. The scavenger receptor has been classified into several subtypes, but the functional activity is not suppressed by progressive internal accumulation of cholesterol (20). The failure of progressively increasing intracellular lipid levels to suppress the scavenger receptor directly contrasts with the hepatic LDL receptor, which is deregulated as the degree of intracellular cholesterol increases. Additionally, the uptake of modified LDL may increase the number or function of scavenger receptors, resulting in a positive feedback system, despite a relentlessly increasing concentration of intracellular cholesterol (21). Progression of the atherosclerotic lesion results in a characteristic deposition of lipid in the core of the plaque but with the potential for differing physical characteristics.

The core of the atherosclerotic plaque consists of cholesterol that may be either in droplet or crystalline form. The crystalline form of cholesterol may impart a degree of structural stability, while the droplet phase is highly thrombogenic. Additionally, other cellular debris and a variable degree of intraplaque fibrous tissue and calcium may provide a degree of plaque stability (22). As the atherosclerotic lesion progresses, the monocyte-macrophage–derived cellular elements gradually deplete because of either apoptosis or the cytotoxic effects of a variety of noxious stimuli. This results in the release of lipids and cellular debris into the plaque that further disrupt plaque stability.

Progressive intraplaque lipid accumulation is not the only role that the monocyte-macrophage system plays in the natural history of atherosclerosis. The secretory function of the macrophage may also be involved in the progression of the atherosclerotic lesion and the degree of plaque vulnerability. The macrophage synthesizes cytotoxic reactive oxygen species and thus plays a significant role in the degree of local intensity of oxidative stress (23). Oxidative stress reduces the availability of nitric oxide, which regulates both platelet function and vasomotor tone, resulting in vasoconstriction and the propensity for increased platelet aggregation.

The macrophage secretes a variety of mediators associated with apoptosis of both smooth muscle and endothelial cells (24). Programmed cell death involving endothelial cells and smooth muscle cells may result in both significant endothelial dysfunction and reduction in plaque stability. The macrophage also secretes a variety of proteolytic enzymes that may be involved in the net balance between intraplaque matrix synthesis and degradation. Collagenase and gelatinase are matrix-metalloproteinases that degrade the matrix protein constituents of the atherosclerotic plaque progressively and increase the risk for plaque rupture due to a reduction in tensile strength of the lesion's fibrous cap (25).

The macrophage also may alter the clinical course during an acute myocardial infarction (MI) or acute coronary syndrome by influencing the balance between clot formation and fibrinolysis. The foam cell may produce procoagulants, such as tissue factor, and thus increases the risk for vascular occlusion by increasing the level of activated clotting factors VII and X (26). The macrophage produces inhibitors of fibrinolysis (27). Plasminogen activator inhibitor (PAI-I) directly antagonizes the ability of either naturally synthesized or exogenously administered tissue plasminogen activator (t-PA) and increases the risk for clot progression due to impaired fibrinolysis.

Lymphocytes

Activated T-lymphocytes play a key role in the immune response system, such as by enhancing antibody synthesis by B-lymphocytes. Additionally, T-lymphocytes may be localized within the atherosclerotic plaque (albeit less prevalently than macrophages) and also are involved in the activation of the monocyte-macrophage system. Lymphocytes are felt to migrate into the lesion-prone area following recognition and binding by VCAM-1 localized on the dysfunctional endothelium.

The putative antigens that potentially provoke the immune response are multiple and a variety of infectious agents have been postulated to play a causal role in the initiation of atherosclerosis. Chlamydia, cytomegalovirus, influenza, enterovirus, and Epstein–Barr virus have all been postulated to potentially be involved in atherogenesis (28). Considerable interest had focused on the role of Chlamydia, because pathologic studies demonstrated the presence of the organism within atherosclerotic plaques (29). The statistical correlations between the degree of atherosclerosis and a variety of infectious agents provided the theoretical basis for the design of clinical trials that employed antibiotic therapy as a means to reduce risk from vascular disease (30). However, the results of the major trials have been generally disappointing (Table 3) (31). The consensus view is that Chlamydia does not currently fulfill criteria for qualifying as an etiologic agent in atherosclerosis (34).

Modified lipoprotein particles and heat shock proteins have also been postulated to be antigens with the potential to generate an immune response by T-lymphocytes. The demonstration of antibodies to oxidized LDL in both serum and within the plaque supports the concept that an immune response directed against altered lipoproteins may play an etiologic role in the initiation and progression of atherosclerosis (35). Studies involving heat shock proteins have presented evidence that support a potential role in atherosclerosis (36). The level of the heat shock proteins is increased during processes that are characterized by cellular injury and are involved in T-cell–dependent antibody synthesis. The levels of heat shock proteins are increased in a variety of autoimmune disorders associated with an increased propensity for atherosclerosis. The presence of heat shock proteins has been positively correlated with the degree of atherosclerosis within the carotid artery of human subjects (37). Additionally, heat shock proteins have been histologically demonstrable within the atherosclerotic plaque (38). The preponderance of evidence supports a role for a localized immune reaction playing a role in both the pathogenesis and the vulnerability of the atherosclerotic plaque although the mechanisms, specific antigens, and pathophysiologic consequences remain controversial.

TABLE 3 Trials of Antibiotics and Cardiovascular Disease

Trial	Population	N	Active treatment	Effect on CVD risk
WIZARD (31)	Stable post-MI	7000	Azithromycin	None
AZACS (32)	ACS	1400	Azithromycin	None
PROVE-IT (33)	ACS	4126	Gatifloxacin	None

Abbreviations: CVD, cardiovascular disease; WIZARD, Weekly Intervention with Zithromax (Azithromycin) for Atherosclerosis and its Related Disorders; AZACS, Azithromycin in Acute Coronary Syndrome; PROVE-IT, Pravastatin or Atorvastatin Evaluation and Infection Therapy; MI, myocardial infarction; ACS, acute coronary syndrome.

Stages of Inflammation

Progressively increasing numbers of inflammatory cells in lesion-prone areas are a major pathologic feature of early atherosclerosis. The process by which inflammatory cells migrate to the subendothelial space is complex and requires recognition, binding, migration, and cellular transformation. Cytokines and chemokines are intimately involved in the movement of inflammatory cells across the endothelial barrier.

Chemokines are small proteins that have been demonstrated to bind heparin but also regulate the transmigration of leukocytes from the plasma compartment to the subendothelial space (39). Chemokines have been classified into four major functional subgroups to identify the approximately 50 variants found in humans (CC, CXC, CXEC, and C) (40). The largest subgroup of the chemokine family is designated CC because of the presence of conserved cysteine residues. The chemokines in this subgroup predominantly function to bind mononuclear cells at the site of inflammation. Monocyte chemoattractant protein-1 (MCP-1) is a member of this family and is a potent agonist for monocyte binding and accumulation within vascular beds that are prone to develop atherosclerosis. The rate and degree of monocyte recruitment is an important early step in the development of CHD (41). The presence of oxidized LDL also induces the production of MCP–1, thus enhancing the accumulation of monocytes in the subendothelial space via a positive feedback mechanism.

Interleukin-8 (IL-8) is a major member of the CXC family and is associated with the accumulation of polymorphonuclear leukocytes. Lymphotactin is the sole member of the C family and attracts lymphocytes to areas of inflammation (42). Fracktaline is a soluble chemokine which has a similar structure to other family members, but is a transmembrane protein with protrusion into the vascular space (43). The various chemokines exhibit multiple functions in the attraction of inflammatory cells to the dysfunctional endothelium and transmigration across the endothelial barrier. Chemokines can also bind directly to circulating white cells and facilitate the attachment to the inflamed endothelium. Additionally, chemokines can contribute directly to adhesion on the endothelium by activating integrins on the cellular membranes that enhance binding.

Adhesion molecules are intimately involved in leukocyte migration into the subendothelial space. As circulating leukocytes come into contact with the inflamed endothelium, a rolling phenomenon is exhibited until they become tightly adherent to the endothelial surface (Fig. 2) (44). Following stable adhesion, the leukocytes migrate across the endothelial barrier. Adhesion molecules play a role in all phases of leukocyte migration. E- and P-selectin are directly involved in the rolling and tethering of inflammatory cells to the dysfunctional endothelium. Additionally, vascular cellular adhesion molecule (VCAM-1) is also involved in this process. The intercellular adhesion molecules (ICAM-1) stabilize the binding process and insure

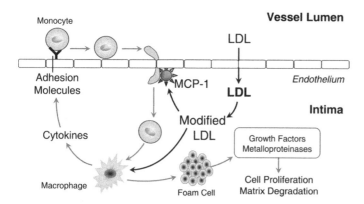

FIGURE 2 Macrophages and foam cells express growth factors and proteinases. Monocytes adhere to the endothelium through cellular adhesion molecules. Migration of these cells into the intima and the action of a variety of cytokines and chemokines results in the transformation of these cells into macrophages, which produce a variety of molecules with proatherogenic effects. Penetration of the intima by low-density lipoprotein results in modification of these particles, which enhances their uptake by the macrophage scavenger receptor and facilitates the formation of the foam cell. *Abbreviations*: LDL, low-density lipoprotein; MCP-1, monocyte chemoattractant protein-1. *Source*: From Ref. 45.

a rigid attachment of the cellular elements to the inflamed endothelium. Adhesion molecules that are directly involved in the transmigration process include ICAM-1, Platelet Endothelial CAM, and CD99. Dyslipidemia is associated with increased expression of both VCAM and ICAM in experimental animal models, thus connecting inflammation and hypercholesterolemia (46). Animal models that do not express VCAM-1 demonstrate a reduction in the severity of atherosclerotic disease despite exposure to diets that lead to high cholesterol levels.

INFLAMMATION AND THE CLASSICAL RISK FACTORS
Obesity

Data have accumulated that link multiple inflammatory markers with an abnormal body mass index (47). Obesity commonly coexists with hypertension, dyslipidemia, and diabetes. Visceral obesity represents a chronic, low-grade inflammatory state, and adipose tissue synthesizes multiple immunomodulating factors, of which leptin, IL-6, tumor necrosis factor (TNF)-alpha, and adiponectin have received the most attention (48).

The adipocyte produces the hormone leptin under genetic control (49). Following secretion by the adipocyte, leptin acts as an afferent signal to the hypothalamus and transmits information relative to the degree of endogenous fat stores. The presence of excessive fat stores results in leptin-mediated reduction of food intake and an increase in energy expenditure. The net result of increased leptin production and receptor recognition is a decrease in body fat and enhanced insulin-sensitive glucose disposal. Obese individuals appear to be resistant to the hypothalamic effects of leptin and catabolic pathways that normally suppress appetite and enhance energy expenditure are not activated. The leptin receptor belongs to the class I cytokine receptor superfamily and orchestrates complex biological effects through signal transduction (50). Leptin may contribute to the pathogenesis of a proinflammatory state, with links to atherosclerosis. Leptin-deficient obese mice that also have a defect in the LDL receptor express severe dyslipidemia and extensive atherosclerosis (51). Experimental and clinical studies support a direct role for leptin in risk for vascular disease.

IL-6 is secreted directly both from adipocytes and from macrophages that are localized within adipose tissue. The rate of synthesis and circulating levels of IL-6 are directly correlated with the degree of obesity (52). Circulating IL-6 is an important factor in the various acute phase reactants that are released following tissue damage or infection. The production of CRP is at least partially regulated by IL-6 levels (53). The relation between IL-6 and CRP suggests that this cytokine makes a major contribution to systemic inflammation in obese subjects.

TNF-alpha is a major factor in the inflammatory state that accompanies chronic obesity. TNF-alpha is synthesized by macrophages, which are localized within adipose tissue (54). Progressive obesity correlates with increasing plasma levels of TNF-alpha and insulin resistance, thus further linking inflammation and obesity. To the contrary, adiponectin is an anti-inflammatory cytokine, which is also produced by adipose tissue (55). The levels of adiponectin are inversely correlated with circulating levels of TNF-alpha, induction of VCAMs, and conversion of the macrophage to the lipid-laden foam cell. Obesity is thus best considered a proinflammatory condition with complex interactions between the classical risk factors and atherosclerosis.

Diabetes Mellitus

The incidence and prevalence of type 2 diabetes mellitus is markedly increasing in the United States, at least partially because of the epidemic of obesity (56). Diabetes has been correlated with multiple inflammatory markers, implying a potentially pathogenic role in atherosclerosis. Inflammatory markers have been evaluated as a means to predict the risk for the development of type 2 diabetes. The Atherosclerosis Risk in Communities (ARIC) study evaluated 10,275 subjects over a nine-year observational period (57). It demonstrated an association between a variety of individual inflammatory markers, including IL-1 and IL-6, fibrinogen, and CRP with the subsequent risk for developing type 2 diabetes. The association increased in obese subjects and was not correlated with markers of pancreatic autoimmunity. The persistence of a chronic inflammatory state in obese subjects may thus perpetuate weight gain and insulin resistance and increase risk for the induction of diabetes.

The degree of control of diabetes as quantitated by the level of glycosylated hemoglobin is correlated with serum inflammatory markers. The NHANES III database was analyzed in a controlled manner for a potential association between glycosylated hemoglobin and CRP (58). High circulating levels of glycosylated hemoglobin were associated with increased levels of CRP when controlled for age, sex, tobacco use, and duration of diabetes. Inflammation may thus be a factor in both the development of diabetes and the degree of glycemic control.

Hypertension

Increased inflammatory tone is also associated with hypertension. Endothelial dysfunction develops early during the course of hypertension and atherosclerosis and is associated with a reduction in the bioactivity of the enzyme nitric oxide synthase, which generates the potent vasodilator and antiplatelet compound nitric oxide (59). The decreased production of nitric oxide in cultured human aortic endothelial cells is associated with increased levels of CRP and may partially explain the correlation between inflammation and hypertension (60).

Angiotensin II is a potent vasoconstrictor and growth promoter that has been correlated with an increased degree of oxidative stress and inflammation. Angiotensin II is linked to nuclear factor kappa B, which is a major mediator of vascular inflammation. The role of angiotensin II as a proinflammatory mediator and promoter of hypertrophy has been examined in both cardiac and renal tissue. Angiotensin-converting enzyme (ACE) inhibition reduces the arterial expression of nuclear factor kappa B-dependent mediators, such as IL-8 and MCP, implying modulation of the renin–angiotensin system decreases inflammation (61). In addition, monocyte infiltration into the renal perivascular space is associated with increased expression of ICAM-1, which is stimulated by angiotensin II and inhibited by ACE inhibitors, angiotensin (AT-1) receptor blockers, and renin inhibitors (62). Angiotensin II also results in increased expression of ICAMs in cardiac perivascular tissue, which results in a significant increase in monocyte infiltration.

The potent vasoconstrictor and growth promoter norepinephrine has also been linked to a proinflammatory state. The tissue remodeling following an acute MI is associated with progressive distortion of ventricular structure and function that leads to congestive heart failure. The rate and degree of the remodeling process have been linked to levels of both norepinephrine and angiotensin II, which cause both progressive hypertrophy and intracardiac fibrosis. The remodeling process is associated with inflammation as documented by increased levels of inflammatory cytokines (63). The level of plasma norepinephrine was linked to these inflammatory markers, implicating an interactive role between sympathetic activation and the enhanced immune response in the development of left ventricular remodeling following acute MI.

Tobacco Use

The consumption of tobacco products is a major modifiable risk factor for CAD. The use of tobacco products increases the risk for coronary atherosclerosis by a variety of mechanisms, including increased procoagulant ability, vasoconstriction, and alteration of lipid parameters (e.g., reduction in HDL-C). Smoking has long been associated with evidence of systemic inflammation. The levels of the acute phase reactant fibrinogen are increased in smokers and have been linked to a variety of inflammatory processes, in addition to the increased risk for hypercoagulability (64). Fibrinolysis is impaired in smoking because of higher levels of plasminogen activator inhibitor (PAI-1), especially in combination with hypercholesterolemia (65). Smokers demonstrate evidence of platelet dysfunction at a young age, including abnormalities in platelet aggregation, glycoprotein IIb/IIIa, abnormal flow of platelet microparticles, and platelet–leukocyte interactions. The markers of platelet dysfunction associated with tobacco use have been correlated with increased risk for recurrent MI (66). Platelet-dependent thrombin generation is significantly increased (67).

Inflammatory markers, such as CRP, have been extensively studied in smokers. The circulating levels of CRP are significantly increased when smokers are compared with nonsmokers, and this is further linked to increased thrombogenicity due to elevated levels of fibrinogen (68). In an 18-year observational study, current smokers were more likely to have increased inflammatory markers (i.e., fibrinogen, ceruloplasmin, haptoglobin, and alpha-1 antitrypsin) than nonsmokers or those who had achieved smoking cessation. The presence of two or more inflammatory markers was associated with a significantly increased risk for MI, suggesting inflammation plays a pathogenic role in atherosclerosis (69).

Dyslipidemia

The role that lipoproteins play in inflammation and atherosclerosis is complex. Multiple inflammatory proteins are correlated with circulating lipoprotein fractions; whether they are simply markers or directly involved in the pathogenesis of atherosclerosis is controversial. Hypertriglyceridemia and low circulating levels of HDL-C are associated with elevated CRP. Within the plasma compartment, CRP is transported free rather than being bound to circulating lipoproteins. However, in the subendothelial space, CRP colocalizes with the monocyte-macrophage system. In vitro, oxidized lipoproteins interact with CRP (70). Also, CRP enhances the generation of proinflammatory cytokines and reactive oxygen species, thereby stimulating the production and subsequent uptake of oxidized LDL by the macrophage scavenger receptor (71,72).

The major apolipoprotein of HDL (apolipoprotein A-1) is not considered to be associated with a proinflammatory state. In fact, elevated levels of HDL-C may protect from a variety of adverse cellular effects associated with inflammation (Fig. 3). For example, high circulating levels of HDL-C are protective from experimental lipopolysaccharide-induced septic shock (74). Also, HDL may have significant anti-inflammatory and antioxidant properties that may partially explain the protection from atherosclerosis by increased circulating levels of this lipoprotein (75).

CRP in the Pathogenesis of Atherosclerosis

CRP is one of a number of immune-response proteins that belongs to the pentraxin family (76). The primary origin of CRP is the liver, and its synthesis is at least partially modulated by IL-6. However, there is evidence that CRP may be produced by cellular elements localized within the atherosclerotic plaque suggesting a potential role in the development of vascular disease. The atherosclerotic plaque is highly cellular in the early phase and is composed primarily of both inflammatory (monocytes and T-lymphocytes) and smooth muscle cells. The smooth muscle cells that migrate into the lesion-prone area undergo conversion from a contractile to a synthetic phenotype. The smooth muscle cell is capable of synthesizing and releasing a variety of molecules, including CRP. Additionally, the production of CRP appears to be relatively enhanced in smooth muscle cells that are localized within vascular beds characterized by atherosclerosis when compared with uninvolved areas (77). Further supportive evidence that CRP has a primary role in the basic pathogenesis of obstructive vascular disease is the demonstration that mRNA for CRP is present within the atherosclerotic plaque, indicating localized protein synthesis within the involved area (78). Staining of the macrophages which are localized within the intima of the atherosclerotic plaque has also been utilized to detect the presence of C reactive protein within the lesion. The co-localization of C-reactive protein with macrophages within the atheroscerotic plaque is compatible with a direct role in intiation and progression of atherosclerosis (79). CRP binds to the Fc gamma receptors CD32 and CD64 and employs these receptors to enter the endothelial cells. CRP colocalizes with the monocyte-macrophage system and thus interacts in multiple pathways that play roles in the atherosclerotic process.

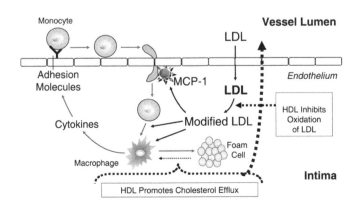

FIGURE 3 Multiple potential antiatherogenic mechanisms of HDL. *Abbreviations*: LDL, low-density lipoprotein; MCP-1, monocyte chemoattractant protein-1; HDL, high-density lipoprotein. *Source*: From Ref. 73.

Inflammation and oxidative stress initiate the process of atherosclerosis by the primary induction of endothelial structural and functional abnormalities. The normally functioning endothelium produces nitric oxide that has multiple antiatherosclerotic functions including vasodilation and antiplatelet activity. The presence of CRP is associated with a dysfunctional endothelium that results in reduction in the synthesis of both nitric oxide and prostacyclin with secondary vasoconstriction and increased platelet aggregation (80). The dysfunctional endothelium also increases the recognition and binding of circulating monocytes with a subsequent increase in the rate of transmigration into the subendothelial space where conversion to the macrophage occurs. CRP has been demonstrated to increase the expression of both endothelial CAMs and MCP-1 (81,82). CRP thus plays a role in the regulation of monocyte migration across the endothelium by increasing the activity of MCP-1–mediated chemotaxis. The CC-chemokine receptor-2 is the major chemotactic receptor on circulating monocytes, and the activity is partially regulated by CRP (83). Following transformation of the monocyte into a macrophage, the scavenger receptor recognizes, binds, and internalizes oxidized LDL. The rate of uptake of oxidized lipoproteins by the macrophage scavenger receptor is enhanced by CRP (84). Neutrophil migration across the endothelium may also be partially regulated by CRP via increased synthesis of IL-8.

Vasoconstricting and growth-promoting mediators such as angiotensin II and endothelin I are directly involved in both inflammation and the atherosclerotic process. Angiotensin II has a variety of proinflammatory activities that are generated following binding to the angiotensin (AT-1) receptor. CRP has been demonstrated to increase the number and activity of the AT-1 receptor and may thus partially mediate the proinflammatory function of this potent vasoconstrictor by increasing signal transduction (85). Increased levels of angiotensin II are also associated with a relative imbalance in the degree of fibrinolytic activity by increasing the activity of plasminogen activator inhibitor (PAI-1) that is associated with a decreased intrinsic capacity to lyse an intravascular clot. CRP has been demonstrated to increase the circulating levels of plasminogen activator inhibitor, which links inflammation with a hypercoagulable state (86).

Tissue factor is a low molecular weight glycoprotein which binds to coagulation factor VII and subsequently activates both factor IX and factor X leading to activation of both the intrinsic and extrinsic coagulation cascades. Tissue factor antigen production and procoagulant activity in monocytes is induced by CRP that might then play an additional role in the hypercoagulable state, which is frequently associated with atherosclerosis (87). However, despite the multiple potential pathogenic mechanisms for CRP in atherosclerosis, the clinical relevance requires more rigorous proof of concept. The levels of CRP should be able to predict the risk for atherosclerosis and ideally the reduction of circulating levels of CRP should demonstrate a decrease in atherosclerotic complications.

INTERVENTIONS THAT MODIFY CRP

Interest has grown concerning the potential role of modification of elevated levels of CRP as a means to decrease risk for atherosclerosis. CRP levels may be modified by either pharmacologic or nonpharmacologic methods, although definite and indisputable prospective controlled clinical evidence that reduction of elevated levels of CRP will independently reduce risk for CHD is currently lacking.

Nonpharmacologic Interventions and CRP

Elevated CRP may be modified by diet, physical activity, and weight loss. Obesity is associated with increased levels of CRP. The intake of fish oil, which is high in the content of omega-3 fatty acids, has been correlated in a variety of epidemiologic studies with a reduction in risk for the complications of atherosclerosis (88,89). Experimental studies have demonstrated that omega-3 fatty acids may also possess anti-inflammatory effects and potentially play a role in the reduction of markers such as CRP (90). However, analysis of the National Health and Nutrition Evaluation Survey (NHANES) database was unable to correlate the consumption of dietary fish oils with alterations in CRP levels (91). The Health Professionals Follow-up Trial demonstrated a trend between CRP levels and consumption of omega-3 fatty acids that did not reach clear statistical significance (92).

The correlation between dietary intake of saturated fat and cholesterol and markers of inflammation is also controversial. The NHANES demonstrated that increased circulating levels of inflammatory markers such as CRP were positively albeit mildly correlated with a diet enriched with saturated fat. However, the association between the degree of total dietary fat and cholesterol content appeared to be unrelated to CRP levels (91). However, the presence of a significant basal inflammatory condition such as obesity may predict the subsequent alteration of inflammatory markers by dietary interventions that reduce cholesterol and saturated fat content as a percent of total calories (93). The institution of a diet restricted in fat and cholesterol in significantly obese women with baseline dyslipidemia did not result in a reduction of an elevated baseline hsCRP.

The risk for developing both type 1 and 2 diabetes may be predicted by inflammatory markers such as CRP (94). Additionally, poor diabetic control is also correlated with the presence of inflammation (95). Dietary interventions have been utilized as a means to improve diabetic control and reduce the inflammatory component associated with abnormal carbohydrate metabolism. Diabetes has been treated with diets that are designed to decrease the availability of rapidly absorbable carbohydrates in an attempt to improve insulin sensitivity by decreasing the glycemic load. The Women's Health Study demonstrated that consumption of a diet composed of readily absorbable carbohydrates was associated impaired glucose levels and an increase in inflammatory markers such as CRP (96).

Pharmacologic Interventions and CRP

Pharmacologic interventions may also alter the levels of CRP, but physicians are cautioned that none has received a clinical indication for this purpose. Although inflammation is an attractive target for intervention, trials of antibiotic treatments have been largely unremarkable, and the enhanced cardiovascular risks observed with the COX-2 inhibitors serve as a warning that biological plausibility alone does not translate into clinical benefit (Table 4). The anti-inflammatory effects of such drugs must be considered secondary to the primary clinical uses of these treatments. Hypolipidemic agents have been studied extensively for both their role in the optimization of the lipid profile and a variety of plea and trophic effects including reduction of inflammatory markers. Additionally, a variety of other pharmocologic agents, including nicotinic acid, anti-platelet therapy, their brick acid derivatives, and hypologlycemic agents have also been demonstrated to improve inflammatory markers.

Statins

Statin therapy reduces cardiovascular morbidity and mortality across a spectrum of at-risk cohorts. Statins are indicated for the reduction of LDL-C with a relatively modest side effect profile. The magnitude of the statin-mediated reduction in CRP levels is variable, not specific to any particular drug within the class, and may be at least partially dependent on the pretreatment concentration. However, the administration of statin therapy is generally associated with a reduction in hsCRP levels in the range of 15% to 25% (99). The impact of statin therapy on CRP levels occurs relatively rapidly and can be documented within six weeks following the institution of therapy (100). The role of CRP as a marker of therapeutic efficacy has been evaluated in a variety of trials utilizing statin therapy.

Primary Prevention and CRP (Experimental Statin Studies)

The role of CRP as a marker for inflammation and predictor of risk for coronary atherosclerosis has also been analyzed in several primary-prevention trials that used statin therapy to reduce the incidence of cardiac events. Statin therapy is associated with multiple nonlipid or pleiotropic effects, of which a major facet is the reduction of inflammatory markers. The effect of statin therapy on circulating levels of CRP and dyslipidemia has been demonstrated in these pivotal trials and has been correlated with cardiovascular event rates.

Air Force/Texas Coronary Atherosclerosis Prevention Study

In the Air Force/Texas Coronary Atherosclerosis Prevention Study (AFCAPS/TEXCAPS), lovastatin, 20 to 40 mg/day, reduced the risk for acute major coronary events by 37% compared

TABLE 4 Trials of COX-2 Inhibitors and Cardiovascular Disease

Trial	Population	N	Agent	Effect on CVD risk
Meta-analysis (97)	Arthritis/chronic pain	20742	Rofecoxib	Increase
APC (98)	Colon cancer	2026	Celecoxib	Increase

Abbreviations: CVD, cardiovascular disease; APC, Adenoma Prevention with Celecoxib.

with placebo in 6605 low-to-moderate coronary risk men and women with average LDL-C, but below average HDL-C (101). In 5742 participants, hsCRP was measured at baseline in the AFCAPS/TEXCAPS and following one year of randomized therapy (102). While hsCRP concentration was only minimally correlated with lipid levels at the origin of the study, the risk for developing coronary events was significantly correlated with increasing levels of hsCRP. Lovastatin also demonstrated a direct anti-inflammatory effect that was independent of its effect on lipids by reducing circulating levels of hsCRP by 14.8%, while no effect on CRP was seen in the placebo group. When the cohort was divided into subgroups based on the median levels of LDL-C and hsCRP, an intriguing trend toward benefit was observed with lovastatin in the subgroup with LDL-C lower than the median, but hsCRP above the median level (Fig. 4).

West of Scotland Coronary Prevention Study

In the West of Scotland Coronary Prevention Study (WOSCOPS), pravastatin, 40 mg/day, reduced fatal and nonfatal MI by 31% compared with placebo in 6595 male subjects with moderately severe hypercholesterolemia (103). In the WOSCOPS, subjects identified with the metabolic syndrome had significantly higher levels of hsCRP when compared with individuals who did not fulfill the prespecified diagnostic criteria (104). The elevation of hsCRP (defined as greater than 3 mg/L) in the WOSCOPS also predicted the incidence of both CHD events and diabetes independently.

Justification for the Use of Statins in Primary Prevention: Evaluating Rosuvastatin

The Justification for the Use of Statins in Primary Prevention: Evaluating Rosuvastatin (JUPITER) study will randomize 15,000 primary-prevention subjects with LDL-C less than 130 mg/dL but with an elevated CRP greater than or equal to 2 mg/L to rosuvastatin versus placebo (105). If the JUPITER trial proves to be positive in the reduction of primary risk for the development of vascular disease, it would justify an aggressive approach with statin therapy in individuals with evidence of inflammation in the presence of relatively normal LDL-C levels.

Secondary Prevention and CRP (Experimental Statin Studies)

Secondary prevention is defined as the presence of documented atherosclerosis or a previous MI. The role of inflammatory markers has been analyzed in a variety of secondary-prevention trials utilizing statin therapy that encompassed a broad range of risk categories.

Cholesterol and Recurrent Events

In the Cholesterol and Recurrent Events (CARE) trial, 40 mg/day of pravastatin versus placebo in 4159 subjects, post-acute MI reduced the risk for recurrent CHD events (106). A nested case–control study evaluated the ability of the inflammatory markers hsCRP and SAA, which had been measured in the prerandomization blood samples obtained from 391 participants who subsequently developed a recurrent acute MI, to predict the incidence of recurrent cardiovascular

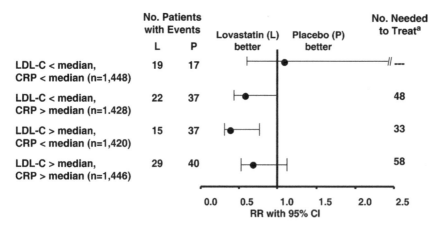

FIGURE 4 AFCAPS/TexCAPS: RR of acute coronary events by median LDL-C and CRP Level. *Note*: Median, LDL-C = 149 mg/dL; median CRP = 0.16 mg/dL. [a]Calculated on five patient years, at risk to prevent one event. *Abbreviations*: CRP, C-reactive protein; LDL, low-density lipoprotein; RR, relative risk; CI, confidence interval. *Source*: From Ref. 102.

events (107). These patients were compared with an age- and sex-matched cohort who remained free of complications of atherosclerosis during the trial. The levels of hsCRP and SAA were positively correlated with the risk for recurrent acute MI, and the predictive value was independent of the use of tobacco products and baseline lipid values in multivariate analysis.

While the measurement of inflammatory markers predicted the risk for recurrent events among subjects who were randomly assigned to placebo, the risk was attenuated and lost statistical significance in individuals who received statin therapy (Fig. 5). These findings imply not only that individuals who have suffered an acute MI with relatively normal lipid values can be stratified into risk categories on the basis of levels of CRP and SAA, but also that statin therapy may exert potentially valuable anti-inflammatory effects independent of the reduction in circulating lipid concentrations.

Pravastatin or Atorvastatin Evaluation and Infection Therapy

In a 2 × 2 design, the PROVE-IT study tested the role of an aggressive LDL-C reduction regimen versus moderate LDL-C reduction and also antibiotic treatment versus placebo on cardiovascular events in 4162 subjects with an acute coronary syndrome (108). The patients who were randomized to aggressive therapy received 80 mg of atorvastatin versus a matched cohort treated with 40 mg of pravastatin per day. The antibiotic treatment was gatifloxacin and yielded no benefit (33). However, aggressive statin therapy achieved not only significantly lower LDL-C levels than moderate therapy, but also greater cardiovascular benefit than a moderate approach.

The role of inflammatory markers as manifest by changes in hsCRP was also analyzed in the PROVE-IT trial (109) The levels of CRP were elevated at baseline in the study because of the association of inflammation with acute coronary syndromes. Standard and aggressive therapeutic regimens were both associated with a reduction in levels of CRP. The results of the PROVE-IT trial were stratified on the basis of achieved LDL-C and changes in hsCRP. Subjects who achieved an LDL-C level less than 70 mg/dL had a significant reduction in coronary events when compared with less optimal LDL-C levels (2.7 vs. 4.0 events per 100 patient years). Interestingly, a virtually identical relative clinical benefit was observed in the subjects whose CRP levels fell to less than 2 mg/L following the administration of statin therapy when compared with individuals with higher levels (2.8 vs. 3.9 events per 100 patient years) (Fig. 6). The lowest cardiac event rate was documented in subjects who achieved an LDL-C level of less than 70 mg/dL and an hsCRP level of less than 2 mg/L, thus providing further evidence for utilization of both lipid and inflammatory parameters to guide the intensity of therapy.

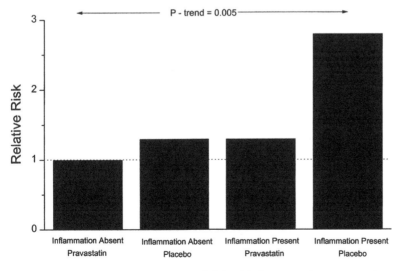

FIGURE 5 Cholesterol and recurrent events: Relative risks for recurrent coronary events among post-myocardial infarction patients according to presence (both CRP and SAA levels ≥90th percentile) or absence (both CRP and SAA levels <90th percentile) of evidence of inflammation and by randomized pravastatin assignment. *Abbreviations*: CRP, C-reactive protein; LDL, low-density lipoprotein. *Source:* From Ref. 106.

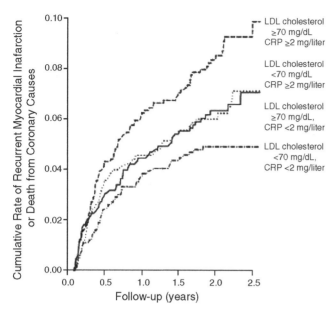

FIGURE 6 Pravastatin or atorvastatin evaluation and infection therapy: interrelation of LDL-C and hsCRP among Patients with ACS. In PROVE-IT, patients achieving LDL-C greater than 70 mg/dL had a greater number of events than those who achieved LDL-C less than 70 mg/dL. Patients achieving CRP greater than 2 mg/L had a greater number of events than those who achieved less than 2 mg/L. There was no correlation ($R = 0.18$) between achieved LDL-C and CRP. Based on these data, the investigators suggested a "Dual Goal Therapy" approach, moving CRP from being not only a predictor of risk but also a hypothetical therapeutic target. *Abbreviations*: CRP, C-reactive protein; CHD, coronary heart disease. *Source*: From Ref. 108.

Reversal of Atherosclerosis with Aggressive Lipid Lowering

The Reversal of Atherosclerosis with Aggressive Lipid Lowering (REVERSAL) trial demonstrated that aggressive statin therapy could halt atherosclerotic progression compared with a moderate regiment in a cohort of 654 subjects with documented CHD who were clinically stable to receive either an aggressive or conventional lipid-lowering regimen and were evaluated with intravascular ultrasonography (110). The role of CRP was also analyzed in the REVERSAL trial. The analysis of the total study (recipients of both atorvastatin and pravastatin) population demonstrated a decrease in the geometric mean CRP level from 2.9 to 2.3 mg/L, which was weakly correlated with reductions in LDL-C. Progression of atherosclerosis was analyzed in univariate analysis and was correlated with the percent change in apolipoprotein B-100, non-HDL-C, LDL-C and CRP. The effect of CRP on atheroma volume was adjusted for changes in lipid levels and reduction of inflammation was both independently and significantly related to progression rates. Subjects who demonstrated greater reduction in CRP levels had the most significant improvement in the rate of coronary ultrasonographically demonstrable atherosclerotic progression. The slowest rate of progression was documented in individuals with optimal reductions in both lipid levels and inflammatory markers.

Nicotinic Acid

The use of nicotinic acid as a widely employed pharmacologic intervention to improve dyslipidemia has been hampered by the side effect profile which includes a variety of troublesome side effects including flushing, pruritus, worsening of glucose tolerance, exacerbation of gout, and induction of peptic ulcer disease. The role of nicotinic acid as an anti-inflammatory agent in general and specifically the effect on CRP lacks the broad database accumulated with statins. Diabetic subjects frequently have elevated CRP levels, and nicotinic acid has been demonstrated to improve the inflammatory markers significantly despite the potential for the worsening of glucose tolerance in a relatively small study of subjects with diabetes (111,112).

Fibric Acid Derivatives

Fibric acid derivatives have been demonstrated to have effects on several inflammatory markers in subjects with dyslipidemia (113). However, similar to nicotinic acid, the clinical experience with fibric acid derivatives in inflammation is relatively modest. Fenofibrate reduces circulating levels of hsCRP, although the effect on inflammatory markers is not as rapid as relative to that of statins (114). Gemfibrozil has been demonstrated to reduce CRP levels (115).

Antiplatelet Therapy

Aspirin has significant antiplatelet activity through inhibition of cyclo-oxygenase and has been demonstrated to reduce morbidity and mortality in a variety of acute coronary syndromes. Additionally, aspirin has significant anti-inflammatory activity when used at a relatively high dose. The large-scale Physicians' Health Study, which utilized aspirin on alternate days at a dose of 325 mg, demonstrated a reduction in cardiovascular events in primary prevention (6). Although CRP predicted cardiovascular events, it is difficult to separate the relative quantitative clinical benefits of aspirin, especially when used at a dose that is not considered to have a major anti-inflammatory action.

Hypoglycemic Agents

Diabetes is considered to have a major inflammatory component especially when combined with obesity or the metabolic syndrome. Several classes of medications used as oral hypoglycemic agents have been demonstrated to reduce circulating levels of CRP, although the clinical relevance is unclear. The glitazones are PPAR gamma agonists and increase insulin sensitivity, resulting in improved glycemic control (116). Rosiglitazone has been evaluated in human subjects as a potential intervention that would alter not only insulin sensitivity, but also inflammatory markers. In one study, rosiglitazone decreased the circulating levels of both CRP and matrix metalloproteinase-9 (117). Rosiglitazone may thus have potential beneficial effects on plaque stability.

OTHER EMERGING MARKERS OF INFLAMMATION

Besides CRP, considerable interest has been generated concerning the ability of other markers of inflammation to further enhance the assessment of cardiovascular risk and response to therapy. Multiple emerging markers of inflammation have been identified, including fibrinogen, vascular and endothelial CAMs, SAA, TNF alpha, and a variety of ILs. However, the most substantial clinical database has accumulated concerning myeloperoxidase and Lp-PLA$_2$ in atherosclerosis.

Myeloperoxidase

Myeloperoxidase is a glycosylated basic heme protein localized within granules of circulating leukocytes (118). Myeloperoxidase is released when leukocytes degranulate, and this enzyme may thus be involved in a variety of host defense mechanisms that are mediated through the formation and release of toxic free radicals. Myeloperoxidase activity is associated with a reduction in nitric oxide levels (119). Myeloperoxidase has been inversely related to brachial artery flow-mediated dilatation as a noninvasive indicator of endothelial dysfunction (120). Clinical interest in the role of myeloperoxidase as a marker for atherosclerosis began with the finding that this enzyme localizes within atherosclerotic plaque (121). Myeloperoxidase increases oxidative stress by producing a variety of reactive oxygen species. Myeloperoxidase has been linked to cardiovascular risk in case–control studies, even when evaluated in multivariate analysis, which controlled for age, sex, diabetes, hypertension, consumption of tobacco products, and lipid subfractions (122). Additionally, localized production of myeloperoxidase may be involved in increased plaque vulnerability and rupture with an increased risk of generating an acute occlusive intravascular thrombus. The presence of myeloperoxidase in culprit lesions of subjects with sudden cardiac death may play a role in plaque rupture with the subsequent generation of a malignant arrhythmia (123). Myeloperoxidase may be a useful marker for the presence and severity of atherosclerosis, but no available therapeutic interventions is able to reduce the activity of this enzyme.

Lipoprotein-Associated Phospholipase A$_2$

Lp-PLA$_2$ is a member of a family of inflammatory proteins that hydrolyze phospholipids and subsequently generate both lysophospholipids and fatty acids (124). Clinical studies positively correlate type II secretory phospholipase with the pathogenesis of atherosclerosis and as a marker for the subsequent development of CHD. The enzyme has been linked to other mediators of inflammation and circulates in the plasma bound to LDL. Lp-PLA$_2$ may be directly linked to atherosclerosis by enzymatically generating catabolic products from phospholipids that are carried within the LDL fraction, that could potentially induce endothelial dysfunction or direct vascular damage.

The roles of Lp-PLA$_2$ and hsCRP have been analyzed for their possible role in CHD in the ARIC study (10). A prospective case cohort study was performed in 12,819 healthy men and women who were stratified for traditional risk factors and inflammatory markers over a six-year trial duration. A proportional hazards model was created and stratified by the levels of LDL-C. The levels of Lp-PLA$_2$ and hsCRP levels were higher in the subjects who suffered an acute MI when compared with matched controls. The hazard ratio following adjustment for age, sex, and race was 1.784 for Lp-PLA$_2$ and 2.53 for CRP. Analysis of subjects whose LDL-C levels fell below the median of 130 mg/dL demonstrated that both inflammatory markers were significantly and independently associated with increased risk for CHD in fully adjusted models. The results of the ARIC study imply a clinical role for stratification by inflammatory markers even in the presence of relatively normal LDL-C.

The role of Lp-PLA$_2$ and CRP as potential markers for the prediction of cardiovascular risk was also analyzed in WOSCOPS (125). In WOSCOPS, fibrinogen, white blood cell count, and CRP all predicted subsequent cardiovascular risk. Additionally, Lp-PLA$_2$ had a positive association with the risk for development of CHD that was independent of other markers of inflammation and conventional risk factors. The findings in the ARIC and WOSCOPS further substantiate the role of inflammation as being directly involved in the atherosclerotic process, although the clinical utility of measuring Lp-PLA$_2$ will require further investigation.

CLINICAL RECOMMENDATIONS

To maximize reproducibility and clinical utility, hsCRP levels should be measured on at least two separate occasions with a 14-day interval between the obtaining of the samples. The patient should be evaluated for the presence of clinical conditions associated with elevations of CRP levels, such as acute or chronic infection, collagen vascular disease, estrogen administration, or tobacco usage. While significant elevations of hsCRP may occur in clinical situations, it is relatively uncommon for a persistent elevation in excess of 15 mg/L to be documented.

Guidelines for the usage of inflammatory and other novel markers have been put forth by the American Heart Association and the Centers for Disease Control (126). In essence, inflammatory markers may be most useful in guiding treatment decisions in patients at intermediate risk for near-term CHD (10–20% Framingham risk over the next decade), especially in cases where the risk level appears to be on the borderline based on the traditional risk factors alone. In these patients, the presence of an abnormal hsCRP level may encourage the physician to intensify treatment.

The measurement of circulating levels of hsCRP allows the stratification of subjects into low-, intermediate-, and high-risk groups (Table 5). Levels of hsCRP appear to have far more sensitivity for the prediction for cardiovascular events than noncardiovascular mortality (79). Additionally, even within the accepted range of risk prediction categories for hsCRP, further stratification is possible. Individuals whose levels fall below 0.5 mg/L are at extremely low risk for the subsequent development of a cardiovascular event. In contrast, subjects who demonstrate sustained elevations of CRP in excess of 10 mg/L are at extremely high cardiovascular risk, assuming that other causes of chronic inflammation have been excluded and the measurement is reproducible.

TABLE 5 Centers for Disease Control/American Heart Association Workshop Guidelines for Interpretation of High-Sensitivity C-Reactive Protein

hsCRP is the analyte of first choice based on assay precision, accuracy, availability, and standardized assay calibrations

Low risk	<1.0 mg/L
Average risk	1.0 to 3.0 mg/L
High risk	>3.0 mg/L

hsCRP >10 mg/L should precipitate search for non-CV causes of inflammation

Abbreviation: hsCRP, high-sensitivity C-reactive protein.
Source: From Ref. 126.

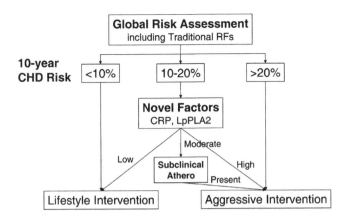

FIGURE 7 Potential use of novel risk factors and inflammatory markers in clinical practice. *Source:* Adapted from Ref. 127.

The cost of an hsCRP determination is roughly equivalent to that of a lipid profile and thus is not prohibitive as a diagnostic modality in the primary evaluation for cardiovascular risk.

Packard has also put forth a hypothetical treatment algorithm based on Lp-PLA2 that demonstrates the place for inflammatory markers (Fig. 7) (127).

CONCLUSIONS

The argument has been made that CRP should be included in the assessment of global cardiovascular risk (128). The Framingham Risk score has been a valuable addition to the assessment of a 10-year risk and there is mounting clinical evidence that CRP independently adds to the predictive value of the standard calculated score. Additional evidence has accumulated that CRP measurements also correlates with and adds prognostic information to the formal definition of the metabolic syndrome. Prognostic information obtained by measuring CRP appears to be consistent in epidemiologic and experimental studies that analyzed sex, ethnicity, and various risk categories in a variety of populations. Additionally, the data obtained from the large-scale statin trials also support the utilization of CRP both as a prognostic marker and as a therapeutic target.

A large body of data from epidemiologic, pathologic, basic science, and interventional trials has implicated the role of inflammation as major factor in the initiation of atherosclerosis (129). Additionally, the measurement of inflammatory markers can be utilized in all phases of atherosclerosis as a means to stratify the subsequent risk for complications related to obstructive vascular disease. The most promising marker is CRP and a variety of studies have demonstrated the clinical utility of this inflammatory marker both as a means to predict vascular risk and possibly as a therapeutic target. Further studies will be necessary to establish the role of the utilization of this promising marker to stratify individuals for risk at coronary disease and monitor response to therapy.

REFERENCES

1. Heart Disease and Stroke Statistics. Update, American Heart Association, 2005.
2. Lloyd-Jones DM, Wilson PW, Larson MG, et al. Framingham risk score and prediction of lifetime risk for CHD. Am J Cardiol 2004; 94(1):20–24.
3. Michos ED, Vasamreddy CR, Becker DM, et al. Women with a low Framingham risk score and a family history of premature coronary heart disease have a high prevalence of subclinical coronary atherosclerosis. Am Heart J 2005; 150(6):1276–1281.
4. Brindle PM, McConnachie A, Upton MN, et al. The accuracy of the Framingham risk-score in different socioeconomic groups: a prospective study. Br J Gen Pract 2005; 55(520):838–845.
5. Tice JA, Browner W, Tracy RP, Cummings SR. The relation of CRP levels to total and cardiovascular mortality in older U.S. women. Am J Med 2003; 114(3):119–205.
6. Ridker PM, Cushman M, Stampfer MJ, et al. Inflammation, aspirin, and the risk of cardiovascular disease in apparently healthy men. N Engl J Med 1997; 336(14):973–979.
7. Ridker PM, Buring JE, Shih J, et al. Prospective study of CRP and the risk of future cardiovascular events among apparently healthy women. Circulation 1998; 98(8):731–733.

8. Danesh J, Wheeler JG, Hirshfield GM, et al. CRP and other circulating markers of inflammation in the prediction of CHD. N Engl J Med 2004; 350(14):1387–1397.

9. Sakkinen P, Abbott RD, Curb JD, et al. CRP and myocardial infarction. J Clin Epidemiol 2002; 55(5):445–451.

10. Ballantyne CM, Hoogeveen RC, Bang H, et al. Lipoprotein-associated phospholipase A2, high-sensitivity CRP, and risk for incident coronary heart disease in middle-aged men and women in the Atherosclerosis Risk in Communities (ARIC) study. Circulation 2004; 109(7):837–842.

11. Tommasi S, Carluccio E, Bentivoglio M, et al. CRP as a marker for cardiac ischemic events in the year after a first, uncomplicated myocardial infarction. Am J Cardiol 1999; 83(12):1595–1599.

12. Ross R. Atherosclerosis is an inflammatory disease. Am Heart J 1999; 138(5 pt 2):S419–S420.

13. Li H, Cybulsky MI, Gimbrone MA Jr., Libby P. An atherogenic diet rapidly induces VCAM-1, a cytokine-regulatable mononuclear leukocyte adhesion molecule, in rabbit aortic endothelium. Arterioscler Thromb 1993; 13(2):197–204.

14. van Furth R. Human monocytes and cytokines. Res Immunol 1998; 149(7–8):719–720.

15. Wijffels JF, de Rover Z, Kraal G, Beelen RH. Macrophage phenotype regulation by colony-stimulating factors at bone marrow level. J Leukoc Biol 1993; 53(3):249–255.

16. Adams DO, Hamilton TA. The cell biology of macrophage activation. Annu Rev Immunol 1984; 2:283–318.

17. Gown AM, Tsukada T, Ross R. Human atherosclerosis. II. Immunocytochemical analysis of the cellular composition of human atherosclerotic lesions. Am J Pathol 1986; 125(1):191–207.

18. Goldstein JL, Brown MS. Lipoprotein receptors and the control of plasma LDL-C levels. Eur Heart J 1992; 13(suppl B):34–36.

19. Nishino T, Horii Y, Shiiki H, et al. Immunohistochemical detection of advanced glycosylation end products within the vascular lesions and glomeruli in diabetic nephropathy. Hum Pathol 1995; 26(3):308–313.

20. Fogelman AM, Haberland ME, Seager J, et al. Factors regulating the activities of the low-density lipoprotein receptor and the scavenger receptor on human monocyte-macrophages. J Lipid Res 1981; 22(7):1131–1141.

21. Han J, Hajjar DP, Tauras JM, Nicholson AC. Cellular cholesterol regulates expression of the macrophage type B scavenger receptor, CD36. J Lipid Res 1999; 40(5):830–838.

22. Ravn HB, Falk E. Histopathology of plaque rupture. Cardiol Clin 1999; 17(2):263–270.

23. Heinecke JW. Mechanisms of oxidative damage by myeloperoxidase in atherosclerosis and other inflammatory disorders. J Lab Clin Med 1999; 1333(4):321–325.

24. Geng YJ, Hernderson LE, Levesque EB, et al. Fas is expressed in human atherosclerotic intima and promotes apoptosis of cytokine-primed human vascular smooth muscles cells. Arterioscler Thromb Vasc Biol 1997; 17(10):2200–2208.

25. Galis ZS, Sukhova GK, Lark MW, Libby P. Increased expression of matrix metalloproteinases and matrix degrading activity in vulnerable regions of human atherosclerotic plaques. J Clin Invest 1994; 94(6):2493–2503.

26. Puddu GM, Cravero E, Arnone G, et al. Molecular aspects of atherogenesis: new insights and unsolved questions. J Biomed Sci 2005; 12(6):839–853.

27. Takahashi K, Takeya M, Sakashita N. Multifunctional roles of macrophages in the development and progression of atherosclerosis in humans and experimental animals. Med Electron Microsc 2002; 35(4):179–203.

28. Danesh J, Collins R, Peto R. Chronic infections and CHD: is there a link? Lancet 1997; 350(9075):430–436.

29. Kaplan M, Yavuz SS, Cinar B, et al. Detection of Chlamydia pneumoniae and Helicobactor pylori in atherosclerotic plaques of carotid artery by polymerase chain reaction. Int J Infect Dis 2005; 10(2):116–123.

30. Gupta S, Leatham EW, Carrington D, et al. Elevated Chlamydia pneumoniae antibodies, cardiovascular events, and azithromycin in male survivors of myocardial infarction. Circulation 1997; 96(2):404–407.

31. O'Connor CM, Dunne MW, Pfeffer MA, et al. Azithromycin for the secondary prevention of CHD events: the WIZARD study: a randomized controlled trial. JAMA 2003; 290(11):1459–1466.

32. Cercek B, Shah PK, Noc M, et al. Effect of short-term treatment with azithromycin on recurrent ischaemic events in patients with acute coronary syndrome in the Azithromycin in Acute Coronary Syndrome (AZACS) trial: a randomised controlled trial. Lancet 2003; 361(9360):809–813.

33. Cannon CP, Braunwald E, McCabe CH, et al. Antibiotic treatment of Chlamydia pneumoniae after acute coronary syndrome. N Engl J Med 2005; 352(16):1646–1654.

34. Andraws R, Berger JS, Brown DL. Effects of antibiotic therapy on outcomes of patients with CHD: a meta-analysis of randomized controlled trials. JAMA 2005; 293(21):2641–2647.

35. Salonen JT, Yla-Herttuala S, Yamamoto R, et al. Autoantibody against oxidized LDL and progression of carotid atherosclerosis. Lancet 1992; 339(8798):883–887.

36. Ghayour-Mobarhan M, Lamb DJ, Lovell DP, et al. Plasma antibody titres to heat shock proteins-60, -65 and -70: their relationship to coronary risk factors in dyslipidemic patients and healthy individuals. Scand J Clin Lab Invest 2005; 65(7):601–614.

37. Hansson GK. Immune mechanisms in atherosclerosis. Arterioscler Thromb Vasc Biol 2001; 21(12):1876–1890.

38. Xiao Q, Mandal K, Schett G, et al. Association of serum-soluble heat shock protein 60 with carotid atherosclerosis: clinical significance determined in a follow-up study. Stroke 2005; 36(12):2571–2576.
39. Baggiolini M. Chemokines and leukocyte traffic. Nature 1998; 392(6676):565–568.
40. Gerard C, Rollins BJ. Chemokines and disease. Nat Immunol 2001; 2(2):108–115.
41. Gerrity RG. The role of the monocyte in atherogenesis: I. Transition of blood-borne monocytes into foam cells in fatty lesions. Am J Pathol 1981; 103(2):181–190.
42. Hoefer IE, Grundmann S, van Royen N, et al. Leukocyte subpopulations and arteriogenesis: specific role of monocytes, lymphocytes and granulocytes. Atherosclerosis 2005; 181(2):285–293.
43. Boisvert WA. Modulation of atherogenesis by chemokines. Trends Cardiovasc Med 2004; 14(4):161–165.
44. Gimbrone MA Jr. Endothelial dysfunction, hemodynamic forces, and atherosclerosis. Thromb Haemost 1999; 82(2):722–726.
45. Ross R. Atherosclerosis—an inflammation disease. N Engl J Med 1999; 340:115–126.
46. Iiyama K, Hajra L, Iiyama M, et al. Patterns of vascular cell adhesion molecule-1 and intercellular adhesion molecule-1 expression in rabbit and mouse atherosclerotic lesions and at sites predisposed to lesion formation. Circ Res 1999; 85(2):199–207.
47. Wisse BE. The inflammatory syndrome: the role of adipose tissue cytokines in metabolic disorders linked to obesity. J Am Soc Nephrol 2004; 15(11):2792–2800.
48. Koerner A, Kratzsch J, Kiess W. Adipocytokines: leptin-the classical, resistin-the controversial, adiponectin-the promising, and more to come. Best Pract Res Clin Endocrinol Metab 2005; 19(4):525–546.
49. Considine RV. Human leptin: an adipocyte hormone with weight-regulatory and endocrine functions. Semin Vasc Med 2005; 5(1):15–24.
50. Zhang F, Chen Y, Heiman M, Dimarchi R. Leptin: structure, function and biology. Vitam Horm 2005; 71:345–372.
51. Hasty AH, Shimano H, Osuga J, et al. Severe hypercholesterolemia, hypertriglyceridemia, and athero-sclerosis in mice lacking both leptin and the low density lipoprotein receptor. J Biol Chem 2001; 276(40):37402–37408.
52. Fried SK, Bunkin DA, Greenberg AS. Omental and subcutaneous adipose tissues of obese subjects release interleukin-6: depot difference and regulation by glucocorticoid. J Clin Endocrinol Metab 1998; 83(3):847–850.
53. Heinrich PC, Castell JV, Andus T. Interleukin-6 and the acute phase response. Biochem J 1990; 265(3):621–636.
54. Weisberg SP, McCann D, Desai M, et al. Obesity is associated with macrophage accumulation in adi-pose tissue. J Clin Invest 2003; 112(12):1796–1808.
55. Kadowaki T, Yamauchi T. Adiponectin and adiponectin receptors. Endocr Rev 2005; 26(3):439–451.
56. Wild S, Roglic G, Green A, et al. Global prevalence of diabetes: estimates for the year 2000 and projec-tions for 2030. Diabetes Care 2004; 27(5):1047–1053.
57. Duncan BB, Schmidt MI, Pankow JS, et al. Low-grade systemic inflammation and the development of type 2 diabetes: the Atherosclerosis Risk in Communities study. Diabetes 2003; 52(7):1799–1805.
58. King DE, Mainous AG III, Buchanan TA, Pearson WS. C-reactive protein and glycemic control in adults with diabetes. Diabetes Care 2003; 26(5):1535–1539.
59. Bautista LE. Inflammation, endothelial dysfunction, and the risk of high blood pressure: epidemio-logic and biological evidence. J Human Hypertension 2003; 17:223–230.
60. Venugopal SK, Devaraj S, Yuhanna I, Shaul P, Jialal I. Demonstration that CRP decreases eNOS expres-sion and bioactivity in human aortic endothelial cells. Circulation 2002; 106(12):1439–1441.
61. Hernandez-Preza MA, Bustos C, Ortego M, Tunon J, Ortega L, Egido J. ACE inhibitor quinapril reduces the arterial expression on NF-kappaB-dependent proinflammatory factors but not of collagen I in a rabbit model of atherosclerosis. Am J Pathol 1998; 153(6):1825–1837.
62. Mervaala EM, Muller DN, Park JK, et al. Monocyte infiltration and adhesion molecules in a rat model of high human rennin hypertension. Hypertension 1999; 33(1 pt 2):389–395.
63. Sekiguchi K, Li X, Coker M, et al. Cross-regulation between the rennin-angiotensin system and inflam-matory mediators in cardiac hypertrophy and failure. Cardiovasc Res 2004; 63(3):433–442.
64. Hunter KA, Garlick PJ, Broom I, Anderson SE, McNurlan MA. Effects of smoking and abstention from smoking on fibrinogen synthesis in humans. Clin Sci (Lond) 2001; 100(4):459–465.
65. Antoniades C, Tousoulis D, Vasiliadou C, et al. Combined effects of smoking and hypercholes-terolemia on inflammatory process, thrombosis/fibrinolysis system, and forearm hyperemic response. Am J Cardiol 2004; 94(9):1181–1184.
66. Casey RG, Joyce M, Roche-Nagle G, et al. Young male smokers have altered platelets and endothelium that precedes atherosclerosis. J Surg Res 2004; 116(2):227–233.
67. Hioki H, Aoki N, Kawano K, et al. Acute effects of cigarette smoking on platelet-dependent thrombin generation. Eur Heart J 2001; 22(1):56–61.
68. Yasue H, Hirai N, Mizuno Y, et al. Low-grade inflammation, thrombogenicity, and atherogenic lipid profile in cigarette smokers. Circ J 2006; 70(1):8–13.
69. Lind P, Engstrom G, Stavenow L, et al. Risk of myocardial infarction and stroke in smokers is related to plasma levels of inflammation-sensitive proteins. Arterioscler Thromb Vasc Biol 2004; 24(3):577–582.

70. Chang MK, Binder CJ, Torzewski M, Witztum JL. CRP binds to both oxidized LDL and apoptotic cells through recognition of a common ligand: phosphorylcholine of oxidized phospholipids. Proc Natl Aced Sci USA 2002; 99(20):13043–13048.

71. Tebo JM, Mortensen RE. Internalization and degradation of receptor bound CRP by U-937 cells: induction of H2O2 production and tumoricidal activity. Biochem Biophys Acta 1991; 1095(3):210–216.

72. Ballou SP, Lozanski G. Induction of inflammatory cytokine release from cultured human monocytes by CRP. Cytokine 1992; 4(5):361–368.

73. Barter PJ, Nicholls S, Rye K-A, et al. Antiinflammatory Properties of HDL. Circ Res 2004; 95(8):764–772.

74. Wu A, Hinds CJ, Thiermermann C. HDLs in sepsis and septic shock: metabolism, actions, and therapeutic applications. Shock 2004; 21(3):210–221.

75. Navab M, Anantharamaiah GM, Fogelman AM. The role of HDL in inflammation. Trends Cardiovasc Med 2005; 15(4):158–161.

76. Bottazzi B, Garlanda C, Salvatori G, et al. Pentraxins as a key component of innate immunity. Curr Opin Immunol 2006; 18(1):10–15.

77. Jabs WJ, Theissing E, Nitschke M, et al. Local generation of CRP in disease coronary artery venous bypass grafts and normal vascular tissue. Circulation 2003; 108(12):1428–1431.

78. Yasojima K, Schwab C, McGeer EG, McGeer PL. Generation of CRP and complement components in atherosclerotic plaques. Am J Pathol 2001; 158(3):1039–1051.

79. Devaraj S, Du Clos TW, Jialal I. Binding and internalization of CRP by Fcgamma receptors on human aortic endothelial cells mediates biological effects. Arterioscler Thromb Vasc Biol 2005; 25(7): 1359–1363.

80. Venugopal SK, Devaraj S, Jialal I. CRP decreases prostacyclin release from human aortic endothelial cells. Circulation 2003; 108(14):1676–1678.

81. Pasceri V, Willerson JT, Yeh ET. Direct proinflammatory effect of CRP on human endothelial cells. Circulation 2001; 104(9):E46.

82. Pasceri V, Cheng JS, Willerson JT, Yeh ET. Modulation of CRP-mediated monocyte chemoattractant protein-1 induction in human endothelial cells by anti-atherosclerosis drugs. Circulation 2001; 103(21):2531–2534.

83. Han KH, Hong KH, Park JH, et al. CRP promotes monocyte chemoattractant protein-1-mediated chemotaxis through upregulating CC chemokine receptor 2 expression in human monocytes. Circulation 2004; 109(21):2566–2571.

84. Ji SR, Wu Y, Potempa LA, et al. Interactions of CRP with low-density lipoproteins: Implications for an active role of modified CRP in atherosclerosis. Int J Biochem Cell Biol 2006; 38(4):648–661.

85. Wang CH, Li SH, Weisel RD, et al. CRP upregulates angiotensin type 1 receptors in vascular smooth muscle. Circulation 2003; 107(13):1783–1790.

86. Singh U, Devaraj S, Jialal I. CRP decreases tissue plasminogen activator activity in human aortic endothelial cells: evidence that CRP is a procoagulant. Arterioscler Thromb Vasc Biol 2005; 25(10):2216–2221.

87. Carter AM. Inflammation, thrombosis and acute coronary syndromes. Diab Vasc Dis Res 2005; 2(3):113–121.

88. Hu FB, Bronner L, Willet WC, et al. Fish and omega-3 fatty acid intake and risk of CHD in women. JAMA 2002; 287(14):1815–1821.

89. Harper CR, Jacobson TA. The fats of life: the role of omega-3 fatty acids in the prevention of CHD. Arch Intern Med 2001; 161(18):2185–2192.

90. James MJ, Gibson RA, Cleland LG. Dietary polyunsaturated fatty acids and inflammatory mediator production. Am J Clin Nutr 2000; 7(suppl 1):343S–348S.

91. King DE, Egan BM, Geesey ME. Relation of dietary fat and fiber to elevation of CRP. Am J Cardiol 2003; 92(11):1335–1339.

92. Pischon T, Hankinson SE, Hotamisligil GS, Rifai N, et al. Habitual dietary intake of n-3 and n-6 fatty acids in relation to inflammatory markers among US men and women. Circulation 2003; 108(2): 155–160.

93. Erlinger TP, Miller ER III, Charleston J, Appel LJ. Inflammation modifies the effects of a reduced-fat low-cholesterol diet on lipids: results from the DASH-sodium trial. Circulation 2003; 108(2): 150–154.

94. Chase HP, Cooper S, Osberg J, et al. Elevated CRP levels in the development of type 1 diabetes. Diabetes 2004; 53(10):2569–2573.

95. Bahceci M, Tuzcu A, Ogun C, Canorue N, et al. Is serum CRP concentration correlated with HbA1c and insulin resistance in Type 2 diabetic men with or without CHD? J Endocrinol Invest 2005; 28(2):145–150.

96. Liu S, Manson JE, Buring JE, et al. Relation between a diet with a high glycemic load and plasma concentrations of high-sensitivity CRP in middle-aged women. Am J Clin Nutr 2002; 75(3):492–498.

97. Juni P, Nartey L, Reichenbach S, et al. Risk of cardiovascular events and rofecoxib: cumulative meta-analysis. Lancet 2004; 364(9450):2021–2029.

98. Topol EJ. Arthritis medicines and cardiovascular events-"house of coxibs." JAMA 2005; 293(3):366–368.

99. Balk EM, Lau J, Goudas LC, et al. Effects of statins on nonlipid serum markers associated with cardiovascular disease: a systematic review. Ann Intern Med 2003; 139(8):670–682.

100. Ray KK, Cannon CP. Early time to benefit with intensive statin treatment: could it be the pleiotropic effects? Am J Cardiol 2005; 96(5A):54F–60F.
101. Downs JR, Clearfield M, Weis S, et al. Primary prevention of acute coronary events with lovastatin in men and women with average cholesterol levels: results of AFCAPS/TexCAPS. Air Force/Texas Coronary Atherosclerosis Prevention Study. JAMA 1998; 279(20):1615–1622.
102. Ridker PM, Rifai N, Clearfield M, et al. Measurement of CRP for the targeting of statin therapy in the primary prevention of acute coronary events. N Engl J Med 2001; 344(26):1959–1965.
103. Shepherd J, Cobbe SM, Ford I, et al. Prevention of CHD with pravastatin in men with hypercholesterolemia. West of Scotland Coronary Prevention Study Group. N Engl J Med 1995; 333(20): 1301–1307.
104. Sattar N, Gaw A, Scherbakova O, et al. Metabolic syndrome with and without CRP as a predictor of CHD and diabetes in the West of Scotland Coronary Prevention Study. Circulation 2003; 108(4):414–419.
105. Ridker PM. JUPITER Study Group. Rosuvastatin in the primary prevention of cardiovascular disease among patients with low levels of LDL-C and elevated high-sensitivity CRP: rationale and design of the JUPITER trial. Circulation 2003; 108(19):2292–2297.
106. Sacks FM, Pfeffer MA, Moye LA, et al. The effect of pravastatin on coronary events after myocardial infarction in patients with average cholesterol levels. Cholesterol and Recurrent Events Trial investigators. N Engl J Med 1996; 335(14):1001–1009.
107. Ridker PM, Rifai N, Pfeffer MA, et al. Inflammation, pravastatin, and the risk of coronary events after myocardial infarction in patients with average cholesterol levels. Cholesterol and Recurrent Events (CARE) Investigators. Circulation 1998; 98(9):839–844.
108. Cannon CP, Braunwald E, McCabe CH, et al. Intensive versus moderate lipid lowering with statins after acute coronary syndromes. N Engl J Med 2004; 350(15):1495–1504.
109. Ridker PM, Cannon CP, Morrow D, et al. CRP levels and outcomes after statin therapy. N Engl J Med 2005; 352(1):20–28.
110. Nissen SE, Tuzcu EM, Schoenhagen P, et al. Statin therapy, LDL-C, CRP, and CHD. N Engl J Med 2005; 352(1):29–38.
111. Grundy SM, Vega GL, McGovern ME, et al. Efficacy, safety, and tolerability of once-daily niacin for the treatment of dyslipidemia associated with type 2 diabetes: results of the assessment of diabetes control and evaluation of the efficacy of Niaspan trial. Arch Intern Med 2002; 162(14):1568–1576.
112. Backes JM, Howard PA, Moriarty PM. Role of CRP in cardiovascular disease. Ann Pharmacother 2004; 38(1):110–118.
113. Fruchart JC, Staels B, Duriez P. PPARS, metabolic disease and atherosclerosis. Pharmacol Res 2001; 44(5):345–352.
114. Undas A, Celinska-Lowenhoff M, Domagala TB, et al. Early antithrombotic and anti-inflammatory effects of simvastatin versus fenofibrate in patients with hypercholesterolemia. Thromb Haemost 2005; 94(1):193–199.
115. Despres JP, Lemieux I, Pascot A, et al. Gemfibrozil reduces plasma CRP levels in abdominally obese men with the atherogenic dyslipidemia of the metabolic syndrome. Arterioscler Thromb Vasc Biol 2003; 23(4):702–703.
116. Campbell IW. The clinical significance of PPAR gamma agonism. Curr Mol Med 2005; 5(3):349–363.
117. Haffner SM, Greenberg AS, Weston WM, et al. Effect of rosiglitazone treatment on nontraditional markers of cardiovascular disease in patients with type 2 diabetes mellitus. Circulation 2002; 106:679–684.
118. Nauseef WM, Malech HL. Analysis of the peptide subunits of human neutrophil myeloperoxidase. Blood 1986; 67(5):1504–1507.
119. Eiserich JP, Baldus S, Brennen ML, et al. Myeolperoxidase, a leukocyte-derived vascular NO oxidase. Science 2002; 296(5577):2391–2394.
120. Vita JA, Brennan ML, Gokee N, et al. Serum myeloperoxidase levels independently predict endothelial dysfunction in humans. Circulation 2004; 110(9):1134–1139.
121. Daugherty A, Dunn JL, Rateri DL, Heinecke JW. Myelooeroxidase, a catalyst for lipoprotein oxidation, is expressed in human atherosclerotic lesions. J Clin Invest 1994; 94(1):437–444.
122. Zhang R, Brennan ML, Fu X, et al. Association between myeloperoxidase levels and risk of CHD. JAMA 2001; 286(17):2154–2156.
123. Sugiyama S, Okada Y, Sukhova GK, et al. Macrophage myeloperoxidase regulation by granulocyte macrophage colony-stimulating factor in human atherosclerosis and implications in acute coronary syndromes. Am J Pathol 2001; 158(3):879–891.
124. Leitinger N, Watson AD, Hama SY, et al. Role of group II secretory phopholipase A2 in atherosclerosis: 2. Potential involvement of biologically active oxidized phospholipids. Arterioscler Thromb Vasc Biol 1999; 19(5):1291–1298.
125. Packard CJ, O'Reilly DS, Caslake MJ, et al. Lipoprotein-associated phospholipase A2 as an independent predictor of CHD. West of Scotland Coronary Prevention Study Group. N Engl J Med 2000; 343(16):1148–1182.
126. Pearson TA, Mensah GA, Hong Y, et al. CDC/AHA Workshop on Markers of Inflammation and Cardiovascular Disease: Application to Clinical and Public Health Practice: overview. Circulation 2004; 110(25):e543–e544.

127. Caslake MJ, Packard CJ. Lipoprotein-associated phospholipase A2 as a biomarker for coronary disease and stroke. Nat Clin Pract Cardiovasc Med 2005; 2(10):529–535.
128. Ridker PM, Wilson PW, Grundy SM. Should CRP be added to metabolic syndrome and to assessment of global cardiovascular risk? Circulation 2004; 109(23):2818–2825.
129. Ceriello A, Motz E. Is oxidative stress the pathogenic mechanism underlying insulin resistance, diabetes, and cardiovascular disease? The common soil hypothesis revisited. Arterioscler Thromb Vasc Biol 2004; 24(5):816–823.

13 | Chronic Kidney Disease

Nelson Kopyt

Department of Medicine, Temple University, Philadelphia, and
Lehigh Valley Hospital, Allentown, Pennsylvania, U.S.A.

KEY POINTS

- CKD is a major public health problem affecting approximately 20 million adults in the United States.
- All patients at risk for CKD (especially diabetics, elderly, hypertensives, family history of kidney disease) should have a basic metabolic profile, calculate a glomerular filtration rate, do a urine analysis, and a spot urine for protein to creatinine ratio, and then stage their CKD if it is present.
- The presence of CKD should be considered a cardiovascular disease (CVD) equivalent.
- The presence of CKD indicates the need for an aggressive global cardiovascular risk reduction program.
- Proteinuria is more then a marker for CKD: it is a contributor to the progressive loss of kidney function especially at high levels as well as an independent predictor of increased risk for CVD and death.
- In addition to aggressive cardiovascular risk reduction, patients with CKD and/or proteinuria should be strongly considered for therapy with an angiotensin converting enzyme inhibitor or an angiotensin receptor blocker especially in the face of significant proteinuria.
- Patients with CKD and estimated GFR below $60 \, mL/min/1.73 \, m^2$ should also be assessed for anemia, parathyroid, mineral, and vitamin D abnormalities in addition to traditional cardiovascular risk assessment.

CASE

RL is a 65-year-old male with a 20-year history of hypertension, 15-year history of type 2 diabetes and hyperlipidemia, obesity. He is status post–three vessel coronary artery bypass surgery eight years ago. Concomitant medical problems include gout, osteoarthritis, asymptomatic carotid bruits and peripheral vascular disease with two-block claudication. A serum creatinine of 1.5 was found in 1998, 1.8 in 2000, and currently his creatinine is 2.2. Urinalysis shows 3 plus protein. Electrocardiogram (EKG) demonstrates left ventricular hypertrophy (LVH). Review of systems is positive for dyspnea on exertion, orthopnea, edema, visual complaints, and the claudication. Medications include metoprolol (25 mg), hydrochlorthiazide (12.5 mg), lisinopril (10 mg), simvastatin (10 mg), glipizide (10 mg), aspirin (81 mg), allopurinol (300 mg) and occasional naprosyn. Physical examination demonstrates a pulse of 104, blood pressure (BP) 168/70, and a body mass index (BMI) of 32. Diabetic and atherosclerotic retinopathy, bilateral carotid bruits, diffuse point of maximal impulse (PMI) with a systolic murmur, rales at the bases, aortic, and femoral bruits, and 2 plus edema. The patient was unaware of his renal disease.

CHRONIC KIDNEY DISEASE: WHAT IS THE CRISIS?

The crisis regarding chronic kidney disease (CKD) is that it is "underdiagnosed, undertreated," and the relationship to cardiovascular disease (CVD) "underrecognized." As is typified in the above case history, many physicians and their patients are unaware of the enormity and diversity of renal disease. Many physicians are not aware that patients like this are more likely to die of events related to CVD than of consequences of progression of their renal disease per se (1–3). CVD is the main cause of death in patients with CKD. It is now estimated that one in every nine adults (approximately 20–30 million Americans) has CKD and most are not aware of it. CKD is more common in the elderly, affecting one out of every four people over the age of 65. End-stage renal disease (ESRD) prevalence is expected to double by 2010 to 630,000 patients at a projected cost per year of 28.3 billion dollars (4). Nor are they aware of the significant impact that early CKD has on the cardiovascular state of an individual, as well as the tremendous increase in cardiovascular risk that this chapter will address. Prevention of renal impairment is an urgent challenge facing the medical profession. No treatment other than kidney transplantation effectively restores renal function once ESRD develops, and CVD is the leading cause of death among patients with ESRD (4). Progression along the continuum from early renal impairment to ESRD involves interactions of risk factors and deleterious conditions with increasing cardiovascular and renal risk (Fig. 1) (5).

The purpose of this review is to define CKD, how to adequately assess renal function as well as provide recent, representative data reinforcing the observation that increased cardiovascular risk is prevalent in all stages of CKD and to stress the importance of aggressive traditional interventions along with the possible benefits of nontraditional interventions to reduce this risk. I will show data demonstrating that the relation between reduced glomerular filtration and cardiovascular risk has been shown in the general population, hypertensive patients, individuals at high cardiovascular risk, and patients with cardiac dysfunction, specifically congestive heart failure (CHF) with the cardio-renal syndrome. Also, I review data demonstrating that during and after acute cardiac ischemic events, the survival is strongly dependent on renal function.

To determine the presence of CKD, one first must determine the level of renal function that classically is defined by the glomerular filtration rate (GFR). Most physicians focus on ESRD, the most visible consequence of CKD. Early CKD, which is frequently asymptomatic, has received little attention. The underestimation of renal function, which historically has been assessed by the serum creatinine, is the primary reason for this. It is not uncommon, such as in the case of our patient, to see patients with serum creatinine levels of 1.5 to 2.5 mg/dL and erroneously assume that they have relatively persevered renal function. What were frequently overlooked were important variables such as age, sex, race, and body mass. Once renal function is assessed by either a measured or calculated GFR or creatinine clearance (CrCl), it becomes apparent how severe their renal function is. The GFR or the CrCl provides an alternative to the serum creatinine, and is a much more reliable indicator of the level of kidney function. It is often not feasible to measure a GFR, which is quite time consuming and costly, and a 24-hour urine collection for the measurement of a CrCl is frequently difficult and inaccurate. Numerous formulas have been developed to estimate the GFR or CrCl from a serum creatinine and other variables. A commonly used formula to predict CrCl (mL/min per 1.73 m^2) is the

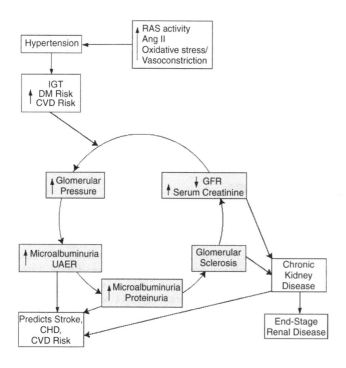

FIGURE 1 The renal continuum. *Abbreviations*: Ang II, angiotensin II; CHD, coronary heart disease; CVD, cardiovascular disease; DM, diabetes mellitus; GFR, glomerular filtration rate; IGT, impaired glucose tolerance; RAS, renin–angiotensin system; UAER, urinary albumin excretion rate. Source: Ref. 5.

Cockroft–Gault equation from serum creatinine, age, weight, and height (1). CrCl measured by a 24-hour urine collection or calculated by the Cockroft–Gault equation unfortunately over-estimated GFR by 19% and 16%, respectively (6). The Modification of Diet in Renal Disease (MDRD) study equation provides useful approximations of the GFR (7). This equation has been modified several times, and the correlation of the GFR predicted from the "six-variable equation" was excellent ($R^2 = 90.3\%$) (8).

Both the Cockroft–Gault and the MDRD study equations offer a fairly accurate estimate of renal function, which is defined as the GFR. In patients with CKD, the MDRD study equation appears to provide a more accurate and precise estimate of GFR than either the Cockroft–Gault equation or a measured creatinine clearance. These equations are only accurate in the study populations that were utilized to validate them. They should be used with caution in subgroups of the population not included in the development or validation of these equations such as children (below the age of 16), the elderly, pregnant women, and patients with reduced muscle mass, liver disease, or malnutrition. In these populations, we still have to rely on a measured 24-hour urine creatinine clearance until a more accurate method is verified or these equations are validated in these groups. Serum creatinine utilized in these calculations also must be in a steady state of creatinine balance. In principle, a calculated GFR would be lower than predicted if the serum creatinine is rising (such as in acute kidney failure), and it would be higher than predicted if the serum creatinine is falling.

Cockcroft–Gault (1976): $CrCl = IBW \times [(140\text{–age})/72 \times S_{Cr}]$ males = X1 females = X0.85 where IBW is ideal body weight

MDRD (four variable equation): $GFR = 186 \times S^{-1.154} \times age^{-0.203} \times 0.742$ if female $\times 1.210$ if African-American

MDRD (six variable equation): $GFR = 170 \times S^{-0.999} \times age^{-0.176} \times BUN^{-0.170} \times Alb^{\pm 0.318} \times 0.762$ if female $\times 1.180$ if African-American

We are constantly looking for a more accurate marker than the serum creatinine to assess GFR in our patients. On the horizon, Cystatin C may prove to be a more accurate index of the level of GFR (9,10). Cystatin C is a cysteine protease inhibitor that is produced and secreted by all nucleated cells, filtered by the kidney, and degraded by the proximal tubule. Its levels are not dependent on muscle mass (11). Concentrations of Cystatin C are almost totally dependent on GFR making it a potential candidate as a marker for renal function. Cystatin C may afford an opportunity to better characterize the association of kidney function with mortality risk. Two studies have demonstrated that Cystatin C is a stronger and more linear predictor of CVD mortality and heart failure than estimated GFR or serum creatinine (12,13). The risk for noncardiac deaths attributed to pulmonary disease, infection, cancer, and other causes was similarly associated with Cystatin C levels (14).

The National Kidney Foundation's guidelines for CKD make the following recommendations about assessment of kidney function (15).

- Estimates of GFR are the best overall indices of the level of kidney function.
- The level of GFR should be estimated from prediction equations that take into account the serum creatinine concentration and some or all of the following variables: age, gender, race, and body size. In adults, the MDRD study and Cockroft–Gault equations provide useful estimates of GFR. In children, the Schwartz and Counahan–Barratt equations are useful.
- The serum creatinine concentration should not be used alone to assess the level of kidney function.
- Clinical laboratories should report an estimate of GFR using a prediction equation, in addition to reporting the creatinine measurements.
- Auto-analyzer manufacturers and clinical laboratories should calibrate serum creatinine assays using an international standard.
- Measurement of CrCl using timed (e.g., 24-hour) urine collections does not improve the estimate of GFR over that provided by prediction equations. A 24-hour urine sample provides useful information for estimation of GFR in individuals with exceptional dietary intake (vegetarian diet, use of creatine supplements) or muscle mass (amputation, malnutrition, muscle wasting). It is also useful for assessment of diet and nutritional status and need to start dialysis.

DEFINITION OF CHRONIC KIDNEY DISEASE

Prior to 2002, the nomenclature commonly associated with kidney disease was quite confusing with no unified accepted definition. The publication in 2002 of the National Kidney Foundation's (NKF's) Kidney Disease Outcome Quality Initiative (K/DOQI) clinical practice guidelines for the evaluation, classification, and risk stratification of CKD has facilitated the identification and classification of CKD and is now universally accepted (8). CKD is persistent kidney damage and/or GFR <60 mL/min/1.73 m² for at least three months. Kidney damage may be confirmed by renal biopsy or markers of damage, such as abnormal blood tests, urine tests, or imaging studies. Based on the degree of decrease in the GFR, CKD is classified into five stages and associated with each stage is an appropriate action plan (Table 1) (8,16). Qualitatively, stages 1 and 2 represent kidney damage, stage 3 is moderately decreased kidney function, stage 4 is severely decreased kidney function, and stage 5 is kidney failure, usually with signs and symptoms of uremia requiring such kidney replacement therapies as dialysis or transplantation.

National Kidney Foundation (10)

Definition of CKD
- GFR <60 mL/min/1.73m² for ≥3 mo with or without kidney damage or
- Kidney damage for ≥3 mo, with or without decreased glomerular filtration rate (GFR), manifested by either
  - Pathologic abnormalities
  - Markers of kidney damage, e.g., proteinuria

Early Chronic Kidney Disease a Major Health Problem

Analysis of the Third National Health and Nutrition Examination Survey (NHANES III, 1988–1994) suggests that CKD is a major public health problem that is estimated to afflict 20 million adults (11% of the population) in the United States (8,17). Using the K/DOQI definition of CKD, it has become apparent that the disease is more common than previously recognized. Half with exclusively kidney damage manifested by microalbuminuria/proteinuria (stages 1 and 2), and half with a GFR less the 60 mL/min/1.73 m² (stages 3 and 4). The prevalence of early stages of disease (stages 1 to 4; 10.8%) is more than 100 times greater than the prevalence of kidney failure (stage 5; 0.1%). The prevalence of the five stages of CKD in the United States and this dramatic decrease in the prevalence of CKD from stage 3 to 4 and 5 is depicted in Figure 2. Aging further increases the incidence of CKD with prevalence in patient's age greater than 70 of 25% (19). The assumption can be made that any older patient with a serum creatinine of >1.0 mg/dL will have a GFR of <60 mL/min/1.73 m² and, by definition, CKD. In addition to age, hypertension and diabetes are also important predictors of CKD. In a study performed by the Kaiser Permanente's center for Health Research, a large not for profit Health Maintenance Organization (HMO) in California, the natural history of CKD was examined in 27,998 adults with a follow up of five years (20). Based on the five stages of severity of CKD from the NKF-K/DOQI guidelines, the five-year mortality rates for stages 2, 3, and 4 were

TABLE 1 Classification of Chronic Kidney Disease According to Glomerular Filtration Rate

Stage	Description	GFR (mL/min/1.73 m²)	Action
1	Kidney damage with normal or ↑ GFR	≥90	Diagnose and treat Treat comorbid conditions Slow progression
2	Kidney damage with mild ↓ GFR	60–89	Estimate progression
3	Moderate ↓ GFR	30–59	Evaluate and treat complications
4	Severe ↓ GFR	15–29	Prepare for kidney replacement therapy
5	Kidney failure	<15 (or dialysis)	Kidney replacement If uremia is present

Note: Prevalence for stage 5 is from the U.S. Renal Data System (1998); prevalence for stages 1 to 4 is from the Third National Health and Nutrition Examination Survey (1988 to 1994).
Source: From Ref. 16.

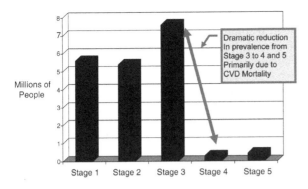

FIGURE 2 Dramatic reduction in prevalence of CKD between stage 3 and stage 4 or 5 CKD. *Abbreviations:* CKD, chronic kidney disease; CVD, cardiovascular disease. *Source:* From United States Renal Disease System (USRDS) 2004 Annual data report and Ref. 18.

19.5%, 24.3%, and 45.7%, respectively, whereas the frequency of renal replacement therapy (RRT) was much lower at 1.1%, 1.3%, and 19.9%, respectively. RL, in our case presentation above with stage 3 CKD, the most prevalent stage, has an 18.7-fold greater likelihood of mortality than progression to ESRD. Even in stage 4 CKD, twice as many patients died than progressed on to ESRD, with the primary cause of death being CVD.

With a uniform and widely accepted definition and classification of CKD, we can now easily screen our patients for CKD by simply measuring serum creatinine, calculating an estimated GFR with the modified MDRD equation, and obtaining spot urinary total protein to creatinine ratio. Many laboratories and hospitals are now offering estimated GFR values along with serum creatinine concentrations as well as an easy to use GFR calculator utilizing the MDRD equation on the National Kidney Foundation website (21). After the GFR is calculated the stage of CKD can be identified and the appropriate action plan instituted as is defined in Table 1. After identifying the appropriate stage and instituting an action plan to decrease CVD risk as well as the progression of CKD [including aggressive control of BP to less than 130/80 and the use of angiotensin-modulating therapy (angiotensin-converting enzyme inhibitors (ACE-Is) or angiotensin-receptor blockers (ARBs)], we hope the majority of patients will stabilize at that stage of CKD. It is also important to continue to track the patient's stage of CKD over time with serial calculations of GFR to make sure that they are stable and not progressing.

Factors that increase the risk of progression of CKD through the five stages to ESRD include low GFR, hypertension, diabetes, proteinuria, congenital low nephron number (as is seen in low-birth-weight infants), anemia, hyperlipidemia, smoking, obesity, and chronic use of nephrotoxins (i.e., analgesics). These factors should be identified in all patients with CKD and managed aggressively to impact the epidemic of CKD/ESRD and CVD.

The number of ESRD patients in the United States is expected to increase by 48% from 1998 to 2010 (3). As of 2003, the United States Renal Data System (USRDS) report indicated a prevalent ESRD population in the United States of 406,081 with 292,215 undergoing dialysis and 113,866 with transplantation. With growth fueled by the aging of the baby boomer population and the increasing burden of diabetes in the United States, by 2030 the ESRD population could increase by 460,000 new cases per year and is predicted to reach a total population of 2.24 million people, with two-thirds of these new patients having diabetes as a primary cause for their ESRD (22). Greater than half of the 2030 ESRD population is predicted to be age 65 or older and races other than white (23).

Utilizing the NHANES 1999–2000, Nickolas et al., characterized the demographics and health care access of patients with stages 1 through 4 CKD (24). Awareness levels for stage 5 CKD, as would be expected, was 100%, whereas those for stages 1 through 4 were below 50% (24). Only 22% of the 7.6 million Americans with stage 3 CKD are aware that they have CKD, thus indicating the tremendous need for educating both the medical community and the general public.

The ever increasing evidence that CKD is recognized as a major CVD risk factor, with a hazard risk ratio for morbidity and mortality several fold greater than seen with other risk factors, forces us to screen our patients for CKD more aggressively. Unfortunately, CKD is frequently silent as is noted in the NHANES data above. Even in family members of ESRD patients, where one would expect an increased awareness of CKD, a recent study demonstrated only 13% awareness of having CKD, and despite the fact that 83% had seen a physician in the past six-month, only 7.9% of those were aware of the presence of CKD (25). This stresses the need for improved awareness by the medical community for the need to screen for CKD and to communicate these results to their patients. The screening process is not difficult (Table 2) and includes a basic metabolic profile, a calculated GFR, a urine analysis, and a urine protein to creatinine ratio. With this information we can then determine the presence of CKD and appropriately stage its severity utilizing the information in Table 1.

IS CHRONIC KIDNEY DISEASE ASSOCIATED WITH INCREASED CARDIOVASCULAR DISEASE RISK?

The burden of CVD in early CKD has now clearly been demonstrated by both retrospective and prospective studies, some of which will now be reviewed. It is now apparent that CKD is a CVD equivalent.

The Hypertension Detection and Follow-up Program (HDFP), a community-based, randomized, controlled trial of two antihypertensive treatment strategies in 10,940 participants between 1975 and 1980, was the first clinical hypertensive trial to include data on serum creatinine values (26). These investigators noted an eight-year all-cause mortality risk increased in a stepwise manner according to serum creatinine value between <0.7 and >2.5 mg/dL. A fivefold increase in mortality was noted between the groups with the lowest and highest creatinine values with CVD as the major cause of death and kidney disease representing an uncommon cause of death. From this report to the most current reports, it has become evident though not widely appreciated that the major threat to patients with CKD is CV death rather than ESRD and that the enhanced risk begins at the earliest stages of CKD and therefore associated with a tremendous increase in mortality after initiating dialysis therapy.

In the Hypertension Optimal Treatment (HOT) clinical trial, patients with a serum creatinine level >1.5 mg/dL at baseline were significantly more likely to be male and older, and to have more severe systolic hypertension and a history of myocardial infarction, stroke, or diabetes (27). Because of the increased prevalence of myocardial infarction, LVH, and heart failure in this group, the relative risk for cardiovascular death was 3.24 among patients with reduced renal function at baseline (17).

In a cohort of 6223 patients enrolled in the Framingham Heart Study, 9% of men and 8% of women were found to have mild chronic renal impairment (28). In both men and women, the prevalence of CVD, coronary heart disease (CHD), heart failure, and LVH were greater in those with mild renal impairment than in those with normal serum creatinine values (23). The Framingham data, gathered during slightly more than 11 years of follow-up, indicate that even mild renal impairment is associated with risk for adverse outcomes, especially in men, and is strongly associated with coexisting CVD and risk factors for CVD (28).

TABLE 2 Chronic Kidney Disease Screening

- During routine health encounter assess risk via sociodemographic characteristics, past medical history, family history, and measured blood pressure
- Who should be screened:
  - Diabetics
  - Older individuals
  - Family history of kidney disease
  - High blood pressure
  - Autoimmune diseases
  - Reduction in kidney mass
  - History of recovery from acute renal failure
  - History of low birth weight
  - Exposure to certain drugs
  - African-Americans, American-Indians, Hispanic, Asian, or Pacific Islanders
  - Chronic use of potentially nephrotoxic medications
  - Metabolic syndrome
- How to screen:
  - Basic metabolic profile
  - Calculate a GFR
  - Urine analysis
  - Spot urine protein to creatinine ration or albumin to creatinine ratio
- Define stage of CKD and develop an action plan

Abbreviation: GFR, glomerular filtration rate.

The Hoorn study was a population-based cohort study of glucose tolerance and other CVD risk factors in a Caucasian population aged 50 to 75 (29). Baseline measurements were obtained from 1989 to 1992 with a 10.2-year follow-up ($n = 631$). The eGFR utilizing the MDRD formula ranged from 16.8 to 116.9 mL/min/1.73 m^2. Forty-three percent of the 117 deaths were from cardiovascular causes. Renal function was inversely associated with all-cause and CVD mortality, with a decrease of GFR by 5 mL/min/1.73 m^2 being associated with a 26% increase in risk of cardiovascular death even after adjustment for baseline hypertension, diabetes mellitus, age, sex, and other traditional risk factors for CVD. Based on GFR tertiles, the lowest survival rate was noted in the cohort with worst renal function. In this study, a decrease in GFR from 90 to 60 mL/min/1.73 m^2 was associated with a fourfold increase in risk of CVD mortality. These investigators also reported that even mild impairment of renal function is associated with adverse changes in left ventricular structure with an increase in left ventricular mass in men but not in women (30).

The Cardiovascular Health Study, a prospective population-based study of persons older than 65 with a median follow-up of 7.3 years, demonstrated that all-cause mortality and CVD mortality was increased almost twofold in patients with renal insufficiency (31). Renal insufficiency was defined as a serum creatinine level of 1.5 mg/dL or higher in men and 1.3 mg/dL or higher in women. In addition, there was a linear increase in the risk of CVD, peripheral vascular disease, and CHF with an increasing serum creatinine level. In the same cohort of patients, Shlipak et al. (32) demonstrated that the prevalence of clinical and subclinical CVD was 64% in patients with CKD, as compared with 43% in those with normal renal function.

In a study of the natural history of the various stages of diabetic nephropathy, the U.K. Prospective Diabetes Study (UKPDS 64) demonstrated the tremendous impact of progressive CKD on mortality (33). In this study, the annual transition rates through the stages of nephropathy and to death from any cause were analyzed. With no nephropathy present slightly more patients progressed on to microalbuminuria then died (2% vs. 1.4%, respectively). With microalbuminuria present, roughly the same progressed on to overt albuminuria as died (2.8% vs. 3%, respectively). Of the albuminuria group, twice as many patients died as progressed on to an elevated serum creatinine or the need for renal replacement therapy (RRT) (4.6% died vs. 2.3% progressing on). With the development of an elevated serum creatinine or the need for RRT the mortality was 19.2%.

A subgroup analysis of the 9287 persons in the Heart Outcome and Prevention Evaluation (HOPE) study (34) with renal insufficiency (serum creatinine $\geq$ 1.4 mg/dL) demonstrated a greater cumulative incidence of each primary outcome measure (CVD death, myocardial infarction, or stroke).

The relationships between serum creatinine concentration and the risk of major events related to ischemic heart disease and stroke and all-cause mortality were examined in the British Population–Based Study, a prospective study of middle aged men (aged 49 to 59 years old) from 24 British towns with an average follow-up of 14.75 years ($N = 7690$) (35). Stroke risk was significantly increased with serum creatinines above 1.3 mg/dL even after adjustment for a wide range of CVD risk factors (relative risk, 1.6). Both all-cause mortality and overall CVD mortality were significantly increased in those with a serum creatinine level above 1.5 mg/dL. These investigators concluded that even borderline increases in serum creatinine concentration are associated with increased risk of cerebrovascular death in both normotensive and hypertensive people.

The prevalence of CKD in older hypertensive patients was evaluated in the 40,514 participants 55 years or older who were enrolled in the Antihypertensive and Lipid-Lowering Treatment to Prevent Heart Attack Trial (ALLHAT) (36). Original entry criteria for the ALLHAT trial included a serum creatinine of less than 2 mg/dL. The simplified MDRD equation was used to calculate the estimated GFR and determine the baseline renal function in this cohort of patients. The prevalence of CVD was then assessed at the different levels of GFR. Fifty-seven percent of patients had mild [60–89 mL/min/1.73 m^2 (stage 2 CKD)], 17.2% had moderate [30–59 mL/min/1.73 m^2 (stage 3 CKD)], and 0.6% had severe [29 mL/min/1.73 m^2 (stage 4 CKD)] reductions in GFR. A history of previous acute myocardial infarctions (AMIs) and stroke was present in 19.2%, 23.4%, 28.7%, and 26.9% of persons with stage 2, 3, 4, and 5 CKD, respectively. A history of coronary bypass surgery or angioplasty or other revascularization procedure was noted in 9.2%, 13.6%, 17.2%, and 14.4% of patients with stage 2 to 5 CKD, respectively. A history of CHD was present in 21.2%, 26.4%, 31.3%, and 28.7% of patients with stage 2 to 5

CKD strata, respectively. At the time of enrollment, EKG criteria for LVH were noted in 3.9%, 4.2%, 6.0%, and 11.2% of patients with stages 2 to 5 CKD, respectively.

These investigators concluded that the prevalence of reduced GFR is high in older hypertensive patients. Patients with moderate or severe reduction in GFR are more likely to have a history of CVD and EKG-LVH. Even modest reductions in GFR are independently associated with a higher prevalence of CVD and EKG-LVH (30). The greater prevalence of moderate CKD (following the definition of K/DOQI practice guidelines: eGFR <60 mL/min/1.73 m^2) in the ALLHAT cohort (18%) at the time of randomization as compared to 4.6% in the NHANES III cohort of the general adult population may be explained by the overall greater age of the patients in the ALLHAT at the time of enrollment (1). These findings provide evidence-based data that CKD is a CVD equivalent.

Two recent, large studies of managed care populations have also corroborated these findings (19,37). CHF, coronary artery disease (CAD), and diabetes were more prevalent in the group that died suggesting perhaps that the primary therapeutic focus in patients with CKD may be on these diseases and modifying risk factors such as obesity, lack of exercise, smoking, hyperlipidemia, and hypertension rather than the progression of CKD itself (37). An analysis of the rates of atherosclerotic vascular disease (ASVD), CHF, RRT and death was performed in a 5% sampling of Medicare patients ($n = 1,091,201$) (38). With use of Cox regression, the corresponding adjusted hazards in the nondiabetic non-CKD, diabetic without CKD, CKD without diabetes and both diabetes and CKD populations were as follows: ASVD, 1, 1.30, 1.16, and 1.41 ($P < 0.0001$); CHF, 1, 1.44, 1.28, and 1.79 ($P < 0.0001$); RRT, 1, 2.52, 23.1, and 38.9 ($P < 0.0001$); and death, 1, 1.21, 1.38, and 1.56, respectively ($P < 0.0001$). This study again corroborates the fact that in patients with CKD, the risks of ASVD and CHF are much greater than the risk for RRT.

Go et al. recently published their results of the outcomes analysis in 1,120,295 adults with CKD enrolled in Kaiser Permanente of Northern California (39). Figure 3 demonstrates the age-standardized rates for all-cause mortality and for cardiovascular events following a stepwise reduction in GFR from less than 60 mL/min (stage 3 CKD) to less than 15 mL/min (stage 5 CKD).

Collectively, now with well over 1 million patients in these databases, clearly they corroborate the observations of the HDFP that patients with CKD have increased rates of all-cause mortality and cardiovascular events that are demonstrable at all stages of CKD and progress with advancing stages of CKD. This risk develops well before ESRD and with a much greater frequency of nonrenal over renal outcomes (40).

Effect of CKD on CV Secondary Outcomes

More than 50% of deaths among patients with ESRD are due to cardiovascular events (41). Two subsequent reports then demonstrated that the risk of subsequent cardiovascular events is higher among patients with CKD than among patients with normal renal function (42,43).

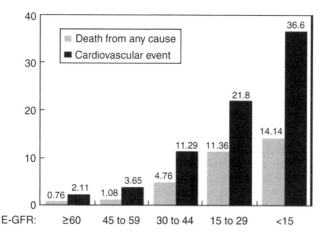

FIGURE 3   Age-standardized rates for all-cause mortality and for cardiovascular events in 1,120,295 adults who were enrolled in Kaiser Permanente of Northern California. During this follow-up period of 2.84 years only 0.28% of patients started dialysis and 0.03% underwent renal transplantation. *Source*: From Ref. 20.

A recent statement paper by the American Heart Association Councils on Kidney in Cardiovascular Disease, High Blood Pressure Research, Clinical Cardiology, and Epidemiology and Prevention (44) reported that the two-year mortality rate after myocardial infarction among patients with end-stage renal disease is approximately 50%, which is twice the mortality rate after myocardial infarction in the general population.

Until recently, limited information existed on the risks associated with lesser degrees of CKD in patients with post-AMIs. The Valsartan in Acute Myocardial Infarction Trial (VALIANT) examined the relative effects of captopril, valsartan, or both in 14,527 patients who sustained an AMI complicated by CHF, left ventricular dysfunction (LVEF), or both (45). The study excluded patients with initial serum creatinine values of 2.5 mg/dL or greater. These investigators demonstrated that the prevalence of coexisting risk factors and prior CVD was greatest among patients with a reduced estimated GFR (less than 45.0 ml/min/1.73 m^2) and the use of the therapies that would have the greatest impact on reducing morbidity and mortality (aspirin, β blockers, statins, and coronary-revascularization procedures) was lowest in this group. The risk of death or the composite end point of death from cardiovascular causes, reinfarction, CHF, stroke, or resuscitation after cardiac arrest increased with declining estimated GFRs. In this study a decrease in GFR from greater than 75 to less than 45 mL/min resulted in a increase in death from any cause and the composite end point of approximately 27% and 34%, respectively. Although the rate of renal events increased with declining estimated GFRs, the adverse outcomes were predominantly cardiovascular. These investigators also demonstrated that CKD is more common than suspected (33.5% of the 14,527 patients in the VALIANT study had an estimated GFR of less than 60 mL/min/1.73 m^2) and is clearly a significant independent risk factor for cardiovascular events among patients who have had a myocardial infarction complicated by heart failure, left ventricular systolic dysfunction, or both, as compared with patients with preserved renal function. This risk is progressive and with an estimated GFR below 81.0 mL/min/1.73 m^2, each reduction of the estimated GFR by 10 units was associated with a 10% increase in the relative risk of death or nonfatal cardiovascular complications (45). This study also further corroborated the repeated finding that the proportion of adverse renal events were relatively small; again patients have a higher risk of cardiovascular events than adverse renal outcomes. Among patients who have had a myocardial infarction, any degree of preexisting renal impairment should be considered a potent, independent, and easily identifiable risk factor for cardiovascular complications. Thus, progressive stages of CKD adversely affect outcomes after an AMI.

As is discussed above, CAD is prevalent and strongly associated with adverse outcomes among patients with ESRD. Mortality in ESRD patients was 19.5% at one year with half due to cardiac disease (46), and increasing to almost 60% during the year after myocardial infarction (47). Joki et al. performed coronary angiography on 24 patients within one month of initiating hemodialysis therapy for ESRD regardless of the presence or absence of angina to assess the incidence of CAD in this population (48). Fifteen patients (62.5%) had significant CAD with 73.3% having multivessel disease. The prevalence of CAD was 72.7% in the symptomatic patients and 53.8% in the asymptomatic patients. Thus the risk associated with CVD begins well before the onset of ESRD, i.e., during the period of early CKD. The 3608 patients enrolled in the Bypass Angioplasty Revascularization Investigation (BARI) Trial with multivessel CAD were assessed with regard to the presence or absence of CKD (49). This was defined as the presence or absence of a preprocedure serum creatinine level of >1.5. Among the 3608 patients enrolled, 76 were found to have CKD. These demonstrated significantly increased seven-year relative risk ratios of 2.2 for all-cause mortality and 2.8 for cardiac mortality as compared with those without CKD. The risk associated with CKD was comparable to and additive to the risk associated with diabetes. These investigators found CKD associated with an increased risk of recurrent hospitalization, subsequent coronary artery bypass graft (CABG), and mortality. With regard to surgical treatments, there is general agreement that patients who have CHD and CKD who warrant intervention appear to do better with coronary artery bypass surgery than with percutaneous coronary angioplasty (50).

CARDIORENAL SYNDROME

The term "cardiorenal syndrome" has been applied to the presence or development of renal dysfunction in patients with heart failure, but the syndrome has not been well described, and its management remains even less well understood (51). Renal insufficiency is common in patients who enter the hospital with heart failure, and carries a grim prognosis. Renal function is affected by CHF and it relates to both cardiovascular and homodynamic properties, as well as having additional prognostic value. The Second Prospective Randomized study of Ibopamine on Mortality and Efficacy (PRIME II) consisted of 1906 patients with CHF [New York Heart Association (NYHA) class III to IV] and evidence of LVEF <0.35. In a subgroup of 372 patients baseline plasma neurohormones were determined and renal function (CrCl) was calculated using the Cockcroft–Gault equation (52). The baseline renal function was the most powerful predictor of mortality; followed by NYHA functional class and the use of ACE-Is. Patients in the lowest quartile of CrCl values (<44 mL/min) had almost three times the risk of mortality (relative risk, 2.85; $P < 0.001$) of patients in the highest quartile (>76 mL/min). In this study, renal function correlated significantly with mortality, and more strongly than impaired cardiac function (LVEF and NYHA class), in advanced CHF, and it is associated with increased levels of N-terminal atrial natriuretic peptide. A stepwise increase in mortality risks with decreasing CrCl and LVEF was noted (Fig. 4). A retrospective analysis of the Studies in Left Ventricular Dysfunction (SOLVD) Treatment Trial and SOLVD Prevention Trial also found that estimated GFR was an important determinant of survival (53). These findings are even more striking because both trials excluded patients with significant elevations of serum creatinine (>2 mg/dL for both the SOLVD Treatment and SOLVD Prevention trials). This underscores the utility of calculating GFR in elderly heart failure patients, as the results of a simple serum creatinine test may seriously underestimate the degree of renal dysfunction, especially in elderly individuals. Once patients are admitted, worsening renal function also signifies a significantly poorer prognosis.

Gottlieb et al. examined outcomes in 1002 patients at university hospitals who had been admitted for acute decompensated heart failure (ADHF), including many with preserved systolic function (54). The majority had some increase in their serum creatinine level, and 30% had at least a 20% rise. Any increase in creatinine level was significant, but an increase of 0.3 mg/dL had a sensitivity of 81% and specificity of 62% for predicting either death or a length of stay of 10 days or more. Similarly, in a series of 412 patients, Smith et al. reported that an increase of 0.2 mg/dL of creatinine predicted a worse outcome during hospitalization (55). In this study a 25% increase in creatinine was a very specific marker for poor prognosis, but lacked sensitivity.

In the Acute Decompensated Heart Failure National Registry (ADHERE®) database of over 100,000 patients, which provides an in-depth look at the treatment and outcomes of patients admitted for ADHF, the mean calculated CrCl by the Cockcroft–Gault equation was 48.9 mL/min/m² for men and 35 mL/min/m² for women (51). Thus the typical patient admitted to the hospital with ADHF has stage 3 CKD according to the NKF-K/DOQI classification. Among women, fewer than 10% have only mild renal dysfunction or a normal GFR, and 46.8% have severe dysfunction or frank renal failure. Renal failure is slightly more prevalent in men; over 60% have at least moderate kidney damage (51). Thus, renal dysfunction is observed in

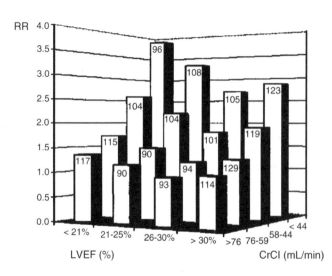

FIGURE 4 Three-dimensional bar graph showing risk of mortality (*vertical axis*) in relation to decreasing quartiles of left ventricular dysfunction (*horizontal axis*) and decreasing quartiles of CrCl as calculated by the Cockcroft–Gault equation (*diagonal axis*). *Source*: From Ref. 52.

most patients with ADHF. It is very likely that progressive renal insufficiency may lead to ADHF and, hence, admission to the hospital.

It is clear that CKD is a significant component of the morbidity and mortality seen in CHF. The cause of heart failure–associated CKD are diverse; but most important, some factors are reversible. Decreased renal perfusion, one of the more common factors, is attributed to hypovolemia (decreased preload), neurohormonally mediated vasoconstriction (increased afterload), and hypotension with preserved cardiac output (vasodilatory shock) or low-output syndrome. Renal dysfunction may also be caused by intrinsic renal disease such as longstanding hypertension and/or diabetes.

The cardiorenal syndrome is defined as moderate or greater renal dysfunction that exists or develops in a patient with heart failure during treatment. Moderate renal dysfunction is defined, in turn, as a GFR of <59 mL/min/m^2 or an increase in serum creatinine of 0.3 mg/dL. In many elderly patients, especially women, this degree of renal dysfunction will exist with a serum creatinine level of <2 mg/dL. Patients with heart failure who are intolerant of ACE-Is or ARBs for reasons other than cough or angioedema should also be considered to have the cardiorenal syndrome.

RELATIONSHIP BETWEEN CKD AND CVD RISK

The at-risk population for both CVD and CKD include patients of advanced age, diabetes mellitus, and high BP. This indicates that there is much overlap between the two groups. Thus, CKD and CVD may be outcomes of the same underlying disorders (Fig. 5).

In a recent review, Menon et al. proposed several reasons for the increased risk of CVD in patients with CKD (57): (i) CKD is associated with increased prevalence of traditional and nontraditional CVD risk factors; (ii) CKD is an independent risk factor for CVD; (iii) many CVD risk factors are also risk factors for progression of CKD; and (iv) the presence of CVD may be a risk factor for CKD. This interrelationship between CVD and CKD, each contributing to the pathogenesis of the other, results in a cycle of cardiovascular and kidney disease progression.

A recent scientific statement from the American Heart Association described two types of CVD risk factors in patients with CKD: traditional and nontraditional (44) [Table 3 (44)]. Traditional CVD risk factors, such as older age, diabetes, greater total cholesterol level, lower high-density lipoprotein (HDL) cholesterol level, LVH, smoking, and greater systolic BP, have been defined in the Framingham Heart Study and used to predict CHD outcomes in the general population (58). Several of these risk factors increase in prevalence as kidney function declines.

Several cross-sectional studies have suggested that the Framingham risk equation is insufficient to capture the extent of CVD risk in patients with CKD (59–61). This may indicate that other nontraditional risk factors listed in Table 2 may play an important role in promoting CVD in patients with CKD or that the traditional risk factors may have a qualitatively or quantitatively different risk relationship with CVD in CKD compared with the general population, i.e., individuals with CKD may have had a longer and more severe exposure to hypertension than subjects without CKD (37).

It has become apparent that as patients progress along the renal continuum of CKD they build on the traditional risk factors with nontraditional risk factors with a resultant exponential increase in CVD risk. Dennis (40) has described a risk pyramid for patients with CKD (Fig. 6) that includes (i) traditional risks, most of which are more prevalent in patients with CKD than in the general population; (ii) common, nontraditional risks that may be more frequent or more intense in CKD; (iii) uncommon, nontraditional risks that are largely unique

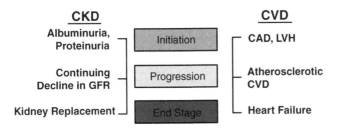

FIGURE 5 Risk factors for progression of CKD parallel those of CVD. Abbreviations: CKD, chronic kidney disease; CVD, cardiovascular disease, GFR, glomerular filtration rate; LVH, left ventricular hypertrophy; CAD, coronary artery disease. *Source*: From Ref. 56.

TABLE 3 Traditional and Nontraditional Cardiovascular Risk Factors in Chronic Kidney Disease

Traditional risk factors	CKD related: nontraditional risk factors
Older age	Albuminuria/proteinuria
Male sex	Homocysteine
Hypertension	Lipoprotein (a) and apolipoprotein (a)
Higher LDL cholesterol isoforms	Lipoprotein remnants
Low HDL cholesterol	Anemia
Diabetes	Abnormal calcium phosphate metabolism
Smoking	Extracellular fluid overload
Physical inactivity	Oxidative stress
Menopause	Inflammation (C-reactive protein)
Family history of CVD	Malnutrition
Left ventricular hypertrophy	Thrombogenic factors
	Sleep disturbances
	Altered nitric oxide/endothelin balance
	Electrolyte imbalance
	Hyperparathyroidism
	Hypovitaminosis D

Abbreviations: LDL, low-density lipoprotein; HDL, high-density lipoprotein CVD, cardiovascular disease.
Source: From Ref. 41.

to CKD, such as azotemia, chronic anemia, and disordered potassium and divalent ion metabolism, and treatment-related factors associated with dialysis or transplantation; and (iv) unknown factors. The connotation of the pyramidal arrangement of these factors is twofold: First, those risks accumulate as CKD progresses and, second, that an intervention aimed at a single risk factor at one level may be thwarted by the cumulative risks at other levels (40).

METABOLIC SYNDROME AND CHRONIC KIDNEY DISEASE

The metabolic syndrome could be considered an intermediate state between normal metabolism and type 2 diabetes mellitus (62,63). It is characterized by a constellation of atherogenic risk factors that include dyslipidemias, hypertension, hyperglycemia, obesity; a susceptible genomic substrate; and superimposed proinflammatory and prothrombotic milieu. Insulin resistance is felt to be a cardinal feature. The metabolic syndrome has been associated with an increased risk for diabetes mellitus and CVD, as well as increased mortality from CVD and all causes (64,65). Considering the relationships outlined above between CKD and CHD raises the suspicion of a relationship with metabolic syndrome as well. Given the prevalence of metabolic syndrome (nearly 20% of the adult U.S. population) and the increased likelihood of developing metabolic syndrome with advancing age, higher BMI, postmenopausal status, smoking, and physical inactivity (66), this possible relationship quite significant.

The association between the metabolic syndrome and the risk for CKD and microalbuminuria was recently studied by Chen et al. in the NHANES III database (67). Utilizing the National Cholesterol Education Program Adult Treatment Panel III (ATP III) definition (an average systolic or diastolic BP of greater than 130/85, an HDL cholesterol of less than 40 mg/dL in men and 50 mg/dL in women, a serum triglyceride of greater than 150 mg/dL, a fasting blood glucose level of greater than 110 mg/dL, and abdominal obesity defined by a waist circumference greater than 102 cm in men or 88 cm in women) (68) these investigators found an overall prevalence of metabolic syndrome in the NHANES III database of 24.7%.

Estimating the GFR with the abbreviated MDRD equation, a strong relationship was identified between the various components of the metabolic syndrome and CKD (67). There was a significant graded relationship between the number of components present and the corresponding prevalence of CKD or microalbuminuria ($P < 0.001$ for each comparison). In the multivariate models, elevated BP level, low HDL-cholesterol level, high triglyceride level, and abdominal obesity were all significantly associated with an increased odds ratio of CKD ($P < 0.05$). Participants with 2, 3, 4, and 5 components of the metabolic syndrome had increased OR of 2.21, 3.38, 4.23, and 5.85, respectively, for CKD, compared with that of those with 0 or 1 component (67). Persons with the metabolic syndrome had 2.60-fold increased odds of CKD compared with their counterparts without the metabolic syndrome. The results were consistent

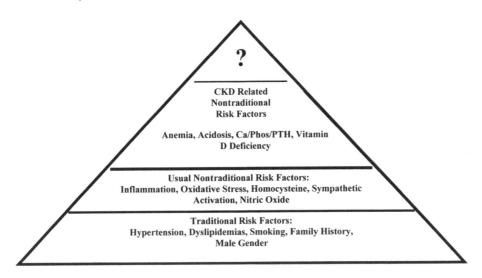

FIGURE 6 Risk pyramid for patients with chronic kidney disease. *Source:* From Ref. 40.

after additional adjustment for BMI. Therefore, the metabolic syndrome is a strong and independent risk factor for CKD and microalbuminuria. In addition, there is a graded relationship between the number of metabolic syndrome components and risk for CKD or microalbuminuria. These findings warrant intervention studies to test the effect of preventing and treating the metabolic syndrome on the risk for CKD and microalbuminuria. These findings suggest that the metabolic syndrome might be an important factor in the cause of CKD.

Further evidence supporting the premise that metabolic syndrome, even after adjusting for diabetes status and BP control, independently contributes to CKD development was provided by Chertow and colleagues utilizing the Atherosclerosis Risk in Communities (ARIC) cohort dataset (69). Of all nondiabetic ARIC participants, 21% ($n = 2110$) met the National cholesterol education program (NCEP) criteria for metabolic syndrome at baseline. Of the 10,096 subjects in the ARIC study with normal baseline renal function and were nondiabetic, 7% developed incident CKD over nine years of follow-up defined as an estimated GFR (abbreviated MDRD equation) of less than 60 mL/min/1.73 m^2. Ten percent of subjects with metabolic syndrome developed CKD compared with 4% of subjects without metabolic syndrome, a difference that remained statistically significant after correction for possible confounding variables and performance of interaction tests to check for modification of the metabolic syndrome–CKD relation. The multivariable adjusted OR of developing CKD in participants with the metabolic syndrome was 1.43 [95% confidence interval (CI), 1.18–1.73]. Compared with participants with no traits of the metabolic syndrome, those with one, two, three, four, or five traits of the metabolic syndrome had OR of CKD of 1.13 (95% CI, 0.89–1.45), 1.53 (95% CI, 1.18–1.98), 1.75 (95% CI, 1.32–2.33), 1.84 (95% CI, 1.27–2.67), and 2.45 (95% CI, 1.32–4.54), respectively. After adjusting for the subsequent development of diabetes and hypertension during the nine-year of follow-up, the OR of incident CKD among participants with the metabolic syndrome was 1.24 (95% CI, 1.01–1.51). Thus, CKD screening, as outlined in Table 2, should be performed at the time of diagnosis and routinely on all patients with metabolic syndrome given the strong relationship between metabolic syndrome and the presence/development of CKD.

The metabolic syndrome is independently associated with an increased risk for incident CKD in nondiabetic adults. Most importantly, these studies remind us of the need to identify and treat factors for cardiovascular risk. Practically, each criterion of the NCEP metabolic syndrome definition identifies a risk factor for CVD that requires intervention independent of its contribution to CKD pathogenesis. The evidence for risk factor management in patients with metabolic syndrome is compelling. Important recent studies demonstrate that alteration of lifestyle is a cost-effective approach to prevent type 2 diabetes (70), a major cause of CVD, CKD, and ESRD (71). Given the prevalence of patients with metabolic syndrome but without diabetes, we need to more effectively identify individuals at risk for CKD.

PROTEINURIA: A RISK FACTOR FOR CHRONIC KIDNEY DISEASE
AND CARDIOVASCULAR DISEASE

The importance of proteinuria and albuminuria as significant risk factors for the progression of CKD was emphasized in a joint consensus conference sponsored by the National Institute of Diabetes and Digestive Kidney Diseases (NIDDK) and the NKF, published as an official Position Paper of the NKF in 2003 [Table 4 (72) (72–82)] (83). This Position Paper recommended that for the diagnosis of CKD in adults and post-pubertal children with diabetes, measurement of urinary albumin is preferred to that of total protein. Total protein is more appropriate in children to identify both albuminuria and low-molecular-weight proteinuria. They recommended timed urine collections should not be used. Rather, the ratio of concentrations of urine albumin (in mg/dL) to urine creatinine (in g/dL) on a spot untimed urine specimen should be used (84). Spot urine testing is now an acceptable practice; however, there is still a role for 24-hour urine collections especially in a referral nephrology practice (85). First-morning spot collections are best for children and adolescents to avoid confounding the effect of orthostatic proteinuria [Table 5 (68)]. Because of variability in urinary albumin excretion, two of three specimens collected within a three- to six-month period should be abnormal before considering a patient to have crossed one of these diagnostic thresholds. Exercise within 24 hours, infection, fever, CHF, marked hyperglycemia, marked hypertension, pyuria, and hematuria may elevate urinary albumin excretion over baseline values. Table 6 reviews the diagnostic criteria for albuminuria (86).

Highly sensitive assays for albumin now allow us to test for microgram quantities of albumin in the urine. The definition of microalbuminuria as compared to macroalbuminuria is seen in Table 6. Microalbuminuria is common in the general population with a prevalence of 7.2% in a study of 40,586 inhabitants aged between 28 and 75 in Groningen, the Netherlands (87). The majority of these microalbuminuric subjects (74.9%) have no reported diabetes or hypertension despite the fact that the prevalence was greater in the diabetic and hypertensive people (prevalence in diabetics 16.4%, hypertensives 11.5%, and the nondiabetic nonhypertensives 6.6%).

Cardiovascular risk factors were already elevated at levels of albuminuria currently considered to be normal (15–30 mg per 24 hours). Advanced age, male sex, and the presence of diabetes, hypertension, hyperlipidemia, smoking, myocardial infarction, and stroke were seen more frequently in subjects with increased levels of albuminuria. This cross-sectional study indicates that microalbuminuria is far from being rare and an important indicator for CVD morbidity also in nondiabetic, nonhypertensive subjects.

Little is known, however, about factors that determine the onset of proteinuria. Although hyperglycemia precedes the development of proteinuria among persons with types 1 and 2 diabetes mellitus (33,82), most studies demonstrating a relation between proteinuria and CVD risk factors, including BP, diabetes, cholesterol level, and smoking, are cross-sectional (88–90). Few studies have simultaneously assessed these and other potential predictors of incident proteinuria in the general population (91,92), despite the possibility that CVD and CKD are a result

---

TABLE 4   Facts About Proteinuria

- Even relatively small increases in protein or albumin in the urine are an early sign of kidney injury and often precede any detectable change in the serum creatinine concentration or glomerular filtration rate
- Protein in the urine is more than a marker: persistently high levels damage the kidney and contribute to progressive loss of kidney function
- In persistent proteinuria, the amount of protein excreted bears a direct correlation to the rate of loss of kidney function
- Interventions that reduce the amount of protein in the urine in persistent proteinuria retard the progression of CKD
- Proteinuria is a strong and independent predictor of increased risk for CVD and death, especially in people with diabetes, hypertension, or CKD and the elderly
- The amount of protein excreted shows a strong and close correlation with the risk of death from CVD at all levels of excretion
- Why test for proteinuria?
  - To detect and treat it early, now that therapies are available that can delay the progression of kidney disease (75)
  - To identify people at increased risk for cardiovascular events and treat them for coexistent risk factors such as hypertension, hyperglycemia, and smoking, which improves the risk-benefit ratio of interventional strategies
  - To monitor and to evaluate the effectiveness of treatment

Abbreviations: CKD, chronic kidney disease; CVD, cardiovascular disease.
Source: From Refs. 72–81,83.

TABLE 5 Proteinuria Measurement and Terminology (NKF, NIDDK)

- Albumin is preferred over total protein (except in children)
- Spot urinary albumin to creatinine ratio is preferred over timed collection
- mg /gram (albumin/creatinine) is the preferred unit
- Immunoassays for albumin are sufficiently sensitive

Source: From Ref. 64.

of common etiologic pathways. The Korea Medical Insurance Corporation is a prospective cohort study of 183,634 persons (63% men and 37% women, aged 35–59 years) designed to assess risk factors for chronic diseases. In this setting, the relation between CVD risk factors and incident proteinuria was assessed in a large cohort of 157,377 Korean adults free of proteinuria at baseline (93). Over a 10-year follow-up, proteinuria developed in 3.8% of the men and 2.9% of the women. Fasting glucose and cholesterol levels, BMI, and BP were direct and independent predictors of incident proteinuria in Korean adults. These associations were present even at low levels of exposure, emphasizing the importance of early detection and management of these modifiable risk factors. In the diabetic population, both men and women had a very impressive increase in adjusted relative risk of developing proteinuria of 3.27 and 2.6, respectively.

The Gubbio study comprised of 715 men and 917 women ages 45 to 64 years old with a high prevalence of major CVD risk factors (40.8% hypertension, 39.5% hyperlipidemia, 31.2% cigarette smoking, and 5.3% diabetes mellitus) demonstrated a 4.2% incidence of microalbuminuria and a 0.4% incidence of macroalbuminuria (94–96). This study also demonstrated a greater prevalence of proteinuria in men than women. The prevalence of microalbuminuria was progressively higher with increasing BP, and was higher in men than women at any level of BP. Hyperlipidemia, smoking, and diabetes mellitus also were associated with a high prevalence of microalbuminuria independent of BP and each other. The people with normal urinary albumin excretion had a CHD prevalence (myocardial ischemia or infarction) of 7.5% with a dramatic increase to 21.7% in the presence of microalbuminuria and 33.3% with macroalbuminuria resulting in and odds ration of 3.44 and 6.20, respectively ($p < 0.01$) (96).

Two large studies (the Prevention of Renal and Vascular End-Stage Disease (PREVEND) (97) and the Nord-Trøndelag Health Study [HUNT, Norway 1995–1997) (98)] demonstrated that the incidence of microalbuminuria increases with age, but to a greater extent in men than in women. In the PREVEND study, the prevalence of microalbuminuria was about twofold higher in men. Interestingly, for a given level of any risk factor, urine albumin excretion (UAE) was higher in men than in women. On multivariate analysis with UAE as the dependent variable, an interaction with gender was found for the risk factors age, BMI, and plasma glucose. Thus, for a higher age, BMI, and glucose, the UAE is significantly increased in men when compared with women. It is concluded that gender differences exist in the association between cardiovascular risk factors and UAE. This is consistent with a larger vascular susceptibility to these risk factors in men as compared with women.

In a study of 328 Caucasian patients with non–insulin-dependent diabetes mellitus (NIDDM) followed for five years at the Steno Diabetes Center in Denmark, Parving and colleagues reported a very strong correlation between mortality and the severity of proteinuria (99). After five years 8% of patients with normoalbuminuria, 20% of patients with microalbuminuria, and 35% of patients with macroalbuminuria had died (predominantly from CVD) [$P < 0.01$ (normoalbuminuria vs. micro- and macroalbuminuria) and $P < 0.05$ (microalbuminuria vs. macroalbuminuria)].

TABLE 6 Diagnostic Criteria for Microalbuminuria: Standard Urine Dipsticks Are Not Sensitive Enough to Detect Microalbuminuria

Albuminuria	Timed specimen (μg/min)	Spot specimen (μg/mg Cr)	24-hr timed specimen mg/24 hr
Normo-	<20	<30	<30
Micro-	20–199	30–299	30–299
Macro-	≥200	≥300	≥300

In the HOPE study conducted between 1994 and 1999 (median follow-up 4.5 years) on individuals above 55 years old with a history of CVD ($n = 5545$) or diabetes mellitus and at least one cardiovascular risk factor ($n = 3498$), microalbuminuria was detected in 32.6% of the diabetics and 14.8% of the nondiabetics at baseline. Microalbuminuria increased the adjusted relative risk of a major cardiovascular event by 83% and was associated with a twofold increase in all-cause mortality and a 3.23-fold increase in hospitalization for CHF (100). These investigators found that every 0.4 mg/mmol of microalbuminuria [expressed as the albumin/creatinine ratio (ACR) and microalbuminuria defined as an ACR of greater than 2 mg/mmol] was associated with a 5.9% increase in the adjusted hazard of major cardiovascular events. This would indicate that any degree of albuminuria is a risk factor for cardiovascular events in individuals with or without diabetes; the risk increased with the ACR, starting well below the micro-albuminuria cutoff. Screening for albuminuria identifies people at high risk for these events.

The Losartan Intervention for Endpoint reduction in hypertension (LIFE) study also studied the relation of albuminuria and cardiovascular risk in 8206 hypertensive patients with LVH (101). The risk for the primary composite cardiovascular end point increases continuously from the lowest to the highest decile of baseline urine albumin to creatinine ratio, with a three- to fivefold increase risk noted from the lowest to the highest decile. These investigators also demonstrated a relation of high albumin excretion rate to LVH that was independent of age, BP, diabetes, race, serum creatinine, or smoking, suggesting parallel cardiac organ damage and increased renal albumin excretion rates (102, 100), and may be a marker of generalized hypertensive damage to the vasculature.

Clearly, albuminuria is associated with a significant prediction and risk of CVD events. We are now beginning to see data demonstrating that a reduction in the proteinuria also correlates with a reduction in this risk. In the Reduction of End Points in NIDDM with the Angiotensin II Receptor Antagonist Losartan (RENAAL) study, after control of BP in type 2 diabetic patients with nephropathy, proteinuria, degree of renal failure, serum albumin, and hemoglobin level are independent risk factors that predict renal outcomes. The level of proteinuria proved to be the most important risk for progressive kidney injury in these diabetic patients (104). These investigators also demonstrated that albuminuria is the strongest risk marker for CVD events in type 2 diabetic subjects with nephropathy (105). Both the severe (≥ 3.0 g/g) and moderate ($\geq 1.5 < 3.0$ g/g) proteinuria groups show significantly more cardiovascular events. Controlling for baseline risk markers for CVD, these investigators found an almost linear positive relation between degree of baseline albuminuria and risk for the cardiovascular end point or heart failure. An increase of 1 g/g albuminuria was associated with an increased risk of 17% (95% CI, 12–23%) for the cardiovascular end point and 26% (95% CI, 18–34%) for heart failure. This relation was not influenced by the effect of Losartan therapy on heart failure and was present predominantly in patients with renal events. Interestingly, suppression of the albuminuria was the strongest predictor of long-term protection from cardiovascular events (105). The cardiovascular and heart failure end points occurred more frequently in the groups that had little ($\geq 0 < 30\%$) to no ($< 0\%$) suppression of albuminuria. In contrast, the group that had the greatest reduction in albuminuria ($\geq 30\%$) showed a significant reduction in risk for cardiac events. Every 50% reduction in albuminuria reduces the risk for the cardiovascular end point by 18% (95% CI, 9–25%) and the heart failure end point by 27% (95% CI, 14–38%).

The above studies and others (106–117) have clearly demonstrated that the appearance of trace amounts of albumin (microalbuminuria, 30–300 mg/day) and larger amounts (frank proteinuria, >1 g/day) are associated with an increased risk for renal failure, heart disease, stroke, and cardiovascular mortality. The mechanism by which proteinuria confers increased CVD risk has not been fully elucidated. Possible explanations include the possibility that increased urine protein excretion may adversely affect traditional risk factors [in several trials subjects with albuminuria were more likely to be smokers, have elevated BP, have dyslipidemia (97–99) and demonstrate features of metabolic syndrome, including salt sensitivity and insulin resistance (108)]. Remuzzi has provided compelling evidence that urinary protein is a marker of impaired endothelial function not only in the glomerulus but also throughout the vascular tree (116). This suggests that proteinuria may be a marker of widespread vascular damage, endothelial dysfunction, enhancing pathogenesis, and also appears to be a marker for CVD (108). In these studies, the appearance and disappearance of proteinuria seems to track progression/regression

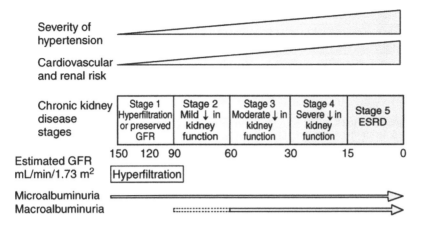

FIGURE 7 Relationship of hypertension severity, cardiovascular and renal risk, and the presence of CKD and increased urinary albumin excretion. *Source*: From Ref. 118. Copyright 2004, with permission from Macmillan Publishers Ltd.

of atherosclerosis. Thus, it is possible that proteinuria completely captures the association between impaired vascular function and progression to cardiovascular events and thereby would serve as an important surrogate marker for progression to CVD. This particular marker is appealing in that it is easily measured and relatively inexpensive, heralding its potentially broad use for cardiovascular risk assessment and as an important marker for monitoring the adequacy of specific interventions (Fig. 7). As the data accumulate from the ongoing trials, and the normal range for urinary albumin excretion in hypertension is better defined, the measurement of UAE rates may serve a dual purpose. First, the presence of albuminuria is a powerful way to identify those patients requiring an integrated intervention on multiple cardiovascular risk factors. Second, a failure to regress albumin excretion in urine may indicate an inadequacy of that intervention (119).

The evidence-based data above provided the basis for the following recommendations by the NKF and NIDDK position paper regarding the monitoring of proteinuria (83).

(i)   Populations at increased risk for CKD as outlined in Table 2 should be screened for microalbuminuria, at least annually, as part of their regular health examination.
(ii) Individuals with documented persistent microalbuminuria (two of three measurements greater than the reference range) who are undergoing treatment for elevated BP, lipid disorders, or both should be retested within six months to determine if treatment goals and reduction in microalbuminuria have been achieved. If treatment has resulted in a significant reduction of microalbuminuria, annual testing for microalbuminuria is recommended. If no reduction in microalbuminuria has occurred, BP and lipid levels should be evaluated to determine: (a) if the targets have been achieved, (b) if specific drugs that interfere with the renin–angiotensin–aldosterone system are part of the antihypertensive therapy, and (c) the treatment regimen should be modified accordingly.
(iii) Based on the available evidence, continued annual surveillance of microalbuminuria is recommended to assess progression of CKD and CVD risk and the response to therapy.

APPROACH TO CKD: NEED FOR COORDINATED MANAGEMENT TO REDUCE CVD RISK (120)

CKD a prevalence of 10% to 20% in most countries world wide, has the clear relation of CKD with CVD documented above. Because of an associated poor outcome from progression of CKD and CVD events, many have advocated for the improved management of CKD. Mild degrees of CKD have been shown to be associated with a series of risk factors or markers that are summarized in Table 7(38). Mortality from CVD in patients with ESRD is 10 to 30 times higher than in the general population, even when adjustments are made for gender, race, and presence of diabetes (35,121). After stratification for age, race, and gender, patients with CKD stage 5 (ESRD) have a dramatically higher rate of cardiovascular morbidity and mortality than

TABLE 7 Cardiovascular Risk Factors or Markers Associated to a Mild Decrease in Estimated Glomeruler Filtration Rate

- Disturbed lipoprotein (a) concentrations
- Insulin resistance and impaired glucose tolerance
- Increased oxidative stress
- Increment in pulse wave velocity
- Increased serum uric acid levels
- Sympathetic overactivity
- Accumulation of ADMA
- Inflammatory and procoagulant biomarkers
- CRP, fibrinogen, interleukin 6, factor VIIc, factor VIIIc, plasmin–antiplasmin complex, and D-dimer
- Obesity and body fat distribution
- Nondipping pattern of ambulatory blood pressure

Abbrevations: ADMA, asymmetric dimethyarginine; CRP, C-reactive protein.
Source: From Ref. 35.

the general population (Fig. 8) (115) CKD is thus a great multiplier of CVD risk. Approximately half of the patients starting hemodialysis have ischemic heart disease and CHF associated with a dramatically rapid progression of atherosclerosis (122). Another indication that the abnormal milieu associated with CKD affects survival is the observation that renal transplantation confers a significant survival benefit over maintenance hemodialysis (123). The exact mechanism of accelerated CVD in CKD is unknown; however, both vascular remodeling and vascular wall calcification have been implicated in the pathogenesis (124). It appears that many of the factors associated with progressive CKD that play a role in this abnormal vascular state begins when the GFR falls below 60 ml/min/m^2. Vascular remodeling can occur as a result of increased tensile stress, leading to medial wall thickening of the artery with subsequent luminal narrowing in small–resistance arteries. The remodeling process may be mediated through endothelial cell production of growth-regulating and vasoactive factors with the renin– angiotensin–aldosterone system perhaps playing a significant role. This may portray another beneficial role for the renin modulation of the renin–angiotensin system (RAS) with ACE-I, ARBs besides their effects on BP and glomerular hemodynamics (16,21,125,126). Coronary calcification is more prevalent in CKD patients than in age- and gender-matched control subjects (128–130). Schwarz et al. (130) has shown that coronary plaques in uremic patients are characterized by marked calcification, increased media thickness, and infiltration and activation of macrophages. The primary difference in the plaques between the renal and nonrenal patients was in the composition of the plaque, not the size. It was initially thought that vascular calcification occurred as a passive process that resulted from calcium–phosphorus crystal deposition as a result of increased calcium–phosphorus ion product and hyperparathyroidism. Recently, it was suggested that calcification is an active cell-mediated process whereby vascular smooth muscle cells assume a bone-forming phenotype (131,132). The exact mechanisms for vascular calcification and the relation between arterial wall calcification and atherosclerosis are poorly understood. It is likely that the excess cardiovascular calcification that is observed in patients with ESRD is a multifactorial process (121). Figure 9 summarizes the plethora of factors that potentially are involved in the pathogenesis, including the CKD-related ones: hyperparathyroidism, hyperphosphatemia, hypertension, abnormal glucose metabolism, treatment with vitamin D analogs, and abnormalities in lipid metabolism. It seems that alterations in mineral metabolism may contribute to the development of vascular calcification (133). Vascular calcification has been associated with increased mortality in patients with ESRD (134,135).

This would mandate an aggressive therapeutic approach in patients with CKD outlined in Table 8. The Joint National Committe VII includes CKD as a "compelling" indication, justifying lower target BP and treatment with specific antihypertensive agents (136).

As one progresses through the stages of CKD, the clear association between morbidity and mortality from CVD events outlined above is far more prevalent than seen in the nonrenal population. This cannot be fully explained by the traditional risk factors outlined in Table 3. Therefore, it is apparent that the nontraditional risk factors may play a more significant role in this CVD risk and association. Data corroborating this, both inferentially and directly, are accumulating at a rapid pace. As the traditional risk factors for CVD have been discussed elsewhere in this book, the remainder of this chapter will deal with the nontraditional risk

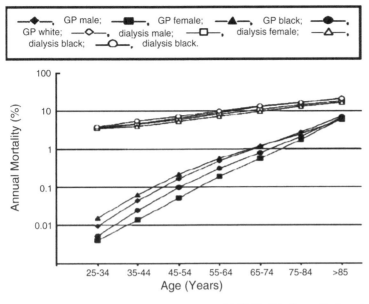

FIGURE 8   Cardiovascular mortality in patients with ESRD. This figure displays the cardiovascular mortality in the general population compared with patients who have renal failure and are treated with either dialysis or renal transplantation. The data are stratified by age, gender, and race. *Source*: From Refs. 115,121.

factors mentioned above. The studies exploring the relation of these nontraditional risk factors with both CKD and CVD risk are presented in the remainder of this chapter, as well as some intriguing data suggesting a role in the pathogenesis of this relation. Many of the nontraditional risk factors impose CVD risk via their effect on vascular calcification, ASVD, and LVH directly.

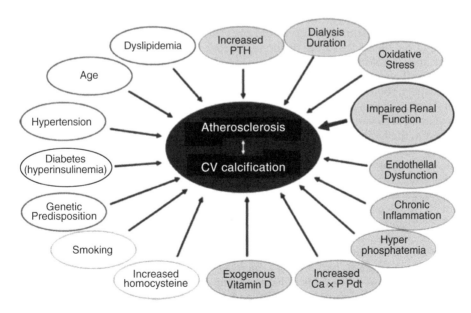

FIGURE 9   Pathogenesis of cardiovascular disease (CVD) in chronic kidney disease. A plethora of factors may be involved in the pathogenesis of CVD in patients with end-stage renal disease (ESRD), including traditional cardiac risk factors (*white ovals*) and kidney disease–related risk factors (*gray ovals*). The importance of a renal dysfunction (absence of normal renal function) cannot be overlooked when assessing mechanisms of CVD in patients with ESRD. *Source*: From Ref. 124.

TABLE 8   Therapeutic Attitudes in Patients with Chronic Kidney Disease and Hypertension

- Lifestyle changes (Salt intake, body weight, and stop smoking)
- Strict blood pressure control (<125/75 mmHg): Combination therapy required in most cases.
    - ACE inhibitor or ARB is required
- Control of associated risk factors
    - Lipids: statins, fibrates
    - Insulin resistance: insulin sensitizers (metformin, glitazones?)
    - Platelet aggregation: aspirins, others?

Abbreviations: ACE, angiotensin-converting enzyme; ARB, angiotensin receptor blocker.

ANEMIA: A CKD-RELATED NONTRADITIONAL CVD RISK FACTOR

Anemia is frequently associated with CKD and when present, serves as an independent risk factor for CVD morbidity and mortality and may negatively affect clinical outcomes (137,138). The deeply negative impact of anemia on cardiac function in CKD patients is caused mostly by its primary role in promoting the development of LVH, the most typical cardiac alteration observed in CKD with 70% of these patients having LVH at the time of initiating dialysis therapy (139). The Canadian Multi-Center Study of Renal Anemia, an echocardiographic analysis of predialysis patients with various degrees of CKD, showed that the prevalence of LVH increases progressively with decreasing renal function, however, 20% already belong to the subgroup of patients with mild renal insufficiency (creatinine clearance, 15–35 mL/min) (140). Horwich and colleagues studied the relation between anemia and mortality in a prospective cohort study in over 1000 patients with advanced heart failure (NYHA class III or IV) (141). They conclude that even mild degrees of anemia, hemoglobin <12.3 g/dL, are associated with a one-year mortality of 44.4%. Lower hemoglobin was associated with an impaired hemodynamic profile, higher blood urea nitrogen and creatinine, and lower albumin, total cholesterol, and BMI. Patients in the lower quartiles were more likely to be NYHA functional class IV ($P < 0.0001$) and have lower peak oxygen consumption ($PKVO_2$) ($P < 0.0001$). Survival at one year was higher with increased hemoglobin quartile (55.6%, 63.9%, 71.4%, and 74.4% for hemoglobin <12.3, 12.3–13.6, 13.7–14.8, and >14.8 g/dL, respectively). The pathogenesis is multifactorial with a predominant and consistent cause being the failure of adequate production of endogenous erythropoietin (EPO) by the kidneys. Kidneys produce EPO in response to low delivery of oxygen (142). EPO stimulates erythroid progenitors in the bone marrow, resulting in increased release of red blood cells from the bone marrow. CKD results in reduction in functional kidney mass and decreased production of endogenous EPO with a resultant decrease in red blood cell mass and anemia. The anemia is seen much earlier in the course of CKD than most physicians suspect, the decline in hemoglobin concentration starting at levels of creatinine clearance of 70 mL/min among men and 50 mL/min among women (143). There are multiple definitions of anemia as can be seen in Table 9 (125,144). The NKF definition of anemia is commonly accepted in the United States.

Even though there is no agreement on the definition of anemia, it is quite prevalent in the CKD population. A recent survey of 5222 patients encompassing the five stages of CKD reviewed the prevalence of anemia (145). Anemia (defined as hemoglobin <12 g/dL) was present in nearly half (47.7%) of the 5222 patients evaluated in a clinical practice setting. These data are consistent with results from an earlier retrospective survey based on data from the Health Care Financing Administration 2728 Form (146). Results from that survey showed a high prevalence of severe anemia (51%), defined as a hematocrit level <28%, as well as hypoalbuminemia (60%) in predialysis patients with CKD. Compared with patients with serum creatinine <1.6 mg/dL, patients with serum creatinine >2.5 mg/dL had a >200% increase in the odds of having hemoglobin <12 g/dL and a >350% increase in the odds of having hemoglobin <10 g/dL (133). This relation was also reflected in the association between GFR and hemoglobin levels. A total of 5.2% of patients with GFRs <60 mL/min/1.73 m^2 had hemoglobin <10 g/dL, compared with 27.2% of patients with GFRs <15 mL/min/1.73 m^2.

Clinical practice guidelines have been published by the NKF-K/DOQI guidelines regarding the evaluation of anemia in CKD (144). These guidelines recommend that patients be evaluated for anemia when their GFR is less than 60 mL/min/1.73 m^2. An anemia workup should

TABLE 9 Multiple Definitions of Anemia

Guidelines	Men (hemoglobin) (g/dL)	Women (hemoglobin) (g/dL)
World Health Organization[a]	<13	<12
NKF Guidelines[b]	<12[c]	<11[d]
European Best Practice Guidelines for the Management of Anemia[e]	<13.5	<11.5

[a]World Health Organization. Available at: http://www.who.int/nut/documents/ida_ assessment_prevention_ control.pdf.
[b]Ref. 139.
[c]In men and postmenopausal women.
[d]Premenopausal women.
[e]Ref.125

be started if the hemoglobin level is below 11 g/dL in premenopausal women and prepubertal patients and less than 12 in adult males and postmenopausal women. If anemia is diagnosed, then additional workup and laboratory monitoring will be required including a complete blood count with indices and reticulocyte count, iron studies [total iron binding capacity (TIBC), iron, transferrin saturation (TSAT), and ferritin], and checking the stool for blood. Workup of the cause of the anemia should be followed as indicated, including such possibilities as CKD, vitamin B_{12} or folate deficiency, and iron deficiency as well as others dictated by the preliminary findings and the history and physical examination. To provide enough iron to support erythropoiesis, the NKF-K/DOQI guidelines recommend that the TSAT level be maintained at 20% to 50% and the serum ferritin be maintained at 100 to 800 ng/mL. If iron deficiency is present then begin with iron replacement therapy and once replete, or if not present, initiate EPO therapy (147). The NKF guidelines recommend target hemoglobin should be between 11 and 12 g/dL (136). Unfortunately, primarily because of the lack of awareness of CKD, as well as the anemia associated with the early stages of CKD, as of 2003, only 29% of patients initiating dialysis have a hemoglobin level at the above mentioned target (136). According to the USRDS 2004 annual report, 68% of anemic CKD patients are not on EPO at the initiation of RRT (148).

EPO was introduced as a standard therapy with the anemia of CKD in 1988 and immediately revolutionized its management. Along with the elimination for the need for repeated transfusions and the dramatic improvements in quality of life was the significant improvement in cardiac function, noted even with the partial correction of anemia. With the recognition of CVD as the leading cause of death among patients with CKD and the role of CKD and anemia in its pathogenesis, it was apparent that more attention needed to be directed toward this powerful and potentially modifiable risk factor. A detailed description of the pathogenesis of CVD from anemia outlined in Figure 10 is beyond the scope of this chapter but can be found in a recent review by Rao and Pereira (142,149). Anemia of CKD associated with a decreased level of EPO results in the hemodynamic adaptations of a high cardiac output state from an increase in cardiac preload and a decrease in systemic vascular resistance resulting in decreased afterload. This leads to initial left ventricular dilatation and increased wall tension, and ventricular remodeling, and hypertrophy is initiated through both hypertrophy of existing myofibrils and realignment of sarcomeres. Although these changes are potentially reversible in a nonuremic milieu, several maladaptive processes in the form of uremia-associated cardiovascular risk factors prevent reversibility over time. Volume expansion, hypertension, persistent activation of the RAS, inflammation, hyperparathyroidism, and diabetes contribute to myocardial fibrosis, calcium deposition, left-ventricular stiffness, arteriosclerosis, and accelerated atherosclerosis (142). It is now well known that EPO is a pleiotropic cytokine with trophic functions beyond erythropoiesis; its anti-apoptotic and angiogenetic effects have direct relevance to myocardial ischemia and vascular disease. The consequences of the anemia of CKD may therefore be mediated by a combination of hemodynamic changes, tissue hypoxia, and absolute and relative EPO deficiency (151).

The temporal relation between CKD and CVD also seems to be true for anemia as well, begins early, and tracks with the decline in GFR and the evolution of CVD. Silverberg has proposed a concept of a cardiorenal anemia syndrome to emphasize that anemia, CKD, and CHF form a self-perpetuating triad (150,152) and interact to translate into mortality multipliers.

Although it is well known that CKD predisposes to CVD and eventually CHF, it is also being appreciated that CHF and anemia are themselves major contributors to the deterioration of kidney function. CHF contributes to diminished kidney tissue perfusion, which activates cascades of kidney tissue injury due to oxidant stress and cytokines. Anemia could accelerate progression of kidney disease by at least two mechanisms, directly by kidney tissue hypoxia and indirectly by inducing cardiac failure, decrease in kidney blood flow, and thereby decreased tissue perfusion and oxygen delivery (142).

Investigators have recently demonstrated a possible new nonhematopoietic role for EPO in CVD pathogenesis. First, it is important to know that EPO receptors are present on endothelial cells (153,154), cardiomyocytes (155), and neurons (156). In a number of studies of a uremic animal model of AMI, deficiency of EPO was associated with excessive infarct size, and acute administration of high doses of EPO diminished infarct size and improved cardiac function (157–162). It has been postulated that part of the mechanism associated with increased morbidity and mortality from CVD events in CKD patients is related to a reduced hypoxia tolerance (154). The finding of main interest, however, was the documentation of the decrease in capillary density seen in the group without EPO (157). This was prevented by EPO, and the density of capillaries was restored to the values seen in sham-operated, untouched animals. A causal relation is suggested, but not proven, by the observation that the capillary density was strongly related to the expression of β-myocyte heavy chain and myocardial contractility, as well as myocardial relaxation (155). Extensive research is now underway studying the potential role that EPO may play with regard to nonhematopoietic mechanisms of angiogenesis rescuing ischemic cardiomyocytes. Clinical trials are also underway to answer this question. Two ongoing trials, The Trial to Reduce Cardiovascular Events with Aranesp Therapy (TREAT) and the Anemia Correction in Diabetes (ACORD) will use darbepoeitin alfa (Aranesp) and epoetin beta (Neo-Recormon), respectively, in diabetics with CKD to correct anemia to a target of 12.0 g/dL or above. The end points are, respectively, cardiovascular events (fatal and nonfatal) and change in left ventricular mass index, and will evaluate the benefits of anemia correction in early diabetic nephropathy on cardiovascular risk reduction (163,164). Anemia, an under-recognized and under-treated concomitant of CKD, is associated with significant clinical and functional consequences. Moreover, during the progression CKD there is strong evidence for detrimental effects on quality of life, exercise tolerance, and related factors that impact activities of daily living. In addition, it is indirectly and perhaps directly linked to cardiac morphologic and functional changes, most specifically LVH and progression of LVMI abnormalities. With the ever growing body of scientific literature on the significant morbidity and mortality associated with the anemia of CKD, a Renal Anemia Management Period (RAMP) has been proposed (165). The RAMP is defined as the time following onset of CKD when anemia develops, and needs early diagnosis and treatment, which would achieve the goals of delaying disease progression, minimizing cardiovascular complications, and enhancing quality of life. If the ongoing trial demonstrates a positive effect of correction of anemia during the earlier stages of CKD before significant cardiac damage has occurred, this would be a significant step forward in perhaps reducing the tremendous burden of CVD morbidity and mortality associated with CKD.

CARDIOVASCULAR CALCIFICATION IN CKD

The dramatic, increased risk of mortality associated with ESRD is demonstrated clearly in Figure 8. It has been known for some time that CVD is common in older adults with ESRD who are undergoing regular dialysis. Vascular calcification, especially arterial calcification, has been recognized for many years as a common complication of CKD (166–168). Blacher et al. in a study of 110 ESRD patients on hemodialysis demonstrated a clear and strong relation between a semiquantitative calcification score and all-cause mortality (135). Within five years, approximately two-thirds of the patients in the highest arterial calcification class had died, compared with none of the patients without calcification. Goodman et al. demonstrated that coronary-artery calcification is common and progressive in young adults with ESRD who are undergoing dialysis (169). None of the 23 patients studied by electron-beam computed tomography (CT) below the age of 20 had evidence of coronary-artery calcification whereas 87.5% (14 out of 16 patients) of those age 20 to 30 years had evidence of coronary-artery calcification, with a mean calcification score of 1157 ± 1996. Only 5% (3 out of 60) of age-matched normal non-CKD controls had calcification. There was a strong statistically significant relation between

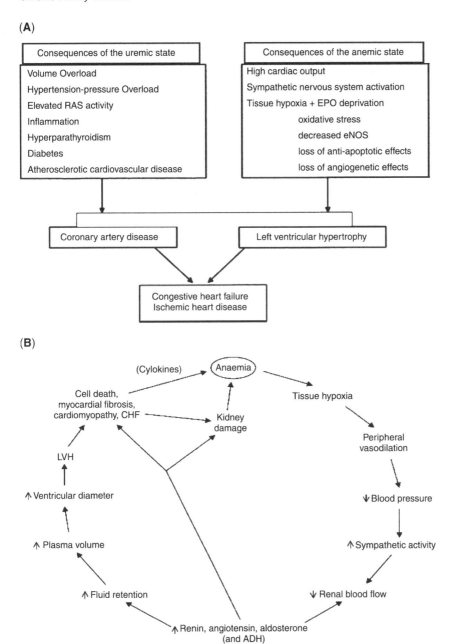

(A)

Consequences of the uremic state
Volume Overload
Hypertension-pressure Overload
Elevated RAS activity
Inflammation
Hyperparathyroidism
Diabetes
Atherosclerotic cardiovascular disease

Consequences of the anemic state
High cardiac output
Sympathetic nervous system activation
Tissue hypoxia + EPO deprivation
oxidative stress
decreased eNOS
loss of anti-apoptotic effects
loss of angiogenetic effects

Coronary artery disease

Left ventricular hypertrophy

Congestive heart failure
Ischemic heart disease

(B)

FIGURE 10 (A) Mechanisms in anemia leading to myocardial damage in chronic kidney disease: combination of factors secondary to diminished glomerular filtration rate and low hemoglobin (149). Consequences of anemia include the hemodynamic compensatory mechanisms that may turn maladaptive, hypoxia-related injury (oxidant stress, endothelial dysfunction) and effects of erythropoietin (EPO) depletion (loss of antiapoptotic and angiogenetic effects of EPO). *Abbreviations*: RAS, rennin–angiotensin system; eNOS, endothelial nitric oxide synthase. (B) The mechanism by which anemia causes heart failure and renal failure. *Source*: From Refs. 149,150.

increasing age, longer duration of dialysis and a higher mean serum phosphorus, calcium phosphorus product, and daily intake of calcium as a phosphorus binder with the group that demonstrated the calcification. The coronary-artery calcification doubled over a 20 ± 3-month period on follow-up CT scanning. Thus providing support for the concept that disturbances of mineral metabolism and possibly parathyroid hormone (PTH) and vitamin D status contribute to coronary-artery calcification in patients with ESRD. Young adults undergoing regular dialysis may harbor clinically silent CAD that is disproportionate to their age (48,135). Vascular calcification is predictive of CVD mortality (170,171) and is both common and severe in CKD as is noted above.

The pathogenesis of vascular calcification in CKD remains under investigation, but hyperphosphatemia is an important risk factor for both vascular calcification and CV mortality (172,173). Vascular calcification and CV mortality are also associated with other abnormalities of calcium and phosphate homeostasis, including hypercalcemia, elevated calcium and phosphate ion products, vitamin D therapy, and hyperparathyroidism (171,172), and these findings suggest a link with renal osteodystrophy (ROD). ROD is virtually ubiquitous in CKD, characterized by a spectrum of histological abnormalities of bone that contribute to the biochemical abnormalities described above (174,175). The two ends of the spectrum of ROD include osteitis fibrosa, a high turnover state driven by secondary hyperparathyroidism that ultimately results in a release of calcium and phosphate into the intracellular fluid (176), and adynamic bone disease at the other end of the spectrum characterized by markedly reduced bone turnover and an associated reduction of the ability to buffer calcium and phosphorus in bone and associated with increased postprandial fluctuations as a result (177). Thus, both forms of ROD cause abnormalities in calcium and phosphate homeostasis that are associated with vascular calcification, and it is possible to hypothesize a causative pathologic link among ROD, vascular calcification, and mortality in CKD. Davies et al. have developed an animal model of vascular calcification worsened by CKD and in this model the vascular calcification is prevented by treatment with bone morphogenetic protein-7 (BMP-7) (178). In this model a strong inverse relation was demonstrated between the reduction in bone mineralization and the increase in vascular calcification (173). This observation has now been corroborated in a human study (179). Shulz et al. investigated the relation between CT measures of aortic calcification and values for bone density and the number of fragility fractures in 2348 healthy, postmenopausal women. In a subgroup of 228 women, aortic vascular calcification and bone loss was monitored over time to see if the increase in vascular calcification and the bone loss progress in parallel. When these postmenopausal women with vascular calcification were divided into quartiles based on the percentage change for aortic calcification, a strong graded relation was observed between the progression of vascular calcification and bone loss for each quartile. Women in the highest quartile for gains in aortic calcification had four times greater yearly bone loss (5.3% vs. 1.3% yearly; $P < 0.001$) than women of similar age in the lowest quartile. The renal function of these patients was not mentioned in the paper, however the mean age of the patients with the aortic calcification was 70.6 ± 8.9 years old with estimates of the incidence of CKD in this age group in the general population being approximately 25%. Rix et al. also demonstrated that skeletal changes are initiated at an early stage of CKD (GFR 6–70 mL/min), as estimated from reduced bone mass density and elevated levels of PTH as well as from the biochemical markers of both bone formation and bone resorption (180). A correlation has also been demonstrated between reduced total hip bone mass and all-cause mortality in chronic hemodialysis patients (181) further corroborating the relation between abnormal PTH and vitamin D status, abnormal calcium and phosphorus homeostasis, bone mass density, vascular calcification, and associated CVD mortality.

There is an accumulating body of evidence that vitamin D plays a role in CVD. Abnormal vitamin metabolism, through deficiency of the active form of 1,25-hihydroxyvitamin D_3, and acquired vitamin D resistance through the uremic state have been shown to be important in CKD. Vitamin D has long been known to affect cardiac contractility, vascular tone, cardiac collagen content, and cardiac tissue maturation. The effects of vitamin D are more widespread than the calcium and PTH roles familiar to everyone. Vitamin D has been demonstrated to have biological effects independent of its effect on divalent ions. Abnormalities in endothelial cell function, an increase in plasma renin and angiotensin, and myocardial hypertrophy have been observed in vitamin D receptor knockout mice (182). 1,25-Dihydroxyvitamin D_3 appears to be a negative regulator of the RAS (179,183). Thus, vitamin D deficiency appears to favor a hyperreninemic, hypertensive state with impairment of cardiac contractile function and an increase in myocardial collagen content, a series of abnormalities that could predispose to LVH and CHF. These investigators also demonstrated in this model that administration of vitamin D suppressed renin expression in normal mice. This relation thus lends to a hypothesis that decreased vitamin D receptor activation results in hyperparathyroidism and increased bone loss with all three resulting in arterial calcification. Decreased vitamin D receptor activation has also been associated with insulin resistance and the development of hypertension and LVH.

This associated increase in insulin resistance, hypertension, LVH, and arterial calcification are associated with increased CVD mortality (184). A study of 173 high and moderate risk patients for CAD demonstrated an inverse relation between the levels of 1,25-dihydroxyvitamin D_3 and vascular calcification (185). Vitamin D supplementation in vitamin-D–deficient patients significantly reduces markers of inflammation (186). A small study also demonstrated that low vitamin D status may explain alterations in mineral metabolism as well as myocardial dysfunction in CHF patients and therefore may be a contributing factor to the pathogenesis of CHF (187). In summary, vitamin D has been shown to inhibit inflammatory markers, modulate immune responses, downregulate renin, stimulate cardiomyocytes remodeling, regulate markers of cardiomyocyte hypertrophy, and has been linked to regression of LVH in hemodialysis patients resulting in a potential benefit through the possible association with a reduction in atherosclerosis, reduced myocardial hypertrophy, decreased heart failure, and decreased morbidity and mortality. This will require much more research and investigation to corroborate this hypothesis (181,185,188,189).

The prevalence of vitamin D deficiency in the general population, let alone the early CKD group, is poorly defined. There has been a suggestion that hypovitaminosis D is more prevalent than suspected. Fifty-seven percent of 290 consecutive admissions to the Massachusetts General Hospital were found to be vitamin D deficient (serum concentration of 25-hydroxyvitamin D 15 ng/mL) (190). Only 8% were classified as having renal dysfunction defined as a serum creatinine concentration above 2 mg/dL. This definition clearly may underestimate the true number of patients with CKD in the study. A single center observational study of 43 patients with CKD (defined as a serum creatinine of 1–5 mg/dL; calculated GFR 11–111 mL/min/1.73 m^2) demonstrated that 37 of 43 (86%) had suboptimal levels of 25-hydroxyvitamin D (<30 ng/mL) (191). In a study of 1814 CKD patients by Bakris et al. (192) serum 1,25 dihydroxyvitamin D levels began to fall once the GFR fell below 70 mL/min and PTH was first increased once GFR fell below 50 mL/min. Elevations in serum phosphorus and low serum calcium were not noted until GFR fell to less than 30 and 20 mL/min, respectively. The abnormalities in vitamin D levels and PTH are therefore noted much earlier in the course of CKD than perturbations in calcium and phosphorus, so that waiting for alterations in calcium and phosphorus to indicate a need for evaluating these levels will result in allowing prolonged effects of low vitamin D and elevated PTH on these patients. Another study looking at 312 stage 3 and 4 CKD patients demonstrated that 86% and 89% have 25-hydroxyvitamin D levels less than 35 ng/mL, respectively and 12% of the patients in both stages 3 and 4 have severe deficiency with levels less than 20 ng/mL (243). As we move from stage 3 to stage 4 CKD, the incidence of severe reductions in 1,25-dihydroxyvitamin D_3 level becomes much greater with 65% of stage 4 CKD patients having a severe deficiency in calcetriol with a level below 25 pmol/L as compared to 5% in stage 3 (243). The NKF guidelines therefore recommend that serum levels of calcium, phosphorus, and intact plasma PTH be measured in all patients with GFR <60 mL/min/1.73 m^2 (194). It is recommended that they be monitored on yearly bases and more frequently as the patient progresses through the stages of CKD. Because of the increased morbidity and mortality associated with evaluated phosphorus, calcium and calcium phosphorus product, and intact PTH levels, guidelines for the goal range of these levels were proposed in the 2003 statement paper (Table 10) (183, 194).

Curbing the Promotion of Vascular Calcification in Chronic Kidney Disease

High phosphorus levels stimulate osteoblastic differentiation of vascular smooth muscle cells and directly enhance extracellular calcification by these cells (195). It is therefore conceivable that control of serum phosphorus levels may result in reduced burden of cardiovascular calcification in these patients. As CKD progresses one must begin restricting dietary phosphorus and also utilize phosphate binders once the serum phosphorus increase above the K/DOQI recommendation of 4.6 mg/dL. Calcium binders of phosphate have traditionally been utilized, however, concern over the possible role of calcium loading from these binders in the progression of cardiovascular calcification has been raised. Because of this the K/DOQI recommendations are to limit the use of calcium binders of phosphate to no more than 2 g daily. The concern became more widespread after publication of the Treat to Goal Study (196), which showed a 25% increase in the coronary calcification scores among the patients who were treated with calcium salts compared with a 6% increment in the sevelamer (a noncalcium containing binder of phosphorus) group and a similar difference in aortic artery calcification scores. However, the

TABLE 10   Proposed NKF-K/DOQI™ Bone Metabolism and Disease Guidelines

	Stage 3 and 4	Stage 5
PTH (pg/mL)	35–70 (Stage 3) 70–110 (Stage 4)	150–300
Total corrected serum calcium (mg/dL)	8.4–9.5	8.4–9.5 (preferably toward the lower end)
Serum phosphorus (mg/dL)	2.7–4.6	3.5–5.5
Ca x P (mg^2/dL^2)	<55	<55
Calcium Intake (mg/day)	≤2000	≤2000

Abbreviation: PTH, parathyroid hormone.
Source: From Ref. 1.

mechanism of the beneficial effect of sevelamer on progression of calcification is unknown. One possible mechanism is reduced Ca loading during treatment with the noncalcium binder (197). Sevelamer is also a bile acid sequestrant and therefore is also associated with a reduction in low-density lipoprotein (LDL) cholesterol. Reduced cardiovascular calcification may also result from dramatic reductions in total and LDL cholesterol. Hyperlipidemia, particularly increased LDL-cholesterol, has been implicated in progression of coronary artery calcification (198–200). Callister et al. demonstrated that treatment with 3-hydroxy-3-methylglutaryl CoA reductase inhibitors can reduce the volume of calcified plaque in the coronary arteries. At the follow-up electron beam computed tomography scans, a net reduction in the Ca-volume score of 7% was observed only in treated patients whose final LDL-cholesterol levels were <120 mg/dL ($P < 0.01$) (198). This stresses the need for more aggressive lipid control and use of statin therapy in our CKD patients. Patients who were treated with Sevelamer in the Treat to Goal Study had a significant decrease in their plasma LDL-cholesterol levels from 102 to 65 mg/dL during the study period, whereas the LDL levels did not change in patients who were treated with calcium-containing phosphate binders. Therefore, it is possible that the slower rate of progression of cardiovascular calcification observed in the Treat to Goal Study may have resulted from the significant lowering of the LDL-cholesterol level by sevelamer (197). Two other studies underscore the role of dyslipidemia in the pathogenesis of CV calcification in patients with CKD. Nitta et al. (201) reported the results of their preliminary study from Japan, which showed that progression of aortic calcification in patients with ESRD was significantly retarded during treatment with colistimide (a bile acid sequestrant similar to sevelamer) in combination with atorvastatin compared with the period before treatment was initiated. Tamashiro et al. (202) reported that rapid progression of coronary artery calcification in hemodialysis patients was associated with higher triglycerides and lower HDL-cholesterol levels.

Historically, the treatment of secondary hyperparathyroidism in CKD patients utilized the suppression of PTH secretion by supraphysiologic doses of vitamin D or its analogues in addition to the aggressive control of phosphorus as is mentioned above. Animal studies suggest that perhaps the use of high dose vitamin D is associated with increased vascular calcification because of the stimulation of vitamin D receptors on vascular smooth muscle cells may induce them to manifest osteoblastic phenotypes (197,203) and also have been shown to increase calcification in vascular smooth muscle cell in vitro (204). Moreover, vitamin D therapy enhances the intestinal absorption of calcium and phosphorus and, therefore, often results in hypercalcemia, worsening hyperphosphatemia, and increased calcium X phosphorus product. Thus, although effective in reducing the severity of secondary hyperparathyroidism, excessive dosing of vitamin D may increase the risk for CV calcification. Clearly, however, some vitamin D is required in these patients to circumvent the role of vitamin D deficiency on the progression of CVD in our CKD patients as is discussed above; however the appropriate dose still needs to be determined. It has become clear that the suprapharmacalogic doses utilized in the past for treating hyperparathyroidism may be doing more cardiovascular harm than good. Also, perhaps the utilization of some of the newer analogues of the active form of 1,25 dihydroxy vitamin D that are not associated with as much stimulation of the gut vitamin D receptors may be associated with less morbidity and mortality. Teng et al. demonstrated that use of paricalcitol (an active vitamin D analogue not associated with hypercalcemia because of lack of stimulation of gut vitamin D receptors) was associated with a significant survival advantage over the use of active vitamin D preparation calcetriol (205). The mechanism by which paricalcitol exerts its potential beneficial effect remains to be determined. Some of the possible mechanisms rendered include blunting of the gut absorption and bone resorption of minerals and, in vitro studies, in less sensitization of cells to energy depletion and iron-mediated injury with paricalcitol as compared to calcetriol (205). Also the biologic consequences of vitamin D receptor activation seems to extend beyond the suppression of PTH synthesis, including the suppression of renin expression, modulation of the immune and inflammatory system, and the promotion of vascular endothelial health as discussed above. The need for some vitamin D exposure to these deficient CKD patients was further corroborated by a subsequent study of Teng et al. demonstrating that in a historical cohort study of chronic hemodialysis patients the administration of injectable vitamin D analogues was associated with a significant survival advantage over patients who did not receive any vitamin D therapy (206). Observational studies and randomized trials will be needed to ascertain what the appropriate vitamin D therapy will be in CKD patients and to address what the optimal dose with the greatest survival benefits will be.

The cloning of the calcium-sensing receptor in the parathyroid gland cells (207) allowed for the development of a nonpeptide allosteric modulator of this receptor called calcimimetics. These orally administered compounds could then directly inhibit the release of PTH. The new calcimimetic agent cinacalcet may offer several advantages over vitamin D with respect to CV calcification. They prevent or treat secondary hyperparathyroidism without increasing serum calcium, phosphorus, or calcium X phosphorus product (208). Moreover, they have no adverse effects on vascular calcification. Although no clinical studies have demonstrated such a beneficial effect, preliminary in vitro and in vivo studies indicated that, compared with high doses of vitamin D, calcimimetic agents do not enhance aortic calcification (209–211). Again, more research and data are needed, but the available information seems to indicate that perhaps some combination of therapies at our disposal now utilizing appropriate phosphate binders, vitamin D analogues, and calcimimetic agents can optimize our control of calcium, phosphorus, and PTH levels, improve cardiovascular health, perhaps decrease cardiovascular calcification, and reduce cardiovascular morbidity and mortality in this high risk population.

■ Case Presentation

JS is a 51-year-old Caucasian male with a 15-year history of type 2 diabetes mellitus, hypertension (10 years), hyperlipidemia, gout, and hypothyroidism. He sustained a myocardial infarction at the age of 45 and was diagnosed with a transient ischemic attacks at the age of 49 resulting in the diagnosis of severe right carotid artery stenosis and a carotid artery endarderectomy. Medications include insulin, metoprolol 50 mg, hydralazine 50 mg BID, simvastatin 40 mg, allopurinol 200 mg daily, synthroid 125 mg daily, furosemide 40 mg BID, digoxin, and a long acting nitrate. His current primary complaints are edema, 2 pillow orthopnea, dyspnea on exertion with one block exercise, decreased vision secondary to his diabetic retinopathy, and peripheral neuropathy symptoms. Physical examination revealed an obese male who appeared older than his stated age, BP 130/78, pulse 108, mild jugular vein distention at 90°, decreased breath sounds and rales at the bases on lung exam, benign abdomen, 1 plus edema of the lower extremities, peripheral neuropathy, carotid bruits, an enlarged point of maximal impulse with an S_3 gallop and a soft systolic murmur on cardiac exam. The laboratory studies revealed a sodium 132, potassium 5.2, chloride 106, CO_2 19, blood urea nitrogen (BUN) 42, creatinine 2.8, glucose 186, hemoglobin 10.8, hematocrit 31.6, WBC 12.4, calcium 9.0, phosphorus 3.9, albumin 3.2, urine analysis 3 plus protein on dipstick, total cholesterol 164, HDL 29, LDL 135, and triglycerides 211. Echocardiogram demonstrates LVH with a dilated ventricle, diastolic dysfunction, and a global decrease in systolic function with an ejection fraction of 35%. The estimated GFR by the MDRD equation is 26 mL/min/1.73 m². A 24-hour urine creatinine clearance was 31 mL/min and the protein excretion was 2.6 g/24 hr.

With JS manifesting evidence of overt diabetic nephropathy as well as LVH and evidence of decompensated CHF, he was appropriately started on an ACE-I. One week later his creatinine was 3.1 and his potassium was 5.8. His ACE-I was immediately discontinued, treatment with kayexelate was provided, and he was placed back on his original medical regimen that included traditional therapy for his CHF of digoxin, nitrates, diuretics, and hydralazine. Were these results unexpected and what are the therapeutic options for optimal therapy?

ROLE OF ANGIOTENSIN II MODULATING THERAPY IN CKD/CVD

A large body of clinical trial data provides important evidence for the routine use of angiotensin converting enzyme inhibitor (ACE-I) and angiotensin receptor blockers (ARBs) in the treatment of both diabetic nephropathy and CHF (212–217). Evidence-based data clearly demonstrate that the use of these medications along with β blockers clearly and significantly reduces mortality in patients with decompensated CHF. In addition to protecting against the progression of CKD in diabetic nephropathy, ARB therapy also was reported in the RENAAL and IDNT trial to reduce the incidence of hospitalization for new-onset CHF independent of the effects on BP (213,218).

In the kidney these medications selectively interfere with the effect of angiotensin II on vasoconstriction in the efferent glomerular arteriole. Thus, for any given reduction in systemic BP, the use of these medications will offer a consistently better opportunity to control glomerular capillary pressure associated with mild reductions in GFR (10–20%) as well as urine and albumin excretion.

As was demonstrated in the case above, concern always arises with the observed increase in serum creatinine and associated decrease in GFR with the use of these medications. Bakris and Weir demonstrated that a strong association exists between acute increases in serum creatinine of up to 30% that stabilize within the first two months of ACE-I therapy and long-term preservation of renal function (219). Thus, withdrawal of an ACE-I or ARB should occur only when the rise in creatinine exceeds 30% above baseline within the first two months of initiation of therapy or if hyperkalemia not amenable to appropriate therapy develops. In the above case, one should have tolerated a serum creatinine of up to 3.64 before considering discontinuation of the medication. Serial repeated laboratory studies would have been appropriate in three to four days and one week later to see if the serum creatinine stabilized at a new steady state which is what the majority of patients like JS tend to do. In the RENAAL study only 2% of patients with advanced CKD with diabetic nephropathy had to discontinue Losartan because of a progressive increase in serum creatinine (213). This study also demonstrated that patients with more advanced CKD also benefited from ARB therapy. This suggests that especially in patients with concomitant CHF and CKD, which is a very common occurrence, as is discussed in the cardiorenal section above, one should consider the use of ACE-I or ARB therapy even more aggressively and not be limited by the serum creatinine level unless the expected increase in serum creatinine is greater than 30% over a two-month period. If the serum creatinine does increase by greater than 30%, we need to make sure that the patient is not dehydrated, over diuresed, and also that a bilateral renal artery stenosis or a solitary kidney with renal artery stenosis is not present. Careful history of concomitant medications also needs to be reviewed, especially regarding the use of over the counter nonsteroidal inflammatory medication. Consideration should also be given to a nephrology consult in patients such as this especially with a GFR of less than 30 mL/min/1.73 m^2.

In reviewing JS, electrolytes it is apparent also that he has a type 4 renal tubular acidosis associated with his diabetic kidney disease. One should therefore expect a significant increase in potassium associated with the initiation of angiotensin II-modulating therapy in these patients. It is imperative in such cases to obtain formal dietary counseling with a knowledgeable dietician regarding a low potassium diet to prevent the expected hyperkalemia seen with JS. On further questioning, JS admitted to rather excessive use of orange juice for repeated hypoglycemic episodes and also the use of high potassium foods to supplement the potassium he thought he was losing with the diuretics that he was prescribed. There is also anecdotal evidence suggesting that hyperkalemia occurs more frequently as an adverse effect of ACE-I therapy than with ARBs. Bakris et al. looked at this with a crossover study where CKD patients with GFR rates of 65 ± 5 mL/min/1.73 m^2 received each drug type in random order. They demonstrated that if the GFR was <60 mL/min/1.73 m^2, serum potassium rose to higher levels with the ACE-I, lisinopril, then with the ARB, valsartan (220). One possible explanation for the greater tendency to hyperkalemia with the ACE-I is the greater suppression of plasma aldosterone levels with the ACE-I compared to ARB. Thus if that is a concern in a patient such as JS, then consideration may be given to the use of an ARB that has demonstrated efficacy for the treatment of both diabetic nephropathy and CHF (221–223). In the RENAAL study, only 1% of the patients in the Losartan arm had to discontinue the ARB because of hyperkalemia in a population of patients that were aggressively educated regarding dietary restrictions of potassium (213). Appropriate dietary counseling and education regarding the nonuse of over the counter medications that can increase potassium should significantly increase the successful use of angiotensin II modulating therapy and limit the need for kayexelate use.

In the Ramipril efficacy in nephropathy (REIN) study, maximal renoprotection was achieved when the treatment with an ACE-I was started early in the course of the disease (GFR > 50 mL/min) (224). Treatment is also renoprotective for levels of renal function between 10 and 30 mL/min, indicating the need not to withhold ACE inhibitors, even when GFR approximates levels requiring replacement therapy. This message will never be emphasized enough, given the fact that it can be estimated that <20% of patients in need are currently offered this renoprotective treatment, a figure that decreases to 11% to 12% if the GFR is severely impaired (224).

SUMMARY

There is a high prevalence of CVD in patients with CKD. Studies have clearly demonstrated that the presence of CKD, whether it is manifested by proteinuria (albuminuria) or reduced GFR, appears to be an independent risk factor for CVD events. These findings are consistent with the NKF task force and the statement paper by the American Heart Association Council on Kidney in Cardiovascular Disease recommendation that patients with CKD should be considered in the highest-risk group for CVD events. This reinforces the need for early identification and treatment of CKD and its associated comorbid conditions as is discussed above. Also, it is recommended that all patients with CVD be screened for CKD with an estimation of GFR by serum creatinine and prediction equations as well as measurement of spot urine for albumin-to-creatinine ratio or total protein-to-creatinine ratio. This is especially true after admission for acute decompensated CHF, as is discussed above, and also for AMIs (42). The in-hospital mortality after an AMI doubled with a creatinine clearance of 60 mL/min as compared to 100 mL/min and increased eightfold with a creatinine clearance of 30 mL/min.

Once CKD is diagnosed both the traditional and the nontraditional risk factors outlined in Table 3 should be identified and aggressively addressed. Unfortunately, the proportion of patients with CKD who receive appropriate risk-factor modification and intervention is lower than in the general population, a concept termed "therapeutic nihilism." (45,225). Wright et al. observed statistically significantly reduced use of aspirin, β-blockers, ACE-Is, and heparin during hospitalization for AMI in all patients with renal dysfunction. This finding is consistent with previous reports (226,227). Use of aspirin and ACE inhibitors during the initial day of hospitalization was associated with improved short-term survival, and use of aspirin and β-blockers at discharge was associated with improved postdischarge survival across the spectrum of renal failure.

Many databases and registries have shown that this parallels worsening renal function (228,229). Among patients with end-stage renal disease, who are known to be at extreme risk for cardiovascular events, less than 50% are taking a combination of aspirin, beta-blockers, ACE-I or ARBs, and statins (226,230). In the VALIANT trial, a postmyocardial infarction study, patients in the lowest tier of renal function were the least likely to receive risk-modifying cardiovascular medications and to undergo coronary revascularization. Potential reasons include concern about worsening renal function and therapy-related toxic effects related to reduced

TABLE 11 Approach to Chronic Kidney Disease/Cardiovascular Disease

Factor	Marker	Treatment	Goal
Hypertension	BP	Diuretics, CCBs, ACEIs, ARBs, Beta-blockers	<130/80 mmHg
Microvascular disease	Proteinuria	ACEIs, ARBs, stains	<300 mg BP <120/70 mmHg
Glycemia	Glucose, HbA$_{1c}$	Insulin, metformin[a] GTZ, sulfonylureas, etc.	HbA$_{1c}$ <6.5%
Dyslipidema	LDL, TG	Statins, fibrates	LDL <100 mm/dl TG <150 mg/dl
Anemia	Hgb, Fe,	Ethryropoetin, Fe	Hgb >12
Hyperparathyoid	Ca, PO$_4$, PTH	Binders, diet, vit D Calcimimetic	Ca = 9–9.5 PO$_4$ <3.5, PTH <100
Nutrition	Prealbumin	Dietary Council Supplement	Normal prealbumin

[a]Metformin: contraindicated renal insufficiency [serum creatinine concentration above 1.4 mg/dL (124 μmol/L) in women and 1.5 mg/dL (132 μmol/L) in men], or low creatinine clearance.
Abbreviations: BP, blood pressure; ARB, angiotension-receptor blockers; CCB, calcium channel blocker; ACEI, angiotensin converting enzyme inhibitor; GTZ, geitazone; LDL, low-density lipoprotein; PTH, parathyroid hormone; TG, triglyceride; HbA$_{1c}$, Hemoglobin A$_{1c}$; Hgb, hemoglobin.

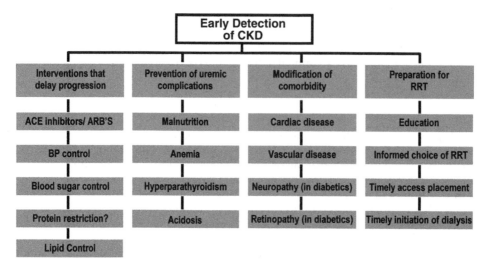

FIGURE 11   Chronic Kidney Disase (CKD): There is a lot to manage. *Source:* From Ref. 15.

clearance (45,231–233). However, studies show that, when appropriately monitored, cardiovascular medications and coronary interventional strategies used in the general population can safely be administered to those with renal impairment and yield similar benefits (29,59,233–236). Our understanding of the efficacy and safety of cardiovascular medications and interventional strategies in these patients is limited, and many cardiovascular trials have excluded patients with renal disease (237).

Increasing data regarding the benefits of addressing some of the nontraditional risk factors have also been reviewed in this chapter. In the case of JS, his hemoglobin is 10.8 classifying him as anemic and studies are now underway to assess the appropriate range for his hemoglobin level. Current thinking with the evidenced-based data available is to address this anemia. His calcium and phosphorus are within acceptable levels when first reviewed; however, when the intact PTH and vitamin D levels were obtained they were significantly abnormal (intact PTH = 289 pg/mL (normal 70–110 pg/mL), 25 hydroxyvitamin D = 10 ng/mL (normal range 50–110 ng/mL) and 1,25 dihydroxyvitamin D_3 of 15 pmol/L (normal range 40–120 pmol/L). Addressing these severe abnormalities also may impact his cardiovascular status as well as perhaps impacting on the progression of his renal disease and renal bone disease.

One could consider JS as the "Perfect Storm" awaiting a CV event and progression to ESRD. The overwhelming likelihood is that he will die of a cardiovascular event before progressing to ESRD and the need for RRT. To delay or circumvent these adverse outcomes will require an aggressive multifaceted approach (Table 11) with a great deal to manage (Fig. 11).

The NKF has developed an interactive clinical action plan available at the NKF web site (126) to assist in the care of these complicated patients. After entering a patient's GFR and comorbid conditions, a clinical action plan will be created that includes the references and guidelines individualized to a given patient.

REFERENCES

1. Wali RK, Henrich WL. Chronic Kidney Disease: A risk factor for Cardiovascular Disease, Cardiol Clin 2005; 23:343–362.
2. Levey AS, Beto JA, Coronado BE, et al. Controlling the epidemic of cardiovascular disease in chronic renal disease: what do we know? what do we need to learn? where do we go from here? National Kidney Foundation Task Force on Cardiovascular Disease. Am J Kidney Dis 1998; 32:853–906.
3. Xue JL, Ma JZ, Louis TA, Collins AJ. Forecast of the number of patients with end-stage renal disease in the United States to the year 2010. J Am Soc Nephrol 2001; 12:2753–2758.
4. Jay L. Xue, Jennie ZMa, Louis TA, Collins AJ. Forecast of the number of patients with end-stage renal disease in the United States to the year 2010. J Am Soc Nephrol 2001; 12:2753–2758.

5. Kopyt NP. Slowing progression along the renal disease continuum, JAOA 2005; 105(4):207.
6. Levey AS, Bosch JP, Lewis JB, et al. A more accurate method to estimate glomerular filtration rate from serum creatinine: a new prediction equation. Modification of Diet in Renal Disease Study Group. Ann Intern Med 1999; 130(6):461–470.
7. Levey AS, Bosch JP, Lewis JB, Greene T, Rogers N, Roth D. A more accurate method to estimate glomerular filtration rate from serum creatinine: A new prediction equation. Modification of Diet in Renal Disease Study Group. Ann Intern Med 1999; 130:461–470.
8. Manjunath G, Sarnak MJ, Levey AS. Estimating the glomerular filtration rate. Do's and don'ts for assessing kidney function, Postgraduate Medicine 2001; 110(6):55–62
9. Coll E, Botey A, Alvarez L, et al. Serum cystatin C as a new marker for noninvasive estimation of glomerular filtration rate and as a marker for early renal impairment. Am J Kidney Dis 2000; 36(1):29–34.
10. Fliser D, Ritz E. Serum cystatin C concentration as a marker of renal dysfunction in the elderly. Am J Kidney Dis 2001; 37:79–83.
11. Vinge E, Lindergard B, Nilsson-Ehle P, Grubb A. Relationships among serum cystatin C, serum creatinine, lean tissue mass and glomerular filtration rate in healthy adults. Scand J Clin Lab Invest 1999; 59:587–592.
12. Shlipak MG, Sarnak MJ, Katz R, et al. Cystatin C and the risk of death and cardiovascular events among elderly persons. N Engl J Med 2005; 352:2049–2060.
13. Sarnak MJ, Katz R, Stehman-Breen CO, et al. Cystatin C concentration as a risk factor for heart failure in older adults. Ann Intern Med 2005; 142:497–505.
14. Fried LF, Katz R, Sarnak MJ, et al. Kidney function as a predictor of noncardiovascular mortality. J Am Soc Nephrol 2005; 16:3728–3735.
15. K/DOQI clinical practice guidelines for chronic kidney disease: evaluation, classification, and stratification. Kidney Disease Outcome Quality Initiative. Am J Kidney Dis 2002; 39:S1–S246. [PMID: 11904577]
16. National Kidney Foundation. Am J Kidey Dis 2002; 39(2 suppl 1):S1–S266.
17. National Kidney Foundation: K/DOQI Clinical Practice Guidelines on Hypertension and Antihypertensive Agents in Chronic Kidney Disease. Am J Kidney Dis 2004; 43(suppl 1):S1–S290.
18. Coresh J, Byrd-Holt D, Astor BC, et al. Chronic Kidney Disease Awareness, Prevalence, and Trends among U.S. Adults, 1999 to 2000. J Am Soc Nephrol 2005; 16:180–188.
19. Keith D, Nichols G, Gullion C, Brown J, Smith D. Mortality of chronic kidney disease (CKD) in a large HMO population. J Am Soc Nephrol 2002; 13:620A (Abstract SU–PO740).
20. Coresh J, Astor BC, Greene T, Eknoyan G, Levey AS. Prevalence of chronic kidney disease and decreased kidney function in the adult US population: Third National Health and Nutrition Examination Survey. Am J Kidney Dis 2003; 41:1–12.
21. www.kidney.org.
22. Collins AJ, Kasiske B, Herzog C, et al. Excerpts from the United States Renal Data System 2003 Annual Data Report: Atlas of End-Stage Renal Disease in the United States. American Journal of Kidney Diseases 2003; 42(6) (Suppl 5).
23. US Renal Data System, Excerpts from the USRDS Annual Data Report. Am J Kidney Dis 2003; 42(suppl 5):S1–S230.
24. Nickolas TL, Frisch GD, Opotowsky AR, Arons R, Radhakrishnan J. Awareness of Kidney Disease in the US Population: Findings From the National Health and Nutrition Examination Survey (NHANES) 1999 to 2000: American Journal of Kidney Diseases 2004; 44(2):185–197.
25. Jirkovitz C, Franch H, Shoham D, Bellenger J, McClellan W. Family Members of Patients Treated for ESRD Have High Rates of Undetected Kidney Disease Am J Kidney Dis 40:1173–1178.
26. Shulman NB, Ford CE, Hall WD, et al. Prognostic value of serum creatinine and effect of treatment of hypertension on renal function. Results from the Hypertension Detection and Follow-up Program (HDFP). The Hypertension Detection and Follow-Up Program Cooperative Group. Hypertension 1989; 13(Suppl):I80–I93.
27. Ruilope LM, Salvetti A, Jamerson K, et al. Renal function and intensive lowering of blood pressure in hypertensive participants of the Hypertension Optimal Treatment (HOT) study. J Am Soc Nephrol 2001; 12:218–225.
28. Culleton BF, Larson MG, Wilson PWF, Evans JC, Parfrey PS, Levy D. Cardiovascular disease and mortality in a community-based cohort with mild renal insufficiency. Kidney Int 1999; 56:2214–2219.
29. Henry RM, Kostense PJ, Bos G, et al. Mild renal insufficiency is associated with increased cardio vascular mortality: the Hoorn study. Kidney Int 2002; 62:1402–1407.
30. Henry RMA, Kamp O, Kostense PF, et al. Mild renal insufficiency is associated with increased left ventricular mass in men, but not in women: An arterial stiffness–related phenomenon-The Hoorn Study, Kidney International 2005; 68:673–679.
31. Fried LF, Shlipak MG, Crump C, et al. Renal insufficiency as a predictor of cardiovascular outcomes and mortality in elderly individuals. J Am Coll Cardiol 2003; 41:1364–1372.
32. Shlipak MG, Fried LF, Crump C, et al. Cardiovascular disease risk status in elderly persons with renal insufficiency. Kidney Int 2002; 62:997–1004.
33. Adler AI, Stevens RJ, Manley SE, Bilous RW, Cull CA, Holman RR. On behalf of the UKPDS Group, Development and progression of nephropathy in type 2 diabetes: The United Kingdom Prospective Diabetes Study (UKPDS 64), Kidney International 2003; 63:225–232.

34. Mann JF, Gerstein HC, Pogue J, Bosch J, Yusuf S. For the HOPE Investigators, Renal insufficiency as a predictor of cardiovascular outcomes and the impact of ramipril: the HOPE randomized trial. Ann Intern Med 2001; 134:629–636.

35. Wannamethee SG, Shaper AG, Perry IJ. Serum creatinine concentration and risk of cardiovascular disease: a possible marker for increased risk of stroke. Stroke 1997; 28:557–563.

36. Rahman M, Brown CD, Coresh J, et al. For the ALLHAT Collaborative Research Group, The Prevalence of Reduced Glomerular Filtration Rate in Older Hypertensive Patients and Its Association With Cardiovascular Disease A Report From the Antihypertensive and Lipid-Lowering Treatment to Prevent Heart Attack Trial, Arch Intern Med 2004; 164:969–976.

37. Keith DS, Nichols GA, Gullion CM, Brown JB, Smith DH. Longitudinal follow-up and outcomes among a population with chronic kidney disease in a large managed care organization. Arch Intern Med 2004; 164:659–663.

38. Foley RN, Murray AM, Li S, et al. Chronic Kidney Disease and the Risk for Cardiovascular Disease, Renal Replacement, and Death in the United States Medicare Population, 1998 to 1999. J Am Soc Nephrol 2005; 16:489–495.

39. Go AS, Chertow GM, Fan D, McCulloch CE, Hsu CY. Chronic kidney disease and the risks of death, cardiovascular events, and hospitalization. N Engl J Med 2004; 351:1296–1305.

40. Dennis VW. Coronary Heart Disease in Patients with Chronic Kidney Disease. J Am Soc Nephrol 2005; 16:S103–S106.

41. Herzog CA, Ma JZ, Collins AJ. Poor long term survival after acute myocardial infarction among patients on long-term dialysis. N Engl J Med 1998; 339:799–805.

42. Wright RS, Reeder GS, Herzog CA, et al. Acute myocardial infarction and renal dysfunction: a high-risk combination. Ann Intern Med 2002; 137:563–570.

43. Al Suwaidi J, Reddan DN, Williams K, et al. Prognostic implications of abnormalities in renal function in patients with acute coronary syndromes. Circulation 2002; 106:974–980.

44. Sarnak MJ, Levey AS, Schoolwerth AC, et al. Kidney disease as a risk factor for development of cardiovascular disease: a statement from the American Heart Association Councils on Kidney in Cardiovascular Disease, High Blood Pressure Research, Clinical Cardiology, and Epidemiology and Prevention. Hypertension 2003; 42:1050–1065.

45. Anavekar NS, McMurray JJ, Velazquez EJ, et al. Relation between renal dysfunction and cardiovascular outcomes after myocardial infarction. N Engl J Med 2004; 351:1285–1295.

46. US Renal Data System: USRDS 2000 Annual Data Report, Bethesda, MD, National Institutes of Health, National Institute of Diabetes and Digestive and Kidney Diseases 2000.

47. Herzog CA, Ma JZ, Collins AJ: Long-term outcome of dialysis patients in the United States with coronary revascularization procedures. Kidney Int 1999; 56: 24–332.

48. Joki N, Hase H, Nakamura R, Yamaguchi T. Onset of coronary artery disease prior to initiation of haemodialysis in patients with end-stage renal disease. Nephrol Dial Transplant 1997; 12:718–723.

49. Szczech LA, Best PJ, Crowley E, et al. Bypass Angioplasty Revascularization Investigation (BARI) investigators. Outcomes of patients with chronic renal insufficiency in the bypass angioplasty revascularization investigation. Circulation 2002; 105:2253–2258.

50. Reddan DN, Szczech LA, Tuttle RH, et al. Chronic kidney disease, mortality, and treatment strategies among patients with clinically significant coronary artery disease. J Am Soc Nephrol 2003; 14:2373–2380.

51. Heywood JT. The Cardiorenal Syndrome: Lessons from the ADHERE Database and Treatment Options. Heart Failure Reviews 2004; 9:195–201.

52. Hillege HL, Girbes ARJ, de Kam PJ, et al. Renal Function, Neurohormonal activation, and Survival in Patients with Chronic Heart Failure. Circulation 2000; 102:203–210.

53. Dries DL, Exner DV, Domanski MJ, Greenberg B, Stevenson LW. The prognostic implications of renal insufficiency in asymptomatic and symptomatic patients with left ventricular systolic dysfunction. J Am Coll Cardiol 2000; 35:681–689.

54. Gottlieb SS, Abraham W, Butler J, et al. The prognostic importance of different definitions of worsening renal function in congestive heart failure. J Card Fail 2002; 8:136–141.

55. Smith GL, Vaccarino V, Kosiborod M, et al. Worsening renal function: What is a clinically meaningful change in creatinine during hospitalization with heart failure? J Card Fail 2003; 9:13–25.

56. Sarnak MJ, Levey AS. Cardiovascular disease and Chronic Renal Disease: A New Paradigm, American. J Kidney Dis 2000; 35(4)(Suppl 1):S117–S131.

57. Menon V, Gul A, Sarnak MJ. Cardiovascular risk factors in chronic Kidney Disease. Kidney Int 2005; 68:1413–1418.

58. Wilson PW, D'Agostino RB, Levy D, et al. Prediction of coronary heart disease using risk factor categories. Circulation 1998; 97:1837–1847.

59. Cheung AK, Sarnak MJ, Yan G, et al. Atherosclerotic cardiovascular disease risks in chronic hemodialysis patients. Kidney Int 2000; 58:353–362.

60. Longenecker JC, Coresh J, Powe NR, et al. Traditional cardiovascular disease risk factors in dialysis patients compared with the general population: the CHOICE Study. J Am Soc Nephrol 2002; 13:1918–1927.

61. Sarnak MJ, Coronado BE, Greene T, et al. Cardiovascular disease risk factors in chronic renal insufficiency. Clin Nephrol 2002;57:327–335.

62. Expert Panel on Detection, Evaluation, and Treatment of High Blood Cholesterol in Adults. Executive summary of the Third Report of the National Cholesterol Education Program (NCEP) Expert Panel on Detection, Evaluation, and Treatment of High Blood Cholesterol.

63. Grundy SM, Brewer HB Jr. Cleeman JI, et al. Definition of metabolic syndrome: report of the National Heart, Lung, and Blood Institute/American Heart Association Conference on Scientific Issues Related to Definition. Circulation 2004; 109:433–438.

64. Lakka HM, Laaksonen DE, Lakka TA, et al. The metabolic syndrome and total and cardiovascular disease mortality in middle-aged men. JAMA 2002; 288:2709–2716.

65. Isomaa B, Almgren P, Tuomi T, et al. Cardiovascular morbidity and mortality associated with the metabolic syndrome. Diabetes Care 2001; 24:683–689.

66. Park YW, Zhu S, Palaniappan L, et al. The metabolic syndrome: prevalence and associated risk factor findings in the US population from the Third National Health and Nutrition Examination Survey, 1988–1994. Arch Intern Med 2003; 163:427–436.

67. Chen J, Muntner P, Hamm LL, et al. The metabolic syndrome and chronic kidney disease in U.S. adults. Ann Intern Med 2004; 140:167–174.

68. National Institutes of Health. Third Report of the National Cholesterol Education Program Expert Panel on Detection, Evaluation, and Treatment of High Blood Cholesterol in Adults (Adult Treatment Panel III). NIH Publication 01-3670. Bethesda, MD: National Institutes of Health, 2001.

69. Kurella M, Lo JC, Chertow GM. Metabolic syndrome and the risk of chronic kidney disease among nondiabetic adults. J Am Soc Nephrol 2005; 16:2134–2140.

70. Sedor JR, Schelling JR. Association of Metabolic Syndrome in Nondiabetic Patients with Increased Risk for Chronic Kidney Disease: The Fat Lady Sings. J Am Soc Nephrol 2005; 16:1880–1882.

71. Jones CA, Krolewski AS, Rogus J, Xue JL, Collins A, Warram JH. Epidemic of end-stage renal disease in people with diabetes in the United States population: Do we know the cause? Kidney Int 2005; 67:1684–1691.

72. Peterson JC, Adler S, Burkart JM, et al. Blood pressure control, proteinuria and the progression of renal disease. The Modification of Diet in Renal Disease Study. Ann Intern Med 1995; 123:754–762.

73. Eknoyan G. On testing for proteinuria: Time for a methodical approach. Cleveland Clinic J Med 2003; 70(6).

74. Keane WF, Eknoyan G. Proteinuria, albuminuria, risk, assessment, detection and elimination (PARADE). A position paper of the National Kidney Foundation. Am J Kidney Dis 1999; 33:1004–1010.

75. Grimm RH Jr., Sandsen KH, Kasiske B, Keane WM, Wahi M. Proteinuria is a risk factor for mortality over 10 years of follow up. MRFIT Research Group. Multiple Risk Factor Intervention Trial. Kidney Int 1997; 63(suppl 63):S10–S14.

76. Mutner P, He J, Hamm L, Loria C, Whelton P. Renal insufficiency and subsequent death resulting from cardiovascular disease in the United States. J Am Soc Nephrol 2002; 13:745–753.

77. SoRelle R. Increases in urinary albumin excretion predict risk of death from all causes as well as those from cardiovascular disease. Circulation 2002; 106:e9037–e9038.

78. Leoncini G, Sacchi G, Viazzi F, et al. Microalbuminuria identifies overall cardiovascular risk in essential hypertension. J Hypertens 2002; 20:1315–1321.

79. Hillege HL, Fidler V, Diercks GF, et al. Urinary albumin excretion predicts cardiovascular and noncardiovascular mortality in the general population. Circulation 2002; 106:1777–1782.

80. Mann JFE, Gerstein HC, Pogue J, Bosch J, Yusuf S. For the HOPE Investigators. Renal insufficiency as a predictor of cardiovascular outcomes and the impact of ramipril: The HOPE randomized trial. Ann Intern Med 2001; 134:629–636.

81. Keane WF. Proteinuria: Its clinical importance and role in progressive renal disease. Am J Kidney Dis 2000; 35:(suppl 1):S97–S105.

82. Diabetes Control and Complications Trial Research Group. The effect of intensive treatment of diabetes on the development and progression of long-term complications in insulin-dependent diabetes mellitus. N Engl J Med 1993; 329:977–986.

83. Eknoyan G, Hostetter T, Bakris G, et al. Proteinuria and Other Markers of Chronic Kidney Disease: A Position Statement of the National Kidney Foundation (NKF) and the National Institute of Diabetes and Digestive and Kidney Diseases (NIDDK). Am J Kidney Dis 2003; 42(4):617–622.

84. Gaspari F, Perico N, Remuzzi G. Timed Urine Collections Are Not Needed to Measure Urine Protein Excretion in Clinical Practice, Am J Kidney Dis 2006; 47(1).

85. Shidham G, Hebert LA. Timed Urine Collections Are Not Needed to Measure Urine Protein Excretion in Clinical Practice, Am J Kidney Dis 2006.

86. Position Statement: Diabetic Nephropathy, American Diabetes Association. Diabetes Care 2002; 34(suppl 1):S85–S89.

87. Hillege HL, Janssen WMT, Bak AAA, et al. For the Prevend Study Group, Microalbuminuria is common, also in a nondiabetic, nonhypertensive population, and an independent indicator of cardiovascular risk factors and cardiovascular morbidity, J Int Med 2001; 249:519–526.

88. Briganti EM, Branley P, Chadban SJ, et al. Smoking is associated with renal impairment and proteinuria in the normal population: the Aus Diab Kidney Study: Australian Diabetes, Obesity and Lifestyle Study. Am J Kidney Dis 2002; 40:704–712.

89. Hoehner CM, Greenlund KJ, Rith-Najarian S, Casper ML, McClellan WM. Association of the insulin resistance syndrome and microalbuminuria among nondiabetic native Americans: the Inter-Tribal Heart Project. J Am Soc Nephrol 2002; 13:1626–1634.

90. Garg AX, Kiberd BA, Clark WF, Haynes RB, Clase CM. Albuminuria and renal insufficiency preva-
     lence guides population screening: results from the NHANES III. Kidney Int 2002; 61:2165–2175.
91. Chelliah R, Sagnella GA, Markandu ND, MacGregor GA. Urinary protein and essential hypertension
     in black and in white people. Hypertension. 2002; 39:1064–1070.
92. Tozawa M, Iseki K, Iseki C, Oshiro S, Ikemiya Y, Takishita S. Influence of smoking and obesity on the
     development of proteinuria. Kidney Int 2002; 62:956–962.
93. Jee SH, Boulware LE, Guallar E, Suh I, Appel LJ, Miller ER. Direct, Progressive Association of
     Cardiovascular Risk Factors With Incident Proteinuria. Arch Intern Med 2005; 165:2299–2304
94. Cirillo M, Senigalliesi L, Laurenzi M, et al. Microalbuminuria in nondiabetic adults: Relation of blood
     pressure, body mass, plasma cholesterol, and smoking-The Gubbio Population Study. Arch Intern
     Med 1998; 158:1933–1939.
95. Cirillo M, Stellato D, Laurenzi M, et al. Pulse pressure and isolated systolic hypertension: association
     with microalbuminuria. Kidney Int 2000; 58:1211–1218.
96. Cirillo M, Laurenzi M, Panarelli P, et al. Relation of urinary albumin excretion to coronary heart
     disease and low renal function: Role of blood pressure. Kidney Int 2004; 65:2290–2297.
97. Verhave JC, Hellege HL, Burgerhof JGM, Navis G, de Zeeuw D. Cardiovascular Risk Factors Are
     Differently Associated with Urinary Albumin Excretion in Men and Women. J Am Soc Nephrol 2003;
     14:1330–1335.
98. Romundstad S, Holmen J, Hallan H, Kvenild K, Kruger O, Nidthjell K. Microalbuminuria, car-
     diovascular disease and risk factors in a nondiabetic/nonhypertensive population. The Nord-
     Trndelag Health Study (HUNT, 1995–97), Norway. Journal of Internal Medicine 2002;
     252:164–172.
99. Gall MA, Borch-Johnsen KB, Hougaard P, Nielsen FS, Parving HH. Albuminuria and poor glycemic
     control predict mortality in NIDDM. Diabetes 1995; 44:1303–1309.
100. Gerstein HC, Mann JFE, Yi Q, et al. For the HOPE Study Investigators, Albuminuria and Risk of
     Cardiovascular events, death, and heart failure in diabetic and nondiabetic individuals. JAMA 2001;
     286:421–426.
101. Ibsen H, Wachtell K, Olsen MH, et al. Albuminuria and cardiovascular risk in hypertensive patients
     with left ventricular hypertrophy: The LIFE study, Kidney International 2004; 66(s92):S56–S58.
102. Wachtell K, Olsen MH, Dahlof B, et al. Microalbuminuria in hypertensive patients with electrocardio-
     graphic left ventricular hypertrophy: The Life Study. J Hyperten 2002; 20(3):405–412.
103. Wachtell K, Plamieri V, Olsen MH, et al. Urine albumin/creatinine ratio and echocardiographic left
     ventricular structure and function in hypertensive patients with electrocardiographic left ventricular
     hypertrophy: The LIFE study. Am Heart J 2002; 143:319–326
104. Kean WF, Brenner BM, de Zeeuw D, et al. For the RENAAL study investigators. The risk of develop-
     ing end-stage renal disease in patients with type 2 diabetes and nephropathy: The RENAAL Study.
     Kidney Int 2003; 63:1499–1507.
105. de Zeeuw D, Remuzzi G, Parving HH, et al. Albuminuria, a Therapeutic Target for Cardiovascular
     Protection in Type 2 Diabetic Patients With Nephropathy. Circulation 2004; 110:921–927.
106. Borch-Johnsen K, Feldt-Rasmussen B, Strandgaard S, et al. Urinary albumin excretion: an independ-
     ent predictor of ischemic heart disease. Arterioscler Throm Vasc Biol 1999; 19:1992–1997.
107. Miettinen H, Haffner SM, Lehto S, et al. Proteinuria predicts stroke and other atherosclerotic vas-
     cular disease events in nondiabetic and noninsulin-dependent diabetic subjects. Stroke 1996;
     27:2033–2039.
108. Morgensen CE. Microalbuminuria predicts clinical proteinuria and early mortality in maturity-onset
     diabetes. N Engl J Med 1984; 310:356–360.
109. Nelson RG, Pettitt DJ, Carraher MJ, et al. Effect of proteinuria on mortality in NIDDM. Diabetes 1988;
     37:1499–1504.
110. Mattock MB, Morrish NJ, Viberti GC, et al. Prospective study of microalbuminuria as predictor of
     mortality in NIDDM. Diabetes 1992; 41:735–741.
111. Damsgaard EM, Froland A, Jorgensen OD, et al. Eight to nine year mortality in known non-insulin
     dependent diabetics and controls. Kidney Int 1992; 41:731–735.
112. Neil A, Hawkins M, Potok M, et al. A prospective population-based study of microalbuminuria as a
     predictor of mortality in NIDDM. Diabetes Care 1993; 16:996–1003.
113. MacLeod JM, Lutale J, Marshall SM. Albumin excretion and vascular deaths in NIDDM. Diabetologia
     1995; 38:610–616.
114. Ballard DJ, Humphrey LL, Melton J III, et al. Epidemiology of persistent proteinuria in type II
     diabetes mellitus: population-based study in Rochester, Minnesota. Diabetes 1988; 37:405–412.
115. African Am Study of Kidney Disease and Hypertension (AASK) Study Group. Effect of ramipril vs.
     amlodipine on renal outcomes in hypertensive nephrosclerosis: a randomized controlled trial. JAMA
     2001; 285:2719–2728.
116. Remuzzi G, Bertani T. Pathophysiology of progressive nephropathies. N Engl J Med 1998;
     339:1448–1456.
117. Zandi-Nejad K, Eddy AA, Glassock RJ, Brenner BM. Why is proteinuria an ominous biomarker of
     progressive kidney disease? Kidney International 2004 66(suppl 92):S76–S89.
118. Segura J, Campo C, Ruilope LM. Effect of proteinuria and glomerular filtration rate on cardiovascu-
     lar risk in essential hypertension. Kidney Int 2004; 66(s92):S45–S49.

119. Redon J, Williams B. Microalbuminuria in essential hypertension: Redefining the threshold. J Hypertens 2002; 20:353–355.
120. Levin A. The need for optimal and coordinated management of CKD, Kidney International 2005; 68(Suppl 99):S7–S10.
121. Foley RN, Pargrey PS, Sarnak MJ. Clinical epidemiology of cardiovascular disease in chronic renal disease. Am J Kidney Disease 1998; 32(5)(Suppl 3):S112–S119.
122. Lindner A, Chatta B, Sherrark DI, Scribner BF. Accelerated atherosclerosis in prolonged maintenance hemodialysis. NEJM 1974; 290:697–701.
123. Wolfe RA, Ashby VB, Molford EL, et al. Comparison of mortality in all patients on dialysis, patients on dialysis awaiting transplantation, and recipients of a first cadaveric transplant. NEJM 1999; 341:1725–1730.
124. Nolan CR. Strategies for improving long-term survival in patients with ESRD. J Am Soc Nephrol 2005; 16:S120–S127.
125. Locatelli, Francesco. Revised European best practice guidelines for the management of anaemia in patients with chronic renal failure. Nephrol Dial Transplant 2004; 19(suppl 2):ii1–ii47.
126. http://www.kidney.org/professionals/KDOQI/cap.cfm.
128. Goodman WG, London G, Amann K, et al. Vascular calcificaton in chronic kidney disease. Am J Kidney Dis 2004; 43:572–579.
129. Raggi P, Boulay A, Chasan-Taber S, et al. Cardiac calcification in adult hemodialysis patients. A link between end-stage renal disease and cardiovascular disease? J Am Coll Cardiol 2002; 39:695–701.
130. Schwarz U, Buzello M, Ritz E, et al. Morphology of coronary atherosclerotic lesions in patients with end-stage renal failure. Nephrol Dial Transplant 2000; 15:218–223.
131. Schinke T, McKee MD, Kiviranta R, Karsenty G. Molecular determinants of arterial calcification. Ann Med 1998; 30:538–541.
132. Proudfoot D, Shanahan CM. Biology of calcification in vascular cells: Intima versus media. Herz 2001; 26:245–251.
133. Goodman WG, Goldin J, Kuizon BD, et al. Coronary-artery calcification in young adults with end-stage renal disease who are undergoing dialysis. N Engl J Med 2000; 342:1478–1483.
134. London GM, Guerin AP, Marchais SJ, Metivier F, Pannier B, Adda H. Arterial media calcification in end-stage renal disease: Impact on all-cause and cardiovascular mortality. Nephrol Dial Transplant 2003; 18:1731–1740.
135. Blacher J, Guerin AP, Pannier B, Marchais SJ, London GM. Arterial calcifications, arterial stiffness, and cardiovascular risk in end-stage renal disease. Hypertension 2001; 38:938–942.
136. The Seventh Report of the Joint National Committee on Prevention, Detection, Evaluation, and Treatment of High Blood Pressure: The JNC 7 report. JAMA 2003; 289:2560–2572.
137. Anand IS, Kuskowski MA, Rector TS, et al. Anemia and change in hemoglobin over time related to mortality and morbidity in patients with chronic heart failure: Results from Val-HeFT. Circulation 2005; 112:1121–1127.
138. Wu WC, Rathore SS, Wang Y, Radford MJ, Krumholz HM. Blood transfusion in elderly patients with acute myocardial infarction. N Engl J Med 2001; 345:1230–1236.
139. Foley RN, Parfrey PS, Harnett JD, et al. Clinical and echocardiographic disease n patients starting end-stage renal disease therapy. Kidney Int 1995; 47:186–192.
140. Levin A, Thompson CR, Ethier J, et al. Left ventricular mass index increases in early renal disease: Impact of decline in hemoglobin. Am J Kidney Disease 1999; 34:125–134.
141. Tamara B, Horwich, Gregg C, et al. Anemia is associated with worse symptoms, greater impairment in functional capacity and a significant increase in mortality in patients with advanced heart failure. J Am Coll Cardiol 2002; 39:1780–1786.
142. Hillman RS. Anemia. In: Fauci AS, Braunwald E, Isselbacher KJ, et al, eds. Harrison's Prinicples of Internal Medicine. New York, NY: McGraw-Hill; 1998:334–339
143. Hsu CJ, McCulloch CE, Curhan GC. Epidemiology of anemia associated with chronic renal insufficiency among adults in the United States: Results from the Third National Health and Nutrition Examination Survey. J Am Soc Nephrol 2002; 13:504–510.
144. National Kidney Foundation. K/DOQI clinical practice guidelines for anemia of chronic kidney disease, 2000. Am J Kidney Dis 2001; 37(suppl 1):S182–S238.
145. McClellan W, Aronoff SL, Bolton WD, et al. The prevalence of anemia in patients with chronic kidney disease, CURRENT MEDICAL RESEARCH AND OPINION 2004; 20(9):1501–1510.
146. Obrador GT, Roberts, T, St. Peter WL, et al. Trends in anemia at initiation of dialysis in the United States. Kidney Int 2001; 60:1875–1884.
147. Schwartz AB, Prasad V, Garcha J. Anemia of chronic kidney disease: a combined effect of marginal iron stores and erythropoietin deficiency. Dialysis Transplant 2004; 33:758–767.
148. United states Renal Data System. 2004 Annual Data Report Atlas of End-Stage Renal Disease in the United States. Bethesda: Md, 2004. Available at: http://www.usrds.org.
149. Rao M, Pereira BJG. Optimal anemia management reduces cardiovascular morbidity, mortality, and costs in chronic kidney disease, Kidney International 2005; 68:1432–1438.
150. Silverberg D. Outcomes of anaemia management in renal insufficiency and cardiac disease. Nephrol Dial Transplant 2003; 18(Suppl 2):ii7–ii12.
151. van der Meer P, Voors AA, Lipsic E, van Gilst WH, van Veldhuisen DJ. Erythropoietin in cardiovascualr diseases, European Heart Journal 2004; 25:285–291.

152. Silverberg D, Wexler D, Blum M, Wollman Y, Iaina A. The cardio–renal anaemia syndrome: does it exist? Nephrol. Dial. Transplant 18(Suppl 8):viii 7-viii12.

153. Haller H, Christel C, Dannenberg L, Thiele P, Lindschau C, Luft FC. Signal transduction of erythropoietin in endothelial cells. Kidney Int 1996; 50:481–488.

154. Chong ZZ, Kang JQ, Maiese K. Erythropoietin is a novel vascular protectant through activation of Akt1 and mitochondrial modulation of cysteine proteases. Circulation 2002; 106:2973–2979.

155. Wright GL, Hanlon P, Amin K, Steenbergen C, Murphy E, Arcasoy MO. Erythropoietin receptor expression in adult rat cardiomyocytes is associated with an acute cardioprotective effect for recombinant erythropoietin during ischemia-reperfusion injury. FASEB J 2004; 18:1031–1033.

156. Grasso G, Sfacteria A, Cerami A, Brines M. Erythropoietin as a tissue-protective cytokine in brain injury: What do we know and where do we go? Neuroscientist 2004; 10:93–98.

157. van der Meer P, Lipsic E, Henning RH, et al. Erythropoietin induces neovascularization and improves cardiac function in rats with heart failure after myocardial infarction. J Am Coll Cardiol 2005; 46:125–133.

158. Parsa CJ, Matsumoto A, Kim J, et al. A novel protective effect of erythropoietin in the infracted heart. J Clin Invest 2003; 112:999–1007.

159. Lipsic E, van der Meer P, Henning RH, et al. Timing of erythropoietin treatment for cardioprotection in ischemia/reperfusion. J Cardiovasc Pharmacol 2004; 44:473–479.

160. van der Meer P, Lipsic E, Henning RH, et al. Erythropoietin improves left ventricular function and coronary flow in an experimental model of ischemia-reperfusion injury. Eur J Heart Fail 2004; 6:853–859.

161. Dikow R, Kihm LP, Zeier M, et al. Increased infarct size in uremic rats: Reduced ischemia tolerance? J Am Soc Nephrol 2004; 15:1530–1536.

162. Ritz E. Heart Failure after Myocardial Infarction-Benefit beyond Hemoglobin from Erythropoetin, J Am Soc Nephrol 2005; 16:3449–3454.

163. Rao M, Pereira B. Prospective trials on anemia of chronic disease: The Trial to Reduce Cardiovascular Events with Aranesp Therapy (TREAT). Kidney Int 2003; (Suppl 87):S12–S19.

164. Laville M. New strategies in anaemia management: ACORD (Anaemia CORrection in Diabetes) trial. Acta Diabetol 2004; 41:S18–S22.

165. Besarab A, Levin A. Defining a renal anemia management period. Am J Kidney Dis 2000; 36 (Suppl 3):S13–S23.

166. Ibels LS, Stewart JH, Mahony JF, et al. Occlusive arterial disease in uraemic and haemodialysis patients and renal transplant recipients. A study of the incidence of arterial disease and of the prevalence of risk factors implicated in the pathogenesis of arteriosclerosis. Q J Med 1977; 46:197–214.

167. Davies MR, Hruska KA. Pathophysiological mechanisms of vascular calcification in end-stage renal disease. Kidney Int 2001; 60:472–479.

168. Salusky IB, Goodman WG. Cardiovascular calcification in end-stage renal disease. Nephrol Dial Transplant 2002; 17:336–339.

169. Goodman WG, Goldin J, Kuizon BD, et al. Coronary-artery calcification in young adults with end-stage renal disease who are undergoing dialysis. N Engl J Med 2000; 342:1478–1483.

170. London GM, Guerin AP, Marchais SJ, Metivier F, Pannier B, Adda H. Arterial media calcification in end-stage renal diseases: Impact on all-cause and cardiovascular mortality. Nephrol Dial Transplant 2003; 18:1731–1740.

171. Raggi P, Boulay A, Chasan-Taber S, et al. Cardiac calcification in adult hemodialysis patients. A link between end-stage renal disease and cardiovascular disease? J Am Coll Cardiol 2002; 39:695–701.

172. Block GA, Port FK. Re-evaluation of risks associated with hyperphosphatemia and hyperparathyroidism in dialysis patients: Recommendations for a change in management. Am J Kidney Dis 2000; 35:1226–1237.

173. Ganesh SK, Stack AG, Levin NW, Hulbert-Shearon T, Port FK. Association of elevated serum PO4, Ca X PO4 product, and parathyroid hormone with cardiac mortality risk inchronic hemodialysis patients. J Am Soc Nephrol 2001; 12:2131–2138.

174. Davies MR, Lund RJ, Mathew S, Hruska KA. Low Turnover Osteodystrophy and Vascular Calcification Are Amenable to Skeletal Anabolism in an Animal Model of Chronic Kidney Disease and the Metabolic Syndrome. J Am Soc Nephrol 2005; 16:917–928.

175. Llach F, Bover J. Renal osteodystrophies. In: Brenner BM, eds. The Kidney. Philadelphia: W.B. Saunders, 2000:2103–2186

176. Gonzalez EA, Lund RJ, Martin KJ, et al. Treatment of a murine model of high-turnover renal osteodystrophy by exogenous BMP-7. Kidney Int 2002; 61:1322–1331.

177. Lund RJ, Davies MR, Brown AJ, Hruska KA. Successful ctreatment of an adynamic bone disorder with bone morphogenetic protein-7 in a renal ablation model. J Am Soc Nephrol 2004; 15:359–369.

178. Davies MR, Lund RJ, Hruska KA. BMP-7 is an efficacious treatment of vascular calcification in a murine model of atherosclerosis and chronic renal failure. J Am Soc Nephrol 2003; 14:1559–1567.

179. Schulz E, Kiumars A, Liu X, Sayre J, Gilsanz V. Aortic Calcification and the Risk of Osteoporosis and Fractures. J Clin Endocrinol Metab 2004; 89:4246–4253.

180. Rix M, Andreassen H, Eskildsen P, Langdahl B, and Olgaard K, Bone mineral density and biochemical markers of bone turnover in patients with predialysis chronic renal failure. Kidney Int 1999; 56:1084–1093.
181. Taal MW, Roe S, Masud T, Green D, Porter C, Cassidy MJD. Total hip bone mass predicts survival in chronic hemodialysis patients. Kidney Int 2003; 63:1116–1120
182. Li YC, Kong J, Wei M, et al. 1,25-Dihydroxyvitamin D3 is a negative endocrine regulator of the renin-angiotensin system. J Clin Invest 2002 110:229–238.
183. Weishaar RE, Simpson RU. the involvement of the endocrine system I regulating cardiovascular function: Emphasis on vitamin D_3. Endocrine Rev 1989; 10:351–365.
184. Andress D. Vitamin D in chronic kidney disease: A systemic role for selective vitamin D receptor activation. Kidney Int 2006; 69(1):33–43.
185. Watson KE, Abrolat ML, Malone LL, et al. Active Serum Vitamin D Levels Are Inversely Correlated with Coronary Calcification. Circulation 1997; 96:1755–1760.
186. Timms PM, Mannan N, Hitman GA, et al. Circulating MMP9, vitamin D and variation in the TIMP-1 response with VDR genotype: mechanisms for inflammatory damage in chronic disorders? Q J Medicine 2002; 95:787–796.
187. Zimmerman A, Schulze Schleithoff S, Tenderich G, Berthold HK, Korfer R, Stehle P. Low vitamin D status: a contributing factor in the pathogenesis of congestive heart failure? J Am Coll Cardiol 2003; 41:105–112.
188. Mathieu C, Adorini L. The coming of age of 1,25-dihydroxyvitamin D_3 analogs as immunomodulatory agents. Trends Mol Med 2002; 8:174–179.
189. Park CW, Oh YS, Shin YS, et al. Intravenous calcitriol regresses myocardial hypertrophy in hemodialysis patients with secondary hyperparathyroidism. Am J Kidney Dis 1999; 33:73–81.
190. Thomas MK, Lloyd-Jones DM, Thadhani RI, et al. Hypovitaminosis D in Medical Inpatients. NEJM 1998; 338(12):777–783.
191. Gonzalez EA, Sachdeva A, Oliver DA, Martin KJ. Vitamin D insufficiency and deficiency in chronic kidney disease. A single center observational study. J Am Soc Nephrol 2004; 24(5):503–510.
192. Bakris GL, Levin A, Molitch M, et al. Disturbances of 1,25 Dihydroxyvitamin D3 (1,25 D) in Patients with Chronic Kidney Disease. J Am Soc Nephrol 2005; 16:495a, abstract F-P0732.
194. National Kidney Foundation. K/KOQI clinical practice guidelines for bone metabolism and disease in chronic kidney disease. AM J Kidney Dis 2003; 42(suppl 3):S1–S201.
195. Jono S, McKee MD, Murry CE, et al. Phosphate regulation of vascular smooth muscle cell calcification. Circ Res 2000; 87:e10–e17.
196. Chertow GM, Burke SK, Raggi P. For the Treat to Goal Working Group: Sevelamer attenuates the progression of coronary and aortic calcification in hemodialysis patients. Kidney Int 2002; 62:245–252.
197. Qunibi WY, Reducing the Burden of Cardiovascular Calcification in Patients with Chronic Kidney Disease. J Am Soc Nephrol 2005; 16:S95–S102.
198. Budoff MJ, Lane KL, Bakhsheshi H, et al. Rates of progression of coronary calcium by electron beam tomography. Am J Cardiol 2000; 86:8–11.
199. Callister TQ, Raggi P, Cooil B, Lippolis NJ, Russo DJ. Effect of HMG-CoA reductase inhibitors on coronary artery disease as assessed by electron-beam computed tomography. N Engl J Med 1998; 339:1972–1978.
200. Achenbach S, Ropers D, Pohle K, et al. Influence of lipid-lowering therapy on the progression of coronary artery calcification: A prospective evaluation. Circulation 2002; 106:1077–1082.
201. Nitta K, Akiba T, Nihei H. Colestimide co-administered with atorvastatin attenuates the progression of vascular calcification in hemodialysis patients. Nephrol Dial Transplant 2004; 19:2156.
202. Nitta K, Akiba T, Nihei H. Colestimide co-administered with atorvastatin attenuates the progression of vascular calcification in hemodialysis patients. Nephrol Dial Transplant 2004; 19:2156.
203. Merke J, Hofmann W, Goldschmidt D, Ritz E. Demonstration of 1,25(OH)2 vitamin D_3 receptors and actions in vascular smooth muscle cells in vitro. Calcif Tissue Int 1987; 41:112–114.
204. Jono S, Nishizawa Y, Shioi A, Morii H. 1,25-dihydroxyvitamin D_3 increases in vitro vascular calcification by modulating secretion of endogenous parathyroid hormone-related peptide. Circulation 1998; 98:1302–1306.
205. Teng M, Wolf M, Lowrie E, Ofsthun N, Lazarus JM, Thadhani R. Survival of Patients Undergoing Hemodialysis with Paricalcitol or Calcitriol Therapy. N Engl J Med 2003; 349:446–456.
206. Teng M, Wolf M, Ofsthun N, et al. Activated Injectable Vitamin D and Hemodialysis Survival: A Historical Cohort Study. J Am Soc Nephrol 2005; 16:1115–1125.
207. Edward M, Brown, Gerardo Gamba, et al. Cloning and characterization of an extracellular Ca2+- sensing receptor from bovine parathyroid. Nature 1993; 366:575–580.
208. Block GA, Martin KJ, de Francisco AL, et al. Cinacalcet for secondary hyperparathyroidism in patients receiving hemodialysis. N Engl J Med 2004; 350:1516–1525.
209. Shalhoub V, Shatzan E, Lacey D, Martin D. Calcification of bovine vascular smooth muscle cells in vitro by calcitriol and paricalcitol but not the calcimimetic. J Am Soc Nephrol 2004; 15:281A.
210. Henley C, Colloton M, Cattley R, et al. 1,25-Dihydroxyvitamin D_3 but not cinacalcet HCl (Sensipar/Mimpara) mediates aortic mineralization in a rat model of secondary hyperparathyroidism. Nephrol Dial Transplant 2005; 20:1370–1377.

211. Rodriguez M, Mendoza FC, Aguilera-Tejero E, et al. The calcimimetic NPS R-568 decreases vascular calcification in uremic rats treated with calcitriol. J Am Soc Nephrol 2004; 15:279A.

212. Lewis EJ, Hunsicker LG, Bain RP, Rohde RD. The effect of angiotensin-converting-enzyme inhibition on diabetic nephropathy. The Collaborative Study Group. N Engl J Med 1993; 329:1456–1462.

213. Brenner BM, Cooper ME, de Zeeuw D, et al. Effects of losartan on renal and cardiovascular outcomes in patients with type 2 diabetes and nephropathy. N Engl J Med 2001; 345:861–869.

214. Lewis EJ, Hunsicker LG, Clarke WR, et al. Renoprotective effect of the angiotensin-receptor antagonist irbesartan in patients with nephropathy due to type 2 diabetes. N Engl J Med 2001; 345:851–860.

215. The SOLVD investigators. Effect of enalapril on mortality and the development of heart failure in asymptomatic patients with reduced left ventricular efection fractions. N Engl J Med 1992; 327:685.

216. Jong P, Yusuf S, Rousseau MF, et al. Effect of enalapril on 12-year survival and life expectancy in patients with left ventricular systolic dysfunction:a follow-up study. Lancet 2003; 361:1843.

217. Kleber FX, Niemoller L, Doering W. Impact of converting enzyme inhibition on progression of chronic heart failure: Results of the Munich Mild Heart Failure Trial. Br Heart J 1992; 67:289.

218. Berl T, Hunsicker LG, Lewis JB, et al. Cardiovascular outcomes in the Irbesartan Diabetic Nephropathy Trial of patients with type 2 diabetes and overt nephropathy. Ann Intern Med 2003; 138:542–549.

219. Bakris GL, Weir MR. Angiotensin-converting enzyme inhibitor-associated elevations in serum creatinine: is this a cause for concern? Arch Intern Med 2000; 160(5):685–693.

220. Bakris GL, Siomos M, Richardson D, et al. ACE inhibition or angiotensin receptor blockade: impact on potassium in renal failure. Kidney Int 2000; 58(5):2084–2092.

221. Pitt B, Poole-Wilson PA, Segal R, et al. Effect of losartan compared with captopril on mortality in patients with symptomatic heart failure: randomised trial—the Losartan Heart Failure Survival Study ELITE II. Lancet 2000; 355(9215):1582–1587.

222. Maggioni AP, Anand I, Gottlieb SO, Latini R, Tognoni G, Cohn JN. Effects of valsartan on morbidity and mortality in patients with heart failure not receiving angiotensin-converting enzyme inhibitors. J Am Coll Cardiol 2002; 40(8):1414–1421.

223. Granger CB, McMurray JJ, Yusuf S, et al. Effects of candesartan in patients with chronic heart failure and reduced left-ventricular systolic function intolerant to angiotensin-converting-enzyme inhibitors: the CHARM-Alternative trial. Lancet 2003; 362(9386):772–776.

224. Ruggenenti P, Perna A, Remuzzi G, et al. ACE inhibitors to prevent end-stage renal disease: when to start and why possibly never to stop: a post hoc analysis of the REIN trial results. J Am Soc Nephrol 2001; 12:2832–2837.

225. United States Renal Data System. USRDS 1999 annual data report. Bethesda: Md. National Institute of Diabetes and Digestive and Kidney Diseases, 1999. (Also available at http://www.usrds.org/adr_1999.htm.)

226. Beattie JN, Soman SS, Sandberg KR, Yee J, Borzak S, Garg M, et al. Determinants of mortality after myocardial infarction in patients with advanced renal dysfunction. Am J Kidney Dis. 2001; 37:1191–1200.

227. Medication use among dialysis patients in the DMMS. In: U.S. Renal Data System 1998 Annual Report. Bethesda, MD: National Institute of Diabetes and Digestive and Kidney Diseases; 1998:51–60.

228. Manjunath G, Tighiouart H, Ibrahim H, et al. Level of kidney function as a risk factor for atherosclerotic cardiovascular outcomes in the community. J Am Coll Cardiol 2003; 41:47–55.

229. Al-Ahmad A, Rand WM, Manjunath G, et al. Reduced kidney function and anemia as risk factors for mortality in patients with left ventricular dysfunction. J Am Coll Cardiol 2001; 38:955–962.

230. Shlipak MG, Heidenreich PA, Noguchi H, Chertow GM, Browner WS, McClennan MD. Association of renal insufficiency with treatment and outcomes after myocardial infarction in elderly patients. Ann Intern Med 2002; 137:555–562.

231. Walsh CR, O'Donnell CJ, Camargo CA Jr., Giugliano RP, Lloyd-Jones DM. Elevated serum creatinine is associated with 1-year mortality after acute myocardial infarction. Am Heart J 2002; 144:1003–1011.

232. McCullough PA, Sandberg KR, Borzak S, Hudson MP, Garg M, Manley HJ. Benefits of aspirin and beta-blockade after myocardial infarction in patients with chronic kidney disease. Am Heart J 2002; 144:226–232.

233. Berger AK, Duval S, Krumholz HM. Aspirin, beta-blocker, and angiotensin-converting enzyme inhibitor therapy in patients with end-stage renal disease and an acute myocardial infarction. J Am Coll Cardiol 2003; 42:201–208.

234. McCullough PA, Wolyn R, Rocher LL, Levin RN, O'Neill WW. Acute renal failure after coronary intervention: incidence, risk factors, and relationship to mortality. Am J Med 1997; 103:368–375.

235. Tonelli M, Moyé L, Sacks FM, et al. Effect of pravastatin on loss of renal function in people with moderate chronic renal insufficiency and cardiovascular disease. J Am Soc Nephrol 2003; 14:1605–1613.

236. Holdaas H, Fellstrom B, Jardine AG, et al. Effect of fluvastatin on cardiac outcomes in renal transplant recipients: a multicentre, randomized, placebo-controlled trial. Lancet 2003; 361:2024–2031.

237. Keeley EC, Kadakia R, Soman S, Borzak S, McCullough PA. Analysis of long-term survival after revascularization in patients with chronic kidney disease presenting with acute coronary syndromes. Am J Cardiol 2003; 92:509–514.

14 | Anticoagulation and Antiplatelet Agents

Adnan K. Chhatriwalla and Deepak L. Bhatt
Department of Cardiovascular Medicine, Cleveland Clinic, Cleveland, Ohio, U.S.A.

KEY POINTS

Pathogenesis of Thrombosis

The clotting process occurs in four phases:

- Formation of the platelet plug
- Thrombus propagation by the coagulation cascade
- Termination
- Fibrinolysis

Acute Coronary Syndrome

- Rupture of an atherosclerotic plaque is generally the inciting event in acute coronary syndrome (ACS)
- Aspirin should be given in an initial loading dose to all ACS patients and continued indefinitely unless there is a contraindication
- IV unfractionated heparin or subcutaneous low molecular weight heparin should be administered in addition to antiplatelet therapy in ACS
- In high-risk ACS patients, the use of GP IIb/IIIa inhibitor therapy should be considered
- The addition of clopidogrel to aspirin therapy in ACS reduces the risk of adverse cardiovascular outcomes in patients with ACS

Percutaneous Coronary Intervention (PCI)

- High doses of aspirin have not shown increased efficacy when compared to standard doses.
- Routine heparin has fallen out of use after PCI due to lack of efficacy.
- Warfarin therapy in combination with aspirin results in slightly lower risk of cardiovascular events; however, this is outweighed by increased hemorrhagic complications.
- Pretreatment with clopidogrel 300 to 600 mg as little as two hours prior to PCI improves short-term and long-term outcomes.
- GP IIb/IIIa inhibitor use results in reduced 30 day and six-month mortality.
- Evidence suggests that bivalirudin therapy is equivalent to heparin + GP IIb/IIIa inhibitor use during PCI with less bleeding complications.

Primary and Secondary Prevention of Myocardial Infarction

- Aspirin use reduces the risk of a first myocardial infarction by about one-third.
- Risk–benefit outcomes may vary when applied to different populations.
- High-dose aspirin therapy has not been shown to offer additional benefit when compared to standard-dose aspirin therapy for the secondary prevention of MI.
- Aspirin resistance has been reported from 5.5% to 56.8% in various studies.
- Clopidogrel therapy in combination with aspirin is being evaluated in secondary prevention and high-risk primary prevention of cardiovascular events.
- Preliminary data demonstrate a benefit to ximelagatran therapy for the secondary prevention of cardiovascular events.

Atrial Fibrillation and Atrial Flutter

- Antithrombotic strategies for atrial fibrillation and atrial flutter are identical.
- Adjusted-dose warfarin therapy has demonstrated significant benefit in the primary prevention of stroke in the setting of atrial fibrillation.
- Aspirin therapy is somewhat less effective than warfarin for stroke prevention.

- Ximelagatran therapy has been demonstrated to be as effective as warfarin therapy in the primary prevention of stroke.
- Advanced age, prior stroke, or TIA, hypertension, and diabetes are independent risk factors for stroke in the setting of atrial fibrillation.
- Warfarin therapy is recommended for the primary prevention of stroke in high-risk patients with atrial fibrillation.
- Warfarin or full-dose aspirin therapy are acceptable for the primary prevention of stroke in moderate-risk patients with atrial fibrillation.
- Full-dose aspirin therapy is recommended for the primary prevention of stroke in low-risk patients with atrial fibrillation.

Dilated Cardiomyopathy

- Some evidence points to a benefit of aspirin therapy for the prevention of cardiovascular events in patients with CHF.
- No reduction in thromboembolic events has been observed with the routine use of warfarin anticoagulation in patients with CHF.
- Further data are necessary to determine the benefit of antithrombotic strategies in patients with nonischemic CHF.

Deep Venous Thrombosis and Pulmonary Embolism

- Weight-based dosing of UFH is effective in the prevention of recurrent thromboembolism.
- Low molecular weight heparin administration is at least as effective as UFH in the prevention of recurrent thromboembolism, and may be more cost-effective.
- Preliminary data suggest that ximelagatran therapy is noninferior to low molecular weight heparin and warfarin combination therapy in the prevention of recurrent thromboembolism.
- The length of treatment for DVT/PE is determined by the risk-factor profile of the patient.
  - Three months duration for a first episode associated with a reversible cause
  - Six to 12 months duration for an idiopathic first episode
  - Lifelong therapy for patients with a hypercoagulable state or recurrent episodes of DVT/PE
- Anticoagulant-based prophylaxis for DVT is more effective that aspirin alone.
- Preliminary data suggest that Ximelagatran therapy is equivalent to warfarin or LMWH for DVT prophylaxis.

Peripheral Vascular Disease

- Aspirin therapy has been shown to decrease cardiovascular events in patients with PAD; however, its benefit on PAD itself is unclear.
- Clopidogrel is somewhat more effective than aspirin in decreasing cardiovascular events in patients with PAD.
- Conflicting data exist regarding the benefits of pentoxifylline in the symptomatic treatment of PAD.
- Cilostazol is superior to pentoxifylline in the symptomatic treatment of PAD.

OVERVIEW

Antithrombotic therapy is a mainstay in treatment of many cardiovascular disorders, and the evolution of cardiovascular care has in many ways been accelerated by novel antithrombotic regimens. In this chapter, we will begin by describing the pathogenesis of thrombosis and thrombolysis, and proceed to a discussion of the issues pertinent to antithrombotic therapy in various cardiovascular states. We will address preventive strategies as well as acute management of cardiovascular complications, and we will finish by discussing the future direction of antithrombotic therapy in the management of cardiovascular disease.

PATHOGENESIS OF THROMBOSIS

The clotting process is a dynamic interrelation of multiple processes, which can be viewed as occurring in four phases: initiation and formation of the platelet plug, thrombus propagation by the coagulation cascade, termination by antithrombotic control mechanisms, and removal of the thrombus by fibrinolysis. Initial platelet activation at the site of vascular injury results from a number of physiologic stimuli, including potent stimuli such as collagen and thrombin and weaker stimuli such as adenosine diphosphate (ADP) and epinephrine (Fig. 1). The response of activated platelets to vascular injury involves four processes: adhesion, aggregation, degranulation, and procoagulant activity. Platelet adhesion is mediated by the formation of pseudopods during platelet activation and the binding of von Willebrand factor (VWF) in the subendothelial matrix to platelet surface receptors. Platelet aggregation occurs in conjunction with conformational changes in glycoprotein (GP) IIb/IIIa, the most abundant receptor on platelet surfaces. During platelet activation, GP IIb/IIIa is converted from a low-affinity to a high-affinity fibrinogen receptor, allowing fibrinogen to serve as a bridge for aggregation of activated platelets. Platelet degranulation during activation results in the secretion of a variety of substances, including the following:

- Fibrinogen, which participates in platelet aggregation and thrombus propagation by the coagulation cascade
- ADP and thromboxane A_2 (TXA_2), which stimulate platelet activation and aggregation
- Fibronectin and thrombospondin, which may stabilize platelet aggregates
- Growth factors, which mediate tissue repair

Platelet procoagulant activity involves the exposure of phospholipids on the platelet surface, integral for formation of enzyme complexes in the coagulation cascade. Thrombus propagation through the coagulation cascade involves the sequential activation of a series of proenzymes and inactive precursor proteins in stepwise fashion, resulting in significant signal amplification (Fig. 2). The extrinsic pathway is activated in the presence of tissue factor (TF) and thromboplastin, exposed after endothelial damage. The intrinsic pathway is activated by contact with negatively charged surfaces. The common end point of both pathways involves the activation of prothrombin to thrombin, an enzyme that converts plasma-soluble fibrinogen to fibrin, an insoluble protein that polymerizes as a component in the forming thrombus. The formation of the prothrombinase complex, i.e., Factor Xa, Factor Va, calcium, phospholipid, and Factor II (prothrombin) is approximately 300,000 times more efficient in thrombin generation than factor Xa and prothrombin alone, with the net result that thrombin generation and fibrin deposition is localized to activated platelets at sites of vascular injury (1).

Termination of the coagulation cascade is mediated by a variety of factors, most notably through antithrombin (AT) (previously antithrombin III), Proteins C and S, and tissue factor

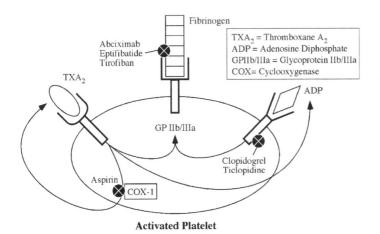

FIGURE 1 Binding of TXA_2 to its receptor results in platelet degranulation and release of ADP and TXA_2. Platelet activation by ADP and TXA_2 results in subsequent expression of the GP IIb/IIIa receptor. *Abbreviations*: TXA_2 thromboxane A2; ADP, adenosine diphosphate; GP IIb/IIIa, glycoprotein IIb/IIIa; COX, cyclooxegenase.

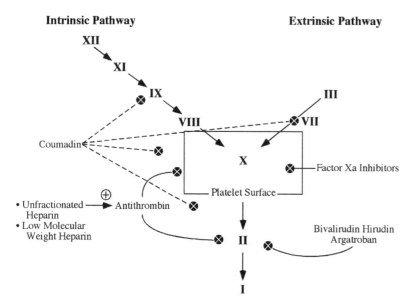

FIGURE 2   Coumadin inhibits the synthesis of Factors II, VII, IX, and X. Unfractionated heparin and low molecular weight heparin differ in their relative inhibition of Factors II and X. Factor II: thrombin; Factor I: fibrin.

pathway inhibitor (TFPI). AT is a circulating plasma protease inhibitor that neutralizes thrombin and Factors Xa, IXa, XIa and XIIa. The binding of heparin to AT accelerates its activity up to 4000-fold (2). Activated protein C (APC), in combination with protein S, inactivates Factors Va and VIIIa. TFPI, present in low concentrations in circulating plasma, directly inhibits Factor Xa and, in complex with Factor Xa, inhibits TF/Factor VIIa and the activation of the extrinsic pathway.

Thrombolysis refers to the process by which thrombus is organized and removed to restore vessel patency following the activation of the coagulation cascade. This is accomplished through the action of plasmin, an enzyme with broad activity, activated from the proenzyme plasminogen. Tissue-type plasminogen activator (tPA) and urokinase are the two physiologic plasminogen activators. tPA is the major activator for intravascular thrombolysis and its activity is increased several hundred-fold in the presence of thrombin (3). Urokinase is largely responsible for thrombolysis in the extravascular compartment.

■ Case 1

A 56-year-old male with hypertension and hyperlipidemia presents to the emergency room with substernal chest pressure worsened by exertion, mild shortness of breath, and diaphoresis. The patient's chest radiograph is unremarkable and electrocardiogram is within normal limits. The patient's symptoms respond to sublingual nitroglycerin administration and he is placed on cardiac monitor in the chest pain unit. Initial blood work reveals elevations in the cardiac troponin and creatine kinase levels.

● *Question 1: What are the data for the benefit of aspirin and heparin therapy in acute coronary syndrome (ACS)?*
● *Question 2: Which patients may benefit from addition of clopidogrel and GP IIb/IIIa inhibitor therapy?*

ACUTE CORONARY SYNDROME

Rupture of an atherosclerotic plaque is generally the inciting event in ACS. Both superficial and deep intimal injury result in exposure of collagen, VWF and TF, leading to platelet activation and stimulation of the coagulation cascade as described in the previous section. Aggregating platelets form the core of the growing thrombus, with upstream and/or downstream clot propagation secondary to fibrin deposition. Although this process can be viewed as "physiological" and ultimately contributing to repair of the injured vessel, the formation of intraluminal thrombosis and vascular occlusion may result in myocardial ischemia or infarction. Antiplatelet and anticoagulation agents in this setting have been extensively studied and shown to be of clinical benefit, and the use of these agents has substantially contributed to the decrease in morbidity and mortality associated with ACS over the past two decades.

Aspirin

Aspirin (acetylsalicylic acid, ASA) irreversibly inhibits cyclooxygenase-1 in platelets and megakaryo-cytes and blocks the formation of TXA_2 via arachidonic acid metabolism. Aspirin thereby inhibits platelet aggregability for the life of the platelet (7–10 days). Aspirin is an effective antithrombotic agent over a wide dosing range and in fact, there has been much debate as to the ideal dose of aspirin in treatment and prevention of cardiovascular events. Aspirin has been postulated to have additional benefits in the prevention of cardiovascular disease, including an anti-inflammatory effect and an antiatherogenic effect (4–6); however, these have been difficult to prove in the clinical setting. Aspirin use is associated with an increased risk of nonfatal extracranial hemorrhage which corresponds to an absolute risk of approximately one to two patients per 1000 treated patients per year, and an increased risk of intracranial hemorrhage of approximately one patient per 1000 treated patients over three years (7). Dose-dependent gastrointestinal (GI) side effects include nausea, heartburn, and GI bleeding secondary to impairment of prostaglandin-mediated cytoprotection in the GI mucosa. The increased risk of GI bleeding seems largely due to platelet inactivation in as much as similar increases in GI bleeding have been seen with the use of other antiplatelet agents, which do not inhibit prostaglandin production.

A number of randomized clinical trials have established the efficacy of aspirin in patients with ACS, which encompasses unstable angina (USA) and non-ST elevation myocardial infarction (NSTEMI). Aspirin administration resulted in a 71% reduction in mortality and a 51% reduction in the combined end point of death and nonfatal myocardial infarction (MI) compared to placebo administration in the Canadian Multicenter Trial (8). In the RISC trial, low-dose aspirin administration (75 mg) was shown to significantly reduce the combined end point of death and acute MI when compared to intravenous (IV) heparin and placebo at 5, 30, 90 days, and one year follow-up (9). The 2002 American College of Cardiology/American Heart Association (ACC/AHA) guidelines for management of USA or NSTEMI indicate the prompt initiation of antiplatelet therapy with aspirin as a Class I recommendation (level of evidence A) (10). Based upon these recommendations, aspirin should be given in an initial loading dose of 162.5 to 325 mg to all patients with ACS unless there is a contraindication. Patients are often directed to chew or crush tablets to achieve a more rapid antithrombotic effect. Aspirin administration should then be continued indefinitely at a daily dose of 75 to 325 mg daily. Given the increased risk of hemorrhage at higher aspirin doses (1), there has been much debate about the optimal dosing of aspirin to achieve the antithrombotic benefits with a minimal risk of side effects. We will further discuss this topic later in this chapter.

Indirect Thrombin Inhibitors

Heparin is an indirect thrombin inhibitor, which acts by binding to the heparin-binding site on AT to increase its activity 4000-fold (2). Heparin is an effective antithrombotic agent for a number of indications. The adverse effects of heparin include an increased risk of hemorrhage and heparin-induced thrombocytopenia (HIT). The risk of hemorrhage with heparin use has been reported as high as 10%; however the risk of major bleeding is approximately 2%, similar to other antithrombotic agents (11). HIT occurs in approximately 1% of patients treated for three days, and 5% to 10% of patients treated for five or more days; however, the incidence is less with low-molecular-weight heparin (LMWH) use (12).

The efficacy of unfractionated heparin (UFH) in ACS has been established by a number of randomized clinical trials. The heparin-atenolol trial was the first to show a statistically significant reduction in the incidence of transmural MI in patients receiving heparin therapy (2% vs. 17% for placebo) (13). The rationale for combination therapy with aspirin in ACS centers around the fact that these two agents inhibit thrombus formation at different points in the coagulation pathway. Initial trials evaluating the addition of heparin to aspirin therapy in ACS were underpowered. In the heparin-aspirin trial, the incidence of MI was reduced (0.8% vs. 3.3% with aspirin alone) but no mortality benefit was observed (11). In the RISC trial, although the group of patients receiving heparin and aspirin therapy had the lowest incidence of events, the risk reduction was not significant (9). Further studies showed that heparin administration by continuous infusion rather than intermittent bolus (as in the RISC trial) led to improved outcomes (14). A meta-analysis of six early small trials established the efficacy of heparin in addition to aspirin in ACS, revealing an odds ratio of 0.67 for death or acute MI during combined therapy (15).

A number of studies using LMWH in ACS have been performed; however, only enoxaparin (administered 1 mg/kg subcutaneously every 12 hours) has consistently been shown to improve outcomes in ACS in comparison to UFH. The advantage of LMWH compared to UFH is the use of a weight-adjusted dosing regimen that allows for clinical use without monitoring of the anticoagulant effect. In the ESSENCE trial, combination therapy with enoxaparin plus aspirin was superior to the combination of UFH and aspirin in 3171 patients with ACS with respect to the combined end point of death, MI and recurrent angina (19.8% vs. 23.3%) (16). A reduction was also seen in the rate of repeat revascularization at one year (32% vs. 36%) (17) and the risks of major bleeding and thrombocytopenia were similar in the two groups (18). Further cost–benefit analysis showed that therapy with enoxaparin resulted in an in-hospital cost savings of US $763 per patient compared with UFH, and a savings of US $1172 per patient at one year (19). Enoxaparin was further shown to be superior to UFH in the combined end point of death, MI and urgent revascularization (12.4% vs. 14.5%) in the Thrombolysis in myocardial infarction 11B (TIMI IIB) trial (20). There has been concern regarding the use of LMWH in patients with ACS scheduled for cardiac catheterization, because of inability to monitor or fully reverse the anticoagulation effect. In the Superior SYNERGY Yield of the New strategy of Enoxaparin, Revascularization and Glycoprotein IIb/IIIa inhibitors trial, the use of enoxaparin was evaluated in patients with planned cardiac catheterization and coronary intervention. In comparison to UFH, patients treated with enoxaparin had no significant difference in stent thrombosis (1.3% vs. 1.7%), unsuccessful coronary intervention (3.6% vs. 3.4%) or emergency coronary artery bypass graft surgery (CABG) (0.3% vs. 0.3%) and no difference was observed in the primary end point of death or nonfatal MI at 30 days (14.0% vs. 14.5%) (21). A small but significant increase in major bleeding was noted (9.1% vs. 7.6%), but there was no difference in the need for blood transfusion between groups.

The 2002 ACC/AHA guidelines for management of USA or NSTEMI list anticoagulation with subcutaneous LMWH or IV UFH in addition to antiplatelet therapy as a Class I recommendation (level of evidence A) (10). This should be continued for at least 48 hours, or until cardiac catheterization and percutaneous coronary intervention (PCI) if an early interventional approach is planned.

Glycoprotein IIb/IIIa Receptor Antagonists

GP IIb/IIIa receptor antagonists block the final common pathway for platelet aggregation through crosslinking with fibrinogen (22). Abciximab is the Fab fragment of the chimeric humanized mouse monoclonal antibody 7E3, with a high affinity for the GP IIb/IIIa receptor. Tirofiban and eptifibatide are molecules that mimic part of the structure of fibrinogen, thus leading to competitive inhibition of binding of fibrinogen to the IIb/IIIa receptor. A variety of other proteins, including fibronectin, VWF and vitronectin, are capable of binding to platelets via the IIb/IIIa receptor; however, fibrinogen dominates due to its high plasma concentration.

Abciximab is an IV agent with an initial half-life of less than 10 minutes and a secondary half-life of 30 minutes, secondary to rapid receptor binding. Abciximab remains in the circulation for up to 10 days; however, platelet function generally recovers clinically 48 hours after cessation of the drug. Administration of abciximab in doses ranging from 0.15 to 0.30 mg/kg produces a rapid inhibition of platelet function, with 80% of platelet IIb/IIIa receptors occupied at the highest dose. Sustained inhibition is attained with prolonged infusions. Patients undergoing coronary intervention are typically treated with a 0.25 mg/kg IV bolus followed by 0.125 mcg/kg/min infusion up to a maximum of 10 mcg/min. In cases where coronary intervention is delayed, the abciximab bolus and infusion may be initiated 18 to 24 hours prior to intervention. The major safety concerns in the use of abciximab involve the risk of thrombocytopenia and excess bleeding. In the EPIC trial, major hemorrhage and transfusion requirement was increased twofold with abciximab administration (23). The bleeding risk was significantly lower in the EPILOG trial, with lower dose heparin use (24). Thrombocytopenia can be observed with abciximab administration, and this effect may be rapid and severe. A pooled analysis of eight placebo-controlled trials revealed an increased incidence of mild (4.2% vs. 2%) and severe (1% vs. 0.4%) thrombocytopenia with abciximab use, and both were more frequent with bolus administration prior to sustained infusion (25). Thrombocytopenia following abciximab therapy may be seen more rapidly than with other forms of drug-induced thrombocytopenia (14–21 days), and has been reported within several hours of use. Pseudothrombocytopenia may also be seen with abciximab use, and in one review accounted for 36% of low platelet counts with abciximab therapy (26). Pseudothrombocytopenia is not associated with adverse outcomes.

Tirofiban is an IV agent with a half-life of approximately two hours. Initial studies performed using tirofiban revealed dose-dependent ex vivo inhibition of platelet aggregation within minutes of IV bolus administration. Continuous infusion results in sustained inhibition of platelet aggregation, with normalization of platelet function four to eight hours following discontinuation. Tirofiban can be administered via a 0.4 mcg/kg/min IV infusion over 30 minutes followed by a 0.1 mcg/kg/min sustained IV infusion in patients with normal renal function. The safety profile of tirofiban is favorable compared to other cardiovascular agents. No significant increase in the risk of thrombocytopenia (1.17% vs. 0.9% for placebo) or major bleeding (5.3% vs. 3.7%) was observed in the RESTORE trial (27), and no increase in thrombocytopenia was observed with tirofiban use in a pooled analysis (25).

Eptifibatide is an IV agent with a plasma half-life of 10 to 15 minutes. A pilot study demonstrated that IV bolus administration resulted in greater than 80% inhibition of platelet aggregation within 15 minutes in greater than 75% of patients (28). This effect was maintained for 24 hours during a continuous IV infusion. Eptifibatide can be administered via a 180 mcg/kg IV bolus followed by a 2 mcg/kg/min IV infusion up to 72 hours in patients with normal renal function. In patients undergoing coronary intervention, a second 180 mcg/kg IV bolus can be given 10 minutes after the first bolus. Eptifibatide has a favorable safety profile compared to other antiplatelet agents. The incidence of major bleeding was only slightly elevated when compared to placebo in the PURSUIT trial (10.6% vs. 9.1%) (29). A pooled analysis of randomized placebo-controlled trials found that eptifibatide did not increase the incidence of thrombocytopenia (25).

Most of the initial trials of GP IIb/IIIa inhibition in ACS were performed using abciximab. The GUSTO IV-ACS trial was performed in patients with ACS not undergoing coronary intervention. Patients randomized to receive either of two regimens of abciximab in addition to aspirin and heparin showed no benefit with comparison to placebo for the primary end point of death or MI at 30 days (30). Furthermore, the rate of revascularization at 30 days was the same (30%) in each group. No survival benefit was observed with abciximab therapy at one year, and increased mortality was reported in the subset of patients with negative serum troponin or elevated C-reactive protein at baseline (31). Several trials investigating the use of abciximab in ACS patients undergoing PCI have shown benefits in outcome and will be reviewed later in this chapter.

Clopidogrel

Clopidogrel is a thienopyridine derivative that is metabolized by the liver to form a compound that binds to platelet ADP $P2Y_{12}$ receptors to inhibit platelet activation, with no direct effect on arachidonic acid metabolism. Clopidogrel administration is associated with a reduction in ADP binding sites, with no change in ADP binding affinity. An oral loading dose of 300 mg detectably inhibits platelet aggregability in two hours, with maximal effect observed six hours after loading (7). As with aspirin, platelet function returns to normal in approximately seven days after a loading dose. Compared to aspirin alone, the thienopyridines are associated with a lower risk of GI hemorrhage and upper GI symptoms (7). The addition of clopidogrel to aspirin was associated with a significant increase in major (3.7% vs. 2.7%) and minor (5.1% vs. 2.4%) bleeding, but not life-threatening bleeding events, in the Clopidogrel in Unstable Angina to Prevent Recurrent Events (CURE) trial (32). A greater bleeding risk was seen in the subset of ACS patients who proceeded to CABG. This finding has led to some reluctance to administer clopidogrel in the setting of ACS before the coronary anatomy is defined, to minimize the risk of bleeding should the patient require CABG. However, a recent review article suggests that the benefit of aspirin and clopidogrel therapy in maintaining vessel and graft patency may outweigh the increased perioperative bleeding risks (33).

The efficacy of clopidogrel in ACS was established in the CURE trial. When compared to aspirin therapy alone, the combination of aspirin and clopidogrel therapy resulted in a significant reduction in the primary end point of cardiovascular death, MI or stroke in high-risk patients with ACS (9.3% vs. 11.4%) (32). Further analysis of the CURE data showed that this benefit began to emerge within 24 hours of treatment with clopidogrel, and that the magnitude of the benefit continued to increase from 1 to 30 days and from 31 days to 1 year following treatment (34). The total cardiovascular benefit at one year (22 events per 1000 patients) greatly outweighed the increased risk in major bleeding (five events per 1000 patients). The 2002 ACC/AHA guidelines for management of USA or NSTEMI indicate the administration of antiplatelet therapy with clopidogrel as a Class I recommendation for patients with aspirin insensitivity, for hospitalized patients for whom PCI is planned, and for hospitalized patients in whom a noninvasive approach is planned (10). Based on these recommendations, clopidogrel should be administered at a loading dose of 300 mg promptly and continued at a daily dose of 75 mg for at least one month, and for nine months to one year depending on the clinical situation. The benefit of clopidogrel on cardiovascular events may be present for longer than one year after treatment; however, this has not been adequately studied as of yet, though clinical investigation is ongoing (35).

▣ Case 2

A 60-year-old male with a prior history of coronary artery disease and hypertension is referred for left heart catheterization due to symptoms of worsening angina. An exercise stress test performed prior to catheterization was consistent with ischemia in the inferior wall. Left heart catheterization reveals mild diffuse coronary artery disease in all three coronary territories, and a 90% focal stenosis in the mid-right coronary artery. The lesion is deemed amenable to PCI and stenting.
- *Question 1: What constitutes appropriate antithrombotic therapy in the peri-interventional setting?*
- *Question 2: What are the benefits of GP IIb/IIIa inhibitor therapy in the setting of PCI?*
- *Question 3: Are direct thrombin inhibitors as effective as GP IIb/IIIa inhibitors in the prevention of adverse cardiovascular outcomes following PCI?*

PERCUTANEOUS CORONARY INTERVENTION

The advent of coronary angioplasty and stent deployment has been limited by two major factors: acute or subacute vessel thrombosis, and restenosis. Coronary stents are generally made of metal alloys and are thrombogenic. Early studies reported acute (<24 hours) and subacute (within several days) thrombosis at an incidence of approximately 18% (36). Due to such high complication rates, several aggressive antithrombotic regimens have been investigated and refined over time to optimize benefit and to reduce risk in patients undergoing PCI. Initial trials involved high-dose aspirin therapy and dipyridamole; however further research showed no difference in outcome in patients treated with aspirin alone compared to combination therapy (37). A later trial comparing aspirin at doses of 80 or 1500 mg per day found no difference between groups with respect to MI (3.6% vs. 3.9%) and need for surgical revascularization (3.6% vs. 3.7%) (38).

Anticoagulation with heparin was fairly standard with the early use of PCI and coronary stent implantation. However, a study randomizing patients to heparin or no heparin following successful PCI (and stent placement in one-third of patients) showed no difference in cardiac complications between groups (4% vs. 3%) (39). Routine heparin use has since fallen out of favor in the post-PCI setting. The use of additional antithrombotic agents in combination with aspirin has been evaluated in a number of trials.

Warfarin

Warfarin is an oral anticoagulant whose action is mediated through inhibition of the vitamin K–dependent synthesis of coagulation factors II, VII, IX, and X. However, warfarin also inhibits the vitamin K–dependent proteins C and S, which results in competing anticoagulant and thrombogenic effects of warfarin therapy. The full anticoagulant effect of warfarin does not occur until the normal clotting factors are cleared from the circulation, some 36 to 72 hours after administration. Therefore, the initiation of heparin and warfarin therapy is generally overlapped for four to five days in patients with thrombotic disease. The half-life of warfarin is approximately 36 hours. The prothrombin time (PT), which is sensitive to the reduced activity of factors II, VII, and X, has been utilized to follow the anticoagulant effect of warfarin therapy. The international standardized ratio (INR) complements the PT and is meant to standardize the PT by comparison to a universal standard. The risk of bleeding with warfarin therapy is dependent on the level of anticoagulation and the presence of patient-specific risk factors. If needed, reversal of the anticoagulant effect can be accomplished with administration of vitamin K, fresh frozen plasma, or recombinant factor VIIa, depending on the urgency of the clinical situation. The incidence of warfarin skin necrosis has been reported following initiation of warfarin therapy, and is due to rapid reduction in protein C levels upon warfarin administration and induction of a hypercoagulable state. Skin lesions are characterized by rapid margination from an erythematous macule on the extremities, breasts and trunk. Skin biopsy reveals fibrin thrombi in cutaneous vessels with interstitial hemorrhage. Treatment involves discontinuation of warfarin, administration of vitamin K and institution of heparin at therapeutic doses.

The combination of warfarin and aspirin therapy has been shown to slightly reduce the risk of cardiovascular events; however, this has been accompanied by a significant increase in the risk of hemorrhagic complications (40). Short-term therapy with ticlopidine in addition to long-term aspirin was shown to have significant benefit in the STARS trial, which compared aspirin/ticlopidine therapy to aspirin/warfarin and aspirin alone. The incidence of a combined end point of death, emergency CABG, MI and stent thrombosis was 0.5%, 2.7%, and 3.6%, respectively, in the three groups (41). The risk of bleeding complications was observed as 6.2% with warfarin, 5.5% with ticlopidine, and 1.8% with aspirin alone. Although ticlopidine has been shown to be very effective, the severe complication of thrombotic thrombocytopenic purpura associated with ticlopidine use led to investigation evaluating clopidogrel–aspirin combination therapy in PCI. Clopidogrel (at 75 mg per day following a 300 mg loading dose) has been shown to have at least equal efficacy to ticlopidine in the CLASSICS (42) trial as well as a meta-analysis (43). These data are summarized in Table 1 below. Recent evidence shows that pretreating patients with clopidogrel as little as two hours prior to PCI is associated with reduced short-term and long-term cardiovascular end points, and that these benefits are observed up to one year with long-term therapy (45–47). Furthermore, an increased clopidogrel loading dose of 600 mg appears to reduce the incidence of cardiovascular complications when compared to a 300 mg loading dose (48).

Glycoprotein IIb/IIIa Antagonists

A large body of data has demonstrated that the use of GP IIb/IIIa antagonists improves outcomes following PCI, with similar benefits observed in patients with or without stent placement. A meta-analysis of 19 randomized trials showed a significant reduction in mortality at 30 days (RR 0.69) and six months (RR 0.79) with GP IIb/IIIa inhibitor use (49). This benefit was observed to be greater in high-risk patients, i.e., in acute MI, than in low-risk patients undergoing elective PCI. The incidence of MI was similarly reduced at 30 days (RR 0.67) and six months (RR 0.63). The EPISTENT trial demonstrated the benefit of abciximab therapy following elective PCI at one year (RR 0.48 for death or large MI), and showed a mortality benefit still present at three years (50–53). The major trials demonstrating the benefits of GP IIb/IIIa inhibitors in the setting of PCI are outlined in Table 2.

Direct Thrombin Inhibitors

The group of direct thrombin inhibitors includes the drugs bivalirudin, lepirudin, and argatroban. The first two agents are hirudin analogs derived from the medicinal leech Hirudo Medicinalis. These agents bind to the active site of thrombin as well as the fibrinogen-binding site to inhibit both clot-bound thrombin and circulating thrombin. Lepirudin has a Food and Drug Administration (FDA) indication for treatment in patients with HIT and thromboembolic disease; bivalirudin has an FDA indication for PCI. Argatroban is a reversible synthetic direct thrombin inhibitor, which binds to the active site of thrombin, inhibiting both free and clot-bound thrombin. Argatroban has FDA indications for the prophylaxis and treatment of thrombosis in patients

TABLE 1 Clopidogrel vs. Ticlopidine Following Percutaneous Coronary Intervention

Trial	N	Treatment	Outcome	Incidence (%)	p
CLASSICS (42)	102	Clopidogrel	MACE	1.2	$p \geq 0.555$
		Ticlopidine		0.9	
		Clopidogrel	Adverse events: major bleeding, thrombocytopenia, neutropenia or drug discontinuation	4.6	$p = 0.005$
		Ticlopidine		9.1	
Bhatt, et al. (43)	13,955	Clopidogrel	MACE	2.1	$p = 0.002$
		Ticlopidine		4.0	
Moussa, et al. (44)	283	Clopidogrel	MACE	2.4	$p = 0.85$
	1406	Ticlopidine		3.1	

Abbreviation: CLASSICS, Double-blind study of the safety of clopidogrel with and without a loading dose in combination with aspirin compared with ticlopidine in combination with aspirin after coronary stenting; the clopidogrel aspirin stent international cooperative study.

with HIT as well as for anticoagulation in patients with HIT undergoing PCI. Unlike the hirudin analogs, argatroban is hepatically cleared. The direct thrombin inhibitors are not associated with thrombocytopenia and activity is monitored by measurement of the activated partial thromboplastin time. No reversal agents exist; however, argatroban in particular has a short half-life

TABLE 2 Glycoprotein IIb/IIIa Inhibitor Use in Percutaneous Coronary Intervention

Trial	n	Regimen	Outcome (follow-up)	Incidence (%)	*p*-value
EPISTENT (50)	2399	Stent + placebo	Death, MI	11.4	
		Stent + abciximab	(six months)	5.6	$p < 0.001$
		POBA + abciximab		7.8	$p = 0.01$
ESPRIT (54)	2064	Stent + placebo	Death, MI,	10.5	$p = 0.0015$
		Stent + eptifibatide	urgent target vessel revascularization, thrombotic bailout IIb/IIIa inhibitor therapy (48 hr)	6.6	
CADILLAC (55)	2082	POBA POBA + abciximab Stent Stent + abciximab	Death, reinfarction, disabling stroke, ischemia-driven target vessel revascularization (6 mo)	20 16.5 11.5 10.2	$p < 0.001$
ADMIRAL (56)	300	Stent + placebo Stent + abciximab	Death, reinfarction, urgent target vessel revascularization (30 days, three months)	14.6 15.9 6.0 7.4	$p = 0.01, 0.02$
ISAR-REACT (57)	2159	600 mg clopidogrel + placebo 600 mg clopidogrel + abciximab	Death, MI, urgent target vessel revascularization (30 days)	4 4	$p = 0.82$
EPIC (23)	2099	POBA + placebo POBA + abciximab	Death, nonfatal MI, unplanned surgical revascularization, repeat PCI, stent placement, IABP insertion (30 days)	12.8 8.3	$p = 0.008$
EPILOG (24)	2792	Placebo + standard heparin Abciximab + standard heparin Abciximab + low-dose heparin	Death, MI, urgent revascularization (30 days)	11.7 5.4 5.2	$p < 0.001$ $p < 0.001$
TARGET (58)	4809	Abciximab Tirofiban	Death, infarction, need for urgent revascularization (30 days)	6 7.6	$p = 0.038$

Abbreviations: EPISTENT, Evaluation of Platelet IIb/IIIa Inhibition in Stenting Investigators; ESPRIT, Enhanced Suppression of the Platelet IIb/IIIA Receptor with Integrillin Therapy; CADILLAC, Comparison of angioplasty with stenting, with or without abciximab, in acute MI; ADMIRAL, Platelet glycoprotein IIb/IIIA inhibition with coronary stenting for acute MI; ISAR-REACT, A clinical trial of abciximab in elective percutaneous coronary intervention after pretreatment with clopidogrel; EPIC, Use of a monoclonal antibody directed against the platelet glycoprotein IIb/IIIa receptor in high-risk coronary angioplasty; EPILOG, Platelet glycoprotein IIb/IIIa receptor blockade and low-dose heparin during percutaneous coronary revascularization; TARGET, Comparison of two platelet glycoprotein IIb/IIIa inhibitors, tirofiban and abciximab, for the prevention of ischemic events with percutaneous coronary revascularization.

TABLE 3 Bivalirudin Therapy in Percutaneous Coronary Intervention

Trial	*n*	Treatment	Outcomes	Incidence (%)	*p*-value
REPLACE-1 (59)	1056	Heparin ± GP IIb/IIIa inhibitor	Death, MI repeat revascularization within 48 hours or hospital discharge	6.9	
			Major bleeding	2.7	
		Bivalirudin ± GP IIb/IIIa inhibitor	Death, MI, repeat revascularization within 48 hours or hospital discharge	5.6	*p* = 0.40
			Major bleeding	2.1	*p* = 0.52
REPLACE-2 (61)	6010	Heparin + GP IIb/IIIa inhibitor	Death (6 and 12 mo) MI (6 mo) Repeat revascularization (6 mo)	1.4, 2.5 7.4 11.4	
		Bivalirudin ± GP IIb/IIIa inhibitor	Death (6 and 12 mo) MI (6 mo) Repeat revascularization (6 mo)	1.0, 1.9 8.2 12.1	*p* = 0.15, 0.16 *p* = 0.24 *p* = 0.45

Abbreviations: REPLACE, Randomized Evaluation of PCI Linking Angiomax to Reduced Clinical Events; GP, glycoprotein.

leading to rapid clearance upon discontinuation of IV infusion. Reports of rare cases of anaphylaxis to lepirudin have led to recommendations against repeat exposure to this agent. The bleeding risks with direct thrombin inhibitors are similar to those with other anticoagulation agents, with a 2.1% incidence of major bleeding with bivalirudin in the REPLACE-1 trial (59).

Reported outcomes with the use of argatroban in patients with HIT during PCI are comparable to established data using standard therapy; therefore, argatroban provides a reasonable therapeutic option in this setting (60). The majority of data regarding the use of direct thrombin inhibitors in PCI involves the use of bivalirudin. The REPLACE-1 (59) and REPLACE-2 (61) trials have established the efficacy and safety of bivalirudin therapy, and are summarized in Table 3 below. Subset analysis from these trials has demonstrated the safety and efficacy of bivalirudin in patients with renal insufficiency (62) and diabetes (63). Retrospective analysis of data from the Cleveland Clinic demonstrates a lower incidence of bleeding (1.7% vs. 4.0%) and no difference in long-term survival in patients treated with bivalirudin alone compared to heparin in combination with a GP IIb/IIIa inhibitor (64). A modest cost benefit (US $400 saved per patient) (65) and a decreased length of stay in the recovery area (36 minutes) (66) have been demonstrated with bivalirudin therapy compared to heparin and GP IIb/IIIa combination therapy, outcomes which may prove important to patient flow at busy interventional centers. A trial of bivalirudin therapy in ACS patients is ongoing (67).

▪ Case 3

A 65-year-old female patient returns to your clinic six months after undergoing primary angioplasty to the left anterior descending artery following a MI. The patient has been clinically well, and is undergoing treatment for her cardiovascular risk factors, including hypertension and hyperlipidemia. She is accompanied by her sister, who has no history of coronary artery disease, but is concerned about their strong family history of coronary disease. The sisters wish to know if there are any additional ways to reduce their risk of future cardiovascular events.

● *Question 1: What is the benefit of aspirin therapy in the primary and secondary prevention of MI?*
● *Question 2: Who should receive preventative therapy, and what doses of aspirin are appropriate for prevention?*
● *Question 3: Do all patients derive a benefit from aspirin therapy?*
● *Question 4: What additional antithrombotic agents are of benefit in the prevention of MI?*

PRIMARY AND SECONDARY PREVENTION OF MI

Data from several large-scale trials conclusively indicate that aspirin use reduces the risk of a first MI by approximately 1/3. These are listed in Table 4 below. The decision to prescribe aspirin therapy in the primary prevention of MI involves an assessment of the patient's cardiovascular risk. This is well illustrated in the recent Women's Health Study, which showed that the benefits of aspirin therapy in the prevention of a first major cardiovascular event in healthy women aged 45 or older were confined to the subgroup of patients aged 65 or older (68). The American Heart Association guidelines recommend the use of aspirin prophylaxis in individuals with a 10-year risk of cardiovascular disease of 10% or more (74), while the United States Preventive Services Task Force (USPSTF) recommends the

TABLE 4 Aspirin in Primary Prevention of Cardiovascular Events

Trial	*n*	Aspirin dose	Outcome	Risk reduction (%)	*p*-value
Women's Health Study (68)	39,876	100 mg QOD	First major CV event (8.2–10.9 years)	9	$p = 0.13$
Physicians' Health Study (69)	22,071	325 mg QOD	First MI (five years)	44	$p < 0.00001$
British Doctor's Trial (70)	5139	500 mg QD	MI, stroke, CV death (six years)	1.2	$p = $ NS
Hypertension Optimal Treatment Trial (71)	18,790	75 mg QD	First MI	36	$p = 0.002$
			MACE	15	$p = 0.03$
Primary Prevention Project (72)	4495	100 mg QD	Cardiovascular mortality MACE	44	$p = 0.049$
				23	$p = 0.014$
Thrombosis Prevention Trial (73)	6085	75 mg QD	Nonfatal MI	32	$p = 0.004$

discussion of aspirin prophylaxis with patients who have a 10-year cardiovascular risk of 6% (75). Ten-year cardiovascular risk may be estimated using the Framingham models for men and women (76). It is important to understand that these US guidelines are based on data accumulated in large part from the United States and Europe, and that risk–benefit outcomes may be different when applied to different populations. A recent study investigating the use of the USPSTF guidelines to a Japanese population recommended that the threshold for initiating antiplatelet therapy in the primary prevention of cardiovascular events should be two to five times higher in this population, due to a lower estimated incidence of coronary heart disease in middle-aged men and a higher risk of hemorrhagic stroke (77).

A number of antithrombotic agents have been used in the secondary prevention of MI in patients with preexisting cardiovascular disease. Strong evidence exists for aspirin therapy in the secondary prevention of MI, and warfarin and ximelagatran have been extensively studied as well. The benefit of aspirin is best established by the Antithrombotic Trialists' Collaboration (ATC). A meta-analysis of 25 trials of antiplatelet therapy (in which the majority of patients were treated with aspirin) showed significant reductions in subsequent MI (32%), nonfatal stroke (27%), and vascular death (15%) (78). The optimal dose of aspirin in secondary prevention has been widely studied. The ATC analyses have shown no benefit to higher dose (up to 1500 mg) aspirin therapy when compared to "medium" dose therapy (75–325 mg per day) (78–80). A stratified study based on aspirin dosing indicated that patients treated with 75 to 150 mg per day of aspirin had more benefit than those treated with less than 75 mg per day or greater than 500 mg per day; however, these findings were not significant (80). Meta-regression models have indicated that aspirin dosing at 81 mg per day may result in a 1.2% decrease in ischemic events at 30 days when compared to 325 mg per day dosing (81); however, debate regarding optimal aspirin dosing continues.

There has existed concern regarding the use of nonaspirin NSAIDs in combination with aspirin in patients with cardiovascular disease, with some preliminary evidence suggesting that these medications might diminish the benefit of aspirin prophylaxis for the secondary prevention of cardiovascular events. Concern regarding the use of nonaspirin NSAIDs in conjunction with aspirin stems from reported reductions in platelet inhibition in patients treated with ibuprofen (82) and naproxen (83) (but not acetaminophen or diclofenac) in addition to aspirin. Attempts to link these findings to clinical outcomes have yielded contradictory results. A retrospective analysis of 7107 patients with cardiovascular disease demonstrated increases in all-cause mortality and cardiovascular mortality in patients treated with ibuprofen in addition to aspirin [hazard ratio (HR) 1.93 and 1.73, respectively] (84); however, a more recent study of 3589 patients (with or without cardiovascular disease) showed no increase in the risk of MI with ibuprofen use in addition to aspirin (85). Given these contradictory findings and the lack of prospective data, firm recommendations against the use of nonsteroidal anti-inflammatory drugs (NSAIDs) in combination with aspirin cannot be made at this time.

Despite the well-established benefits of aspirin therapy, treatment failures are common. This has led to much investigation into the issue of biochemical "aspirin resistance," which is a separate entity from treatment failure secondary to nonadherence, comorbid conditions or drug interactions (86). Although several studies have investigated the prevalence of biochemical aspirin resistance through measurement of platelet function, small sample sizes and differences in measurement technique have led to varying results. The prevalence of aspirin resistance has been reported as ranging from 5.5% to 56.8% in various studies (87). Several studies have shown an increase in cardiovascular and cerebrovascular events in patients with aspirin resistance, although the definitions of resistance have varied across studies. In one study, aspirin resistance was partially overcome with increased aspirin dosing (88); however, sufficient data are not available to make recommendations regarding aspirin therapy in patients with documented resistance.

The CAPRIE (89) trial established the efficacy of clopidogrel in the secondary prevention of cardiovascular events. At a mean follow-up of two years, patients treated with a combination of aspirin (325 mg per day) and clopidogrel (75 mg per day) were observed to have a decreased incidence of MI when compared to patients treated with aspirin alone [4.2% vs. 5.0%, relative risk reduction (RRR) 19.2%] (90). Subset analysis of the CAPRIE data revealed that high-risk patients derived particular benefit from clopidogrel therapy, including patients with diabetes mellitus (91), prior ischemic events (92) or prior cardiac surgery (93). As with aspirin, treatment failure with clopidogrel has been described, with reports of lack of platelet response to clopidogrel varying from 4% to 30% across studies (94,95). Treatment failure with clopidogrel may be secondary to drug interactions as well as receptor polymorphisms, resulting in "clopidogrel resistance." A small study reported an increased incidence of recurrent cardiovascular events in patients with a decreased platelet response to clopidogrel therapy following acute MI; however, this study was underpowered to draw any firm conclusions regarding the clinical ramifications of clopidogrel resistance (96).

Other antiplatelet agents have been investigated for the secondary prevention of cardiovascular events. Most notably, interest in the class of oral GP IIb/IIIa inhibitors was lost after the BRAVO trial, which showed an increase in mortality (3.0% vs. 2.3%) with lotrafiban compared to placebo in 9190 patients with unstable coronary or cerebrovascular disease, or a stable combination of peripheral, coronary or cerebrovascular disease (97). A meta-analysis of oral GP IIb/IIIa inhibitors also showed an excess in mortality (98).

The use of oral anticoagulation in addition to aspirin therapy in the secondary prevention of cardiovascular events has shown modest benefit. Three recent trials investigating warfarin therapy in addition to aspirin therapy are summarized below (Table 5), and indicate that there exists a small incremental benefit to combination therapy. However, the increased risk of bleeding observed with the addition of anticoagulant therapy to aspirin (15% in the ASPECT-2 trial) (99) has largely precluded its use for the secondary prevention or MI.

Ximelagatran

The emergence of ximelagatran as an oral alternative to warfarin therapy in Europe led to its study as an agent for the secondary prevention of cardiovascular events. Ximelagatran

TABLE 5 Aspirin vs. Warfarin for Secondary Prevention of Cardiovascular Events

Trial	N	Treatment	Outcome	Incidence (%)	p-value
ASPECT-2 Study (99)	336	Aspirin	MI, stroke, or death	9	
	325	Warfarin (INR 3.0–4.0)		5	p = 0.0479
	332	Aspirin + warfarin (INR 2.0–2.5)		5	p = 0.03
CHAMP Study (100)	2537	Aspirin	Death	17.3	
	2522	Aspirin + warfarin (INR 1.5–2.5)	MI	13.1	
			Death	17.6	p = 0.76
			MI	13.3	p = 0.78
Hurlen, M et al. (101)	1206	Aspirin	Death, MI, stroke	20.0	
	1216	Warfarin (INR 2.8–4.2)		16.7	p = 0.03
	1208	Aspirin + warfarin (INR 2.0–2.5)		15.0	p = 0.001

Abbreviations: ASPECT-2, Aspirin and Coumadin after acute coronary syndromes; CHAMP, Cooperative Studies Program clinical trial comparing combined warfarin and aspirin with aspirin alone in survivors of acute MI; INR, international standardized ratio.

is an oral direct thrombin inhibitor that is rapidly absorbed and cleared renally with a half-life of approximately five hours. Potential advantages of ximelagatran therapy include fixed oral dosing, low incidence of drug interactions and the lack of need for therapeutic monitoring of anticoagulation. Ximelagatran carries a small but significant risk of liver toxicity manifested by elevations in serum transaminase levels and its bleeding risk is similar to that of other anticoagulants (1.3% risk of major bleeding in the THRIVE trial) (102). The ESTEEM Trial compared Ximelagatran treatment at four different doses to placebo in addition to aspirin for the secondary prevention of cardiovascular events. Addition of ximelagatran to aspirin resulted in a reduction in the composite end point of death, nonfatal MI and severe recurrent ischemia (12.7% vs. 16.3%), with a nonsignificant increase in the risk of major bleeding (1.8% vs. 0.9%) (103). Concerns regarding the side effect profile of ximelagatran have prevented its approval in the United States at this time. Yet because ximelagatran does not require dose adjustment or anticoagulation monitoring, similar compounds may provide an attractive future option for prophylaxis following MI pending further study.

The 2002 ACC/AHA guidelines recommend lifelong antiplatelet therapy following a MI with aspirin at doses of 75 to 325 mg per day, or clopidogrel in cases of aspirin intolerance (10). The use of oral anticoagulants, i.e., warfarin and ximelagatran, is not addressed and has not been established as the standard of care.

■ Case 4

A 70-year-old retired male medical malpractice attorney with controlled hypertension is referred to your clinic for management of atrial fibrillation, which was recently diagnosed on a screening electrocardiogram. The patient denies a history of palpitations, and on arrival the patient has no complaints. Although the patient has not previously undergone rigorous cardiovascular examination, he has no history of coronary artery disease or structural heart disease. After you obtain the patient's history, he tells you that he feels fine, and does not wish to take medication to treat an asymptomatic condition.
- *Question 1: Which patients with atrial fibrillation benefit from antithrombotic therapy?*
- *Question 2: What antithrombotic therapies are acceptable in the management of atrial fibrillation?*

ATRIAL FIBRILLATION AND ATRIAL FLUTTER

Atrial fibrillation is the most common cardiac rhythm disorder, affecting approximately 2.5 million people in the United States (104), and is an independent risk factor for ischemic stroke. Thrombogenesis in atrial fibrillation may be multifactorial. The effects of blood stasis in a dilated and dysfunctional left atrium are well described, however the presence of endothelial dysfunction, inflammation, platelet activation, and a hypercoagulable state have been postulated in atrial fibrillation as well (105). Overall, atrial fibrillation accounts for approximately 15% of strokes in the United States (106), with an average risk of 4.5% per year in patients not treated with antithrombotic therapy. A meta-analysis of five randomized, controlled trials studying the use of adjusted-dose warfarin in patients with atrial fibrillation showed a RRR of 68% (1.4% vs. 4.5% for control) for the primary prevention of stroke (Table 6) (112). This corresponds to a number needed to treat of 32 patients per year to prevent one stroke. The majority of strokes occurring in the warfarin arms in these trials occurred in patients with subtherapeutic anticoagulation or in those in whom warfarin had been stopped.

The evidence for aspirin prophylaxis in atrial fibrillation is weaker than that for warfarin. A pooled analysis of three trials reported a 21% RRR with aspirin therapy compared to placebo, with results that were of borderline statistical significance (113). A similar result (22% RRR) was seen with aspirin therapy in a meta-analysis (114). A large meta-analysis comparing aspirin therapy to oral vitamin K antagonist (VKA) therapy found a 46% RRR for all stroke and 52% RRR for ischemic stroke with VKA's, with a 1.7-fold increased rate of major hemorrhage (115). For 1000 patients treated, this corresponds to 23 fewer ischemic strokes at the expense of nine additional major bleeding episodes.

Two large trials, SPORTIF III (116) and SPORTIF V (117), have compared fixed-dose ximelagatran to adjusted-dose warfarin prophylaxis for stroke in atrial fibrillation (Table 7) Both trials were designed to demonstrate the "noninferiority" of ximelagatran therapy. The evidence from both trials supports the notion that ximelagatran therapy is equivalent to warfarin therapy; however, a cost-effectiveness analysis performed on the data from these trials demonstrated that

TABLE 6 Warfarin in Atrial Fibrillation

Trial	*N*	INR range	Outcome	Incidence (%)
AFASAK (107)	1007	2.8–4.2 + aspirin	Stroke, systemic embolism, TIA, intracranial hemorrhage	2.7
SPAF (108)	1330	2.0–4.5 + aspirin	Stroke, systemic embolism	2.3
BAATAF (109)	420	1.5–2.7	Stroke	0.4
CAFA (110)	383	2.0–3.0	Stroke, systemic embolism, intracranial or fatal hemorrhage	3.4
SPINAF (111)	525	1.4–2.8	Stroke	0.9

Abbreviations: AFASAK, Placebo-controlled, randomized trial of warfarin and aspirin for prevention of thromboembolic complications in chronic atrial fibrillation; SPAF, Stroke Prevention in Atrial Fibrillation study; BAATAF, Boston Area Anticoagulation Trial for Atrial Fibrillation Investigators; CAFA, Canadian atrial fibrillation anticoagulation study; SPINAF, Warfarin in the prevention of stroke associated with nonrheumatic atrial fibrillation; INR, international standardized ratio; TIA, Transientischemic attack.

ximelagatran therapy was unlikely to provide a cost–benefit savings over warfarin in intermediate-risk patients (118). Concerns regarding the side effect profile of ximelagatran have prevented its approval in the United States at this time. Yet because ximelagatran does not require dose adjustment or anticoagulation monitoring, similar compounds may provide an attractive future option for prophylaxis in atrial fibrillation.

Guidelines for stroke prophylaxis in atrial fibrillation are dependent on individual patients' risk-factor profiles, with more aggressive medical regimens recommended for patients at higher risk for stroke. An analysis of pooled data by the Atrial Fibrillation Investigators group identified age (RR 1.4 per decade), prior stroke or transient ischemic attack (TIA) (RR 2.5), hypertension (RR 1.6) and diabetes (RR 1.7) as independent risk factors for stroke (112). The 2004 American College of Chest Physicians (ACCP) guidelines recommend anticoagulation with adjusted-dose warfarin (target INR 2.0–3.0) for patients at high risk for stroke, i.e., patients with persistent atrial fibrillation or patients with paroxysmal atrial fibrillation and any of the following risk factors: prior ischemic stroke, TIA, systemic embolism, age greater than 75 years, moderately or severely impaired left ventricular function, hypertension, or diabetes mellitus (106). Antithrombotic therapy with warfarin or aspirin (325 mg per day) is acceptable for patients at intermediate risk for stroke, i.e., patients aged between 65 and 75 with no additional risk factors. Aspirin therapy alone is recommended for patients less than 65 years of age with no additional risk factors. Clopidogrel plus aspirin combination therapy is currently being evaluated for stroke prophylaxis in atrial fibrillation.

Two recent trials, AFFIRM (119) and RACE (120), have demonstrated no difference in the incidence of ischemic events in patients randomized to a rhythm-control versus rate-control strategy for atrial fibrillation. Based on this evidence, long-term antithrombotic therapy is recommended for high-risk patients even if normal sinus rhythm is restored. Guidelines for the management of atrial flutter mirror those for atrial fibrillation, and antithrombotic strategies for the two disorders should be identical (121).

■ Case 5

A 28-year-old female with postpartum cardiomyopathy presents for one-year follow-up. Despite clinical improvement on a regimen including angiotensin-converting enzyme inhibitors (ACE-Is), beta-blockers, and diuretics, her ejection fraction remains 25% on recent transthoracic echocardiogram. She feels generally well at this time.

● *Question 1: Does antithrombotic therapy reduce the incidence of cardiovascular events in patients with congestive heart failure (CHF)?*

TABLE 7 Ximelagatran in Atrial Fibrillation

Trial	*N*	Regimen	Outcome	Incidence (%)	*p*-value
SPORTIF III (116)	1704	Ximelagatran 36 mg b.i.d.	Stroke, systemic embolism	1.6	*p* = 0.10
	1703	Warfarin		2.3	
SPORTIF V (117)	1960	Ximelagatran 36 mg b.i.d.	Stroke, systemic embolism	1.6	*p* < 0.001 for
	1962	Warfarin (INR 2.0–3.0)		1.2	noninferiority

Abbreviations: SPORTIF, Stroke prevention with the oral direct thrombin inhibitor Ximelagatran compared with warfarin in patients with nonvalvular atrial fibrillation; INR, international standardized ratio.

DILATED CARDIOMYOPATHY

CHF has been associated with a prothrombotic state in several studies, and some data have suggested that CHF patients are at increased risk of MI, stroke, and thromboembolism (122–124). The benefit of antithrombotic therapy in patients with CHF has been examined in several large retrospective studies; however, to date only one prospective randomized controlled trial examining this issue has been performed (125).

Retrospective data from the V-HeFT trials has been contradictory, showing a benefit to antiplatelet therapy with aspirin, dipyridamole or both (0.5 vs. 2.7 thromboembolic events per 100 patient-years) in the V-HeFT I trial, but no such benefit in the V-HeFT II trial (1.6 vs. 2.1 events per 100 patient years) (126). Post-hoc analysis from the SOLVD trial demonstrated that CHF patients treated with antiplatelet therapy (with aspirin in greater than 95% of patients) had reduced mortality (HR 0.82) and a lower risk of sudden cardiac death (HR 0.78) (127). In the SAVE trial, CHF patients treated with antiplatelet therapy were observed to have a decreased incidence of stroke (124). The use of clopidogrel in addition to aspirin therapy in heart failure was shown to result in greater platelet inactivation in the PLUTO-CHF trial; however clinical outcomes with combination therapy in CHF are not yet available (128).

Retrospective analysis demonstrated no reduction in thromboembolic events with warfarin anticoagulation therapy in V-HeFT I or V-HeFT II (126). Analysis of the SOLVD data demonstrated benefits in mortality (HR 0.76) and in the combined end point of death and hospital admission for heart failure (HR 0.82) with warfarin anticoagulation (129); however, no direct comparison was made between CHF patients treated with antiplatelet therapy and warfarin. The Warfarin/Aspirin Study in Heart failure (WASH) trial is a randomized controlled trial performed to examine aspirin versus warfarin therapy in CHF (130). In WASH, no benefit was observed with either therapy with respect to the primary end point of death, MI, or stroke; however this was a small trial enrolling only 279 patients. The larger WATCH trial was designed to further examine this question, but has been prematurely terminated before providing a conclusive answer. At present, no guidelines exist which recommend the use of warfarin anticoagulation for primary prophylaxis of thromboembolic events in CHF. Aspirin therapy should be employed based on preexisting risk factors for coronary artery disease and stroke, as in patients with normal ventricular function.

There has existed concern regarding the use of ACE-I's in combination with aspirin in patients with heart failure, with some preliminary evidence suggesting that aspirin may interfere with the benefits of ACE-I's. This question has been studied extensively using retrospective data. However, a recent study in France showed no interaction between aspirin and ACE-I's in 755 patients with left ventricular dysfunction (131), and there are currently no recommendations to avoid the combination of aspirin and ACE-I therapy in patients with heart failure.

■ Case 6

A 40-year-old female presents to the emergency room for evaluation of left lower extremity swelling and pain which has progressed over three days. The patient takes oral contraceptives and smokes one pack of cigarettes daily. Physical examination reveals unilateral nonpitting edema and mild erythema of the left lower extremity below the knee. No palpable cord is present and arterial pulses are intact. Deep venous thrombosis (DVT) is suspected and the diagnosis is confirmed with Doppler ultrasound.

- *Question 1: What is the therapeutic goal in management of DVT and/or pulmonary embolism (PE)?*
- Question 2: What are the optimal inpatient and outpatient regimens for management of thromboembolic disease?
- Question 3: What factors influence the optimal duration of therapy for thromboembolic disease?

DEEP VENOUS THROMBOSIS AND PULMONARY EMBOLISM

Venous thromboembolic disease, which encompasses deep-venoas-thrombosis (DVT) and pulmonary embolism (PE), has an incidence of approximately 1.9 per 1000 patient-years in patients greater than 45 years of age, with higher incidence with increasing age (132). Risk factors for venous thromboembolic disease include extremity immobilization, lower extremity trauma, prolonged hospitalization, oral contraceptive use, pregnancy, obesity, stroke, hormone replacement therapy, and malignancy.

The clinical manifestations of DVT include unilateral swelling, warmth, and erythema of the involved extremity. A palpable cord may be present along the length of the involved vein, and distension of superficial veins may be present. The diagnosis of DVT may be made through a number of noninvasive means, including duplex venous ultrasonography, magnetic resonance imaging, and impedance plethysmography. Duplex ultrasound examination is the most common means of diagnosis, and involves evaluation for venous flow abnormalities suggestive of thrombosis, carrying a positive predictive value approaching 95% for proximal DVT. In rare cases, contrast venography may be utilized for diagnosis of DVT; however, this invasive test carries a measurable risk and is generally avoided in favor of the noninvasive tests.

Therapy for DVT is directed at minimizing clot propagation, PE and long-term complications such as recurrent DVT, thrombophlebitis, postphlebitic syndrome, or pulmonary hypertension secondary to thromboembolic disease. The diagnosis of PE is often difficult. Clinical manifestations of PE include pleuritic chest pain, dyspnea, and hypoxia; however, chest radiography, electrocardiography, and echocardiography findings are generally nonspecific. Elevation of the serum D-dimer level is very sensitive but not specific. Pulmonary artery angiography has remained the gold standard for diagnosis of PE; however, improvements in noninvasive diagnostic testing continue to be made. Pulmonary ventilation or perfusion scans have been shown to be of diagnostic benefit when used in conjunction with a clinical prediction model (133). Computed tomography of the pulmonary arteries was shown in initial studies to have a sensitivity and specificity of approximately 90% for the diagnosis of PE (134), and technologic advances in image resolution continue to improve its diagnostic accuracy such that at some centers it is the diagnostic procedure of choice.

The benefit of anticoagulation in the treatment of DVT and PE has been established in several randomized clinical trials (135). Heparin therapy is usually initiated simultaneously with warfarin therapy; this is necessary because during the first few days of warfarin therapy, the prolongation of the INR is mainly secondary to a decrease in factor VII, which results in suppression of the extrinsic coagulation pathway but not the intrinsic pathway. The use of a weight-based dosing protocol for UFH therapy has been shown to be superior in achieving therapeutic levels within 24 hours (97% vs. 77% for standard therapy) and resulted in an 80% relative risk reduction for recurrent thromboembolism (136). A five-day regimen of combination therapy with UFH and warfarin has been shown to be as effective as 10 days of therapy in reducing the risk of recurrent thromboembolic disease (7.1% vs. 7.0%) (137). LMWH have been compared to UFH for the treatment proximal DVT in a number of trials. One meta-analysis reported lower rates of recurrent DVT with LMWH use compared to heparin (2.7% vs. 7.0%) and less major bleeding (0.9% vs. 3.2%) (138). As in ACS LMWH use has been associated with a cost-benefit when compared to UFH. One trial reported a savings of US \$40,149 per 100 patients treated in the hospital, and a potential savings of US \$91,332 if 37% of these patients were candidates for outpatient therapy with LMWH (139). For the treatment of DVT, enoxaparin may be administered 1 mg/kg subcutaneously every 12 hours. Ximelagatran therapy has been recently evaluated for the treatment of DVT and was shown to be noninferior to LMWH and warfarin combination therapy [2.1% vs. 2.0% incidence of recurrent venous thromboembolism (VTE)] (102). Concerns regarding the side effect profile of ximelagatran have prevented its approval in the United States at this time. Yet because ximelagatran does not require dose adjustment or anticoagulation monitoring, other oral thrombin inhibitors or Factor Xa inhibitors may provide an attractive future option for treatment and prophylaxis for DVT and PE.

The length of anticoagulation therapy for VTE is determined by the risk profile of the patient, with patients at higher risk of recurrent thromboembolic disease receiving longer treatment regimens. The Seventh ACCP Conference on Antithrombotic and Thrombolytic Therapy guidelines recommends three months of anticoagulation therapy for patients with a first episode of DVT associated with a reversible risk factor, and at least 6 to 12 months of therapy for patients with an idiopathic first episode of DVT (140). Lifelong therapy is suggested for patients with a first episode of DVT and documented hypercoagulable states, two or more thrombophilic conditions, or two or more episodes of DVT. Further recommendations are made for anticoagulation with LMWH for the first three to six months of long-term therapy for patients with DVT and cancer.

DVT prophylaxis is often warranted for hospitalized patients due to many risk factors, including advanced age, surgical procedures, and extremity immobilization. DVT is often clinically silent in these patients, but may still lead to significant morbidity if untreated, with DVT incidence ranging from 10% to 20% in general medical patients to up to 80% of patients with major trauma, spinal cord injury, or in critical care units (141). A number of prophylactic strategies have been investigated, including mechanical means of reducing venous stasis (e.g., graduated compression stockings and intermittent pneumatic compression devices) and pharmaceutical therapies (e.g., low dose UFH and low dose LMWH). The methods of mechanical prophylaxis have been studied less exhaustively than the anticoagulant means of prophylaxis, and no method of mechanical prophylaxis has been shown to decrease the risk of death or PE (142). Therefore, mechanical prophylaxis is generally recommended only in low-to-moderate risk patients, in combination with anticoagulant prophylaxis, or in patients at high risk for bleeding complications.

Anticoagulant-based prophylaxis for thromboembolic disease has been shown to have significant efficacy when compared to placebo or with aspirin administration, with a 63% reduction in the incidence of thromboembolic disease when compared to aspirin alone in one trial (142). The use of low dose LMWH has been shown to reduce thromboembolic events in a number of trials, and in some cases low dose LMWH has been shown to deliver incremental benefit over UFH (141). Enoxaparin can be administered 30 mg subcutaneously twice daily or 40 mg subcutaneously once daily for this indication. Several trials have shown similar efficacy with ximelagatran prophylactic therapy following orthopedic surgery, when compared to LMWH or warfarin (143). The recommendations outlined by the ACCP and published in September 2004 are useful in guiding prophylactic therapy for thromboembolic disease (141).

Case 7

A 71-year-old female with diabetes, hypertension, chronic renal insufficiency, and coronary artery disease presents for routine follow-up with a chief complaint of severe calf pain with walking, which is relieved with rest. The patient has moderately diminished arterial pulses in both lower extremities. You suspect that these symptoms represent claudication and refer the patient for a more thorough vascular evaluation.

● *Question 1: What are the benefits of antithrombotic therapy in peripheral arterial disease (PAD)?*

PERIPHERAL ARTERIAL DISEASE

The incidence of PAD parallels that of coronary artery disease, and the two conditions are associated with the same risk factors, i.e., tobacco use, diabetes mellitus, hypertension, and hyperlipidemia. Patients with PAD limiting blood flow to the extremities most commonly present with claudication, defined as a reproducible pain in a specific muscle group, which is induced by exercise and relieved with rest. As in cardiac angina, symptoms are related to an imbalance between supply and demand of blood flow, and therefore oxygen delivery. As with cardiovascular disease, the use of antithrombotic agents has been essential to medical management of PAD. The ATC overview reported a 23% reduction in the risk of nonfatal MI, nonfatal stroke or vascular death with aspirin therapy in 9214 patients with PAD treated with aspirin, however the benefit of aspirin use on peripheral vascular disease itself is not clear from these data (80). In the Physicians' Health Study, aspirin use (325 mg per day) was observed to decrease the need for peripheral arterial surgery, but no reduction in the incidence of claudication was observed (144). Clopidogrel therapy was shown to substantially reduce the risk of cardiovascular death, stroke or MI when compared to aspirin alone in patients with PAD enrolled in the CAPRIE trial (89).

Pentoxifylline

Pentoxifylline is a rheological modifier whose benefits are derived through decreases in platelet aggregability, fibrinogen levels, whole-blood viscosity and an increase in erythrocyte deformity. Conflicting data exist regarding the benefits of pentoxifylline in the symptomatic treatment of PAD. A meta-analysis of randomized controlled trials demonstrated a modest improvement in walking distance with pentoxifylline compared to placebo (29 m) (145); however, in a head-to-head trial comparing pentoxifylline to cilostazol, no benefit was seen over placebo (146).

Cilostazol

Cilostazol is a phosphodiesterase inhibitor, which promotes arterial vasodilation and inhibits platelet aggregation. A meta-analysis of eight randomized, placebo-controlled trials demonstrated the efficacy of cilostazol in increasing maximum and pain-free walking distances by 50% and 67%, respectively (147). A randomized, placebo-controlled trial demonstrated the superiority of cilostazol therapy to pentoxifylline, with a benefit in maximal walking distance with cilostazol (54% increase) and no benefit with pentoxifylline (30% increase) compared to placebo (34% increase) (146). Reports of increased mortality in patients with CHF treated with phosphodiesterase inhibitors preclude cilostazol use in patients with CHF.

Anticoagulation therapy with heparin and warfarin has been evaluated for patients with peripheral vascular disease, and has shown little promise as the small benefits observed with anticoagulation therapy appear to be completely outweighed by the increased bleeding risks (148).

FUTURE DIRECTIONS

Further investigation into patient characteristics which may portend increased or decreased benefit to specific antiplatelet agents or anticoagulants offers promise for patient-specific therapy in the future (149). Novel ADP receptor antagonists are also in Phase 2 and Phase 3 testing. For example, the thienopyridine Prasugrel is being compared against clopidogrel in a 13,000 patient ACS trial. Cangrelor is an IV ADP antagonist that holds promise in ACS and PCI. Continued investigation into new agents for anticoagulation may change the scope of the field in the near future as well. Several novel agents will likely find increased use in the near future, including direct Factor Xa inhibitors, such as fondaparinux. Fondaparinux results in factor Xa inhibition through AT with no effect on thrombin, and carries indications for treatment and prophylaxis in DVT. Oral agents in development directly bind to the active site of Factor Xa to inhibit its activity independent of AT. Also under investigation are recombinant TFPI, inhibitors of factor V and VIII and APC.

REFERENCES

1. Sims PJ, Wiedmer T, Esmon CT, et al. Assembly of the platelet prothrombinase complex is linked to the vesiculation of the platelet plasma membranes. Studies in Scott syndrome: an isolated defect in platelet procoagulant activity. J Biol Chem 1989; 264:17049–17057.
2. Marcum JA, McKenney JB and Rosenberg RD. Acceleration of thrombin-antithrombin complex formation in rat hindquarters via heparin-like molecules bound to the endothelium. J Clin Invest 1984; 74:341–350.
3. Hoylaerts M, Rijken DC, Lijnen HR, et al. Kinetics of the activation of plasminogen by human tissue plasminogen activator. Role of fibrin. J Biol Chem 1982; 257:2912–2919.
4. Ikonomidis I, Andreotti F, Economu E, et al. Increased proinflammatory cytokines in patients with chronic stable angina and their reduction by aspirin. Circulation 1999; 100:793–798.
5. Feldman M, Jialal I, Devaraj S and Cryer B. Effects of low-dose aspirin on serum C-reactive protein and thromboxane B2 concentrations: a placebo-controlled study using a highly sensitive C-eactive protein assay. J Am Coll Cardiol 2001; 37:2036–2041.
6. Ridker PM, Cushman M, Stampfer MJ, et al. Inflammation, aspirin, and the risk of cardiovascular disease in apparently healthy men [published erratum appears in N Engl J Med 1997; 337(5):356]. N Eng J Med 1997; 336:973–979.
7. Hankey GJ, Eikelboom JW. New Drugs, old drugs: antiplatelet drugs. MJA 2003; 178:568–574.
8. Cairns JA, Gent M, Singer J, et al. Aspirin, sulfinpyrazone, or both in unstable angina. Results of a Canadian multicenter trial. N Engl J Med 1985; 313:1369–1375.
9. Risk of MI and death during treatment with low dose aspirin and intravenous heparin in men with unstable coronary artery disease. The RISC group. Lancet 1990; 336:827–830.
10. Braunwald E, Antman E, Beasley J, et al. ACC/AHA 2002 guideline update for the management of patients with unstable angina and non-ST-segment elevation MI-summary article. A report of the American college of cardiology/american heart association task force on practice guideline (committee on the management of patient with unstable angina). J Am Coll Cardiol 2002; 40:1366–1374.
11. Theroux P, Ouimet H, McCans J, et al. Aspirin, heparin, or both to treat acute unstable angina. N Engl J Med 1988; 319:1105–1111.
12. Warkentin TE, Levine MN, Hirsh J, et al. Heparin-induced thrombocytopenia in patients treated with low-molecular-weight heparin or unfractionated heparin. N Engl J Med 1995; 332:1330–1335.
13. Telford AM, Wilson C. Trial of heparin versus atenolol in prevention of MI in intermittent coronary syndrome. Lancet 1981; 1:1225–1228.
14. Neri Serneri GG, Gensini GF, Poggesi L, et al. Effect of heparin, aspirin, or alteplase in reduction of myocardial ischemia in refractory unstable angina. Lancet 1990; 335:615–618.
15. Oler A, Whooley MA, Oler J, and Grady, D. Adding heparin to aspirin reduces the incidence of MI and death in patients with unstable angina. JAMA 1996; 276:811–815.

16. Cohen M, Demers C, Gurfinkel EP, et al. For the efficacy and safety of subcutaneous enoxaparin in Non-Q wave coronary events study group. A comparison of low-molecular weight heparin with unfractionated heparin for unstable coronary artery disease. N Engl J Med 1997; 337:447–452.

17. Goodman SG, Cohen M, Bigonzi F, et al. Randomized trial of low molecular weight heparin (enoxaparin) versus unfractionated heparin for unstable coronary artery disease: one-year results of the ESSENCE study. Efficacy and safety of subcutaneous enoxaparin in Non–Q wave coronary events. J Am Coll Cardiol 2000; 36:693–698.

18. Berkowitz SD, Stinnett S, Cohen M, et al. Prospective comparison of hemorrhagic complications after treatment with enoxaparin versus unfractionated heparin for unstable angina pectoris or non-T-segment elevation acute MI. Am J Cardiol 2001; 88:1230–1234.

19. Mark DB, Cowper PA, Berkowitz SD, et al. Economic assessment of low-molecular-weight heparin (enoxaparin) versus unfractionated heparin in acute coronary syndrome patients: results from the ESSENCE randomized trial. Circulation 1998; 97:1702–1707.

20. Antman EM, McCabe CH, Gurfinkel EP, et al. Enoxaparin prevents death and cardiac ischemic events in unstable Angina/Non-Q-wave MI: results of the thrombolysis in MI (TIMI) 11B trial. Circulation 1999; 100:1593.

21. Ferguson JJ, Califf RM, Antmen EM, et al. Enoxaparin vs unfractionated heparin in high-risk patients with non-ST-segment elevation acute coronary syndromes managed with an intended early invasive strategy: primary results of the SYNERGY randomized trial. JAMA 2004; 292:45–54.

22. Bhatt DL, Topol EJ. Current role of platelet glycoprotein IIb/IIIa inhibitors in acute coronary syndromes. JAMA 2000; 284:1549–1558.

23. The EPIC investigators. Use of a monoclonal antibody directed against the platelet glycoprotein IIb/IIIa receptor in high-risk coronary angioplasty. The epic investigation. N Engl J Med 1994; 330:956–961.

24. The EPILOG investigators. Platelet glycoprotein IIb/IIIa receptor blockade and low-dose heparin during percutaneous coronary revascularization. N Engl J Med 1997; 336:1689–1696.

25. Dasgupta H, Blankenship JC, Wood GC, et al. Thrombocytopenia complicating treatment with intravenous glycoprotein IIb/IIIa receptor inhibitors: a pooled analysis. Am Heart J 2000; 140:206–211.

26. Sane DC, Damaraju LV, and Topol EJ. Occurrence and clinical significance of pseudothrombocytopenia during abciximab therapy. J Am Coll Cardiol 2000; 36:75–83.

27. Effects of platelet glycoprotein IIb/IIIa blockade with tirofiban on adverse cardiac events in patients with unstable angina or acute MI undergoing coronary angioplasty. The RESTORE Investigators. Randomized efficacy study of tirofiban for outcomes and restenosis. Circulation 1997; 96:1445–1453.

28. Harrington RA, Kleiman NS, Kottke-Marchant K, et al. Immediate and reversible platelet inhibition after intravenous administration of a peptide glycoprotein IIb/IIIa inhibitor during percutaneous coronary intervention. Am J Cardiol 1995; 76:1222–1227.

29. The PURSUIT trial investigators. Inhibition of platelet glycoprotein IIb/IIIa with eptifibatide in patients with acute coronary syndromes. New Engl J Med 1998; 339:436–443.

30. Simoons ML. Effect of glycoprotein IIb/IIIa receptor blocker abciximab on outcome in patients with acute coronary syndromes without early coronary revascularization: the GUSTO IV-ACS randomised trial. Lancet 2001; 357:1915–1924.

31. Ottervanger JP, Armstrong P, Barnathan ES, et al. Long-term results after the glycoprotein IIb/IIIa inhibitor abciximab in unstable angina: One-year survival in the GUSTO IV-ACS (Global use of strategies to open occluded coronary arteries IV-acute coronary syndrome) Trial. Circulation 2003; 107:437–442.

32. The clopidogrel in unstable angina to prevent recurrent events (CURE) trial investigators. Effects of clopidogrel in addition to aspirin in patients with acute coronary syndromes without ST-segment elevation. N Engl J Med 2001; 345:494–502.

33. Merritt JC, Bhatt DL. The efficacy and safety of perioperative antiplatelet therapy. J Thromb Thrombolysis 2004; 17:21–27.

34. Yusuf S, Mehta SR, Zhao F, et al. on behalf of the CURE (Clopidogrel in unstable angina to prevent recurrent events) trial investigators. Early and late effects of clopidogrel in patients with acute coronary syndromes. Circulation 2003; 107:966–972.

35. Bhatt DL, Topol EJ. On behalf of the CHARISMA Executive committee. Clopidogrel added to aspirin versus aspirin alone in secondary prevention and high-risk primary prevention: Rationale and design of the clopidogrel for high atherothrombotic risk and ischemic stabilization, management and avoidance (CHARISMA) trial. Am Heart J 2004; 148:263–268.

36. Tan K, Sulke N, Taub N, Sowton E. Clinical and lesion morphologic determinants of coronary angioplasty success and complications: current experience. J Am Coll Cardiol 1995; 25:855–865.

37. Lembo NJ, Black AJ, Roubin GS, et al. Effect of pretreatment with aspirin versus aspirin plus dipyridamole on frequency and type of acute complications of percutaneous transluminal coronary angioplasty. Am J Cardiol 1990; 65:422–426.

38. Mufson L, Black A, Roubin G, et al. A randomized trial of aspirin in PCI: effect of high dose versus low dose aspirin on major complications and restenosis. J Am Coll Cardiol 1988; 11:236A.

39. Garachemani AR, Kaufmann U, Fleisch M, et al. Prolonged heparin after uncomplicated coronary interventions: a prospective, randomized trial. Am Heart J 1998; 136:352–356.

40. Serruys PW, de Jaegere P, Kiemeneij F, et al. A comparison of balloon-expandable-stent implantation with balloon angioplasty in patients with coronary artery disease. N Engl J Med 1994; 331: 89–495.

41. Leon MB, Baim DS, Popma JJ, et al. For the stent anticoagulation restenosis study investigators. A clinical trial comparing three antithrombotic-drug regimens after coronary artery stenting. N Engl J Med 1998; 339:1665–1671.

42. Bertrand ME, Rupprecht HJ, Urban P, et al. Double-blind study of the safety of clopidogrel with and without a loading dose in combination with aspirin compared with ticlopidine in combination with aspirin after coronary stenting; the clopidogrel aspirin stent international cooperative study (CLASSICS). Circulation 2000; 102:624–629.

43. Bhatt DL, Bertrand ME, Berger PB, et al. Meta-analysis of randomized and registry comparisons of ticlopidine with clopidogrel after stenting. J Am Coll Cardiol 2002; 39:9–14.

44. Moussa I, Oetgen M, Roubin G, et al. Effectiveness of clopidogrel and aspirin versus ticlopidine and aspirin in preventing stent thrombosis after coronary stent implantation. Circulation 1999; 99:2364–2366.

45. Mehta SR, Yusuf S, Peters RJ, et al. Effects of pretreatment with clopidogrel and aspirin followed by long-term therapy in patients undergoing percutaneous coronary intervention: the PCI-CURE study. Lancet 2001; 358:527–533.

46. Steinhubl ST, Berger PB, Mann JT III, et al. Early and sustained dual oral antiplatelet therapy following percutaneous coronary intervention: a randomized controlled trial. JAMA 2002; 288:2411–2420.

47. Kandzari DE, Berger PB, Kastrati A, et al. Influence of treatment duration with a 600-mg dose of clopidogrel before percutaneous coronary revascularization. J Am Coll Cardiol 2004; 44:2133–2136.

48. Patti G, Colonna G, Pasceri V, et al. Randomized trial of high loading dose of clopidogrel for reduction of periprocedural MI in patients undergoing coronary intervention: results from the ARMYDA-2 (Antiplatelet therapy for reduction of myocardial damage during angioplasty) study. Circulation 2005; 111:2099–2106.

49. Karvouni E, Katritsis DG, Ioannidis JP. Intravenous glycoprotein IIb/IIIa receptor antagonists reduce mortality after percutaneous coronary interventions. J Am Coll Cardiol 2003; 41:26–32.

50. Lincoff AM, Calleff RM, Moliterno DJ, et al. For the evaluation of platelet IIb/IIIa inhibition in stenting investigators. Complimentary clinical benefits of coronary — artery stenting and blockade of platelet glycoprotein IIb/IIIa receptors. N Engl J Med 1999; 341:319–327.

51. Topol EJ, Mark DB, Lincoff AM, et al. Outcomes at 1 year and economic implication of platelet glycoprotein IIb/IIIa blockade in patients undergoing coronary stenting: results from a multicentre randomized trial. EPISTENT investigators. Evaluation of platelet IIb/IIIa inhibitor for stenting. lancet 1999; 354:2019–2024.

52. Topol EJ, Lincoff AM, Kereiakes DJ, et al. Multi-year follow-up of abciximab therapy in three randomized, placebo-controlled trials of percutaneous coronary revascularization. Am J Med 2002; 113:1–6.

53. Bhatt DL, Marso SP, Lincoff AM, et al. Abciximab reduces mortality in diabetics following percutaneous coronary intervention. J Am Coll Cardiol 2000; 35:922–928.

54. Novel dosing regimen of eptifibatide in planned coronary stent implantation (ESPRIT): a randomized, placebo-controlled trial. The ESPRIT Investigators. Enhanced suppression of the platelet IIb/IIIA receptor with integrillin therapy. Lancet 2000; 356:2037–2044.

55. Stone GW, Grines CL, Cox DA, et al. Comparison of angioplasty with stenting, with or without abciximab, in acute MI. N Engl J Med 2002; 346:957–966.

56. Montalescot G, Barragan P, Wittenberg O, et al. For the ADMIRAL investigators. Platelet glycoprotein IIb/IIIA inhibition with coronary stenting for acute MI. N Engl J Med 2001; 344:1895–1903.

57. Kastrati A, Mehilli J, Schuhlen H, et al. A clinical trial of abciximab in elective percutaneous coronary intervention after pretreatment with clopidogrel. N Engl J Med 2004; 350:232–238.

58. Topol EJ, Moliterno DJ, Herrmann HC, et al. For the TARGET investigators. Comparison of two platelet glycoprotein IIb/IIIa inhibitors, tirofiban and abciximab, for the prevention of ischemic events with percutaneous coronary revascularization. N Engl J Med 2001; 344:1888–1894.

59. Lincoff AM, Bittle JA, Kleiman NS, et al. For the REPLACE–1 investigators. Comparison of bivalirudin versus heparin during percutaneous coronary intervention (the randomized evaluation of PCI linking Angiomax to reduced clinical events [REPLACE]–1 trial). Am J Cardiol 2004; 93:1092–1096.

60. Lewis BE, Matthai WH, Cohen M, et al. for the ARG-216/310/311 study investigators. Coronary intervention in patients with heparin-induced thrombocytopenia. Cathet Cardiovasc Intervent 2002; 57:177–184.

61. Lincoff AM, Kleiman NS, Kereiakes DJ, et al. For the REPLACE–2 investigators. Long-term efficacy of bivalirudin and provisional glycoprotein IIb/IIIa blockade vs heparin and planned glycoprotein IIb/IIIa blockade during percutaneous coronary revascularization: REPLACE–2 randomized trial. JAMA 2004; 292:696–703.

62. Chew DP, Lincoff AM, Gurm H, et al. Bivalirudin versus heparin and glycoprotein IIb/IIIa inhibition among patients with renal impairment undergoing percutaneous coronary intervention (A subanalysis of the REPLACE-2 trial). Am J Cardiol 2005; 95: 581–585.

63. Gurm HS, Sarembock IJ, Kereiakis DJ, et al. Use of bivalirudin during percutaneous coronary intervention in patients with diabetes mellitus. J Am Coll Cardiol 2005; 45: 1932–1938.

64. Gurm HS, Rajagopal V, Fathi R, et al. Effectiveness and safety of bivalirudin during percutaneous coronary intervention in a single medical center. Am J Cardiol 2005; 95: 16–721.

65. Cohen DJ, Lincoff AM, Lavelle TA, et al. On behalf of the REPLACE–2 investigators. Economic evaluation of bivalirudin with provisional glycoprotein IIb/IIIa inhibition versus heparin with routine glycoprotein IIb/IIIa inhibition for percutaneous coronary intervention: results from the REPLACE–2 trial. J Am Coll Cardiol 2004; 44:1792–1800.

66. Schussler JM, Cameron CS, Azam A, et al. Effect of bivalirudin on length of stay in the recovery area after percutaneous coronary intervention compared with heparin alone, heparin + abciximab, or heparin + eptifibatide. Am J Cardiol 2004; 94:1417–1419.

67. Stone GW, Bertrand M, Colombo A, et al. Acute catheterization and urgent intervention triage strategY (ACUITY) trial: study design and rationale. Am Heart J 2004; 148:764–765.

68. Ridker PM, Cook NR, Lee IM, et al. A randomized trial of low-dose aspirin in the primary prevention of cardiovascular disease in women. New Engl J Med 2005; 352:293–1304.

69. Steering committee of the physicians' health study research group. Final report on the aspirin component of the ongoing physician's health study. N Engl J Med 1989; 321:129–135.

70. Peto R, Gray R, Collins R, et al. Randomised trial of prophylactic daily aspirin in British male doctors. Br Med J (Clin Res Ed) 1988; 296: 313–316.

71. Hansson L, Zanchett A, Carruthers SG, et al. Effects of intensive blood-pressure lowering and low-dose aspirin in patients with hypertension: principal results of the hypertension optimal treatment (HOT) randomized trial. Lancet 1998; 351:1755–1762.

72. Low-dose aspirin and vitamin E in people at cardiovascular risk: a randomized trial in general practice. Collaborative group of the primary prevention project. Lancet 2001; 357:89–95.

73. Thrombosis prevention trial: randomized trial of low-intensity oral anticoagulation with warfarin and low-dose aspirin in the primary prevention of ischaemic heart disease in men at increased risk. The medical research council's general practice research framework. Lancet 1998; 351:233–241.

74. Pearson TA, Blear SN, Daniels ST, et al. AHA Guideline for primary prevention of cardiovascular disease and stroke: 2002 update: consensus panel guide to comprehensive risk reduction for adult patients without coronary or other atherosclerotic vascular diseases. American heart association science advisory and coordinating committee. Circulation 2002; 106:388.

75. US preventive services task force. Guide to clinical preventive services, 3rd ed, 2000–2002. http://www.ahrq.gov/clinic/prevnew.htm

76. Wilson PW, D'Agostino R, Levy D, et al. Prediction of coronary heart disease using risk factor categories. Circulation 1998; 97:1837–1847.

77. Morimoto T, Fukui T, Lee T and Matsui K. Application of U.S. guidelines in other countries: aspirin for the primary prevention of cardiovascular events in Japan. Amer J Med 2004; 117:459–468.

78. Antithrombotic trialists' collaboration. secondary prevention of vascular events by prolonged antiplatelet therapy. BMJ 1988; 296:320–331.

79. Antiplatelet trialists' collaboration. Collaborative overview of randomised trials of antiplatelet therapy: I. prevention of death, MI, and stroke by prolonged antiplatelet therapy in various categories of patients. BMJ 1994; 308(6291):81–106.

80. Antithrombotic trialists' collaboration. Collaborative meta-analysis of randomized trials of antiplatelet therapy for prevention of death, MI, and stroke in high risk patients. BMJ 2002; 324(7329):71–86.

81. Kong D. Aspirin in cardiovascular disorders. What is the optimum dose? Am J Cardiovasc Drugs 2004; 4(3):151–158.

82. Catella-Lawson F, Reilly M, Kapoor S, et al. Cyclooxygenase inhibitors and the antiplatelet effects of aspirin. N Engl J Med 2001; 345 (25):1809–1817.

83. Capone ML, Sciulli MG, Tacconelli ST, et al. Pharmacodynamic interaction of naproxen with low-dose aspirin in healthy subjects. J Am Coll Card 2005; 45:1295–1301.

84. MacDonald TM, Wei L. Effect of ibuprofen on cardioprotective effect of aspirin. Lancet 2003; 361:573–574.

85. Patel TN, Goldberg KC. Use of aspirin and ibuprofen compared with aspirin alone and the risk of MI. Arch Intern Med 2004; 164:852–856.

86. Bhatt DL. Aspirin resistance: more than just a laboratory curiosity. J Am Coll Cardiol 2004; 43:1127–1129.

87. Sanderson S, Emery J, Baglin T, et al. Narrative review: aspirin resistance and its clinical implications. Ann Int Med 2005; 142:370–380.

88. Roller RE, Dorr A, Ulrish S, Pilger E. Effect of aspirin treatment in patients with peripheral arterial disease monitored with the platelet function analyzer PFA-100. Blood Coagul Fibrinolysis 2002; 13:277–281.

89. The CAPRIE steering committee. A randomized, blinded, trial of clopidogrel versus aspirin in patients at risk of ischemic events (CAPRIE). Lancet 1996; 348:1329–1339.

90. Cannon CP, on behalf of the CAPRIE investigators. Effectiveness of clopidogrel versus aspirin in preventing acute MI in patients with symptomatic atherothrombosis (CAPRIE trial). Am J Cardiol 2002; 90:760–762.

91. Bhatt DL, Marso SP, Hirsch AT, et al. Amplified benefit of clopidogrel versus aspirin in patients with diabetes mellitus. Am J Cardiol 2002; 90:625–628.

92. Ringleb PA, Bhatt DL, Hirsch AT, et al. Benefit of clopidogrel over aspirin is amplified in patients with a history of ischemic events. Stroke 2004; 35:528–532.

93. Bhatt DL, Chew DP, Hirsch AT, et al. Superiority of clopidogrel versus aspirin in patients with prior cardiac surgery. Circulation 2001; 103:363–368.

94. Nguyen TA, Diodati JG, Pharand C. Resistance to clopidogrel: a review of the evidence. J Am Coll Cardiol 2005; 45:1157–1164.

95. Serebruany VL, Steinhubl SR, Berger PB, et al. Variability in platelet responsiveness to clopidogrel in 544 patients. J Am Coll Cardiol 2005; 45:246–251.

96. Matetzky S, Shenkman B, Guetta V, et al. Clopidogrel resistance is associated with increased risk of recurrent atherothrombotic events in patients with acute MI. Circulation 2004; 109:3171–3175.

97. Topol EJ, Easton D, Harrington RA, et al. On behalf of the blockade of the glycoprotein IIb/IIIa receptor to avoid vascular occlusion (BRAVO) trial investigators. Randomized, double-blind, placebo-controlled, international trial of the oral IIb/IIIa antagonist Lotrafiban in coronary and cerebrovascular disease. Circulation 2003; 108:399–406.

98. Chew DP, Bhatt DL, Sapp S, et al. Increased mortality with oral platelet glycoprotein IIb/IIIa antagonists: a meta-analysis of phase III multicenter randomized trials. Circulation 2001; 103:201–206.

99. van Es RF, Jonker JJ, Verheugt FWA, et al. Aspirin and Coumadin after acute coronary syndromes (the ASPECT-2 study): a randomised controlled trial. Lancet 2002; 360:109–113.

100. Fiore LD, Ezekowirz MD, Brophy MT, et al. Department of veterans affairs cooperative studies program clinical trial comparing combined warfarin and aspirin with aspirin alone in survivors of acute MI. Primary results of the CHAMP study. Circulation 2002; 105:557–563.

101. Hurlen M, Abdelnoor M, Smith P, et al. Warfarin, aspirin or both after MI. N Engl J Med 2002; 347:969–974.

102. Fiessinger JN, Huisman MV, Davidson BL, et al. For the THRIVE treatment study investigators. Ximelagatran vs. low-molecular-weight heparin and warfarin for the treatment of deep vein thrombosis: a randomized trial. JAMA 2005; 293:681–689.

103. Wallentin L, Wilcox RG, Weaver WD, et al. Oral Ximelagatran for secondary prophylaxis after MI: the ESTEEM randomised controlled trial. Lancet 2003; 362:789–797.

104. Go AS, Hylek EM, Phillips JA, et al. Prevalence of diagnosed atrial fibrillation in adults: national implications for rhythm management and stroke prevention: the anticoagulation and risk factors in atrial fibrillation (ATRIA) study. JAMA 2001; 285:2370–2375.

105. Lip GY. Does atrial fibrillation confer a hypercoagulable state? Lancet 1995; 346:1313–1314.

106. Singer DE, Albers GW, Dalen JE, et al. Antithrombotic therapy in atrial fibrillation: the seventh ACCP conference on antithrombotic and thrombolytic therapy. Chest 2004; 126:429S–456S.

107. Peterson P, Boysen G, Godtfredsen J et al. Placebo-controlled, randomized trial of warfarin and aspirin for prevention of thromboembolic complications in chronic atrial fibrillation. Lancet 1989; 1:175–179.

108. Stroke prevention in atrial fibrillation investigators. Stroke prevention in atrial fibrillation study: final results. Circulation 1991; 84:527–539.

109. Boston area anticoagulation trial for atrial fibrillation investigators. The effect of low-dose warfarin on the risk of stroke in patients with nonrheumatic atrial fibrillation. N Engl J Med 1990; 323:1505–1511.

110. Connolly SJ, Laupacis A, Gent M, et al. Canadian atrial fibrillation anticoagulation (CAFA) study. J Am Coll Cardiol 1991; 18:349–355.

111. Ezekowitz MD, Bridgers SL, James KE, et al. Warfarin in the prevention of stroke associated with nonrheumatic atrial fibrillation. N Engl J Med 1992; 327:1406–1412.

112. Atrial fibrillation investigators. Risk factors for stroke and efficacy of antithrombotic therapy in atrial fibrillation: analysis of pooled data from five randomized controlled trials. Arch Intern Med 1994; 154:1449–1457.

113. Atrial fibrillation investigators. The efficacy of aspirin in patients with atrial fibrillation: analysis of pooled data from 3 randomized trials. Arch Intern Med 1997; 157:1237–1240.

114. Hart RG, Benavente O, McBride R, et al. Antithrombotic therapy to prevent stroke in patients with atrial fibrillation: a meta-analysis. Ann Intern Med 1999; 131:492–501.

115. van Walraven C, Hart RG, Singer DE, et al. Oral anticoagulants vs. aspirin in nonvalvular atrial fibrillation-an individual patient meta-analysis. JAMA 2002; 288:2441–2448.

116. The executive steering committee on behalf of the SPORTIF III investigators. Stroke prevention with the oral direct thrombin inhibitor Ximelagatran compared with warfarin in patients with non-valvular atrial fibrillation (SPORTIF III): randomised controlled trial. Lancet 2003; 362:1691–1698.

117. The executive steering committee on behalf of the SPORTIF V investigators. Ximelagatran vs warfarin for stroke prevention in patients with nonvalvular atrial fibrillation: a randomized trial. JAMA 2005; 293:690–698.

118. O'Brien CL and Gage BF. Costs and effectiveness of Ximelagatran for stroke prophylaxis in chronic atrial fibrillation. JAMA 2005; 293:699–706.

119. AFFIRM investigators. A comparison of rate control and rhythm control in patients with atrial fibrillation. N Engl J Med 2002; 347:1825–1833.

120. Van Gelder IC, Hegens VE, Bosker HA, et al. A comparison of rate control and rhythm control in patients with recurrent persistent atrial fibrillation. N Engl J Med 2002; 347:1834–1840.

121. Jordaens L, Missault L, Germonpre E, et al. Delayed restoration of atrial function after conversion of atrial flutter by pacing or electrical cardioversion. Am J Cardiol 1993; 71:63–67.

122. Fuster V, Gersh BT, Giuliani ER, et al. The natural history of idiopathic dilated cardiomyopathy. Am J Cardiol 1981; 47:525–531.

123. Lip GY, Gibbs CR. Does heart failure confer a hypercoagulable state? Virchow's triad revisited. J Am Coll Card 1999; 33:1424–1426.

124. Loh E, Sutton MS, Wun C-CC, et al. Ventricular dysfunction and the risk of stroke after MI. N Engl J Med 1997; 336:251–257.

125. Lip GY, Gibbs CR. Antiplatelet agents versus control or anticoagulation for heart failure in sinus rhythm: a Cochran systematic review. QJM 2002; 95:461–468.

126. Dunkman, WB, Johnson GR, Carson PE, et al. For the V–HeFT VA cooperative studies group. Incidence of thromboembolic events in congestive heart failure. Circulation 1993; 87(Suppl. VI):VI94–VI101.

127. Al-Khadra AS, Salem DN, Rand WM, et al. Antiplatelet agents and survival: a cohort analysis from the studies of left ventricular dysfunction (SOLVD) trial. J Am Coll Card 1998; 32:419–425.

128. Serebruany VL, Malinin AI, Jerome SD, et al. Effects of clopidogrel and aspirin combination versus aspirin alone on platelet aggregation and major receptor expression in patients with heart failure: the Plavix use for treatment of congestive heart failure (PLUTO-CHF) trial. Am Heart J 2003; 146:713–720.

129. Al-Khadra AS, Salem DN, Rand WM, et al. Warfarin anticoagulation and survival: a cohort analysis from the studies of left ventricular dysfunction. J Am Coll Card 1998; 31:749–753.

130. Cleland JG, Findlay I, Jafri S, et al. The Warfarin/Aspirin study in heart failure (WASH): a randomized trial comparing antithrombotic strategies for patients with heart failure. Am Heart J 2004; 148:157–164.

131. Aumegeat V, Lamblin N, de Groote P, et al. Aspirin does not adversely affect survival in patient with stable congestive heart failure treated with angiotensin-converting enzyme inhibitors. Chest 2003; 124:1250–1258.

132. Cushman M, Tsai AW, White RH, et al. Deep vein thrombosis and pulmonary embolism in two cohorts: the longitudinal investigation of thromboembolism etiology. Am J Med 2004; 117:19–25.

133. Wells, et al. Thromb Haemost 2000; 83:416–420.

134. Qanadli SD, El Hajjam M, Mesurolle B, et al. Pulmonary embolism detection: prospective evaluation of dual-section helical CT versus selective pulmonary arteriography in 157 patients. Radiology 2000; 217:447–455.

135. Hirsh J, Bates SM. Clinical trials that have influenced the treatment of venous thromboembolism: a historical perspective. Ann Intern Med 2001; 134:409–417.

136. Raschke RA, Reilly BM, Guidry JR, et al. The weight-based heparin dosing nomogram compared with a "standard care" nomogram. Ann Intern Med 1993; 119:874–881.

137. Hull RD, Raskob GE, Rosenbloom D, et al. Heparin for 5 days as compared with 10 days in the initial treatment of proximal venous thrombosis. New Eng J Med 1990; 322:1260–1264.

138. Siragusa S, Cosmi B, Piovella F, et al. Low molecular weight heparins and unfractionated heparin in the treatment of patients with acute venous thromboembolism: results of a meta-analysis. Am J Med 1996; 100:269–277.

139. Hull RD, Raskob GE, Rosenbloom D, et al. Treatment of proximal vein thrombosis with subcutaneous low molecular weight heparin vs intravenous heparin. An economic perspective. Arch Intern Med 1997; 157:289–294.

140. Buller HR, Agnelli G, Hull R, et al. Antithrombotic therapy for venous thromboembolic disease: The seventh ACCP conference on antithrombotic and thrombolytic therapy. Chest 2004; 126:401S–428S.

141. Geerts WH, Pineo GF, Heit JA, et al. Prevention of venous thromboembolism: the seventh ACCP conference on antithrombotic and thrombolytic therapy. Chest 2004; 126: 338S–400S.

142. Graor RA, Stewart JH, Lotke PA, et al. RD heparin (ardeparin sodium) vs. aspirin to prevent deep venous thrombosis after hip or knee replacement surgery [abstract]. Chest 1992; 102:118S.

143. Evans HC, Perry CM, and Faulds D. Ximelagatran/melagatran: a review of its use in the prevention of venous thromboembolism in orthopedic surgery. Drugs 2004; 64:649–678.

144. Goldhaber SZ, Monson JE, Stampfer MJ, et al. Low-dose aspirin and subsequent peripheral arterial surgery in the physicians' health study. Lancet 1992; 340:143–145.

145. Hood SC, Moher D, Barber GG. Management of intermittent claudication with pentoxifylline: meta-analysis of randomized controlled trials. CMAJ 1996; 155:1053–1059.

146. Dawson DL, Cutler BS, Hiatt WR, et al. A comparison of Cilostazol and pentoxifylline for treating intermittent claudication. Am J Med 2000; 109:523–530.

147. Thompson PD, Zimet R, Forbes WP, Zhang P. Meta-analysis of results from eight randomized, placebo-controlled trials on the effect of Cilostazol on patients with intermittent claudication. Am J Cardiol 2002; 90:1314–1319.

148. Visseren FL, Eikkelboom BC. Oral anticoagulant therapy in patients with peripheral artery disease. Sem Vasc Med 2003; 3:339–344.

149. Conde ID, Kleiman NS. Patient-specific antiplatelet therapy. J Thromb Thrombolysis 2004; 17:63–77.

150. Serebruany VL, Steinhubl SR, Berger PB, et al. Analysis of risk of bleeding complications after different doses of aspirin in 192,036 patients enrolled in 31 randomized controlled trials. Am J Cardiol 2005; 95:1218–1222.

15 | Congestive Heart Failure: Epidemiology, Pathophysiology, and Current Therapies

Nicolas W. Shammas
Midwest Cardiovascular Research Foundation, Cardiovascular Medicine, P.C., Davenport, Iowa and University of Iowa Hospitals and Clinics, Iowa City, Iowa, U.S.A.

KEY POINTS

- Modifiable pathophysiologic mechanisms for congestive heart failure (CHF) include the sympathetic nervous system (SNS) and the renin–angiotensin–aldosterone system (RAAS).
- Risk factors for development of CHF including diabetes, coronary artery disease (CAD), and hypertension need to be aggressively managed to reduce left ventricular systolic and/or diastolic dysfunction.
- Treatment of chronic symptomatic CHF consists of diuretics, beta-blockers, angiotensin-converting enzyme inhibitors (ACEIs) [or angiotensin receptor blockers (ARB) as an alternative], and aldosterone antagonists.
- The use of intravenous (IV) inotropes in acute decompensated heart failure should be discouraged except to achieve hemodynamic stability.
- Mechanical devices to treat CHF include biventricular pacing, implantable cardioverter defibrillator (ICD), or left ventricular assist device (LVAD), and need to be considered for eligible patients.
- Diastolic dysfunction needs to be considered as a cause of heart failure when CHF is present in the setting of normal left ventricular systolic function. Treatment consists of diuresis, beta-blockers or verapamil, and an ACEI.

EPIDEMIOLOGY OF CHF

CHF is a clinical syndrome resulting from the inability of the heart to pump adequate amount of blood to meet the demands of the body. It can be caused by an impaired left ventricular (LV) systolic function (systolic failure) or a reduced ability of the heart to relax despite normal systolic function (diastolic failure).

CHF is highly prevalent in the United States and is a leading cause of hospitalization in the elderly (1). Over 500,000 new cases are diagnosed annually costing our health-care system US $40 billion (2) with subsequent high mortality (3). Although systolic failure has been the main focus of CHF studies, diastolic failure occurs in approximately 30% to 35% and 55% in all patients and in the elderly with CHF, respectively (4,5). We tend to separate systolic failure from diastolic failure, but it should be noted that this division is arbitrary as patients with systolic failure can have diastolic failure and vice versa (6).

The number of hospitalization for CHF in the United States is rising in both males and females (2), and is partly due to the high prevalence of hypertension, diabetes, and obesity (7). Recent advances in the management of CHF have not had a significant impact on the incidence of patients with CHF, at least as practiced in the community (8). Survival from heart failure over the past two decades might be improving after diagnosis mostly among men and younger persons with less improvement in the elderly and women (9). Data from the Framingham Heart Study suggested that survival, however, might be improving in both sexes over the past 50 years (10). The continued rise in CHF incidence will pose a significant burden on our society, unless drastic changes are undertaken in prevention and therapy (11).

PATHOPHYSIOLOGY OF CHF

CHF results from several potential injuries to the myocardium (12,13) including CAD, hypertension, valvular heart disease, diabetes, congenital heart defects, anemia, and alcoholism. Injury to the LV leads to LV remodeling defined as stretching and dilatation of the LV cavity size with subsequent reduction in ejection fraction (EF). LV remodeling following injury is an attempt to reduce wall stress and increase cardiac output by hypertrophy of viable myocytes

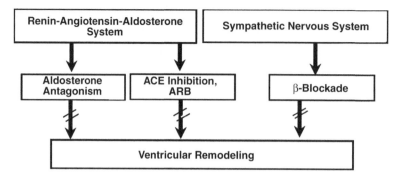

FIGURE 1   The renin-angiotensin-aldosterone system and the sympathetic nervous system promote ventricular remodeling, a process that can be reversed with aldosterone antagonism, ACEI and beta blockers.

(increase in cell length more than width). However, this process leads to an increase in mass-to-volume ratio and subsequently the vicious cycle of further increase in wall stress and premature myocyte cell death occurs (14). The reduction in EF leads to the symptoms of CHF including dyspnea, orthopnea, paroxysmal nocturnal dyspnea, chest pain, fatigue, and overall reduced functional capacity. Also the reduction in EF is a prognostic indicator of increased mortality, arrhythmias, and sudden cardiac death (15,16).

The RAAS and SNS play a major role in the cardiac remodeling process (Fig. 1). Activation of the RAAS system leads to (i) endothelial damage; (ii) sodium retention and myocardial fibrosis mediated by angiotensin II (AII) and aldosterone; (iii) peripheral vasoconstriction; and (iv) a rise in AII (17), which leads to programmed cell death (apoptosis), hypertrophy, and fibrosis. AII also promotes aldosterone secretion. In addition, a rise in endothelin-1 production, reduced synthesis and release of nitric oxide (NO), increased degradation of NO, and formation of reactive oxygen species occur and contribute to vasoconstriction (17–19). Furthermore, inflammatory markers and cytokines are increased thereby further exacerbating endothelial dysfunction (18,20,21).

Elevated sympathetic tone is also an integral part of heart failure. A rise in circulating levels of catecholamines in response to SNS activation leads to suppression of adrenergic receptors (22), has direct toxic effects on the myocardium (23), increases myocardial oxygen consumption and coronary blood flow requirements, decreases myocardial mechanical efficiency, induces LV hypertrophy, and precipitates potentially debilitating and fatal arrhythmias (24). Catecholamines mediate toxicity as a result of beta-adrenoceptor–mediated cyclic adenosine monophosphate–dependent calcium overload of cardiac myocytes (25).

Pharmacologic interventions that block neurohormonal activation can reduce mortality and morbidity in patients with CHF. Blocking AII and catecholamines alone is not optimal because aldosterone "escapes" angiotensin suppression (26) and needs to be selectively blocked for additional reduction in mortality and morbidity (27,28) (Fig. 2). Data also suggests that beta-adrenergic blockade may diminish activity of the RAAS and vice versa (29) thereby reducing the harmful effects of the neurohormonal cycle in CHF. Other therapies have been considered in CHF and include vasopeptidase inhibitors, endothelin antagonists, immunomodulating agents, and growth hormone (30), all of which have shown conflicting results. In this chapter, we will focus primarily on proven therapies that alter morbidity and mortality of patients with CHF.

ACC/AHA CLASSIFICATION OF CHF

A relatively new classification for CHF was recently proposed by the American College of Cardiology/American Heart Association (ACC)/(AHA) (3), which takes into account the pathophysiology of CHF. This new classification complements the New York Heart Classification (NYHC) and is not intended to replace it (31). Four stages have been proposed and include the following:

Stage A: Asymptomatic patients with no LV dysfunction are at risk of developing CHF. Over 60 million people fall in this category and include those with CAD, hypertension,

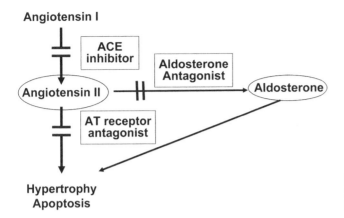

Angiotensin I

Hypertrophy
Apoptosis

FIGURE 2 Pharmacologic interventions that block the renin-angiotension-aldosterone system.

diabetes mellitus, and a family history of cardiomyopathy (CM). Stage A is not represented in the NYHC.

Stage B: Asymptomatic patients with LV dysfunction. This is equivalent to class I of the NYHC. In the United States, there are about 10 million people in stage B.

Stage C: Symptomatic patients with exertion and with LV dysfunction. This is equivalent to the NYHC class II and class III and includes about five million people in the United States.

Stage D: Symptomatic patients at rest. This is equivalent to class IV of the NYHC and includes about 200,000 people in the United States.

The ACC/AHA classification focuses on the pathophysiology of CHF, emphasizing the importance of recognizing its risk factors. The new classification helps physicians treating patients with hypertension and diabetes as early CHF patients where aggressive management of these risk factors is expected to reduce the evolution to symptomatic failure.

PHARMACOLOGIC THERAPY OF CHF
Diastolic Dysfunction

Diastolic dysfunction is a problem of relaxation of the LV. It is caused by conditions that typically reduce LV compliance such as CAD, hypertension, valvular disease, and age (32). In addition, elevated triglyceride levels have been associated with diastolic dysfunction, possibly related to intracellular lipid accumulation (33). Furthermore, sleep apnea has been shown to correlate with impairment of LV relaxation and might be linked to increased aortic stiffness (34). Finally, hypertrophic CM leads to diastolic dysfunction caused by myocyte hypertrophy and fibrosis. In nonobstructive CM, treatment with losartan for six months did not change LV cavity size or mass, but yielded some improvement in diastolic function (35).

Isolated diastolic dysfunction is uncommon. In the absence of valvular disease and CAD, the incidence of diastolic dysfunction in patients with CHF and normal LV systolic function was 11.5% as identified by echocardiography (36). In this study, diastolic dysfunction was evaluated based on measurement of early (E) and late (A) transmitral velocities and E wave deceleration time, and accounting for pseudonormal filling.

Predictors of diastolic dysfunction in patients with normal LV function and suspected heart failure include left atrial volume index and N-terminal pro B-type natriuretic peptide (37). Different LV geometric patterns also lead to varying degree of diastolic dysfunction (38).

Patients with LV diastolic dysfunction need to be treated with aggressive blood pressure control and with the use of diuretics, beta-blockade, or nondihydropyridine calcium channel blockers (diltiazem or verapamil) (39). ACEI or ARBs can have long-term value in reducing LV hypertrophy and theoretically may improve LV compliance (40). Even in the absence of hypertrophy, ACEIs have been shown to improve diastolic dysfunction in contrast to hydralazine and hydrochlorothiazide (41). Spironolactone might also be effective in improving diastolic function in the elderly, possibly by reducing myocardial fibrosis (42). The Effect of Losartan and Amlodipine on Left Ventricular Diastolic Function in Patients with Mild-to-Moderate Hypertension (J-ELAN) is a multicenter, randomized and prospective trial that will evaluate the effects of amlodipine and losartan in patients with hypertension and LV diastolic dysfunction (43). The follow-up period in this study will be 18 months.

Impaired glucose tolerance and insulin resistance in patients with type II diabetes is associated with impaired diastolic function of the LV (44). In asymptomatic patients with type II diabetes, an association between diastolic dysfunction and endothelial dysfunction and abnormalities on stress myocardial single-photon emission computed tomography has been seen (45). Tight glycemic control also has a favorable effect on diastolic dysfunction. In a small prospective study in patients with poorly controlled Type I diabetes and no clinically detectable heart disease, patients were treated aggressively with insulin and followed for up to a year. After 12 months, the mean values of all blood pressure, metabolic and LV parameters were unchanged, but diastolic parameters were inversely correlated with percent changes of glycated hemoglobin (46).

In conclusion, diastolic dysfunction is an important cause of heart failure that requires aggressive therapy of risk factors including hypertension, diabetes, sleep apnea, elevated triglycerides, CAD, and valvular disease. Cardiovascular drugs such as ACEI and ARB are important in reducing LV hypertrophy and improving LV compliance. Also, drugs that improve diastolic function such as beta-blockers and calcium channel blockers are important therapies and need to be considered. Diuretics are important to reduce LV filling pressure and improve symptoms.

Asymptomatic Left Ventricular Systolic Dysfunction

More patients with reduced LV function have been identified, partly because of objective echocardiographic measurements of LV function rather than just relying on the emergence of symptoms for diagnosis (47). In a recent study, the prevalence of asymptomatic LV systolic dysfunction (EF $\leq$ 50%) was 6.0% in men and 0.8% in women with a hazard ratio (HR) for CHF of 4.7 at 12 years of follow-up (48).

Patients with *asymptomatic* LV systolic dysfunction (stage B, ACC/AHA classification) require aggressive treatment of their hypertension, diabetes, and lipid disorders. Smoking cessation, reducing alcohol intake or illicit drug use, and routine exercise are important interventions. In patients with supraventricular arrhythmias, treatment of fast heart rate is essential to reduce tachycardia-induced CM. Revascularization in patients with ischemic heart disease (49) and corrective valvular surgery in patients with severe mitral or aortic valve insufficiency or aortic valve stenosis is a necessary first step toward LV recovery. Correction of anemia is also important in patients with asymptomatic LV dysfunction as a hematocrit less than or equal to 40% is associated with progression to symptomatic heart failure, first heart failure hospitalization, and death or the development of heart failure symptoms compared with patients with hematocrit greater than 46% (50). Neurohormonal activation does occur in patients with asymptomatic LV dysfunction and is also responsible for the continued deterioration of EF and progression to symptomatic failure (51).

ACE inhibitors and beta-blockers are important in patients with reduced LV function (EF $\leq$ 45%), irrespective of etiology, including postmyocardial infarction patients (52,53). Chronic ACEI treatment reduces or reverses LV remodeling by reducing LV dilatation and improving EF (54). In the Studies of Left Ventricular Dysfunction (SOLVD) trial (SOLVD investigators, 1999), asymptomatic patients with reduced LV function (EF < 35%) were randomized to enalapril (n = 2117) versus placebo (n = 2111) and followed for an average of 37.4 months. The reduction in cardiovascular mortality was larger in the enalapril group than placebo group (risk reduction of 12%, p = 0.12). Also, the combined end point of death and heart failure was 36% lower in the enalapril group (p < 0.001). Furthermore, current guidelines also emphasize the use of ACEI in patients with asymptomatic LV dysfunction and history of myocardial infarction (MI). These patients are at high risk of developing LV remodeling and CHF several months after the initial insult (55).

ARBs are a reasonable alternative in stage B patients who are intolerant to ACEI (56). There is no data to support the use of calcium channel blockers or digoxin in patients with asymptomatic LV dysfunction. Also, the dual endothelin A/B receptor antagonist enrasentan (60–90 mg/day) had an adverse impact on LV remodeling when compared to enalapril (10–20 mg/day) at six months follow-up (57). In this randomized, double-blind, parallel group study of 72 asymptomatic patients of enrasertan versus enalapril, enrasertan did increase resting cardiac index, but was associated with more serious adverse events (16.7% and 2.8%, respectively, $p = 0.02$).

Patients with asymptomatic LV dysfunction, post-MI, and an EF of less than or equal to 30% despite optimal medical therapy for at least 40 days post-MI (58) need to be considered for an ICD without requiring screening for ventricular arrhythmias whether occurring spontaneously or induced by electrophysiologic testing (59–61). ICD therapy in this population yielded a 31% reduction in mortality during an average follow-up of 20 months (62).

Periodic follow-up of patients with asymptomatic LV dysfunction is indicated with serial assessment of LV function using echocardiography or isotope ventriculography. Patients with familial CM need to have their immediate family members screened for asymptomatic LV dysfunction (58).

Symptomatic Left Ventricular Systolic Dysfunction

Symptomatic LV systolic dysfunction (stage C, ACC/AHA classification) requires intense pharmacologic treatment (Table 1) and close follow-up. In addition to aggressively managing the similar risk factors discussed above for asymptomatic LV dysfunction, patients will need to be treated with pharmacologic and mechanical means to improve their quality of life and survival. A close monitoring of heart function with echocardiography or isotope ventriculography is needed to assess response to therapy and continue to closely monitor EF. A summary of therapies that are proven to positively impact morbidity and mortality in patients with stage C CHF is given below.

Angiotensin-Converting Enzyme Inhibitors

ACEIs are important therapy for CHF, leading to a mortality reduction of 15% to 20% in patients with LV systolic dysfunction (EF < 40%). In addition, ACEIs reduce the combined end point of morbidity (mostly heart failure hospitalizations) and mortality by 30% to 35%.

The Cooperative North Scandinavian Enalapril Survival Study compared the effects of enalapril versus placebo on mortality in patients with severe CHF. Enalapril reduced mortality by 31% at one year ($p = 0.001$) as well as CHF hospitalization (63). In the SOLVD trial, patients receiving conventional treatment for class II and III heart failure were randomly assigned to receive either placebo ($n = 1284$) or enalapril ($n = 1285$). Enalapril reduced mortality by 16%

TABLE 1   Commonly Used Drugs in the Treatment of Congestive Heart Failure

Angiotensin-converting enzyme inhibitors	
Accupril	5–40 mg PO Q.d., max 40 mg/day, start 5–10 mg PO Q.d.
Captopril	12.5–50 mg PO t.i.d., max 150 mg/day, start 6.25–12.5 mg PO t.i.d.
Enalapril	2.5–20 mg PO b.i.d., max 40 mg/day, start at 2.5 mg Q.d.
Lisinopril	5–20 mg PO Q.d., max 40 mg/day, start 2.5–5 mg PO Q.d.
Monopril	10–40 mg PO Q.d./b.i.d., max 80 mg/day, start 10 mg PO Q.d.
Perindopril	4–16 mg PO Q.d., max 16 mg/day, start 2 mg PO Q.d.
Ramipril	5 mg PO b.i.d., max 10 mg/day, start at 2.5 mg PO b.i.d.
Angiotensin receptor blockers	
Losartan	25–100 mg PO Q.d., max 100 mg/day, start 25–50 mg PO Q.d.[a]
Candesartan	8–32 mg PO Q.d., max 32 mg/day, start 16 mg PO Q.d.[a]
Valsartan	40–160 mg PO b.i.d., max 320 mg/day, start 40 mg PO b.i.d.
Irbesartan	75–300 mg PO Q.d., max 300 mg/day, start 75 mg PO Q.d.[a]
Beta-blockers	
Carvedilol	3.125–25 mg PO b.i.d., max 50 mg PO Q.d., start 3.125 mg PO b.i.d.
Metoprolol succinate	12.5–200 mg PO Q.d., max 200 mg/day, start 12.5 mg PO Q.d.
Bisoprolol	5–10 mg PO Q.d., max 10 mg PO Q.d., start 2.5 mg PO Q.d.[a]
Aldosterone antagonists	
Spironolactone	12.5–25 mg PO b.i.d., max 50 mg/day, start 12.5 mg PO b.i.d.
Eplerenone	50 mg PO Q.d., max 50 mg/day, start 25 mg PO Q.d.[b]

[a]Off label use
[b]For congestive heart failure patients postmyocardial infarction

($p = 0.0036$) and mortality and CHF by 26% ($p < 0.0001$) at an average follow-up of 41.4 months (64,65). Furthermore, enalapril reduced development of heart failure by 37% and hospitalization from heart failure by 36% ($p < 0.001$) (66). Finally, data from the SOLVD trial showed that enalapril attenuates progressive increases of LV dilatation and hypertrophy in patients with reduced LV function (67).

Several trials have noted a mortality reduction with ACEI in patients with clinical evidence of CHF after sustaining an MI. The Acute Infarction Ramipril Efficacy Study showed a 27% ($p = 0.002$) reduction in the 30-month cumulative mortality with ramipril over placebo in post-MI CHF patients. In addition, in the Trandolapril Cardiac Evaluation Study, trandolapril reduced mortality by 22% ($p = 0.01$) in patients with reduced LV function after an MI. Trandolapril reduced overall mortality from cardiovascular causes, sudden death, and the development of severe heart failure (68). Furthermore, in the Survival and Ventricular Enlargement trial, captopril was administered 3 to 16 days after MI in patients with asymptomatic LV dysfunction (EF < 40%) and followed for an average of 42 months. Long-term administration of captopril was associated with an improvement in survival (risk reduction was 19%, $p = 0.019$) and reduced morbidity and mortality due to major cardiovascular events. These benefits were observed in patients irrespective of whether they received thrombolytic therapy, aspirin, or beta-blockers. Finally, in the Survival of MI Long-Term Evaluation Study (69), the effect of the ACEI zofenopril on mortality and morbidity after anterior MI was studied. Patients were randomly assigned within 24 hours after the onset of symptoms of acute anterior MI to receive either placebo (784 patients) or zofenopril (772 patients) for six weeks. At six weeks, the cumulative reduction in the risk of death or severe CHF was 34% ($p = 0.018$). At one year, the reduction in mortality risk was 29% ($p = 0.011$). Zofenopril significantly improved both short-term and long-term outcome when initiated within 24 hours of MI and continued for six weeks.

Outpatient's utilization of ACEIs is currently not optimal. A recent study has shown that there is a significant decline in the use of ACEIs following hospital discharge. It is more likely for patients to be on ACEIs as outpatients if they were initiated on ACEIs during their hospital stay. Therefore, early initiation of therapy and close outpatient follow-up is needed to ensure continuation of this effective therapy (70).

Angiotensin Receptor Blockers

Early studies comparing ARBs and ACEI in the management of CHF patients suggested that ARB was safe and effective in these patients. In the Randomized Evaluation of Strategies for Left Ventricular Dysfunction (RESOLVD) pilot study (26), 768 patients in NYHC II to IV and EF less than 40% received candesartan, candesartan plus enalapril, or enalapril alone for 43 weeks. LV cavity size increased less and BNP levels decreased more with combination therapy compared to ARB or ACEI alone. The RESOLVD trial, however, showed no significant differences in clinical events among ACE inhibitor, ARB, and their combination (56). The study was not powered, however, to evaluate clinical events.

In another small study, the Evaluation of Losartan in the Elderly (ELITE) trial (71), 722 patients with EF less than or equal to 40%, 65 years of age or more, and in NYHC class II to IV were included. The primary end point was death and/or hospital admission for heart failure, and was 9.4% in the losartan group compared to 13.2% in the captopril group (risk reduction 32%, $p = 0.075$). This risk reduction was primarily due to a decrease in all-cause mortality (4.8% vs. 8.7%; risk reduction 46%, $p = 0.035$) with similar rate of hospital admissions in both groups (5.7%). The ELITE trial led to a larger study, the Losartan Heart Failure Survival Study ELITE II (72) trial, in an attempt to confirm the findings of ELITE I. In ELITE II, 3152 patients aged 60 years or older with NYHC II to IV and EF of less than 40% were randomly assigned to losartan ($n = 1578$) titrated to 50 mg q.d, or captopril ($n = 1574$) titrated to 50 mg t.i.d. Surprisingly, there were no differences in all-cause mortality or sudden death between the two groups emphasizing the importance of larger trials to assess outcome in heart failure patients. ELITE II also confirmed that ARB could be a potential substitute to an ACEI because ARB did not lead to inferior outcome in this study.

The Valsartan in Heart Failure trial (Val-HeFT) (73) randomized 5010 patients with heart failure of New York Heart Association (NYHA) class II, III, or IV to receive 160 mg of valsartan or placebo b.i.d. The primary outcomes were mortality and the combined end point of mortality and morbidity, defined as the incidence of cardiac arrest with resuscitation, hospitalization for heart failure, or receipt of IV inotropic or vasodilator therapy for at least four hours. Mortality was similar in both groups but the combined end point of morbidity and mortality was reduced by 13.2% with valsartan ($p = 0.009$) predominantly driven by reduction in heart failure hospitalizations (13.8% vs. 18.2%, $p < 0.001$). In a subset of the Val-HeFT trial of patients intolerant to ACEI, valsartan (titrated to 160 mg b.i.d) reduced both all-cause mortality and combined mortality and morbidity compared with placebo (17.3% vs. 27.1%, $p = 0.017$, and 24.9% vs. 42.5%, $p < 0.001$, respectively) (74). Furthermore, an echocardiographic substudy of the Val-HeFT study included 5010 patients with moderate CHF and showed that valsartan taken with either ACEI or beta-blockers reversed LV remodeling (75). It should be noted, however, that in a post hoc analysis of the Val-HeFT trial, valsartan had a favorable effect in patients receiving either a beta-blocker or ACEIs (76), but an adverse effect in patients receiving both types of drugs (73), raising concerns about the safety of combining an ARB with an ACEI and a betablocker. This concern could not be validated in the Candesartan in Heart Failure Assessment of Reduction in Mortality and morbidity (CHARM) trial discussed below.

The CHARM is a randomized, double-blind, placebo-controlled, multicenter, international trial program that included heart failure patients, NYHC class II to IV. This trial had three complementary arms: (i) CHARM-added; candesartan (titrated to 32 mg q.d.) is added to an ACEI, (ii) CHARM-alternative; candesartan administered to patients who cannot tolerate ACEIs, and (iii) CHARM-preserved; candesartan is administered to patients with preserved LV function irrespective of whether they are on ACEI or not. In the CHARM-added and CHARM-alternative arms, patients with EF less than or equal to 40% were included. In the "overall program" of this study, which included both preserved and reduced LV function, total mortality was not reduced compared to placebo. However, in a subset analysis, patients with symptomatic heart failure and reduced LV function, candesartan significantly reduced all-cause mortality (28% vs. 31%, $p = 0.0018$), cardiovascular death (22.8% vs. 26.2%, $p = 0.005$), and CHF hospitalizations (22.5% vs. 28.1%, $p < 0.001$) when added to standard therapies including ACEI, beta-blockers, and aldosterone antagonists (77). Candesartan also reduced progression to diabetes (78), sudden cardiac death, and death from worsening heart failure in patients with symptomatic failure (79).

The Valsartan in Acute MI Trial (80) randomized patients 0.5 to 10 days after an acute MI, with reduced LV function to valsartan (4909 patients) titrated to 160 mg t.i.d., valsartan (80 mg t.i.d.) plus captopril (50 mg b.i.d.) (4885 patients), or captopril (4909 patients) alone titrated to 50 mg t.i.d. in addition to standard therapy. The primary end point of the study was all-cause mortality at a median follow-up of 24.7 months. Valsartan was equally effective to captopril in reducing all cause mortality. Also combining valsartan with captopril increased the rate of adverse events without improving survival.

In the Optimal Trial in MI with Angiotensin II Antagonist Losartan (OPTIMAAL), patients after an acute MI were randomized to losartan versus captopril. The primary end point was reduction in all cause mortality at a mean follow-up of 2.7 years. A nonsignificant difference was seen in total mortality in favor of captopril (18% vs. 16% in the losartan vs. captopril, respectively, $p = 0.07$). However, there were significantly more cardiovascular deaths with losartan (15%) than with captopril (13%) ($p = 0.03$) (81). Losartan was better tolerated than captopril with fewer patients discontinuing their medications (17% vs. 23%, $p < 0.0001$) (82). An echocardiographic substudy of the OPTIMAAL trial has shown that both losartan and captopril improve systolic function after an acute MI, but the benefit is greater for captopril (83).

Currently the recommendation is to use an ACEI as a first-line therapy to treat CHF patients. However, a growing body of evidence suggests that an ARB can be an alternative to an ACEI, if patients cannot tolerate the latter (58).

Aldosterone Blockers

Aldosterone is secreted by the zona glomerulosa of the adrenal gland and is induced by AII, adrenocorticotropic hormone, and potassium. Aldosterone leads to sodium and water absorption and the excretion of potassium. Although AII is a dominant stimulus of aldosterone

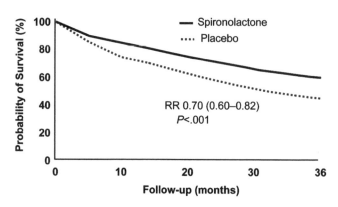

FIGURE 3 Data from the RALES trial showed that at 36 months follow-up, spironolactone reduced mortality by 30% when added to conventional therepy in patients with symptomatic congestive heart failure. *Source*: From Ref. 27.

secretion (84), ACEI or ARB is not sufficient to block aldosterone secretion (26,85,86). Recent data also suggests that ARB reduces plasma aldosterone level but, as seen in the Val-HeFT trial, this reduction occurs in various subgroups including those taking beta-blockers and ACEIs despite differing clinical outcomes (87). Although it is unclear whether aldosterone levels relate to heart failure progression, recent data confirms that aldosterone blockers are important to improve morbidity and mortality in patients with CHF and reduced LV systolic function. Recent data also suggest that aldosterone blockade reduces ventricular remodeling and myocardial fibrosis and has important effects on autonomic balance, fibrinolysis, oxidative stress, and activation of the nuclear factor kappa B and activating protein-1 signaling pathways (88).

Two large trials have been recently published to evaluate the role of aldosterone antagonism in CHF management. The Randomized Aldactone Evaluation Study (RALES) (27) randomized patients ($n = 1663$) with advanced CHF and EF less than or equal to 35% to spironolactone 25 mg daily ($n = 822$) or placebo ($n = 841$) including ACEI, digoxin, and diuretics. After a mean follow-up of 24 months, the trial was stopped early. Spironolactone reduced the primary end point of mortality by 30% (46% vs. 35%, $p < 0.001$) primarily due to reduction of progression of CHF and sudden cardiac death (Fig. 3). In addition, spironolactone significantly improved the symptoms of heart failure as assessed by the NYHA functional class ($p < 0.001$) and reduced recurrent hospitalization due to worsening CHF by 35% ($p < 0.001$). The use of spironolactone not only markedly increase following the publication of the RALES study, but also the risk of hyperkalemia (89). Spironolactone-induced hyperkalemia accounted for an increase in hospitalization from 2.4 per 1000 patients in 1994 to 11.0 per 1000 patients in 2001 ($p < 0.001$), and a mortality increase from 0.3 per 1000 to 2.0 per 1000 patients ($p < 0.001$) (90). Patients with elevated potassium levels (>5 mEq/L) and high baseline creatinine (>2.0) should not be initiated on spironolactone to avoid serious hyperkalemia problem. Close monitoring of potassium levels is needed when patients are started on an aldosterone antagonist.

Another recent trial, Eplerenone Post-AMI Heart Failure Efficacy and Survival Study (EPHESUS) (28) randomized patients with CHF and an EF less than 40%, 3 to 14 days post-MI, to eplerenone (25–50 mg daily) or placebo. At a mean follow-up of 27 months, eplerenone, a competitive, relatively selective mineralocorticoid receptor antagonist, reduced total mortality by 15% ($p = 0.008$), cardiovascular mortality or cardiovascular hospitalizations by 13% ($p = 0.002$), and sudden cardiac death by 21% ($p = 0.03$). The EPHESUS study established the importance of aldosterone antagonism in post-MI patients with reduced LV function irrespective of the degree of failure. Based on these trials, aldosterone antagonists are now considered to be a primary therapy in patients with LV dysfunction and CHF.

Beta-Blockade in Heart Failure

The activation of the SNS in patients with reduced LV function leads to excess catecholamine secretion, which adversely affects the myocardium and contributes to LV remodeling and progression to CHF.

Multiple beta-blockers have been shown to reduce mortality and morbidity in patients with heart failure and reduced LV systolic function (Fig. 4). Current data support the use of carvedilol, metoprolol succinate, and bisoprolol to treat patients with CHF. Beta-blockers reduce mortality by approximately 35% when added to standard therapy in mild-to-moderate

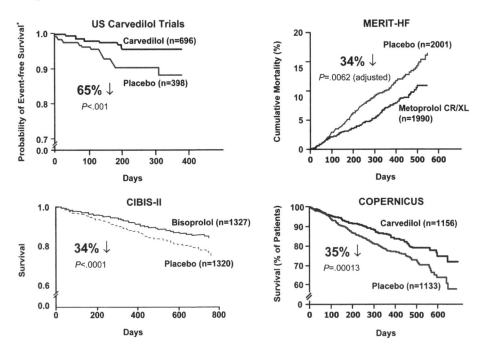

FIGURE 4 Various beta-blockers have shown a significant reduction in mortality in patients with symptomatic congestive heart failure. *Source*: From Refs. 91–94.

(91–93) or advanced CHF (94). Beta-blockers also reduce hospitalizations by 33% to 38% (91,92,95) and reduce cardiac remodeling, reduce cavity size, and improve EF (96).

In the U.S. Carvedilol Heart Failure study (91), 1094 patients were enrolled in a double-blind, placebo-controlled, stratified program in which they received one of four treatment protocols based on their exercise capacity. Patients with heart failure were randomized to placebo ($n = 398$) or carvedilol ($n = 696$) on top of conventional therapy. The overall mortality at six-month follow-up was reduced by 65% with carvedilol ($p < 0.001$), which led to early termination of the study by the Data and Safety Monitoring Board. Carvedilol also reduced hospitalization for cardiovascular causes by 27% ($p = 0.036$), and the combined risk for hospitalization and death by 38% ($p < 0.001$). This effect was seen in both black and nonblack patients with heart failure (97). Carvedilol also reduced length of hospital stay and length of stay in the intensive care unit leading to a 57% lower inpatient care costs for cardiovascular admissions ($p = 0.016$) and 81% lower costs for heart failure admissions ($p = 0.022$) (95). Finally, among patients with severe heart failure (EF < 22%, markedly reduced six-minute corridor walk test, and severe impairment of quality of life), carvedilol improved LV function compared to placebo ($p = 0.004$) with a trend in symptoms improvement. Because the number of patients with severe CHF was small in the U.S. Carvedilol Heart Failure Study, it was not possible to make any firm conclusions about the long-term outcome of patients with severe heart failure management in this study (98). In the Carvedilol Prospective Randomized Cumulative Survival Study Group (99), 2289 patients with severe heart failure symptoms were randomly assigned to receive carvedilol ($n = 1156$) or placebo ($n = 1133$). The carvedilol group experienced no increase in cardiovascular risk and had fewer patients who died [19 vs. 25; HR, 0.75; 95% confidence interval (CI), 0.41–1.35] or who died and were hospitalized (134 vs. 153; HR, 0.85; 95% CI, 0.67–1.07). Carvedilol was well tolerated in euvolemic patients, with fewer patients withdrawn from treatment than placebo.

In the Metoprolol CR/XL Randomized Intervention Trial in Congestive Heart Failure study, 3991 patients with chronic heart failure in NYHC II to IV and EF less than or equal to 40% were enrolled in a double-blind, randomized, placebo-controlled study of metoprolol CR/XL versus placebo (92). All cause mortality and sudden death were reduced by 34% ($p = 0.00009$) and 41% ($p = 0.0002$) in the metoprolol group. Also, metoprolol CR/XL reduced the number of hospitalizations due to worsening heart failure ($p < 0.001$) and number of days in hospital due to worsening heart failure ($p < 0.001$) (100). In post-MI patients with symptomatic CHF and an EF less than or equal to 40% and receiving contemporary management, metoprolol CR/XL reduced total mortality by 40% ($p = 0.0004$) and sudden death by 50% ($p = 0.0004$) (101).

The Cardiac Insufficiency Bisoprolol II (CIBIS-II) study was a double-blind, placebo-controlled trial in Europe that enrolled 2647 symptomatic patient with Class III or IV heart failure and an EF less than or equal to 35% randomized to bisoprolol or placebo. At 1.3 years, all cause mortality and sudden death were reduced by 34% ($p < 0.0001$) and 44% ($p = 0.0011$), respectively, with bisoprolol. Also, bisoprolol resulted in fewer hospital admissions per patient hospitalized, fewer hospital admissions overall, fewer days spent in hospital or intensive care unit leading to a reduction in the cost of care by 5% to 10% compared to placebo (102).

Beta-blockers are a heterogenous group of drugs with differences in antiadrenergic actions. The Carvedilol or Metoprolol European Trial (103,104) is the only randomized trial that compared two beta-blockers in a randomized, double-blind study in the management of CHF patients. About 3029 patients with class II to IV heart failure were recruited at 317 centers in 15 European countries. At 58 months, there was a 17% reduction in mortality with carvedilol compared to metoprolol tartrate ($p = 0.0017$). Recently, carvedilol (6.25–25 mg b.i.d.) was also shown in The Glycemic Effects in Diabetes Mellitus: Carvedilol-Metoprolol Comparison in Hypertensives study not to alter glycemic control in diabetics when compared to metoprolol tartrate (50–200 mg t.i.d.). Furthermore, it did improve some components of the metabolic syndrome such as improving insulin sensitivity (105).

Currently recommended beta-blockers in the management of CHF are carvedilol, metoprolol succinate, and bisoprolol (58). Beta-blockade is still underutilized in patients with CHF despite the overwhelming data to their effectiveness and safety (106). Educational efforts need to continue to focus on promoting guidelines in heart failure management in order to improve the overall outcome of these patients.

Aggressive titration of beta-blockers is needed in patients with CHF. Higher levels of beta-blockade and ACEI are associated with better improvement of EF and greater reductions in cardiovascular hospitalizations (107–109). In a substudy of the Assessment of Treatment with Lisinopril and Survival trial, the composite end point of mortality or hospitalization decreased incrementally with the use of high-dose ACE inhibitors ($n = 475$) [adjusted odds ratio (OR), 0.93; $p = $ not significant], high-dose ACE inhibitors plus beta-blockers ($n = 72$) (OR, 0.89; $p = $ not significant), and high-dose ACE inhibitors plus beta-blockers plus digoxin ($n = 77$) (OR, 0.47; $p = 0.006$) compared with low-dose ACE inhibitors ($n = 471$) (109). A stepwise approach in titration of beta-blockade is generally followed with an increase in the dose every two weeks as tolerated until achieving the maximum tolerable dose.

Digoxin Therapy in CHF

Digoxin is over 250 years old and was introduced by William Withering (110). Although digoxin is very effective in controlling heart rate in patients with atrial fibrillation, a controversy exists about its role in the treatment of patients with CHF (111).

The Digitalis Investigation Group (DIG) (112) is a randomized, double-blind clinical trial that studied the effects of digoxin on mortality and hospitalization in patients with CHF and followed for an average of 37 months. In this trial, digoxin had no effect on mortality but did reduce the rate of hospitalization both overall and for worsening heart failure. A comprehensive post hoc analysis of the DIG showed that digoxin at a serum concentration of 0.5–0.9 ng/mL did reduce mortality [29% vs. 33%, Adjusted HR (AHR) of 0.77] and heart failure hospitalizations (23% vs. 33%, AHR of 0.68) in all heart failure patients with no interaction with EF greater than 45% ($p = 0.834$) or sex ($p = 0.917$) (113). This post hoc analysis is hypothesis generating and will need to be prospectively validated. In another substudy of the DIG trial, there was no statistically significant difference in perceived health, quality of life measures, and the six-minute walk test between the digoxin and the placebo group in patients in normal sinus rhythm at 12-month follow-up (114). Furthermore, digoxin efficacy did not appear to be affected by the glomerular filtration rate (GFR), although renal dysfunction was a very strong predictor of mortality particularly in patients with GFR less than 50 mL/min (151).

Patients on digoxin and receiving standard treatment for CHF might experience a slight reduction in EF (115–117,145), worsening maximal exercise capacity, and increased incidences of treatment failure upon withdrawal of this drug (116,117).

Currently, digoxin is indicated for the treatment of chronic heart failure in patients with LV dysfunction and NYHC class II to III despite optimal medical treatment with ACEI, beta-blockers, and diuretics (ACC/AHA Class IIa indication). Digoxin is not indicated for the acute treatment of CHF, and serial measurements of digoxin levels are currently considered unnecessary. When digoxin is administered with amiodarone, the dose should be reduced (118).

Mechanical Treatment of Stage C Heart Failure
Cardiac Resynchronization Therapy

Patients with advanced heart failure symptoms despite optimal medical management, an EF less than 35%, and a wide QRS complex greater than or equal to 130 msec qualify for cardiac resynchronization therapy (CRT). The outcomes of CRT system implantation in 2078 patients from a multicenter study program showed that the procedure is safe, well tolerated, and has a high success rate (119).

In the Multicenter InSync Randomized Clinical Evaluation (MIRACLE) trial (7), 369 patients with EF less than or equal to 35%, QRS duration is equal to 130 msec or greater, and class III to IV NYHC despite optimal medical treatment were randomized to controls ($n = 182$, ICD activated, CRT off) and the CRT group ($n = 187$, ICD activated, CRT on). CRT improved quality of life, functional status, and exercise capacity without adversely influencing ICD function. In addition, in the InSync III study (120), a multicenter, prospective, nonrandomized, six-month trial of 422 patients with wide QRS complex and a class III or IV heart failure, sequential CRT therapy provided a modest increase in stroke volume, improved exercise capacity, but had no change in functional status or quality of life compared to a historic control from the MIRACLE trial. Furthermore, CRT has also been shown to induce opposite changes in QRS duration and LV function helping in the process of reverse remodeling, a process more apparent in patients with nonischemic heart failure and less severe mitral insufficiency (121). Finally, in the Comparison of Medical Therapy, Pacing, and Defibrillation in Heart Failure (COMPANION) trial, the risk of the combined end point of death from or hospitalization for heart failure was reduced by 34% ($p < 0.002$) and the secondary end point of death from any cause by 24% ($p = 0.059$) in the pacemaker group compared to the pharmacologic therapy alone (122). In this trial, the addition of a defibrillator reduced mortality beyond that achieved with CRT therapy alone.

Current guidelines recommend CRT therapy in patients with advanced heart failure symptoms and wide QRS complex, who are already optimized on medical treatment with the goal to improve exercise capacity, functional status, and quality of life and to help reversing the remodeling process (58).

Implantable Cardioverter Defibrillators

Sudden death is a major cause of mortality in patients with LV dysfunction. ICDs are currently indicated in patients with moderate CHF and reduced EF less than 30% on optimal medical therapy who (i) are at least 40 days post-MI, (ii) have nonischemic CM, or (iii) have had a serious arrhythmia such as ventricular fibrillation, ventricular tachycardia, or cardiac arrest (60–62,123).

In the Sudden Cardiac Death in Heart Failure trial, 2521 patients with moderate heart failure and an EF less than or equal to 35% were randomized to conventional therapy for CHF plus placebo, conventional therapy plus amiodarone, or conventional therapy plus ICD. Amiodarone had no favorable effect on survival whereas ICD reduced overall mortality by 23% at 45.5 months mean follow-up (123). In addition, the COMPANION (122) trial showed that ICD therapy can reduce death by 36% ($p = 0.003$) in patients with advanced heart failure due to ischemic or nonischemic CM and a QRS greater than or equal to 120 msec when compared to optimal medical therapy. The Multicenter Automatic Defibrillator Implantation Trial II (MADIT-II) randomized 1232 patients with EF less than or equal to 30% to ICD or conventional medical therapy. Death was the primary end point and the average follow-up was 20 months. The mortality rates were 19.8% in the conventional therapy group and 14.2% in the defibrillator group (HR for the risk of death in the ICD group was 0.69, $p = 0.016$) (61,62). A long-term follow-up study from MADIT-II showed that the probability of survival after successful therapy by an ICD for ventricular fibrillation or tachycardia was 80% at one year, and these patients will be subsequently at an increased risk of heart failure and nonsudden cardiac death (124). Although advanced heart failure patients have a poorer prognosis than those with less severe failure, analysis from the MADIT-II trial indicated that benefit from ICD therapy is similar among all the different heart failure subgroups (59). Currently the MADIT-CRT trial is ongoing and is testing whether CRT-D will reduce the risk of mortality in patients with reduced EF ($\leq$30%), prolonged QRS equal to 130 msec or greater, and NYHC Class I–II (125).

Miscellaneous Therapy

In addition to pharmacologic therapy, CHF patients should be instructed on dietary salt restriction (2 gm sodium/day), daily weight monitoring, fluid restriction, smoking cessation, regular exercise, avoidance of alcohol intake and aggressive treatment of hypertension and lipid disorders. Supplemental oxygen is needed in patients with oxygen saturation of less than 92% on room air after ambulation. Finally, sleep apnea has been associated with CHF, and these patients need to be screened and aggressively treated for moderate-to-severe apnea (126). CHF patients also should avoid nonsteroidal anti-inflammatory drugs, most calcium channel blockers, and antiarrhythmics. They also should not receive the combination of an ARB, ACEI, and spironolactone to minimize the risk of severe hyperkalemia. Long-term administration of positive inotropes is also discouraged except for palliative reasons. Finally, exercise testing in these patients is also important to determine an appropriate exercise program.

Management of the ACC/AHA Stage D CHF

Acutely decompensated CHF patients with severe LV dysfunction require intense pharmacologic and mechanical management. Patients with advanced decompensated failure have a poor short-term prognosis. In the Initiation Management Predischarge Assessment of Carvedilol Heart Failure registry (127), mortality and rehospitalization rate was 31% at 60-day follow-up.

Positive inotropic agents such as dopamine and milrinone might be utilized for palliative reasons because they improve symptoms and increase functional capacity, but they could worsen arrhythmias and possibly increase the risk of mortality (128,129). In a randomized trial of milrinone versus placebo in patients with decompensated CHF, 951 patients on standard therapy were included. Milrinone caused more sustained hypotension and atrial arrhythmias compared to placebo, with no positive impact on mortality, 60-day mortality, or composite incidence of death or admission (130). An analysis from the Acute Decompensated Heart Failure National Registry, a large retrospective registry of patients with acute decompensated CHF, showed that patients who received milrinone and dobutamine had a higher in-hospital mortality than those who received nitroglycerin and nesiritide. Both nesiritide and nitroglycerin had similar in-hospital mortality (131). Current ACC/AHA guidelines consider the use of intermittent positive inotropic agents for the management of decompensated heart failure as a class III indication, indicating that their use should be discouraged.

Data on IV nesiritide suggests that this drug is effective in lowering wedge pressure and improving patient's symptoms. Nesiritide is a 32 amino acid sequence recombinant human B-type natriuretic peptide that was shown to reduce both preload and afterload and increase cardiac index with no effect on heart rate (132). In the Vasodilatation in the Management of Acute CHF (VMAC) trial, 489 inpatients with decompensated CHF were enrolled in a randomized trial of nesiritide versus nitroglycerin or placebo for three hours followed by nesiritide or nitroglycerin for 24 hours. The primary and secondary outcomes of the study are pulmonary capillary wedge pressure (PCWP) at three hours and 24 hours, respectively. IV nesiritide was administered as a bolus of 2 mcg/kg followed by continuous infusion of 0.01 mcg/kg/min. At three hours, dyspnea improved with nesiritide compared with placebo ($p = 0.03$) but there was no difference compared to nitroglycerin. At 24 hours, the reduction in PCWP was greater in the nesiritide group (−8.2 mm Hg) than in the nitroglycerin group (−6.3 mm Hg), with a modest improvement in clinical status (VMAC investigators). In VMAC, there was no significant difference between nesiritide and nitroglycerin subjects in six-month mortality and more side effects have been reported with nitroglycerin than with nesiritide. The hemodynamic benefits and safety of nesiritide in patients with acutely decompensated CHF are maintained in patients receiving chronic beta-blockers (133).

In the Prospective Randomized Evaluation of Cardiac Ectopy with Dobutamine or Natrecor Therapy, 255 patients were randomized to dobutamine or nesiritide in the management of decompensated CHF. Dobutamine was associated with arrhythmia and tachycardia

TABLE 2 Percent 30-Day Mortality in Seven Nesiritide Trials

Trial	Natrecor (%)	Control (%)	Hazard ratio	Confidence interval
Mills et al.	2.70	7.50	0.38	0.05,2.67
PRECEDENT	3.70	6.10	0.6	0.18,1.97
VMAC	5.90	5.80	1.25	0.24,6.45
PROACTION	6.90	4.90	1.43	0.53,3.97
FUSION I	8.10	5.10	1.56	0.75,3.24
Pooled (all)	4.20	0.90	4.99	0.58,42.73
	1.40	2.90	0.49	0.07,3.47
	5.30	4.30	1.27	0.81,2.01

Abbreviations: PRECDENT, Prospective Randomized Evaluation of Cardial Ectopy with Dobytamine or Natrecor Therpy; VMAC, Efficacy Comparative Vasodilation in the Management of Acute Congestive Heart Failure; PROACTION, Prospective Randomized Outcomes Study of Acutely Decompensated Congestive Heart Failure Treated Initially as Outpatients with Natrecor, FUSION, Follow-up Serial Infusions of Natrecor.

whereas nesiritide reduced ventricular ectopy and did not increase heart rate suggesting a safer profile of nesiritide over dobutamine (134).

Nesiritide has not been studied in a trial powered enough to evaluate its effects on mortality. The 30-day mortality from pooled data from seven clinical trials (Table 2) (132,135,138) was 5.3% for Natrecor and 4.3% for control [HR 1.27 (0.81–2.01)]. In a recent pooled analysis of three randomized studies (1) that met the following inclusion criteria: randomized double-blind study of patients with acutely decompensated heart failure, therapy administered as single infusion (six hours or more), inotrope not mandated as control, and reported 30-day mortality, 485 patients were randomized to nesiritide and 377 to control therapy. Death at 30 days occurred more in nesiritide than in placebo (7.2% vs. 4%, $p = 0.059$). This analysis suggested that nesiritide might increase mortality, and that an adequately powered and controlled trial is needed for nesiritide in patients with acute decompensated CHF.

Mechanical Support of the Failing Heart

The Randomized Evaluation of Mechanical Assistance in Treatment of Chronic Heart Failure trial (139,140) randomized 129 patients with end-stage heart failure, who were ineligible for cardiac transplantation to receive a LV-assist device ($n = 68$) or optimal medical management ($n = 61$). Survival (52% vs. 25%, $p = 0.002$) and quality of life were significantly improved with the device compared to medical therapy at one year. Serious adverse events did occur in the group when compared to medical therapy and included infection, bleeding, and device malfunction. In this trial, patients undergoing inotropic support derived major mortality and quality of life benefits from the assist device compared to patients receiving medical therapy. Also, patients not undergoing inotropic support had an overall better survival rates both with and without the assist device, but differences did not reach significance.

Recent improvements in the HeartMate VE LVAD to the HeartMate XVE LVAD have recently led to significant improvements in outcomes (141) indicating that as technology and experience with LVAD evolve, this therapy might become more accessible to the class IV heart failure patient who is ineligible for cardiac transplantation.

CONCLUSION

Treatment of heart failure starts with controlling risk factors, management of asymptomatic systolic dysfunction, and aggressive treatment of symptomatic failure with diuretics, beta-blockers, ACEI (or ARB as an alternative), and aldosterone antagonists. The use of IV inotropes should be discouraged except for hemodynamic stability. IV nesiritide can be utilized for acute symptomatic relief of inpatients with acute decompensated CHF. Mechanical devices including biventricular pacing, ICD, or LVAD need to be considered for eligible patients. Diastolic dysfunction is often a neglected cause of CHF, and diagnosis needs to be considered when CHF is present in the setting of normal LV systolic function. Treatment relies on reducing LV filling with diuresis, enhancing LV relaxation with beta-blockers and verapamil, and reducing long-term hypertrophy with ACEI.

■ Case 1

AJ is a 72-year-old male with history of coronary artery bypass surgery, ischemic CM, and an ejection fraction (EF) of 20%. The patient's shortness of breath has been progressive and over the past three months it has been occurring with minimal exertion, placing him in a Class III NYHC for CHF. The patient has been on Coreg 25mg PO b.i.d., enalapril 10mg PO b.i.d., spironolactone 25mg PO q.d. and digoxin 0.125mg PO q.d. In addition, the patient is on furosemide 80mg PO b.i.d.. The patient is euvolemic on his current medical regimen. His electrocardiogram showed a normal sinus rhythm with a left bundle branch block and a QRS complex duration of 140msec. The patient was referred to the electrophysiology service to consider biventricular pacing with an internal defibrillator. This was performed successfully. Two weeks subsequent to the procedure, the patient's symptoms markedly improved and he was reclassified as NYHC Class II. Cardiac rehabilitation was initiated and at three-month follow-up he was asymptomatic with a moderate level of exertion, leading a near-normal lifestyle. EF was reassessed and was 32%.

■ Case 2

HJ is a 25-year-old female with postpartum, nonischemic CM, an ejection fraction (EF) of 25%, and class III NYHC symptoms. Transesophageal echocardiogram revealed severe mitral insufficiency. The patient was started on Coreg 3.125mg PO b.i.d., digoxin 0.25mg PO daily, and enalapril 2.5mg PO b.i.d. In addition, a low dose of furosemide was started at 20mg PO daily. Over the course of 12 weeks, Coreg was titrated to 25mg PO b.i.d. and enalapril to 20mg PO b.i.d. Spironolactone was added at 25mg PO b.i.d. After three months of optimal therapy, the patient's EF was reassessed and was found to be 35%. Mitral insufficiency continued to be in the severe range. Surgical consultation was obtained and mitral valve repair was performed successfully. The patient was kept on these medications postoperatively, and at six-month follow-up her EF improved to 45%. She was completely asymptomatic.

REFERENCES

1. Haney S, Sur D, Xu Z. A review and primary care perspective. J Am Board Fam Pract 2005; 18:189–198.
2. O'Connell JB, Bristow M. Economic impact of heart failure in the United States: time for a different approach. J Heart Lung Transplant 1993; 13:S107–S112.
3. Hunt SA, Baker DW, Chin MH, et al. American College of Cardiology/American Heart Association Task Force on Practice Guidelines (Committee to Revise the 1995 Guidelines for the Evaluation and Management of Heart Failure); International Society for Heart and Lung Transplantation; Heart Failure Society of America. ACC/AHA Guidelines for the Evaluation and Management of Chronic Heart Failure in the Adult: executive summary a report of the American College of Cardiology/American Heart Association Task Force on Practice Guidelines (Committee to Revise the 1995 Guidelines for the Evaluation and Management of Heart Failure): developed in collaboration with the International Society for Heart and Lung Transplantation; endorsed by the Heart Failure Society of America. Circulation 2001; 104(24):2996–3007.
4. Senni M, Tribouilloy CM, Rodeheffer RJ, et al. Congestive heart failure in the community. A study of al incident cases in Olmsted County, Minnesota, in 1991. Circulation 1998; 98:2282–2289.
5. Kitzman DW, Gardin JM, Gottdiener JS, et al. Importance of Heart Failure with Preserved Systolic Function in Patients 65 years of age. Am J Cardiol 2001; 87:413–419.
6. Brush C. Doppler Tissue Analysis of Mitral Annular Velocities: Evidence for Systolic Abnormalities in Patients with Diastolic Heart Failure. J Am Soc Echocardiogr 2003; 16(10):1031–1036.
7. Young JB. The Global Epidemiology of Heart Failure. Med Clin North Am 2004; 88(5):1135–1143, ix.
8. Senni M, Tribouilloy CM, Rodeheffer RJ, et al. Congestive Heart Failure in the Community: Trends in Incidence and Survival in a 10-year Period. Arch Intern Med 1999; 159(1):29–34.
9. Roger VL, Weston SA, Redfield MM, et al. Trends in Heart Failure Incidence and Survival in a Community-based Population. JAMA 2004; 292(3):344–350.
10. Levy D, Kenchaiah S, Larson MG, et al. Long-term Trends in The Incidence of and Survival with Heart Failure. N Engl J Med 2002; 347(18):1397–1402.
11. Stewart S, MacIntyre K, Capewell S, McMurray JJ. Heart Failure and the Aging Populationsan Increasing Burden in the 21st Century? Heart 2003; 89(1):49–53.
12. Levy D, Larson MG, Vasan RS, et al. The Progression From Hypertension to Congestive Heart Failure. JAMA 1996; 275(20):1557–1562.
13. Kannel WB, Ho K, Thom T. Changing Epidemiological Features of Cardiac Failure. Br Heart J 1994; 72(suppl 2):S3–S9.
14. Blaufarb IS, Sonnenblick EH. The Rennin-angiotensin System in Left Ventricular Remodeling. Am J Cardiol 1996; 77(13):8C–16C.
15. Solomon SD, Anavekar N, Skali H, et al. For the Candesartan in Heart Failure Reduction in Mortality (CHARM) Investigators. Influence of Ejection Fraction on Cardiovascular Outcomes in a Broad Spectrum of Heart Failure Patients. Circulation 2005; 112(24):3738–3744.
16. Curtis JP, Sokol SI, Wang Y, et al. The Association of Left Ventricular Ejection Fraction, Mortality, and Cause of Death in Stable Outpatients with Heart Failure. J Am Coll Cardiol 2003; 42(4):736–742.
17. Opie LH. The Neuroendocrinology of Congestive Heart Failure. Cardiovasc J S Afr 2002; 13(4):171–178.

18. Tousoulis D, Charakida M, Stefanadis C. Inflammation and Endothelial Dysfunction as Therapeutic Targets in Patients With Heart Failure. Int J Cardiol 2005; 100(3):347–353.

19. Bauersachs J, Schafer A. Endothelial Dysfunction in Heart Failure: Mechanisms and Therapeutic approaches. Curr Vasc Pharmacol 2004; 2(2):115–124.

20. Francis GS. Neurohumoral Activation and Progression of Heart Failure: hypothetical and Clinical considerations. J Cardiovasc Pharmacol 1998; 32(Suppl 1):S16–S21.

21. Blum A, Miller H. Pathophysiological Role of Cytokines in Congestive Heart Failure. Annu Rev Med 2001; 52:15–27.

22. Bristow MR. Changes in Myocardial and Vascular Receptors in Heart Failure. J Am Coll Cardiol 1993; 22(4 Suppl A):61A–71A.

23. Mann DL, Kent RL, Parsons B, Cooper G, IV. Adrenergic Effects on The Biology of The Adult Mammalian cardiocyte. Circulation 1992; 85(2):790–804.

24. Nikolaidis LA, Trumble D, Hentosz, et al. Catecholamines Restore Myocardial Contractility in Dilated Cardiomyopathy at the Expense of Increased Coronary Blood Flow and Myocardial Oxygen Consumption (MvO2 cost of catecholamines in heart failure). Eur J Heart Fail 2004; 6(4):409–419.

25. Mann DL. Basic Mechanisms of Disease Progression in the Failing Heart: the Role of Excessive Adrenergic drive. Prog Cardiovasc Dis 1998; 41(1 Suppl 1):1–8.

26. McKelvie RS, Yusuf S, Pericak D, et al. Comparison of Candesartan, Enalapril, and Their Combination in Congestive Heart Failure: Randomized Evaluation of Strategies for Left Ventricular Dysfunction (RESOLVD) pilot study. The RESOLVD pilot study investigators. Circulation 1999; 100(10):1056–1064.

27. Pitt B, Zannad F, Remme WJ, et al. The Effect of Spironolactone on Morbidity and Mortality in Patients with severe Heart Failure. Randomized Aldactone Evaluation Study Investigators. N Engl J Med 1999; 341:709–717.

28. Pitt B, Williams G, Remme W, et al. The EPHESUS Trial: Eplerenone in Patients with Heart Failure Due To Systolic Dysfunction Complicating Acute Myocardial Infarction. Eplerenone Post-AMI Heart Failure Efficacy and Survival Study. Cardiovasc Drugs Ther 2001; 15: 79–87.

29. Goldsmith SR. Interactions Between the Sympathetic Nervous System and The RAAS in Heart Failure. Curr Heart Fail Rep 2004; 1(2):45–50.

30. van de Wal RM, Voors AA, Plokker HW, van Gilst WH, van Veldhuisen DJ. New Pharmacological Strategies in Chronic Heart Failure. Cardiovasc Drugs Ther 2004; 18(6):491–501.

31. Ahmed A. American college of Cardiology/American Heart Association Chronic Heart Failure Evaluation and Management Guidelines: relevance to the geriatric practice. J Am Geriatr Soc 2003; 51(1):123–126.

32. Ewy GA. Diastolic Dysfunction. J Insur Med 2004; 36(4):292–297.

33. de Las Fuentes L, Waggoner AD, Brown AL, Davila-Roman VG. Plasma triglyceride Level is an Independent Predictor of Altered Left Ventricular Relaxation. J Am Soc Echocardiogr 2005; 18(12):1285–1291.

34. Kasikcioglu HA, Karasulu L, Durgun E, Oflaz H, Kasikcioglu E, Cuhadaroglu C. Aortic Elastic Properties and Left Ventricular Diastolic Dysfunction in Patients With Obstructive Sleep Apnea. Heart Vessels. 2005; 20(6):239–44.

35. Araujo AQ, Arteaga E, Ianni BM, Buck PC, Rabello R, Mady C. Effect of Losartan on Left Ventricular Diastolic Function in Patients with Nonobstructive Hypertrophic Cardiomyopathy. Am J Cardiol 2005; 96(11):1563–1567.

36. Mottram PM, Short L, Baglin T, Marwick TH. Is 'Diastolic Heart Failure' a Diagnosis of Exclusion? Echocardiographic Parameters of Diastolic Dysfunction in Patients with Heart Failure and Normal systolic function. Heart Lung Circ 2003; 12(3):127–134.

37. Lim TK, Ashrafian H, Dwivedi G, Collinson PO, Senior R. Increased Left Atrial Volume Index is an Independent Predictor of Raised Serum Natriuretic Peptide in Patients with Suspected Heart Failure but Normal Left Ventricular Ejection Fraction: Implication for Diagnosis of Diastolic Heart Failure. Eur J Heart Fail 2005.

38. Qu P, Ding Y, Xia D, Wang H, Tian X. Variations in Cardiac Diastolic Function in Hypertensive Patients with Different Left Ventricular Geometric Patterns. Hypertens Res 2001; 24(5):601–604.

39. Morris SA, Van Swol M, Udani B. The Less Familiar Side of Heart Failure: Symptomatic Diastolic dysfunction. J Fam Pract 2005; 54(6):501–511.

40. Mandinov L, Eberli FR, Seiler C, Hess OM. Diastolic Heart Failure. Cardiovasc Res 2000; 45(4):813–825.

41. Chang NC, Shih CM, Bi WF, Lai ZY, Lin MS, Wang TC. Fosinopril Improves Left Ventricular Diastolic Function in Young mildly Hypertensive Patients Without Hypertrophy. Cardiovasc Drugs Ther 2002; 16(2): 141–147.

42. Roongsritong C, Sutthiwan P, Bradley J, Simoni J, Power S, Meyerrose GE. Spironolactone Improves Diastolic Function in the Elderly. Clin Cardiol 2005; 28(10):484–487.

43. The J-ELAN investigators. Effect of Losartan and Amlodipine on Left Ventricular Diastolic Function in Patients with Mild-To-Moderate Hypertension (J-ELAN). Circ J 2006; 70(1):124–128.

44. Bajraktari G, Koltai MS, Ademaj F, et al. Relationship Between Insulin Resistance and Left Ventricular Diastolic Dysfunction in Patients with Impaired Glucose Tolerance and Type 2 Diabetes. Int J Cardiol 2005.

45. Charvat J, Michalova K, Chlumsky J, Valenta Z, Kvapil M. The Association Between Left Ventricle Diastolic Dysfunction and Endothelial Dysfunction and the Results of Stress Myocardial SPECT in asymptomatic patients with type 2 diabetes. J Int Med Res 2005; 33(5):473–482.
46. Grandi AM, Piantanida E, Franzetti I, et al. Effect of Glycemic Control on Left Ventricular Diastolic Function in Type 1 diabetes mellitus. Am J Cardiol 2006; 97(1):71–76.
47. Rodeheffer RJ. The New Epidemiology of Heart Failure. Curr Cardiol Rep 2003; 5(3):181–186.
48. Wang TJ, Evans JC, Benjamin EJ, et al. Natural History of Left Ventricular Systolic Dysfunction in the Community. Circulation 2003; 108(8):977–982.
49. Das SR, Drazner MH, Yancy CW, Stevenson LW, Gersh BJ, Dries DL. Effects of Diabetes Mellitus and ischemic Heart Disease on the Progression from Asymptomatic Left Ventricular Dysfunction to Symptomatic heart failure: a retrospective analysis from the studies of left ventricular dysfunction (SOLVD) prevention trial. Am Heart J 2004; 148(5):883–888.
50. Das SR, Dries DL, Drazner MH, Yancy CW, Chae CU. Relation of Lower Hematocrit to Progression From Asymptomatic Left Ventricular Dysfunction to Symptomatic Heart Failure (from the studies of left ventricular dysfunction prevention trial). Am J Cardiol 2005; 96(6):827–831.
51. Francis GS, Benedict C, Johnstone DE, et al. Comparison of Neuroendocrine Activation in Patients With Left Ventricular Dysfunction with and without Congestive Heart Failure. A Substudy of the Studies of Left Ventricular Dysfunction (SOLVD). Circulation 1990; 82(5):1724–1729.
52. Philippides GJ. Managing The Post-Myocardial Infarction Patient with Asymptomatic Left Ventricular Dysfunction. Cardiology 2005; 105(2):95–107.
53. Dries DL, Strong MH, Cooper RS, Drazner MH. Efficacy of Angiotensin-converting Enzyme Inhibition in Reducing Progression from Asymptomatic Left Ventricular Dysfunction to Symptomatic Heart Failure in Black and White Patients. J Am Coll Cardiol 2002; 40(2):311–317.
54. Konstam MA, Kronenberg MW, Rousseau MF, et al. Effects of the Angiotensin Converting Enzyme Inhibitor Enalapril on the Long-term Progression of Left Ventricular Dilatation in Patients with Asymptomatic Systolic Dysfunction. SOLVD (Studies of Left Ventricular Dysfunction) Investigators. Circulation 1993; 88(5 Pt 1):2277–2283.
55. Jessup M, Brozena S. Heart Failure. N Engl J Med 2003; 348(20):2007–2018.
56. Eisenberg MJ, Gioia LC. Angiotensin II Receptor Blockers in Congestive Heart Failure. Cardiol Rev 2006; 14(1):26–34.
57. Prasad SK, Dargie HJ, Smith GC, et al. Comparison of the Dual Receptor Endothelin Antagonist Enrasentan with Enalapril in Asymptomatic Left Ventricular Systolic Dysfunction: a Cardiovascular magnetic Resonance Study. Heart 2005.
58. ACC/AHA 2005 Guideline Update. Diagnosis and Management of Chronic Heart Failure in the Adult. August 2005.
59. Zareba W, Piotrowicz K, McNitt S, Moss AJ. MADIT II investigators. Implantable Cardioverter-Defibrillator Efficacy in Patients with Heart Failure and Left Ventricular Dysfunction (from the MADIT II population). Am J Cardiol 2005; 95(12):1487–1491.
60. Moss AJ. MADIT–I and MADIT–II. J Cardiovasc Electrophysiol 2003; 14(suppl 9):S96–S98.
61. Moss AJ, Daubert J, Zareba W. MADIT–II: Clinical Implications. Card Electrophysiol Rev 2002; 6(4):463–465.
62. Moss AJ, Zareba W, Hall WJ, et al. Multicenter Automatic Defibrillator Implantation Trial II Investigators. Prophylactic Implantation of a Defibrillator in Patients with Myocardial Infarction and Reduced Ejection Fraction. N Engl J Med 2002; 346(12):877–883.
63. CONSENSUS Trial Study Group. Effects of Enalapril on Mortality in Severe Congestive Heart Failure. Results of the Cooperative North Scandinavian Enalapril Survival Study (CONSENSUS). N Engl J Med 1987; 316(23):1429–1435.
64. SOLVD investigators. Effect of Enalapril on Survival in Patients with Reduced Left Ventricular Ejection Fractions and Congestive Heart Failure. N Engl J Med 1991; 325(5):293–302.
65. SOLVD investigators. Effect of Enalapril on Mortality and the Development of Heart Failure in Asymptomatic Patients with Reduced Left Ventricular Ejection Fractions. The SOLVD investigators. N Engl J Med 1992; 327(10):685–691.
66. Pitt B. Use of Converting Enzyme Inhibitors in Patients With Asymptomatic Left Ventricular Dysfunction. J Am Coll Cardiol 1993; 22(4 Suppl A):158A–161A.
67. Greenberg B, Quinones MA, Koilpillai C, et al. Effects of Long-term Enalapril Therapy on Cardiac Structure and Function in Patients with Left Ventricular Dysfunction. Results of the SOLVD Echocardiography Substudy. Circulation. 1995; 91(10):2573–2581.
68. Kober L, Torp-Pedersen C, Carlsen JE, et al. A Clinical Trial of the Angiotensin-converting-enzyme Inhibitor Trandolapril in Patients with Left Ventricular Dysfunction After Myocardial Infarction. Trandolapril cardiac evaluation (TRACE) study group. N Engl J Med 1995; 333(25):1670–1676.
69. Ambrosioni E, Borghi C, Magnani B. The Effect Of the Angiotensin-converting-enzyme Inhibitor Zofenopril on Mortality and Morbidity After Anterior Myocardial Infarction. The Survival of Myocardial Infarction Long-term Evaluation (SMILE) Study Investigators. N Engl J Med 1995; 332(2):80–85.
70. Butler J, Arbogast PG, Daugherty J, Jain MK, Ray WA, Griffin MR. Outpatient Utilization of Angiotensin-converting Enzyme Inhibitors Among Heart Failure Patients After Hospital Discharge. J Am Coll Cardiol 2004; 43(11):2036–2043.

71. Pitt B, Segal R, Martinez FA, et al. Randomised Trial of Losartan versus Captopril in Patients Over 65 with Heart Failure (Evaluation of losartan in the elderly study, ELITE). Lancet 1997; 349(9054):747–752.

72. Pitt B, Poole-Wilson PA, Segal R, et al. Effect of Losartan Compared with Captopril on Mortality in Patients with Symptomatic Heart Failure: Randomised Trial — The Losartan Heart Failure Survival Study ELITE II. Lancet 2000; 355(9215):1582–1587.

73. Cohn JN, Tognoni G. valsartan Heart Failure Trial Investigators. A Randomized Trial of the Angiotensin-Receptor Blocker Valsartan in Chronic Heart Failure. N Engl J Med 2001; 345(23):1667–1675.

74. Maggioni AP, Anand I, Gottlieb SO, et al. Effects of Valsartan on Morbidity and Mortality in Patients with Heart Failure Not Receiving Angiotensin-converting Enzyme Inhibitors. J Am Coll Cardiol 2002; 40(8):1414–1421.

75. Wong M, Staszewsky L, Latini R, et al. Val-HeFT Hart Failure Trial Investigators. Valsartan Benefits Left Ventricular Structure and Function in Heart Failure: Val-HeFT Echocardiographic study. J Am Coll Cardiol 2002; 40(5):970–975.

76. Krum H, Carson P, Farsang C, et al. Effect of Valsartan Added to Background ACE Inhibitor Therapy in Patients with Heart Failure: Results from Val-HeFT. Eur J Heart Fail 2004; 6(7):937–945.

77. Young JB, Dunlap ME, Pfeffer MA, et al. Mortality and Morbidity Reduction with Candesartan in Patients with Chronic Heart Failure and left Ventricular Systolic Dysfunction: Results of the CHARM Low-left Ventricular Ejection Fraction Trials. Circulation 2004; 110(7):2618–2626.

78. Yusuf S, Ostergren JB, Gerstein HC, et al. Candesartan in Heart Failure-assessment of Reduction in Mortality and Morbidity Program Investigators. Effects of Candesartan on the Development of a New Diagnosis of Diabetes Mellitus in Patients with Heart Failure. Circulation 2005; 112(1):48–53.

79. Solomon SD, Wang D, Finn P, et al. Effect of Candesartan on Cause-specific Mortality in Heart Failure Patients: the Candesartan in Heart Failure Assessment Of Reduction in Mortality and Morbidity (CHARM) Program. Circulation 2004; 110(15):2180–2183.

80. Pfeffer MA, McMurray JJ, Velazquez EJ, et al. Valsartan, Captopril, or Both in Myocardial Infarction Complicated by Heart Failure, Left Ventricular dysfunction, or Both. N Engl J Med 2003; 349(20):1893-1906.

81. Doggrell SA. ACE Inhibitors or AT-1 Antagonists - Which is OPTIMAAL After Acute Myocardial Infarction? Expert Opin Pharmacother 2003; 4(3):407–409.

82. Dickstein K, Kjekshus J. OPTIMAAL Steering Committee of the OPTIMAAL Study Group. Effects of losartan and captopril on mortality and morbidity in high-risk patients after acute myocardial infarction: the OPTIMAAL randomised trial. Optimal trial in myocardial infarction with angiotensin II antagonist losartan. Lancet 2002; 360(9335):752–760.

83. Moller JE, Dahlstrom U, Gotzsche O, et al. OPTIMAAL Study Group. Effects of losartan and captopril on left ventricular systolic and diastolic function after acute myocardial infarction: results of the optimal trial in myocardial infarction with angiotensin II antagonist losartan (OPTIMAAL) echocardiographic substudy. Am Heart J 2004; 147(3):494–501.

84. Weber KT. Aldosterone in Congestive Heart Failure. N Engl J Med 2001; 345(23):1689–1697.

85. Schjoedt KJ, Andersen S, Rossing P, et al. Aldosterone Escape During Blockade Of the Rennin-angiotensin-aldosterone System in Diabetic Nephropathy is Associated with Enhanced Decline in Glomerular Filtration Rate. Diabetologia 2004; 47(11):1936–1939.

86. Deswal A, Yao D. Aldosterone Receptor Blockers in the Treatment of Heart Failure. Curr Treat Options Cardiovasc Med 2004; 6(4):327–334.

87. Cohn JN, Anand IS, Latini R, Masson S, Chiang YT, Glazer R; Valsartan Heart Failure Trial Investigators. sustained reduction of aldosterone in response to the angiotensin receptor blocker valsartan in patients with chronic heart failure: results from the valsartan heart failure trial. Circulation 2003; 108(11):1306–1309.

88. Pitt B. Effect of aldosterone blockade in patients with systolic left ventricular dysfunction: Implications of the RALES and EPHESUS Studies. Mol Cell Endocrinol 2004; 217(1–2):53–8.

89. Masoudi FA, Gross CP, Wang Y, et al. Adoption of Spironolactone Therapy for Older Patients With Heart Failure And Left Ventricular Systolic Dysfunction in the United States, 1998–2001. Circulation 2005; 112(1):39–47.

90. Juurlink DN, Mamdani MM, Lee DS, et al. Rates of hyperkalemia after publication of the Randomized Aldactone Evaluation Study. N Engl J Med 2004; 351(6):543–551.

91. Packer M, Bristow MR, Cohn JN, et al. The effect of carvedilol on morbidity and mortality in patients with chronic heart failure. U.S. Carvedilol Heart Failure Study Group. N Engl J Med 1996; 334:1349–1355.

92. MERIT-HF study group. Effect of metoprolol CR/XL in chronic heart failure: metoprolol CR/XL randomised Intervention Trial in Congestive Heart Failure (MERIT-HF). Lancet 1999; 253:2001–2007.

93. CIBIS–II Investigators. The Cardiac Insufficiency Bisoprolol Study II (CIBIS–II): a randomised trial. Lancet 1999; 353:9–13.

94. Packer M, Coats AJ, Fowler MB, et al. Carvedilol Prospective Randomized Cumulative Survival Study Group. Effect of carvedilol on survival in severe chronic heart failure. N Engl J Med 2001; 344:1651–1658.

95. Fowler MB, Vera-Llonch M, Oster G, et al. Influence of carvedilol on hospitalizations in heart failure: incidence, resource utilization and costs. U.S. Carvedilol Heart Failure Study Group. J Am Coll Cardiol 2001; 37:1692–1699.

96. Remme WJ, Riegger G, Hildebrandt P, et al. The benefits of early combination treatment of carvedilol and an ACE-inhibitor in mild heart failure and left ventricular systolic dysfunction. The Carvedilol

and ACE-Inhibitor Remodeling Mild Heart Failure Evaluation Trial (CARMEN). Cardiovasc Drugs Ther 2004; 18(1):57–66.

97. Yancy CW, Fowler MB, Colucci WS, et al. Carvedilol Heart Failure Study Group. Race and the response to adrenergic blockade with carvedilol in patients with chronic heart failure. N Engl J Med 2001; 344(18):1358–1365.

98. Cohn JN, Fowler MB, Bristow MR, et al. Safety and efficacy of carvedilol in severe heart failure. The U.S. Carvedilol Heart Failure Study Group. J Card Fail 1997; 3(3):173–179.

99. Krum H, Roecker EB, Mohacsi P, et al. Carvedilol Prospective Randomized Cumulative Survival (COPERNICUS) Study Group. Effects of initiating carvedilol in patients with severe chronic heart failure: results from the COPERNICUS study. JAMA 2003; 289(6):712–718.

100. Hjalmarson A, Goldstein S, Fagerberg B, et al. Effects of controlled-release metoprolol on total mortality, hospitalizations, and well-being in patients with heart failure: The Metoprolol CR/XL Randomized Intervention Trial in Congestive Heart Failure (MERIT-HF). MERIT-HF Study Group. JAMA 2000; 283(10):1295–1302.

101. Janosi A, Ghali JK, Herlitz J, et al. MERIT-HF study group. Metoprolol CR/XL in Postmyocardial infarction Patients With Chronic Heart Failure: Experiences From MERIT-HF. Am Heart J 2003; 146(4):721–728.

102. CIBIS–II investigators. Reduced Costs with Bisoprolol Treatment For Heart Failure: An Economic Analysis of The Second Cardiac Insufficiency Bisoprolol study (CIBIS–II). Eur Heart J 2001; 22(12):1021–1031.

103. Torp-Pedersen C, Poole-Wilson PA, Swedberg K, et al. Effects of metoprolol and carvedilol on cause-specific mortality and morbidity in patients with chronic heart failure—COMET. Am Heart J 2005; 149(2): 370–376.

104. Poole-Wilson PA, Swedberg K, Cleland JG, et al. Comparison of Carvedilol and Metoprolol on Clinical Outcomes in Patients with Chronic Heart Failure in the Carvedilol or Metoprolol European Trial (COMET): Randomised Controlled Trial. Lancet 2003; 362(9377): 7–13.

105. Bakris GL, Fonseca V, Katholi RE, et al. Metabolic effects of carvedilol vs metoprolol in patients with type 2 diabetes mellitus and hypertension: A Randomized Controlled trial. JAMA 2004; 292(18):2227–2236.

106. Lenzen MJ, Boersma E, Scholte Op Reimer WJ, et al. Under-utilization of evidence-based drug treatment in patients with heart failure is only partially explained by dissimilarity to patients enrolled in landmark trials: a report from The Euro Heart Survey on Heart Failure. Eur Heart J 2005; 26(24):2706–2713.

107. Hori M, Sasayama S, Kitabatake A, et al. Low-dose carvedilol improves left ventricular function and reduces cardiovascular hospitalization in japanese patients with chronic heart failure: The Multicenter Carvedilol Heart Failure Dose Assessment (MUCHA) trial. Am Heart J 2004; 147(2):324–330.

108. Bristow MR, Gilbert EM, Abraham WT, et al. Carvedilol Produces Dose-related Improvements in Left Ventricular Function and Survival in Subjects with Chronic Heart Failure. MOCHA investigators. Circulation 1996; 94(11):2807–2816.

109. Majumdar SR, McAlister FA, Cree M. Do evidence-based treatments provide incremental benefits to patients with congestive heart failure already receiving angiotensin-converting enzyme inhibitors? A Secondary Analysis of One-year Outcomes From the Assessment of Treatment with Lisinopril and Survival (ATLAS) study. Clin Ther 2004; 26(5):694–703.

110. Wade OL. Digoxin 1785–1985.   I. Two Hundred Years of Digitalis. J Clin Hosp Pharm 1986; 11(1):3–9.

111. Poole-Wilson PA, Robinson K. Digoxin—a redundant drug in congestive cardiac failure. Cardiovasc Drugs Ther. 1989; 2(6):733–741.

112. Digitalis Investigation Group. The effect of digoxin on mortality and morbidity in patients with heart failure. The Digitalis Investigation Group. N Engl J Med 1997; 336(8):525–533.

113. Ahmed A, Rich MW, Love TE, et al. Digoxin and reduction in mortality and hospitalization in heart failure: a comprehensive post hoc analysis of the DIG trial. Eur Heart J 2006; 27(2):178–186.

114. Lader E, Egan D, Hunsberger S, Garg R, Czajkowski S, McSherry F. The effect of digoxin on the quality of life in patients with heart failure. J Card Fail 2003; 9(1):4–12.

115. Shammas NW, Harris ML, McKinney D, Hauber WJ. Digoxin withdrawal in patients with dilated cardiomyopathy following normalization of ejection fraction with beta blockers. Clin Cardiol 2001; 24(12):786–787.

116. Uretsky BF, Young JB, Shahidi FE, Yellen LG, Harrison MC, Jolly MK. Randomized Study Assessing The Effect of Digoxin Withdrawal in Patients with Mild to Moderate Chronic Congestive Heart Failure: Results of the PROVED trial. PROVED investigative group. J Am Coll Cardiol 1993; 22(4):955–962.

117. Packer M, Gheorghiade M, Young JB, et al. Withdrawal of digoxin from patients with chronic heart failure treated with angiotensin-converting-enzyme inhibitors. RADIANCE Study. N Engl J Med 1993; 329(1):1–7.

118. Dec GW. Digoxin remains useful in the management of chronic heart failure. Med Clin North Am 2003; 87(2):317–337.

119. Leon AR, Abraham WT, Brozena S, et al. InSync III Clinical Study Investigators. Cardiac resynchronization with sequential biventricular pacing for the treatment of moderate-to-severe heart failure. J Am Coll Cardiol 2005; 46(12):2298–2304.

120. Leon AR, Abraham WT, Curtis AB, et al. MIRACLE Study Program. Safety of Transvenous Cardiac Resynchronization System Implantation in Patients with Chronic Heart Failure: Combined Results of over 2,000 Patients From a Multicenter Study Program. J Am Coll Cardiol 2005; 46(12):2348–2356.

121. Woo GW, Petersen-Stejskal S, Johnson JW, Conti JB, Aranda JA Jr, Curtis AB. Ventricular reverse remodeling and 6-month outcomes in patients receiving cardiac resynchronization therapy: Analysis of the MIRACLE Study. J Interv Card Electrophysiol 2005; 12(2):107–113.

122. Bristow MR, Saxon LA, Boehmer J, et al. Comparison of Medical Therapy, Pacing, and Defibrillation in Heart Failure (COMPANION) Investigators. Cardiac-Resynchronization Therapy with or without an Implantable Defibrillator in Advanced Chronic Heart failure. N Engl J Med 2004; 350(21):2140–2150.

123. Bardy GH, Lee KL, Mark DB, et al. Sudden Cardiac Death in Heart Failure Trial (SCD-HeFT) Investigators. Amiodarone or an implantable cardioverter-defibrillator for congestive heart failure. N Engl J Med 2005; 352(3):225–237.

124. Moss AJ, Greenberg H, Case RB, et al. Multicenter Automatic Defibrillator Implantation Trial–II (MADIT–II) Research Group. Long-term Clinical Course of Patients After Termination of Ventricular Tachyarrhythmia by an Implanted Defibrillator. Circulation 2004; 110(25):3760–3765.

125. Moss AJ, Brown MW, Cannom DS, et al. Multicenter Automatic Defibrillator Implantation Trial-Cardiac Resynchronization Therapy (MADIT-CRT): Design and Clinical Protocol. Ann Noninvasive Electrocardiol 2005; 10(suppl 4):34–43.

126. Naughton MT. The Link Between Obstructive Sleep Apnea and Heart Failure: Underappreciated Opportunity for Treatment. Curr Cardiol Rep 2005; 7(3):211–215.

127. O'Connor CM, Stough WG, Gallup DS, Hasselblad V, Gheorghiade M. Demographics, Clinical characteristics, and Outcomes of Patients Hospitalized for Decompensated Heart Failure: Observations from the IMPACT-HF Registry. J Card Fail 2005; 11(3):200–205.

128. Levine BS. Intermittent Positive Inotrope Infusion in the Management of End-stage, Low-output Heart Failure. J Cardiovasc Nurs 2000; 14(4):76–93.

129. Felker GM, O'Connor CM. Inotropic Therapy for Heart Failure: An Evidence-based Approach. Am Heart J 2001; 142(3):393–401.

130. Cuffe MS, Califf RM, Adams KF Jr, et al. Outcomes of a Prospective Trial of Intravenous Milrinone for Exacerbations of Chronic Heart Failure (OPTIME-CHF) Investigators. Short-term Intravenous Milrinone for Acute Exacerbation of Chronic Heart Failure: a Randomized Controlled Trial. JAMA 2002; 287(12):1541–1547.

131. Abraham WT, Adams KF, Fonarow GC, et al. ADHERE Scientific Advisory Committee and Investigators; ADHERE Study Group. In-hospital Mortality in Patients with Acute Decompensated Heart Failure requiring intravenous vasoactive medications: an analysis from the acute decompensated heart failure National Registry (ADHERE). J Am Coll Cardiol 2005; 46(1):57–64

132. Colucci WS, Elkayam U, Horton DP, et al. Intravenous Nesiritide, a Natriuretic Peptide, in the Treatment of Decompensated Congestive Heart Failure. Nesiritide Study Group. N Engl J Med 2000; 343(4):246–253.

133. Abraham WT, Cheng ML, Smoluk G. Vasodilation in the Management of Acute Congestive Heart Failure (VMAC) Study Group. Clinical and Hemodynamic Effects of Nesiritide (B-type natriuretic peptide) in Patients with Decompensated Heart Failure Receiving Beta Blockers. Congest Heart Fail 2005; 11(2):59–64

134. Burger AJ, Horton DP, LeJemtel T, et al. Prospective Randomized Evaluation of Cardiac Ectopy with Dobutamine or Natrecor Therapy. Effect of Nesiritide (B–type natriuretic peptide) and Dobutamine on Ventricular Arrhythmias in The Treatment of Patients with Acutely Decompensated Congestive Heart Failure: the PRECEDENT study. Am Heart J 2002; 144(6):1102–1108.

135. Mills RM, LeJemtel TH, Horton DP, et al. Sustained Hemodynamic Effects of an Infusion of Nesiritide (Human b-type Natriuretic peptide) in Heart Failure: a Randomized, Double-blind, Placebo-controlled Clinical trial. Natrecor Study Group. J Am Coll Cardiol 1999; 34(1):155–162.

136. VMAC Investigators (Vasodilatation in the Management of Acute CHF). Intravenous Nesiritide vs Nitroglycerin for Treatment of Decompensated Congestive Heart Failure: a Randomized Controlled Trial. JAMA 2002; 287(12):1531–1540.

137. Peacock WF, Emerman CL, Silver MA. Nesiritide Added to Standard Care Favorably Reduces Systolic Blood Pressure Compared with Standard Care Alone in Patients With Acute Decompensated Heart Failure. Am J Emerg Med 2005; 23(3):327–331.

138. Yancy CW, Saltzberg MT, Berkowitz RL, et al. Safety and feasibility of Using Serial Infusions of Nesiritide for Heart Failure in an Outpatient Setting (from the FUSION I trial). Am J Cardiol 2004; 94(5):595–601.

139. Rose EA, Gelijns AC, Moskowitz AJ, et al. Randomized Evaluation of Mechanical Assistance For the Treatment of Congestive Heart Failure (REMATCH) Study Group. Long-term Mechanical Left Ventricular Assistance for end-stage Heart failure. N Engl J Med 2001; 345(20):1435–1443.

140. Stevenson LW, Miller LW, Desvigne-Nickens P, et al. REMATCH Investigators. Left Ventricular Assist Device as Destination for Patients Undergoing Intravenous Inotropic Therapy: a Subset Analysis From REMATCH (Randomized Evaluation of Mechanical Assistance in Treatment of Chronic Heart Failure). Circulation 2004; 110(8):975–981.

141. Long JW, Kfoury AG, Slaughter MS, et al. Long-term Destination Therapy with the Heartmate XVE Left Ventricular Assist Device: Improved Outcomes Since The REMATCH Study. Congest Heart Fail 2005; 11(3):133–138.

142. AIRE Investigators. Effect of Ramipril on Mortality and Morbidity of Survivors of Acute Myocardial Infarction with Clinical Evidence of Heart Failure. The Acute Infarction Ramipril Efficacy (AIRE) Study Investigators. Lancet 1993; 342:821–828.

143. Braunwald E, Ross J Jr, Sonnenblick EH. Mechanisms of contraction of the normal and failing heart. 2nd ed. Boston: Little, Brown, 1976:417.

144. Cohn JN. The management of Chronic Heart Failure. N Engl J Med 1996; 335:490–498.

145. DiBianco R, Shabetai R, Kostuk W, Moran J, Schlant RC, Wright R. A Comparison of Oral Milrinone, Digoxin, and Their Combination in the Treatment of Patients With Chronic Heart Failure. N Engl J Med 1989; 320(11):677–683.

146. Francis GS. Pathophysiology of Chronic Heart Failure. Am J Med 2001; 110(Suppl 7A):37S–46S.

147. Keating GM, Goa KL. Nesiritide: a Review of its Use in Acute Decompensated Heart Failure. Drugs 2003; 63(1):47–70

148. Pfeffer MA, Braunwald E, Moye LA, et al. Effect of Captopril on Mortality and Morbidity in Patients with Left Ventricular Dysfunction After Myocardial Infarction. Results of the Survival and Ventricular Enlargement Trial. The SAVE Investigators. N Engl J Med 1992; 327(10):669–677.

149. Packer M, Cohn JN, Abraham WT, et al. Consensus Recommendations for the Management of Chronic Heart Failure. Am J Cardiol 1999; 83:1A–38A.

150. Pfeffer MA, Swedberg K, Granger CB, et al. Effects of Candesartan on Mortality and Morbidity in Patients with Chronic Heart Failure: the CHARM-Overall Programme. Lancet 2003; 362(9386):759–766.

151. Shlipak MG, Smith GL, Rathore SS, Massie BM, Krumholz HM. Renal Function, Digoxin Therapy, and Heart Failure Outcomes: Evidence From the Digoxin Intervention Group Trial. J Am Soc Nephrol 2004; 15(8):2195–2203.

152. Vasan RS, Levy D. The role of Hypertension in the Pathogenesis of Heart Failure. A Clinical Mechanistic Overview. Arch Intern Med 1996; 156(16):1789–1796.

16 | Stroke Prevention

Shyam Prabhakaran, Bernardo Liberato, and Ralph L. Sacco
Stroke and Critical Care Division, The Neurological Institute, Columbia University, New York, New York, U.S.A.

KEY POINTS

- Primary stroke prevention is the single most effective and widely applicable approach in the management of high-risk patients.
- Transient ischemic attack is associated with a high early risk (often within two days) of ischemic stroke and represents a unique opportunity to intervene urgently.
- Atrial fibrillation and severe carotid stenosis are associated with considerable stroke risk and warrant specific treatments including anticoagulation (warfarin) and carotid endarterectomy in appropriate cases.
- For lacunar stroke, intracranial atherosclerotic stroke, and cryptogenic stroke, antiplatelet therapy (aspirin, clopidogrel, or extended-release dipyirdamole-aspirin) is indicated to prevent stroke recurrence.
- Emerging risk markers include elevated homocysteine levels, and chronic inflammation/infection, and the use of surrogate markers such as carotid intima-media thickness or silent strokes may prove valuable in the future.

INTRODUCTION

Stroke is defined by the World Health Organization as "sudden onset of signs of focal or global disturbance of cerebral function lasting more than 24 hours (unless interrupted by surgery or death), with no apparent nonvascular cause" (1). Despite a decline in stroke mortality since the middle of the last century, it remains a major cause of morbidity and mortality worldwide, ranking second behind heart disease in mortality. In addition, it is a leading cause of disability, exerting psychological, physical, and financial burdens to the patient, community, and society. The direct and indirect costs related to stroke in the United States in 2005 is estimated to be nearly 57 billion dollars (2). The public health impact of stroke cannot be overstated, especially with the growing elderly population in most developed countries.

A basic assumption of stroke preventive measures is that a reduction in prevalence of risk factors should decrease stroke prevalence and incidence. A study comparing two time periods (1981–1984 vs. 2002–2004) in Oxfordshire demonstrated the benefits of population level changes in multiple risk factors over time (3). This study found that reductions in smoking, cholesterol, blood pressure (BP), and increases in premorbid antiplatelet, lipid lowering, and BP medications were associated with lower overall stroke incidence in 2002–2004 compared to 1981–1984. Prevention is, therefore, crucial in the public health battle against stroke, especially given the relatively few successful acute stroke treatments. Furthermore, since risk factors contribute to stroke risk over years and decades, there is a significantly greater window of opportunity for stroke prevention compared with acute stroke treatment.

Stroke prevention is contingent upon identifying individuals and/or communities at risk. Some risk factors may be nonmodifiable, such as age, sex, race-ethnicity, and heredity. However, there are also multiple modifiable risk factors with opportunities of intervention. This chapter outlines the epidemiology of stroke, risk factors, primary and secondary prevention strategies and treatments, and finally, novel and emerging risk factors.

OVERVIEW OF ISCHEMIC STROKE

Stroke prevention strategies are often hindered by the heterogeneity of stroke. Hemorrhage stroke, which constitutes approximately 15% to 20% of all strokes, is further divided into subarachnoid hemorrhage (SAH) and intracerebral hemorrhage (ICH). These disease entities, while sharing some risk factors with ischemic stroke, have specific patterns of presentation and management strategies

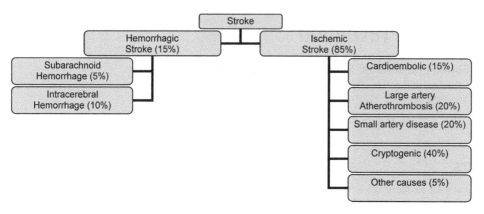

FIGURE 1 Classification of stroke.

that differ dramatically from ischemic stroke. Therefore, this chapter will introduce ischemic stroke subtypes and transient ischemic attack (TIA), focusing on ischemic stroke prevention only.

Ischemic Stroke Subtype Classification

Even in ischemic stroke, considerable heterogeneity exists and treatment strategies are guided by determination of stroke subtype. Subtype classification schemes have been developed, with the Trial of Org 10172 in Acute Stroke (TOAST) classification being the most widely used clinically (4). Derived from TOAST, five distinct categories of ischemic stroke are recognized: cardioembolisom, large artery atherosclerosis (LAA), small artery disease, undetermined or cryptogenic stroke, and other specified-cause stroke (Fig. 1).

Cardioembolic Stroke

Documented cardiac sources of embolism account for 15% of all ischemic strokes in most modern registries and databases (5–7). Syndromes of cardioembolic stroke (CE) characteristically begin suddenly, occasionally with swift improvement suggesting rapid recanalization. The latter is sometimes associated with petechial hemorrhagic conversion of a bland infarction. The most common cardiac sources are atrial fibrillation (AF) with atrial thrombus, left ventricular thrombus after myocardial infarction (MI), cardiomyopathy with depressed ejection fraction (EF), and valvular heart disease.

Large Artery Atherosclerosis

Large artery thrombosis and occlusion occurs in 20% of ischemic strokes. Two mechanisms are often implicated: perfusion failure and artery-to-artery embolism. The former depends on the presence of intracranial collaterals and if they are absent, it can result in classic deep internal borderzone infarction when the internal carotid artery (ICA) or middle cerebral artery (MCA) is affected. Artery-to-artery embolism implies the release of thrombotic debris from a proximal plaque to a more distal branch vessel resulting in occlusion and tissue infarction.

Small Artery Disease

Lacunar stroke, accounting for 20% of infarctions, arises from arterial lipohyalinization and often produces stroke syndromes with fairly stereotyped presentations. These include pure motor hemiparesis from internal capsular or basis pontis infarction, pure sensory stroke from thalamic infarction, dysarthric-clumsy hand syndrome from deep pontine or white matter infarction, and ataxia-hemiparesis also from deep pontine infarction.

Undetermined or Cryptogenic Stroke

Despite modern technological advances in the evaluation of stroke, this remains the most common stroke subtype (40%). Hypotheses regarding the exact mechanisms in these unexplained strokes include occult embolism such as paradoxical embolus via a patent foramen ovale (PFO) and prothrombotic states such as antiphospholipid antibody syndrome.

Other Determined Cause

These strokes are the result of rare but well-known causes of stroke often in the young such as migraine, cervical arterial dissection, and cerebral venous thrombosis. Stroke of other determined cause only accounts for lesser than 5% ischemic strokes.

Transient Ischemic Attack

TIA lies on one end of the spectrum of focal brain ischemia, the other being complete brain infarction or ischemic stroke. While TIA symptoms are, by definition, reversible, the risk factors and risk of stroke following TIA are similar to that of ischemic stroke and warrant urgent evaluation and intervention. Some studies suggest that TIA might actually be a higher risk state in the acute period. This sense of urgency is apparent in the newly proposed definition of TIA, changing the duration criteria from less than 24 hours to less than one hour. The TIA Working Group expert panel's new definition of TIA is "a brief episode of neurologic dysfunction caused by focal brain or retinal ischemia, with clinical symptoms lasting less than one hour and without evidence of infarction on brain imaging" (8).

EPIDEMIOLOGY OF STROKE
Mortality

According to the Centers for Disease Control and Prevention, the decline in deaths due to coronary heart disease (CHD) and stroke were among the 10 great public health achievements in the United States during the last century (9). The decline in stroke mortality from 88.8 deaths to 26.5 deaths per 100,000 from 1950 to 1999 (73% decrease) is a remarkable achievement. Credit for this dramatic change has been given to improved risk factor modification, especially hypertension control and smoking cessation. Internationally, however, stroke mortality continues to be very high, with minimal rates of decline. The lowest rates are found in North America and Western Europe while Eastern Europe, Asia, and South America continue to have very high mortality rates (10).

Incidence

While there has been a decline in stroke mortality during the last century, most studies have found steady or slightly increasing stroke incidence rates during this same period (11–13). However, two more recent studies have found that incidence of stroke during the last decade is declining (3,14).

Population-based studies have observed that the age- and sex-adjusted incidence of ischemic stroke per 100,000 ranges from 88 to 162 among Caucasians (3,6,15–17), 149 to 168 among Hispanics (15,16), and 191 to 246 among African-Americans (15,18). These data suggest that a race-ethnic difference exists, with a greater burden of stroke incidence among African-Americans and Hispanics.

Prevalence

In terms of public health burden, stroke prevalence has far greater implications than incidence rates. As stroke mortality declines and average lifespan continues to increase, the number of individuals surviving from strokes has been increasing and will probably continue to rise. It has been estimated that in the United States, there are over four million stroke survivors with nearly 12% of the population over 75 years of age being affected (2).

RISK FACTORS FOR ISCHEMIC STROKE

Several factors that elevate stroke risk cannot be modified by treatment regimens and may be better termed "risk markers." These include age, gender, race-ethnicity, geography, and genetics/heredity (Table 1). Certain other biologic and lifestyle determinants have been associated with elevated stroke risk (Table 2). As modifiable risk factors, these represent opportunities for clinicians to intervene and thereby lower stroke risk in high-risk patients. The Stroke Council of the American Heart Association (AHA) in its statement, "Primary prevention of ischemic stroke," has outlined the goals of risk factor management (20).

Nonmodifiable Risk Factors
Age

The incidence of stroke is known to increase with advancing age, doubling each decade after 55 years; the most dramatic risk elevations occur in the group of individuals over 75 years.

TABLE 1 Nonmodifiable Risk Factors for Ischemic Stroke

Risk factor	Effect on stroke incidence
Age	Doubles per decade over age 55
Sex	1.4-fold increase for men
Race-ethnicity	2.4-fold increase for African Americans
	2.0-fold increase for Hispanics
Heredity	1.9-fold increase among first degree relatives

Source: From Ref. 19.

Furthermore, stroke mortality increases with age due to increased incidence rates or higher case fatality. The adjusted relative risk (RR) associated with increase in age of every decade was estimated to be 1.66 in men and 1.93 in women (21). In the Cardiovascular Heart Study, the RR of stroke was 1.81 in the 70 to 74 age group, 2.96 in the 75 to 79 age group, and 3.55 in the 80 to 85 age group compared to the 65 to 69 age group (22). As incidence increases with age, there is also a substantial increase in the number of survivors (prevalence) in the older population (2,4).

Gender

Age-adjusted stroke incidence and mortality appear to be higher among men compared to women. In terms of stroke-related mortality over the past 25 years, there is a persistently higher risk among men compared to women, about 14% to 20% increase in whites and 21% to 34% increase in blacks (4). This risk difference lessens with increasing age and is reversed in the age group over 85, where women have a slightly higher risk of death from stroke. Likewise, stroke incidence appears to be higher among males, a finding that is also most striking in the younger age groups and dissipates with advancing age (Fig. 2) (15,22).

However, several studies have shown that women, over a lifetime, are more likely to suffer a stroke with worse functional outcomes at three and six months after stroke (23–26). This has been attributed to the longer average lifespan of women compared to men, leading to an over representation of women in the age group over 85, where risk of stroke is highest. Some studies have suggested a difference in management by the sexes, with less intense diagnostic evaluation in women with stroke (27–29). In contrast, others have observed a gender difference favoring women after intravenous thrombolysis for ischemic stroke (30,31).

Race and Ethnicity

National statistics have shown that African-Americans have nearly double the mortality from stroke compared to Caucasians. This difference is magnified in the younger age groups (nearly four times higher among African-Americans) and is less apparent in the elderly (32). Although

TABLE 2 Established Modifiable Risk Factors for Ischemic Stroke

Risk factor	Prevalence in the United States (%)	Relative risk	Risk reduction with treatment
Smoking	23	1.9	50% in 1 yr, baseline in 5 yr
Hypertension			35–40%
50–59 yr	20	4.0	
60–69 yr	30	3.0	
70–79 yr	40	2.0	
80–89 yr	55	1.4	
90 + yr	60	1.0	
Diabetes	20	1.5–3.0	No direct reduction in stroke risk
Dyslipidemia	20–45	1.0–1.4	16–30%
Atrial fibrillation			68% (warfarin)
50–59 yr	0.5	4.0	21% (aspirin)
60–69 yr	1.8	2.6	
70–70 yr	4.8	3.3	
80–89 yr	8.8	4.5	

Source: From Ref. 20.

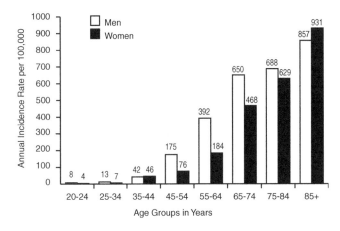

FIGURE 2   Incidence of stroke by age group and gender. *Source*: From Ref. 15.

a small increase of stroke mortality exists for Hispanics compared to Caucasians, it also dissipates with age.

Incidence of stroke among different race-ethnic groups has also been studied, again showing race-ethnic disparities most prominently in the younger age groups (<65). In the Greater Cincinnati/Northern Kentucky Stroke Study (GCNKSS), the age- and sex-adjusted incidence of first stroke among African-Americans was 288 per 100,000 person-years, nearly twice that seen in the predominantly white population of Rochester, Minnesota (18) and 246 per 100,000 for first ischemic stroke (33). A similar pattern was seen in the Northern Manhattan Stroke Study (NOMASS), where African-Americans had a 2.4-fold and Caribbean Hispanics a 2-fold increase in stroke incidence compared with whites (Fig. 3) (15). Mexican-Hispanics in The Brain Attack Surveillance in Corpus Christi Project also had a higher incidence of stroke compared to non-Hispanic Caucasians (16). These data suggest that the increased stroke mortality seen in minorities, particularly in young African-Americans, is partly explained by the increased stroke incidence.

In terms of stroke subtype, several studies have found that the overall increased incidence in minority groups seems to be from an increase in all subtypes of stroke. In Northern Manhattan, African-Americans and Hispanics had higher rates of all subtypes, but most dramatically in the intracranial atherosclerotic and lacunar subtypes of ischemic stroke and less so in cardioembolic and cryptogenic strokes (CS) (34). In GCNKSS, all subtypes had higher incidence rates among African-Americans compared to Caucasians, with the highest risk ratios (RR 1.9) in lacunar stroke and CS subtypes (7).

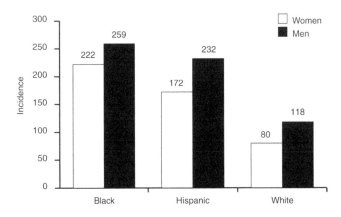

Age-adjusted stroke incidence for white, black, and Hispanic northern Manhattan residents over age 20

FIGURE 3   Incidence of stroke by race-ethnicity and gender. *Source*: From Ref. 15.

Geography

The concept of a "stroke belt" has been known since at least 1940 and refers to the southeastern United States: North Carolina, South Carolina, Georgia, Mississippi, Alabama, Tennessee, Louisiana, and Arkansas. The excess stroke mortality in this region is thought to be 1.3 to 1.5 times more than the rest of the United States. Within this region, a "super stroke belt" or "stroke buckle" has been identified to exist in the Carolinas and Georgia with even higher mortality than other "stroke belt" states (35). In recent years, with the decline of stroke mortality across the United States, there has been a shift in this geographic distribution with Oregon and Washington forming a satellite of the "stroke belt," and Mississippi and Alabama falling out the highest stroke mortality group (36).

While its causes are debated, there is less debate regarding the existence of a "stroke belt" or regional variations in stroke mortality (37). Although some of the excess mortality seems to be related to a higher proportion of African-Americans (in whom stroke mortality is known to be higher) living in the "stroke belt," this is unlikely to explain the entire difference. Furthermore, the difference in stroke mortality has been shown to exist across age, gender, and race-ethnic groups and does not seem to reflect differences in diagnostic accuracy, standards of care, certification practices, or incidence rates (37). Other potential explanations include regional variations in stroke risk factors (hypertension, diabetes, etc.), lifestyle differences (smoking, alcohol, and exercise), societal factors such as socioeconomic status, dietary and micronutrient factors, and genetic variation by region (35,37).

Genetics

Large epidemiological studies have shown that family history of stroke, MI, or both were associated with stroke at a younger age. By subtype, family history of stroke was associated with all subtypes though less pronounced in CE (38). Genetic susceptibility to other risk factors such as hypertension, hyperlipidemia, and diabetes may be potential confounders in this relationship. There are also aggregation studies that show clustering of risk in families, sometimes on the basis of twin studies showing higher concordance among monozygotic twins compared to dizygotic. Furthermore, animal and human genetic studies have begun to identify putative "stroke genes."

Although rare, several Mendelian stroke disorders have been identified: cerebral autosomal dominant arteriopathy with subcortical infarcts and leukoencephalopathy, homocystinuria, familial hypercholestrolemia, Tangier disease, sickle cell disease, Fabry disease, protein C and S deficiency, Factor V Leiden and prothrombin gene mutations, mitochondial disorders, fibromuscular dysplasia, and Marfan's syndrome. These should be considered in childhood and young adults presenting with ischemic stroke. However, more recent evidence suggests that the majority of ischemic stroke may be a complex, polygenic disorder with multiple gene–environment interactions and unlikely to result from single gene mutations (39).

Modifiable Risk Factors
Lifestyle/Behavioral Risk Factors
Cigarette Smoking

Tobacco use, most commonly cigarette smoking, is a major public health problem in the United States, with 50 million (23%) Americans still smoking (40). Although longitudinal trends suggest an overall decline in smoking, this is belied by the increase seen in certain groups of the population, particularly young women. Cigarette smoking is an independent risk factor for stroke that is readily amenable to modification. A meta-analysis of 32 studies found an RR of stroke for smokers of 1.9, with greater impact among younger individuals and perhaps in women (41). The population-attributable risk is 12% to 18%. A dose–response relationship exists, with increased stroke risk in heavy smokers compared with light smokers (42). Smoking also exerts its impact differentially on stroke, being most dramatic in SAH, intermediate in ischemic stroke, and lowest in ICH. The effects of passive cigarette smoking exposure also increase the risk of progression of atherosclerosis and risk of ischemic stroke (43–45). urrogate stroke risk markers, such as carotid atherosclerosis, are clearly linked to smoking (46). It may also increase stroke risk by increasing carotid intima-medial thickness (IMT) and arterial stiffness (47). Current smoking status was associated with a 50% increase in progression of IMT (43). Other mechanisms by which smoking increases ischemic stroke risk include activation of blood viscosity, hypercoaguability and enhanced platelet aggregation, decreased high-density lipoprotein cholesterol (HDL-C) levels, and elevation of BP (48).

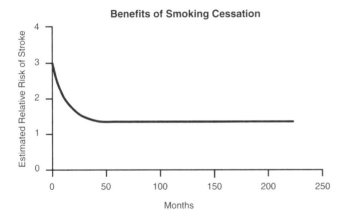

FIGURE 4 Stroke risk reduction with smoking cessation. *Source*: From Ref. 49.

Treatment and Recommendations. Smoking cessation is associated with marked reduction in stroke risk. Observational studies have noted that significant lowering of risk occurs within two to five years after smoking cessation, with 50% risk reduction at one year. In fact, the risk of stroke among former smokers reduces to that of nonsmokers within five years of smoking cessation (Fig. 4) (49). The potential impact of eliminating smoking in the United States has been estimated to reduce strokes by 61,500 per year and save 3.08 billion dollars in stroke-related health care costs (50).

Based on the Cochrane Tobacco Addiction Review Group, physician advice alone increased the odds of quitting by 1.7, as were nurses' counseling and individual and group therapy. All forms of nicotine replacement therapy (gum, patch, inhaler, and nasal spray) were equally effective in smoking cessation with an OR of 1.7. The same review found that buproprion and nortriptyline increase cessation rates (51). In a randomized controlled trial, combination therapy with buproprion and nicotine were more effective at maintaining abstinence at 12 months compared with either treatment alone (52). Current guidelines, therefore, support smoking cessation to lower cardiovascular and cerebrovascular risk. The use of counseling, various nicotine substitutes, and buproprion, in combination has been recommended (53). The AHA Stroke Council recommends smoking cessation for all current smokers (20).

Alcohol

Although alcohol poses health risks and is readily modifiable, the relationship between alcohol and ischemic stroke has been less straightforward. Studies have shown an increased risk of hemorrhagic stroke with increasing levels of alcohol consumption (54,55). However, the Nurses' Health Study found a protective effect of mild alcohol consumption (up to 1.2 drinks per day) for ischemic stroke (56). In a large study of male physicians, moderate alcohol consumption was again protective for ischemic stroke (57). Other prospective cohort studies have failed to confirm this relationship (58,59).

In NOMASS, a J-shaped relationship between alcohol and ischemic stroke was found with an elevated stroke risk for heavy alcohol consumption (greater than 5 drinks per day) and a protective effect in light to moderate drinkers (2 or fewer drinks per day) when compared to nondrinkers (Fig. 5) (60). In a meta-analysis of 35 observational studies, greater than 60g of daily alcohol intake was associated with an RR of 1.69 for ischemic stroke. Furthermore, moderate consumption (0–12 and 12–24 g/day) was associated with reduced ischemic stroke risk (RR 0.80 and 0.72, respectively) (61).

Alcohol, therefore, may have both beneficial and deleterious effects, depending on the quantity consumed. The various mechanisms through which alcohol may increase the risk of stroke include hypertension, hypercoagulable states, cardiac arrhythmias, and cerebral blood flow reductions. However, there is also evidence that light to moderate drinking can increase HDL-C levels, reduce the risk of coronary artery disease (CAD), and increase endogenous tissue plasminogen activator, stabilize plaques, and improve endothelial function (62).

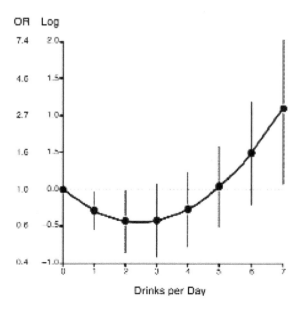

FIGURE 5 Alcohol consumption and risk of stroke. *Source*: From Ref. 60.

Treatment and Recommendations. Recommendations for alcohol consumption reflect this J-shaped relationship regarding stroke risk. Heavy drinking (>5 drinks per day) and binge drinking should be discouraged and moderate drinking (up to 2 drinks per day for men and 1 drink per day for nonpregnant women) may be recommended for those who wish to drink (20). Extensive promotion of alcohol intake to the general population, however, cannot be justified given the adverse effects to other organ systems and the potential for alcohol abuse and addiction (63). Although no randomized studies exist due to ethical concerns, the Physicians Health Study (PHS) did show that in the cohort of physicians who increased their consumption from less than 1 drink per week to 1 to 6 drinks per week, there was a 29% decrease in cardiovascular events (64).

Physical Inactivity
The 2000–2001 Behavioral Risk Factor Surveillance Survey found that 26% Americans report no leisure-time physical activity and 55% adults did not achieve the recommended amount of physical activity, a majority of who were in the lower income and educational levels (65). Moreover, these include a significant proportion of elderly who are unlikely or unable to participate in physical activity at the recommended levels (66). The prevalence of this risk factor will, therefore, undoubtedly increase as the population ages.

Regular moderate exercise is known to reduce mortality and cardiovascular disease (67,68), but the relationship to stroke is more controversial. Studies have evaluated the association between physical activity and the risk of stroke, and the preponderance of evidence supports this association. Older middle-aged Japanese-American men in the Honolulu Heart Study with habitual physical activity had lower risk of thromboembolic stroke, an effect found only in nonsmokers (69). The Framingham Study showed that physical activity lowered stroke risk in men, but not in women (70). However, both the Copenhagen City Heart Study and the Nurses' Health Study of women 40 to 65 years old demonstrated that increased physical activity was also associated with lower stroke risk in women (71,72). In the NOMASS, leisure-time physical activity was protective for stroke (OR 0.37) among all ages, genders, and race-ethnic subgroups (73). In addition, heavy exercise for an extended duration afforded added benefit over light or moderate forms for lesser duration. In the PHS, increasing physical activity, showed a trend for decreasing stroke risk (74). A meta-analysis of 23 studies of physical activity and stroke risk found that highly active people had a 27% lower risk of stroke or mortality compared with less active people (75).

The protective effect of physical activity may be mediated by, or partly confounded by, the effect of exercise on various other risk factors like hypertension, diabetes, dyslipidemia, and obesity. Other than control of risk factors, biological mechanisms such as increased HDL-C and reduced homocysteine levels and platelet activity may also explain the protective effects of physical activity (76–78).

Treatment and Recommendations. Given these data, public health goals should emphasize physical activity particularly among those over 65 years of age, who are at highest risk for stroke and cardiovascular disease. Current recommendations from the AHA Stroke Council encourage all physically capable and medically cleared patients to engage in at least 30 minutes of moderate-intense physical activity (i.e., brisk walking or 40–60% maximum capacity) on most and preferably all days of the week. Vigorous or intensive exercise (>60% maximum capacity) for 20 to 40 minutes three to five days per week can add further cardiovascular health benefits (20).

Diet

Earlier studies suggested that excess fat intake might lead to increased risk of both CHD and stroke (79). The Framingham Study, however, produced conflicting results with an inverse association between dietary fat and ischemic stroke in men (80). Similarly, a large prospective study of Japanese found that higher animal fat and cholesterol intake were associated with lower stroke mortality (81) Another large prospective study of over 40,000 male health professionals did not find an association between total fat or any type of fat (saturated, unsaturated, and trans fats) with ischemic stroke (82). In the Northern Manhattan Study, fat intake above 65 g/day was associated with increased risk of incident stroke (unpublished data).

Increased intake of fruits and vegetables is associated with lower ischemic stroke risk, even after controlling for standard risk factors. Cruciferous and green leafy vegetables as well as citrus fruits were associated with greater protective effects (83). These foods may have a protective effect in stroke because of their antioxidant content that reduces atherogenesis. One study found that higher levels of carotenoids (antioxidants found in fruits and vegetables) were inversely associated with ischemic stroke risk (84). Other dietary factors that have been associated with a reduced risk of stroke include consumption of milk and calcium (85), cereal fiber (86), whole grain (87), and fish (88,89). Diet is probably an important risk factor for stroke but it may be mediated through other traditional risk factors. For example, high daily dietary intake of fat may act as an independent risk factor or may affect other stroke risk factors such as hypertension, diabetes, dyslipidemia, obesity, and cardiac disease.

Treatment and Recommendations. The AHA Stroke Council recommends an overall healthy diet as a goal in the prevention of cardiovascular disease and stroke, including five servings of fruits and vegetables per day. The AHA Step I diet recommends lesser than 10% calories from saturated fats, lesser than 300 mg/day of cholesterol intake, salt intake of lesser than 6 g/day, and substituting unsaturated fatty acids for trans-fatty acids (90). Reduced salt and increased potassium intake are also recommended to reduce hypertension, a known risk factor for stroke.

Obesity

Six of 10 Americans are overweight or obese (body mass index, BMI $\geq$ 25 kg/m^2), a prevalence that increases with age (40). Large studies have shown that abdominal obesity [defined by National Cholesterol Education Program Adult Treatment Panel III (NCEP ATP III) as >40 in. in men, >37 in. in women], rather than general obesity or BMI, is an independent risk factor for ischemic stroke (91). A case–control study from Northern Manhattan found men with waist–hip ratios (WHR) greater than 0.93 and women with WHR greater than 0.86 were at higher risk of stroke. Men had a greater risk than women with an odds ratio of 3.8 versus 2.5. The WHR had a greater effect on stroke risk in younger patients (<65 years) than in older patients (>65 years). This risk was independent of BMI and other known risk factors (92). In a prospective study of women, obesity as measured by BMI ($\geq$30 kg/m^2) also increased the risk of ischemic stroke (93).

Treatment and Recommendations. Current AHA recommendations encourage weight reduction on the basis of reducing associated comorbidities with desirable BMI goal of 18.5 to 24.9 kg/m^2 (90). Suitable interventions include diet and nutritional consultations to reduce caloric intake and increase caloric expenditure via exercise. The roles of bariatric procedures and medications to promote weight loss are still uncertain.

Medical Risk Factors

Hypertension

Hypertension is the most important modifiable risk factor for stroke. The risk of stroke increases in direct proportion to increasing BP. Elevated BP causes shear stresses on blood vessels and predisposes them to arteriosclerotic changes. Hypertension and the newly coined prehypertension affect over 100 million people in the United States (94). Because of its high prevalence, the population-attributable risk (etiologic fraction) for stroke is nearly 40% depending on the age group (20). The prevalence of hypertension also differs by race-ethnic group leading to vastly different race-specific attributable risks for stroke. Given its high etiologic fraction, even modest control of hypertension could result in substantial lowering of stroke incidence and prevalence (95).

In the Framingham Study, hypertension (defined as >160/95 mmHg) was associated with an age-adjusted stroke RR of 3.1 for men and 2.9 for women (96). Using this cohort, a risk factor profile has been generated showing that for every 10-mmHg increase in systolic blood pressure (SBP), the RR for stroke was 1.9 for men and 1.7 for women. Even borderline hypertension compared to normal BP confers an RR of 1.5.

Isolated systolic hypertension, which affects two-thirds of elderly patients, is also an independent risk factor for stroke, adjusting for age and diastolic blood pressure (DBP) (97). Several prospective studies have found that increase in DBP also substantially increase stroke risk. In a meta-analysis of nine prospective studies, stroke risk increased by 46% for every 7.5-mmHg increase in DBP (98). In a Dutch population–based study of stroke, untreated hypertension (defined as >160/95 mmHg) was associated with an RR of stroke of 1.76 compared with hypertensive patients who were treated and "controlled." BP control in this study was defined by Dutch guidelines as less than 160/90 mmHg (99).

Past definitions of hypertension have undergone changes in recent years. The risk of stroke has a direct and continuous relationship with BP elevation (Fig. 6) (100), an association that is apparent even at pressures as low as 115/75 mmHg (101). The Joint National Committee (JNC 7) on Prevention, Detection, Evaluation, and Treatment of High Blood Pressure Report redefined categories of hypertension based on these data. The current definition of normal BP is SBP that is lesser than 120 mmHg and DBP that is lesser than 80 mmHg. Furthermore, they created a new category of "prehypertension," with BP of 120 to 139/80 to 89 mmHg. This category identifies patients who are at higher risk of developing hypertension. If other compelling reasons exist, these individuals should also begin antihypertensive therapy (102).

Treatment and Recommendations. Prospective studies and randomized controlled trials have consistently found that treatment of hypertension reduces stroke risk in all age groups.

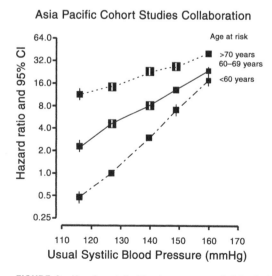
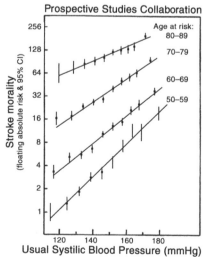

FIGURE 6 Usual systolic blood pressure and risk of stroke by age, with data from prospective cohort study overviews. *Source*: From Ref. 100.

Lowering SBP has been shown to be beneficial in reducing stroke risk in all age groups, particularly in elderly populations. The Swedish Trial in Old Patients with Hypertension (STOP)-Hypertension program of 1600 patients aged 70 to 84 years showed that active treatment significantly reduced the number of stroke, MI, and also stroke morbidity and mortality compared to placebo (103). The Systolic Hypertension in the Elderly Program trial observed a 36% lower stroke incidence with hypertensive therapy, a benefit that was seen across all stroke subtypes (104). The Syst-Eur trial showed that treatment of isolated systolic hypertension resulted in 42% reduction in stroke risk (105).

The STOP-2 trial found similar stroke rates among different antihypertensive agents: 22% for conventional agents, 20% for angiotensin-converting enzyme (ACE) inhibitors, and 20% for calcium channel blockers (106). The Antihypertensive and Lipid Lowering Heart Attack Trial shed more light on relative differences between these agents in terms of cardiovascular protection. For both black and nonblack populations, diuretic-based treatment and ACE-based treatment were both equally protective in terms of most cardiovascular outcomes, except for a lower risk of heart failure in the diuretic group. Among blacks, the risk of stroke was less in the diuretic group (107).

In a meta-analysis of 14 treatment trials, a mean SBP reduction of 5 to 6 mmHg was associated with 35% to 40% decreased stroke incidence, regardless of the level of baseline pressure (108). Furthermore, as no lower threshold seems to exist and benefit extends to those with normal BP, antihypertensive therapy should be considered for all patients who are considered to be at a high risk for stroke (109). Despite convincing evidence, awareness and treatment of the condition are far from optimal. Only 70% of hypertensive patients were aware of the diagnosis, 59% were being actively treated with medications, and only 34% were controlled to the goal of less than 140/90 mmHg (102).

Despite many studies addressing the benefits of adequate BP control in primary stroke prevention, fewer studies are available that demonstrate the impact of BP control in secondary stroke prevention. The Heart Outcomes Prevention Evaluation (HOPE) Study investigated ramipril (10 mg/day vs. placebo) among 9297 patients, of whom 11% in both groups had a history of prior stroke. Statistically significant treatment benefits were seen for combined outcomes (MI, stroke, and vascular events) and stroke (110). The benefit was observed regardless of the degree of BP lowering (111).

The Perindopril Protection Against Recurrent Stroke Study was conducted to investigate stroke outcomes in hypertensive and nonhypertensive patients with a prior stroke or TIA treated with the ACE-I, perindopril. After four years of follow-up, there was a 43% RR reduction in stroke risk in the treatment group (perindopril +/− indapamide) compared to placebo; the use of perindopril alone had no discernible effect in stroke risk reduction (112). Whether the results observed were secondary to BP control or to a direct effect of both the ACE inhibitor and the diuretic remains unknown.

Angiotensin receptor blockers (ARB) also afford stroke benefit as assessed in the Study on COgnition and Prognosis in the Elderly (SCOPE, candesartan) and Losartan Intervention For Endpoint reduction in hypertension study (losartan) trials, where 42% and 25% stroke risk reductions were seen with ARB versus other antihypertensive agents (113,114). Although these results are more applicable to primary stroke prevention in high-risk patients, they strongly support the use of ACE-inhibitor or ARB therapy in secondary stroke prevention, regardless of the baseline BP.

The current JNC 7 recommendations support the use of antihypertensive medications for the treatment of most individuals with uncomplicated hypertension, as nonpharmacologic measures are less effective. Attempts to control BP with lifestyle modifications may be considered in those with lower risk. The latter include weight loss, sodium restriction, potassium supplementation, restriction of alcohol, stress reduction, and other mineral supplements such as calcium and magnesium. The target should be less than 140/90 mmHg in everyone and less than 130/80 mmHg in diabetics and renal patients (102).

Diabetes Mellitus
The number of Americans diagnosed with type-II diabetes in 2000 was estimated at 11.8 million, with perhaps another 4.9 million with impaired glucose tolerance (115). Amongst those with stroke, the prevalence of diabetes mellitus (DM) was shown to be 22% and 20% among elderly blacks and Hispanics in northern Manhattan (116).

Numerous studies have shown that DM is an independent risk factor for stroke, with an RR ranging from 1.5 to 3.0. In addition, stroke mortality is significantly greater in those with elevated blood sugars. In the Honolulu Heart Program, the adjusted RR of stroke was two times higher in Japanese diabetic men compared with nondiabetics (117). In the Atherosclerosis Risk In Communities (ARIC) Study of over 14,000 subjects, diabetes (defined as a fasting glucose =140 mg/dL) had an adjusted RR of ischemic stroke of 2.26. In addition, insulin resistance in the ARIC study, as measured by elevated fasting insulin levels in nondiabetic patients, was also associated with increased risk of stroke (RR 1.19 per 50 pmol/L increase) (118).

Some studies have suggested a gender difference in the stroke risk from diabetes. One study suggested diabetic women had a greater risk of stroke than diabetic men (119). There may be race-ethnic differences in the prevalence and risk from diabetes. In NOMASS, DM was associated with an OR of 1.7 with attributable risks of 13% and 20% among blacks and Hispanics, respectively (116).

Treatment and Recommendations.   The accumulating evidence on diabetes and cardiovascular risk was critical in the decision to make it a CHD equivalent and a high-risk state that requires aggressive management. Intensive glycemic control aimed at maintaining normal glucose levels in both type-I and type-II diabetics has been shown to reduce microvascular complications such as retinopathy, nephropathy, and neuropathy but has not been shown to alter macrovascular complications, including stroke (120–122). However, using carotid IMT as a surrogate, the Diabetes Control and Complications Study found that intensive glycemic control slowed IMT progression compared to conventional treatment (123). Acute treatment of hyperglycemia was evaluated in the Glucose Insulin in Stroke Trial study, where there was no significant difference in the four-week mortality in the insulin-euglycemic group compared to the control group (124).

Aggressive treatment of elevated BP in diabetics has, however, been shown to decrease the risk of stroke (105,125,126). In the UK Prospective Diabetes Study, active treatment of hypertension with tight control (goal <150/85 mmHg) resulted in a 44% stroke risk reduction among diabetics (126). In the Hypertension Optimal Treatment (HOT) study, tighter DBP control (<80 mmHg) was associated with 30% stroke risk reduction compared to the groups with DBP lesser than 90 mmHg (127). ACE inhibitors may be even more beneficial in diabetics, as demonstrated in the MICRO-HOPE sub–study that found a 33% stroke risk reduction with ramipril, independent of BP reduction (128).

Among diabetics in most lipid lowering drug trials, there was no significant benefit of statin therapy in lowering stroke risk (129,130). However, in the Heart Protection Study (HPS), diabetics treated with simvistatin showed a 28% reduction ($p = 0.01$) in ischemic stroke risk compared to placebo (131). In the Collaborative Atorvastatin Diabetes Study, type-II diabetics with at least one additional risk factor (retinopathy, albuminuria, current smoking, or hypertension) treated with atorvastatin had a 48% stroke risk reduction (132). Based on the above studies, NCEP ATP III guidelines consider DM a CAD equivalent with low-density lipoprotein cholesterol (LDL-C) target of lesser than 100 mg/dL and a non–HDL-C target of lesser than 130 mg/dL (among diabetic patients with a baseline triglyceride that exceeds 200 mg/dL) (133). The guidelines from the American Diabetes Association set a HDL-C target above 40 mg/dL for men and above 50 mg/dL for women (134).

Current AHA recommendations for primary stroke prevention are to maintain BP goal as lesser than 130/80 mmHg among diabetics; the use of ACE-I and ARB may add further benefit over other antihypertensive medications (20). The AHA guidelines also support tighter glycemic control in diabetics with ischemic stroke or TIA to reduce microvascular and possibly macrovascular complications with a goal HgA1c of less than 7% (90). Despite the known risks of uncontrolled diabetes, glycemic control is inadequate in 30% to 50% of diabetics, a public health barometer that calls for stronger interventions.

Dyslipidemia

Elevated serum triglyceride, total cholesterol, and LDL and reduced HDL are known risk factors for vascular disease, CHD in particular. The relationship between dyslipidemia and stroke has not been as consistent in observational studies. The Multiple Risk Factor Intervention Trial showed that mortality from ischemic stroke was greater among men with high total cholesterol (135). In the Honolulu Heart Program, the highest quartile of

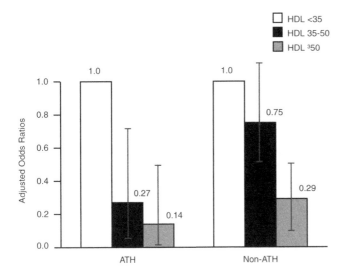

FIGURE 7 HDL and risk of stroke in the Northern Manhattan Stroke Study. *Abbreviations*: HDL, high-density lipoprotein; DM, diabetes mellitus; BMI, body mass index; LDL, low-density lipoprotein. *Source*: From Ref. 142.

total cholesterol compared to lowest quartile was associated with an RR of 1.4, with a trend for a continuous relationship with thromboembolic stroke risk (136). Large meta-analyses including over 450,000 people, however, found no association between cholesterol and stroke (137).

The heterogeneity of ischemic stroke in comparison to CAD may partly explain these inconsistent findings. Stroke subtypes related to atherosclerosis (LAA) may have a closer link with lipid levels; elevated cholesterol levels have been associated with stroke caused by large vessel disease (138). Studies have also shown that elevated total cholesterol and LDL-C levels correlate with the degree and progression of carotid atherosclerosis on ultrasound (139), while increased HDL-C is protective (140,141). A dose–response effect was seen in NOMASS with higher HDL-C levels conferring greater protection, especially in the atherosclerotic stroke subtype (Fig. 7) (142). Likewise, in the Oxfordshire community study, HDL-C was inversely related to risk of TIA or minor stroke (143).

Other lipid markers such as lipoprotein(a) may be a risk factor in individuals with evidence of early onset of atherosclerosis and stroke (144). In NOMASS, individuals with abnormal lipoprotein(a) levels of more than 30 mg/dL were at an increased risk (RR 1.6) for stroke when adjusted for hypertension, diabetes, CHD, smoking, education, age, gender, and race (145). In addition, the risk for stroke appeared to increase with higher lipoprotein(a) levels (>50 mg/dL). Lipoprotein(a) levels can be reduced by 25% with niacin therapy (146) but studies of the outcome are lacking. Other markers such as apolipoprotein a1 (Apo a1) and apolipoprotein b (Apo b), may also have an impact on stroke risk. Studies have shown that the presence of carotid plaque is linked to Apo b and may be inversely related to Apo a1 (147).

Treatment and Recommendations. Despite less convincing prospective data, accumulating evidence from clinical trials using 3-hydroxy-3-methylglutaryl coenzyme A (HMG-CoA) reductase inhibitors, or "statins," has shown significant reductions in stroke risk among those with CAD or atherosclerosis. The Scandinavian Simvistatin Survival Study (4S), the Cholesterol and Recurrent Events study, the Long-term Intervention with Pravastatin in Ischemic Disease all showed significant risk reductions in fatal and nonfatal strokes (148–150). Meta-analyses of large randomized controlled trials found a 16% to 30% reduction in stroke risk and 22% reduction in overall mortality with statin use (151,152). Carotid ultrasound studies have also observed plaque regression with statin use (153–157). Nonstatin agents have also been studied. The veterans affairs high-density lipoprotein intervention trial (VA-HIT) study showed that fibrates produced a 25% stroke risk reduction and 59% for TIA (158). In the Coronary Drug Project, niacin afforded a 24% reduction in TIA or stroke (159).

Despite these results suggesting that statins are effective for primary prevention of stroke, data specifically addressing secondary stroke prevention are lacking. In HPS, comparing simvistatin (40 mg/day) versus placebo for the prevention of vascular events in high-risk patients (defined as prior occlusive arterial disease, presence of diabetes, or elevated cholesterol), more than 3000 of the total 20,000 patients had a history of ischemic stroke or TIA. Over five years, the mean total cholesterol was reduced by 20%, with a significant stroke risk reduction of 25% (160). The ongoing Stroke Prevention by Aggressive Reduction in Cholesterol Levels Study may provide more evidence concerning the benefit of lipid-lowering therapy in preventing recurrence of stroke (161).

Current NCEP guidelines support lipid analysis in those with cholesterol over 200 mg/dL and cardiovascular risk factors. Risk factors include cigarette smoking, hypertension (>140/90 mmHg or on medication), low HDL-C (<40 mg/dL), family history of premature CHD, and age (men >45 years, women >55 years). NCEP ATP III guidelines support the use of lipid-lowering therapies including therapeutic lifestyle modifications and statins to achieve LDL-C below 100 mg/dL in those with CHD, stroke or TIA due to carotid stenosis over 50%, or over 20%, 10-year risk or other CHD equivalents including diabetes; lesser than 130 mg/dL in those with 2+ CHD risk factors and 10% to 20% 10-year risk; and lesser than 160 mg/dL in those with 2+ CHD risk factors and lesser than 10%, 10-year risk or 0 to 1 CHD risk factors (Table 3) (133). But when the risk is deemed very high, an LDL-C goal less than 70 mg/dL is a therapeutic option on the basis of available clinical trial evidence (162). Suggested management of those with CAD and low HDL-C includes weight loss, exercise, cessation of smoking, and possibly niacin or fibrates. The AHA guidelines similarly support the aggressive management of dyslipidemia with lipid lowering therapy in patients with atherosclerotic heart disease and elevated LDL-C (20).

Atrial Fibrillation

Over two million individuals in the United States have AF, a prevalence that increases with age (163,164). The prevalence among those older than 65 years is close to 6%, with more whites affected than blacks (165). Over 75,000 cases of stroke per year are attributed to AF, and the number is predicted to increase as the population ages. Hence, its attributable risk of stroke is highest in the older age groups (166). Other risk factors for AF include age above 65, male gender, white race, cardiac disease, hypertension, diabetes, and enlarged left atrium (167).

Chronic AF is a powerful risk factor for stroke, accounting for 50% of embolic strokes (20). In the Framingham Study, the risk of stroke was 20 times greater in patients with AF with valvular disease, and five times greater in patients with nonvalvular AF (168). This elevated risk was independent of age, hypertension, and other cardiac abnormalities.

The Stroke Prevention in Atrial Fibrillation (SPAF) trials involved 3950 patients with nonvalvular AF. SPAF I randomized patients to placebo, aspirin, or adjusted-dose warfarin. Patients on placebo had an annual stroke incidence of 6%. SPAF I further identified patients with AF at high risk for stroke: those with hypertension, congestive heart failure (CHF), prior stroke, TIA, or systemic emboli, diabetes, and prosthetic valves, and women over 75. Left ventricular dysfunction and left atrial size also increased stroke risk (169).

SPAF III had a low-risk arm using the risk stratification scheme from SPAF I and found that low-risk patients on aspirin had a stroke rate of 2% per year and 0.8% per year for disabling stroke. Patients with hypertension were considered at moderate risk, with a 3.6% stroke rate per year on aspirin (170). Another risk stratification scheme was developed in 705 subjects from the Framingham Study with the new onset of AF who were not treated with warfarin and censoring for warfarin use during follow-up. A five-year risk of stroke was predicted using this model (Fig. 8) (171).

TABLE 3   Goal LDL Level Stratified by Level of 10-Yr Risk

10-yr risk	LDL goal
>20% (high risk: CAD or equivalent)	<100 mg/dL (optional <70 mg/dL)
10–20% (moderate high risk)	<130 mg/dL
<10%	
2 risk factors (moderate low risk)	<130 mg/dL
<2 risk factors (low risk)	<160 mg/dL

Abbreviations: LDL, low-density lipoprotein; CAD, coronary artery disease.
Source: From Refs. 133, 162.

Step 1

Age, y	Points
55-59	0
60-62	1
63-66	2
67-71	3
72-74	4
75-77	5
78-81	6
82-85	7
86-90	8
91-93	9
>93	10

Step 1

Sex	Points
Men	0
Women	6

Step 1

Systolic Blood Pressure, mm Hg	Points
<120	0
120-139	1
140-159	2
160-179	3
>179	4

Step 1

Diabetes	Points
No	0
Yes	5

Step 1

Prior Stroke or TIA	Points
No	0
Yes	6

Step 1

Add Up Points From Steps 1 Through 5

Look Up Predicted 5-years Risk of Stroke in Table

Predicted 5-year Risk of Stroke

Total Points	5-Year Risk, %
0-1	5
2-3	6
4	7
5	8
6-7	9
8	11
9	12
10	13
11	14
12	16
13	18
14	19
15	21
16	24
17	26
18	28
19	31
2-3	6
21	37
22	41
23	44
24	48
25	51
26	55
27	59
28	63
29	67
30	71
31	75

FIGURE 8 Five-year stroke risk model for atrial fibrillation. *Abbreviation:* TIA, transient ischemic attack. *Source:* From Ref. 171.

Treatment and Recommendations. Several treatment trials have demonstrated that anticoagulant and antiplatelet agents can reduce the risk of stroke from AF. In a meta-analysis of five clinical trials comparing warfarin versus placebo for the primary prevention of stroke, adjusted-dose warfarin resulted in a 68% reduction in stroke risk (172); compared to aspirin, warfarin use effected 45% risk reduction (173). For secondary stroke prevention following TIA or stroke, the European Atrial Fibrillation Trial found that warfarin was associated with a 66% risk reduction compared to placebo and 40% compared to aspirin (174).

Based on the results of SPAF II and III, 325 mg of aspirin has been recommended for those with "lone AF" (i.e., patients <75 years of age without any aforementioned high-risk features), affording a similar risk reduction as warfarin. For the remainder of the patients and following TIA or stroke, the recommended intensity of anticoagulation with warfarin is an International Normalized Ratio (INR) between 2.0 and 3.0, given the increased risk of bleeding with higher levels (175). Cardioversion for new-onset AF and maintenance of sinus rhythm also appreciably lower stroke risk (176). Other management strategies should include control of other high-risk medical comorbidities. Future direct thrombin inhibitors may have a role in stroke prevention in patients with AF (177).

Other Cardiac Risk Factors

CAD is the leading cause of death in the United States (Table 4). Acute MI is known to increase stroke risk in the post-MI period up to four to six weeks. In the Framingham Study, the six-year risk of stroke in MI patients was 8% and 11% for men and women, respectively (20). CAD is associated with twice the stroke risk compared with patients without CAD. The presence of left ventricular hypertrophy triples the risk, and associated CHF is associated with four times the risk (168). The attributable risk of stroke from CAD is approximately 12% and ranges from 2.3% to 6.0% for CHF. Antiplatelet therapy is recommended for all patients with CAD to prevent recurrent MI and stroke. For acute MI complicated by left ventricular thrombus, anticoagulation may be reasonable for three months to one year (178).

In a large Medicare cohort, the RR of embolic stroke in those with CHF, compared to those without, was 1.69 (179). Dilated cardiomyopathy predisposes thrombus formation in as high as 50% of the patients and is, therefore, a significant risk factor for CE (3–4% per year). In

TABLE 4 Sources of Cardiac Embolism

Known risk factor	Uncertain risk factor
Atrial fibrillation	Mitral valve prolapse
Mitral stenosis	Mitral annular calcification
Prosthetic mechanical valves	Aortic arch atheroma
Recent myocardial infarction	Patent foramen ovale
Left ventricular thrombus	Atrial septal aneurysm
Dilated cardiomyopathy	
Infective endocarditis	
Marantic endocarditis	

Source: Adapted from Ref. 178.

the Survival and Ventricular Enlargement Study, there was an 18% increase in stroke risk for every 5% decline in EF (180). Currently, the Warfarin versus Aspirin for Reduced Cardiac Ejection Fraction (WARCEF) trial is evaluating the benefits of chronic anticoagulation over the use of aspirin in the rates of stroke and death in patients with severely reduced EF (<35%) (181).

Cardiac valvular abnormalities also increase the risk of stroke. For example, rheumatic mitral stenosis, prosthetic heart valves (182), and endocarditis (183) can all increase the risk of stroke. Mitral annular calcification (MAC) has been associated with increased risk of stroke (RR 2.1) in the Framingham cohort. Stroke incidence appears to increase with the degree of calcification; each millimeter increased the RR by 1.24 (184). Current recommendations support the use of antiplatelet therapy for those with embolic stroke and MAC (185).

For mechanical prosthetic valves, warfarin is recommended with a target INR of 2.5 to 3.5 for the mitral valve versus 2.0 to 3.0 for the aortic valve. For bioprosthetic valves, anticoagulation is optional for the initial three months and antiplatelet therapy is indicated thereafter unless other indications for anticoagulation exist (185). Native valve infective endocarditis is treated with antibiotics with a recommendation against anticoagulants due to risk of intracranial mycotic aneurysm in those with no indication for anticoagulation (186). The continuation of anticoagulants in those with mechanical valve endocarditis is more controversial but the evidence seems to support continuation if there are no contraindications (185). There is less evidence regarding marantic endocarditis, although anecdotal evidence suggests that anticoagulation is better for prevention of embolism, with a preference for heparin or low-molecular weight heparinoids over warfarin in thrombosis associated with cancer (185,187,188). Lastly, rheumatic heart disease is also an indication for warfarin with INR goal of 2.0 to 3.0 (185).

Mitral valve prolapse (MVP) is a common condition in the general population. Despite 6% female and 4% male prevalence, MVP has been associated with an extremely low stroke incidence, estimated at 1/6000 per year (189). A community based cohort study of over 700 patients with MVP followed for a mean of 5.5 years found an RR of stroke of 2.2 in patients with MVP. However, the excess risk of stroke was primarily in older patients (greater than 50 years of age). Patients with other risk factors such as mitral valve thickening, left atrial enlargement, and AF with MVP were also at higher risk. These other risk factors may account for the excess risk of stroke, but these conditions may arise directly from MVP (190). The current American College of Chest Physicians (ACCP) recommendations do not support antithrombotic therapy in those without evidence of embolism. However, in those with embolism, antiplatelet agents are first-line therapy and anticoagulation is reserved for embolism despite antiplatelet therapy (178).

Aortic Arch Atheroma

Complex aortic arch atheromas may also be a risk factor for stroke. Using transesophageal echocardiography (TEE) in a French case–control study, atheromas of 4 mm or above in thickness in the ascending aorta or proximal arch were significantly associated with stroke with an adjusted OR of 9.1 (191). In another case–control study, complex (ulcerated or mobile) atheromas (adjusted OR 17.1) were more strongly linked with stroke compared to noncomplex large (≥4 mm) atheromas (adjusted OR 2.4) (192). Prospective studies have also confirmed high stroke risk among those with complex aortic arch plaques including mobile or pedunculated elements (193,194). From these studies, the annual stroke risk ranges from 11.9% to 33%, 3.5% to 7%, and 2.8% for plaque above 4 mm, below 4 mm, and no aortic plaque, respectively.

Treatment and Recommendations. There have been no randomized studies addressing antithrombotic therapies for aortic arch disease. Two retrospective and nonrandomized studies showed a benefit of oral anticoagulant therapy over aspirin in patients with mobile thrombi in the aortic arch (195,196). However, hemorrhagic complications possibly outweighed the benefits of the anticoagulants. One other retrospective study of 519 patients with aortic plaques below 4 mm found that statins, but not oral anticoagulation or antiplatelet therapy, had a significant protective effect against recurrent embolism (197). Concerns also exist regarding the possibility that anticoagulation might increase the risk of cholesterol embolism (198). Further studies are needed to determine the optimal treatment for aortic arch atheroma. ACCP guidelines currently support antiplatelet agents in those with stroke and antiplatelet or anticoagulant therapy for those with CS associated with mobile plaque (178). The ongoing Aortic Arch Related Cerebral Hazard trial is comparing warfarin with aspirin plus clopidogrel (199).

Patent Foramen Ovale

There is growing epidemiologic evidence that PFO is a risk factor for stroke, especially cryptogenic infarction in the young. This venous to arterial pathway can occasionally result in paradoxical embolism to the brain. Numerous retrospective and case-control studies suggest that PFO is a risk factor for CS (200,201). However, no prospective cohort studies have evaluated the question of whether a PFO increases the risk of stroke in stroke-free individuals. Prospective data does exist on the risk of recurrent stroke in patients with PFO and other atrial septal anomalies.

Treatment and Recommendations. In patients with a CS and a documented PFO, the best strategy for secondary prevention has been a matter of intense debate. The results of a prospective study evaluating young patients (<55 years) with CS and a PFO, found an extremely elevated risk of recurrent stroke with PFO plus atrial septal aneurysm (ASA). The hazard ratio with the two anomalies combined was 4.2, whereas either anomaly alone did not increase recurrent stroke risk (202).

The Patent Foramen Ovale in Cryptogenic Stroke Study (PICSS), a sub–study of Warfarin-Aspirin Recurrent Stroke Study (WARSS), is the only randomized, double-blind study to investigate the best medical management in patients with stroke and PFO (203). Of the 630 patients from WARSS who underwent TEE (an older cohort compared to PFO-ASA study), a PFO was found in 39% of the patients with CSs and in 29.9% of the patients with other known causes. In PICSS, PFO alone did not confer increased recurrence risk. In addition, the size of the PFO and the presence of an associated ASA were not determinants of recurrent stroke. After two years of follow-up, the rates of recurrent stroke or death were similar between the group treated with warfarin and the aspirin-treated patients (16.5% and 13.2%). These results do not support one therapy over the other in unselected patients with CS and PFO.

The current ACCP guidelines recommend that for CS with PFO, antiplatelet therapy is the preferred treatment unless there is evidence of deep venous thrombosis (DVT) or stroke recurrence despite antiplatelet therapy, for which warfarin is recommended (178). The role for endovascular or surgical PFO closure is currently being investigated by clinical trials and cannot be routinely recommended at this point (204).

Asymptomatic Carotid Atherosclerotic Disease

Carotid stenosis is a well-established risk factor for recurrent stroke. In the North American Symptomatic Carotid Endarterectomy Trial (NASCET) study, patients with symptomatic carotid stenosis had a 26% two-year risk of recurrent stroke with medical treatment after a TIA or minor stroke and an ipsilateral carotid stenosis of 70% or more (205). However, the risk of first stroke with asymptomatic carotid artery disease is lower and has been reported to be 1.3% annually in those with 75% stenosis or less, and 3.3% annually in those with stenosis more than 75% (206). The combined TIA and stroke risk was 10.5% per year in those with more than 75% carotid stenosis. The prevalence of asymptomatic carotid disease increases with age, occurring in over 50% of the subjects 65 to 94 years of age in some studies (207), and is an increasingly common condition that deserves careful consideration.

Treatment and Recommendations. In the Asymptomatic Carotid Artery Stenosis (ACAS) Study, a large randomized trial of endarterectomy in asymptomatic carotid stenosis

(60–99%), 1662 patients were randomized to surgery plus best medical therapy or to best medical therapy alone (208). Angiographic complications occurred in 1.2% and the periop-erative stroke risk was 2.3%, much lower than in NASCET or the European Carotid Surgery Trial (ECST). After a median followup of 2.7 years, the study was stopped early because of a significant surgical benefit. The rate of ipsilateral stroke, any perioperative stroke or death in surgically treated patients was estimated at 5% over five years while in medically treated patients, the rate was 11% (53% risk reduction, $p < 0.004$). Unlike NASCET, the benefit was most notable among men compared to women, the women having a 3.6% complication rate compared to 1.7% in men, and there was no gradation of benefit with degree of carotid artery stenosis.

Another large randomized trial recently showed that in subjects <75 years of age with >60% carotid stenosis, the five-year stroke risks for medically treated and surgically treated patients (11% and 3.8%, respectively) were very similar to those observed in ACAS. The immediate 30-day risk of stroke or death after endarterectomy was 3.1%. In contrast to ACAS, the surgical benefits extended to both men and women. Based on both ACAS and Asymptomatic Carolid Surgery Trial (ACST), carotid endarterectomy (CEA) may be consid-ered in those with 60 to 99% asymptomatic carotid stenosis if performed by a surgeon with lesser than 3% surgical complication rate. Patient selection criteria regarding comorbid con-ditions, life expectancy, and demographics including gender are crucial (20).

Transient Ischemic Attack

The yearly stroke-risk following TIA ranges from 1% to 15% depending greatly on multiple variables including how recent the TIA was, the underlying etiology, clinical syndrome, and associated radiologic features (210). In hospital-referred patients, the average annual risk of stroke, MI, or death was 7.5% after TIA (211). The largest study to evaluate the short-term prognosis after a TIA reported the 90-day risk of stroke to be 10.5%, with 50% of those occur-ring within the first 48 hours after the event (212). Other epidemiological studies have found similar stroke risk following TIA (213–215). These studies suggest an increased early stroke risk following TIA (with the first 48 hours being the highest risk period) and underscore the urgency with which TIA should be evaluated and preventive measures implemented.

Age greater than 60 years, the presence of diabetes, symptom duration of more than 10 minutes, weakness, and speech impairment—each conferred an increased risk of stroke in the following three months, with odds ratios between 1.5 and 2.3. The 90-day risk of stroke was as low as 0% with none of these risk factors and as high as 34% with all five risk factors (212). Features associated with less risk include transient monocular blindness, with a 10.3% three-year risk of stroke compared to hemispheric TIA patients (216), and isolated sensory or visual symptoms were associated with lower 90-day stroke risk (217).

Treatment and Recommendations. TIA represents a unique opportunity for evaluation and inter-vention. Rapid screening for the above vascular risk factors with laboratory and radiographic tests is recommended. The AHA recommendations for stroke prevention in patients with TIA are based on the underlying mechanism of TIA (90). For noncardioembolic TIA, antiplatelet therapy is the first-line therapy, while warfarin is indicated for select causes of cardioembolism (see below).

SECONDARY PREVENTION OF STROKE

Studies addressing prevention of stroke recurrence in those with prior TIA or stroke have largely been antiplatelet and anticoagulant trials. In addition, large studies on interventional treatments including CEA have helped guide current practice parameters.

Antiplatelet Therapy

Aspirin

An irreversible blocker of the thromboxane pathway in platelet aggregation, aspirin has been found in multiple clinical trials to be beneficial for secondary stroke prevention. Collectively in the French, British, European, and Canadian trials, aspirin benefit ranged from 20% to 30% risk reduction in stroke and vascular death. The Antithrombotic Trialists Collaboration found that aspirin was associated with a 22% RR reduction in vascular events (stroke, MI, vascular death) among patients with a prior TIA/stroke. The absolute benefit offered by aspirin, when all doses where analyzed, was a modest 2.5% (218).

The optimal dose of aspirin has been an area of intense debate. The Dutch TIA Study showed equal benefit from very low and moderate doses of salicylates (30 mg vs. 283 mg a day) (219). The UK-TIA trial used very different dosing schedules and found similar results (300 mg/day vs. 1300 mg/day) (220). Given the potential side effects mainly from gastrointestinal bleeding and ulceration, lower dose aspirin (50–325 mg/day) is a reasonable strategy for long-term secondary stroke prevention (221).

Clopidogrel

Through its inhibitory effects on adenosine diphosphate-induced platelet aggregation, clopidogrel is another drug used to decrease cardiovascular risk. The efficacy of clopidogrel in the prevention of ischemic strokes has been analyzed in the Clopidogrel versus Aspirin in Patients at Risk of Ischemic Events (CAPRIE) study where patients with nondisabling ischemic strokes, recent MI, and symptomatic peripheral arterial disease were randomized to aspirin (325 mg/day) or clopidogrel (75 mg/day) (222). In terms of combined vascular outcomes, there was an 8.7% RR reduction in favor of clopidogrel. This overall benefit was driven primarily by the peripheral arterial disease group (RR reduction 23.8%), but was less apparent in the group with a prior ischemic stroke, where an insignificant RR reduction of 7.3% in favor of clopidogrel was observed. The rates of intracranial hemorrhage were similar between the two groups but gastrointestinal hemorrhage occurred less in the clopidogrel group (1.99% vs. 2.66%). Although thrombotic thrombocytopenic purpura (TTP) has been reported with the use of clopidogrel, the CAPRIE study did not show a higher risk of fatal thrombocytopenia compared with the use of aspirin.

Ticlopidine

Even though two large trials revealed a benefit from ticlopidine in secondary stroke prevention with RR reduction as high as 30%, the risk of severe neutropenia (0.8%) and reports of TTP caused this drug to virtually disappear from current neurological practice (223,224). Moreover, the African American Aspirin Stroke Prevention Study compared aspirin (650 mg/day) with ticlopidine in black patients with non-CEs and found no significant difference between the two groups in the combined outcome of stroke, MI, and vascular death (225).

Extended-Release Dipyridamole and Aspirin

The European Stroke Prevention Study II was a double-blind randomized study evaluating the efficacy of placebo compared with aspirin (25 mg twice daily), extended-release dipyridamole (200 mg twice daily), and the combination of aspirin and extended-release dipyridamole. The outcomes of stroke and/or death were measured in a follow-up period of two years. There was a 23% RR reduction favoring the combination therapy when compared to aspirin alone and 37% RR reduction when compared to placebo (Fig. 9) (226). There was no significant difference in mortality between the groups despite a higher risk of moderate to severe bleeding events in the aspirin-containing arms. The most common side effect due to extended release dipyridamole/aspirin combination is headache.

Clopidogrel and Aspirin

The Management of Atherothrombosis with Clopidogrel in High-Risk Patients with Recent Transient Ischemic or Ischemic Stroke (MATCH) trial randomized 7599 patients with a recent TIA or stroke (and at least one other risk factor) to clopidogrel (75 mg/day) plus an additional agent (aspirin or placebo) (227). After 18 months, the primary endpoint (composite of ischemic stroke, MI, vascular death, or hospitalization for acute ischemic event) occurred in 15.7% of the combination group and 16.7% of the clopidogrel group. The RR reduction was 6.6% ($p = 0.32$) and offset also by higher rates of life-threatening bleeding episodes in the combination group (3% vs. 1%, $p < 0.0001$). Given this elevated risk of hemorrhage and no clear ischemic stroke protection, combination therapy of clopidogrel and aspirin is not recommended for secondary stroke prevention in patients considered to be at high risk for cerebrovascular events.

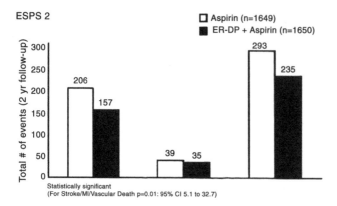

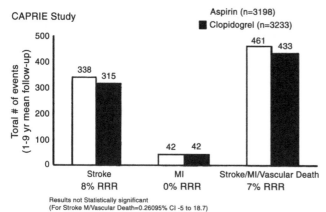

FIGURE 9 Results from the EPSS-2 and CAPRIE trials. *Abbreviations*: RRR, *Source*: From Ref. 178.

Recommendations

Aspirin, clopidogrel, and aspirin/extended-release dipyridamole are all acceptable first-line options in the prevention of recurrent stroke among patients with non-CE. Factors that should be considered in deciding the appropriate antiplatelet therapy in stroke and TIA patients include cost, side effect profile, and other comorbidities. Aspirin is cheaper, but has more gastrointestinal side effects than clopidogrel. While the combination of clopidogrel and aspirin may provide benefit in those with acute coronary syndrome or coronary stents (228), it is not recommended for ischemic stroke patients based on the results of the MATCH trial. Until further studies comparing the efficacy of other combination therapies, aspirin/extended-release dipyridamole is the only available combination therapy recommended as a first-line option for secondary prevention after a non-CE.

Oral Anticoagulation

There is strong evidence supporting the efficacy of warfarin in primary and secondary prevention of certain types of CE. This was covered in detail in the section on AF and cardiac risk factors. However, the use of oral anticoagulation for non-CE has been an area of debate. Long-term anticoagulation was sometimes utilized in patients with non-CE in whom secondary prevention with aspirin was not effective (i.e., "aspirin failure"), occult embolism was inferred (i.e., CS with PFO), or intracranial atherosclerosis was the etiology.

Several pivotal randomized controlled trials have changed the way non-CE is managed. The WARSS randomized 2200 patients to receive either aspirin (325 mg/day) or warfarin for a target INR of 1.4 to 2.8. The two-year risk of recurrent stroke or death was similar in the warfarin group compared to the aspirin group (17.8% vs. 16%), with comparable bleeding complications (2.22% per year for warfarin and 1.49% per year for aspirin). The final conclusion of the study was that aspirin and warfarin had equivalent efficacy in secondary prevention after non-CE with comparable and relatively low risk of bleeding complications (229).

The risk of recurrent stroke in large vessel intracranial atherosclerosis can be as high as 10% per year. The retrospective arm of the Warfarin Aspirin for Symptomatic Intracranial Disease (WASID) trial evaluated the efficacy of anticoagulation compared with antiplatelet therapy for the secondary prevention of strokes attributable to posterior circulation intracranial atherosclerosis (230). Given the results of their retrospective analysis showing annual recurrence rates of 10.4% in the aspirin group and 3.6% in the warfarin group, a prospective trial was performed. The prospective part of the WASID study was a double-blind randomized trial that enrolled patients with symptomatic, angiographically proven, high-degree (>50%) intracranial stenosis. Patients were assigned to receive either warfarin (INR goal of 2.0–3.0) or aspirin (1300 mg/day). The study was prematurely stopped after a mean follow-up of 1.8 years given the higher rates of major hemorrhagic complications in the warfarin-treated group (8.3% for warfarin vs. 3.2% for aspirin). The rates for all strokes or vascular death were similar in both groups (21.8% for warfarin vs. 22.1% for aspirin). These results offer evidence against the widely used practice of chronic anticoagulation for symptomatic patients with large artery intracranial atherosclerosis (231).

Further evidence for the nonsuperiority of warfarin over aspirin is provided by a recent Cochrane review (232). The authors analyzed five trials (over 4000 patients) on the efficacy of anticoagulation compared to antiplatelet therapy for the secondary prevention of non-CEs. The rates of recurrent stroke were similar with all levels of anticoagulation (INR ranges 1.4–2.8, 2.1–3.6, and 3–4.5) when compared with antiplatelet agents. The major bleeding rates were significantly higher in the high-intensity anticoagulation group but similar between the low- and medium-intensity anticoagulation compared with antiplatelets.

Recommendations

Current recommendations limit warfarin use to clearly indicated cases of cardiac embolism such as AF or mechanical valves (178). Antiplatelet therapy is recommended for others with non-CE including CS with PFO and intracranial atherosclerosis.

Interventional Strategies for Secondary Prevention

Carotid Endarterectomy (Table 5)

In NASCET, patients with severe stenosis (70–99%) benefited from CEA with a 65% RR reduction in any ipsilateral stroke over five years. This benefit had a graded effect across different degrees of severe stenosis, with the 90% to 99% group showing the maximal risk reduction, the 80% to 89% group, moderate risk reduction, and the 70% to 79% group, the lowest benefit. In the 50% to 69% stenosis group (moderate stenosis), the ipsilateral stroke risk reduction was less significant (29% RR reduction, $p = 0.05$), with the greatest benefit seen in men, those with stroke rather than TIAs, and hemispheric rather than retinal symptoms (205,233). In those with stenosis below 50%, surgery offered no benefit over medical therapy.

TABLE 5 Evidence for Treatment of Carotid Stenosis

Trial	Degree stenosis (%)[a]	Perioperative stroke or death (%)	5-yr risk of perioperative stroke, ipsilateral stroke, or death		Relative risk reduction (%)	p value	Absolute risk reduction (%)	NNT to prevent 1 stroke in 5 yr
			Surgical group (%)	Medical group (%)				
NASCET	≥70	5.0	13.0	26.2	51	<0.001	13.2	8
	50–69	6.9	15.7	22.2	29	0.045	6.5	15
	<50	6.7	14.9	18.7	20	0.16	3.8	26
ECST	≥70	4.5	9.6	24.7	61	0.001	15.1	7
	50–69	9.1	15.0	9.4	−54	NS	−5.6	–
	<50	6.9	13.3	8.3	−60	NS	−5.0	–
VA	>50	4.7	4.7	9.4	50	0.08	4.7	21
ACAS	>60[b]	2.3	5.1	11.0	53	0.004	5.9	17
ACST	>60	2.6	6.4	11.8	45	<0.001	5.5	–

[a]Using NASCET criteria.
[b]Using Doppler criteria.
Abbreviations: NNT, number needed to treat; NASCET, North American Symptomatic Carotid Endarterectomy Trial; ECST, European Carotid Surgery Trial; VA, vertebral artery; ACAS, asymptomatic carotid artery stenosis; ACST, Asymptomatic Carolid Surgery Trial.

The Veterans Affairs Cooperative Study showed an absolute risk reduction of 11.7% for surgery versus medical therapy in patients with ICA stenosis of 50% to 99% at one year of follow-up. Similar to NASCET, their results showed a greater benefit for patients with higher degrees of stenosis and surgical complication and mortality rate near 5% (234). The ECST evaluated the benefit of CEA for symptomatic patients with ICA stenosis (235,236). In comparison with NASCET, there were some differences that led to slightly different results. The main methodological differences were in the angiographic criteria for determining the degree of stenosis (ECST method overestimated the stenosis compared to the NASCET method) and the definition of stroke as a deficit persistent for more than seven days compared to that from NASCET, a neurological deficit persisting for over 24 hours. ECST found an absolute benefit for surgery of 11.6% in three-year risk of stroke or death (14.9% vs. 26.5%) among patients with a symptomatic stenosis over 80%. The risk of major stroke or death complicating surgery was 7%. When the results of ECST were reanalyzed and the degree of stenosis was recalculated using the NASCET method, the absolute risk reduction in the five-year risk of stroke or death was 21.2% for CEA compared to medical treatment in patients with a 70% to 99% ICA stenosis (237).

In a recent pooled analysis of NASCET, ECST, and the vertebral artery (VA) trial, surgery was found to be detrimental in those with stenosis below 30%, not efficacious in those with 30% to 49% stenosis, of marginal benefit for those with 50% to 69% stenosis (RR 0.75, 95% CI 0.56–0.94), and highly beneficial in those with 70% to 99% stenosis without near occlusion (RR 0.39, 95% CI 0.28–0.51). This post hoc analysis suggested that benefit seemed to diminish in the small subgroup with near-total occlusion or "string sign" (238). Despite a higher surgical risk, those with contralateral carotid occlusion still had better outcomes with surgery compared to medical treatment alone (22% vs. 69% two-year ipsilateral stroke risk) (239). Among 210 NASCET patients presenting with probable lacunar stroke, with 50% to 99% ipsilateral carotid stenosis, the risk reduction with CEA was less clear (RRR 35%, $p = 0.53$) (240).

The margin of surgical benefit is related to the surgical complication rate, with an estimated 20% reduction in five-year benefit for every 2% increase in complication rate above 6% to 7% (241). Factors that increase surgical risk include history of hemispheric TIA, left compared to right-sided CEA, irregular or ulcerated plaque, contralateral carotid occlusion, and lack of collateral circulation to the ipsilateral hemisphere (242,243). The timing of surgery after TIA or stroke is sometimes delayed by four to six weeks because of concerns of hemorrhagic conversion of an acute infarct. However, pooled data from NACSET and ESCT suggest that after minor, nondisabling stroke or TIA, the benefit was greater for those treated within two weeks (244).

Angioplasty and Stenting

In the last decade, interventional techniques have been developed to offer noninvasive alternatives to surgical CEA. Advocates of carotid angioplasty and stenting (CAS) cite its less-invasive nature, reduced cranial nerve and wound complications, utility in high-risk patients unsuitable for general anesthesia and surgery, and ability to access lesions more cephalad along the carotid artery. In addition, it may be preferable in those with prior neck surgery or radiation due to the difficulty of CEA in these scenarios. However, unlike CEA, the long-term outcomes from CAS have not been well studied. Critics also emphasize that CAS may have higher rates of procedure-related strokes, vessel dissection, and a greater potential for restenosis.

Trials addressing the efficacy and safety of CAS have shown mixed results. The Carotid and Vertebral Artery Transluminal Angioplasty Study (CAVATAS) randomized 504 patients to CEA versus CAS (74% received balloon angioplasty alone) (245). The results showed that 30-day and three-year stroke outcomes were similar in the two groups but complications such as cranial neuropathies and groin or neck hematomas were less frequent in the CAS group (1.2% vs. 6.7%). Restenosis was more common in the CAS group (14% vs. 4%).

With the advent of distal protection devices that have further reduced the risks of embolic stroke during the procedure, more recent studies have suggested that short-term stroke risk with CAS may be lower than CEA, especially in high-risk individuals. The Stenting and Angioplasty with Protection in Patients at High Risk for Endarterectomy study was designed to test the hypothesis that CAS was not inferior to CEA in patients considered at high risk for carotid surgery (246). Those included in this study and considered at a high risk for CEA included those with clinically significant cardiac disease, severe pulmonary disease, contralateral carotid occlusion, contralateral laryngeal-nerve palsy, previous radical neck surgery or radiation therapy to the neck, recurrent stenosis after endarterectomy, and age above 80 years. The study found trends for less vascular events in the CAS group at 30 days (4.8% vs. 9.8%, $p = 0.09$) and cumulative vascular events at one year (12.2% vs. 21.1%, $p = 0.05$). In addition, fewer patients required repeat revascularization at one year in the CAS group (0.6% vs. 4.3%, $p = 0.04$).

Some methodological concerns have been raised. These include the high percentage (22%) of patients enrolled with CEA restenosis, a condition due to intimal hyperplasia rather than atherosclerosis and likely to respond better to CAS. In addition, nearly 80% were asymptomatic patients with stenosis above 80% in the trial, a group that showed less benefit from CEA than symptomatic patients from prior studies. Lastly, the endpoint of MI, which was not included in the CEA trials, seems to have been driving the trend towards CAS superiority. Further studies comparing CAS to CEA in lower-risk individuals (similar to those enrolled in NASCET, ECST, ACAS, and ACST) are needed before any further conclusions can be made regarding the safety, efficacy, and long-term durability of carotid stenting and angioplasty.

Studies on intracranial and vertebro-basilar endovascular revascularization are more limited. While surgical treatment of VA stenosis is an option, it is not preferred due to the technical difficulty of the operation (247). Therefore, the preferred treatments are medical management and possibly endovascular revascularization in those with recurrent events despite maximal medical therapy (248,249). Larger studies are necessary before stronger statements regarding endovascular treatment of VB stenosis can be made.

Symptomatic intracranial atherosclerosis accounts for approximately 8% of ischemic strokes. Although the optimal medical management of this group currently supports antiplatelet therapy over warfarin (231), there is still debate as to whether alternative treatment strategies have a role in those who fail medical therapy. Given the high rate of recurrent stroke in this population, attempts to apply endovascular techniques have been advocated (231,250). Small case series have suggested that procedure-related stroke occurs in 8% to 50% and vessel dissection in 38% when patients are treated with balloon angioplasty for intracranial stenosis (251–253). Stent-assisted technology and development of undersized stents may be an option that reduces vessel recoil and dissection as well as rates of restenosis (254,255).

In the Stenting of Symptomatic Atherosclerotic Lesions in the Vertebral or Intracranial Artery Study, successful delivery of a stainless-steel stent with enhanced flexibility occurred in 95% of the cases, with 32.4% six-month restenosis rate, 6.1% stroke risk at 30 days, 14% stroke risk at one year (all posterior circulation strokes), and no deaths (256). However, in the setting of acute stroke combined with perfusion failure secondary to intracranial stenosis, the rates of peri-procedural complications may be nearly 50% (257). Careful patient selection, therefore, is required before considering intracranial angioplasty for symptomatic atherosclerotic lesions failing maximal medical therapy.

In strokes secondary to complete ICA occlusion, there is no clear advantage to surgical bypass in unselected patients. The extracranial–intracranial (EC–IC) bypass trial failed to show a benefit from the surgical procedure due to high rates of complication and is not currently recommended (258). However, the elevated risks of recurrent stroke in this patient population (as high as 14% per year in some studies), argued for another trial that might select more appropriate surgical candidates using preoperative evaluation of hemodynamic reserve, using methods such as positron-emission tomography (PET). The Carotid Occlusion Surgery Study is an ongoing trial to determine whether EC–IC bypass is superior to medical therapy in patients with recently symptomatic unilateral ICA occlusion, and PET scan criteria of exhausted hemodynamic reserve (elevated oxygen extraction fraction in the under-perfused brain region). Currently, risk factor modification and antiplatelet medications are the recommended treatment modalities for carotid occlusion.

Treatment Recommendations

Carotid revascularization with CEA (in addition to antiplatelet therapy and aggressive risk factor modification) is supported for symptomatic severe stenosis (70–99%) and should be performed within two weeks of ipsilateral nondisabling stroke or TIA by a surgeon with less than 6% morbidity and mortality rate (Fig. 10). For carotid stenosis of 50% to 69% and ipsilateral stroke or TIA, CEA is recommended but careful consideration for age, stroke severity, and

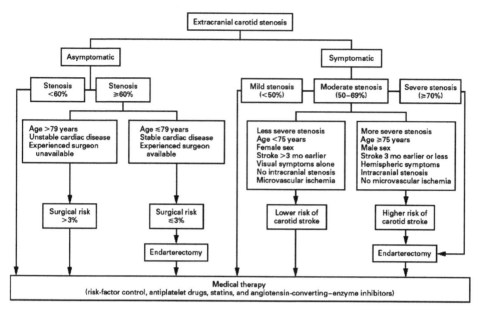

FIGURE 10   Algorithm for management of extracranial carotid stenosis. *Source*: From Ref. 259.

other comorbidities should be undertaken. The situations in which CAS is currently considered preferable to surgery are cases of high surgical risk, ICA stenosis secondary to prior radiation therapy to the neck, previous CEA with recurrent stenosis, contralateral ICA occlusion, and surgically inaccessible high CCA bifurcation (260). Its efficacy compared with the well-established role of CEA among lower risk patients remains to be determined by ongoing trials (CAVATAS-2). Data on vertebro-basilar and intracranial angioplasty is limited and should be considered only when maximal medical therapy fails, given the high degree of complications from procedure-related strokes and dissections. Pending ongoing trial data, there is no evidence to support EC/IC bypass for carotid occlusion.

OTHER PUTATIVE STROKE RISK FACTORS
Homocysteine

Hyperhomocysteinemia may act to promote or accelerate atherosclerosis (261). In over 100 case–control, cross-sectional, and prospective studies, an association between homocysteine levels and vascular disease has been observed (262,263). Regarding stroke risk, the evidence is still emerging. Trends for an association of the highest quartile of homocysteine and stroke have been seen in the Framingham Study as well as British Regional Heart Study (264,265). In the Northern Manhattan Study, levels greater than 15 μmol/L were strongly associated with vascular death, combined vascular outcomes, and with ischemic stroke in a tri-ethnic population. The link between moderate homocysteine elevations (10–15 μmol/L) and ischemic stroke were less dramatic (Fig. 11) (266). The Homocysteine Collaborative Group's meta-analysis of the data concluded that a moderate independent association existed with a 25% lower level being associated with about a 20% lower stroke and cardiac risk in asymptomatic persons (267).

Serum homocysteine levels can be modulated by diet. The Framingham study found that deficiencies in folate, B_{12}, and pyridoxine levels accounted for the majority of elevated homocysteine levels (268) and multivitamin therapy has been shown to lower homocysteine levels even among those who are not vitamin–deficient (269). No primary stroke prevention trials for homocysteine exist. However, the large prospective Vitamin in Stroke Protection Trial failed to show any benefit from homocysteine-lowering therapy (B_6, B_{12}, and folate) in preventing recurrent stroke despite reduction in homocysteine levels (270). Further clinical trials such as the Vitamins To Prevent Stroke (VITATOPS) study may help address these lingering questions (271). Preliminary results from VITATOPS revealed no significant reduction in markers of vascular inflammation [C-reactive protein (CRP)] or hypercoaguability (prothrombin fragments,

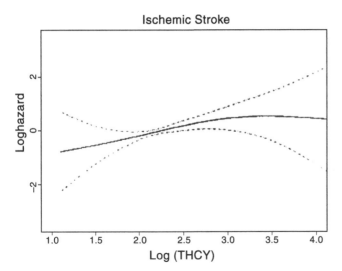

FIGURE 11 Homocysteine and risk of ischemic stroke in Northern Manhattan Stroke Study: the estimated log of the hazard ratio (HR) plotted as a function of the log of total baseline homocysteine value with the 95% confidence margins shown with the *dashed lines*. HR 1.0 is equivalent to log hazard of 0; HR 1.3 indicates log HR of 0.26, tHcy of 10 μmol/L indicates log tHcy of 2.3; tHcy 15 μmol/L, log tHcy of 2.7. *Source:* From Ref. 266.

d-dimer) despite reduction in total homocysteine levels (272). Homocysteine may be a marker of overall vascular disease rather than a direct etiological contributor to stroke.

Exogenous Estrogens

The relationship between exogenous estrogens and stroke has been studied in both younger women on oral contraceptives pills (OCP) as well as in older women taking hormone replacement therapy (HRT). The effects of estrogen are different in these different physiological states.

The Women's Health Initiative study on HRT and stroke showed an increased risk of stroke in women taking estrogen with hazard ratio of 1.31 (273). The Women's Estrogen for Stroke Trial evaluated the use of HRT compared to placebo in menopausal women with a history of a prior TIA/stroke and found an increased risk of fatal strokes among HRT patients (OR 2.8). Although the trial found comparable rates of minor strokes, the strokes occurring in the HRT group were associated with slightly worse neurologic and functional deficits (274).

Oral contraceptives with high estrogen content have also been shown to increase the risk of stroke. Newer OCP formulations contain significantly lower amounts of estrogen. A large case–control study did not find an increased risk of stroke in women who used oral contraceptives with estrogen content less than 50 mg (275). A meta-analysis of 16 studies did find an RR of 2.7 for stroke in oral contraceptive users (276). These authors also found that lower estrogen doses were associated with lower risk of stroke (RR 1.65). However, since women taking oral contraceptives are generally young and without significant vascular risk factors, the absolute risk is still low. The increased risk of stroke amounts to one additional stroke in 24,000 non-smoking, nonhypertensive women. It is not clear if the risk is higher in women who smoke, have other vascular risk factors, or have migraine.

Chronic Infection and Inflammation

The association between inflammatory conditions (infections such as *Chlamydia*, periodontal disease, elevations in sedimentation rate, CRP, white blood count, and other immunological markers) and ischemic stroke has been recently reported (277–280). *Chlamydia pneumoniae* and other causes of chronic infection may cause endothelial injury and increase the risk of vascular disease. CRP as a marker of inflammation has been associated with an increased risk of cardiovascular disease (281). Elevated CRP levels may also be a risk factor for stroke (282). In the PHS, men who developed ischemic stroke had higher levels of baseline CRP than those who did not have stroke (283).

In a case–control study of 89 stroke cases and 89 controls from the Northern Manhattan Study, chronic infection with *C. pneumoniae* was found to be an independent risk factor for stroke (277). Patients with stroke were more likely to have antibodies to *C. pneumoniae*. Serum IgA titers were more associated with stroke than IgG, suggesting IgA may be a better marker.

Further studies of chronic infections and inflammatory markers will help elucidate the underlying pathophysiology.

Periodontal disease, one of the most common human infections affecting as many as 45% of individuals over 65 years (284), is now recognized to be strongly linked to carotid atherosclerosis and stroke. In the NHANES I, periodontal disease was found to be strongly associated with stroke with an adjusted OR of 2.1 (285). Oral pathogens have been found in carotid plaques (286). Chronic infections, including periodontal disease, were independently associated with carotid IMT, even after adjusting for CRP level (287). Although much is still unexplained or unknown, the weight of current evidence suggests that an inflammatory component along with environmental and genetic factors may be a potential determinant of atherosclerosis and target for intervention (280).

Metabolic Syndrome

As a constellation of abnormalities that are related to insulin resistance, MetS (defined as three or more of the following: elevated triglyceride level, low HDL-C, elevated fasting glucose, high BP, and high waist circumference) is gaining popularity as an independent and strong risk factor for cardiovascular disease and stroke (133,288–290). In the ARIC Study, there was an overall 30% prevalence of MetS in baseline nondiabetics without cardiac disease. The twofold increased cardiovascular risk was significant in women, not in men, suggesting a gender interaction (291). Another large prospective study found that MetS was associated with RR of 1.39 in men and 2.10 in women (292). Others have also demonstrated an association with carotid atherosclerosis and MetS (293,294). Whether certain components are more powerful than others and whether early treatment of MetS reduces risk await further study.

Carotid Intima-Medial Thickness

Carotid intima-media thickness has been associated with systemic atherosclerosis and is potentially an early marker and subclinical predictor of stroke and MI. The ARIC study, Rotterdam Study, the British Regional Heart Study, and the Cardiovascular Health Study demonstrated the strong positive association of carotid IMT and incident stroke risk, adjusting for conventional vascular risk factors (295–298). Moreover, some recent studies have also shown that carotid IMT is a risk factor for stroke and cardiovascular events, independent of carotid plaque (299).

Several hypotheses have been proposed regarding the role of IMT in atherosclerosis. One hypothesis is that carotid IMT is an intermediate stage in the causal pathway of plaque formation. Others, however, have commented that carotid IMT and carotid plaque might represent different phenotypic expressions of atherosclerosis with divergent risk factors and predictive values. Lipid lowering therapies appear to have some benefit in retarding IMT progression (153–155). However, there is still a great deal of debate regarding the power of IMT measurements to predict future vascular events beyond those derived from traditional and more readily obtainable risk factor assessments (300).

Silent Infarcts

Silent brain infarcts are frequently observed on brain imaging of elderly individuals and are likely related to traditional stroke risk factors (301). Furthermore, it may serve as a marker for vascular disease and may have value in predicting subsequent stroke risk and vascular dementia. In longitudinal studies, the presence of silent brain infarctions has been shown to increase the risk of subsequent stroke (302,303). In one study from Japan involving 933 healthy subjects, the risk of stroke was increased 10-fold among those with silent infarcts (304). In the Cardiovascular Health study of over 3300 subjects over 65 years of age, the RR of stroke was 1.9 in those with silent infarctions (305). Whether aggressive risk factor modification and antithrombotic therapy are beneficial approaches remain to be elucidated.

White Matter Hyperintensity

There is evidence that periventricular white matter lesions or leukoariosis, on brain magnetic resonance imaging (MRI) correlate with increased risk of cardiovascular death (306). In addition, white matter hyperintensity (WMH) has been shown in prospective studies to increase the risk of stroke, particularly lacunar stroke (307–309). It is likely that WMH and lacunar strokes share a similar pathophysiology: lipohyalinotic vasculopathy of the small perforating blood vessels (310).

CONCLUSIONS

Ischemic stroke is a complex disease with considerable heterogeneity that has proven more challenging and perhaps more difficult to treat than other vascular diseases. The most convincing data in stroke prevention with the most robust findings come from studies of single stroke subtypes (i.e., SPAF and NASCET), suggesting that underlying pathogenesis and mechanism should be a strong consideration in planning future stroke prevention trials. Stroke may be too disparate to "lump" into a single category for analysis or treatment and "splitting" may yield more important results.

Nevertheless, the pharmacological armamentarium for stroke prevention is ever expanding and the optimal management of high-risk individuals is an evolving arena that requires individualized care and multimodal therapies. Stroke preventive measures continue to improve with numerous studies showing major benefits from risk factor modifications and treatments. It is hopeful that more widespread use of these stroke prevention strategies will have a lasting impact on reducing the future incidence, prevalence, and mortality associated with stroke (Fig. 12).

■ Case 1

A 71-year-old Caucasian man presents to the Emergency Room with 24-hour history of stuttering, right hemiparesis, dysarthria, and word-finding difficulty. Stroke risk factors include age, hypertension, and current cigarette smoking. Examination reveals mild transcortical motor aphasia with dysarthria and mild-moderate right hemiparesis involving face, arm, and leg equally. BP is 195/100 mmHg.

a. Localization: Left MCA territory involving deep white matter and frontal language connections.
b. Labs tests: Fasting cholesterol 220 mg/dL, LDL-C 125 mg/dL, and HDL-C 41 mg/dL.
c. Radiology: MRI shows multiple small–diffusion-weighted imaging (DWI) lesions in left corona radiata and some distal MCA cortical lesions, magnetic resonance angiogram shows left ICA stenosis of 70% to 95% at bifurcation. Carotid Doppler shows plaque at left ICA bifurcation with 70% stenosis; right ICA below 40% stenosis.
d. Diagnosis: acute ischemic stroke involving left ICA internal watershed territory.
e. Subtype/etiology: LAA with likely perfusion failure 1/2 artery–artery embolism.
f. Treatment—multimodal approach addressing the following:

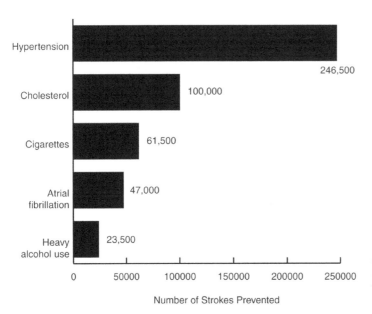

FIGURE 12 Number of strokes prevented with risk factor elimination or modification. *Source*: From Ref. 311.

i. Symptomatic left carotid stenosis—if no high-risk features are found in presurgical evaluation, proceed with CEA. Timing of surgery is to be preferably within two weeks given small infarcts. Monitor patient for complications, specifically cranial neuropathies, perioperative stroke, and hyperperfusion syndrome.

ii. Antithrombotic therapy—in addition to carotid revascularization, antiplatelet therapy is indicated. Options include aspirin, clopidogrel, or extended-release dipyridamole/aspirin depending on tolerability, costs, and other comorbidities. All would be reasonable in this patient.

iii. Dyslipidemia—initiate lipid-lowering therapy with HMG-CoA reductase inhibitors ("statins") with goal LDL below 100mg/dL (option for 70mg/dL) and HDL above 40mg/dL.

iv. Smoking—cessation should be encouraged and assistance offered. Options include counseling, drugs (nicotine replacement), and buproprion.

v. Hypertension—acute management of BP favors permissive hypertension (up to 220/120mmHg during acute period) to assist in perfusion and limit infarct progression. Following CEA, initiation of anti–hypertensive medication is indicated with a preference for ACE-I or ARB with goal BP below 120/80mmHg.

vi. Rehabilitation—speech and physical therapy should be offered to improve functional outcome and limit disability following stroke.

■ Case 2

A 65-year-old African-American woman presents with dysarthria and left face, arm, and leg weakness for 30 minutes. Stroke risk factors include age, race, diabetes, hypertension, and occasional binge drinking. Medications include aspirin daily. Neurological examination is normal.

a. Localization: Right subcortical white matter.
b. Labs tests: Glycosylated hemoglobin 9.0%, glucose 210 mg/dL, LDL-C 105 mg/dL.
c. Radiology: MRI is negative for acute stroke, but shows moderate periventricular T2 white matter hyperintensities.
d. Diagnosis: Right subcortical TIA.
e. Subtype/etiology: Likely small vessel disease from DM and HTN.
f. Treatment—multimodal approach addressing the following:

i. TIA—90-day risk for stroke is almost 35% given age, motor, speech symptoms, duration above 10 minutes, and diabetes with half of the risk during first 48 hours. Urgent evaluation, admission for observation is to be recommended.

ii. Antithrombotic therapy—for stroke prevention, consider switching to extended-release dipyridamole plus aspirin or clopidogrel alone given already on aspirin daily.

iii. Dyslipidemia—initiate lipid-lowering therapy with HMG-CoA reductase inhibitors ("statins") with goal LDL-C below 100mg/dL (option for 70mg/dL) and HDL-C above 40mg/dL.

iv. Hyperglycemia—consultation to achieve better glycemic control.

v. Hypertension—among diabetics, ACE-I or ARB are preferable for vascular risk reduction with goal BP below 130/80mmHg.

vi. Alcohol use—discourage binge or heavy drinking and recommend moderation if possible (<1 drink per day for woman).

vii. White matter hyperintensities—current evidence suggests that white matter hyperintensities may increase risk of stroke and dementia. Recommend risk factor reduction as above.

■ Case 3

75-year-old white man presents with acute left side visual loss. Risk factors include age, sex, CAD, and hypercholesterolemia on statin therapy. Examination reveals a dense left homonymous hemianopia, irregularly irregular pulse, and BP of 155/60mmHg.

a. Localization: Right occipital lobe.
b. Labs tests: Fasting cholesterol 180mg/dL, LDL-C 103mg/dL, and HDL-C 45mg/dL. Electrocardiogram showed AF.
c. Radiology: MRI shows right occipital pole acute DWI lesion.
d. Diagnosis: acute right Posterior cerebral astery infarct.
e. Subtype/etiology: cardioembolism secondary to new onset AF.
f. Treatment—multimodal approach addressing the following:

i. AF—risk of recurrent stroke is 18% over five years.

ii. Antithrombotic therapy—long-term anticoagulation with warfarin is warranted.

iii. Dyslipidemia—increase statin dose with goal LDL-C below 100 mg/dL (option for 70mg/dL) and HDL-C above 40mg/dL.

iv. Hypertension—acute management of BP favors permissive hypertension (up to 220/120mmHg during acute period) to improve perfusion and limit infarct progression. Upon discharge, initiate anti-hypertensive therapy with ACE-I with goal BP below 140/90mmHg.

g. Rehabilitation—visual rehabilitation can be considered; driving should be restricted with subsequent serial visual field testing to assess for improvement.

REFERENCES

1. WHO Task Force on stroke and other cerebrovascular disorders: stroke. Recommendations on stroke prevention, diagnosis and therapy. Stroke 1989; 20:1407–1431.
2. AHA Heart Disease and Stroke Statistics–2005 Update. American Heart Association.
3. Rothwell PM, Coull AJ, Giles MF, et al. Change in stroke incidence, mortality, case fatality, severity, and risk factors in Oxfordshire, UK from 1981 to 2004 (Oxford Vascular Study). Lancet 2004; 363:1925–1933.
4. Adams HP Jr, Bendixen BH, Kappelle LJ, et al (The TOAST investigators). Classification of subtype of acute ischemic stroke: definitions for use in a multicenter clinical trial. Stroke 1993; 24:35–41.
5. Petty GW, Brown RD, Whisnant JP, et al. Ischemic stroke subtypes: a population-based study of incidence and risk factors. Stroke 1999; 30:2513–2516.
6. Kolominsky-Rabas PL, Weber M, Gefeller O, et al. Epidemiology of ischemic stroke subtypes according to TOAST criteria–Incidence, recurrence, and long-term survival in ischemic stroke subtypes: a population-based study. Stroke 2001; 32:2735–2740.
7. Schneider AT, Kissela B, Woo D, et al. Ischemic stroke subtypes: a population-based study of incidence rates among blacks and whites. Stroke 2004; 35:1552.
8. Albers GW, Caplan LR, Easton JD, et al. Transient ischemic attack–proposal for a new definition. N Engl J Med 2002; 347:1713–1716.
9. Centers for Disease Control. Ten great public health achievements–United States, 1900–1999. Morbid Mortal Weekly Rep 1999; 48:241–243.
10. Sarti C, Rastenyte D, Cepaitis Z, Tuomilehto J. International trends in mortality from stroke, 1968 to 1994. Stroke. 2000; 31(7):1588–1601.
11. Broderick JP. Stroke trends in Rochester, Minnesota, during 1945 to 1984. Ann Epidemiol 1993; 3:476–479.
12. Wolf PA, D'Agostino RB, O'Neal MA, et al. Secular trends in stroke incidence and mortality. The Framingham Study. Stroke 1992; 23:1551–1555.
13. Howard G, Craven TE, Sanders L, Evans GW. Relationship of hospitalized stroke rate and in-hospital mortality to the decline in US stroke mortality. Neuroepidemiology 1991; 10:251–259.
14. Jamrozik K, Robyn J. Broadhurst RJ, et al. Stroke. Trends in the incidence, severity, and short-term outcome of stroke in Perth, Western Australia. 1999; 30(10):2105–2111.
15. Sacco RL, Boden-Albala B, Gan R, et al. Stroke incidence among white, black, and Hispanic residents of an urban community: the Northern Manhattan Stroke Study. Am J Epidemiol 1998; 147(3):259–268.
16. Morgenstern LB, Smith MA, Lisbeth LD, et al. Excess stroke in Mexican Americans compared with non-Hispanic whites: the Brain Attack Surveillance in Corpus Christi Project. Am J Epidemiol 2004; 160:376–383.
17. Brown RD, Whisant JP, Sicks J, et al. Stroke incidence, prevalence, and survival: secular trends in Rochester, Minnesota through 1989. Stroke 1996; 27:373–380.
18. Broderick J, Brott T, Kothari R, et al. The Greater Cincinnati/Northern Kentucky Stroke Study: preliminary first-ever and total incidence rates of stroke among blacks. Stroke 1998; 29:415–421.
19. Sacco RL. Stroke risk factors: and overview. In: Norris JW, Hachinski V, eds. Stroke Prevention, 2001.
20. Goldstein LB, Adams R, Becker K, et al. Primary prevention of ischemic stroke: a statement for healthcare professionals from the Stroke Council of the American Heart Association. Stroke 2001; 32(1):280–299.
21. Wolf PA, D'Agostino, Belanger AJ, Kannel WB. Probability of stroke: a risk profile from the Framingham Study. Stroke 1991; 22(3):312–318.
22. Manolio TA, Kronmal RA, Burke GL, et al. Short term predictors of incident stroke in older adults: the Cardiovascular Health Study. Stroke 1996; 27:1479–1486.
23. Bouser MG. Stroke in women: the 1997 Paul Dudley White International Lecture. Circulation 1999; 99(4):463–467.
24. Holyrod-Leduc JM, Kapral MK, Austin PC, Tu JV. Sex differences and similarities in the management and outcome of stroke patients. Stroke 2000; 31(8):1833–1837.
25. Ramani S, Bryne-Logan S, Freund KM, et al. Gender differences in the treatment of cerebrovascular disease. J Am Geriatr Soc 2000; 48(7):741–745.
26. Kapral MK, Fang J, Hill MD, et al. Sex differences in stroke care and outcomes: results from the Registry of the Canadian Stroke Network. Stroke 2005; 36(4):809–814.
27. Roquer J, Campello AR, Gomis M. Sex differences in first-ever acute stroke. Stroke 2003; 34(7):1581–1585.
28. Di Carlo A, Lamassa M, Baldereschi M, et al. Sex differences in the clinical presentation, resource use, and 3-month outcome of acute stroke in Europe: data from a multicenter multinational hospital-based registry. Stroke 2003; 34(5):1114–1119.
29. Glader EL, Stegmayr B, Norrving B, et al. Sex differences in management and outcome after stroke: a Swedish national perspective. Stroke 2003; 34(8):1970–1975.
30. Kent DM, Price LL, Ringleb P, et al. Sex-based differences in response to recombinant tissue plasminogen activator in acute ischemic stroke: a pooled analysis of randomized clinical trials. Stroke 2005; 36(1):62–65.
31. Savitz SI, Schlaug G, Caplan L, Selim M. Arterial occlusive lesions recanalize more frequently in women than in men after intravenous tissue plasminogen activator administration for acute stroke. Stroke 2005; 36(7):1447–1451.

32. Cooper ES. Cardiovascular diseases and stroke in African-Americans: a call for action. J Natl Med Assoc 1993; 85(2):97–100.
33. Woo D, Gebel J, Miller R, et al. Incidence rates of first-ever ischemic stroke subtypes among blacks: a population-based study. Stroke 1999; 30(12):2517–2522.
34. White H, Boden-Albala B, Wang C, et al. Ischemic stroke subtype incidence among whites, blacks, and Hispanics: the Northern Manhattan Study. Circulation 2005; 111(10):1327–1331.
35. Howard G. Why do we have a stroke belt in the southeastern United States? A review of unlikely and uninvestigated potential causes. Am J Med Sci 1999; 317(3):160–167.
36. Howard G, Howard VJ, Katholi C, et al. Decline in US stroke mortality: an analysis of temporal patterns by sex, race, and geographic region. Stroke 2001; 32(10):2213–2220.
37. Lanska DJ, Kuller LH. The geography of stroke mortality in the United States and the concept of a stroke belt. Stroke 1995; 26(7):1145–1149.
38. Schulz UG, Flossmann E, Rothwell PM. Heritability of ischemic stroke in relation to age, vascular risk factors, and subtypes of incident stroke in population-based studies. Stroke 2004; 35(4):819–824.
39. Rubattu S, Giliberti R, Volpe M. Etiology and pathophysiology of stroke as a complex trait. Am J Hypertens 2000; 13(10):1139–1148.
40. Schoenborn CA, Adams PF, Barnes PM, et al. Health behaviors of adults: United States, 1999–2001. Vital Health Stat 10 2004; (219):1–79.
41. Shinton R, Beevers G. Meta-analysis of relation between cigarette smoking and stroke. BMJ 1989; 298(6676):789–794.
42. Gorelick PB, Rodin MB, Langenberg P, et al. Weekly alcohol consumption, cigarette smoking, and the risk of ischemic stroke: results of a case-control study at three urban medical centers in Chicago, Illinois. Neurology 1989; 39(3):339–343.
43. Howard G, Wagenknecht LE, Burke GL, et al., for the ARIC Investigators. Cigarette smoking and progression of atherosclerosis. JAMA 1998; 279:119–124.
44. Bonita R, Duncan J, Truelsen T, et al. Passive smoking as well as active smoking increases the risk of acute stroke. Tob Control 1999; 8(2):156–160.
45. You RX, Thrift AG, McNeill JJ, et al. Ischemic stroke risk and passive exposure to spouses' cigarette smoking. Melbourne Stroke Risk Factor Study (MERFS) Group. Am J Public Health 1999; 89(4):572–575.
46. Sacco RL, Roberts JK, Boden-Albala B, et al. Race-ethnicity and determinants of carotid atherosclerosis in a multiethnic population: the Northern Manhattan Stroke Study. Stroke 1997; 28(5):929–935.
47. Kool MJ, Hoeks AP, Stroijker Boudier HA, et al. Short- and long-term effects of smoking on arterial wall properties in habitual smokers. J Am Coll Cardiol 1993; 22(7):1881–1886.
48. Cruickshank JM, Neil-Dwyer G, Dorrance DE, et al. Acute effects of smoking on blood pressure and cerebral blood flow. J Hum Hypertens 1989; 3(6):443–449.
49. Lightwood JM, Glantz SA. Short-term economic and health benefits of smoking cessation: myocardial infarction and stroke. Circulation 1997; 96:1089–1096.
50. Gorelick PB. Stroke prevention. Arch Neurol 1995; 52(4):347–355.
51. Lancaster T, Stead L, Silagy C, et al for Cochrane Tobacco Addiction Review Group. Effectiveness of interventions to help people stop smoking: findings from the Cochrane Library. Br Med J 2000; 321:355–358.
52. Jorenby DE, Leischow SJ, Nides MA, et al. A controlled trial of sustained-release bupropion, a nicotine patch, or both for smoking cessation. N Eng J Med 1999; 340:685–691.
53. Tobacco Use and Dependence Clinical Practice Guideline Panel, Staff, and Consortium Representatives. A clinical practice guideline for treating tobacco use and dependence: a US Public Health Service report. JAMA 2000; 283:3244–3254.
54. Donahue RP, Abbott RD, Reed DM, Yano K. Alcohol and hemorrhagic stroke: the Honolulu Heart Study. JAMA 1986; 255:2311–2314.
55. Tanaka H, Ueda Y, Hayashi M, et al. Risk factors for cerebral hemorrhage and cerebral infarction in a Japanese rural community. Stroke 1982; 13(1):62–73.
56. Stampfer MJ, Colditz GA, Willett WA, et al. A prospective study of moderate alcohol consumption and the risk of coronary disease and stroke in women. N Engl J Med 1988; 319:267–273.
57. Berger K, Ajani UA, Kase CS, et al. Light-to-moderate alcohol consumption and risk of stroke among U.S. male physicians. N Engl J Med 1999; 341(21):1557–1564.
58. Harmsen P, Rosengren A, Tsipogianni A, Wilhelmsen L. Risk factors for stroke in middle-aged men in Goteborg, sweden. stroke 1990; 21:223–229.
59. Kono S, Ikeda M, Tokudome S, Nishizumi M, Kuratsune M. Alcohol and mortality: a cohort study of male Japanese physicians. Int J Epidemiol 1986; 15:527–532.
60. Sacco RL, Elkind M, Boden-Albala B, et al. The protective effect of moderate alcohol consumption on ischemic stroke. JAMA 1999; 281:53–60.
61. Reynolds K, Lewis B, Nolen JD, et al. Alcohol consumption and risk of stroke: a meta-analysis. JAMA 2003; 289(5):579–588.
62. Thornton J, Symes C, Heaton K. Moderate alcohol intake reduces bile cholesterol saturation and raises HDL cholesterol. Lancet 1983; 2(8354):819–822.
63. Wannamethee SG, Sharper AG. Alcohol, coronary heart disease and stroke: an examination of the J-shaped curve. Neuroepidemiology 1998; 17(6):288–295.
64. Sesso HD, Stampfer MJ, Rosner B, et al. Seven-year changes in alcohol consumption and subsequent risk of cardiovascular disease in men. Arch Intern Med 2000; 160(17):2605–2612.

65. Centers for Disease Control and Prevention. Prevalence of physical activity, including lifestyle activities among adults–United States, 2000–2001. MMWR Morb Mortal Wkly Rep 2003; 52(32):764–769.
66. US Department of Health and Human Services. Physical Activity and Health: A Report of the Surgeon General. Atlanta, GA: US Department of Health and Human Services, Center for Disease Control and Prevention, National Center Chronic Disease Prevention and Health Promotion, 1996.
67. Blair SN, Kohl HW III, Barlow CE, et al. Changes in physical fitness and all-cause mortality. A prospective study of healthy and unhealthy men. JAMA 1995; 273(14):1093–1098.
68. Fischer HG, Koenig W. Physical activity and coronary heart disease. Cardiologia 1998; 43(10):1027–1035.
69. Abbott RD, Rodriguez BL, Burchfiel CM, Curb JD. Physical activity in older middle-aged men and reduced risk of stroke: the Honolulu Heart Program. Am J Epidemiol 1994; 139:881–893.
70. Kiely DK, Wolf PA, Cupples LA, Beiser AS, Kannel WB. Physical activity and stroke risk: the Framingham Study. Am J Epidemiol 1994; 140:608–620.
71. Lindenstrom E, Boysen G, Nyboe J. Lifestyle factors and risk of cerebrovascular disease in women. The Copenhagen City Heart Study. Stroke 1993; 24(10):1468–1472.
72. Hu FB, Stampfer MJ, Colditz GA, et al. Physical activity and risk of stroke in women. JAMA 2000; 283(22):2961–2967.
73. Sacco RL, Gan R, Boden-Albala B, et al. Leisure-time physical activity and ischemic stroke risk: the Northern Manhattan Stroke Study. Stroke 1998; 29:380–387.
74. Lee IM, Hennekens CH, Berger K, et al. Exercise and risk of stroke in male physicians. Stroke 1999; 30(1):1–6.
75. Lee CD, Folsom AR, Blair SN. Physical activity and stroke risk: a meta analysis. Stroke 2003; 34:2475–2482.
76. Williams PT. High-density lipoprotein cholesterol and other risk factors for coronary heart disease in female runners. N Engl J Med 1996; 334(20):1298–1303.
77. Wang JS, Jen CJ, Chen HI. Effects of exercise training and deconditioning on platelet function in men. Arterioscler Thromb Vas Biol 1995; 15:1668–1674.
78. Nygard O, Vollset SE, Refsum H, et al. Total plasma homocysteine and cardiovascular risk profile–the Hordaland Homocysteine Study. JAMA 1995; 274:1526–1533.
79. Takeya Y, Popper JS, Schmimizu, et al. Epidemiologic studies of coronary heart disease and stroke in Japanese men living in Japan, Hawaii and California. Stroke 1984; 15:15–23.
80. Gillman MW, Cupples A, Millen B, et al. Inverse association of dietary fat with development of ischemic stroke in men. JAMA 1997; 278:2145–2150.
81. Sauvaget C, Nagano J, Hayashi M, Yamada M. Animal protein, animal fat, and cholesterol intakes and risk of cerebral infarction mortality in the Adult Health Study. Stroke 2004; 35:1531–1537.
82. He K, Merchant A, Rimm E, et al. Dietary fat intake and risk of stroke in male US healthcare professionals: 14 year prospective cohort study. BMJ 2003; 327:777–782.
83. Joshipura KJ, Ascherio A, Manson JE, et al. Fruit and vegetable intake in relation to risk of ischemic stroke. JAMA 1999; 282:1233–1239.
84. Hak AE, Ma J, Powell CB, et al. Prospective study of plasma carotenoids and tocopherols in relation to risk of ischemic stroke. Stroke 2004; 35:1584–1588.
85. Abbott RD, Curb D, Rodriguez BL, et al. Effect of dietary calcium and milk consumption on risk of thromboembolic stroke in older middle-aged men. The Honolulu Heart Study. Stroke 1996; 27:813–818.
86. Mozaffarian D, Kumanyika SK, Lemaitre RN, et al. Cereal, fruit, and vegetable fiber intake and the risk of cardiovascular disease in elderly individuals. JAMA 2003; 289:1659–1666.
87. Liu S, Manson JE, Stampfer MJ, et al. Whole grain consumption and risk of ischemic stroke in women: a prospective study. JAMA 2000; 284(12):1534–1540.
88. Iso H, Rexrode KM, Stampfer MJ, et al. Intake of fish and omega-3 fatty acids and risk of stroke in women. JAMA 2001; 285(3):304–312.
89. He K, Song Y, Daviglus M, et al. Fish consumption and incidence of stroke: a meta analysis of cohort studies. Stroke 2004; 35:1538–1542.
90. Pearson TA, Blair SN, Daniels SR, et al. AHA Guidelines for Primary Prevention of Cardiovascular Disease and Stroke—2002 Update. Consensus Panel Guide to Comprehensive Risk Reduction for Adult Patients Without Coronary or Other Atherosclerotic Vascular Diseases. American Heart Association Science Advisory and Coordinating Committee. Circulation 2002; 106(3):388–391.
91. Walker SP, Rimm EB, Ascherio A, et al. Body size and fat distribution as predictors of stroke among US men. Am J Epidemiol 1996; 144(12):1143–1150.
92. Suk SH, Sacco RL, Boden-Albala B, et al. Abdominal obesity and risk of ischemic stroke: the Northern Manhattan Stroke Study. Stroke 2003; 34:1586–1592.
93. Rexrode KM, Hennekens CH, Willett WC, et al. A prospective study of body mass index, weight change, and risk of stroke in women. JAMA 1997; 277:1539–1545.
94. Qureshi AI, Suri FK, Kirmani JF, Diavni AA. Prevalence and trends of prehypertension and hypertension in United States: National Health and Nutrition Examination Surveys 1976 to 2000. Med Sci Monit 2005; 11(9):CR403–CR409.
95. MacMahon S, Rodgers A. The epidemiological association between blood pressure and stroke: implications for primary and secondary prevention. Hypertens Res 1994; 17:S23–S32.
96. Kannel WB, Wolf PA, Verter J, McNamara PM. Epidemiologic assessment of the role of blood pressure in stroke. The Framingham Study. JAMA 1970; 214:301–310.

97. Kannel WB, Wolf PA, McGee DL, et al. Systolic blood pressure, arterial rigidity, and risk of stroke: the Framingham Study. JAMA 1981; 245:1225–1229.
98. MacMahon S, Peto R, Cutler J, et al. Blood pressure, stroke, and coronary heart disease. Part 1, Prolonged differences in blood pressure: prospective observational studies corrected for the regression dilution bias. Lancet 1990; 335(8692):765–774.
99. Klungel O, Stricker B, Paes A, et al. Excess stroke among hypertensive men and women attributable to undertreatment of hypertension. Stroke 1999; 30:1312–1318.
100. Lawes CM, Bennett DA, Feigin VL, Rodgers A. Blood pressure and stroke: an overview of published reviews. Stroke 2004; 35:776–785.
101. Lewington S, Clarke R, Qizilbash N, Peto R, Collins R. Age specific relevance of usual blood pressure to vascular mortality: a meta-analysis of individual data for one million adults in 61 prospective studies. Lancet 2002; 360:1903–1913.
102. Chobanian AV, Bakris GL, Black HR, et al. The Seventh Report of the Joint National Committee on Prevention, Detection, Evaluation, and Treatment of High Blood Pressure: the JNC 7 report. JAMA 2003; 289:2560–2572.
103. Dahlof B, Linholm L, Hansson L, et al. Morbidity and mortality in the Swedish Trial in Old Patients with Hypertension (STOP-Hypertension). Lancet 1991; 338:1281–1285.
104. SHEP Cooperative Research Group. Prevention of stroke by antihypertensive drug treatment in older persons with isolated systolic hypertension: final results of the Systolic Hypertension in the Elderly Program (SHEP). JAMA 1991; 265:3255–3264.
105. Staessen JA, Fagard R, Thijs L, et al. Randomized double-blind comparison of placebo and active treatment for older persons with systolic hypertension. Lancet 1997; 350:757–764.
106. Hansson L, Lindholm LH, Ekbom T, et al. Randomized trial of old and new antihypertensive drugs in elderly patients: cardiovascular mortality and morbidity; the Swedish Trial in Old Patients with Hypertension-2 Study. Lancet 2000; 354:1744–1745.
107. Wright JT Jr, Dunn JK, Cutler JA, et al. Outcomes in hypertensive black and nonblack patients treated with chlorthalidone, amlodipine, and lisinopril. JAMA 2005; 293(13):1595–1608.
108. Collins R, Peto R, MacMahon S, et al. Blood pressure, stroke, and coronary heart disease. Part 2, Short-term reductions in blood pressure: overview of randomised drug trials in their epidemiological context. Lancet 1990; 335(8693):827–838.
109. Dunbabin DW, Sandercock PA. Preventing stroke by the modification of risk factors. Stroke 1990; 21(12 Suppl):IV36–IV39.
110. Bosch J, Salim Y, Pogue J, et al. Use of ramipril in preventing stroke: double blind randomized trial. BMJ 2002; 324:699–704.
111. HOPE Study Investigators. Effects of angiotensin-converting-enzyme inhibitor, ramipril on cardiovascular events in high-risk patients. N Engl J Med 2000; 342:145–153.
112. PROGRESS Collaborative group. Randomised trial of a perindopril-based blood pressure-lowering regimen among 6105 individuals with previous stroke or transient ischemic attack. Lancet 2001; 358:1033–1041.
113. Lithell H, Hansson L, Skoog I, et al. The Study on Cognition and Prognosis in the Elderly (SCOPE): principal results of a randomized double-blind intervention trial. J Hypertens 2003; 21:875–886.
114. Dahlof B, Devereux RB, Kjeldsen SE, et al. Cardiovascular morbidity and mortality in the Losartan Intervention For Endpoint reduction in hypertension study (LIFE): a randomised trial against atenolol. Lancet 2002; 359:995–1003.
115. Mokdad AH, Ford ES, Bowman EA, et al. Prevalence of obesity, diabetes, and obesity-related health risk factors, 2001. JAMA 2003; 289(1):76–79.
116. Sacco RL, Boden-Albala B, Abel G, et al. Race-ethnic disparities in the impact of stroke risk factors: the northern Manhattan stroke study. Stroke 2001; 32:1725–1731.
117. Abbott RD, Donahue RP, MacMahon SW, Reed DM, Yano K. Diabetes and the risk of stroke. The Honolulu Heart Program. JAMA 1987; 257:949–952.
118. Folsom A, Rasmussen M, Chambless L, et al. Prospective associations of fasting insulin, body fat distribution, and diabetes with risk of ischemic stroke. Diabetes Care 1999; 22:1077–1083.
119. Lindegard B, Hillbom M. Associations between brain infarction, diabetes, and alcoholism: observations from the Gothenberg population cohort study. Acta Neurol Scand 1987; 75:195–200.
120. The Diabetes Control and Complications Trial/Epidemiology of Diabetes Interventions and Complications Research Group. Retinopathy and nephropathy in patients with type 1 diabetes four years after a trial of intensive therapy. N Engl J Med 2000; 342(6):381–389.
121. UKPDS Group. Intensive glucose control with sulfonylureaas on insulin compared with conventional treatment and role of complications with type 2 diabetes (UKPDS 33). Lancet 1998; 352:837–853.
122. Alter M, Lai SM, Friday G, et al. Stroke recurrence in diabetics. Does control of blood glucose reduce risk? Stroke 1997; 28(6):1153–1157.
123. Nathan DM, Lachin J, Cleary P, et al. Intensive diabetes therapy and carotid intima-media thickness in type 1 diabetes mellitus. N Engl J Med 2003; 348(23):2294–2303.
124. Scott JF, Robinson GM, French JM, et al. Glucose potassium insulin infusions in the treatment of acute stroke patients with mild to moderate hyperglycemia: the Glucose Insulin in Stroke Trial (GIST). Stroke 1999; 30(4):793–799.

125. Curb JD, Pressel SL, Cutler JA, et al. Effect of diuretic-based antihypertensive treatment on cardiovascular disease risk in older diabetic patients with isolated systolic hypertension. Systolic Hypertension in the Elderly Program Cooperative Research Group. JAMA 1996; 276(23): 1886–1892.

126. Adler A, Stratton IM, Neil HA, et al. Association of systolic blood pressure with macrovascular and microvascular complications of type 2 diabetes (UKPDS36): prospective observational study. Br Med J 2000; 321:412–419.

127. Hansson L, Zanchetti A, Carruthers SG, et al. Effects of intensive blood-pressure lowering and low-dose aspirin in patients with hypertension: principal results of the Hypertension Optimal Treatment (HOT) randomised trial. Lancet 1998; 315:1755–1762.

128. Heart Outcomes Prevention Evaluation (HOPE) Study Investigators. Effects of ramipril on cardiovascular and microvascular outcomes in people with diabetes mellitus: results of the HOPE study and MICRO-HOPE substudy. Lancet 2000; 355:253–259.

129. Sever PS, Dahlof B, Poulter NR, et al. Prevention of coronary and stroke events with atorvastatin in hypertensive patients who have average or lower-than-average cholesterol concentrations in the Anglo-Scandinavian Cardiac Outcomes Trial—Lipid Lowering Arm (ASCOT-LLA): a multicentre randomised controlled trial. Lancet 2003; 361:1149–1158.

130. Goldberg RB, Mellies MJ, Sacks FM, et al. Cardiovascular events and their reduction with pravastatin in diabetic and glucose-intolerant myocardial infarction survivors with average cholesterol levels: subgroup analyses in the cholesterol and recurrent events (CARE) trial. The CARE investigators. Circulation 1998; 98:2513–2519.

131. Collins R, Armitage J, Parish S, et al. MRC/BHF Heart Protection Study of cholesterol-lowering with simvistatin in 5963 people with diabetes: a randomised placebo-controlled trial. Lancet 2003; 361:2005–2016.

132. Colhoun HM, Betteridge DJ, Durrington PN, et al. Primary prevention of cardiovascular disease with atorvastatin in type 2 diabetes in the Collaborative Atorvastatin Diabetes Study (CARDS): multicentre randomised placebo-controlled trial. Lancet 2004; 364:685–696.

133. Adult Treatment Panel III. Executive Summary of the Third Report of The National Cholesterol Education Program (NCEP) Expert Panel on Detection, Evaluation, and Treatment of High Blood Cholesterol in Adults (Adult Treatment Panel III). JAMA 2001; 285:2486–2497.

134. American Diabetes Association. Dyslipidemia management in adults with diabetes. Diab Care 2004; 27:S68–S71.

135. Iso H, Jacobs DR, Wentworth D, et al. Serum cholesterol levels and six year mortality from stroke in 350,977 men screened for the multiple risk factor intervention trial. N Engl J Med 1989; 320:904–910.

136. Benfante R, Yano K, Hwang LJ, et al. Elevated serum cholesterol is a risk factor for both coronary heart disease and thromboembolic stroke in Hawaiian Japanese men: implications of shared risk. Stroke 1994; 25:814–820.

137. Qizilbash N, Lewington S, Duffy S, et al. Cholesterol, diastolic blood pressure, and stroke: 13,000 strokes in 450,000 people in 45 prospective cohorts: Prospective studies collaboration. Lancet 1995; 346:1647–1653.

138. Schulz UGR, Rothwell PM. Differences in vascular risk factors between etiological subtypes of ischemic stroke: importance of population-based studies. Stroke 2003; 34:2050–2059.

139. van der Meer IM, Iglesias del Sol A, Hak AE, et al. Risk factors for progression of atherosclerosis measured at multiple sites in the arterial tree: the Rotterdam Study. Stroke 2003; 34:2374–2379.

140. O'Leary DH, Anderson KM, Wolf PA, et al. Cholesterol and carotid atherosclerosis in older persons: the Framingham Study. Ann Epidemiol 1992; 2(1–2):147–153.

141. Salonen R, Nyyssonen K, Porkkala E, et al. Kuopio Atherosclerosis Prevention Study (KAPS): a population-based primary prevention trial of the effect of LDL lowering on atherosclerotic progression in carotid and femoral arteries. Circulation 1995; 92:1758–1764.

142. Sacco RL, Benson RT, Kargman DE, et al. High density lipoprotein cholesterol and ischemic stroke in the elderly. The Northern Manhattan Stroke Study. JAMA 2001; 285:2729–2735.

143. Wannamethee SG, Sharper AG, Ebrahim S. HDL-Cholesterol, total cholesterol, and the risk of stroke in middle-aged British men. Stroke 2000; 31(8):1882–1888.

144. Shintani S, Kikuchi S, Hamaguchi H, Shiigai T. High serum lipoprotein(a) levels are an independent risk factor for cerebral infarction. Stroke 1993; 24(7):965–969.

145. Kargman DE, Berglund LF, Boden-Albala B, et al. Increased stroke risk and lipoprotein (a) in a racially mixed area: the Northern Manhattan Stroke Study. Stroke 1999; 30:251.

146. Guyton AJ, Capuzzi DM. Efficacy and safety of an extended-release niacin (Niaspan): a long-term study. Am J Cardiol 1998; 82:74–86.

147. Jeng JS, Sacco RL, Lui RC, et al. Association of apolipoproteins to carotid artery atherosclerosis: the Northern Manhattan Stroke Study. Stroke 1999; 30:251.

148. Scandinavian Simvastatin Survival Study Group. Randomized trial of cholesterol lowering in 4444 patients with coronary heart disease: the Scandinavian Simvastatin Survival Study (4S). Lancet 1994; 344:1383–1389.

149. Sacks FM, Pfeffer MA, Moye LA, et al. for the Cholesterol and Recurrent Events Trial Investigators. The effects of pravastatin on coronary events after myocardial infarction in patients with average cholesterol levels. NEJM 1996; 335:1000–1009.

150. The Long-term Intervention with Pravastatin in Ischemic Disease (LIPID) Study Group. Prevention of cardiovascular events and death with pravastatin in patients with coronary heart disease and a board range of initial cholesterol levels. NEJM 1998; 339:1349–1357.

151. Blauw GJ, Lagaay AM, Smelt AH, Westendorp RG. Stroke, statins, and cholesterol. A meta-analysis of randomized, placebo-controlled, double-blind trials with HMG-CoA reductase inhibitors. Stroke 1997; 28:946–950.

152. DiMascio R, Marchioli R, Tognoni G. Cholesterol reduction and stroke occurrence: an overview of randomized clinical trials. Cerebrovasc Dis 2000; 10(2):85–92.

153. Blackenhorn DH, Selzer RH, Crawford DW, et al. Beneficial effects of colestipol-niacin therapy on the common carotid artery. Two and four-year reduction of carotid intimal-media thickness measured by ultrasound. Circulation 1993; 88:20–28.

154. Furberg CD, Adams HP, Applegate WB, et al. for the Asymptomatic Carotid Artery progression Study (ACAPS) Research Group. Effects of lovastatin on early carotid atherosclerosis and cardiovascular events. Circulation 1994; 90:1679–1687.

155. Hodis HN, Mack WJ, LaBree L, et al. Reduction in carotid arterial wall thickness using lovastatin and dietary therapy: randomized, controlled clinical trial. Ann Intern Med 1996; 124:548–556.

156. MacMahon S, Sharp N, Gamble G, et al. Effects of lowering average of below-average cholesterol levels on the progression of carotid atherosclerosis: results of the LIPID Atherosclerosis Substudy. LIPID Trial Research Group. Circulation 1998; 97(18):1784–1790.

157. Crouse JR, Byington RP, Bond MA, et al. Pravastatin, Lipids, and Atherosclerosis in the Carotid Arteries (PLAC-II). Am J Cardiol 1995; 75:455–459.

158. Rubins HB, Robins SJ, Collins D, et al. Gemfibrozil for the secondary prevention of coronary heart disease in men with low levels of high-density lipoprotein cholesterol. NEJM 1999; 341:410–418.

159. Coronary Drug Project Group. Clofibrate and niacin in coronary heart disease. JAMA 1975; 231:360–381.

160. Heart Protection Study Collaborative Group. MRC/BHF Heart Protection Study of cholesterol lowering with simvastatin in 20,536 high-risk individuals: a randomized placebo-controlled trial. Lancet 2002; 360:7–22.

161. The SPARCL Investigators. Design and baseline characteristics of Stroke Prevention by Aggressive Reduction in Cholesterol Levels (SPARCL) Study. Cerebrovasc Dis 2003; 16:389–395.

162. Grundy SM, Cleeman JI, Bairey Merz N, et al. Implications of recent clinical trials for the National Cholesterol Education Program Adult Treatment Panel III Guidelines. Circulation 2004; 110:227–239.

163. Kannel WB, Abbott DR, Savage DD, McNamara PM. Epidemiologic features of chronic atrial fibrillation. NEJM 1982; 306:1018–1022.

164. Benjamin EJ, Plehn JF, D'Agostino RB, et al. Mitral annular calcification and the risk of stroke in an elderly cohort. N Engl J Med 1992; 327:374–379.

165. Go AS, Hylek EM, Phillips KA, et al. Prevalence of diagnosed atrial fibrillation in adults: national implications for rhythm management and stroke prevention: the AnTicoagulation and Risk Factors in Atrial Fibrillation (ATRIA) Study. JAMA 2001; 285(18):2370–2375.

166. Sacco RL, Benjamin EJ, Broderick JP, et al. Risk factors. Stroke 1997; 28:1507–1517.

167. Psaty BM, Manolia TA, Kuller LH, et al. Incidence of and risk factors for atrial fibrillation in older adults. Circulation 1997; 96(7):2455–2461.

168. Wolf PA, Abbott RD, Kannel WB. Atrial fibrillation as an independent risk factor for stroke: the Framingham Study. Stroke 1991; 22:983–988.

169. Stroke Prevention in Atrial Fibrillation Study. Circulation 1991; 84:527–539.

170. Hart RG, Halperin JL, Pearce LA, et al. Lessons from the Stroke Prevention in Atrial Fibrillation trials. Ann Intern Med 2003; 138:831–838.

171. Wang TJ, Massaro JM, Levy D, et al. A risk score for predicting stroke or death in individuals with new-onset atrial fibrillation in the community: the Framingham Heart Study. JAMA 2003; 290:1049–1056.

172. Hart RG, Benavente O, McBride R, Pearce LA. Antithrombotic therapy to prevent stroke in patients with atrial fibrillation: a meta-analysis. Ann Intern Med 1999; 131:492–501.

173. van Walraven C, Hart RG, Singer DE, et al. Oral anticoagulants vs aspirin in nonvalvular atrial fibrillation: an individual patient meta-analysis. JAMA 2002; 288(19):2441–2448.

174. EAFT (European Atrial Fibrillation Trial) Study Group. Secondary prevention in non-rheumatic atrial fibrillation after transient ischaemic attack or minor stroke. Lancet 1993; 342(8882):1255–1262.

175. SPIRIT study: a randomized trial of anticoagulants versus aspirin after cerebral ischemia of presumed arterial origin. The Stroke Prevention in Reversible Ischemia Trial (SPIRIT) Study Group. Ann Neurol 1997; 42:857–865.

176. Allessie MA, Boyden PA, Camm AJ, et al. Pathophysiology and prevention of atrial fibrillation. Circulation 2001; 103(5):769–777.

177. Olsson SB; Executive Steering Committee on behalf of the SPORTIF III Investigators. Stroke prevention with the oral direct thrombin inhibitor ximelagatran compared with warfarin in patients with non-valvular atrial fibrillation (SPORTIF III): randomized controlled trial. Lancet 2003; 362:1691–1698.

178. Albers GW, Amarenco P, Easton JD, et al. Antithrombotic and thrombolytic therapy for ischemic stroke: the Seventh ACCP Conference on Antithrombotic and Thrombolytic Therapy. Chest 2004; 126(3 Suppl):483S–512S.

179. Yuan Z, Bowlin S, Einstadter D, et al. Atrial fibrillation as a risk factor for stroke: a retrospective cohort study of hospitalized medicare beneficiaries. Am J Public Health 1998; 88(3):395–400.

180. Pfeffer MA, Braunwald E, Moye LA, et al. Effect of captopril on mortality and morbidity in patients with left ventricular dysfunction after myocardial infarction. Results of the survival and ventricular enlargement trial. The SAVE Investigators. N Engl J Med 1992; 327(10):669–677.
181. Pullicino PM, Halperin JL, Thompson JL. Stroke in patients with heart failure and reduced left ventricular ejection fraction. Neurology 2000; 54:288–294.
182. Cerebral Embolism Task Force. Cardiogenic brain embolism. Arch Neurol 1986; 443:71–84.
183. Salgado AV, Furlan AJ, Keys TF, Nichols TR, Beck GJ. Neurologic complications of endocarditis: a 12 year experience. Neurology 1989; 39:173–178.
184. Benjamin EJ, Levy D, Vaziri SM, et al. Independent risk factors for atrial fibrillation in a population based cohort: the Framingham Heart Study. JAMA 1994; 271:840–844.
185. Salem DM, Stein PD, Al-Ahmad A, et al. The Seventh ACCP Conference on Antithrombotic and Thrombolytic Therapy. Antithrombotic therapy in valvular heart disease—native and prosthetic valves. Chest 2004; 126:457S–482S.
186. Paschalis C, Pugsley W, John R, Harrison MJ. Rate of cerebral embolic events in relation to antibiotic and anticoagulant therapy in patients with bacterial endocarditis. Eur Neurol 1990; 30:87–89.
187. Rogers LR. Cerebrovascular complications in cancer patients. Neurol Clin 2003; 21(1):167–192.
188. Lee AY, Levine MN, Baker RI, et al. Low-molecular-weight heparin versus a coumarin for the prevention of recurrent venous thromboembolism in patients with cancer. N Engl J Med 2003; 349(2):146–153.
189. Hart RG, Easton JD. Mitral valve prolapse and cerebral infarction. Stroke 1982; 13(4):429–430.
190. Avierinos JF, Brown RD, Foley DA, et al. Cerebral ischemic events after diagnosis of mitral valve prolapse. Stroke 2003; 34:1339–1345.
191. Amarenco P, Cohen A, Tzourio C, et al. Atherosclerotic disease of the aortic arch and the risk of ischemic stroke. NEJM 1994; 331:1474–1479.
192. Di Tullio MR, Sacco RL, Savoia MT, et al. Aortic atheroma morphology and the risk of ischemic stroke in a multiethnic population. Am Heart J 2000; 139:329–336.
193. Mitusch R, Doherty C, Wucherpfennig H, et al. Vascular events during follow-up in patients with aortic arch atherosclerosis. Stroke 1997; 28(1):36–39.
194. Davila-Roman VG, Murphy SF, Nickerson NJ, et al. Atherosclerosis of the ascending aorta is an independent predictor of long-term neurologic events and mortality. J Am Coll Cardiol 1999; 33(5):1308–1316.
195. Dressler FA, Craig WR, Castello R, Labovitz AJ. Mobile aortic atheroma and systemic emboli: efficacy of anticoagulation and influence of plaque morphology on recurrent stroke. J Am Coll Cardiol 1998; 31(1):134–138.
196. Ferrari E, Vidal R, Chevallier T, Baudouy M. Atherosclerosis of the thoracic aorta and aortic debris as a marker of poor prognosis: benefit of oral anticoagulants. J Am Coll Cardiol 1999; 33(5):1317–1322.
197. Tunick PA, Nayar AC, Goodkin GM, et al. Effect of treatment on the incidence of stroke and other emboli in 519 patients with severe thoracic aortic plaque. Am J Cardiol 2002; 90(12):1320–1325.
198. Hollier LH, Kazmier FJ, Ochsner J, et al. "Shaggy" aorta syndrome with atheromatous embolization to visceral vessels. Ann Vasc Surg 1991; 5(5):439–444.
199. Powers WJ. Oral anticoagulant therapy for the prevention of stroke. N Engl J Med 2001; 345(20):1493–1495.
200. Di Tullio M, Sacco RL, Gopal A, Mohr JP, Homma S. Patent foramen ovale as a risk factor for cryptogenic stroke. Ann Intern Med 1992; 117:461–465.
201. Overell JR, Bone I, Lees KI. Interatrial septal abnormalities and stroke: a meta-analysis of case-control studies. Neurology 2000; 55(8):1172–1179.
202. Mas J, Arquizan C, Lamy C, et al. Recurrent cerebrovascular events associated with patent foramen ovale, atrial septal aneurysm, or both. N Engl J Med 2001; 345:1740–1746.
203. Homma S, Sacco RL, Di Tullio MR, et al. Effect of medical treatment in stroke patients with patent foramen ovale: patent foramen ovale in Cryptogenic Stroke Study. Circulation 2002; 105:2625–2631.
204. Maisel WH, Laskey WK. Patent foramen ovale closure devices: moving beyond equipoise. JAMA 2005; 294(3):366–369.
205. North American Symptomatic Carotid Endarterectomy Trial Collaborators. Beneficial effect of carotid endarterectomy in symptomatic patients with high-grade stenosis. N Engl J Med 1991; 325:445–453.
206. Norris JW, Zhu CZ, Bornstein NM, Chambers BR. Vascular risks of asymptomatic carotid stenosis. Stroke 1991; 22:1485–1490.
207. Pujia A, Rubba P, Spencer MP. Prevalence of extracranial carotid artery disease detectable by echo-Doppler in an elderly population. Stroke 1992; 23:818–822.
208. ACAS Executive Committee. Endarterectomy for asymptomatic carotid artery stenosis. JAMA 1995; 273:1421–1428.
209. ACST Collaborative Group. Prevention of disabling and fatal strokes by successful carotid endarterectomy in patients without recent neurological symptoms: randomized controlled trial. Lancet 2004; 363:1491–1502.
210. Sacco RL. Risk factors for TIA and TIA as a risk factor for stroke. Neurology 2004; 62:S7–S11.
211. Hankey GJ, Slattery JM, Warlow CP. The prognosis of hospital-referred transient ischaemic attacks. J Neurol Neurosurg Psychiatry 1991; 54:793–802.
212. Johnston SC, Gress DR, Browner WS, Sidney S. Short-term prognosis after emergency department diagnosis of TIA. JAMA 2001; 284:2901–2906.

213. Lovett JK, Dennis MS, Sandercock PA, et al. Short-term prognosis following acute cerebral ischemia. Stroke 2003; 34:e138–e142.
214. Panagos PD, Pancioli AM, Khoury J, et al. Short-term prognosis after emergency department diagnosis and evaluation of transient ischemic attack (TIA). Acad Emerg Med 2003; 10(5):432–433.
215. Hill MD, Yiannakoulias N, Jeerakathil T, et al. The high risk of stroke immediately after transient ischemic attack. Neurology 2004; 62:2015–2020.
216. Benavente O, Eliasziw M, Streifler JY, et al. Prognosis afer transient monocular blindness associated with carotid artery stenosis. N Engl J Med 2001; 345:1084–1090.
217. Johnston SC, Sidney S, Bernstein AL, et al. A comparison of risk factors for recurrent TIA and stroke in patients diagnosed with TIA. Neurology 2003; 60:280–285.
218. Antithrombotic Trialists' Collaboration. Collaborative meta-analysis of randomized trials of antiplatelet therapy for the prevention of death, MI, and stroke in high risk patients. BMJ 2002; 324:71–86.
219. The Dutch TIA Trial Study Group. A comparison of two doses of aspirin (30 mg vs. 283 mg a day) in patients after a transient ischemic attack or minor ischemic stroke. N Engl J Med 1991; 325(18):1261–1266.
220. Farrell B, Godwin J, Richards S, et al. The United Kingdom transient ischaemic attack (UK-TIA) aspirin trial: final results. J Neurol Neurosurg Psychiatry 1991; 54:1044–1054.
221. Algra A, van Gijn J. Aspirin at any dose above 30 mg offers only modest protection after cerebral ischaemia. J Neurol Neurosurg Psychiatry 1996; 60:197–199.
222. CAPRIE Steering Committee. A randomized, blinded, trial of clopidogrel versus aspirin in patients at risk of ischaemic events. Lancet 1996; 348:1329–1339.
223. Hass WK, Easton JD, Adams HP Jr, et al. A randomized trial comparing ticlopidine hydrochloride with aspirin for the prevention of stroke in high-risk patients. Ticlopidine Aspirin Stroke Study Group. N Engl J Med 1989; 321:501–507.
224. Gent M, Blakeley JA, Easton DA. The Canadian American Ticlopidine Study (CATS) in thromboembolic stroke. Lancet 1989; 1:1215–1220.
225. Gorelick PB, Richardson D, Kelly M, et al. Aspirin and ticlopidine for prevention of recurrent stroke in black patients: a randomized trial. JAMA 2003; 289:2947–2957.
226. Diener HC, Cunha L, Forbes C, et al. European Stroke Prevention Study: 2. Dipyridamole and acetylsalicylic acid in the secondary prevention of stroke. J Neurol Sci 1996; 143:1–13.
227. Diener HC, Bogousslavsky J, Brass LM, et al. on behalf of the MATCH investigators. Aspirin and clopidogrel vs clopidogrel alone after recent ischemic stroke or transient ischemic attack in high-risk patients (MATCH): randomised, double-blind, placebo-controlled trial. Lancet 2004; 364:331–337.
228. The Clopidogrel in Unstable Angina to Prevent Recurrent Events Trial Investigators. Effects of clopidogrel in addition to aspirin in patients with acute coronary syndromes without ST-segment elevation. N Engl J Med 2001; 345:494–502.
229. Mohr JP, Thompson JL, Lazar RM, et al. A comparison of warfarin and aspirin for the prevention of recurrent ischemic stroke. N Engl J Med 2001; 345:1444–1451.
230. Chimowitz MI, Kokkinos J, Strong J, et al. The Warfarin-Aspirin Symptomatic Intracranial Disease Study. Neurology 1995; 45:1488–1493.
231. Chimowitz MI, Lynn MJ, Howlett-Smith H, et al. Comparison of warfarin and aspirin for symptomatic intracranial arterial stenosis. N Engl J Med 2005; 352:1305–1316.
232. Algra A, De Schryver ELLM, van Gijn, et al. Oral anticoagulants versus antiplatelet therapy for preventing further vascular events after transient ischemic attack or minor stroke of presumed arterial origin. The Cochrane Library 2004.
233. Barnett HJ, Taylor DW, Eliasziw M, et al. Benefit of carotid endarterectomy in patients with symptomatic moderate or severe stenosis. North American Symptomatic Carotid Endarterectomy Trial Collaborators. N Engl J Med 1998; 339(20):1415–1425.
234. Mayberg MR, Wilson SE, Yatsu F, et al. Veterans Affairs Cooperative Studies Program 309 Trialist Group. Carotid endarterectomy and prevention of cerebral ischemia in symptomatic carotid stenosis. JAMA 1991; 266:3289–3294.
235. European Carotid Surgery Trialists Collaborative Group. MRC European Carotid Surgery Trial: interim results for symptomatic patients with severe (70–99%) or mild (0–29%) carotid stenosis. Lancet 1991; 337:1235–1243.
236. European Carotid Surgery Trialists' Collaborative Group. Randomised trial of endarterectomy for recently symptomatic carotid stenosis: final results of the MRC European Surgery Trial (ECST). Lancet 1998; 351:1379–1387.
237. Rothwell PM, Gutnikov SA, Warlow CP. Reanalysis of the final results of the European Carotid Surgery Trial. Stroke 2003; 34:514–523.
238. Rothwell PM, Eliasziw M, Gutnikov SA, et al. Analysis of pooled data from the randomised controlled trials of endarterectomy for symptomatic carotid stenosis. Lancet 2003; 361(9352):107–116.
239. Gasecki AP, Eliasziw M, Ferguson GG, et al. Long-term prognosis and effect of endarterectomy in patients with symptomatic severe carotid stenosis and contralateral carotid stenosis or occlusion: results from NASCET. J Neurosurg 1995; 83:778–782.
240. Inzitari D, Eliasziw M, Sharpe BL, et al. Risk factors and outcome of patients with carotid artery stenosis presenting with lacunar stroke. North American Symptomatic Carotid Endarterectomy Trial Group. Neurology 2000; 54:660–666.
241. Chassin MR. Appropriate use of carotid endarterectomy. NEJM 1998; 339:1441–1471.

242. Ferguson GG, Eliasziw M, Barr HW, et al. The North American Symptomatic Carotid Endarterectomy Trial: surgical results in 1415 patients. Stroke 1999; 30(9):1751–1758.
243. Henderson RD, Eliasziw M, Fox AJ, et al. Angiographically defined collateral circulation and risk of stroke in patients with severe carotid artery stenosis. North American Symptomatic Carotid Endarterectomy Trial (NASCET) Group. Stroke 2000; 3(1):128–132.
244. Rothwell PM, Eliasziw M, Gutnikov SA, et al. Endarterectomy for symptomatic carotid stenosis in relation to clinical subgroups and timing of surgery. Lancet 2004; 363(9413):915–924.
245. Endovascular versus surgical treatment in patients with carotid stenosis in the Carotid and Vertebral Artery Transluminal Angioplasty Study (CAVATAS): a randomized trial. Lancet 2001; 357:1729–1737.
246. Yadav JS, Wholey MH, Kuntz RE, et al. Protected carotid-artery stenting versus endarterectomy in high-risk patients. N Engl J Med 2004; 351:1493–1501.
247. Berger R, Flynn LM, Kline RA, Caplan L. Surgical reconstruction of the extracranial vertebral artery: management and outcome. J Vasc Surg 2000; 31:9–18.
248. Coward LJ, Watt H, Featherstone RL, et al. Endovascular versus medical treatment in patients with vertebral artery stenosis in the Carotid and Vertebral Artery Transluminal Angioplasty Study (CAVATAS): a randomised trial. European Stroke Conference 2004.
249. Flossmann E, Rothwell PM. Prognosis of vertebrobasilar transient ischaemic attack and minor stroke. Brain 2003; 126:1940–1954.
250. Thijs VN, Albers GW. Symptomatic intracranial atherosclerosis: outcome of patients who fail antithrombotic therapy. Neurology 2000; 55:490–497.
251. Alazzaz A, Thornton J, Aletich VA, et al. Intracranial percutaneous transluminal angioplasty for atherosclerotic stenosis. Arch Neurol 2000; 57:1625–1630.
252. McKenzie JD, Wallace RC, Dean BL, et al. Preliminary results of intracranial angioplasty for vascular stenosis caused by atherosclerosis and vasculitis. AJNR 1996; 82:953–960.
253. Takis C, Kwan ES, Pessin MS, et al. Intracranial angioplasty: experience and complications. AJNR 1997; 18:1661–1668.
254. Levy EI, Hanel RA, Bendok BR, et al. Staged stent-assisted angioplasty for symptomatic intracranial vertebrobasilar artery stenosis. J Neurosurg 2002; 97:1294–1301.
255. De Rochemont, Rdu M, Turowski B, et al. Recurrent symptomatic high-grade intracranial stenoses: safety and efficacy of undersized stents—initial experience. Radiology 2004; 231(1):45–49.
256. SSYLVIA Study Investigators. Stenting of Symptomatic Atherosclerotic Lesions in the Vertebral or Intracranial Arteries (SSYLVIA): study results. Stroke 2004; 35:1388–1392.
257. Gupta R, Schumacher HC, Mangla S, et al. Urgent endovascular revascularization for symptomatic intracranial atherosclerotic stenosis. Neurology 2003; 61:1729–1735.
258. The EC/IC Bypass Study Group. Failure of extracranial-intracranial arterial bypass to reduce the risk of ischemic stroke: results of an international randomized trial. NEJM 1985; 313:1191–1200.
259. Sacco RL. NEJM 2001.
260. Brott TG, Brown RD, Meyer FB, et al. Carotid revascularization for prevention of stroke: carotid endarterectomy and carotid artery stenting. Mayo Clin Proc 2004; 79:1197–1208.
261. Duan J, Murohara T, Ikeda H, et al. Hyperhomocysteinemia impairs angiogenesis in response to hindlimb ischemia. Arterioscler Thromb Vasc Biol 2000; 20(12):2579–2585.
262. Clarke R, Daly L, Robinson K, et al. Hyperhomocysteinemia: an independent risk factor for vascular disease. N Engl J Med 1991; 324(17):1149–1155.
263. Boushey CJ, Beresford SA, Omenn GS, Motulsky AG. A quantitative assessment of plasma homocysteine as a risk factor for vascular disease. Probable benefits of increasing folic acid intakes. JAMA 1995; 274:1049–1057.
264. Bostom AG, Rosenberg IH, Sibershatz H, et al. Nonfasting plasma homocysteine levels and stroke incidence in elderly persons: the Framingham Study. Ann Intern Med 1999; 131:352–355.
265. Pery IJ, Refsum H, Morris RW, et al. Prospective study of serum total homocysteine concentration and risk of stroke in middle aged British men. Lancet 1995; 346:1395–1398.
266. Sacco RL, Anand K, Lee HS, et al. Homocysteine and the risk of ischemic stroke in a triethnic cohort: the Northern Manhattan Study. Stroke 2004; 35:2263–2269.
267. Homocysteine Studies Collaboration. Homocysteine and the risk of ischemic heart disease and stroke: a meta analysis. JAMA 2002; 288:2015–2022.
268. Selhub J, Jacques PF, Wilson PW, et al. Vitamin status and intake as primary determinants of homocysteinemia in an elderly population. JAMA 1993; 270(22):2693–2698.
269. Homocysteine Lowering Trialists' Collaboration. Lowering blood homocysteine with folic acid based supplements: meta-analysis of randomized trials. BMJ 1998; 316:894–898.
270. Toole JF, Malinow MR, Chambless LE, et al. Lowering homocysteine in patients with ischemic stroke to prevent recurrent stroke, myocardial infarction, and death: the Vitamin Intervention for Stroke Prevention (VISP) randomized controlled trial. JAMA 2004; 291:565–575.
271. The VITATOPS Trial Study Group. The VITATOPS (vitamins to prevent stroke) Trial: rationale and design of an international, large, simple, randomised trial of homocysteine-lowering multivitamin therapy in patients with recent transient ischaemic attack or stroke. Cerebrovasc Dis 2002; 13:120–126.
272. Dusitanond P, Eikelboom JW, Hankey GJ, et al. Homocysteine-lowering treatment with folic acid, cobalamin, and pyridoxine does not reduce blood markers of inflammation, endothelial dysfunction,

or hypercoagulability in patients with previous transient ischemic attack or stroke: a randomized substudy of the VITATOPS trial. Stroke 2005; 36:144–146.

273. Wassertheil-Smoller S, Hendrix SL, Limacher M, et al. Effect of estrogen plus progestin on stroke in postmenopausal women. The women's health initiative: a randomized trial. JAMA 2003; 289:2673–2684.

274. Viscoli CM, Brass LM, Kernan WN, et al. A clinical trial of estrogen-replacement therapy after ischemic stroke. N Engl J Med 2001; 345:1243–1249.

275. Petitti DB, Sidney S, Bernstein A, et al. Stroke in users of low-dose oral contraceptives. N Engl J Med 1996; 335:8–15.

276. Gillum LA, Mamidipudi SK, Johnston SC. Ischemic stroke risk with oral contraceptives: a meta-analysis. JAMA 2000; 284:72–78.

277. Elkind MS, Lin IF, Grayston JT, Sacco RL. Chlamydia pneumoniae and the risk of first ischemic stroke: the Norterhn Manhattan Stroke Study. Stroke 2000; 31:1521–1525.

278. Elkind MS, Cheng J, Boden-Albala B, et al. Elevated white blood cell count and carotid plaque thickness: the Northern Manhattan Stroke Study. Stroke 2001; 32(4):842–849.

279. Grau AJ, Boddy AW, Dukovic DA, et al. Leukocyte count as an independent predictor of recurrent ischemic events. Stroke 2004; 35(5):1147–1152.

280. Lindsberg PJ, Grau AJ. Inflammation and infections as risk factors for ischemic stroke. Stroke 2003; 34(10):2518–2532.

281. Ridker PM, Hennekens CH, Buring JE, Rifai N. C-reactive protein and other markers of inflammation in the prediction of cardiovascular disease in women. N Eng J Med 2000; 342:836–843.

282. Rost NS, Wolf PA, Kase CS, et al. Plasma concentration of C-reactive protein and risk of ischemic stroke and transient ischemic attack: the Framingham study. Stroke 2001; 32(11):2575–2579.

283. Ridker PM, Cushman M, Stampfer MJ, Tracy RP, Hennekens CH. Inflammation, aspirin, and the risk of cardiovascular disease in apparently healthy men. N Engl J Med 1997; 336:973–979.

284. Brown LJ, Brunelle JA, Kingman A. Periodontal status in the United States, 1988–1991: prevalence, extent, and demographic variation. J Dent Res 1996; 75:672–683.

285. Wu T, Trevisan M, Genco RJ, et al. Periodontal disease and risk of cerebrovascular disease: the first national health and nutrition examination survey and its follow-up study. Arch Intern Med 2000; 160(18):2749–2755.

286. Chiu B. Multiple infections in carotid atherosclerotic plaques. Am Heart J 1999; 138:S534–S536.

287. Desvarieux M, Demmer RT, Rundek T, et al. Periodontal microbiota and carotid intima-media thickness: the Oral Infections and Vascular Disease Epidemiology Study (INVEST). Circulation 2005; 111(5):576–582.

288. Lakka HM, Laaksonen DE, Lakka TA, et al. The metabolic syndrome and total and cardiovascular disease mortality in middle-aged men. JAMA 2002; 288(21):2709–2716.

289. Bonora E, Kiechl S, Willeit J, et al. Carotid atherosclerosis and coronary heart disease in the metabolic syndrome: prospective data from the Bruneck study. Diabetes Care 2003; 26(4):1251–1257.

290. Ninomiya JK, L'Italien G, Criqui MH, et al. Association of the metabolic syndrome with history of myocardial infarction and stroke in the Third National Health and Nutrition Examination Survey. Circulation 2004; 109(1):42–46.

291. McNeil AM, Rosamond WD, Girman CJ, et al. The metabolic syndrome and 11-year risk of incident cardiovascular disease in the atherosclerosis risk in communities study. Diabetes Care 2005; 28(2):385–390.

292. Koren-Morag N, Goldbourt U, Tanne D. Relation between the metabolic syndrome and ischemic stroke or transient ischemic attack: a prospective cohort study in patients with atherosclerotic cardiovascular disease. Stroke 2005; 36(7):1366–1371.

293. McNeil AM, Rosamond WD, Girman CJ, et al. Prevalence of coronary heart disease and carotid arterial thickening in patients with the metabolic syndrome (the ARIC Study). Am J Cardiol 2004; 94(10):1249–1254.

294. Gorter PM, Olijhoek JK, van der Graaf, et al. Prevalence of the metabolic syndrome in patients with coronary heart disease, cerebrovascular disease, peripheral arterial disease or abdominal aortic aneurysm. Atherosclerosis 2004; 173(2):363–369.

295. Bots ML, Hoes AW, Koudstaal PJ, et al. Common carotid intima-media thickness and risk of stroke and myocardial infarction: the Rotterdam Study. Circulation 1997; 96(5):1432–1437.

296. O'Leary DH, Polak JF, Knonmal RA, et al. Carotid-artery intima and media thickness as a risk factor for myocardial infarction and stroke in older adults. Cardiovascular Health Study Collaborative Research Group. N Engl J Med 1999; 340(1):14–22.

297. Ebrahim S, Papacosta O, Whincup P, et al. Carotid plaque, intima media thickness, cardiovascular risk factors, and prevalent cardiovascular disease in men and women: the British Regional Heart Study. Stroke 1999; 30(4):841–850.

298. Chambless LE, Folsom AR, Clegg LX, et al. Carotid wall thickness is predictive of incident clinical stroke: the Atherosclerosis Risk in Communities (ARIC) study. Am J Epidemiol 2000; 151(5):478–487.

299. Rosvall M, Janzon L, Berglund G, et al. Incidence of stroke is related to carotid IMT even in the absence of plaque. Atherosclerosis 2005; 179(2):325–331.

300. del Sol AI, Moon KG, Hollander M, et al. Is carotid intima-media thickness useful in cardiovascular disease risk assessment? The Rotterdam Study. Stroke 2001; 32(7):1532–1538.

301. Vermeer SE, Koudstaal PJ, Oudkerk M, et al. Prevalence and risk factors of silent brain infarcts in the population-based Rotterdam Scan Study. Stroke 2002; 33(1):21–25.
302. Longstreth WT Jr, Bernick C, Manolio TA, et al. Lacunar infarcts defined by magnetic resonance imaging of 3660 elderly people: the Cardiovascular Health Study. Arch Neurol 1998; 55(9):1217–1225.
303. Vermeer SE, Hollander M, van Dijk EJ, et al. Silent brain infarcts and white matter lesions increase stroke risk in the general population: the Rotterdam Scan Study. Stroke 2003; 34(5):1126–1129.
304. Kobayashi S, Okada K, Koide H, et al. Subcortical silent brain infarction as a risk factor for clinical stroke. Stroke 1997; 28(10):1932–1939.
305. Bernick C, Kuller L, Dulberg C, et al. Silent MRI infarcts and the risk of future stroke: the cardiovascular health study. Neurology 2001; 57(7):1222–1229.
306. Tarvonen-Schroder S, Kurki T, Raiha I, Sourander L. Leukoaraiosis and cause of death: a five year follow-up. JNNP 1995; 58:586–589.
307. Kuller LH, Longstreth WT Jr, Arnold AM, et al. White matter hyperintensity on cranial magnetic resonance imaging: a predictor of stroke. Stroke 2004; 35(8):1821–1825.
308. Miyao S, Takano A, Teramoto J, Takahashi A. Leukoaraiosis in relation to prognosis for patients with lacunar infarction. Stroke 1992; 23(10):1434–1438.
309. Inzitari D, DiCarlo A, Mascalchi M, et al. The cardiovascular outcome of patients with motor impairment and extensive leukoaraiosis. Arch Neurol 1995; 52(7):687–691.
310. Inzitari D. Leukoaraiosis: an independent risk factor for stroke? Stroke 2003; 34(8):2067–2071.
311. Gorelick PB. Stroke prevention: windows of opportunity and failed expectations? A discussion of modifiable cardiovascular risk factors and a prevention proposal. Neuroepidemiology 1997; 16(4):163–173.

17 | Peripheral Arterial Disease

Stanley G. Rockson and Emil M. deGoma
Division of Cardiovascular Medicine, Stanford University School of Medicine, Stanford, California, U.S.A.

KEY POINTS

- Screening for peripheral arterial disease (PAD) should be conducted in all patients with suggestive symptoms, physical findings, preexisting atherosclerotic disease in another vascular territory, or risk factors, such as age >70 years, tobacco use, or diabetes.
- The initial, cost-effective test of choice is the ankle-brachial index (ABI). If revascularization is planned, imaging is recommended to further characterize stenoses.
- Management of global atherothrombotic disease is paramount in the treatment of PAD patients. Risk factor optimization involves permanent smoking cessation, antihypertensive therapy with goal blood pressures below 130/85, lipid lowering with statins to achieve an low-density lipoprotein (LDL)-cholesterol below 70 to 100 mg/dL, and glucose control to maintain a HbA1c below 7%. All PAD patients should receive lifelong antiplatelet therapy, with aspirin 75 to 325 mg daily as first-line therapy or, and when contraindicated, clopidogrel 75 mg daily.
- For symptomatic PAD patients, medical management should be attempted first with exercise rehabilitation and, if desired, cilostazol 100 mg twice daily in the absence of contraindications.
- Revascularization through surgical or endovascular procedures can be employed in selected cases of refractory claudication.

INTRODUCTION

Peripheral arterial disease (PAD) represents a critical, but often overlooked, manifestation of atherosclerosis, a surrogate marker for plaque progression in the vital coronary and cerebral vasculature. Inclusive anatomic definitions of PAD encompass numerous vascular territories, namely carotid, renal, mesenteric, and extremity arteries as well as the aorta. The following discussion focuses on the clinical presentation, evaluation, and management of lower limb arterial disease.

EPIDEMIOLOGY

Based on current epidemiologic projections, approximately 27 million people in Europe and North America have PAD (1), with the United States comprising an estimated 8 to 12 million people (Fig. 1) (2,3). Prevalence increases dramatically with age. PAD affects 12% to 20% of U.S. residents age 65 and older, or an estimated four to eight million people (5). With the aging of the population, by 2050, the U.S.A prevalence may exceed 15 million among those over the age of 65 and 19 million overall (5). Analysis of the Asian continent reveals similar prevalence statistics (6,7).

PAD shares the same risk factors as other atherosclerotic diseases such as coronary artery disease (CAD), namely, old age, diabetes mellitus, smoking, hypertension, and hyperlipidemia (Fig. 2) (8–10). Tobacco use and diabetes confer the highest risk of PAD with odds ratios of two to three. Blacks represent the highest risk ethnic group, exhibiting three times the prevalence of PAD compared to non-Hispanic whites (11). Epidemiologic data supports the growing importance of prothrombotic measures and inflammatory markers. Elevated serum levels of lipoprotein a (12), homocysteine (13,14), fibrinogen (15,16), and C-reactive protein have been associated with the development of PAD (17,18).

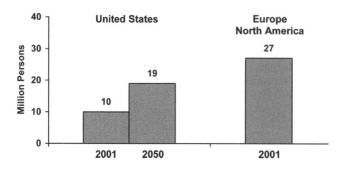

FIGURE 1 Prevalence of peripheral arterial disease. *Source*: From Refs. 1, 2, 4.

PROGNOSTIC SIGNIFICANCE

While PAD itself can lead to debilitating claudication and, rarely, life-threatening limb ischemia (9,19), the burden of disease arises not from peripheral pathology but from coexistent CAD and cerebrovascular disease (CVD). Analysis of patients in a long-term health care facility 62 years and older demonstrated that 58% of the patients with symptomatic PAD had evidence of CAD by history or ECG, and 34% had evidence of CVD by examination or imaging (20). Similarly, a large, multicenter trial revealed that 56% of the patients with PAD documented by ankle-brachial index (ABI) or prior revascularization also had a history of atherosclerotic coronary, cerebral, or aortic aneurysmal disease (3). Pooling together available evidence, approximately 60% of the patients with PAD have significant CAD, CVD, or both (Fig. 3).

Coexisting CAD and CVD result in significantly increased mortality among PAD patients. The San Diego Artery Study, a 10-year prospective investigation, followed patients with PAD identified through segmental blood pressure analysis and Doppler ultrasonography. The study demonstrated that PAD conferred threefold increase in risk of all-cause mortality, a sixfold increase in the risk of death from cardiovascular disease, and a sevenfold increase in the risk of death from CAD (Fig. 4) (2). Among subjects with severe, symptomatic PAD, mortality from CVD increased 15-fold. Subgroup analysis of the Systolic Hypertension in the Elderly Program showed that the incidence of CVD morbidity and mortality was three times higher in men and women with PAD diagnosed by ABI when followed over a one- to two-year period (21). Even when clinically silent, PAD exacts a striking toll. Subjects enrolled with asymptomatic large-vessel PAD in the San Diego Artery Study, experienced significantly higher rates of all-cause mortality compared to normal subjects (Fig. 5) (2). In absolute terms, individuals with PAD share the same risk of CAD mortality as patients with a history of myocardial infarction exceeding 20% over a 10-year period. The Multicenter Study of Osteoporotic Fractures demonstrated an annual CAD mortality rate of

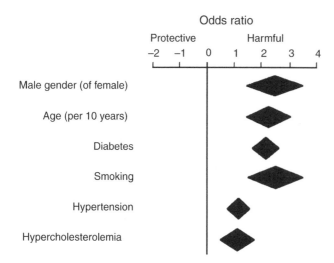

FIGURE 2 Risk factors for peripheral arterial disease. *Source*: From Ref. 9.

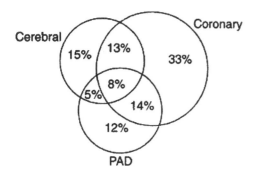

FIGURE 3 Coexistent coronary artery disease and cerebrovascular disease. *Abbreviation*: PAD, peripheral arterial disease. *Source*: From Ref. 38.

2.9% among women diagnosed with PAD without a prior history of CAD (23). In the San Diego Artery Study, men with PAD without a prior history of CAD had a CAD mortality outcome per year of 2.5% (2). As a result, the National Cholesterol Education Panel deemed PAD a CAD-risk equivalent in the Adult Treatment Panel III (ATP III) guidelines published in 2002 (24).

PATHOPHYSIOLOGY

Atherothrombosis, the same pathophysiologic process that contributes to the progression of CAD and CVD, gives rise to PAD. Confluence of lipid-laden macrophages or foam cells in the intimal layer of the endothelium gives rise to fatty streaks. Subsequent evolution into a fatty plaque results from continued cholesterol deposition, migration and proliferation of smooth muscle cells, and production of a fibrous cap from extracellular connective tissue. As with disease in other arterial territories, peripheral atheromata limit flow and perturb the balance of oxygen supply and demand. Moderate stenoses manifest an oxygen deficit with exertion, resulting in claudication when increased oxygen consumption exceeds distal delivery. With severe stenoses, an oxygen deficit may exist even in the absence of activity, engendering symptoms at rest. The most catastrophic presentation of PAD arises from plaque rupture. Degradation of the fibrous cap exposes thrombogenic factors, inducing platelet plug formation and activating the coagulation cascade, leading to sudden total occlusion and complete absence of distal flow. Unless urgent measures are undertaken to lyse or bypass the thrombus, critical limb ischemia followed by infarction is the consequence. Within the lower extremity, the superficial femoral artery, at the level of the adductor canal, represents the most frequent site of hemodynamically significant stenosis, followed by the popliteal and iliac arteries (25,26).

CLINICAL MANIFESTATIONS
Symptomatology

Claudication represents the sympotmatic manifestation of PAD arising as a consequence of oxygen imbalance in the lower limbs. As defined by the World Health Organization/Rose Questionnaire, classic claudication can be characterized as leg pain that occurs in one or both

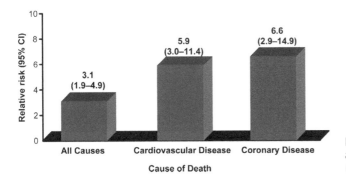

FIGURE 4 Increased risk of coronary artery disease and cerebrovascular disease–related mortality. *Source*: From Ref. 2.

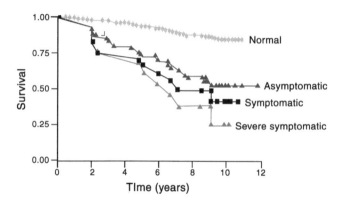

FIGURE 5 Kaplan–Meier survival curves based on mortality from all causes among normal subjects and subjects with peripheral arterial disease. *Source*: From Refs. 2, 22.

calves, present during walking but absent at rest. This discomfort prompts cessation or slowing of activity, and resolves after resting for 10 minutes or less (Table 1) (27). As in myocardial ischemia where 30% of the patients lack typical complaints of substernal chest pressure (29), patients with PAD rarely fulfill all of the Rose criteria.

In a large population of subjects with the aggregate risk factors of age, smoking, or diabetes, only 6% of those who manifest PAD (defined by the ABI) experienced classic intermittent claudication (3). This estimate is consistent with other analyses (30). Forty-six percent of the PAD subjects presented an atypical constellation of symptoms, while the remaining 48% were entirely asymptomatic (3,4,31,32). The low sensitivity of typical claudication symptoms for the detection of clinically significant PAD was similarly demonstrated in a survey of 50 patients with PAD in the Systolic Hypertension in the Elderly Program (33).

As might be inferred from the derivation of claudication from the Latin *claudicatio*, "to limp," this symptom presentation deserves consideration as a spectrum of symptoms not simply limited to calf pain. Firstly, discomfort occurs at sites other than the gastrocnemius and soleus. Aortoiliac disease, for example, may give rise to pain in the buttocks and thighs. In addition, patients may experience symptoms other than muscle pain; some report leg stiffness, others arthalgias or limb weakness (34). One study of 163 patients with PAD identified by ABI identified older age, diabetes mellitus, and male gender as risk factors for atypical presentation (35). More research is needed to appropriately expand the definition of claudication and incorporate common nonclassic symptoms to increase the predictive value of clinical history.

Physical Examination

Inspection and palpation of the lower extremities can yield important clues to the presence of PAD (Table 2) (36). The absence of both the pedal pulses in a single extremity suggests the

TABLE 1 World Health Organization/Rose Questionnaire

a. Do you get pain in either leg upon walking?	Y	N	
b. Does this pain ever begin when you are standing still or sitting?	Y	N	
c. Do you get this pain in your calf (or calves)?	Y	N	
d. Do you get it when you walk uphill or hurry?	Y	N	
e. Do you get it when you walk at an ordinary pace on the level?	Y	N	
f. Does the pain ever disappear while you are still walking?	Y	N	
g. What do you do if you get it when you are walking?	A Stop	B Slow down	C Continue at the same pace
h. What happens to it if you stand still?	A Usually continues for more than 10 min		B Usually disappears in 10 min or lesser

Intermittent claudication: "Yes" to a, "no" to b, "yes" to c and d, e is intentional, "no" to f, "stop" or "slow down" to g, and "usually disappears in 10 min or lesser" to h.
Source: From Ref. 28.

TABLE 2 Physical Examination Findings in Peripheral Arterial Disease

Sign	Se (%)	Sp (%)	LR+	LR−
Absent pedal pulses	63–72	92–99	14.9	0.3
Absent femoral pulse	7	99	6.1	NS
Limb bruit	20–50	95–99	7.3	0.7
Asymmetric limb coolness	10	98	6.1	0.9
Wounds or sores	2	100	7.0	NS
Atrophic skin	50	70	1.7	NS
Hairless lower limb	48	71	1.7	NS
Prolonged capillary refill	28	85	1.9	NS

Abbreviations: Se, sensitivity; Sp, specificity; LR+, positive likelihood ratio; LR−, negative likelihood ratio; NS, not significant.
Source: From Ref. 36.

presence of PAD with a specificity of 92% to 99% and a positive likelihood ratio of 15. Importantly, the absence of either the dorsalis pedis or the posterior tibial pulse alone is not indicative of disease as up to 10% to 14% of healthy individuals have an isolated nonpalpable pedal pulse. Other signs suggestive of PAD include an absent femoral pulse, the presence of a bruit, asymmetric coolness, and wounds or sores on the foot. The only finding that has argue-ments against PAD is the presence of one or both pedal pulses, with a likelihood ratio of 0.3; however, studies indicate that up to one in three patients with PAD has at least one palpable pedal pulse. Signs with little discriminatory power include atrophic skin, hairless lower limbs, and a prolonged capillary refill time. Overall, the utility of the physical examination is limited by the low sensitivity of physical findings.

CLINICAL CLASSIFICATION

Clinical severity can be graded using either the Rutherford or Fontaine classification systems (Table 3). Rutherford Category 0 represents asymptomatic disease. Categories 1, 2, and 3 indi-cate mild, moderate, and severe claudication, respectively. Those with ischemic rest pain are designated as Category 4. Finally, Categories 5 and 6 represent minor or major tissue loss from ulcers and gangrene (37).

DIAGNOSTIC EVALUATION
Ankle-Brachial Index

Simple to perform and of high yield, the ABI, a bedside approximation of the ratio of perfusion pressures in lower: upper extremities, is the primary screening test for PAD (Fig. 6). With the patient lying supine, a handheld Doppler probe is used to measure systolic pressures in the brachial, posterior tibial, and dorsalis pedis arteries. Dividing the greater of the ankle systolic pressures by the greater of two systolic brachial pressures yields the index. The threshold ABI for the diagnosis of PAD is 0.9. Patients experiencing claudication symptoms typically have

TABLE 3 Rutherford and Fontaine Classification of Peripheral Arterial Disease

Rutherford		Fontaine	
Grade	Category	Stage	Description
0	0	I	Asymptomatic
I	1	II	Mild claudication
	2		Moderate claudication
	3		Severe claudication
II	4	III	Rest pain
III	5	IV	Minor tissue loss
	6		Major tissue loss

Source: From Refs. 37, 38.

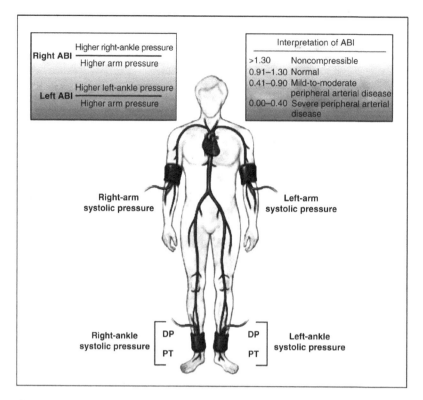

Right ABI $\dfrac{\text{Higher right-ankle pressure}}{\text{Higher arm pressure}}$

Left ABI $\dfrac{\text{Higher left-ankle pressure}}{\text{Higher arm pressure}}$

Interpretation of ABI

>1.30	Noncompressible
0.91–1.30	Normal
0.41–0.90	Mild-to-moderate peripheral arterial disease
0.00–0.40	Severe peripheral arterial disease

Right-arm systolic pressure

Left-arm systolic pressure

Right-ankle systolic pressure   DP   PT

DP   PT   Left-ankle systolic pressure

FIGURE 6   Ankle-brachial index (ABI). *Source*: From Ref. 39.

ABI values ranging from 0.41 to 0.90, and those with critical leg ischemia have values of 0.40 or less (39). A resting value less than 0.9 has a sensitivity of 95% and a specificity of 100% for the presence of angiographic disease, defined as at least one stenosis greater than or equal to 50% within a major lower limb artery (40). Lower extremity exercise using treadmill protocols or repeated active pedal plantar flexion reduces ankle systolic pressures in individuals with PAD, thereby increasing test sensitivity (41).

The utility of the ABI lies not only as a cutoff for detection of PAD but also as a reliable prognostic indicator. Analysis of 744 patients who had undergone testing for PAD demonstrated that subjects with ABI values between 0.4 and 0.85 carried a relative risk of mortality of 2.0 compared to those with ABI values above 0.85, while patients with ABI values less than 0.4 suffered an even higher relative risk of mortality of 3.4 (42).

Despite having excellent overall test characteristics, important limitations to the ABI exist. In two circumstances most frequently encountered in the diabetic population, the ABI may yield false negatives. Noncompressible calcified tibial and peroneal arteries elevate measured ankle systolic pressures, resulting in spurious normal-to-elevated ABI values despite the possible coexistence of significant atherosclerosis. Brachial pressures obtained in patients with subclavian artery stenosis underestimate true central systolic pressures, inappropriately lowering the internal reference to which lower extremity pressures are compared; as a result, the calculated ABI may conceal existing vascular disease. In these cases, evaluation of PAD requires noninvasive imaging or angiography (1).

Segmental Blood Pressure Measurement and Volume Plethysmography

Once the diagnosis of PAD has been established using ABI measurements at rest or following exercise, segmental pressure and volume recordings can be evaluated in the vascular laboratory to further characterize the location and severity of stenoses (Fig. 7). These two noninvasive modalities used in combination achieve 95% accuracy as compared with the gold standard, angiography (1,9).

(A)

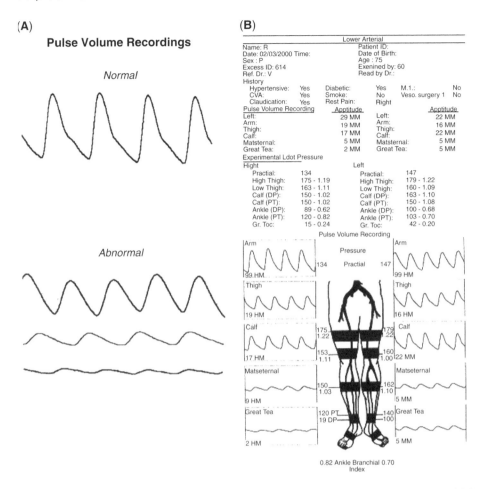

FIGURE 7 (**A**) Pulse volume waveforms. (**B**) Volume plethysmography demonstrating bilateral infrapopliteal disease. *Source*: From Ref. 38.

Analysis of segmental lower limb pressures involves the measurement of systolic blood pressures at the proximal and distal thigh, calf, ankle, transmetatarsal region of the foot, and toe using a Doppler probe placed over the appropriate arterial vessel. A drop in pressure between two contiguous segments exceeding 30 mmHg suggests significant proximal disease. For example, a decrease in systolic pressure at the distal thigh reflects superficial femoral artery disease, while a drop in pressure at the calf signifies popliteal disease. Comparison of the left and right limb at the same level also yields important information. Asymmetric systolic pressures with discrepancies greater than 20 to 30 mmHg indicate arterial occlusive disease proximal to the site with the lower pressure (43).

Segmental volume plethysmography utilizes a series of pneumatic cuffs placed along the leg to measure volume changes induced by the propagating pulse. Pressure transducers translate alterations in cuff size to generate waveforms for different segments of each lower extremity (1,43). The normal pulse volume contour consists of a sharp systolic peak followed by a downstroke with a prominent dicrotic notch. Mild arterial disease proximal to the measured site results in obliteration of the dicrotic notch, and more significant occlusion progressively diminishes pulse amplitude.

Doppler Ultrasonography

Ultrasound provides sensitive (92%) and specific (97%) detection of PAD and elucidates the morphology and hemodynamic consequences of arterial lesions (44). B-mode provides topographic information useful for characterizing native arteries, bypass grafts, and stented vessels (45). Doppler sonography yields functional data in the form of blood velocities. PAD manifests as increased peak systolic velocities and abnormal velocity waveforms (46). Vessels free of disease present a triphasic velocity waveform due to initial forward flow in systole, reversal of flow in early diastole, and resumption of forward flow in late diastole (47,48). Absent reverse flow indicates mild arterial occlusion, while a dampened systolic flow signal signifies advanced disease (49).

Magnetic Resonance Angiography

Magnetic resonance angiography (MRA) has emerged as the imaging modality-of-choice to visualize arterial occlusions and to identify potential bypass targets prior to revascularization (50,51). Contrast-enhanced MRA using gadolinium achieves a sensitivity of 98% and a specificity of 96% for detecting stenoses exceeding 50% (52,53). This high degree of accuracy permits safe and cost-effective surgical planning on the basis of MRA alone, without preoperative invasive angiography (54–56).

Computed Tomographic Angiography

Suboptimal resolution of small diameter vessels and the need for nephrotoxic contrast agents limit the utility of computed tomographic angiography (CTA) for routine evaluation of PAD, most frequently, to patients with contraindications to MRA (46,57). Wider availability of scanners, the ability to visualize calification, and the ability to image patients with pacemakers and other metallic implants represent the few advantages of CTA (46,57).

Angiography

Although the last decade has witnessed significant advancements in noninvasive imaging, angiography remains the gold standard for evaluation of PAD. Catheterization yields the highest resolution images and permits direct measurement of pressure gradients across stenoses, providing insight into their physiologic significance (46). For lesions amenable to percutaneous intervention, angiography serves as the platform for angioplasty and stent deployment.

Summary

Screening for PAD should be conducted in all patients with suggestive symptoms, physical findings, preexisting atherosclerotic disease in another vascular territory, or risk factors such as old age, smoking, or diabetes (Fig. 8) (39). The initial, cost-effective test of choice is the ABI. An ABI less than 0.9 establishes the diagnosis of PAD. If the ABI exceeds 1.3, suggesting noncompressible calcified infrapopliteal arteries, further studies are required to determine the presence or absence of PAD. For high-risk patients with resting values within the normal range, exercise testing is recommended to increase the sensitivity of the ABI. Repeated active plantar flexion or treadmill testing lowers ankle systolic pressures and may elicit an abnormal ABI. Finally, once the diagnosis of PAD has been established, imaging is recommended to further characterize stenoses if revascularization is planned.

MANAGEMENT OF ATHEROTHROMBOTIC DISEASE

Antiplatelet therapy and aggressive risk factor reduction form the cornerstones of PAD management, improving survival and decreasing the incidence of myocardial infarction and cerebrovascular events.

Antiplatelet Therapy

Considerable data support the use of antiplatelet agents as one of the component, pivotal therapies to decrease morbidity and mortality in patients with PAD (Table 4). To date, two landmark meta-analyses have examined the effects of platelet inhibition on serious vascular events, defined as heart attack, stroke, or vascular-related death. The Antiplatelet Trialists' Collaborative project examined 42 trials conducted between 1990 and September 1997, with enrollment of a total of 9214 patients with PAD (58). The meta-analysis conducted by Robless reviewed 24 trials conducted between 1966 and January 1999 enrolling 6036 PAD patients (61). Both studies demonstrated that compared to placebo, antiplatelet therapy reduced the relative risk of

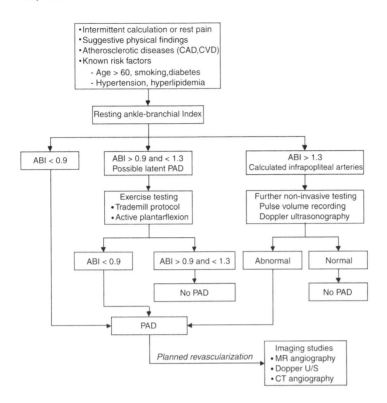

FIGURE 8   Algorithm for evaluation of peripheral arterial disease. *Source*: From Ref. 39.

serious vascular events by 22% to 23% and the absolute risk by 1.3% to 1.6%, yielding a number needed to treat of 63–77.

Antiplatelet agents exert their effects through numerous mechanisms, thus reflecting the complex interaction between platelets, the coagulation cascade, and the vessel wall. Clearly, inhibition of platelet aggregation, the final, catastrophic event in atherothrombotic disease, represents one mode of action. Evidence suggests that antiplatelet agents improve cardiovascular outcomes by modifying earlier atherosclerotic processes, as well (62–65). In one mouse model of premature atherosclerosis, platelet adhesion preceded the development of manifest atheroma and prolonged blockade of platelet adhesion attenuated plaque formation in multiple vascular territories (66). In another study, administration of activated platelets promoted monocyte arrest on plaque surfaces and increased the size of atherosclerotic lesions (67). Mechanisms for platelet-mediated atherogenesis include platelet granule release of vascular and leukocyte mitogens and chemokines such as platelet factor 4, induction of chemoattractant synthesis and secretion by the vascular wall, and promotion of low-density lipoprotein (LDL-cholesterol) accumulation (65).

Aspirin
Aspirin antagonizes platelet function by decreasing synthesis of thromboxane A2 (TxA2), a potent platelet-aggregating agent and vasoconstrictor, through irreversible inhibition of cyclo-oxygenase-1–mediated metabolism of arachadonic acid (68). Among a population of patients with atherosclerotic disease involving at least one vascular territory, treatment with aspirin yields a significant 23% odds reduction and 3.1% absolute risk reduction in serious vascular events (58). However, limited data exist to firmly establish the benefit of aspirin among patients with PAD in the absence of additional vascular disease. Only six double-blind, randomized controlled trials have compared aspirin to placebo, the majority of which tested high doses of aspirin, 975 to 1500 mg/day, and examined peripheral vascular outcomes such as graft patency or need for subsequent revascularization or amputation (61). For patients with PAD alone, the efficacy of aspirin in reducing the incidence of heart attack and

TABLE 4 Comparison of Antiplatelet Efficacy in Atherosclerotic Disease

Prior history	Comparison	RRR (%)	ARR (%)	NNT	References
CAD, CVD, or PAD	Antiplatelet vs. placebo	22	2.5	40	(58)
	ASA vs. placebo	23	3.1	33	(59)
	Clopidogrel vs. ASA	9	0.5	200	(60)
	Antiplatelet vs. placebo	22–23	1.3–1.6	63–77	(59,61)
PAD	ASA vs. placebo	N/A	N/A	N/A	
	Clopidogrel vs. ASA	24	1.2	83	(60)

Note: There is insufficient data comparing aspirin to placebo in patients with PAD alone.
Abbreviations: RRR, relative risk ratio; ARR, adjusted relative risk; NNT, number needed to treat; CAD, coronary artery disease; CVD, cerebrovascular disease; PAD, peripheral arterial disease; ASA, aspirin; N/A, not available.

stroke has largely been extrapolated from studies examining patients with preexisting CAD or CVD (61).

There is some indirect evidence that aspirin may be an inadequate platelet inhibitor in PAD. In contrast to recent meta-analyses (58,61), no significant reduction in serious vascular events was observed with antiplatelet therapy in a review published by the Antithrombotic Trialists' Collaboration in 1994 (69). Although the study ultimately recommended aspirin, based upon the absence of heterogeneity between subgroups, others interpreted the data as insufficient to recommend aspirin in view of a small and statistically uncertain effect (70). The primary difference between the meta-analyses published in 1994 and 2001 to 2002 was the inclusion of recent trials using clopidogrel and picotamide, suggesting that agents other than aspirin account for the significantly different outcomes. In vitro data also suggest the need for more potent antiplatelet therapy. Despite aspirin use, platelets harvested from 20 PAD patients demonstrated significantly higher aggregation than controls in the absence of antiplatelet therapy (71).

Suboptimal outcomes can largely be attributed to platelet activation via TxA2-independent pathways. Clinical treatment failure may also arise from "true" aspirin resistance, exhibited by inappropriately high TxA2 synthesis (68). Potential mechanisms include decreased aspirin bioavailability, accelerated platelet turnover, TxA2 production by cyclooxygenase (COX)-2, platelet synthesis of TxA2 from precursors produced by other cells, and variant COX-1 that is less susceptible to aspirin inhibition (68). A case–control study of 976 patients with prior vascular disease taking aspirin demonstrated a progressively increased risk of major vascular events with each increased quartile of urinary 11-dehydrothromboxane B2, a marker of in vivo TxA2 production (72). Compared to the lowest quartile, the highest quartile suffered a 3.5-fold increase in the risk of cardiovascular death during five years of follow-up.

Clopidogrel

Clopidogrel irreversibly inhibits platelet aggregation induced by the binding of adenosine diphosphate to its receptor, P2Y12, on the platelet surface. Compared to aspirin, clopidogrel achieved better vascular outcomes in a large, randomized trial of 19,185 patients with recent ischemic stroke, myocardial infarction, or symptomatic peripheral disease (60). In the Clopidogrel versus Aspirin in Patients at Risk of Ischemic Events trial, an annual 5.3% risk of serious vascular events was observed in the group receiving clopidogrel compared to 5.8% in the aspirin-treated group. Clopidogrel therapy resulted in a statistically significant relative risk reduction of 9%, but the absolute risk reduction of 0.5% coupled with a substantially higher cost has called into question the clinical significance of these results.

For patients with PAD, the benefit of clopidogrel was more pronounced. Among 6452 patients with symptomatic PAD, an annual 3.7% risk of vascular events was observed in patients receiving clopidogrel compared to 4.9% in the aspirin-treated arm (60). Treatment with clopidogrel in patients with PAD yielded a relative risk reduction of 24% and absolute risk reduction of 1.2%, yielding a number needed to treat of 83 (Fig. 9). One cost-effective analysis of clopidogrel in this subgroup revealed an increase in quality-adjusted life expectancy at a cost comparable to other accepted health care interventions (73).

Addition of clopidogrel to aspirin therapy has been evaluated in patients presenting with acute coronary syndrome or undergoing percutaneous coronary intervention. In Clopidogrel

Relative-risk reduction (%)

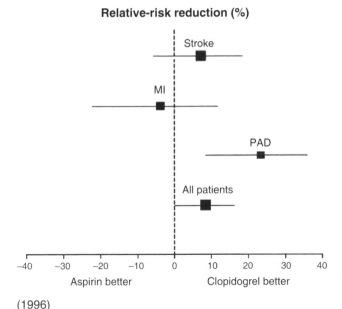

(1996)

FIGURE 9 Clopidogrel versus aspirin in the reduction of major vascular events. *Abbreviation*: PAD, peripheral arterial disease. *Source*: From Ref. 60.

in Unstable Angina to Prevent Recurrent Events trial and Clopidogrel for the Reduction of Events During Observation trial, dual antiplatelet therapy achieved statistically significant relative risk reductions in vascular events of 20% and 27%, respectively, compared to aspirin alone (74,75). Conclusions regarding coadministration of clopidogrel and aspirin in PAD patients, however, await the results of the ongoing Clopidogrel for High Atherothrombotic Risk and Ischemic Stabilization, Management, and Avoidance (CHARISMA) trial (76).

Recommendations

Recent guidelines put forward by three separate groups recommend lifelong antiplatelet therapy in all PAD patients, with aspirin as first-line treatment (9,77,78). These organizations acknowledged the superior clopidogrel data but concluded that additional studies are necessary to firmly establish a cost-effective benefit. Currently, clopidogrel is recommended for PAD patients with a contraindication to aspirin therapy. The recommended dose of aspirin in PAD patients is 75 to 325 mg daily. Higher doses have not been associated with improved outcomes but incur a higher risk of bleeding (58,69). The recommended dose of clopidogrel is 75 mg daily.

Risk Factor Management
Tobacco Use

Smoking is a potent risk factor for the development and progression of PAD. In one meta-analysis of 17 studies, tobacco use increased the prevalence of symptomatic PAD in a dose-dependent manner, 2.3-fold overall among current smokers compared to nonsmokers (79). In patients with existing PAD, smoking is associated with an increased risk of death (80), amputation (81,82), life-threatening ischemia (83), and failed revascularization (84) as well as worsened claudication and exercise performance (85).

Smoking cessation has been associated with a significant reduction in overall mortality (80,86), the risk of myocardial infarction (86), and the incidence of graft reocclusion (79). Efficacy in relieving claudication symptoms, however, has been inconsistent and observed benefits have been modest (87,88).

Cessation of tobacco use remains a difficult challenge, particularly among PAD patients who achieve lower success rates than those with CAD (86,89). Structured physician advice is recommended at each patient encounter through the application of the five As (Table 5) (90–92). In conjunction with counseling, nicotine replacement therapy and buproprion are recommended to maximize the success of permanent smoking cessation (92,93).

TABLE 5 The Five A's of Smoking Cessation

Ask	At every patient contact episode enquire about current and past smoking status, previous quit and previous experience with NRT
Advise	Strongly advise all smokers to quit, Educate all smokers about the risks of continued smoking and benefits of cessation
Assess	Identify the smoker's current stage in the transtheoretical model
Assist	All patients in the preparation stage should be targeted for further intervention and offered NRI bupropion
Arrange	Suitable follow-up needs to be arranged and referral to a smoking cessation clinic needs to be on Conside

Abbreviation: NRT, nicotine replacement therapy.
Source: From Hobbs and Bradbury 2003.

Hypertension

In the Framingham Study, hypertension increased the risk of developing symptomatic PAD 2.5-fold in men and 3.9-fold in women (94). High blood pressure significantly increases the risk of all-cause mortality in patients with manifest PAD but does not appear to worsen local disease (9). The Heart Outcomes Prevention Evaluation (HOPE) study represents the largest trial to date examining the benefits of antihypertensive therapy in the PAD population. Among the 4051 PAD patients enrolled, administration of ramipril 10 mg daily for 4.5 years was associated with a 22% relative risk reduction in myocardial infarction, stroke, or vascular-related death (Fig. 10) (95,96). Trials of commonly used antihypertensive drugs, including angiotensin converting enzyme (ACE) inhibitors, calcium channel blockers, alpha-blockers, and beta-blockers, have failed to show a benefit on PAD progression or claudication symptoms (97–100).

No clear evidence supports the use of a particular drug class in the management of hypertension in patients with PAD. The dramatic findings from the HOPE trial were initially attributed to possible effects specific to ACE-inhibitors independent of blood pressure lowering. More thorough analysis using 24-hour ambulatory blood pressure monitoring, however, demonstrated large reductions in blood pressure, mitigating enthusiasm for ACEI-mediated pleiotropic effects (101).

Early case reports in PAD raised concern over symptom exacerbation and the precipitation of critical limb ischemia with beta-blocker use (102). Reduction in lower extremity blood flow was thought to arise through depressed cardiac contractility or unopposed alpha-mediated vasoconstriction (103). Subsequent studies did not show an adverse effect on surrogate markers of disease severity, such as lower extremity blood flow, or clinical endpoints, including claudication severity and exercise capacity (103–105). As a result, a meta-analysis and review concluded that beta-blockers are safe except in cases of severe disease, and might be present in patients with rest pain and tissue loss (39,103–105).

The optimal blood pressure goal for patients with PAD remains controversial. The 2003 Seventh Report of the U.S.A Joint National Committee (JNC VII) and the 2004 American College of Cardiology/American Heart Association Guidelines, recommend maintaining blood pressure below 140/90 in patients with PAD (106,107). However, the HOPE trial and EURopean trial On reduction of cardiac events with Perindopril in stable caronary Artery disease (EUROPA) trial showed a significant reduction in major vascular events in high-risk patients with mean baseline blood pressures of 139/79 and 137/82 mmHg, respectively (95,108). Based on these results, the

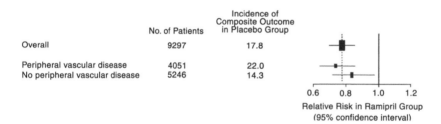

FIGURE 10 Evidence for the benefit of ACE inhibitors in peripheral arterial disease from the Heart Outcomes Prevention Evaluation study. *Source*: From Ref. 95.

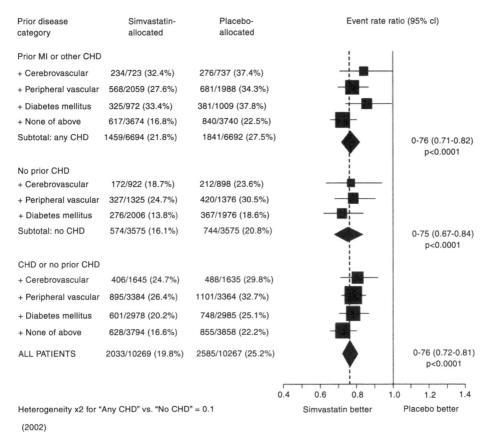

Prior disease category	Simvastatin-allocated	Placebo-allocated	Event rate ratio (95% cl)
Prior MI or other CHD			
+ Cerebrovascular	234/723 (32.4%)	276/737 (37.4%)	
+ Peripheral vascular	568/2059 (27.6%)	681/1988 (34.3%)	
+ Diabetes mellitus	325/972 (33.4%)	381/1009 (37.8%)	
+ None of above	617/3674 (16.8%)	840/3740 (22.5%)	
Subtotal: any CHD	1459/6694 (21.8%)	1841/6692 (27.5%)	0·76 (0.71–0.82) p<0.0001
No prior CHD			
+ Cerebrovascular	172/922 (18.7%)	212/898 (23.6%)	
+ Peripheral vascular	327/1325 (24.7%)	420/1376 (30.5%)	
+ Diabetes mellitus	276/2006 (13.8%)	367/1976 (18.6%)	
Subtotal: no CHD	574/3575 (16.1%)	744/3575 (20.8%)	0·75 (0.67–0.84) p<0.0001
CHD or no prior CHD			
+ Cerebrovascular	406/1645 (24.7%)	488/1635 (29.8%)	
+ Peripheral vascular	895/3384 (26.4%)	1101/3364 (32.7%)	
+ Diabetes mellitus	601/2978 (20.2%)	748/2985 (25.1%)	
+ None of above	628/3794 (16.6%)	855/3858 (22.2%)	
ALL PATIENTS	2033/10269 (19.8%)	2585/10267 (25.2%)	0·76 (0.72–0.81) p<0.0001

0.4   0.6   0.8   1.0   1.2   1.4

Heterogeneity x2 for "Any CHD" vs. "No CHD" = 0.1   Simvastatin better   Placebo better

(2002)

FIGURE 11   Evidence for the benefit of statins in peripheral arterial disease from the Heart Protection Study. *Source*: From Ref. 59. Copyright 2002.

2003 European Society of Hypertension-European Society of Cardiology and others recommend a more aggressive target blood pressure below 130/85 (39,109).

Hyperlipidemia

Treatment of hyperlipidemia, particularly through statin use, is a critical element of risk factor management to minimize the risk of atherothrombotic disease in patients with PAD. Among 6748 PAD patients enrolled in the landmark Heart Protection Study, treatment with simvastatin 40 mg daily resulted in a significant relative risk reduction of 24% in major vascular events, and an absolute risk reduction of 5.8%, yielding a number needed to treat of 17 (59) (Fig. 11). A smaller study that evaluated atorvastatin for symptomatic relief of claudication, although insufficiently powered to assess the effect of therapy on vascular events, did demonstrate congruous benefits (110).

The ATPIII Guidelines recommend a target LDL-cholesterol level below 100 mg/dL for patients with PAD, a CAD-risk equivalent (111). Based on the results of four trials that followed the 2001 publication (59,112–115), the National Cholesterol Panel in 2004 put forward an optional, more aggressive target of less than 70 mg/dL for those considered at "very high risk" (116). This new category consists of patients with known atherosclerotic vascular disease and at least one of the following: (i) multiple major risk factors, especially diabetes mellitus, (ii) severe and poorly controlled risk factors, especially continued smoking, (iii) the metabolic syndrome, or (iv) acute coronary syndromes (116).

Diabetes Mellitus

Diabetes mellitus has been associated with a twofold increased risk of developing PAD as well as more aggressive disease, manifesting as critical ischemia and the need for revascularization or limb amputation (9). Even among patients without diabetes, higher levels of hemoglobin A1c have been associated with an increased risk of PAD, suggesting an important role for glycemic control (117). Randomized controlled trials, however, have not established a benefit of aggressive glucose lowering on macrovascular outcomes. In the Diabetes Control and Complications Trial and the U.K. Prospective Diabetes Study, intensive hyperglycemic therapy did not reduce the incidence of mortality, myocardial infarction, stroke, or peripheral vascular events among type 1 and type 2 diabetics (118–120). Subgroup analysis of patients treated with metformin revealed a statistically significant 30% relative risk reduction for serious macrovascular events compared to conservative management (119). In addition, rates of all-cause mortality and myocardial infarction were reduced by 36% and 39%, respectively, suggesting that not all diabetic therapies are equivalent.

Based on improvements in microvascular outcomes of retinopathy, nephropathy, and neuropathy, the 2005 American Diabetes Association Guidelines recommends a treatment hemoglobin A1c goal of less than 7.0% with metformin as first-line oral therapy (121). The recently conceived International Diabetes Federation Global Guidelines recommends maintaining a hemoglobin A1c below 6.5%. It remains unclear whether achieving these targets will yield a reduction in myocardial infarction, stroke, and vascular-related death for PAD patients.

MANAGEMENT OF INTERMITTENT CLAUDICATION

Few options exist to effectively address the presenting concerns of patients with PAD. Exercise training, cilostazol therapy, and revascularization have demonstrated the greatest benefit in ameliorating claudication symptoms and associated functional limitations (Table 6).

Exercise Rehabilitation

Exercise rehabilitation remains the mainstay of therapy since the first randomized controlled trial in 1966 demonstrated a significant improvement in treadmill walking activity (124,125). In contrast to the general activity recommendations for cardiovascular disease prevention—moderate intensity aerobic exercise for 30 minutes most days of the week (126)—exercise prescription for PAD involves structured, symptom-based, progressive lower extremity endurance training. A typical exercise program starts by determining the training intensity usually in terms of treadmill speed and grade that provokes claudication within five minutes (127). Patients walk at this workload until moderately severe claudication occurs, rest for a brief period to allow symptoms to subside, and subsequently resume exercise (128). Alternating periods of activity and rest continue for a target duration of 30 to 60 minutes. Training sessions scheduled three to five times per week gradually increase workload intensity or duration as permitted by symptoms.

Significant clinical improvement occurs following four weeks of training (127), peaks after four months (129), and persists, provided the patients continue lower extremity exercise (130). One review of 571 patients enrolled in 18 nonrandomized and three randomized studies

TABLE 6 Medical Therapy for Intermittent Claudication

	Exercise rehabilitation	**Cilostazol**
Therapy	Walk to elicit claudication of moderate severity, then rest until symptoms subside	100 mg twice daily 50 mg twice daily with concurrent use of CYP3A4 or CYP2C19 inhibitors
	Alternate walk-rest-walk pattern for 30 to 60 min Repeat sessions three times weekly, gradually increasing activity intensity and duration	
Efficacy	Maximal distance: +122% Pain-free distance: +179%	Maximal distance: +50% Pain-free distance: +67%
Limitations	High degree of motivation required to achieve appropriate intensity	Contraindicated in heart failure due to increased mortality observed with PDE III inhibitors
	Uncertain benefit in unmonitored setting Limited insurance coverage in the United States	

Compared to baseline; for cilostazol 100 mg twice daily.
Source: From Refs. 122, 123.

demonstrated that exercise rehabilitation increased distance to onset of pain by 179% and maximal walking distance by 122% (122). In a review limited to randomized trials, analysis of 250 patients in 10 studies revealed an overall improvement in walking ability of 150% (131). Importantly, objective benefits in walking distance translated into significant improvements in self-reported functional ability and perception of general health and well-being (132,133).

Several mechanisms involving both sides of the oxygen demand-supply relationship, likely account for the observed relief of claudication symptoms (127). Oxygen delivery may be augmented at the level of the peripheral microcirculation through enhanced nitric oxide–mediated endothelial vasodilatation (134,135) and decreased blood viscosity (136). Exercise rehabilitation may also alter oxidative muscle metabolism (137,138) and walking biomechanics (139) to improve myocyte oxygen extraction and utilization. Studies do not suggest a significant role of angiogenesis and improved collateral circulation in the observed symptomatic benefit of exercise training (127).

In addition to improving symptoms and functional performance, exercise rehabilitation serves to further optimize risk factor management. In a study of 34 patients with intermittent claudication, a six-month rehabilitation program significantly reduced mean LDL-cholesterol by 8% and systolic blood pressure by 6% (140).

Despite their demonstrated efficacy, supervised exercise programs remain underutilized. In a European study of two academic general practice networks, 32% of the patients suffering from claudication engaged in monitored exercise training (141). Enrollment in the United States suffers from limited insurance coverage for hospital- or clinic-based rehabilitation despite initial cost-effectiveness data suggesting superiority to angioplasty (142). Unsupervised, home-based programs have not shown a consistent benefit, the failure likely arising from suboptimal intensity, duration, and frequency of training (133). Nonetheless, for highly motivated individuals, a detailed exercise prescription as described above may serve as a viable option even in an unmonitored environment (143).

Pharmacologic Therapy
Cilostazol

Cilostazol is the only widely used pharmacologic therapy approved for intermittent claudication (144). Numerous potentially beneficial effects have been elucidated (145), including arterial vasodilatation (146) and platelet inhibition (147) through increased levels of cyclic-adenosine monophosphate, as well as reduction in vascular smooth muscle proliferation (148) and increased circulating high-density lipoprotein–cholesterol (149). How cilostazol ultimately achieves relief of claudication symptoms, however, remains unknown.

A recent meta-analysis (123) of eight major randomized, placebo-controlled trials in the United States and the United Kingdom (149–154) examined the efficacy of cilostazol in patients with intermittent claudication. Administration of cilostazol, 50 and 100 mg twice daily, for 12 to 24 weeks increased maximum walking distance by 44% and 50%, respectively; this was significantly greater than the 21% increase observed with placebo (123). Pain-free walking distance rose by 60% and 67% from baseline with cilostazol 50 and 100 mg twice daily, compared to a rise of 40% with placebo. Importantly, these treadmill results translated into enhanced patient perceptions of physical well being as assessed by two validated quality-of-life questionnaires (123). Based on the above studies, the recommended dose for the treatment of claudication is 100 mg twice daily.

In the eight major U.S.A/U.K. cilostazol trials, the minor side effects that occurred significantly more frequently in the cilostazol-treated group compared to placebo included headache (32% vs. 13%), diarrhea (17% vs. 7%), rhinitis (8% vs. 5%), and peripheral edema (6% vs. 4%) (123). These symptoms rarely required drug discontinuation, either resolving spontaneously or responding to symptomatic treatment or dose reduction (144).

As a type III phosphodiesterase inhibitor, cilostazol is contraindicated in patients with heart failure. Chronic use of milrinone and other phosphodiesterase III inhibitors in heart failure patients has been associated with increased mortality from ventricular arrhythmias (155,156). Overall, cilostazol has achieved a safe cardiovascular record. U.S./U.K. clinical trials, with enrollment of 1441 cilostazol-treated patients, and U.S.A postmarketing surveillance totaling 70,340 patient-years of exposure, have demonstrated no increase in adverse cardiovascular outcomes compared to placebo (157). Long-term clinical experience in Japan, where cilostazol was first developed and used for vascular disorders, has produced comparable safety data (158).

Although no direct evidence indicates worsened outcomes among heart failure patients treated with cilostazol, insufficient data precludes sound determination of safety in the high-risk, heart failure subgroup (157). Cilostazol does have both an inotropic (159) and consistent chronotropic effect, increasing heart rate by five to seven beats per minute (157), suggesting that avoidance in the heart failure population remains prudent.

Despite its platelet-inhibition properties, cilostazol use is not a contraindication to concomitant aspirin or clopidogrel therapy. One study of 21 patients with PAD demonstrated no change in bleeding time with concurrent administration of cilostazol and aspirin, clopidogrel, or a combination of the two (160). Examination of four randomized, controlled trials revealed no increased risk of hemorrhagic events among 201 patients receiving both cilostazol and aspirin (144).

Significant interactions occur with drugs inhibiting the predominant metabolic pathways of cilostazol, CYP3A4 and CYP2C19. Inhibitors of CYP3A4 such as ketoconazole and erythromycin (161,162), and inhibitors of CYP2C19, such as omeprazole (163), have been shown to increase cilostazol plasma concentrations. Therefore, a lower dose of cilostazol, 50 mg twice daily, is recommended in patients using medications known to inhibit these cytochromes.

Pentoxifylline

The first drug available for the management of PAD symptoms, pentoxifylline, is no longer recommended for routine use (164). Purported to improve microcirculatory flow through enhanced erythrocyte deformability and decreased blood viscosity (165–167), initial enthusiasm for pentoxifylline has waned based upon data indicating an insignificant and inconsistent benefit compared to placebo. One meta-analysis of randomized and nonrandomized studies (88) and another limited to randomized, controlled trials (168) demonstrated an increase in pain-free walking distance of 21.0 to 29.4 m and an increase in total walking distance of 43.8 to 48.4 m. This effect-size is significantly less than that observed with exercise rehabilitation (88) and less than the benefit achieved with cilostazol therapy. One randomized trial of 54 patients demonstrated a lower mean increase in maximum walking distance in the pentoxifylline group (30%) compared to the cilostazol group (57%) (153). Moreover, this study (153) and others (169,170) revealed no difference in walking distance between patients treated with pentoxifylline and those administered placebo. Further supporting a limited clinical effect, withdrawal of pentoxifylline in one trial yielded no adverse outcomes in walking ability, in contrast to cessation of cilostazol therapy (171).

Statins

Statins, in addition to playing a critical role in risk factor management, may alleviate the symptoms of PAD (172). Post hoc analysis of the Scandinavian Simvastatin Survival Study (4S) demonstrated a significant 38% relative risk reduction and 1.3% absolute risk reduction in new or worsening intermittent claudication compared to placebo (173). One randomized, placebo-controlled study of 86 patients demonstrated that simvastatin administration for six months increased mean pain-free walking distance by 164% compared to baseline, or five times that of placebo (174). Total walking distance rose by 140% compared to baseline, significantly more than the 12% increase observed in the placebo group (174). In another study, treadmill exercise time until onset of symptoms increased by 42% after 12 months of simvastatin therapy among 31 PAD subjects already treated with cilostazol (175). An insignificant decrease in walking ability was observed in the control group. The precise pharmacologic pathways of statin-induced symptom relief are yet to be elucidated but plausible mechanisms involve pleiotropic effects such as the reversal of endothelial dysfunction (174,176).

Revascularization

Revascularization for chronic PAD is indicated either for debilitating claudication that fails to respond to medical therapy or for lower extremity tissue loss indicated by gangrene or recurrent ulcers (9,177,178). The decision to pursue a surgical versus an endovascular approach depends upon the extent of disease and lesion morphology (9). Though limited comparative data exist, shorter, more focal stenoses favor angioplasty and stenting, with bypass reserved for more diffuse disease. More proximal revascularization at the level of the aorta, iliac, and femoral arteries achieves higher long-term patency rates compared to distal, infrapopliteal

OUTCOME OF PTA AND BYPASS IN CLAUDICATION

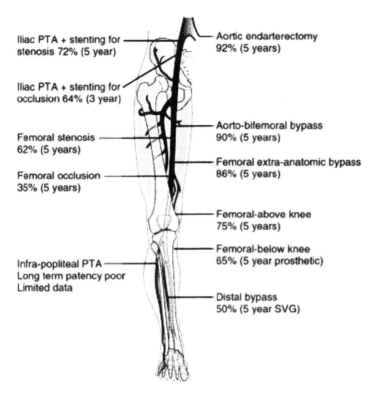

Iliac PTA + stenting for stenosis 72% (5 year)

Iliac PTA + stenting for occlusion 64% (3 year)

Femoral stenosis 62% (5 years)

Femoral occlusion 35% (5 years)

Infra-popliteal PTA Long term patency poor Limited data

Aortic endarterectomy 92% (5 years)

Aorto-bifemoral bypass 90% (5 years)

Femoral extra-anatomic bypass 86% (5 years)

Femoral-above knee 75% (5 years)

Femoral-below knee 65% (5 year prosthetic)

Distal bypass 50% (5 year SVG)

FIGURE 12   Patency rates following angioplasty and bypass *Source*: From Ref. 7.

intervention (9). Restenosis rates following revascularization are minimized with appropriate risk factor management and antiplatelet therapy (77). The benefit of aspirin, aspirin and dipyridamole, and ticlopidine are well described (179,180). Relevant data for clopidogrel could not be obtained from the planned Clopidogrel and Aspirin in the Management of Peripheral Endovascular Revascularization trial due to frequent use in high-risk cardiovascular patients (180). Anticoagulation with heparin and coumadin may improve outcomes in selected cases such as patients undergoing vein graft bypass and femoropopliteal angioplasty (179,180) (Fig. 12).

The Detection and Treatment Gap

Suboptimal management of PAD persists despite a wealth of data indicating its associated morbidity and mortality and the availability of medical therapy to reduce cardiovascular risk. Detection is complicated by the frequently asymptomatic nature of PAD. In a large population with risk factors of age, smoking, or diabetes, only 10% of the people with PAD detected by ABI experienced classic intermittent claudication defined as exercise-induced calf pain requiring cessation of walking and resolving within 10 minutes (3). Because classic claudication symptoms represent the exception rather than the rule, appropriate management of PAD requires proactive screening of high-risk populations in combination with heightened public awareness. Unfortunately, surveys demonstrate that only 32% of people older than 50 years are familiar with the term "peripheral arterial disease," and fewer can accurately describe the symptomatology, prognostic significance, risk factors, and treatment options (181,182). The Walking and Leg Circulation Study demonstrated that PAD participants' assessment of their risk of cardiovascular events was comparable with that of patients with no heart disease (176). Hindered by limited public and physician awareness, PAD is diagnosed in only a minority of the patients with the disease (3,5).

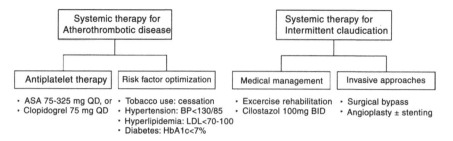

FIGURE 13 Overview of the management of peripheral arterial disease. *Abbreviation:* LDL, low-density lipoprotein.

When PAD is recognized, the proper, potentially life-saving interventions are frequently not instituted. Numerous studies conducted in a variety of populations including high-risk patients following revascularization, expose a significant treatment gap. Antiplatelet therapy was reported in 38% to 85% of the patients with established PAD (3,183–189). Among subjects with hypertension, hyperlipidemia, and diabetes, targeted therapy was initiated in 81% to 86%, 46% to 68%, and 83% of the patients, respectively (3,183,189). Despite similar prognostic implications, appropriate medication use is lower among PAD patients compared to CAD patients. In one retrospective chart review, the absence of CAD or CVD reduced the observed prevalence of antiplatelet, antihypertensive, and statin use among PAD patients by 34%, 22%, and 41%, respectively, a significant discrepancy shown by other studies (185,189).

In studies that examine not only drug utlilization but also achievement of risk factor modification goals, compliance rates with current guidelines for hypertension, hyperlipidemia, and diabetes were appallingly low. Appropriate reductions in blood pressure, defined as lower than 140/90 by the JNC VII guidelines, were observed in 26% to 66% of the PAD patients (188–190). Twenty-three percent to 47% of the patients achieved LDL-cholesterol levels less than 100 mg/dL, the goal established by the National Cholesterol Education Panel ATPIII (189,190). Target hemoglobin A1C below 7% was achieved by 33% to 52% (188–190). Moreover, hypertension and hyperlipidemia were not detected at all in 14% and 21% to 27% of PAD patients, respectively, and were ultimately diagnosed only during the study protocol (185,189).

■ Case 1: Medical Management

Mr. A is a 64-year-old man who presents to clinic with bilateral exertional calf pain precipitated by walking one block. His past medical history is notable for type II diabetes mellitus, hypertension, and hyperlipidemia. His father and older brother were diagnosed with CAD in their 50s. He reports having smoked one to two packs per day for the past 40 years and expresses interest in quitting. His current medications include metformin 1000 mg b.i.d., lisinopril 10 mg q.d., simvastatin 20 mg q.d., and aspirin 81 mg q.d.. At the clinic visit, his blood pressure is 156/92 and his heart rate is 88, consistent with measurements taken at home. Examination reveals cool lower extremities and diminished dorsalis pedis and posterior tibialis pulses. Popliteal pulses are 1+ bilaterally and a prominent systolic bruit is heard over the left femoral artery. Blood tests performed two months before show a hemoglobin A1c of 8.2% and an LDL-C of 128 mg/dL. Other laboratory studies, including an AST, ALT, and creatinine, are normal. Upper and lower extremity blood pressure measurements reveal an ankle-brachial index of 0.78 on the right and 0.82 on the left.

How Should Management of Mr. A's Newly Diagnosed PAD Proceed?

Comprehensive medical management relies on antiplatelet therapy and aggressive risk factor reduction to improve survival and minimize the incidence of heart attack and stroke, as well as exercise training and cilostazol to relieve symptoms.

Adding clopidogrel 75 mg daily to aspirin therapy reduces the absolute risk of myocardial infarction, stroke, or vascular-related death by 1.2%, according to the CAPRIE trial. Expressing interest in smoking cessation places Mr. A in the completative stage of behavioral change. He should be educated regarding the risks of continued tobacco use, offered nicotine replacement therapy, and referred to a smoking cessation program. Mr. A's blood pressure exceeds the targets established by American and European organizations of 140/90 and 130/85, respectively. The ACE inhibitor should first be maximized, given the patient's concurrent diabetes. He will undoubtedly require a second antihypertensive agent for adequate blood pressure control. A thiazide, beta-blocker, or calcium channel blocker would all be acceptable choices. According to NCEP ATP III guidelines, Mr. A's goal LDL-C should be at least less than 100 mg/dL if not less than 70 mg/dL, given the presence of numerous risk factors including two CAD-risk equivalents, diabetes and PAD. The statin should be titrated appropriately. An additional agent such as ezetimibe may be needed to achieve optimal LDL reduction. Mr. A's hemoglobin A1c of 8.2% exceeds the recommended target of 7.0%, warranting addition of a sulfonylurea.

For ameloriation of claudication, the patient should be enrolled in a structured walking program. Given the risk of coexistent CAD, a pharmacologic stress test is recommended prior to initiation of exercise rehabilitation. Provided he has no evidence of systolic dysfunction, cilostazol 100 mg b.i.d. can be started as adjunctive pharmacologic therapy for symptom relief.

■ Case 2: Emergent Thrombolysis

Mr. B is a 71-year-old man, status post left femoral-popliteal bypass, who presents to the emergency department with worsening left lower extremity pain. At baseline, he reports persistent left greater than right claudication symptoms. Over the past 12 hours, he has noted increasing left leg pain at rest. On examination, the left leg is pale and cool to the touch below the knee. Popliteal, dorsalis pedis, and posterior tibialis pulses are absent on the left and present on the right.

How Should Management of Mr. B's Acute Limb Ischemia Proceed?

Treatment for presumed acute peripheral arterial occlusion begins with immediate anticoagulation. In the absence of contraindications, heparin should be initiated with a goal PTT of two times control. Subsequent management depends on whether the underlying etiology of ischemia is embolic or thrombotic in origin. Most cases of acute embolic disease are associated with severe ischemia, necessitating rapid reperfusion best established through open surgical thromboembolectomy (179). Less severe ischemia due to peripheral arterial thrombosis may be amenable to endovascular therapy with intra-arterial thrombolysis. In this case, clinical history suggests a thrombotic origin of acute limb ischemia. As a result, Mr. B underwent urgent contrast angiography, which revealed abrupt termination of contrast flow in the femoral-popliteal bypass graft, as well as an occluded native superficial femoral artery. A guidewire was inserted into the occluded graft and intra-arterial alteplase was infused for 18 hours. Repeat angiography revealed a patent graft and identified the likely etiology of graft failure, a high-grade distal anastomotic stricture that was subsequently repaired by vein patch angioplasty (179).

■ Case 3: Revascularization

Mr. C is a 60-year-old man with severe PAD who reports right thigh pain at rest despite maximal medical therapy. MRA reveals a 90% right common iliac stenosis measuring 4 cm in length and diffuse moderate disease less than 50% in the right superficial femoral artery.

How Should Management of Mr. C's Refractory PAD Proceed?

Revascularization for chronic PAD is indicated for debilitating claudication that fails to respond to medical therapy or for lower extremity tissue loss indicated by gangrene or recurrent ulcers. The TransAtlantic Inter-Society Consensus Working Group (TASC) has developed a comprehensive morphologic stratification for iliac lesions (Table 6) (7). Based on the TASC classification, Mr. C has a type B iliac lesion for which angioplasty and stenting are frequently performed despite the absence of definitive evidence.

SUMMARY

Management of global atherothrombotic disease is paramount in the treatment of PAD patients (Fig. 13). Risk factor optimization involves permanent smoking cessation, antihypertensive therapy with goal blood pressures below 130/85, lipid lowering with statins to achieve an LDL-cholesterol below 70 to 100 mg/dL, and glucose control to maintain an HbA1c below 7%. All PAD patients should receive lifelong antiplatelet therapy, with aspirin 75 to 325 mg daily as first-line therapy or, when contraindicated, clopidogrel 75 mg daily. For symptomatic

TABLE 6

TASC type and recommendations	Iliac lesions
Type A: endovascular treatment of choice	• Single stenosis of CIA or EIA <3cm

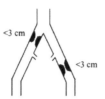

Type B: endovascular treatment more often used, but insufficient evidence	• Single CIA or EIA stenosis 3–10 cm; two CIA and/or EIA stenoses <5 cm; single CIA occlusions (lesions not extending into CFA)

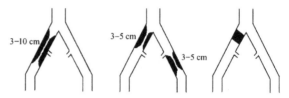

Type C: surgical treatment more often used, but insufficient evidence	• Bilateral long segment (5–10 cm) stenoses of CIA and/or EIA that do not extend into CFA; unilateral EIA occlusion not extending into CFA; unilateral EIA stenosis extending into CFA; bilateral CIA occlusions

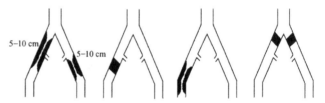

Type D: surgical treatment of choice	• Diffuse multiple stenoses of CIA, EIA, and CFA; unilateral CIA and EIA occlusions; bilateral EIA occlusions; coexistent aortic aneurysm or other condition requiring aortic or iliac surgery

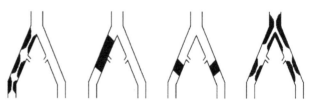

Abbreviation: CIA, common iliac artery; EIA, external iliac artery; CFA, common femoral artery.
Source: From Ref. 180.

PAD patients, medical management should be attempted first with exercise rehabilitation and cilostazol 100 mg twice daily. Revascularization via surgical or endovascular procedures can be employed in rare cases of refractory claudication.

REFERENCES

1. Mohler ER III. Peripheral arterial disease: identification and implications. Arch Intern Med 2003; 163(19):2306–2314.
2. Criqui MH, Langer RD, et al. Mortality over a period of 10 years in patients with peripheral arterial disease. N Engl J Med 1992; 326(6):381–386.
3. Hirsch AT, Criqui MH, et al. Peripheral arterial disease detection, awareness, and treatment in primary care. JAMA 2001; 286(11):1317–1324.

4. Criqui MH, Fronek A, et al. The sensitivity, specificity, and predictive value of traditional clinical evaluation of peripheral arterial disease: results from noninvasive testing in a defined population. Circulation 1985; 71(3):516–522.
5. Becker GJ, McClenny TE, et al. The importance of increasing public and physician awareness of peripheral arterial disease. J Vasc Interv Radiol 2002; 13(1):7–11.
6. Amudha K, Chee KH, et al. Prevalence of peripheral artery disease in urban high-risk Malaysian patients. Int J Clin Pract 2003; 57(5):369–372.
7. Wang J, Li XY, et al. A cross-sectional study of peripheral arterial occlusive disease in Wanshoulu area, Beijing. Zhonghua Liu Xing Bing Xue Za Zhi 2004; 25(3):221–224.
8. Murabito JM, D'Agostino RB, et al. Intermittent claudication. A risk profile from The Framingham Heart Study. Circulation 1997; 96(1):44–49.
9. Dormandy JA, Rutherford RB. Management of peripheral arterial disease (PAD). TASC Working Group. TransAtlantic Inter-Society Concensus (TASC). J Vasc Surg 2000; 31(1 Pt 2):S1–S296.
10. Selvin E, Erlinger TP. Prevalence of and risk factors for peripheral arterial disease in the United States: results from the National Health and Nutrition Examination Survey, 1999–2000. Circulation 2004; 110(6):738–743.
11. Kullo IJ, Bailey KR, et al. Ethnic differences in peripheral arterial disease in the NHLBI Genetic Epidemiology Network of Arteriopathy (GENOA) study. Vasc Med 2003; 8(4):237–242.
12. Price JF, Lee AJ, et al. Lipoprotein (a) and development of intermittent claudication and major cardiovascular events in men and women: the Edinburgh Artery Study. Atherosclerosis 2001; 157(1):241–249.
13. Falk E, Zhou J, et al. Homocysteine and atherothrombosis. Lipids 2001; 36(suppl):S3–S11.
14. Taylor LM Jr. Elevated plasma homocysteine as risk factor for peripheral arterial disease—what is the evidence? Semin Vasc Surg 2003; 16(3):215–222.
15. Doweik L, Maca T, et al. Fibrinogen predicts mortality in high-risk patients with peripheral artery disease. Eur J Vasc Endovasc Surg 2003; 26(4):381–386.
16. McDermott MM, Greenland P, et al. Inflammatory markers, D-dimer, pro-thrombotic factors, and physical activity levels in patients with peripheral arterial disease. Vasc Med 2004; 9(2):107–115.
17. Ridker PM, Stampfer MJ, et al. Novel risk factors for systemic atherosclerosis: a comparison of C-reactive protein, fibrinogen, homocysteine, lipoprotein(a), and standard cholesterol screening as predictors of peripheral arterial disease. JAMA 2001; 285(19):2481–2485.
18. Unlu Y, Karapolat S, et al. Comparison of levels of inflammatory markers and hemostatic factors in the patients with and without peripheral arterial disease. Thromb Res 2006; 117(4):357–364.
19. Dormandy J, Heeck L, et al. The natural history of claudication: risk to life and limb. Semin Vasc Surg 1999; 12(2):123–137.
20. Aronow WS, Ahn C. Prevalence of coexistence of coronary artery disease, peripheral arterial disease, and atherothrombotic brain infarction in men and women > or = 62 years of age. Am J Cardiol 1994; 74(1):64–65.
21. Newman AB, Sutton-Tyrrell K, et al. Morbidity and mortality in hypertensive adults with a low ankle/arm blood pressure index. JAMA 1993; 270(4):487–489.
22. Hackam DG, Goodman SG, et al. Management of risk in peripheral artery disease: recent therapeutic advances. Am Heart J 2005; 150(1):35–40.
23. Vogt MT, Cauley JA, et al. Decreased ankle/arm blood pressure index and mortality in elderly women. JAMA 1993; 270(4):465–469.
24. Program NCE. Third report of the National cholesterol Education Program (NCEP). Expert panel on detection, evaluation, and treatment of high blood cholesterol in adults. Final Report, discussion paper. National Heart, Lung, and Blood Institute, 2002.
25. Mannick JA. Current concepts in diagnostic methods. Evaluation of chronic lower-extremity ischemia. N Engl J Med 1983; 309(14):841–843.
26. Townsend CM, Beauchamp DR, Evers BM, Mattox KL. Sabiston Textbook of Surgery. Elsevier, 2004.
27. Rose GA. The diagnosis of ischaemic heart pain and intermittent claudication in field surveys. Bull World Health Organ 1962; 27:645–658.
28. Criqui MH, Denenberg JO, et al. The correlation between symptoms and non-invasive test results in patients referred for peripheral arterial disease testing. Vasc Med 1996; 1(1):65–71.
29. Brieger D, Eagle KA, et al. Acute coronary syndromes without chest pain, an underdiagnosed and undertreated high-risk group: insights from the Global Registry of Acute Coronary Events. Chest 2004; 126(2):461–469.
30. Fowkes FG, Housley E, et al. Edinburgh Artery Study: prevalence of asymptomatic and symptomatic peripheral arterial disease in the general population. Int J Epidemiol 1991; 20(2):384–392.
31. McDaniel MD, Cronenwett JL. Basic data related to the natural history of intermittent claudication. Ann Vasc Surg 1989; 3(3):273–277.
32. American Heart Association. Heart disease and stroke statistics, 2005.
33. Newman AB, Sutton-Tyrrell K, et al. Lower extremity arterial disease in elderly subjects with systolic hypertension. J Clin Epidemiol 1991; 44(1):15–20.
34. McDermott MM, Greenland P, et al. Leg symptoms in peripheral arterial disease: associated clinical characteristics and functional impairment. JAMA 2001; 286(13):1599–1606.
35. McDermott MM, Mehta S, et al. Exertional leg symptoms other than intermittent claudication are common in peripheral arterial disease. Arch Intern Med 1999; 159(4):387–392.

36. McGee S. Evidence-Based Physical Diagnosis. Philadelphia: Saunders, 2001.
37. Dieter RS, Chu WW, et al. The significance of lower extremity peripheral arterial disease. Clin Cardiol 2002; 25(1):3–10.
38. Schmieder FA, Comerota AJ. Intermittent claudication: magnitude of the problem, patient evaluation, and therapeutic strategies. Am J Cardiol 2001; 87(12A):3D–13D.
39. Hiatt WR. Medical treatment of peripheral arterial disease and claudication. N Engl J Med 2001; 344(21):1608–1621.
40. Belch JJ, Topol EJ, et al. Critical issues in peripheral arterial disease detection and management: a call to action. Arch Intern Med 2003; 163(8):884–892.
41. McPhail IR, Spittell PC, et al. Intermittent claudication: an objective office-based assessment. J Am Coll Cardiol 2001; 37(5):1381–1385.
42. McKenna M, Wolfson S, et al. The ratio of ankle and arm arterial pressure as an independent predictor of mortality. Atherosclerosis 1991; 87(2–3):119–128.
43. Jaff MR. Diagnosis of peripheral arterial disease: utility of the vascular laboratory. Clin Cornerstone 2002; 4(5):16–25.
44. Whelan JF, Barry MH, et al. Color flow Doppler ultrasonography: comparison with peripheral arteriography for the investigation of peripheral vascular disease. J Clin Ultrasound 1992; 20(6):369–374.
45. Reimer P, Landwehr P. Non-invasive vascular imaging of peripheral vessels. Eur Radiol 1998; 8(6):858–872.
46. Olin JW, Kaufman JA, et al. Atherosclerotic Vascular Disease Conference. Writing Group IV: imaging. Circulation 2004; 109(21):2626–2633.
47. Kohler TR, Nance DR, et al. Duplex scanning for diagnosis of aortoiliac and femoropopliteal disease: a prospective study. Circulation 1987; 76(5):1074–1080.
48. Zierler RE. Duplex and color-flow imaging of the lower extremity arterial circulation. Semin Ultrasound CT MR 1990; 11(2):168–179.
49. Mohler ER III. Noninvasive diagnosis of peripheral vascular disease. Uptodate. 2004.
50. Rajagopalan S, Prince M. Magnetic resonance angiographic techniques for the diagnosis of arterial disease. Cardiol Clin 2002; 20(4):501–512.
51. Auerbach EG, Martin ET. Magnetic resonance imaging of the peripheral vasculature. Am Heart J 2004; 148(5):755–763.
52. Visser K, Hunink MG. Peripheral arterial disease: gadolinium-enhanced MR angiography versus color-guided duplex US-a meta-analysis. Radiology 2000; 216(1):67–77.
53. Eiberg JP, Lundorf E, et al. Peripheral vascular surgery and magnetic resonance arteriography-a review. Eur J Vasc Endovasc Surg 2001; 22(5):396–402.
54. Cambria RP, Yucel EK, et al. The potential for lower extremity revascularization without contrast arteriography: experience with magnetic resonance angiography. J Vasc Surg 1993; 17(6):1050–1056; discussion 1056–1057.
55. Carpenter JP, Baum RA, et al. Peripheral vascular surgery with magnetic resonance angiography as the sole preoperative imaging modality. J Vasc Surg 1994; 20(6):861–869; discussion 869–871.
56. Huber TS, Back MR, et al. Utility of magnetic resonance arteriography for distal lower extremity revascularization. J Vasc Surg 1997; 26(3):415–423; discussion 423–424.
57. Portugaller HR, Schoellnast H, et al. Multislice spiral CT angiography in peripheral arterial occlusive disease: a valuable tool in detecting significant arterial lumen narrowing? Eur Radiol 2004; 14(9):1681–1687.
58. Collaborative meta-analysis of randomised trials of antiplatelet therapy for prevention of death, myocardial infarction, and stroke in high-risk patients. BMJ 324(7329):71–86.
59. MRC/BHF Heart Protection Study of cholesterol lowering with simvastatin in 20,536 high-risk individuals: a randomised placebo-controlled trial. Lancet 2002; 360(9326):7–22.
60. A randomised, blinded, trial of clopidogrel versus aspirin in patients at risk of ischaemic events (CAPRIE). CAPRIE Steering Committee. Lancet 1996; 348(9038):1329–1339.
61. Robless P, Mikhailidis DP, et al. Systematic review of antiplatelet therapy for the prevention of myocardial infarction, stroke, or vascular death in patients with peripheral vascular disease. Br J Surg 2001; 88(6):787–800.
62. Chesterman CN, Berndt MC. Platelet and vessel wall interaction and the genesis of atherosclerosis. Clin Haematol 1986; 15(2):323–353.
63. DiCorleto PE. Cellular mechanisms of atherogenesis. Am J Hypertens 1993; 6(11 Pt 2):314S–318S.
64. Cassar K, Bachoo P, et al. The role of platelets in peripheral vascular disease. Eur J Vasc Endovasc Surg 2003; 25(1):6–15.
65. Weber C. Platelets and chemokines in atherosclerosis: partners in crime. Circ Res 2005; 96(6):612–616.
66. Massberg S, Brand K, et al. A critical role of platelet adhesion in the initiation of atherosclerotic lesion formation. J Exp Med 2002; 196(7):887–896.
67. Huo Y, Schober A, et al. Circulating activated platelets exacerbate atherosclerosis in mice deficient in apolipoprotein E. Nat Med 2003; 9(1):61–67.
68. Cattaneo M. Aspirin and clopidogrel: efficacy, safety, and the issue of drug resistance. Arterioscler Thromb Vasc Biol 2004; 24(11):1980–1987.
69. Collaborative overview of randomised trials of antiplatelet therapy—I: Prevention of death, myocardial infarction, and stroke by prolonged antiplatelet therapy in various categories of patients. Antiplatelet Trialists' Collaboration. BMJ 1994; 308(6921):81–106.

70. Eccles M, Freemantle N, et al. North of England evidence based guideline development project: guideline on the use of aspirin as secondary prophylaxis for vascular disease in primary care. North of England Aspirin Guideline Development Group. BMJ 1998; 316(7140):1303–1309.
71. Robless PA, Okonko D, et al. Increased platelet aggregation and activation in peripheral arterial disease. Eur J Vasc Endovasc Surg 2003; 25(1):16–22.
72. Eikelboom JW, Hirsh J, et al. Aspirin-resistant thromboxane biosynthesis and the risk of myocardial infarction, stroke, or cardiovascular death in patients at high risk for cardiovascular events. Circulation 2002; 105(14):1650–1655.
73. Schleinitz MD, Weiss J, et al. Clopidogrel versus aspirin for secondary prophylaxis of vascular events: a cost-effectiveness analysis. Am J Med 2004; 116(12):797–806.
74. Yusuf S, Zhao F, et al. Effects of clopidogrel in addition to aspirin in patients with acute coronary syndromes without ST-segment elevation. N Engl J Med 2001; 345(7):494–502.
75. Beinart SC, Kolm P, et al. Long-term cost effectiveness of early and sustained dual oral antiplatelet therapy with clopidogrel given for up to one year after percutaneous coronary intervention results from the Clopidogrel for the Reduction of Events During Observation (CREDO) Trial. J Am Coll Cardiol 2005; 46(5):761–769.
76. Bhatt DL, Topol EJ. Clopidogrel added to aspirin versus aspirin alone in secondary prevention and high-risk primary prevention: rationale and design of the Clopidogrel for High Atherothrombotic Risk and Ischemic Stabilization, Management, and Avoidance (CHARISMA) trial. Am Heart J 2004; 148(2):263–268.
77. Clagett GP, Sobel M, et al. Antithrombotic therapy in peripheral arterial occlusive disease: the Seventh ACCP Conference on Antithrombotic and Thrombolytic Therapy. Chest 2004; 126(suppl 3):609S–626S.
78. Antiplatelet therapy in peripheral arterial disease. Consensus statement. Eur J Vasc Endovasc Surg 26(1):1–16.
79. Willigendael EM, Teijink JA, et al. Influence of smoking on incidence and prevalence of peripheral arterial disease. J Vasc Surg 2004; 40(6):1158–1165.
80. Faulkner KW, House AK, et al. The effect of cessation of smoking on the accumulative survival rates of patients with symptomatic peripheral vascular disease. Med J Aust 1983; 1(5):217–219.
81. Stewart CP. The influence of smoking on the level of lower limb amputation. Prosthet Orthot Int 1987; 11(3):113–116.
82. Leng GC, Papacosta O, et al. Femoral atherosclerosis in an older British population: prevalence and risk factors. Atherosclerosis 2000; 152(1):167–174.
83. Jonason T, Ringqvist I. Factors of prognostic importance for subsequent rest pain in patients with intermittent claudication. Acta Med Scand 1985; 218(1):27–33.
84. Ameli FM, Stein M, et al. The effect of postoperative smoking on femoropopliteal bypass grafts. Ann Vasc Surg 1989; 3(1):20–25.
85. Gardner AW. The effect of cigarette smoking on exercise capacity in patients with intermittent claudication. Vasc Med 1996; 1(3):181–186.
86. Jonason T, Bergstrom R. Cessation of smoking in patients with intermittent claudication. Effects on the risk of peripheral vascular complications, myocardial infarction and mortality. Acta Med Scand 1987; 221(3):253–260.
87. Quick CR, Cotton LT. The measured effect of stopping smoking on intermittent claudication. Br J Surg 1982; 69(suppl):S24–S26.
88. Girolami B, Bernardi E, et al. Treatment of intermittent claudication with physical training, smoking cessation, pentoxifylline, or nafronyl: a meta-analysis. Arch Intern Med 1999; 159(4):337–345.
89. Terry ML, Berkowitz HD, et al. Tobacco. Its impact on vascular disease. Surg Clin North Am 1998; 78(3):409–429.
90. Anderson JE, Jorenby DE, et al. Treating tobacco use and dependence: an evidence-based clinical practice guideline for tobacco cessation. Chest 2002; 121(3):932–941.
91. Karnath B. Smoking cessation. Am J Med 2002; 112(5):399–405.
92. Hobbs SD, Bradbury AW. Smoking cessation strategies in patients with peripheral arterial disease: an evidence-based approach. Eur J Vasc Endovasc Surg 2003; 26(4):341–347.
93. Hiatt WR. Pharmacologic therapy for peripheral arterial disease and claudication. J Vasc Surg 2002; 36(6):1283–1291.
94. Kannel WB, McGee DL. Update on some epidemiologic features of intermittent claudication: the Framingham Study. J Am Geriatr Soc 1985; 33(1):13–18.
95. Yusuf S, Sleight P, et al. Effects of an angiotensin-converting-enzyme inhibitor, ramipril, on cardiovascular events in high-risk patients. The Heart Outcomes Prevention Evaluation Study Investigators. N Engl J Med 2000; 342(3):145–153.
96. Ostergren J, Sleight P, et al. Impact of ramipril in patients with evidence of clinical or subclinical peripheral arterial disease. Eur Heart J 2004; 25(1):17–24.
97. Coffman JD. Drug therapy: vasodilator drugs in peripheral vascular disease. N Engl J Med 1979; 300(13):713–717.
98. Roberts DH, Tsao Y, et al. Placebo-controlled comparison of captopril, atenolol, labetalol, and pindolol in hypertension complicated by intermittent claudication. Lancet 1987; 2(8560):650–653.
99. Solomon SA, Ramsay LE, et al. beta blockade and intermittent claudication: placebo controlled trial of atenolol and nifedipine and their combination. BMJ 1991; 303(6810):1100–1104.

100. Lip GY, Makin AJ. Treatment of hypertension in peripheral arterial disease. Cochrane Database Syst 2003; Rev(4):CD003075.
101. Svensson P, de Faire U, et al. Comparative effects of ramipril on ambulatory and office blood pressures: a HOPE substudy. Hypertension 2001; 38(6):E28–E32.
102. Frohlich ED, Tarazi RC, et al. Peripheral arterial insufficiency. A complication of beta-adrenergic blocking therapy. JAMA 1969; 208(13):2471–2472.
103. Thadani U, Whitsett TL. Beta-adrenergic blockers and intermittent claudication. Time for reappraisal. Arch Intern Med 1991; 151(9):1705–1707.
104. Radack K, Deck C. Beta-adrenergic blocker therapy does not worsen intermittent claudication in subjects with peripheral arterial disease. A meta-analysis of randomized controlled trials. Arch Intern Med 1991; 151(9):1769–1776.
105. Heintzen MP, Strauer BE. Peripheral vascular effects of beta-blockers. Eur Heart J 1994; 15 (suppl C):2–7.
106. Chobanian AV, Bakris GL, et al. Seventh report of the Joint National Committee on Prevention, Detection, Evaluation, and Treatment of High Blood Pressure. Hypertension 2003; 42(6):1206–1252.
107. Antman EM, Anbe DT, et al. ACC/AHA guidelines for the management of patients with ST-elevation myocardial infarction-executive summary: a report of the American College of Cardiology/American Heart Association Task Force on Practice Guidelines (Writing Committee to Revise the 1999 Guidelines for the Management of Patients With Acute Myocardial Infarction). Circulation 2004; 110(5):588–636.
108. Fox KM. Efficacy of perindopril in reduction of cardiovascular events among patients with stable coronary artery disease: randomised, double-blind, placebo-controlled, multicentre trial (the EUROPA study). Lancet 2003; 362(9386):782–788.
109. European Society of Hypertension-European Society of Cardiology guidelines for the management of arterial hypertension. J Hypertens 21(6):1011–1053.
110. Mohler ER III, Hiatt WR, et al. Cholesterol reduction with atorvastatin improves walking distance in patients with peripheral arterial disease. Circulation 2003; 108(12):1481–1486.
111. The Third Report of The National Cholesterol Education Program (NCEP) Expert Panel on Detection, Evaluation, And Treatment of High Blood Cholesterol In Adults (Adult Treatment Panel III). JAMA 2001; 285(19):2486–2497.
112. Cannon CP, McCabe CH, et al. Design of the Pravastatin or Atorvastatin Evaluation and Infection Therapy (PROVE IT)-TIMI 22 trial. Am J Cardiol 2002; 89(7):860–861.
113. Shepherd J, Blauw GJ, et al. Pravastatin in elderly individuals at risk of vascular disease (PROSPER): a randomised controlled trial. Lancet 2002; 360(9346):1623–1630.
114. Huang JC, Hoogwerf RJ. Cholesterol guidelines update: more aggressive therapy for higher-risk patients. Cleve Clin J Med 2005; 72(3):253–262.
115. Major outcomes in moderately hypercholesterolemic, hypertensive patients randomized to pravastatin vs usual care: The Antihypertensive and Lipid-Lowering Treatment to Prevent Heart Attack Trial (ALLHAT-LLT). JAMA 288(23):2998–3007.
116. Grundy SM, Cleeman JI, et al. Implications of recent clinical trials for the National Cholesterol Education Program Adult Treatment Panel III Guidelines. J Am Coll Cardiol 2004; 44(3):720–732.
117. Muntner P, Wildman RP, et al. Relationship between HbA1c level and peripheral arterial disease. Diabetes Care 2005; 28(8):1981–1987.
118. Effect of intensive diabetes management on macrovascular events and risk factors in the Diabetes Control and Complications Trial. Am J Cardiol 75(14):894–903.
119. Effect of intensive blood-glucose control with metformin on complications in overweight patients with type 2 diabetes (UKPDS 34). UK Prospective Diabetes Study (UKPDS) Group. Lancet 1998; 352(9131):854–865.
120. Intensive blood-glucose control with sulphonylureas or insulin compared with conventional treatment and risk of complications in patients with type 2 diabetes (UKPDS 33). UK Prospective Diabetes Study (UKPDS) Group. Lancet 1998; 352(9131):837–853.
121. Standards of medical care in diabetes. Diabetes Care 2005; 28(suppl 1):S4–S36.
122. Gardner AW, Poehlman ET. Exercise rehabilitation programs for the treatment of claudication pain. A meta-analysis. JAMA 1995; 274(12):975–980.
123. Thompson PD, Zimet R, et al. Meta-analysis of results from eight randomized, placebo-controlled trials on the effect of cilostazol on patients with intermittent claudication. Am J Cardiol 2002; 90(12):1314–1319.
124. Larsen OA, Lassen NA. Effect of daily muscular exercise in patients with intermittent claudication. Scand J Clin Lab Invest 1967; 99(suppl):168–171.
125. Regensteiner JG, Hiatt WR. Current medical therapies for patients with peripheral arterial disease: a critical review. Am J Med 2002; 112(1):49–57.
126. Fletcher GF, Balady G, et al. Statement on exercise: benefits and recommendations for physical activity programs for all Americans. A statement for health professionals by the Committee on Exercise and Cardiac Rehabilitation of the Council on Clinical Cardiology, American Heart Association. Circulation 1996; 94(4):857–862.
127. Stewart KJ, Hiatt WR, et al. Exercise training for claudication. N Engl J Med 2002; 347(24):1941–1951.
128. Nehler MR, Hiatt WR. Exercise therapy for claudication. Ann Vasc Surg 1999; 13(1):109–114.

129. Bulmer AC, Coombes JS. Optimising exercise training in peripheral arterial disease. Sports Med 2004; 34(14):983–1003.
130. Menard JR, Smith HE, et al. Long-term results of peripheral arterial disease rehabilitation. J Vasc Surg 2004; 39(6):1186–1192.
131. Leng GC, Fowler B, et al. Exercise for intermittent claudication. Cochrane Database Syst Rev 2000; (2):CD000990.
132. Regensteiner JG, Steiner JF, et al. Exercise training improves functional status in patients with peripheral arterial disease. J Vasc Surg 1996; 23(1):104–115.
133. Regensteiner JG, Meyer TJ, et al. Hospital vs home-based exercise rehabilitation for patients with peripheral arterial occlusive disease. Angiology 1997; 48(4):291–300.
134. Arosio E, Cuzzolin L, et al. Increased endogenous nitric oxide production induced by physical exercise in peripheral arterial occlusive disease patients. Life Sci 1999; 65(26):2815–2822.
135. Brendle DC, Joseph LJ, et al. Effects of exercise rehabilitation on endothelial reactivity in older patients with peripheral arterial disease. Am J Cardiol 2001; 87(3):324–329.
136. Ernst EE, Matrai A. Intermittent claudication, exercise, and blood rheology. Circulation 1987; 76(5):1110–1114.
137. Hiatt WR, Regensteiner JG, et al. Benefit of exercise conditioning for patients with peripheral arterial disease. Circulation 1990; 81(2):602–609.
138. Hiatt WR, Regensteiner JG, et al. Effect of exercise training on skeletal muscle histology and metabolism in peripheral arterial disease. J Appl Physiol 1996; 81(2):780–788.
139. Womack CJ, Sieminski DJ, et al. Improved walking economy in patients with peripheral arterial occlusive disease. Med Sci Sports Exerc 1997; 29(10):1286–1290.
140. Izquierdo-Porrera AM, Gardner AW, et al. Effects of exercise rehabilitation on cardiovascular risk factors in older patients with peripheral arterial occlusive disease. J Vasc Surg 2000; 31(4): 670–677.
141. Bartelink ML, Stoffers HE, et al. Walking exercise in patients with intermittent claudication. Experience in routine clinical practice. Br J Gen Pract 2004; 54(500):196–200.
142. Treesak C, Kasemsup V, et al. Cost-effectiveness of exercise training to improve claudication symptoms in patients with peripheral arterial disease. Vasc Med 2004; 9(4):279–285.
143. Wolosker N, Nakano L, et al. Evaluation of walking capacity over time in 500 patients with intermittent claudication who underwent clinical treatment. Arch Intern Med 2003; 163(19):2296–2300.
144. Reilly MP, Mohler ER III. Cilostazol: treatment of intermittent claudication. Ann Pharmacother 2001; 35(1):48–56.
145. Schror K. The pharmacology of cilostazol. Diabetes Obes Metab 2002; 4(suppl 2):S14–S19.
146. Oida K, Ebata K, et al. Effect of cilostazol on impaired vasodilatory response of the brachial artery to ischemia in smokers. J Atheroscler Thromb 2003; 10(2):93–98.
147. Kohda N, Tani T, et al. Effect of cilostazol, a phosphodiesterase III inhibitor, on experimental thrombosis in the porcine carotid artery. Thromb Res 1999; 96(4):261–268.
148. Tsuchikane E, Katoh O, et al. Impact of cilostazol on intimal proliferation after directional coronary atherectomy. Am Heart J 1998; 135(3):495–502.
149. Elam MB, Heckman J, et al. Effect of the novel antiplatelet agent cilostazol on plasma lipoproteins in patients with intermittent claudication. Arterioscler Thromb Vasc Biol 1998; 18(12):1942–1947.
150. Dawson DL, Cutler BS, et al. Cilostazol has beneficial effects in treatment of intermittent claudication: results from a multicenter, randomized, prospective, double-blind trial. Circulation 1998; 98(7):678–686.
151. Money SR, Herd JA, et al. Effect of cilostazol on walking distances in patients with intermittent claudication caused by peripheral vascular disease. J Vasc Surg 1998; 27(2):267–274; discussion 274–275.
152. Beebe HG, Dawson DL, et al. A new pharmacological treatment for intermittent claudication: results of a randomized, multicenter trial. Arch Intern Med 1999; 159(17):2041–2050.
153. Dawson DL, Cutler BS, et al. A comparison of cilostazol and pentoxifylline for treating intermittent claudication. Am J Med 2000; 109(7):523–530.
154. Strandness DE Jr., Dalman RL, et al. Effect of cilostazol in patients with intermittent claudication: a randomized, double-blind, placebo-controlled study. Vasc Endovascular Surg 2002; 36(2):83–91.
155. Packer M, Carver JR, et al. Effect of oral milrinone on mortality in severe chronic heart failure. The PROMISE Study Research Group. N Engl J Med 1991; 325(21):1468–1475.
156. Nony P, Boissel JP, et al. Evaluation of the effect of phosphodiesterase inhibitors on mortality in chronic heart failure patients. A meta-analysis. Eur J Clin Pharmacol 1994; 46(3):191–196.
157. Pratt CM. Analysis of the cilostazol safety database. Am J Cardiol 2001; 87(12A):28D–33D.
158. Donnelly, R. Evidence-based symptom relief of intermittent claudication: efficacy and safety of cilostazol. Diabetes Obes Metab 2002; 4(suppl 2):S20–S25.
159. Cone J, Wang S, et al. Comparison of the effects of cilostazol and milrinone on intracellular cAMP levels and cellular function in platelets and cardiac cells. J Cardiovasc Pharmacol 1999; 34(4):497–504.
160. Wilhite DB, Comerota AJ, et al. Managing PAD with multiple platelet inhibitors: the effect of combination therapy on bleeding time. J Vasc Surg 2003; 38(4):710–713.
161. Suri A, Forbes WP, et al. Effects of CYP3A inhibition on the metabolism of cilostazol. Clin Pharmacokinet 1999; 37(suppl 2):61–68.

162. Abbas R, Chow CP, et al. In vitro metabolism and interaction of cilostazol with human hepatic cytochrome P450 isoforms. Hum Exp Toxicol 2000; 19(3):178–184.

163. Suri A, Bramer SL. Effect of omeprazole on the metabolism of cilostazol. Clin Pharmacokinet 1999; 37(suppl 2):53–59.

164. Jackson MR, Clagett GP. Antithrombotic therapy in peripheral arterial occlusive disease. Chest 1998; 114(suppl 5):666S–682S.

165. Aviado DM, Porter JM. Pentoxifylline: a new drug for the treatment of intermittent claudication. Mechanism of action, pharmacokinetics, clinical efficacy and adverse effects. Pharmacotherapy 1984; 4(6):297–307.

166. Di Perri T, Carandente O, et al. Studies of the clinical pharmacology and therapeutic efficacy of pentoxifylline in peripheral obstructive arterial disease. Angiology 1984; 35(7):427–435.

167. Creager MA. Medical management of peripheral arterial disease. Cardiol Rev 2001; 9(4):238–245.

168. Hood SC, Moher D, et al. Management of intermittent claudication with pentoxifylline: meta-analysis of randomized controlled trials. Cmaj 1996; 155(8):1053–1059.

169. Porter JM, Cutler BS, et al. Pentoxifylline efficacy in the treatment of intermittent claudication: multicenter controlled double-blind trial with objective assessment of chronic occlusive arterial disease patients. Am Heart J 1982; 104(1):66–72.

170. Lindgarde F, Jelnes R, et al. Conservative drug treatment in patients with moderately severe chronic occlusive peripheral arterial disease. Scandinavian Study Group. Circulation 1989; 80(6):1549–1556.

171. Dawson DL, DeMaioribus CA, et al. The effect of withdrawal of drugs treating intermittent claudication. Am J Surg 1999; 178(2):141–146.

172. McDermott MM, Guralnik JM, et al. Statin use and leg functioning in patients with and without lower-extremity peripheral arterial disease. Circulation 2003; 107(5):757–761.

173. Pedersen TR, Kjekshus J, et al. Effect of simvastatin on ischemic signs and symptoms in the Scandinavian simvastatin survival study (4S). Am J Cardiol 1998; 81(3):333–335.

174. Mondillo S, Ballo P, et al. Effects of simvastatin on walking performance and symptoms of intermittent claudication in hypercholesterolemic patients with peripheral vascular disease. Am J Med 2003; 114(5):359–364.

175. Aronow WS, Nayak D, et al. Effect of simvastatin versus placebo on treadmill exercise time until the onset of intermittent claudication in older patients with peripheral arterial disease at six months and at one year after treatment. Am J Cardiol 2003; 92(6):711–712.

176. McDermott MM, Mandapat AL, et al. Knowledge and attitudes regarding cardiovascular disease risk and prevention in patients with coronary or peripheral arterial disease. Arch Intern Med 2003; 163(18):2157–2162.

177. Comerota AJ. Endovascular and surgical revascularization for patients with intermittent claudication. Am J Cardiol 2001; 87(12A):34D–43D.

178. Brook RD, Weder AB, et al. Management of intermittent claudication. Cardiol Clin 2002; 20(4):521–534.

179. Dorffler-Melly J, Koopman MM, et al. Antiplatelet agents for preventing thrombosis after peripheral arterial bypass surgery. Cochrane Database Syst Rev 2003; (3):CD000535.

180. Dorffler-Melly J, Koopman MM, et al. Antiplatelet and anticoagulant drugs for prevention of restenosis/reocclusion following peripheral endovascular treatment. Cochrane Database Syst Rev 2005; (1):CD002071.

181. International, O. R. C. Awareness of Peripheral Vascular Disease, 2000.

182. Intersearch, T. N. S. Peripheral arterial disease study, 2001.

183. McDermott MM, Mehta S, et al. Atherosclerotic risk factors are less intensively treated in patients with peripheral arterial disease than in patients with coronary artery disease. J Gen Intern Med 1997; 12(4):209–215.

184. Anand SS, Kundi A, et al. Low rates of preventive practices in patients with peripheral vascular disease. Can J Cardiol 1999; 15(11):1259–1263.

185. Clark AL, Byrne JC, et al. Cholesterol in peripheral vascular disease-a suitable case for treatment? QJM 1999; 92(4):219–222.

186. Bismuth J, Klitfod L, et al. The lack of cardiovascular risk factor management in patients with critical limb ischaemia. Eur J Vasc Endovasc Surg 2001; 21(2):143–146.

187. Gen Teh L, Sieunarine K, et al. Suboptimal preventive practices in patients with carotid and peripheral vascular occlusive disease in a tertiary referral setting. ANZ J Surg 2003; 73(11):932–927.

188. Ness J, Aronow WS, et al. Prevalence of symptomatic peripheral arterial disease, modifiable risk factors, and appropriate use of drugs in the treatment of peripheral arterial disease in older persons seen in a university general medicine clinic. J Gerontol A Biol Sci Med Sci 2005; 60(2):255–257.

189. Okaa RK, Umoh E, et al. Suboptimal intensity of risk factor modification in PAD. Vasc Med 2005; 10(2):91–96.

190. Rehring TF, Sandhoff BG, et al. Atherosclerotic risk factor control in patients with peripheral arterial disease. J Vasc Surg 2005; 41(5):816–822.

18 Acute Myocardial Infarction

James T. Willerson
University of Texas Health Science Center and Texas Heart Institute, Houston, Texas, U.S.A.

Paul W. Armstrong
University of Alberta Hospital Heart Function Clinic, University of Alberta, Edmonton, Alberta, Canada

KEY POINTS

- Acute myocardial infarction (AMI) occurs when there are severe and prolonged reductions in coronary blood flow and myocardial oxygen delivery usually associated with coronary artery thrombosis. Myocardial infarction (MI) begins on the inner wall of the heart and is confined there in the first 30 minutes to one to two hours. Referred to as non-Q wave MI (NQMI) or non-ST segment elevation MI (NSTEMI), most of these infarcts are limited to the subendocardial region. With longer periods of severely reduced coronary blood flow, the infarct progresses vertically outward to become an ST elevation MI (STEMI) or Q wave MI that is often transmural in extent.
- Most MIs are caused by thrombosis of a coronary artery in which an atherosclerotic plaque has fissured or ruptured, exposing the subendothelium to flowing blood and allowing platelets to adhere and aggregate, subsequently joined by white cells and red blood cells in the development of a thrombus.
- The platelet adherence and aggregation at sites of atherosclerotic plaque fissuring or ulceration also results in the local accumulation of mediators that promote the growth of a thrombus and cause dynamic vasoconstriction, including thromboxane A2, serotonin, adenosine diphosphate (ADP), thrombin, platelet activating factor (PAF), oxygen-derived free radicals, and endothelin. At sites of coronary artery atherosclerosis, there is also a local decrease or absence of the normally present endothelial vasoprotective substances, including prostacyclin, nitric oxide, and tissue plasminogen activator (tPA), which, when present, inhibit or diminish arterial vasoconstriction, inflammation, and thrombosis with vascular injury.
- The TIMI 18 study suggests that patients with NSTEMI (and those with unstable angina) who have elevations in serum CRP or Troponin levels on admission and those with a TIMI Risk Factor Score of 3 or greater have reductions in subsequent risk of death, MI, and need for future intervention when treated by percutaneous coronary intervention procedure (PCI) or CABG. Women with ACS seem particularly likely to benefit from interventional therapy when admitted with elevated serum CRP and troponin-I.
- Statin therapy should be initiated in patients with AMIs beginning on admission to the hospital in a dose sufficient to markedly lower serum Low-density lipoprotein (LDL) concentrations rapidly.
- When faced with STEMI, the physician should ask the following questions: What is the time from symptom onset to first medical contact? What is the risk of thrombolytic therapy? What is the time required to transport the patient and achieve PCI by a skilled operator? PCI is superior to thrombolytic therapy where there is immediate access to skilled facilities and physician/healthcare teams.

PATHOPHYSIOLOGY

The coronary heart disease syndromes are listed in Table 1.

ACUTE MYOCARDIAL INFARCTION

Acute myocardial infarction (AMI) occurs when there are severe and prolonged reductions in coronary blood flow and myocardial oxygen delivery usually associated with coronary artery thrombosis. MI begins on the inner wall or subendocardium of the heart and is confined there

TABLE 1   Coronary Heart Disease Syndromes

Stable angina pectoris
Unstable angina pectoris
Variant angina ("Prinzmetal's angina")
Acute myocardial infarction
"Non-ST segment elevation" (NSTEMI) or non-Q wave (usually
nontransmural infarcts) (NQMI)
"ST segment elevation" (STEMI) or Q wave MI (usually transmural MI)

in the first 30 minutes to one to two hours and is referred to as a non-Q wave (NQMI) or non-ST segment elevation MI (NSTEMI); most, but not all, of these infarcts are limited to the subendocardial region of the heart. With longer periods of severe reductions in coronary blood flow, the infarct progresses vertically outward to become an ST elevation MI (STEMI) or usually Q wave MI that is often transmural in extent.

Most MIs are caused by thrombosis of a coronary artery in which an atherosclerotic plaque has fissured or ruptured exposing the subendothelium to flowing blood and allowing platelets to adhere and aggregate subsequently joined by white cells and red blood cells in the development of a thrombus (1–7). The platelet adherence and aggregation at sites of atherosclerotic plaque fissuring or ulceration also results in the local accumulation of mediators that promote the growth of a thrombus and cause dynamic vasoconstriction, including thromboxane A_2, serotonin, adenosine diphosphate (ADP), thrombin, platelet activating factor (PAF), oxygen-derived free radicals, and endothelin (Fig. 1) (8,9–22). At sites of coronary artery atherosclerosis, there is also a local decrease or absence of the normally present endothelial vasoprotective substances, including prostacyclin, nitric oxide, and tissue plasminogen activator (tPA), which when present inhibit or diminish arterial vasoconstriction, inflammation, and thrombosis with vascular injury (Fig. 1).

Herrick (2) described acute MI caused by coronary artery thrombosis in 1912. Subsequently, the role of coronary artery thrombosis in leading to MI was debated until studies by DeWood et al. (6) demonstrated by coronary arteriography that coronary artery thrombosis is almost always the cause of acute STEMIs. Buja and Willerson (7) confirmed the association between thrombosis of the infarct-related coronary artery and the development of acute STEMI by detailed clinicopathologic correlations. Ninety percent or more of STEMIs have prolonged occlusive coronary artery thrombosis in the infarct-related artery (6). Occasionally, however, increased myocardial oxygen demand above the ability of a stenosed coronary artery to deliver oxygen causes MI, often NSTEMI. Such increases in myocardial oxygen demand occur in patients with very rapid heart rates and systemic arterial hypertension. Sustained reductions in myocardial oxygen delivery associated with severe systemic arterial hypotension may also cause MI, usually NSTEMI. Approximately 30% of patients with NSTEMI have an occlusive thrombus in the infarct-related artery (7).

We have suggested that unstable angina, NSTEMI, and STEMI represent a continuum pathologically (9,14,15). The process begins with coronary endothelial injury, usually atherosclerotic plaque ulceration or fissuring. Plaque fissuring is more common in women. The degree of coronary artery stenosis where plaque ulceration or fissuring occurs may be mild or severe, but approximately half of the coronary stenoses where plaque fissuring or ulceration occurs are sites of less than 50% luminal diameter narrowing (19,20). We and our associates have further suggested that when platelet-fibrin-rich thrombi and the associated severe vasoconstriction persist for periods of less than 20 to 30 minutes and often recur, the clinical syndrome of unstable angina with brief but repetitive episodes of angina occurring at limited activity or at rest develops (9,14,15). However, when the reduction in coronary blood flow and oxygen delivery to the heart is more prolonged, lasting 20 minutes to one to two hours, a NSTEMI occurs (9,14,15). When the period of inadequate myocardial oxygen delivery persists for more than two hours, STEMI develops. When unstable angina and acute MI are viewed in this manner, it is easy to appreciate that patients with unstable angina and NSTEMIs have "aborted" STEMIs; therefore, they remain at risk for new MI and its consequences in the ensuing several weeks. In these patients, the risk of new MI persists until the

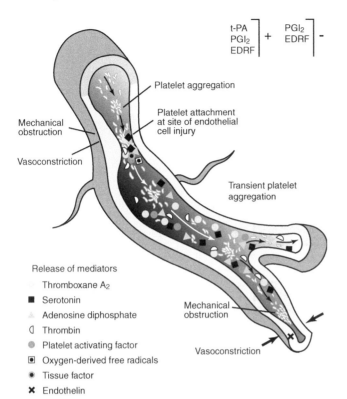

$$\left.\begin{array}{l} \text{t-PA} \\ \text{PGI}_2 \\ \text{EDRF} \end{array}\right] + \left.\begin{array}{l} \text{PGI}_2 \\ \text{EDRF} \end{array}\right] -$$

Platelet aggregation

Platelet attachment at site of endothelial cell injury

Mechanical obstruction

Vasoconstriction

Transient platelet aggregation

Release of mediators

  Thromboxane A_2

■ Serotonin

▲ Adenosine diphosphate

◖ Thrombin

● Platelet activating factor

◙ Oxygen-derived free radicals

● Tissue factor

✖ Endothelin

Mechanical obstruction

Vasoconstriction

FIGURE 1 Schematic diagram suggests probable mechanisms responsible for the conversion from chronic coronary heart disease to acute coronary artery disease syndromes. In this scheme, endothelial injury, generally at sites of atherosclerotic plaques and usually plaque ulceration or fissuring, is associated with platelet adhesion and aggregation and the release and activation of selected mediators, including thromboxane A_2, serotonin, adenosine, diphosphate, platelet-activating factor, thrombin, oxygen-derived free radicals, and endothelin. Local accumulation of thromboxane A_2, serotonin, platelet-activating factor, thrombin, adenosine diphosphate, and tissue factor promotes platelet aggregation. Thromboxane A_2, serotonin, thrombin, and platelet activating factor are vasoconstrictors at sites of endothelial injury. Therefore, the conversion from chronic stable to acute unstable coronary heart disease syndromes is usually associated with endothelial injury, platelet aggregation, accumulation of platelet and other cell-derived mediators, further platelet aggregation, and vasoconstriction, with consequent dynamic narrowing of the coronary artery lumen. In addition to atherosclerotic plaque fissuring or ulceration, other reasons for endothelial injury include flow shear stress, hypertension, immune complex deposition and complement activation, infection, and mechanical injury to the endothelium as it occurs with coronary artery angioplasty and after heart transplantation. Injured endothelial cells have reduced amounts of the normally present vasoprotective substance that when present prevent thrombosis, vasoconstriction, and inflammation, NO, tPA, and prostacyclin. *Abbreviations*: NO, nitric oxide; PGI_2, prostacyclin; t-PA, tissue-type plasminogen activator. *Source*: Modified from Refs. 8,9.

endothelial injury is repaired. Other causes of endothelial injury may also lead to the same sequence of events, including endothelial injury associated with systemic arterial hypertension, flow shear stress, smoking, diabetes, infection, aging, immune complex deposition, substance abuse most especially cocaine, and the placement of a coronary artery catheter or stent into a coronary artery.

Fissuring and ulceration of the plaque often but not always occur in the asymmetric portion or "shoulder region" where there is a thin fibrous cap and a lipid-laden plaque. Inflammation at sites of thin fibrous plaques with adjacent lipid cores best predicts the vulnerable atherosclerotic plaque and the one likely to fissure or ulcerate (4,5,19,20,22). Inflammation is characterized in the unstable plaque by the accumulation of monocyte-derived macrophages, activated T cells, and mast cells. Most likely, proteases released from the infiltrating mononuclear cells contribute to thinning of the fibrous cap through their degradation of collagen and subsequent atherosclerotic plaque fissuring and ulceration (Fig. 2) (22).

(A)

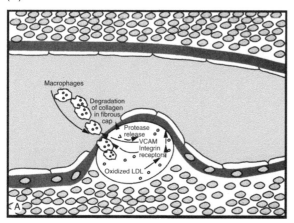

(B)

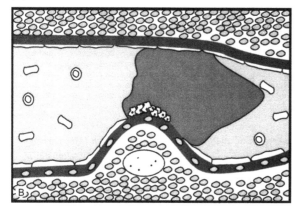

(C)

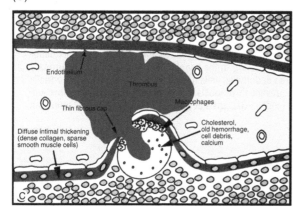

FIGURE 2 (**A**) Potential mechanisms responsible for atherosclerotic plaque fissuring and ulceration. Oxidized low-density lipoprotein (LDL) within the atherosclerotic plaque promotes the upregulation of vascular cell adhesion molecule (VCAM) and other integrins, resulting in the recruitment of inflammatory cells, primarily monocytes-derived macrophages but including activated T cells and mast cells; subsequent protease release from the mononuclear cells; and degradation of collagen in the fibrous cap, leading to its fissuring and ulceration. (**B**) Atherosclerotic plaque fissuring, leading to platelet adhesion and aggregation and thrombosis. (**C**) Atherosclerotic plaque ulceration and thrombosis. *Source*: Courtesy of Dr. Ward Casscells.

CLINICAL DETECTION OF MYOCARDIAL INFARCTION

Patients with MIs typically have severe chest pain, often left precordial and/or substernal, which may or may not radiate into the back, the left arm or sometimes the right arm, the neck, or the jaw. The pain is classically a great heaviness on the chest or "like an elephant on my chest," and is usually associated with diaphoresis and sometimes with nausea and vomiting. On occasion, the pain is located just in the jaw or the neck, the shoulders, the left or right arm, or in the back. Patients with acute MIs usually appear concerned and have a sense of impending doom. However, some patients have painless or "silent" MIs and present with complications of the MI rather than with pain, including heart failure, arrhythmias, a new murmur, hypotension, or sudden death. Patients with diabetes are especially likely to have silent MIs. It is estimated that as many as 20% of diabetics with MIs have silent ones. Similarly, patients after heart transplantation have subsequently silent MIs, if they have an MI. Some seemingly otherwise normal individuals have silent coronary heart disease, including silent MIs.

Electrocardiogram (ECG) of patients with NSTEMI classically shows ST depression and/or T wave flattening or inversion in the leads reflecting alterations in myocardial perfusion of the "culprit" artery. Unfortunately, these ECG changes are not diagnostic and are also seen in patients with stable angina, unstable angina, electrolyte abnormalities most especially hypokalemia; in patients receiving cardiac glycosides; and even in patients with anxiety or fright. The only evolution of these ECG alterations in patients with NSTEMI is a return to the normal pattern. This may occur over hours, days, or even months in some patients. In an occasional patient, one is unable to identify suggestive ECG changes of NSTEMI even though this has occurred. In patients with STEMI, the ECG alterations are generally definitive and allow rapid detection of the event. Classic initial ECG changes include ST segment elevation and T wave inversion. These changes progress to loss of R wave amplitude and development of a Q wave in the subsequent days. In patients with symptoms suggestive of MI, ST segment elevation is important in identifying persistent coronary artery thrombosis and patients that might benefit from either thrombolytic therapy or a percutaneous coronary intervention procedure (PCI), angioplasty (PTCA) and/or the placement of a stent. Other causes of chest pain and ST segment elevation include acute pericarditis, coronary artery spasm, myocardial ischemia in an area of old injury, recent cardioversion, and ventricular aneurysms. In patients with pericarditis, the ST segment elevation is usually generalized. In patients with coronary artery spasm, the ST segment elevation resolves usually within minutes of receiving nitrates or a calcium antagonist without evolution to Q waves. In patients with ventricular aneurysms, the ST segment elevation is persistent over months to years in the ECG leads that reflect the area of the aneurysm. In patients with ST segment elevation after electrical cardioversion, the ST segments return to baseline in the subsequent hours to days without evolution to Q waves.

PHYSICAL EXAMINATION

Patients with small MIs, particularly NSTEMIs, often have no detectable abnormality on physical examination. At the other extreme, patients with extensive damage to the left ventricle, usually those with anterior STEMIs and those with several previous MIs and a new MI with ≥40% irreversible injury of the LV mass, may develop "power-failure" complications of their MIs, including cardiogenic shock, severe LV failure, and/or medically refractory arrhythmias (23–31).

The findings on physical examination in patients with acute MIs depend primarily on the extent of the myocardial damage. Most patients are in obvious discomfort and diaphoretic. Those with extensive myocardial damage develop a reduction in systemic arterial pressure, ranging from mild to severe, including the development of cardiogenic shock. Cardiogenic shock is defined as hypotension resulting from extensive myocardial damage coexisting with evidence that the reduced blood pressure is inadequate for normal systemic perfusion so that cool skin, mental confusion, and oliguria are often present. Patients with extensive LV myocardial necrosis may also have an alternating pulse force (pulsus alternans) and frequent premature ventricular beats. Patients with MI may develop heart block, atrial fibrillation, and/or murmurs of mitral or tricuspid valvular insufficiency. Individuals with acute STEMI may have a precordial "ectopic impulse" which is an abnormally placed impulse over the left precordium, typically along the lower left sternal border or between the left sternal border and the cardiac apex. In patients with acute MI, the heart sounds are generally distant in the hours to days following the event. However, fourth heart sounds may be audible, and when ventricular failure or severe mitral insufficiency occurs, third heart sounds may be heard. When the mitral valve is damaged, a murmur of mitral insufficiency may be audible. These murmurs have variable auscultatory characteristics: they may be ejection in quality, peaking in intensity in mid to late systole, or they may be holosystolic. Intermittent myocardial ischemia with transient dysfunction of the posterior papillary muscle of the mitral valve leads to a murmur of papillary muscle dysfunction typically associated with mild to moderate mitral insufficiency. The murmur of papillary muscle dysfunction usually begins after the first sound, peaks in mid to late systole, and extends up to the second heart sound. Classically, it is heard at the cardiac apex and may radiate toward the left sternal border or into the axilla. If caused by transient myocardial ischemia, the murmur is a temporary one reflecting the transient nature of the mitral insufficiency. If the murmur is caused by MI leading to irreversible injury to a papillary muscle, the murmur is a permanent one. Rupture of a papillary muscle with acute MI causes severe mitral insufficiency, abrupt heart failure, and often cardiogenic shock. In these patients, the apical holosystolic murmur that one expects is often soft and sometimes not even audible. Acute mitral insufficiency occurs most commonly in patients with inferior or lateral STEMIs and in patients with STEMIs (26–28). Rupture of the interventricular septum, i.e., a ventricular septal defect most commonly occurs in patients with acute anterior MIs, although it may also occur in patient with an inferior MI (29–31). The murmur associated with a ventricular septal defect (VSD) is located along the lower left sternal border, is holosystolic, and is often associated with a left sternal border systolic thrill. With the development of pulmonary hypertension associated with a VSD, the systolic murmur becomes shorter, ultimately disappearing altogether with the development of severe pulmonary hypertension. Murmurs of relative mitral or tricuspid insufficiency occur in patients with LV or RV failure as a result of a spatial abnormality in the orientation of the papillary muscles of the mitral or tricuspid valves caused by marked dilatation of the left or right ventricle. Mitral and tricuspid insufficiency occurring in these patients is usually mild to moderate and diminishes in severity with diuresis and unloading therapy.

Abnormally split second heart sounds, i.e., "paradoxical splitting" of the second heart sound is characterized by a widening of the splitting of the second heart sound during expiration in patients with heart failure and in those with left bundle branch block. Left bundle branch block may occur in patients with acute anterior MIs and is generally associated with a large infarct.

Pericardial friction rubs are detected in some patients with STEMIs in the hours to days after the event. They are almost never found in patients with acute NSTEMIs. Patients with audible pericardial friction rubs are usually those with the largest MIs. When pericardial effusions develop in these patients, the heart sounds become distant and the jugular venous pressure elevated. This may progress to sufficient intrapericardial fluid accumulation to result in alteration in ventricular filling and emptying, i.e., the development of cardiac tamponade. When cardiac tamponade develops, the patient has a reduction in systolic blood pressure of >10 mmHg during inspiration ("pulsus paradoxus"), distant heart sounds, elevated jugular venous pressure, and clear lungs. This is a life-threatening occurrence and requires the immediate removal of the pericardial fluid either by catheter or surgical procedure.

Patients with large MIs or extensive myocardial injury from several previous MIs often develop heart failure. Pulmonary edema occurs with acute large anterior MIs and in those with new MIs who have had prior myocardial damage.

MYOCARDIAL STUNNING AND HIBERNATION

Transient myocardial ischemia followed by reperfusion may lead to protracted recovery of segmental ventricular function, known as myocardial stunning (32,33). Stunned myocardial segments may contribute to the development of heart failure when the area of ischemia or infarction is large. Alternatively, persistent ischemia can lead to chronic depression of segmental ventricular function, known as myocardial hibernation (34), which may also contribute to heart failure and can be reversed, thereby correcting severe CHF, in selected patients who undergo coronary artery revascularization either by PCI or coronary artery bypass grafting.

The acute development of left bundle branch block represents a problem in infarct detection electrocardiographically. The left bundle branch block pattern itself mimics what is seen in patients with prior anterior MIs in leads V_1–V_4 of the ECG. However, one may suspect the presence of a new MI in the patient with left bundle branch block when the patient has classic symptoms, and even when a silent MI occurs, when the left bundle branch block pattern is altered by the presence of diminutive R wave voltage, S waves, or initial Q waves in leads I, AVL, and/or V_5–V_6. Abnormal T wave vectors reversed from normal pattern in patients with

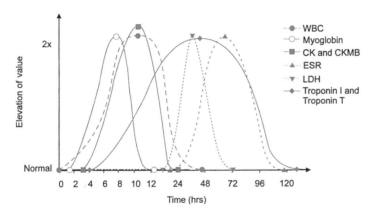

FIGURE 3 Typical changes in several enzymes measured in a patient with an evolving acute MI. Increases in serum myoglobin concentration are the earliest change indicative of MI. Note that the WBC count rises early after infarction and that the serum CK and CK-MB rise before the serum troponin I and T. The ESR and LDH rise relatively late after acute MI. *Abbreviations*: WBC, white blood cell; CK, Creative kinase; CK-MB, MB isoenzymeq CK; ESR, erythrocyte sedimentation rate; LDH, lactic dehydrogenase. *Source*: Modified from Ref. 35.

left bundle branch block, i.e., inverted T waves in V_1–V_3 and/or upright T waves in leads V_4–V_6 may also indicate anterior or lateral ischemia or infarction.

SEROLOGIC TESTS FOR MYOCARDIAL INFARCTION

The relationship of changes in cardiac enzyme concentrations and other intracellular myocardial substances to the development of acute MI is shown in Figure 3. Creatine kinase (CK) usually increases in the sera of patients two to three hours after the onset of acute MI, reaches a peak at 10 to 12 hours, and returns to normal within 24 hours in patients with small infarcts and in those who have reperfusion after endogenous thrombolysis or PCI (36–38). There are three isoenzymes of CK, and the CK-MB isoenzyme is relatively specific for heart muscle injury. In patients with large infarcts, and those who fail to have reperfusion, CK and CK-MB often peak later (18–24 hours after MI) and return to normal 30 to 40 hours after the event (36–38). Stuttering infarcts, defined as repeated episodes of infarction with recurrent chest pain over hours to days, result in repeated elevations of serum CK and CK-MB. Measurements of myoglobin in the peripheral circulation also allow the detection of acute MI, but there is no means to distinguish myoglobin released from the heart and skeletal muscle when both cardiac and skeletal muscle injury occur (39–41). Myoglobin increases occur earlier than CK after MI, i.e., within 30 minutes to two hours, peak earlier, six to eight hours, and return to normal sooner, i.e., within 10 to 12 hours (39–41). Measurement of myoglobin may be very useful in the rapid identification of MI in patients who have not had skeletal muscle injury from trauma, intramuscular injection, recent surgery, cardioversion, heat exposure, consumption of alcohol, or primary skeletal muscle disorders. Recently, however, measurements of cardiac troponins, either troponin I or T have replaced serum measurements of CK and CK-MB as the preferred marker for MI (42–45). Both troponin I and T are released into the systemic circulation within six to eight hours after acute MI or other forms of myocardial injury, and they may remain persistently elevated for at least two to three days after the event. In patients with renal failure, spurious elevations of troponin T and CK-MB have been occasionally found. Previous studies have shown that troponin I accurately reflects myocardial injury even in patients with renal failure (45).

PROGNOSIS

Three-dimensional estimates of the extent of myocardial damage are needed for accurate measurements of infarct size. These may be obtained using contemporary imaging methods, including single photon emission computed tomography (SPECT) (46–50), with magnetic resonance imaging (51), and with three-dimensional echocardiography. Distinction of reversibly ("viable" myocardium) and irreversibly injured myocardium can be made in patients by positron emission tomography (PET imaging) evaluations that combine estimates of myocardial perfusion (rubidium or other PET perfusion marker) and fluorodeoxyglucose studies to identify reversibly injured myocardium as regions with reduced perfusion but persistent metabolic activity. Persistent metabolic activity is indicated by uptake of fluorodeoxyglucose as would be expected to occur at sites of reversible injury when perfusion is markedly reduced or appears to be absent. One may also demonstrate reversible wall motion abnormalities using echocardiography, magnetic resonance imaging, or radionuclide ventriculography when potent inotropic stimuli, such as dobutamine, dopamine, or paired electrical stimulations are used and during low-level exercise five to seven days after myocardial infarction (50,52–55). The extent of myocardial scar may be identified by MR imaging (51).

EVALUATION OF VENTRICULAR FUNCTION

Invasive and noninvasive techniques can be used to allow more precise characterization of ventricular function in patients with reduced systemic arterial blood pressure and uncertain LV functional status. Flow-directed catheters, such as the Swan–Ganz catheter, allow measurement of LV filling pressure.

Measurement of LV filling pressure with the Swan–Ganz catheter enables one to differentiate hypotension caused by hypovolemia from cardiogenic shock and LV failure. Mean pulmonary capillary wedge pressures less than 12 mmHg with hypotension occur with hypovolemia and those ≥15 mmHg are usually associated with cardiogenic shock and LV failure. Cardiac output may be measured with the same catheter. The patient with an acute MI and shock should also have an indwelling arterial cannula placed to allow accurate measurement of systemic arterial pressure and to detect changes in it. The flow-directed pulmonary arterial catheter may also be utilized to help idealize mean pulmonary capillary wedge pressure, either with volume infusion with normal saline when the patient is hypovolemic or by diuresis when the patient is hypervolemic, at values of 15 to 18 mmHg in the hypotensive patient.

LV and RV function after acute MI can be assessed noninvasively with either dynamic myocardial scintigraphy, echocardiography, or magnetic resonance imaging (51,56–60). These methodologies allow measurement of ventricular ejection fraction, ventricular dimensions or volumes, and segmental wall motion. Two-dimensional echocardiography and transesophageal echocardiography with Doppler assessment allow the detection of LV thrombi, VSDs, and mitral insufficiency, as well as an estimation of their severity. Transesophageal echocardiography allows a more precise detection of small intracardiac thrombi than does transthoracic echocardiography.

BIOMARKERS

Several studies have shown that patients with unstable angina and STEMIs with elevated serum C-reactive protein (CRP) levels at hospital discharge, elevations in serum troponin I or T at hospital admission, and/or increases in serum interleukin-6 concentrations or of multiple biomarkers during their hospitalization have an increased risk of future coronary events, presumably reflecting the importance of inflammation in the instability of their unstable atherosclerotic plaques (Fig. 4) (61–80). Table 2 lists biomarkers that have been shown to be predictive of future cardiovascular events in patients with unstable angina and NSTEMI and those with coronary heart disease (61–80).

It has also been shown by Sabatine et al. that elevations in serum troponin, CRP, and brain natriuretic peptide (BNP) each provide unique prognostic information in patients with ACS (80). A relatively simple multimarker strategy that categorizes patients with ACS based on the number of elevated biomarkers at admission allows risk stratification over a range of short- and long-term major cardiac events (Fig. 4) (80).

Berk et al. (65) were among the first to demonstrate the prognostic importance of an increase in CRP in patients with acute coronary heart disease syndromes. Subsequently, several studies, including those by Maseri et al., demonstrated a poorer prognosis in patients with

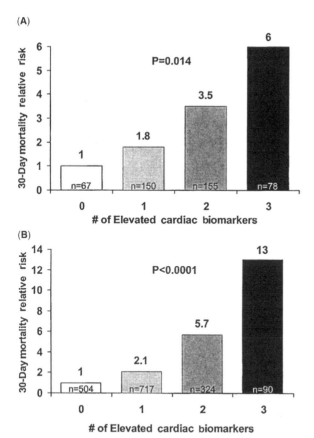

(A)

(B)

FIGURE 4 Relative 30-day mortality risks in OPUS-TIMI 16 and TACTICS-TIMI 18 in patients stratified by the number of elevated cardiac biomarkers. *Source*: Ref. 80, with permission of Lippincott, Williams, and Wilkins.

unstable angina who had increased serum CRP and serum amyloid-A protein values (67). Ridker et al. (71) and Koenig et al. (64) demonstrated that increases in serum CRP predict the development of future coronary events, even in otherwise apparently healthy individuals (64,71,80). In patients with NSTEMIs with CRP values ≥0.3 mg/dL, there is an increased risk of future coronary events, including the need for urgent coronary artery bypass surgery or angioplasty, cardiac death, and MI. Similar data have been provided for patients who have elevated serum fibrinogen values at hospital discharge (68).

Several groups have shown the importance of increases in serum levels of troponin I as prognostic factors indicative of increased risk for patients with ACS. Antman et al. (62) in a

TABLE 2 Biomarkers to Predict Prognosis in Patients with Unstable Angina and NSTEMI

1.	CRP
2.	BNP
3.	CD 40I
4.	Myeloperoxidase
5.	Pregnancy associated protein
6.	SAP
7.	VCAM
8.	ICAM
9.	Interleukin 6
10.	Asymmetric dimethylarginine
11.	Troponins
12.	Phospholipase A_2

Abbreviations: CRP, C-reactive protein; BNP, brain natriuretic peptide; SAP, serum amyloid protein; VCAM, vascular cell adhesion molecule; ICAM, intracellular adhesion molecule.

multicenter study of 1404 symptomatic patients found a relationship between mortality at 42 days and the serum cardiac troponin I levels at patient admission to the hospital (Fig. 5) (62). The mortality rate at 42 days was significantly higher in the 573 patients with cardiac troponin I levels ≥0.4 ng/mL than in the 831 patients with cardiac troponin I levels <0.4 ng/mL. For each increase of 1 ng/mL in the cardiac troponin I level, there was an associated significant increase in the risk ratio for death, after adjustment for baseline characteristics that were independently predictive of mortality. Similar data have been provided for serum values of troponin T in patients with unstable coronary heart disease. Lindahl et al. (61) found that the risk of cardiac events in these patients increased with increasing maximal levels of troponin T obtained in the initial 24 hours after admission. The lowest quartile (<0.06 μg/L) were a low-risk group, the second quartile (0.06–0.18 μg/L) an intermediate group, and the third highest quartile (≥0.18 μg/L) a relatively high-risk group with 4.3%, 10.5%, and 16% risk of either MI or cardiac death, or both, respectively (61). Biasucci et al. (70) demonstrated an increased risk for future coronary events in patients whose serum interleukin-6 levels increased during hospital admission. Other serum markers that when elevated are associated with future vascular and myocardial events include CD40l, serum amyloid protein (SAP), pregnancy associated protein, vascular cell adhesion molecule (VCAM), intracellular adhesion molecule (ICAM), and BNP (Table 2).

Stability of an atherosclerotic plaque depends largely on the structural integrity of its fibrous cap, which is composed primarily of extracellular matrix components rich in collagen. Available evidence supports a role for the release of matrix-degrading enzymes, i.e., matrix metalloproteinases (MMPs) in the catabolism of the structural macromolecules causing a dissolution of the fibrous cap of the plaque (81–85). Available evidence also suggests a probable role for MMP release in excess of their endogenous inhibitors (TIMPs) leading to degradation of collagen in the fibrous cap and the subsequent fissuring and ulceration that predisposes to unstable angina and acute MI. One proposed scheme includes oxidation of low-density lipoprotein (LDL) within the plaque and the chemoattractant influence of oxidized LDL and other oxidation products to promote the expression of adhesion molecules,

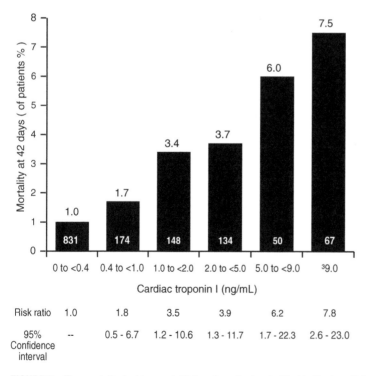

FIGURE 5   The mortality incidence at 42 days in patients admitted to the hospital with unstable angina or NSTEMI (non-Q wave MI) based on their initial cardiac troponin serum levels (nanograms per milligram). The number of patients in each category is shown within each black bar. *Source*: From Ref. 59. Copyright 1996 Massachusetts Medical Society. All rights reserved.

including VCAM and ICAM and the subsequent recruitment of monocyte-derived macrophages, activated T lymphocytes, and mast cells within the plaque. The release of selected MMPs in excess of their TIMP concentrations from monocyte-derived macrophages in the plaque degrades plaque collagen within the fibrous cap causing fissuring and ulceration of the atherosclerotic plaque.

TREATMENT
NSTEMI

Patients with NSTEMI and those with unstable angina are treated similarly. The objective of the treatment should be prevention of coronary artery thrombosis and its associated vasoconstriction at a vulnerable atherosclerotic plaque site where atherosclerotic plaque fissuring or ulceration has occurred. Although each patient should be considered and treated individually, potent antithrombotic therapies are generally used, and those patients that have increased serum levels of CRP and/or of a troponin should be referred for coronary arteriography and PCI or surgical revascularization when their coronary anatomy is appropriate (80,86–91). Recent data also suggest referral of patients for PCI or CABG when they have elevations of multiple serum biomarkers (i.e., CRP, troponin, and BNP) and for those with elevated TIMI risk scores (3–4 or more of the following: age of 65 years or older, at least three risk factors for coronary heart disease, prior coronary artery stenoses of 50% or greater, ST segment deviation on the ECG on presentation, at least two anginal events in the prior 24 hours, use of aspirin in the prior seven days, and elevated serum cardiac markers) (80,86–93). The initial medical treatment of patients with NSTEMI includes administration of aspirin, heparin (either low molecular weight or unfractionated), clopidogrel, and beta blocker if blood pressure or heart rate is elevated. Platelet glycoprotein IIb/IIIa inhibitor may be added for those with continuing angina at rest and/or for those with known or suspected complex coronary artery anatomy and for diabetic patients undergoing PCI. ACE inhibitors and beta blockers are added to the acute and chronic medical management regimen when there are no contraindications.

In patients with NSTEMI or rest angina, immediate hospitalization should occur in a coronary care unit to initiate the therapy mentioned above that might prevent on extend MI. Patients presenting with sustained and more severe chest pain, ECG changes of ST segment deviation, usually depression and T wave flattening or inversion, and elevated serum CK, the MB isoenzyme of CK, and either troponin I or T have NSTEMIs. They are treated in the manner described above and shown in Figure 6. In the medical treatment regimen, one attempts to prevent persistent thrombus formation at the site of an unstable plaque and to relieve the associated vasoconstriction. Aspirin is administered immediately to patients without contraindications. The dosage of aspirin does not appear to be critical, and beneficial results have been reported with both 81 mg and 325 mg given on a daily basis. Intravenous nitroglycerin is initiated beginning at doses of 1 to 2 µg/min with increases in dosage in increments of 5 µg/min to maintain systolic blood pressure in the 100 to 120 mmHg range avoiding systemic arterial hypotension and/or increases in heart rate above 100 beats/min. Pain relief often occurs after complete bed rest and the institution of intravenous nitroglycerin and aspirin. Elevated blood pressure should be controlled with nitrates, an ACE inhibitor, and/or a beta blocker. Patients with rest angina should be given a heparin, unless it is contraindicated. This may be done with unfractionated heparin intravenously, typically beginning with a bolus of approximately 3000 to 5000 units and followed by a sustained infusion of 900 to 1000 U/hour. The partial thromboplastin time (PTT) or activated coagulation time (ACT) is followed at 8 to 12 hour intervals, and the heparin infusion rate is adjusted using a weight-based regimen to maintain the PTT in the 60 to 70 second range or the ACT in the 250 to 350 second range. Alternatively, low-molecular-weight heparin may be given in appropriate dosage subcutaneously. In patients who are allergic to heparin, a direct thrombin inhibitor may be administered. In treating with a heparin or direct thrombin inhibitor, one is attempting to antagonize the effects of thrombin that promote thrombosis and vasoconstriction at sites of vascular injury. ACE inhibitors should be considered in the acute and chronic medical management of these patients when blood pressures and renal function allow. Angiotensin II promotes inflammation in addition to its vasoconstrictor effects and ACE inhibitors may decrease inflammation as they protect

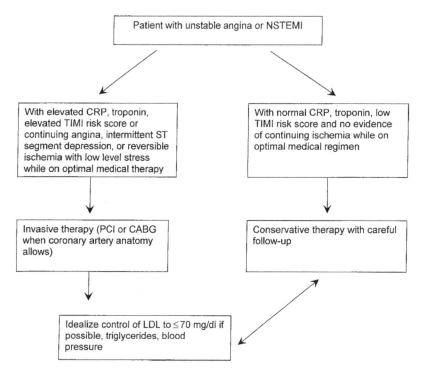

FIGURE 6 Treatment of patients with unstable angina and NSTEMI.

injured coronary arteries (94). However, elevated serum BUN and creatinine values may increase further with ACE therapy, especially in patients with unilateral or bilateral renal artery stenosis, thus limiting their utility. ACE inhibitors may promote potassium retention, and they should be avoided in patients with hyperkalemia. Immediate serum cholesterol and LDL lowering with a statin is also desirable; prompt rapid lowering of total cholesterol and LDL with a statin, such as atorvastatin (Lipitor), has been shown to reduce the risk of future events in patients with acute coronary syndromes (95,96). Beta blockers should be added to this therapy in patients without contraindications who have elevated blood pressure, increased heart rate due to pain or anxiety, or complex ventricular ectopy.

SPECIFIC THERAPIES: EVIDENCE BASED

One to four aspirin per day reduces the risk of death and MI in patients with unstable angina (97–100). However, ASA may not reduce the risk of MI in healthy postmenopausal women (101). Aspirin diminishes platelet aggregation and thromboxane A_2 synthesis and diminishes inflammation and platelet–white blood cell interactions. The combination of aspirin and heparin inhibits the effects of thromboxane A_2 and thrombin as potentiators of platelet aggregation leading to thrombosis and dynamic vasoconstriction. Their inhibition of thromboxane A_2 and thrombin improves regional myocardial blood flow and helps prevent thrombosis. Théroux et al. (97,102) have shown that the administration of heparin often relieves angina and reduces the risk for subsequent MI and death (Fig. 7). In the Théroux study (97), aspirin was also effective in reducing fatal and nonfatal MIs. Others have also shown similar protective effects from aspirin therapy in these patients (98,99). The combination of aspirin and heparin increases the risk of bleeding (97). Abrupt withdrawal of heparin in patients with NSTEMI may be associated with a heparin "rebound," with abrupt worsening of angina, the development of MI, or both (102,103). When heparin and other thrombin inhibitors are discontinued in these patients, it should be done slowly over a period of several hours and with concomitant administration of aspirin or other antiplatelet therapy.

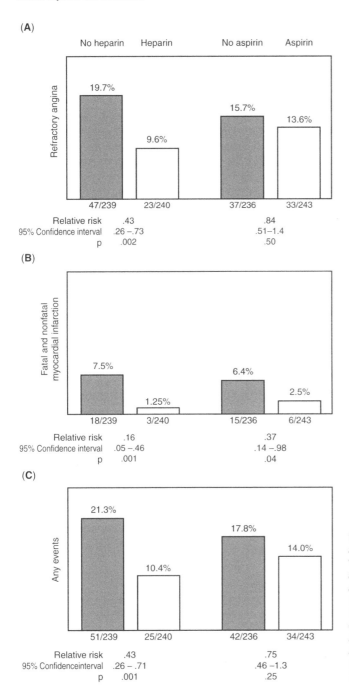

FIGURE 7 (**A–C**) The influence of aspirin and heparin in the treatment of patients with unstable angina pectoris. (**B**) Both aspirin and heparin reduce the risk for fatal and nonfatal myocardial infarction (MI). Heparin also reduces the frequency of important coronary events, including death, fatal and nonfatal MI, and continuing angina. The combination of heparin and aspirin was no more successful than heparin alone in this study. *Source*: From Ref. 97.

Low-molecular-weight heparin acts primarily through antithrombin III-mediated inhibition of factor Xa, but there is also some direct thrombin inhibition. There is evidence that anti-Xa activity relates to survival and efficacy in patients with acute coronary syndromes (104–108). Low anti-Xa activity on enoxaparin treatment was independently associated with a lower mortality rate at 30 days when anti-Xa activity was <0.5 I U /mL (108). As is true of conventional heparin, low-molecular-weight heparin promotes the release of tissue factor pathway inhibitor, which may also contribute to its antithrombotic effects.

Low-molecular-weight heparin is administered subcutaneously. Subcutaneous injections of fixed doses of low-molecular-weight heparin, generally on a two-times-per-day basis, provides a consistent anticoagulant and antithrombin effect. It is usually avoided in patients with elevated serum creatinine values of $\geq 2.5\,mg/dL$ because renal insufficiency potentiates the effect of any particular dose. Instead, unfractionated heparin is given to these patients. In patients with HIT or HITS, low-molecular-weight heparin may still not be safe as there is some cross-reactivity between the heparin antibody and low-molecular-weight heparin. Therefore, a direct acting thrombin inhibitor may be needed if an inhibitor of thrombin is to be used in patients with serum antibodies to heparin.

The influence of low-molecular-weight heparin in patients with NSTEMI was evaluated in the Fragmin during Instability in Coronary Artery Disease (FRISC) study (109). In Table 3, this double-blind trial, 1506 patients were randomly assigned to receive low-molecular-weight heparin, subcutaneous dalteparin (Fragmin), 120 IU/kg body weight with a maximal dose of 10,000 IU given twice daily for six days, and then 7500 IU once daily for the next 35 to 45 days, or placebo. The primary endpoint was the rate of new MI and death during the first six days after initiating treatment. Secondary endpoints were rates of death and new MI after 40 days and 150 days, respectively; the frequency of revascularization procedures; the need for heparin infusion; and a composite endpoint.

Patients were recruited at 23 Swedish hospitals. Eligible patients were men older than 40 years and women more than one year after menopause admitted to the hospital with chest pain in the previous 72 hours. Patients without contraindications received aspirin, 75 mg daily after an initial dose of 300 mg, beta blockers, and calcium antagonists and nitrates as needed. Nitroglycerin was given intravenously at the discretion of the attending physician.

Within the first six days, the rates of new MI and death were lower in the dalteparin group than in the placebo group (1.8% vs. 4.8%, risk ratio 0.37). The frequency of the need for intravenous heparin and revascularization was also reduced by dalteparin treatment. The composite endpoint of death, MI, revascularization, and need for intravenous heparin were also significantly reduced in favor of dalteparin. At 40 days, the differences in rates of MI and death and in the composite endpoint persisted, although subgroup analyses showed that the effect was confined to nonsmokers at this time. Survival analysis showed a risk of reactivation and reinfarction when the dose of dalteparin was decreased; this was especially pronounced in nonsmokers. By four to five months after treatment, there were no significant differences in the rates of death, new MI, or revascularization. This regimen was safe, and patient compliance was good among the treated patients.

This study demonstrated the benefits of thrombin inhibition in the treatment of patients with NSTEMI. However, a potential advantage of low-molecular-weight heparin therapy is the ability to continue it after hospital discharge with continued suppression of thrombin's effects. In this study, the effects of long-term treatment with low-molecular-weight heparin appeared

TABLE 3 Absolute Frequency of Primary and Separate Endpoints for Patients in the FRISC Study

	Placebo ($n = 749$)	Dalteparin ($n = 726$)	Risk ratio (95% CI)	P
Primary endpoints				
Death or MI	116 (15.5%)	102 (14.0%)	0.90 (0.71–1.15)	0.41
Death, MI, or revascularization	326 (43.6%)	296 (40.6%)	0.92 (0.82–1.04)	0.18
Death, MI, revascularization, or intravenous heparin	337 (45.1%)	312 (42.7%)	0.94 (0.84–1.05)	0.28
Exclusion of revascularization for ischemia				
Death, MI, revascularization because of angina	214 (28.7%)	175 (24.1%)	0.84 (0.70–0.99)	0.039
Death, MI, revascularization because of angina, or intravenous heparin	241 (32.3%)	204 (28.1%)	0.87 (0.74–1.01)	0.066
Separate endpoints				
Death[a]	41 (5.5%)	39 (5.4%)	0.98 (0.64–1.50)	
MI[a]	98 (13.4%)	83 (11.7%)	0.86 (0.66–1.14)	0.30
Revascularization	254 (35.5%)	229 (32.9%)	0.92 (0.79–1.06)	0.23
Revascularization because of angina	131 (18.4%)	87 (12.5%)	0.68 (0.53–0.86)	0.002
Heparin infusion	121 (16.7%)	83 (11.9%)	0.71 (0.55–0.91)	0.008

[a]Separate statistical analyses of death and MI not planned in protocol.
Abbreviations: CI, confidence interval; MI, myocardial infarction.
Source: From Ref. 109. Copyright 2001, with permission from Elsevier.

to be primarily confined to nonsmokers, which constituted 80% of the patient population. Efforts at reducing the dose of the low-molecular-weight heparin resulted in a risk of reinfarction that was most pronounced in nonsmokers.

Low-molecular-weight heparin is an alternative to unfractionated heparin in the patient with NSTEMI (109). In patients with unstable angina and NSTEMI, there is an ongoing risk of MI or reinfarction in the subsequent four to six weeks probably related to persistent endothelial injury after plaque ulceration and fissuring and the time required for its repair. The authors believe that as long as the endothelium remains anatomically disrupted and/or dysfunctional the patient has a continuing risk of thrombosis and MI.

In the TIMI 11 study, patients with NSTEMI (and unstable angina) were randomized to receive either (1) unfractionated heparin for approximately three days followed by placebo injections subcutaneously or (2) uninterrupted antithrombin therapy with enoxaparin during the acute phase (104,106). A total of 3910 patients were randomized, and the primary endpoint was death, MI, or urgent revascularization. The primary endpoint occurred by 8 days in 14.5% of patients in the unfractionated heparin group, in 12.4% in the enoxaparin group ($P = 0.048$), by 43 days in 19.7% of patients who received unfractionated heparin, and in 17% of those who received enoxaparin ($P = 0.048$). In the hospital, all patients received aspirin (100–325 mg daily). During the outpatient phase, major hemorrhage occurred in 1.5% of the group treated with placebo and 2.9% of the patients treated with enoxaparin ($P = 0.02$). Thus, the TIMI 11 data suggest that enoxaparin is superior to unfractionated heparin for reducing a composite endpoint of death and serious cardiac ischemic events during the management of patients with NSTEMI (and unstable angina) without a significant increase in the rate of major hemorrhage.

The FRISC and TIMI 11 trials have shown the utility of low-molecular-weight heparin in the treatment of patients with NSTEMI. These trials suggest that low-molecular-weight heparin may be clinically superior to unfractionated heparin in reducing the risk of MI and death and the need for revascularization in patients with NSTEMI. This benefit is achieved at increased risk of minor bleeding and, when continued in the outpatient phase, in minor–major bleeding. Thus, one should seriously consider the use of low-molecular-weight heparin in the treatment of these patients who are not allergic to heparin during the inpatient phase of therapy.

Direct thrombin antagonists will be useful alternatives to heparins in patients who develop thrombocytopenia and/or vascular thrombosis or bleeding as an allergic response to heparin administration—heparin-induced thrombocytopenia (HIT) and heparin-induced thrombosis syndromes (HITS). The direct inhibitors of thrombin have more reliable and consistent effects on PTT than does heparin, allowing much less frequent measurement of PTT or ACT; some patients are managed without follow-up measurements of PTT or ACT.

PLATELET GLYCOPROTEIN IIB/IIIA RECEPTOR ANTAGONISTS

A platelet GP IIb/IIIa receptor antagonist may be added to this therapeutic regimen in patients who continue to have rest angina despite this medical regimen, who will undergo interventional therapy (PCI), percutaneous transluminal coronary angioplasty (PTCA), or stenting. The platelet GP IIb/IIIa inhibitors may be especially useful in diabetic patients (110,111) and in those patients with elevations of a serum troponin, who will undergo PCI (112). Intra-aortic balloon counterpulsation almost always relieves rest pain in the patient with NSTEMI (and unstable angina). In patients with continuing rest angina, proceeding to coronary arteriography and PCI, or CABG is urgently needed. If possible, platelet GP IIb/IIIa inhibitors need to be discontinued several days prior to CABG (usually more than 3 days) to avoid severe intraoperative bleeding that would otherwise occur and that is treated with multiple infusions of fresh platelets from untreated patients.

CLOPIDOGREL

Clopidogrel (Plavix) blocks ADP receptors inhibiting platelet aggregation. Thus, clopidogrel exerts a powerful inhibitory effect on platelet aggregation at sites of atherosclerotic plaque fissuring and ulceration.

Yusuf et al. studied the early and late effects of adding clopidogrel in the treatment of patients with ACS (113). A total of 12,562 patients with ACS were randomized to receive clopidogrel or placebo for 3 to 12 months. Clopidogrel and placebo were added to aspirin therapy in these patients. The proportion of patients experiencing cardiovascular death, MI, or strokes at 30 days was 5.4% in the placebo group and 4.3% in the actively treated group, with a relative risk of 0.79. Beyond 36 days, the corresponding rates were 6.3% versus 5.2% (relative risk 0.82). There was no significant increase in life-threatening bleeding either to 30 days or 12 months, but clopidogrel-treated patients had increased minor and major bleeding and required more blood transfusions. Careful evaluation of the early treatment data showed benefit within 24 hours of treatment with consistently lower rates of adverse outcomes. Thus, clopidogrel should usually be added to aspirin and nitrates and a thrombin inhibitor (a heparin) in the immediate therapy of ACS patients. In patients that are selected for CABG, clopidogrel should be discontinued for at least five days in advance of the surgery with the demonstration of a return to relatively normal platelet aggregation in response to ADP challenge prior to elective or semi-elective CABG. Otherwise, there is a major risk of bleeding intra- and post-operatively. Major bleeding associated with clopidogrel administration is treated with infusions of fresh platelets from untreated patients.

In the CURE trial, there was an approximately 20% reduction in the risk of vascular death, MI, and stroke after nine months of therapy with both aspirin and clopidogrel (113,114). There were 2658 patients who underwent PCI in the CURE trial, a median of 10 days after enrollment. Among these patients, there was a relative reduction in cardiovascular death, MI, or urgent revascularization from the PCI procedure through 30 days of 30% ($P = 0.03$). From the time of the PCI procedure through the remainder of the 12 month follow-up, there was a relative risk reduction of 25% ($P = 0.047$) (113–115).

PLATELET GLYCOPROTEIN IIB/IIIA RECEPTORS

Figure 8 identifies the process of platelet activation and aggregation and the inhibition of platelet aggregation by inhibitors of GP IIb/IIIa receptors. Platelet activation causes changes in the shape of platelets and conformational changes in the GP IIb/IIIa receptors, transforming the receptors from a ligand-unreceptive to a ligand-receptive state. Ligand-receptive GP IIb/IIIa receptors bind fibrinogen molecules, which form bridges between adjacent platelets and facilitate platelet aggregation. Inhibitors of GP IIb/IIIa receptors bind to the GP IIb/IIIa receptors blocking the binding of fibrinogen, thereby preventing platelet aggregation. GP IIb/IIIa receptors are the most abundant on the platelet surface with approximately 50,000 copies per platelet. The most important clinical interaction of the GP IIb/IIIa receptors is with fibrinogen, but this receptor has also been shown to bind other adhesive proteins involved in platelet aggregation, including fibronectin, vitronectin, and von Willebrand factor.

Resting platelets do not express GP IIb/IIIa receptors in a configuration suitable for ligand binding, but with platelet activation, this complex undergoes conformational changes that allow it to bind avidly to fibrinogen (Fig. 8). Once activated, the original platelet mono-layer recruits additional platelets, eventually forming a platelet thrombus through GP IIb/IIIa-fibrinogen–GP IIb/IIIa bridging (Fig. 8). This process continues as new platelets enter the injured vascular bed, become activated by local mediators, express GP IIb/IIIa receptors in the appropriate conformation, and become incorporated into the growing thrombus. An area of previously denuded endothelium resulting from fissuring or ulceration of an atherosclerotic plaque is covered by the growing platelet thrombus (9).

The clinical utility of inhibitors of GP IIb/IIIa receptors in the treatment of patients with ACS, including patients with unstable angina and NSTEMI, has been previously demonstrated (117–125) (Table 5).

PLATELET GLYCOPROTEIN IIB/IIIA RECEPTOR ANTAGONISTS

There are three available platelet GP IIb/IIIa receptor antagonists. They are abciximab (ReoPro), tirofiban (Aggrastat), and eptifibatide (Integrelin) (117–124). Abciximab is a recombinant human-murine chimeric Fab fragment that binds irreversibly to the platelet GP IIb/IIIa receptor with a short plasma half-life of 10 minutes. ReoPro also binds to the $\alpha_2\beta_3$ (vitronectin) receptor and the leukocyte receptor, MAC-1.

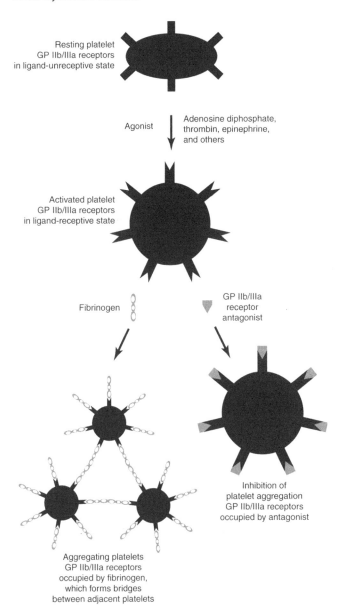

FIGURE 8 (**A**) The activation of platelets, the expression of glycoprotein (GP) IIb/IIIa receptors in a ligand-receptive state, and the protective role played by GP IIb/IIIa receptor antagonists are demonstrated. Platelets aggregate by binding to one another through fibrinogen, which occupies the GP IIb/IIIa receptors, allowing platelets to aggregate in a fibrin mesh. (**B**) Aggregating platelets develop thrombi at sites of endothelial injury. (*Top*): As they aggregate, they degranulate and are transformed into balloon-shaped cells binding to one another through their GP IIb/IIIa-fibrinogen–binding sites. (*Bottom*): A stable thrombus is formed. Source: (**A**) From Ref. 16; (**B**) from Ref. 8.

Tirofiban is a low-molecular-weight non-peptide GP IIb/IIIa receptor antagonist that has a plasma half-life of 1.3 hours and reversible binding to the GP IIb/IIIa receptors. It has no interaction with vitronectin or MAC-1 receptors.

Eptifibatide (Integrelin) is a peptide that competitively inhibits the RGD sequence of GP IIb/IIIa receptors with a long plasma half-life of 150 minutes. Both eptifibatide and tirofiban are cleared by the kidneys and require dose adjustments in patients with renal failure. Eptifibatide, like tirofiban, does not inhibit the vitronectin or MAC-1 receptors.

In the c7E3 Antiplatelet Therapy in Unstable Refractory Angina (CAPTURE) study (125), patients with refractory unstable angina were randomized to receive a monoclonal antibody to the platelet GP IIb/IIIa receptors (abciximab) or placebo for 18–24 hours before PTCA and continuing for one hour afterward. The primary endpoint was the occurrence within 30 days after PTCA of death, MI, or urgent intervention for recurrent ischemia. By 30 days, the primary endpoint had occurred in 71 (11%) of 630 patients who received abciximab compared with 101 (16%) of 635 placebo recipients ($P = 0.01$). The frequency of MI was lower in the abciximab-treated patients than in the placebo-treated patients before PTCA [four patients (0.6%)

compared with 13 patients (2.1%), $P = 0.029$] and during PTCA [16 patients (2.6%) vs. 34 patients (5.5%), $P = 0.009$]. Major bleeding was infrequent, but it occurred more often with abciximab than with placebo [24 patients (3.8%) vs. 12 patients (1.9%), $P = 0.04$]. The protective effect of abciximab was not sustained after therapy, and at six months follow-up, death, MI, or repeat intervention had occurred in 193 patients in each group. This study demonstrated that in patients with refractory unstable angina, abciximab reduces the rate of thrombotic complications, especially MI before, during, and after PTCA, even in patients receiving nitrates and heparin. There was no evidence that this regimen influenced the rate of MI or the need for subsequent revascularization in the days following discontinuation of therapy.

The Platelet Glycoprotein IIb/IIIa in Unstable Angina: Receptor Suppression Using Integrilin Therapy (PURSUIT) trial was the largest done to date involving a GP IIb/IIIa receptor antagonist in patients with unstable angina (119). Ten thousand nine hundred forty-eight patients in 28 countries were randomized to one of two doses of eptifibatide (Integrilin) or placebo. All patients randomized to eptifibatide received a 180 µg/kg bolus and either a 1.3 µg/kg min or a 2.0 µg/kg min infusion for 72 hours. After 1487 patients received a moderate-dose infusion of 1.3 µg/kg min of eptifibatide, this arm was discontinued because the higher-dose arm had a similarly acceptable safety profile. The primary endpoint of the trial was a composite all-cause mortality and nonfatal MI or reinfarction at 30 days after therapy. Secondary endpoints included death and MI or reinfarction at 30 days, the composite at 96 hours and seven days, and safety and efficacy outcome in patients undergoing PCIs. At the time of enrollment, 45% of the patients had NSTEMIs. Aspirin was administered to 93% and heparin to 90% of the patients in the study. Eptifibatide reduced the composite endpoint from 15.7% to 14.2% ($P = 0.03$), a 10% relative reduction in death and nonfatal MI.

In the Platelet Receptor Inhibition in Ischemic Syndrome Management (PRISM) study, 3232 patients with unstable angina were randomized to receive either intravenous tirofiban (a low-molecular-weight, nonpeptide, nonantibody inhibitor of the GP IIb/IIIa receptor) or heparin for 48 hours (Table 4) (120). The primary endpoint was a composite of death, MI, or refractory ischemia. The incidence of the composite endpoint was 32% lower at 48 hours in patients who received tirofiban (3.8% versus 5.6% with heparin). Percutaneous revascularization was performed in 1.9% of the patients during the first 48 hours. At 30 days, the frequency of the composite endpoint with the addition of re-admission for unstable angina was similar in the two groups (15.9% in the tirofiban group vs. 17% in the heparin group). There was a trend toward a reduction in the rate of death or MI with tirofiban, 5.8% compared with 7% in the heparin group, but this did not reach statistical significance. Mortality was 2.3% in the tirofiban group compared with 3.6% in the heparin group ($P = 0.02$). Major bleeding occurred in 0.4% of the patients in both groups. Reversible thrombocytopenia occurred more frequently in tirofiban-treated patients than in heparin-treated ones (1.1% vs. 0.4%, $P = 0.04$).

In the Platelet Receptor in Ischemic Syndrome Management in Patients Limited by Unstable Signs and Symptoms (PRISM-PLUS) study, tirofiban was given to patients with unstable angina and non-Q wave MI in 1915 patients randomly assigned in a double-blind manner to receive tirofiban, heparin, or tirofiban and heparin (121). Patients received aspirin if not contraindicated. The study drugs were infused for a mean of 71 ±20 hours, during which time coronary angiography and angioplasty were performed after 48 hours when clinically indicated. The composite primary endpoint consisted of death, MI, and refractory ischemia within seven days after randomization.

The study was stopped prematurely in the group receiving tirofiban alone because of an excess mortality at seven days, 4.6% compared with 1.1% for the patients treated with heparin alone. The frequency of the composite primary endpoint at seven days was lower among the patients who received tirofiban and heparin than among those who received heparin alone (12.9% vs. 17.9%, risk ratio 0.68, $P = 0.004$). The composite endpoint for the tirofiban plus heparin group was also reduced compared with that in the heparin-only group at 30 days (18.5% vs. 22%, $P = 0.03$) and at six months (27.7% vs. 32%, $P = 0.02$). At seven days, the frequency of death or MI was 4.9% in the tirofiban and heparin group as contrasted with 8% in the heparin-only group ($P = 0.006$). Comparable data at 30 days were 8.7% and 11.9% ($P = 0.03$), respectively, and at six months, 12% and 15% ($P = 0.06$). The protection from tirofiban and heparin was consistent in the various subgroups of patients, both in those treated

TABLE 4 Clinical Outcomes of the PARAGON, PRISM, PRISM-PLUS, and PURSUIT Trials in Which GP IIb/IIIA Antagonists Were Used to Treat Patients with Unstable Angina Pectoris and Non-Q Wave Myocardial Infarction

Characteristic	Paragon			Prism		Prism-plus			Pursuit		
	Placebo	Lamifiban 1 μg/min ± heparin	Lamifiban 5 μg/min ± heparin	Heparin	Tirofiban 0.15 μg/kg min	Heparin	Heparin + tirofiban 0.10 μg/kg min	Tirofiban 0.15 μg/kg min	Placebo	Eptifibatide 1.3 μg/kg min	Eptifibatide 20 μg/kg min
n	758	755	769	1616	1616	797	773	345	4739	1487	4722
30-Day outcome											
Death (%)	2.9	3.0	3.6	3.6	2.3	4.5	3.6	(6.1)	3.7	(3.4)	3.5
Nonfatal MI (%)	10.6	9.4	10.9	4.3	4.1	9.2	6.6	(9.0)	13.5	(12.0)	12.6
Death or MI (%)											
Overall	11.7	10.6	12.0	7.1	5.8	11.9	8.7	(13.6)	15.7	(13.4)	14.2
Relative reduction (%)		9	−6		18		27				10
PTCA patients				9.1	7.2	10.2	5.9		16.8		11.8
Non-PTCA patients				6.2	3.6	7.8	3.6		15.7		14.6
6-Month outcome											
Death (%)	6.6	5.2	6.8			7.0	6.9	(7.2)	6.2		6.4
Nonfatal MI (%)	14.3	10.8	12.9			10.5	8.3	(10.1)	15.7		14.7
Death or MI (%)	17.9	13.7	16.4			15.3	12.3	(15.9)	19.0		17.8
Relative reduction (%)		23	8				20				8
Major bleeding (%)[a]	3.0	3.0	6.0	0.4	0.4	0.8	1.4		1.3		3.0
Intracranial hemorrhage (%)	0	0	0.1	0.1	0.1	0	0		0.1		0.1
RBC transfusion (%)[b]	4.4	4.4	8I7	1.4	2.4	2.8	4.0		1.8		4.4
Thrombocytopenia (%)[c]	1.1	1.5	1.3	0.1	0.4	0.3	0.5		0.4		0.6

[a]Major bleeding as defined by intracranial hemorrhage or decrease in hemoglobin ≤5 g/dL not associated with CABG.
[b]Transfusions reported are not associated with CABG, except for PARAGON.
[c]Thrombocytopenia defined as platelet count ≥50,000 mm.

Abbreviations: MI, myocardial infarction; PARAGON, Platelet IIb/IIIa Antagonism for the Reduction of Acute Coronary Syndrome Events in a Global Organization Network; PRISM, Platelet Receptor Inhibition in Ischemic Syndrome Management; PRISM-PLUS, Platelet Receptor Inhibition in Ischemic Syndrome Management in Patients Limited by Unstable Signs and Symptoms; PTCA, percutaneous transluminal coronary angioplasty; PURSUIT, Platelet Glycoprotein IIb/IIIa in Unstable Angina; Receptor Suppression Using Integrilin Therapy; RBC, red blood cell. Numbers in parentheses are from discontinued treatment arms and are not contemporaneous; these are listed only for completeness, not direct comparisons.
Source: From Ref. 116 with permission.

medically and in those treated with PTCA. Major bleeding occurred in 3% of the patients receiving heparin alone and 4% of the patients receiving combination therapy.

The conclusion of this study is that when administered with heparin and aspirin the platelet GP IIb/IIIa receptor inhibitor, tirofiban, reduces the risk of death or MI in patients with unstable angina and NSTEMI (121).

GP IIb/IIIa receptor antagonists, including the monoclonal antibody (abciximab), synthetic peptide (eptifibatide), and nonpeptide, low-molecular-weight inhibitor (tirofiban), when added to aspirin and heparin in patients with unstable angina pectoris and NSTEMI reduce the risks of MI, death, and need for interventional therapy during their administration. This benefit is particularly apparent in patients having PCI. Recent studies suggest that the platelet GP IIb/IIIa receptor antagonists have their greatest efficacy in patients with unstable angina and NSTEMI with elevated troponin values (112). However, the evidence is compelling that the platelet glycoprotein IIb/IIIa receptor antagonists exert their protective effects primarily in patients with ACS that will have PCI, especially in diabetic patients and those with complex coronary artery lesions (86,111,118,122–124).

In the Evaluation of Platelet IIb/IIIa Inhibitors for Stenting (EPISTENT) study, abciximab therapy reduced the risk of MI, death, and need for subsequent intervention in patients with diabetes mellitus to levels comparable to those found in nondiabetic patients (122). Previously, it had been shown that PCI in patients with diabetes mellitus often fails to provide important long-term beneficial results and have suggested superiority of CABG over PCI in diabetic patients. Thus, this is a potentially important finding of the EPISTENT study; however, not all subsequent studies have confirmed a long-term protective effect for abciximab therapy in patients with diabetes and this needs further evaluation.

The Evaluation of PTCA to Improve Long-term Outcome by the c7E3 GP IIb/IIIa Receptor Blockade (EPILOG) study (123) demonstrated that the benefits of abciximab therapy in patients with coronary heart disease undergoing angioplasty extend to both low- and high-risk patients. The earlier Evaluation of IIb/IIIa Platelet Receptor Antagonist 7E3 in Preventing Ischemic Complications (EPIC) study (124) had shown that abciximab therapy reduced the risk of subsequent MI, death, and need for a second intervention in high-risk patients undergoing PTCA. In the EPIC study, high-risk patients were those with unstable angina, recent NSTEMI, and complicated coronary arterial lesions (124).

In several of the previously mentioned interventional studies using abciximab, composite endpoints were favorably influenced through six months and longer, especially when initial treatment was followed by PCI.

CONSERVATIVE VERSUS INTERVENTIONAL THERAPY

The TIMI 18 study suggests that patients with NSTEMI (and those with unstable angina) who have elevations in serum CRP or troponin levels on admission and those with a TIMI risk factor score of 3 or greater have reductions in subsequent risk of death, MI and need for future intervention when treated by PCI or CABG (Fig. 9) (86,87,89,91,92). Women with ACS seem particularly likely to benefit from interventional therapy when admitted with elevated serum CRP and troponin I (101).

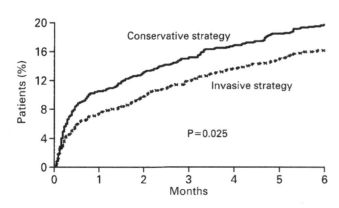

FIGURE 9 Cumulative incidence of the primary endpoint of death, nonfatal MI, or rehospitalization for an acute coronary syndrome during the six-month follow-up. The rate of the primary endpoint was lower in the invasive-strategy group than in the conservative-strategy group (15.9% vs. 19.4%, *p* = 0.025). *Source*: Ref. 126. Copyright © 2001 Massachusetts Medical Society. All rights reserved.

TABLE 5 Summary of Results of Randomized Interventional Trials in Patients with Unstable Angina/Non-Q Wave Myocardial Infarction and Other Patients with Limiting Angina and Complex Coronary Artery Lesions Who Underwent an Interventional Procedure and Were Treated by Glycoprotein IIb/IIIa Antagonists: 30-Day Efficacy Endpoint Figures

	Death (%)	MI (%)	Urgent PCI (%)	Urgent CABG (%)
EPIC trial				
Placebo	1.7	8.6	4.5	3.6
Abciximab bolus	1.3	6.2	3.6	2.3
Abciximab bolus + infusion	1.7	5.2	0.8	2.4
EPILOG trial				
Placebo	0.8	8.7	3.8	1.7
Abciximab + reduced heparin	0.3	3.7	1.2	0.4
Abciximab + standard heparin	0.4	3.8	1.5	0.9
EPISTENT trial				
Placebo + stent	0.6	9.6	1.2	1.1
Abciximab + stent	0.3	4.5	0.6	
Abciximab + PTCA	0.8	5.3	1.3	0.6
IMPACT II trial				
Placebo	1.1	8.1	2.8	2.8
Eptifibatide 135/0.5 dose	0.5	6.6	2.6	1.6
Eptifibatide 135/0.75 dose	0.8	6.9	2.9	2.0
RESTORE trial[a]				
Placebo	0.7	5.7	4.0	1.4
Tirofiban	0.8	4.2	2.3	1.1
CAPTURE trial				
Placebo	1.3	8.2	4.4	1.7
Abciximab	1.0	4.1	3.1	1.0
RAPPORT trial[b]				
Placebo	2.1	4.1	5.4	1.2
Abciximab	2.5	3.3	1.7	0
TARGET trial				
Tirofiban				
Abciximab				

[a]RESTORE trial endpoints listed here are for published post hoc analysis including only *urgent* repeat revascularization for consistency with the other trials. The primary composite endpoint of RESTORE included *urgent or elective* repeat revascularization. RESTORE trial endpoints listed here differ from those of the other trials in that only patients in whom the lesion was successfully crossed with the guidewire were included in the efficacy analysis of RESTORE, providing a "treated patient" analysis rather than the "intention-to-treat" analysis utilized in the other studies.
[b]RAPPORT endpoints listed here are for the secondary composite of death, myocardial reinfarction, and urgent *target vessel* revascularization. This endpoint differs from those of the other trials in that it does not include urgent *nontarget vessel* revascularization procedures.
Abbreviations: CABG, coronary artery bypass graft surgery; CAPTURE, c7E3 Fab Antiplatelet Therapy in Unstable Refractory Angina; EPIC, Evaluation of IIb/IIIa Platelet Receptor Antagonist 7E3 in Preventing Ischemic Complications; EPILOG, Evaluation of PTCA to Improve Long-term Outcome by c7E3 GP IIb/IIIa Receptor Blockade; EPISTENT, Evaluation of Platelet IIb/IIIa Inhibitor for Stenting; IMPACT, Integrilin (eptifibatide) to Minimize Platelet Aggregation and Coronary Thrombosis; MI, myocardial infarction; PCI, percutaneous coronary intervention; RAPPORT, ReoPro and Primary PTCA Organization and Randomized Trial; RESTORE, Randomized Efficacy Study of Tirofiban for Outcomes and REstenosis.
Source: From Ref. 116 with permission.

In the TIMI risk score for patients with NSTEMI (and those with unstable angina) (87,88), patients are risk stratified on the basis of seven baseline characteristics that had been identified earlier in the chapter. On the basis of their TIMI risk scores, they are then categorized as "low risk" (0–2 points), "intermediate risk" (3 or 4 points), or "high risk" (5–7 points). These categories have been shown to have prognostic predictive ability (87,88). A recent study has shown that upstream platelet GP IIb/IIIa inhibition and coronary artery stenting are useful in the invasive management of patients with NSTEMI with intermediate or high risk TIMI scores (OR, 1.39 in low-risk, 0.80 in intermediate-risk, and 0.57 in high-risk patients) (89).

ANGIOTENSIN CONVERTING ENZYME INHIBITORS

Several large-scale clinical trials have demonstrated improved survival with ACE inhibitor therapy begun during acute MI (94). There are data available for 98,496 patients from four clinical trials involving more than 1000 patients each in whom ACE inhibitor therapy was begun in the acute phase (0–36 hours) of MI and continued for four to six weeks (94). Thirty-day mortality was 7%

among patients treated with ACE inhibitors and 7.6% among control patients, i.e., 7% proportional reduction ($P < 0.004$). This represents reductions in deaths of five per 1000 patients. Most of the benefits seen occurred in the first week of treatment. The absolute benefit was more marked in selected high-risk groups, including patients with Killip Class 2 or 3 heart failure, heart rate >100 bpm at entry and in patients with anterior MIs. ACE inhibitor therapy also reduced the incidence of non-fatal CHF, but it was also associated with an excess of persistent hypotension and renal dysfunction (1.3% vs. 0.6%, $P < 0.01$). These data suggest the potential benefit of ACE inhibitors in the early treatment of MIs in patients with anterior MIs, those with CHF, and those at increased risk of MI and death in whom there is no contraindication (94). It should be emphasized, however, that these trials were not conducted exclusively in patients with NSTEMI (and unstable angina), so the application of the data to these select patient groups needs to be done with caution.

Acute Lipid Lowering with a Statin

Waters and coworkers evaluated the effects of high dose atorvastatin given to patients with NSTEMI (and unstable angina) on the incidence of death, nonfatal MI, resuscitated cardiac arrest, or recurrent symptomatic myocardial ischemia (95). The primary endpoint was reduced from 17% in the placebo group to 15% in the Atorvastatin group in the 16 weeks of the trial ($P = 0.048$) (MIRACL Study) (95). This same therapy reduced the overall cerebrovascular accident rate by half and did not cause hemorrhagic stroke (96). We believe that statin therapy should be initiated in these patients beginning on admission to the hospital in a dose sufficient to markedly lower serum LDL concentrations rapidly.

General Considerations

Coronary arteriography should probably be seriously considered for high- and medium-risk patients with NSTEMI and without other severe and life-threatening medical diseases or very advanced age after the angina is controlled medically with aspirin, heparin, and clopidogrel (in patients not likely to need urgent CABG). A platelet GP IIb/IIIa antagonist may be started prior to PCI in patients with an elevated serum troponin, in patients with complex culprit coronary lesions, and in diabetic patients undergoing PCI. Abciximab should probably be the platelet GP IIb/IIIa inhibitor one uses in diabetic patients having PCI as the evidence that a GP IIb/IIIa inhibitor might be protective in the diabetics is strongest for Abciximab.

Coronary arteriography is absolutely indicated in patients with continuing rest angina in whom medical therapy does not prevent their pain. However, medical therapy initially, in patients without the indications mentioned above for interventional therapy, with subsequent referral for coronary arteriography and PCI or CABG of patients with continuing myocardial ischemia at low-level effort despite medical therapy, is a reasonable alternative (Fig. 6). In the patients in whom rest angina recurs despite an appropriate medical regimen, coronary arteriography becomes mandatory.

In patients in whom angina is medically controlled and a conservative regimen is chosen and in those in whom coronary arteriographic findings do not suggest a need for immediate coronary artery revascularization, low-level exercise (or some other form of stress) testing should be obtained. Submaximal exercise tests can usually be safely done several days after the relief of chest pain, followed by more maximal effort studies several weeks later. The addition of some form of nuclear, echocardiographic, or magnetic resonance perfusion or functional imaging with exercise or other stress improves its sensitivity and specificity for the identification of patients with physiologically important CAD. Patients with continuing angina or objective evidence of myocardial ischemia at rest or at low levels of activity despite a good medical regimen and those with significant left main and/or three-vessel coronary stenoses and depressed LV function should undergo coronary artery revascularization (127–129). Diabetic patients with multivessel CAD and need for coronary revascularization appear to benefit more from CABG than PCI with the possible exception that future studies will confirm that PCI with abciximab infusion or one of the drug-eluting stents will be successful in making stent results comparable to those with CABG in these patients.

Treatment of Acute ST Elevation Myocardial Infarction

The major point to stress in the treatment of patients with STEMI is the major impact that the time from symptom onset to effective coronary reperfusion has on patient outcome. Effective reperfusion therapy initiated within the first one hour of symptom onset saves lives. Sixty-five of 1000 patients treated with effective reperfusion are saved, but this benefit declines over time so within the second hour, 37 patients of 1000 treated survive. Less than half the benefit found in the first hour is achieved if reperfusion is delayed 46 hours after symptom onset.

Effective thrombolytic therapy and PCI are administered with antithrombotic therapy, including aspirin, an antithrombin, usually unfractionated heparin or low-molecular-weight heparin and clopidogrel.

When faced with a patient with STEMI, the physician should ask the following questions: What is the time from symptom onset to first medical contact? What is the risk of thrombolytic therapy? What is the time required to transport the patient and achieve PCI by a skilled operator?

PCI is superior to thrombolytic therapy when there is immediate access to skilled facilities and physician/healthcare teams. If this not available, thrombolytic therapy is an effective alternative, usually consisting of either tPA, tenecteplase (TNK-tPA), or reteplase (rPA). Thrombolytic therapy is potentially associated with excessive bleeding, including intracranial hemorrhage in patients with systemic arterial hypertension and those with a prior cerebrovascular accident and with increased bleeding in patients with recent major surgery, prolonged resuscitation attempts, and known bleeding diatheses.

Secondary prevention after MI begins on admission and consists of pharmacologic therapy with statins, aspirin, and usually clopidogrel. Beta blockers should be added in patients with systemic arterial hypertension and anterior MIs in whom there are no contraindications. ACE inhibitors are also useful in patients with elevated blood pressures and in those in whom there is no contraindication to their use. Longer-term, appropriate lifestyle modifications and rehabilitation are important. Guidelines for the management of STEMI have been published by both the European Society of Cardiology and the American College of Cardiology/American Heart Association 2004 STEMI guidelines (130,131).

Thrombolytic Therapy

Although an overall 18% relative risk reduction for thrombolysis over placebo is evident in patients treated later after symptom onset, there is no survival benefit beyond 12 hours after symptom onset (130–133). ACC/AHA guidelines strongly encourage the performance of 12 lead electrocardiograms and consideration of pre-hospital thrombolytic therapy if appropriate personnel and oversight are positioned to deliver it promptly.

At least one-third of the deaths from MI occur prior to hospital arrival. A "chain of survival" program introduced by the AHA emphasizes early recognition and bystander activation of Emergency Medical Services as well as prompt bystander cardiopulmonary resuscitation and defibrillation prior to the provision of advanced cardiac life support.

The objectives of thrombolytic therapy and reperfusion are: (1) The achievement of rapid, high-quality coronary flow; (2) the maintenance of high-quality coronary flow so as to prevent recurrent ischemia and reinfarction; and (3) the enhancement of patient survival and the quality of life. Effective thrombolytic therapy includes an appropriate fibrinolytic agent and concomitant antithrombotic and antiplatelet therapies.

A convenient classification of currently available fibrinolytic agents begins with streptokinase, the originally used fibrinolytic agent employed as a short-term infusion (30–60 minutes) in doses of 1.5×10^6 U. Tissue plasminogen activator is a relatively fibrin-specific prototype, but it has increasingly given way to tPA congeners, TNK-tPA and rPA. These latter agents are characterized by longer plasma half-lives than tPA, thereby permitting bolus injection that not only simplifies administration, but also reduces the potential for medication errors.

When systemic fibrinolytic therapy is administered, procoagulant counterbalancing forces emerge. These relate to fibrinolytic-induced exposure of surface bound thrombin and activation of platelets which, on their surface, provide a source of Factor Xa. These include plasminogen activator inhibitor-1, alpha 2 antiplasmin, platelet factor IV, and prothrombotic and vasoconstrictor substances, such as serotonin and thromboxane A_2.

Antithrombotic agents were discussed earlier in this chapter in the treatment of patients with unstable angina/NSTEMI, but they include aspirin, clopidogrel, and heparin. Confirmation of the safety and efficacy of this form of conjunctive therapy for both tPA and tNK have recently been provided, and they include bolus of unfractionated heparin of 60 U/kg (maximum 4000 U) followed by an infusion of 12 U/kg /hr (maximum 1000 U/hr) with a PTT target of 50 to 70 seconds during the initial 48 hours (134,135). Continuation of the antithrombotic therapy beyond 48 hours should be individualized. Since recurrent ischemia has been noted after sudden cessation of unfractionated heparin, it is wise to gradually withdraw it over a period of several hours (102). During therapy, daily platelet count monitoring should be undertaken to identify heparin-induced thrombocytopenia should it occur. The need for intravenous unfractionated heparin with streptokinase is less certain and there appears to be no obvious advantage over that provided by subcutaneous heparin (136).

Low-molecular-weight heparin given with fibrinolytic therapy is attractive given its ease of administration, relative stability of anticoagulant effect, greater factor Xa inhibition, and lack of need for laboratory monitoring. Consistent reduction in the frequency of reinfarction and refractory ischemia with enoxaparin is evident in clinical trials (136). This benefit comes at the cost of a modest, but significant increase in systemic bleeding (136). However, in the pre-hospital ASSENT III PLUS experience, an excess of intracranial hemorrhage in low-body-weight females >75 years in age has caused caution regarding enoxaparin in small, elderly women (136). Selected direct thrombin inhibitors may also be useful in STEMI patients (137,138). Treatment with streptokinase and bivalirudin compared with UH in patients with MI was done in the Phase III HERO II study (137,138) and compared with bivalirudin and unfractionated heparin in patients receiving streptokinase for STEMI within six hours of symptom onset (138). There was a reduction in the rate of reinfarction in patients treated with bivalirudin, but also a tendency toward excess systemic and intracranial bleeding and no reduction in mortality. Hence, bivalirudin's current role in STEMI treatment appears as an alternative when unfractionated heparin is contraindicated.

The International Study of Infarct Survival II (ISIS-2) showed the important role of aspirin in doses of 162 to 325 mg in enhancing survival, both as solo therapy and when added to streptokinase (139). Chewable aspirin, buccal or oral administration of nonenteric coated aspirin is advisable to ensure rapid initial effect. Subsequently, lifelong therapy with lower dose aspirin, i.e., at least 81 mg enteric coated, is an important part of long-term secondary prevention.

Myocardial perfusion is mediated by microcirculatory and epicardial blood flow, and together they determine infarct size and clinical outcome. Clinical attention has focused on the use of antiplatelet therapy that provides protection over that from aspirin alone (140–149).

The current STEMI ACC/AHA guidelines support the use of the ADP antagonist, clopidogrel, in patients allergic to aspirin (131). New data on the use of clopidogrel have emerged from the CLARITY and COMMIT trials as it relates to the use of clopidogrel in patients with STEMI treated with fibrinolysis and aspirin within 12 hours (142,143). In the CLARITY study, a 300 mg loading dose followed by 75 mg once daily reduced a composite endpoint of death, recurrent MI, or infarct artery occlusion a median of 3.5 days after presentation by approximately 1/3 (odds ratio 0.53–0.76, $P < 0.001$) (142). Importantly, this endpoint was heavily influenced by clopidogrel's impact on angiographic patency; hence, mortality was 2.2% and recurrent MI 3.6% in the placebo group and 2.6% and 2.5%, respectively, in clopidogrel-treated patients. By contrast, the COMMIT study, conducted in 46,000 patients in China, within 24 hours of the onset of STEMI using 75 mg of clopidogrel without a loading dose revealed a 9% relative risk reduction in the composite of death, reinfarction, or stroke at hospital discharge (10.1% vs. 9.3%, $P = 0.002$) (143). Approximately half the patients received fibrinolysis and no age or weight limit was applied. The COMMIT study has not yet been published; thus, its general applicability remains uncertain. It appears that the major contribution from clopidogrel is to reduce reinfarction risk and maintain culprit artery patency.

Platelet GP IIb/IIIa receptor blockers and their efficacy in patients with non-ST elevation acute coronary syndromes led to substantial enthusiasm about their potential role as part of the pharmacologic armamentarium in patients with STEMI (144–149). It was suggested that combining them with reduced dose fibrinolytic one might not only enhance the potential for both macro- and microcirculatory reperfusion, but also reduce the risk of intracranial hemorrhage and systemic bleeding. Extensive Phase II studies evaluating this approach provided evidence of reduced culprit artery reocclusion and more rapid and effective reperfusion (144–149). However, when this concept was first tested in a large Phase III study (GUSTO V) using a combination of half-dose retaplase and full-dose Abciximab as compared with full-dose retaplase, no improvement in mortality was found. There was less reinfarction with combination therapy (149). Subsequently, half-dose tenecteplase with Abciximab was evaluated in the ASSENT III study and a similar benefit on reinfarction and recurrent ischemia was evident as compared with monotherapy with tenecteplase. However, there was no subsequent improvement in mortality (136). In both studies, however, there was an excess of severe bleeding and a trend towards excess intracranial hemorrhage in patients above the age of 75 years with combination GP IIb/IIIa inhibition and fibrinolysis. Therefore, this approach remains largely experimental presently.

INITIAL THERAPY OF STEMI

Supplemental oxygen therapy aimed at limiting the extent of ischemic myocardial injury is part of the initial treatment in the initial hours after STEMI and NSTEMI. Maintenance of an oxygen saturation of at least 94% is desirable.

In patients with persisting ischemic pain, hypertension, or concomitant congestive heart failure, intravenous nitroglycerin beginning at an infusion rate of approximately 5 to 10 mcg/min and titrating upwards to achieve desired response is useful. Caution concerning the use of nitrates, especially given by any route other than intravenously, in patients with AMI is warranted when right ventricular infarction is present. It is also wise to inquire about the prior use of phosphodiesterase inhibitors for erectile dysfunction, since these agents potentiate the blood pressure lowering effect of nitrates and their combination may complicate the clinical course.

In the most recent ACC/AHA guidelines, patients are encouraged to call 911 in five minutes or less from the onset of chest pain and after taking only one sublingual nitroglycerin (131). For patients with established stable angina which is severe and recurrent, two to three nitroglycerin are sometimes necessary and 5 to 10 minutes often required to alleviate their usual ischemic pain. It is our view that this advice should be individualized for patients.

Non-enteric aspirin, 162 to 325 mg, should be administered in a manner that achieves rapid absorption, i.e., chewing, sucking, or swallowing a crushed preparation as quickly as possible after symptom onset.

Having decided to administer fibrinolytic therapy, the clinician has the responsibility to assess the patient's response in the following few hours. Resolution of ischemic chest pain, restoration of hemodynamic stability, and decline in the initial ST segment elevation by at least 50% of its original height are helpful signs of reperfusion (132,150). ST resolution is a good indicator of both macro- and micro-myocardial perfusion and is associated with better recovery of ventricular function, a lesser infarct size, and enhanced clinical outcome (132,150).

An accelerated idioventricular rhythm ("slow V.T.") is uncommon, but is correlated with reperfusion and infarct artery patency. Although a variety of investigative techniques, including contrast echocardiography and magnetic resonance imaging are under investigation, no single technique that is clinically applicable at the bedside has yet emerged to identify reperfusion noninvasively. A systemic algorithm of ST segment monitoring that requires repeat 12 lead electrocardiography at 60 and 90 minutes can be helpful (150,151). Failure to achieve reperfusion may signal the need to proceed with coronary arteriography and consideration of rescue percutaneous intervention (152).

Recurrent ischemic symptoms, if associated with objective evidence of further ST segment shift and/or reinfarction, especially in the first 48 hours after the administration of fibrinolytic therapy, is often an indication for co-intervention with PCI.

Percutaneous Coronary Intervention

The choice of the optimal reperfusion strategy for STEMI has been the subject of controversy for several years. In patients with absolute contraindications to fibrinolysis and those in Killip Class III and IV, primary PCI is the preferred option, provided it can be done in a timely fashion by a skilled operator, in an advanced facility (Fig. 10). Most evidence suggests that PCI is a superior option to thrombolytic therapy, even in patients requiring interhospital transfer.

In the treatment of patients with STEMI, a rapid EMS response, pre-hospital ECG and the capacity for fibrinolysis, appropriate triage of patients in whom primary PCI is preferred, and enhanced state of readiness in the institution that will receive the patient are of major importance. The sensitivity to time is especially important, given the knowledge that coronary thrombus within the first two to three hours is especially sensitive to fibrinolysis and both the CAPTIM and PRAGUE 2 studies demonstrated that fibrinolysis is at least as good, if not superior, to primary PCI in that window (153,154). It is essential that community

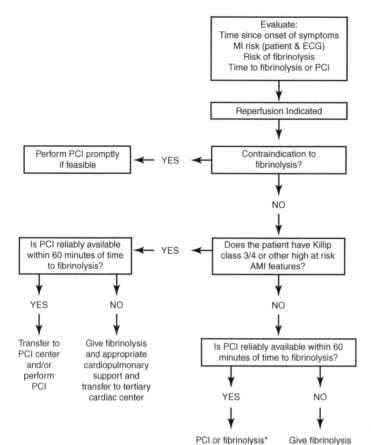

FIGURE 10   PCI treatment of STEMI.
* Use either PCI or fibrinolysis.

hospitals develop or enhance effective communication strategies, with fully equipped tertiary care centers, to ensure that timely transfer of high risk patients and those not responding to fibrinolytic therapy occurs. Since less than 20% of U.S. hospitals have facilities for cardiac catheterization, and even fewer have the capacity for primary PCI, widespread primary PCI therapy for STEMI is not feasible presently. Despite calls for regionalization of care in specialized centers, the potential negative effects on patient care associated with transfer and cardiac care in non-ACS centers as well as the economic implications provide reasons for caution.

The conclusion of the ACC/AHA STEMI Writing Committee on this subject in the following statement expresses the views of the authors: "Given the current literature, it is not possible to say definitively that a particular reperfusion approach is superior for all patients, in all clinical settings, at all times of the day. The main point is that some type of reperfusion therapy should be selected for all appropriate patients with suspected STEMIs. The appropriate and timely use of some reperfusion therapy is likely more important than the choice of therapy, given the current literature and the expanding array of options" (131,151,155).

OTHER CONSIDERATIONS

Although evidence supporting the use of intravenous beta blockers in patients undergoing successful reperfusion is slim and mainly acquired in the pre-reperfusion era, it merits a Class IIa (level of evidence B) (131,156). Intravenous beta blockers may be especially useful in the patients with hypertension, tachycardia, atrial and ventricular arrhythmias, and ongoing ischemic pain. Oral beta blockade most especially with timolol, metoprolol, or propranolol merits a Class Ia recommendation (131).

Inhibition of the renin angiotensin aldosterone system with ACE inhibitors has been extensively studied in patients with STEMIs and has consistently shown a modest but significant effect on short-term mortality (i.e., less than 1%) (94,157). This effect, however as noted earlier in the chapter, is greater in patients with anterior infarcts, pulmonary congestion, and diminished left ventricular ejection fraction where early administration of captopril, lisinopril, or enalapril is especially useful (94,157). Care should be taken, as is the case with beta blockers, in beginning with a low initial dose so as to avoid hypotension. Preference should be given to initiating ACE inhibitors in advance of beta blockers if relative hypotension is of concern, especially in the setting of pulmonary congestion and a large MI. If genuine intolerance to ACE inhibitors exists, angiotensin receptor blockers are an appropriate alternative.

Additional benefit may be provided by aldosterone inhibition. The selective aldosterone blocker, eplerenone, given to patients with left ventricular dysfunction and heart failure complicating MI has been helpful (158). At a mean of 16 months after therapy begun 3 to 14 days after MI, eplerenone significantly reduced each of the two primary endpoints (death 16.7% and cardiovascular death and hospitalization 30.0% with placebo to 14.4% and 26.7% respectively with eplerenone). Patients with elevated serum creatinines were excluded from this study. Special care should be used in monitoring both serum potassium and creatinine levels, if this therapy is employed, and most particularly, with concomitant use of ACE inhibitors. Although eplerenone received a Class Ia recommendation and clearly may be beneficial during the convalescence of STEMI patients (131), less than half of the patients entered in the EPHESUS study received reperfusion therapy, and the actual proportion with ST elevation on admission is unclear (158).

Power-Failure Complications

The development of low cardiac output, pulmonary edema, and shock are serious consequences of STEMI. A first priority requires a systemic screen for correctable causes, such as brady or tachyarrhythmias, hypovolemia, and adverse responses to pharmacotherapy, such as nitrates, beta blockers, and/or ACE inhibitors. Patients with a right ventricular infarction, which occurs in approximately one-third of inferior STEMI patients, present a particular therapeutic challenge (159). Such individuals commonly respond, however, to aggressive volume loading, supplemented with intravenous dobutamine (160). Hemodynamic monitoring with Swan–Ganz catheterization is useful in documenting right- and left-sided filling pressures and guiding appropriate therapy.

Free-wall cardiac rupture with rapid hemodynamic collapse associated with electrical mechanical dissociation is a particularly devastating complication (161). Emergency pericardiocentesis for concomitant pericardial tamponade may, on occasion, salvage the patients but surgical intervention is required. It carries a high mortality but is the only alternative. Occasionally, minor free-wall perforations self seal and give rise to pseudoaneurysm formation.

For patients with cardiogenic shock, without demonstrable mechanical defects, who are <75 years of age with STEMI, compelling data from the SHOCK study exists to proceed with early coronary arteriography and revascularization as is appropriate in individual patients (162,163). Aggressive pharmacologic therapy and the insertion of an intra-aortic balloon are usual preambles to coronary arteriography, and the evidence suggests that this strategy is applicable to patients who develop shock within 36 hours of MI and for whom revascularization can be undertaken within 18 hours of the onset of shock. Such an approach may also be appropriate for selected patients over the age of 75, recognizing that the biologic and chronologic ascertainments of age often differ.

Ventricular Aneurysms

Left ventricular aneurysm formation is an important mechanical complication of MI (164). It occurs in association with transmural necrosis, is associated with infarct thinning and the potential for expansion, and is most common in the anterior wall when the infarct artery is occluded and there are no intercoronary collaterals (164). Although suggested by persisting ST elevation in the setting of Q waves, the diagnosis is best made from echocardiography, SPECT, MRI, or left ventricular angiography. In addition to left ventricular dysfunction and failure, aneurysms may serve as a nidus for mural thrombosis and systemic embolization as well as the substrate for major ventricular arrhythmias. Interrogation of the left ventricular apex for thrombus formation in the early days after a large anterior myocardial infarct is an important investigation. Warfarin therapy is indicated in the presence of acute (or presumed acute) left ventricular thrombosis.

Recurrent Symptoms

Chest pain after STEMI is a common symptom. Concomitant gastrointestinal distress and anxiety may lead to the reporting of previously ignored discomfort and confound the inexperienced diagnostician. Recurrent ischemia and infarction in the first few days after presentation of STEMI is associated with a worsened prognosis (165–169). Recurrent ST elevation in the distribution of the same infarct location as at presentation versus a different region (so-called "ischemia at a distance") are usually indications for early angiography, unless obvious secondary causes or suboptimal medical therapy are discovered. If the discomfort is sustained and associated with recurrent ST elevation and urgent PCI cannot be undertaken in a timely fashion, then repeat fibrinolytic therapy may be appropriate (using a fibrin-specific agent).

Recurrent ischemic pain must be differentiated from that of pericarditis, which is most common in patients with major full thickness myocardial necrosis and extensive infarctions (168,169). The more distinctive characteristics of pericardial pain, exacerbated by respiration and at least partially relieved by the upright position, as well as the occasional physical finding of a pericardial friction rub are useful differential points. More diffuse ST elevation with an upward concavity as well as PR depression are typical electrocardiographic findings. The appreciation of the potential for harm with non-steroidal anti-inflammatory agents and corticosteroids, based on their negative impact on infarct healing, as well as ibuprofen's block of the antiplatelet effect of aspirin have modified prior treatment recommendations (170,171). Aspirin remains the first line of therapy with colchicine 0.6 mg orally every 12 hours and acetaminophen suggested alternatives. Indomethacin is usually effective in pain control and almost always well tolerated clinically. Antithrombotic therapy should be discontinued and careful surveillance for pericardial tamponade undertaken clinically and as required with the aid of echocardiography.

Convalescent Care

In asymptomatic patients, the focal points of subsequent management involve risk stratification, appropriate co-intervention, and the application of secondary prevention through evidence-based medication and lifestyle modification. Fundamental to the risk profile of such patients is an objective evaluation of left ventricular function undertaken either by echocardiography, nuclear imaging studies, or MRI. Patients with severely depressed left ventricular ejection fractions (i.e., <40%) have an increased long-term morbidity and mortality and should be considered for revascularization if appropriate and for AICD placement. As indicated in the earlier section in evaluating patients with NSTEMI, low-level exercise testing with an appropriate imaging procedure, and four to six weeks later, more vigorous exercise or other stress with appropriate cardiac imaging (SPECT, echocardiography, or MRI) help to identify patients at short-term risk for reinfarction and CHF. The ability to perform at least five mets of exercise without early ST depression and with an appropriate rise in systolic blood pressure are useful signs of lower risk.

The controlled environment in the early days after STEMI provides the clinician with a unique opportunity to engage patient and family in aggressive secondary prevention. Appropriate dietary modification to reduce weight and an exercise program developed during rehabilitation are first steps. Smoking cessation, not only for the patient but also those who live in the same household, is especially important. Appropriate therapy to normalize blood glucose in diabetic patients is extremely important. Intense lipid therapy with the early introduction of statins and achieving the lowest possible LDL cholesterol, i.e., one <100 mg/dL and preferably ≤70 mg/dL is important. Recent evidence from the Pravastatin or Atorvastatin Evaluation and Infarction Therapy ("PROVE-IT") indicate that intensive lipid lowering therapy initiated within 10 days after hospital admission of acute coronary syndromes with 80 mg of atorvastatin to achieve an LDL cholesterol of less than 70 mg/dL achieved a 16% reduction (from 26.3% to 22.4%) in composite endpoint of death, MI, unstable angina, requiring re-hospitalization and coronary revascularization, and stroke (172).

Daily walking should be strongly encouraged with a progressive increase in the pace and distance as tolerated. Sexual activity with a usual partner may be resumed within two weeks and is roughly metabolically equivalent to the ability to climb two flights of stairs. Resumption of driving after STEMI is usually subject to a waiting period of between one week to one month for private driving and three months for commercial driving. However, if revascularization has been undertaken, no reversible ischemia is evident, and a good functional status demonstrated, a shorter period of time may be recommended.

Development of an appropriate medical program at the time of hospital discharge and re-evaluation after appropriate uptitration of medical therapy at approximately one month thereafter are important in secondary prevention (173). The successfully reperfused patient is at low risk in the short term. If ACE inhibitors cannot be tolerated, angiotensin receptor blockers should be substituted and long-term aldosterone blockade added for patients with left ventricular dysfunction, i.e., LVEFs <40%.

SUMMARY

The care of patients with STEMI has been transformed in the last decade with a substantial reduction in mortality and morbidity. Perhaps more than in any other acute cardiovascular condition, optimizing therapy highlights the critical dependence on the intersection between the content of evidence-based care and the process and timeliness whereby it is delivered. Enhanced patient education, early emergency response of appropriately trained and equipped paramedical personnel, rapid triage and treatment in the field, and the application of the best reperfusion strategy for the right patient at the right time in the right place are critical components to enhance the care of STEMI patients.

REFERENCES

1. Heberden W. Some account of a disorder of the breast. Med Trans R Coll Phys II London 1786; 59.
2. Herrick JB. Clinical features of sudden obstruction of the coronary arteries. JAMA 1912; 59:2015.
3. Constantinides P. Plaque fissuring in human coronary thrombosis. J Atheroscler Res 1966; 6:1.
4. Davies MJ, Thomas AC. Plaque fissuring—the cause of acute myocardial infarction, sudden ischemic death, and crescendo angina. Br Heart J 1985; 53:363–373.
5. Falk E. Plaque rupture with severe preexisting stenosis precipitating coronary thrombosis: characteristics of coronary atherosclerotic plaques underlying fatal occlusive thrombi. Br Heart J 1983; 50:127–134.
6. DeWood MA, Spores J, Notshe R, et al. Prevalence of total coronary occlusion during the early hours of transmural myocardial infarction. N Engl J Med 1980; 303:897–902.
7. Buja LM, Willerson JT. Clinicopathologic correlates of acute ischemic heart disease syndromes. Am J Cardiol 1981; 47:343–356.
8. Willerson JT. Treatment of Heart Disease. New York: Gower Medical; 1992.
9. Willerson JT, Golino P, Eidt JF, Campbell WB, Buja LM. Specific platelet mediators and unstable coronary artery lesions. Experimental evidence and potential clinical implications. Circulation 1989; 80:198–205.
10. Bush L, Campbell WB, Tilton GD, Buja LM, Willerson JT. Effects of the selective thromboxane synthase inhibitor, dazoxiben, on cyclic flow variations in stenosed canine coronary arteries. Trans Assoc Am Physicians 1983; 96:103–112.
11. Ashton JH, Ogletree ML, Michel IM, et al. Cooperative mediation by serotonin S_2 and thromboxane A_2/prostaglandin H_2 receptor activation of cyclic flow variations in dogs with severe coronary artery stenoses. Circulation 1987; 76:952–959.
12. Golino P, Ashton JH, Buja LM, et al. Local platelet activation causes vasoconstriction of large epicardial canine coronary arteries in vivo: thromboxane A_2 and serotonin are possible mediator. Circulation 1989; 79:154–166.
13. Bush LR, Campbell WB, Kern K, et al. The effects of alpha 2-adrenergic and serotonergic receptor antagonists on cyclic blood flow alterations in stenosed canine coronary arteries. Circ Res 1984; 55:642–652.
14. Willerson JT, Hillis LD, Winniford MD, Buja LM. Speculation regarding mechanisms responsible for acute ischemic heart disease syndromes. J Am Coll Cardiol 1986; 8:245–250.
15. Willerson JT, Campbell WB, Winniford MD, et al. Conversion from chronic to acute coronary artery disease: speculation regarding mechanisms. Am J Cardiol 1984; 54:1349–1354.
16. Hirsh PD, Hillis LD, Campbell WB, Firth BG, Willerson JT. Release of prostaglandins and thromboxane into the coronary circulation in patients with ischemic heart disease. N Engl J Med 1981; 304:685–691.
17. Eidt JF, Allison P, Noble S, et al. Thrombin is an important mediator of platelet aggregation in stenosed and endothelially-injured canine coronary arteries. J Clin Invest 1989; 84:18–27.
18. van den Berg EK, Schmitz JM, Benedict CR, Malloy CR, Willerson JT, Dehmer GJ. Transcardiac serotonin concentration is increased in selected patients with limiting angina and complex coronary lesion morphology. Circulation 1989; 79:116–124.

19. Fuster V, Badimon L, Badimon JJ, Chesebro JH. The pathogenesis of coronary artery disease and the acute coronary syndromes. N Engl J Med 1992; 326:242–250, 310–318.
20. Fuster V, Lewis A. Mechanisms leading to myocardial infarction: insights from studies of vascular biology [Connor Memorial Lecture]. Circulation 1995; 91:256.
21. Carry M, Korley V, Willerson JT, Weigelt L, Ford-Hutchinson AW, Tagari P. Increased urinary leukotriene excretion in patients with cardiac ischemia: in vivo evidence for 5-lipoxygenase activation. Circulation 1992; 85:230–236.
22. Libby P. Molecular bases of the acute coronary syndromes. Circulation 1995; 91:2844–2850.
23. Page DL, Caulfield JB, Kastor JA, DeSanctis RW, Sanders CA. Myocardial changes associated with cardiogenic shock. N Engl J Med 1971; 285:133–137.
24. Alonso DR, Scheidt S, Post M, Killip T. Pathophysiology of cardiogenic shock: quantification of myocardial necrosis, clinical, pathologic, and electrocardiographic correlation. Circulation 1973; 48:588–596.
25. Willerson JT, Curry GC, Watson JT, et al. Intraaortic balloon counterpulsation in patients in cardiogenic shock, medically refractory left ventricular failure, and/or recurrent ventricular tachycardia. Am J Med 1975; 58:183–191.
26. Ballester M, Tasca R, Marin L, Rees S, Rickards A, McDonald L. Different mechanisms of mitral regurgitation in acute and chronic forms of coronary heart disease. Eur Heart J 1983; 4:557–565.
27. Meister SG, Helfant RH. Rapid bedside differentiation of ruptured interventricular septum from acute mitral insufficiency. N Engl J Med 1972; 287:1024–1025.
28. Come PC, Riley MF, Weintraub R, Morgan JP, Nakao S. Echocardiographic detection of complete and partial papillary muscle rupture during acute myocardial infarction. Am J Cardiol 1985; 56:787–789.
29. Moore CA, Mygaard TW, Kaiser DL, Cooper AA, Gibson RS. Post infarction ventricular septal rupture: the importance of location of infarction and right ventricular function in determining survival. Circulation 1986; 74:45–55.
30. Radford MJ, Johnson RA, Daggett WM Jr., et al. Ventricular septal rupture: a review of clinical and physiologic features and an analysis of survival. Circulation 1981; 64:545–553.
31. Mann JM, Roberts WC. Acquired ventricular septal defect during acute myocardial infarction: analysis of 38 unoperated necropsy patients and comparison with 50 unoperated necropsy patients and comparison with 50 unoperated necropsy patients without rupture. Am J Cardiol 1988; 62:8–19.
32. Braunwald E, Kloner RA. The stunned myocardium: prolonged, postischemic ventricular dysfunction. Circulation 1982; 66:1146–1149.
33. Ellis SG, Henschke CI, Sandor T, Wynne J, Braunwald E, Kloner RA. Time course of functional and biochemical recovery of myocardium salvaged by reperfusion. J Am Coll Cardiol 1983; 1:1047–1055.
34. Rahimtoola SH. The hibernating myocardium. Am Heart J 1989; 117:211–221.
35. Willerson JT, Hillis LD, Buja LM. Ischemic Heart Disease: Clinical and Pathophysiological Aspects. New York: Raven, 1982.
36. Roberts R, Sobel BE, Parker CW. Radioimmunoassay of creatinine kinase isoenzymes. Science 1976; 194:855–857.
37. Roberts R, Sobel BE. Isoenzymes of creatine phosphokinase and diagnosis of myocardial infarction. Ann Intern Med 1973; 79; 741–743.
38. Willerson JT, Stone MJ, Ting R, et al. Radioimmunoassay of creatine kinase-B isoenzyme in human sera: results in patients with acute myocardial infarction. Proc Natl Acad Sci USA 1977; 74:1711–1715.
39. Stone MJ, Willerson JT, Gomez-Sanchez CE, Waterman MR. Radioimmunoassay of myoglobin in human serum: results in patients with acute myocardial infarction. J Clin Invest 1975; 56:1334–1339.
40. Stone MJ, Waterman MR, Harimoto D, et al. Serum myoglobin level as diagnostic test in patients with acute myocardial infarction. Br Heart J 1977; 39:375–380.
41. Gilkeson G, Stone MJ, Waterman M, et al. Detection of myoglobin by radioimmunoassay in human sera: its usefulness and limitations as an emergency room screening test for acute myocardial infarction. Am Heart J 1978; 95:70–77.
42. Katus HA, Remppis A, Newmann FJ, et al. Diagnostic efficiency of troponin T measurements in acute myocardial infarction. Circulation 1991; 83:902–912.
43. Mair J, Morandell D, Genser N, Lechleitner P, Dienstl F, Puschendorf B. Equivalent early sensitivities of myoglobin, creatine kinase MB mass, creatine kinase isoform ratios, and cardiac troponins I and T for acute myocardial infarction. Clin Chem 1995; 41:1266–1272.
44. Adams JE III, Bodor GS, Davila-Roman VG, et al. Cardiac troponin I: a marker with high specificity for cardiac injury. Circulation 1993; 88:101–106.
45. Cummins B, Auckland ML, Cummins P. Cardiac-specific troponin I radioimmunoassay in the diagnosis of acute myocardial infarction. Am Heart J 1987; 113:1333–1344.
46. Willerson JT, Parkey RW, Stokely EM, et al. Infarct sizing with technetium-99m stannous pyrophosphate scintigraphy in dogs and man: the relationship between scintigraphic and precordial mapping estimates of infarct size in patients. Cardiovasc Res 1977; 11:291–298.
47. Jansen DE, Corbett JR, Wolfe CL, et al. Quantification of myocardial infarction: a comparison of single photon emission computed tomography with pyrophosphate to serial plasma CK-MB measurements. Circulation 1985; 72:327–333.
48. Wolfe CL, Lewis SE, Corbett JR, Parkey RW, Buja LM, Willerson JT. Measurement of infarction fraction using single photon emission computed tomography. J Am Coll Cardiol 1985; 6:145–151.

49. Corbett JR, Lewis SE, Wolfe CL, et al. Measurement of myocardial infarct size in patients by technetium pyrophosphate single photon tomography. Am J Cardiol 1984; 54:1231–1236.

50. Corbett JR, Nicod P, Lewis SE, Rude RE, Willerson JT. Prognostic value of submaximal exercise radionuclide ventriculography after myocardial infarction. Am J Cardiol 1983; 52:82A–91A.

51. Shan K, Constantine G, Sivananthan M, Flamm SD. Role of cardiac magnetic resonance imaging in the assessment of myocardial viability. Circulation 2004; 109:1328–1334.

52. Dehmer GJ, Lewis SE, Hillis LD, Corbett J, Parkey RW, Willerson JT. Exercise induced alterations in left ventricular volumes and the pressure–volume relationship: a sensitive indicator of left ventricular dysfunction in patients with coronary artery disease. Circulation 1981; 63:1008–1018.

53. Corbett J, Dehmer GJ, Lewis SE, et al. The prognostic value of submaximal exercise testing with radionuclide ventriculography prior to hospital discharge in patients with recent myocardial infarction. Circulation 1981; 64:535–544.

54. Gibson RS, Watson DD, Taylor GJ, et al. Prospective assessment of regional myocardial perfusion before and after coronary revascularization surgery by quantitative thallium-201 scintigraphy. J Am Coll Cardiol 1983; 1:804–815.

55. Melin JA, Wijns W, Keyeux A, et al. Assessment of thallium-201 redistribution versus glucose uptake as predictors of viability after coronary occlusion and reperfusion. Circulation 1988; 77:927–934.

56. Eaton LW, Weiss JL, Bulkley BH, Garrison JB, Weisfeldt ML. Regional cardiac dilatation after acute myocardial infarction. Recognition by two-dimensional echocardiography. N Engl J Med 1979; 300:57–62.

57. McKay RG, Pfeffer MA, Pasternak RC, et al. Left ventricular remodeling after myocardial infarction. A corollary to infarct expansion. Circulation 1986; 74:693–702.

58. Pfeffer MA, Lamas GA, Vaughan DE, Parisi AF, Braunwald E. Effect of captopril on progressive ventricular dilatation. N Engl J Med 1988; 319:80–86.

59. Muller JE, Rude RE, Braunwald E, et al. Myocardial infarct extension: incidence, outcome, and risk factors in the MILIS study. Ann Intern Med 1988; 108:1–6.

60. Corbett JR, Nicod PH, Huxley RL, Lewis SE, Rude RE, Willerson JT. Left ventricular functional alterations at rest and during submaximal exercise in patients with acute myocardial infarction. Am J Med 1983; 74:577.

61. Lindahl B, Venge P, Wallentin L, for the FRISC Study Group. Relation between troponin T and the risk of subsequent cardiac events in unstable coronary artery disease. Circulation 1996; 93:1651–1657.

62. Antman EM, Tanasijevic MJ, Thompson B, et al. Cardiac-specific troponin I levels to predict the risk of mortality in patients with acute coronary syndromes. N Engl J Med 1996; 335:1342–1349.

63. Martin GS, Becker B, Schulman G. Cardiac troponin-I accurately predicts myocardial injury in renal failure. Nephrol Dial Transplant 1998; 13:1709–1712.

64. Koenig W, Sund M, Frölich M, et al. C-reactive protein, a sensitive marker of inflammation, predicts future risk of coronary heart disease in initially healthy middle-aged men. Circulation 1999; 99:237–242.

65. Berk BC, Weintraub WS, Alexander RW. Elevation of C-reactive protein in "acute" coronary artery disease. Am J Cardiol 1990; 65:168–172.

66. Ohman EM, Armstrong PW, Christenson RH, et al. Cardiac troponin T levels for risk stratification in acute myocardial ischemia. N Engl J Med 1996; 335:1333–1341.

67. Liuzzo G, Biasucci LM, Gallimore JR, et al. The prognostic value of C-reactive protein in severe angina. N Engl J Med 1994; 331:417–424.

68. Kruskal JB, Commerford PJ, Franks JJ, Kirsch RE. Fibrin and fibrinogen related antigens in patients with stable and unstable coronary artery disease. N Engl J Med 1987; 317:1361–1365.

69. Haverkate F, Thompson SG, Pyke SD, Gallimore JR, Pepys MB, for the European Concerted Action on Thrombosis and Disabilities Angina Pectoris Study Group. Production of C-reactive protein and risk of coronary events in stable and unstable angina. Lancet 1997; 349:462–466.

70. Biasucci LM, Liuzzo G, Fantuzzi G, et al. Increasing levels of interleukin (IL)-1Ra and IL-6 during the first 2 days of hospitalization in unstable angina are associated with increased risk of in-hospital coronary events. Circulation 1999; 99:2079–2084.

71. Ridker PM, Rifai N, Clearfield M, et al. Measurement of C-reactive protein for the targeting of statin therapy in the primary prevention of acute coronary events. N Engl J Med 2001; 344:1959–1965.

72. de Lemos JA, Morrow DA, Bentley JH, Omland T, Sabatine MS, McCabe CH, et al. The prognostic value of B-type natriuretic peptide in patients with acute coronary syndromes. N Engl J Med 2001; 345:1014–1021.

73. Conde I, Kleiman NS. Soluble CD40 ligand in acute coronary syndromes. N Engl J Med 2003; 348:2575–2577.

74. Freedman JE. CD40 ligand—assessing risk instead of damage? N Engl J Med 2003; 348:1163–1165.

75. Heeschen C, Dimmeler S, Hamm CW, et al. Soluble CD40 ligand in acute coronary syndromes. N Engl J Med 2003; 348:1104–1111.

76. Bayes-Genis A, Conover CA, Overgaard MT, Bailey KR, Christiansen M, Holmes DR Jr, et al. Pregnancy-associated plasma protein A as a marker of acute coronary syndromes. N Engl J Med 2001; 345:1022–1029.

77. Valkonen V-P, Päivä H, Salonen JT, et al. Risk of acute coronary events and serum concentration of asymmetrical dimethylarginine. Lancet 2001; 358:2127–2128.

78. Brennan M-L, Penn MS, Van Lente F, Nambi V, Shishehbor MH. Aviles RJ, et al. Prognostic value of myeloperoxidase in patients with chest pain. N Engl J Med 2003; 349:1595–1604.

79. Morrow DA, Cannon CP, Rifai N, Frey MJ, Vicari R, Lakkis N, et al. Ability of minor elevations of troponins I and T to predict benefit from an early invasive strategy in patients with unstable angina and non-ST elevation myocardial infarction. JAMA 2001; 286:2405–2412.

80. Sabatine MS, Morrow DA, de Lemos JA, Gibson CM, Murphy SA, Rifai N, et al. Multimarker approach to risk stratification in non-ST elevation acute coronary syndromes. Simultaneous assessment of troponin I, C-reactive protein, and B-type natriuretic peptide. Circulation 2002; 105:1760–1763.

81. Henney AM, Wakeley PR, Davies MJ, et al. Localization of stromelysin gene expression in the atherosclerotic plaques by in situ hybridization. Proc Natl Acad Sci USA 1991; 88:8154–8158.

82. Nikkari ST, O'Brien KD, Ferguson M, et al. Interstitial collagenase (MMP-1) expression in human carotid atherosclerosis. Circulation 1995; 92:1393–1398.

83. Sukhova G, Schönbeck U, Rabkin E, et al. Evidence for increased collagenolysis by interstitial collagenases-1 and -3 in vulnerable atheromatous plaques. Circulation 1999; 99:2503–2509.

84. Galis ZS, Muszynski M, Sukhova GK, Simon-Morrissey E, Libby P. Enhanced expression of vascular matrix metalloproteinases induced in vitro by cytokines and in regions of human atherosclerotic lesions. Ann N Y Acad Sci 1995; 748:501–507.

85. Moreno PR, Falk E, Palacios IF, Newell JB, Fuster V, Fallon JT. Macrophage infiltration in acute coronary syndromes. Implications for plaque rupture. Circulation 1994; 90:775–778.

86. Braunwald E, Antman EM, Beasley JW, et al. ACC/AHA 2002 guidelines update for the management of patients with unstable angina and non-ST-segment elevation myocardial infarction: a report of the American College of Cardiology/American Heart Association Task Force on Practice Guidelines. Available at: http://www.acc.org/clinical/guidelines/unstable/unstable.pdf. Accessed April 22, 2002.

87. Antman EM, Cohen M, Bernink PJ, McCabe CH, Horacek T, Papuchis G, et al. The TIMI risk score for unstable angina/non-ST elevation MI: a method for prognostication and therapeutic decision making. JAMA 2000; 284:835–842.

88. Holper EM, Antman EM, McCabe CH, et al. A simple, readily available method for risk stratification of patients with unstable angina or non-Q myocardial infarction: a TIMI 11B substudy. Am J Cardiol. 2001; 87(8):1008–1010.

89. Cannon CP, Weintraub WS, Demepoulos LA, et al. Comparison of early invasive and conservative strategies in patients with unstable coronary syndromes treated with glycoprotein IIb/IIIa inhibitor tirofiban. N Engl J Med 2001; 344:1879–887.

90. Ridker PM, Cannon CP, Morrow D, et al. C-reactive protein levels and outcomes after statin therapy. N Engl J Med 2005; 352:20–28.

91. de Winter RJ, Windhausen F, Cornel JH, Dunselman PHJM, Janus CL, Bendermacher PEF, Michels HR, Sanders GT, Tijssen JGP, Verheugt F. Early invasive versus selectively invasive management for acute coronary syndromes. N Engl J Med 2005; 353:1095–1104.

92. Hamm CW, Bertrand M, Braunwald E. Acute coronary syndrome without ST elevation: implementation of new guidelines. Lancet 2001; 358:1533–1538.

93. Sabatine MS, Morrow DA, Giugliano RP, et al. Implications of upstream glycoprotein IIb/IIIa inhibition and coronary artery stenting in the invasive management of unstable angina/non-ST-elevation myocardial infarction: a comparison of the TIMI IIIB and the Treat Angina with Aggrastat trial. Circulation 2004; 109:874–880.

94. ACE Inhibitor Myocardial Infarction Collaborative Group. Indications for ACE inhibitors in the early treatment of acute myocardial infarction. Systemic overview of individual data from 100,000 patients in randomized trials. Circulation 1998; 97:2202–2212.

95. Schwartz GG, Olsson AG, Ezekowitz MD, Ganz P, Oliver MF, Waters D, et al. Effects of atorvastatin on early recurrent ischemic events in acute coronary syndromes: the MIRACL study: a randomized controlled trial. JAMA 285:1711–1718.

96. Waters DD, Schwartz GG, Olsson AG, Zeiher A, Oliver MF, Ganz P, et al. Effects of atorvastatin on stroke in patients with unstable angina or non-Q-wave myocardial infarction. A myocardial ischemia reduction with aggressive cholesterol lowering (MIRACL) substudy. Circulation 2002; 106:1690–1695.

97. Théroux P, Ouimet H, McCans J, et al. Aspirin, heparin, or both to treat acute unstable angina. N Engl J Med 1988; 319:1105–1111.

98. Cairns JA, Gent M, Singer J, et al. Aspirin, sulfinpyrazone, or both in unstable angina. N Engl J Med 1985; 313:1369–1375.

99. DeCaterina R, Giannessi D, Bernini W, et al. Low-dose aspirin in patients recovering from myocardial infarction: evidence for selective inhibition of thromboxane-related platelet function. Eur Heart J 1985; 6:409–417.

100. Patrono C. Aspirin as an antiplatelet drug. N Engl J Med 1994; 330:1287–1294.

101. Glaser R, Herrmann HC, Murphy SA, et al. Benefit of an early invasive management strategy in women with acute coronary syndromes. JAMA 2002; 288:3124–3129.

102. Théroux P, Waters D, Lam J, Juneau M, McCans J. Reactivation of unstable angina after the discontinuation of heparin. N Engl J Med 1992; 327:141–145.

103. Gold HK, Torres FW, Garabedian HD, et al. Evidence for a rebound coagulation phenomenon after cessation of a 4-hour infusion of a specific thrombin inhibitor in patients with unstable angina pectoris. J Am Coll Cardiol 1993; 21:1039–1047.

104. Peterson JL, Mahaffey KW, Hasselblad V, Antman EM, Cohen M, Goodman SG, et al. Efficacy and bleeding complications among patients randomized to enoxaparin or unfractionated heparin for antithrombin therapy in non-ST-segment elevation acute coronary syndromes: a systemic overview. JAMA 2004; 292:89–96.

105. Ferguson JJ, Califf RM, Antman EM, Cohen M, Grines CL, Goodman S, et al. Enoxaparin vs unfractionated heparin in high-risk patients with non-ST-segment elevation acute coronary syndromes managed with an intended early invasive strategy: primary results of the SYNERGY randomized trial. JAMA 2004; 292:45–54.

106. Wong GC, Giugliano RP, Antman EM. Use of low-molecular-weight heparins in the management of acute coronary artery syndromes and percutaneous coronary intervention. JAMA 2003; 289:331–342.

107. Das P, Moliterno DJ. Fractionating heparins and their clinical data—something for everyone. JAMA 2004; 292:101–103.

108. Montalescot G, Collet JP, Tanguy ML, Ankri A, Payot L, Dumaine R, et al. Anti-Xa activity relates to survival and efficacy in unselected acute coronary syndrome patients treated with enoxaparin. Circulation 2004; 110:392–398.

109. Fragmin during Instability in Coronary Artery Disease (FRISC) Study. Low-molecular-weight heparin during instability in coronary artery disease. Lancet 1996; 347:561–568.

110. Newby LK, Ohman EM, Christenson RH, Moliterno DJ, Harrington RA, White HD, et al. Benefit of glycoprotein IIb/IIIa inhibition in patients with acute coronary syndromes and troponin t-positive status: the paragon-B troponin T substudy. Circulation 2001; 103:2891–2896.

111. Roffi M, Chew DP, Mukherjee D, Bhatt DL, White JA, Heeschen C, et al. Platelet glycoprotein IIb/IIIa inhibitors reduce mortality in diabetic patients with non-ST-segment-elevation acute coronary syndromes. Circulation 2001; 104:2767–2771.

112. Heeschen C, Hamm CW, Goldmann B, Deu A, Langenbrink L, White HD. Troponin concentrations for stratification of patients with acute coronary syndromes in relation to therapeutic efficacy of tirofiban. Lancet 1999; 354:1757–1762.

113. Yusuf S, Mehta SR, Zhao F, Gersh BJ, Commerford PJ, Blumenthal M, et al. on behalf of the CURE Investigators. Early and late effects of clopidogrel in patients with acute coronary syndromes. Circulation 2003; 107:966–972.

114. Yusuf S, Zhao F, Mehta, et al. for the Clopidogrel in Unstable Angina to Prevent Recurrent Events Trial Investigators. Effects of clopidogrel in addition to aspirin in patients with acute coronary syndromes without ST-segment elevation. N Engl J Med 2001; 345:494–502.

115. Berger PB, Steinhubl S. Clinical Implications of Percutaneous Coronary Intervention–Clopidogrel in Unstable Angina to Prevent Recurrent Events (PCI–CURE) study: a US perspective. Circulation 2002; 106:2284–2287.

116. Lincoff AM, Topol EJ, eds. Platelet Glycoprotein IIb/IIIa Inhibitors in Cardiovascular Disease. Totowa, NJ: Humana, 1999.

117. Marcel J, van den Brand BM, Simoons ML. The use of abciximab in therapy resistant unstable angina: clinical and angiographic results of the CAPTURE pilot and the CAPTURE study. In: Lincoff AM, Topol EJ, eds. Platelet Glycoprotein IIb/IIIa Inhibitors in Cardiovascular Disease. Totowa, NJ: Humana, 1999:143–168.

118. The CAPTURE Investigators. Randomized placebo-controlled trial of abciximab before and during coronary intervention in refractory unstable angina: the CAPTURE study. Lancet 1997; 349:1429–1435.

119. The PURSUIT Trial Investigators. Inhibition of platelet glycoprotein IIb/IIIa with eptifibatide in patients with acute coronary syndromes. N Engl J Med 1998; 339:436–443.

120. The Platelet Receptor Inhibition in Ischemic Syndrome Management (PRISM) Study Investigators. A comparison of aspirin plus tirofiban with aspirin plus heparin for unstable angina. N Engl J Med 1998; 338:1498–1505.

121. Platelet Receptor Inhibition in Ischemic Syndrome Management in Patients Limited by Unstable Signs and Symptoms (PRISM-PLUS) Study Investigators. Inhibition of the platelet glycoprotein IIb/IIIa receptor with tirofiban in unstable angina and non-Q-wave myocardial infarction. N Engl J Med 1998; 338:1488–1497.

122. The EPISTENT Investigators. Randomised placebo-controlled and balloon-angioplasty-controlled trial to assess safety of coronary stenting with use of platelet glycoprotein IIb/IIIa blockade. Lancet 1998; 352:87–92.

123. The EPILOG Investigators. Platelet glycoprotein IIb/IIIa blockade with abciximab with low-dose heparin during percutaneous coronary revascularization. N Engl J Med 1997; 336:1689–1696.

124. EPIC Investigators. Use of a monoclonal antibody against the platelet glycoprotein IIb/IIIa receptor in high-risk coronary angioplasty. N Engl J Med 1994; 330:956–961.

125. Hamm CW, Heeschen C, Goldmann B, Vahanian A, Adgey J, Miguel CM, et al. c7E3 Fab Antiplatelet Therapy in Unstable Refractory Angina (CAPTURE) Study Investigators. Benefit of abciximab in patients with refractory unstable angina in relation to serum troponin T levels. N Engl J Med 1999; 340:1623–1629.

126. Cannon CP, Weintraub WS, Demopoulos LA, Vicari R, Frey MJ, Lakkis N, Neumann FJ, Robertson DH, DeLucca PT, DiBattiste PM, Gibson CM, Braunwald E. Comparison of early invasive and conservative strategies in patients with unstable coronary syndromes treated with the glycoprotein IIb/IIIa inhibitor tirofiban. N Engl J Med. 2001; 344:1879–1887.

127. Veterans Administration Coronary Artery Bypass Surgery Cooperative Study Group. Eleven-year survival in the Veterans Administration randomized trial of coronary bypass surgery for stable angina. N Engl J Med 1984; 311:1333–1339.

128. Passamani E, Davis KB, Gillespie MJ, Killip T, and the CASS Principal Investigators and Their Associates. A randomized trial of coronary artery bypass surgery: survival of patients with a low ejection fraction. N Engl J Med 1985; 312:1665–1671.

129. CASS Principal Investigators and Their Associates: Coronary Artery Surgery Study (CASS) a randomized trial of coronary artery bypass surgery: survival data. Circulation 1983; 68:939–950.

130. Armstrong PW, Bogaty P, Buller CE, Dorian P, O'Neill BJ, Canadian Cardiovascular Society Working Group. The 2004 ACC/AHA Guidelines: a perspective and adaptation for Canada by the Canadian Cardiovascular Society Working Group. CJC 2004; 20(11):1075–1079.

131. Antman EM, Anbe DT, Armstrong PW, Bates ER, Green LA, Hand M, Hochman JS, Krumholz HM, Kushner FG, Lamas GA, Mullany CJ, Ornato JP, Pearle DL, Sloan MA, Smith SC. ACC/AHA guidelines for the management of patients with ST-elevation myocardial infarction—executive summary. A report of the American College of Cardiology/American Heart Association Task Force on Practice Guidelines. J Am Coll Cardiol 2004; 44(3):671–719.

132. Boersma E, Maas ACP, Deckers JW, Simoons ML. Early thrombolytic treatment in acute myocardial infarction: reappraisal of the golden hour. Lancet 1996; 348(9030):771–775.

133. Armstrong PW, Collen D, Antman EM. Fibrinolysis for acute myocardial infarction: the future is here and now. Circulation 2003; 107(20):2533–2537.

134. Welsh RC, Armstrong PW. A marriage of enhancement: fibrinolysis and conjunctive therapy. Thromb Haemost 2004; 92(6):1194–1200.

135. Assessment of the Safety and Efficacy of a New Thrombolytic Regimen (ASSENT)-3 Investigators. Efficacy and safety of tenecteplase in combination with enoxaparin, abciximab, or unfractionated heparin: the ASSENT-3 randomised trial in acute myocardial infarction. Lancet 2001; 358(9282):605–613.

136. Wallentin L, Goldstein P, Armstrong PW, Granger CB, Adgey AA, Arntz HR, Bogaerts K, Danays T, Lindahl B, Makijarvi M, Verheugt F, Van de Werf F. Efficacy and safety of tenecteplase in combination with the low-molecular-weight heparin enoxaparin or unfractionated heparin in the prehospital setting: the Assessment of the Safety and Efficacy of a New Thrombolytic Regimen (ASSENT)-3 PLUS randomized trial in acute myocardial infarction. Circulation 2003; 108(2):135–142.

137. White HD, Aylward PE, Frey MJ, Adgey AA, Nair R, Hillis WS, Shalev Y, Brown MA, French JK, Collins R, Maraganore J, Adelman B. Randomized, double-blind comparison of hirulog versus heparin in patients receiving streptokinase and aspirin for acute myocardial infarction (HERO). Circulation 1997; 96(7):2155–2161.

138. White H, Hirulog and Early Reperfusion or Occlusion (HERO)-2 Trial Investigators. Thrombin-specific anticoagulation with bivalirudin versus heparin in patients receiving fibrinolytic therapy for acute myocardial infarction: the HERO-2 randomised trial. Lancet 2001; 358(9296):1855–1863.

139. ISIS-2 Collaborative Group (Second International Study of Infarct Survival). Randomized trial of intravenous streptokinase, oral aspirin, both, or neither among 17,187 cases of suspected acute myocardial infarction: ISIS-2. J Am Coll Cardiol 1988; 12(6 Suppl A):3A–13A.

140. van't Hof AWJ, Liem A, Suryapranata H, Hoorntje JCA, de Boer M-J, Zijlstra F on behalf of the Zwolle Myocardial Infarction Study Group. Angiographic assessment of myocardial reperfusion in patients treated with primary angioplasty for acute myocardial infarction: myocardial blush grade. Circulation 1998; 97(23):2302–2306.

141. Topol EJ. Toward a new frontier in myocardial reperfusion therapy: emerging platelet preeminence. Circulation 1998; 97(2):211–218.

142. Sabatine MS, Cannon CP, Gibson CM, Lopez-Sendon JL, Montalescot G, Theroux P, Claeys MJ, Cools F, Hill KA, Skene AM, McCabe CH, Braunwald E, for the CLARITY-TIMI 28 Investigators. Addition of clopidogrel to aspirin and fibrinolytic therapy for myocardial infarction with ST-segment elevation. N Engl J Med 2005; 352(12):1179–1189.

143. Chen Z. COMMIT/CCS-2: Randomized placebo-controlled trial of adding clopidogrel to aspirin in 46,000 acute myocardial infarction patients. Presentation at ACC 2005, Orlando, FL, U.S.A., 2005.

144. Boersma E, Harrington RA, Moliterno DJ, White H, Theroux P, Van de Werf F, de Torbal A, Armstrong PW, Wallentin LC, Wilcox RG, Simes J, Califf RM, Topol EJ, Simoons ML. Platelet glycoprotein IIb/IIIa inhibitors in acute coronary syndromes: a meta-analysis of all major randomized clinical trials. Lancet 2002; 359(9302):189–198.

145. Armstrong PW. Reperfusion synergism: will it be both sustained and safe? Eur Heart J 2000; 21(23):1913–1916.

146. Antman EM, Gibson CM, de Lemos JA, Giugliano RP, McCabe CH, Coussement P, Menown I, Nienaber CA, Rehders TC, Frey MJ, et al. The Thrombolysis in Myocardial Infarction (TIMI) 14 Investigators. Combination reperfusion therapy with abciximab and reduced dose reteplase: results from TIMI 14. Eur Heart J 2000; 21(23):1944–1953.

147. SPEED Group (Strategies for Patency Enhancement in the Emergency Department). Trial of abciximab with and without low-dose reteplase for acute myocardial infarction. Circulation 2000; 101(24):2788–2794.

148. Brener SJ, Zeymer U, Adgey AA, Vrobel TR, Ellis SG, Neuhaus KL, Juran N, Ivanc TB, Ohman EM, Strony J, Kitt M, Topol EJ. Eptifibatide and low-dose tissue plasminogen activator in acute myocardial

infarction: the integrilin and low-dose thrombolysis in acute myocardial infarction (INTRO AMI) trial. J Am Coll Cardiol 2000; 39(3):377–386.

149. Topol EJ, for the GUSTO V Investigators. Reperfusion therapy for acute myocardial infarction with fibrinolytic therapy or combination reduced fibrinolytic therapy and platelet glycoprotein IIb/IIIa inhibition: the GUSTO V randomised trial. Lancet 2001; 357(9272):1905–1914.

150. de Lemos JA, Braunwald E. ST segment resolution as a tool for assessing the efficacy of reperfusion therapy. J Am Coll Cardiol 2001; 38(5):1283–1294.

151. Armstrong PW, Welsh RC. Tailoring therapy to best suit ST-segment elevation myocardial infarction searching for the right fit. CMAJ 2003; 169(9):925–927.

152. Gershlick AH, Wilcox R, Hughes S, Stevens S, Stephens-Lloyd A, Abrams K, for the REACT Investigators. Rescue Angioplasty Versus Conservative Therapy or Repeat Thrombolysis (REACT) trial for failed reperfusion in AMI. Circulation 2005; 111(13):1728.

153. Steg PG, Bonnefoy E, Chabaud S, Lapostolle F, Dubien PY, Cristofini P, Leizorovicz A, Touboul P, Comparison of Angioplasty and Prehospital Thrombolysis in acute Myocardial Infarction (CAPTIM) Investigators. Impact of time to treatment on mortality after prehospital fibrinolysis or primary angioplasty: data from the CAPTIM randomized clinical trial. Circulation 2003; 108(23):2851–2856.

154. Widimsky P, Budesinsky T, Vorac D, Groch L, Zelisko M, Aschermann M, Branny M, St'asek J, Formanek P, 'PRAGUE' Study Group Investigators. Long distance transport for primary angioplasty vs immediate thrombolysis in acute myocardial infarction. Final results of the randomized national multicentre trial—PRAGUE-2. Eur Heart J 2003; 24(1):94–104.

155. Willerson JT. One size does not fit all Editor's commentary. Circulation 2003; 107(20):2543–2544.

156. Beta-Blocker Heart Attack Study Group. Beta Blocker Heart Attack trial: design features. Controlled clinical trials. JAMA 1981; 2(4):275–285.

157. Latini R, Maggioni AP, Flather M, Sleight P, Tognoni G. ACE inhibitor use in patients with myocardial infarction. Summary of evidence from clinical trials. Circulation 1995; 92(10):3132–3137.

158. Pitt B, Remme W, Zannad F, Neaton J, Martinez F, Roniker B, Bittman R, Hurley S, Kleiman J, Gatlin M. Eplerenone Post-Acute Myocardial Infarction Heart Failure Efficacy and Survival Study Investigators. Eplerenone, a selective aldosterone blocker, in patients with left ventricular dysfunction after myocardial infarction. N Engl J Med 2003; 348(14):1309–1321.

159. Zehender M, Kasper W, Kauder E, Schonthaler M, Geibel A, Olschewski M, Just H. Right ventricular infarction as an independent predictor of prognosis after acute inferior myocardial infarction. N Engl J Med 1993; 328(14):981–988.

160. Dell'Italia LJ, Starling MR, Blumhardt R, Lasher JC, O'Rourke RA. Comparative effects of volume loading, dobutamine, and nitroprusside in patients with predominant right ventricular infarction. Circulation 1985; 72(6):1327–1335.

161. Becker RC, Gore JM, Lambrew CT, Weaver WD, Rubison RM, French WJ, Tiefenbrunn AJ, Bowlby LJ, Rogers WJ. A composite view of cardiac rupture in the United States National Registry of Myocardial Infarction. J Am Coll Cardiol 1996; 27(6):1321–1326.

162. Hochman JS, Sleeper LA, White HD, Dzavik V, Wong SC, Menon V, Webb JG, Steingart R, Picard MH, Menegus MA, et al., SHOCK Investigators. One-year survival following early revascularization for cardiogenic shock. JAMA 2001; 285(2):190–192.

163. Dzavik V, Sleeper LA, Cocke TP, Moscucci M, Saucedo J, Hosat S, Jiang X, Slater J, LeJemtel T, Hochman JS, for the SHOCK Investigators. Early revascularization is associated with improved survival in elderly patients with acute myocardial infarction complicated by cardiogenic shock: a report from the SHOCK Trial Registry. Eur Heart J 2003; 24(9):828–837.

164. Visser CA, Kan G, Meltzer RS, Koolen JJ, Dunning AJ with the technical assistance of Van Corler M, and De Koning H. Incidence, timing and prognostic value of left ventricular aneurysm formation after myocardial infarction: a prospective, Serial echocardiographic study of 158 patients. Am J Cardiol 1986; 57:729–732.

165. Hudson MP, Granger CB, Topol EJ, Pieper KS, Armstrong PW, Barbash GI, Guerci AD, Vahanian A, Califf RM, Ohman EM. Early reinfarction after fibrinolysis: experiences from GUSTO I and GUSTO III trials. Circulation 2001; 104:1229–1235.

166. Armstrong PW, Fu Yuling, Chang WC, Topol EJ, Granger CB, Betriu A, Van de Werf F, Lee KL, Califf RM, for the GUSTO IIb Investigators. Acute coronary syndromes in the GUSTO-IIb trial: prognostic insights and impact of recurrent ischemia. Circulation 1998; 98(18):1860–1868.

167. Schuster EH, Bulkley BH. Early post-infarction angina. Ischemia at a distance and ischemia in the infarct zone. N Engl J Med 1981; 305(19):1101–1105.

168. Oliva PB, Hammill SC. The clinical distinction between regional postinfarction pericarditis and other causes of postinfarction chest pain: ancillary observations regarding the effect of lytic therapy upon the frequency of postinfarction pericarditis, postinfarction angina, and reinfarction. Clinical Cardiology 1994; 17(9):471–478.

169. Tofler GH, Muller JE, Stone PH, Willich SN, Davis VG, Poole WK, Robertson T, Braunwald E. Pericarditis in acute myocardial infarction: characterization and clinical significance. Am Heart J 1989; 117(1):86–92.

170. Bulkley BH, Roberts WC. Steroid therapy during acute myocardial infarction. A cause of delayed healing and of ventricular aneurysm. Am J Med 1974; 56(2):244–250.

171. Catella-Lawson F, Reilly MP, Kapoor SC, Cucchiara AJ, DeMarco S, Tournier B, Vyas SN, FitzGerald GA. Cyclooxygenase inhibitors and the antiplatelet effects of aspirin. N Engl J Med 2001; 345(25):1809–1817.
172. Cannon CP, Braunwald E, McCabe CH, Rader DJ, Rouleau JL, Belder R, Joyal SV, Hill KA, Pfeffer MA, Skene AM, for the Pravastatin or Atorvastatin Evaluation and Infection Therapy—Thrombolysis in Myocardial Infarction 22 Investigators. Intensive versus moderate lipid lowering with statins after acute coronary syndromes. N Engl J Med 2004; 350(15):1495–1504.
173. Ridker PM, Cushman M, Stampfer MJ, Tracy RP, Hennekens CH. Inflammation, aspirin, and the risk of cardiovascular disease in apparently healthy men. N Engl J Med 1997; 336:973–979.

19 | Tobacco and Cardiovascular Disease

Robyn L. Richmond, Nicholas Zwar, and Rowena Ivers

School of Public Health and Community Medicine, The University of New South Wales, Kensington, New South Wales, Australia

KEY POINTS

Demographics and Health Effects of Smoking

- Tobacco is responsible for the death of one in ten adults worldwide.
- Half the people who smoke today, that is, about 650 million people will eventually be killed by tobacco.
- Around 22% of U.S. adults are current smokers (24% of men and 19% of women); 50% of those who had ever smoked were former smokers.
- In developed countries, smoking causes 40% of heart disease deaths among people less than age 65 and 21% of all heart disease deaths.
- Stopping smoking dramatically reduces risk of developing CHD with a 50% reduction after one year compared to continuing smokers.
- In established CHD smokers who quit have a 36% crude relative risk reduction in mortality compared to continuing smokers.
- Nonsmokers living with smokers have an increased risk of heart disease of between 20% and 30%.
- Exposure of nonsmokers to environmental tobacco smoke (ETS) causes an increased risk of lung cancer, in those living with smokers in the region of 20% to 30%.
- The tar, oxidizing gases, and carbon monoxide are the main causative factors in tobacco related diseases.
- Most smokers become dependent on nicotine, which is the addictive drug found in all tobacco products. Nicotine is a highly addictive drug, as addictive as heroin or cocaine.
- There are many health benefits when smoking is ceased, with health benefits existing even for cessation at an advanced age.

Public Health Approaches to Reduce Tobacco Use

- Tax increases are a highly effective way to reduce tobacco consumption.
- Providing information about the health effects and addictive nature of smoking can lead to reduction in cigarette consumption.
- Young people are less responsive to information about the health effects of tobacco than older people, and more educated people respond more quickly to new information than those with minimal education.
- Multiple restrictions on advertising in all media and on promotional activities such as sponsorship of sports and other events, can reduce smoking by more than 6% in high-income countries.
- Restrictions on smoking in public places have reduced tobacco consumption by between 4% and 10%.
- Warning labels can still be effective in motivating smokers to make a quit attempt if they are large on the cigarette pack.
- Antitobacco mass media campaigns can reduce tobacco consumption and increase cessation rates when implemented in conjunction with other public health interventions such as community education and tax increases.
- With a modest price rise, a huge number of premature deaths would be avoided: nine million premature deaths would be avoided in developing countries.
- Implementing multipronged public health strategies have a significant impact on reducing smoking rates in a population, which in turn reduces the number of premature deaths for cigarette related diseases.

Clinical Approaches to Reduce Tobacco Use

- Physicians in both primary care and specialty practice are well placed to treat tobacco dependence and increase rates of smoking cessation as 70% of smokers see a physician each year.

- Other health professionals, such as physician assistants, nurse practitioners, nurses, physical, and occupational therapists can also have a role in smoking cessation.
- Evidence-based guidelines for smoking cessation have been developed and disseminated in many countries including the United States, United Kingdom, Canada, Australia, and New Zealand.
- The majority of guidelines use or have adapted the 5 As approach of the U.S. Clinical Practice Guideline. The 5 As approach includes: asking patients whether they smoke, advising smokers to quit, assessing readiness to stop smoking and level of nicotine dependence, assisting the smoker to quit, and arranging follow up.
- Most patients attempting to quit should be encouraged to use effective pharmacotherapies such as nicotine gum, patch, nasal spray, lozenge, tablet, bupropion, nortriptyline, and clonidine. NRT and bupropion are current first line options for pharmacotherapy.
- NRT is safe in patients with stable CVD.
- Pharmacotherapy should be considered when a pregnant woman is otherwise unable to quit and when the likelihood and benefits of cessation outweigh the risks of NRT and potential continued smoking.
- Bupropion is efficacious in a range of patient populations including those with cardiac and respiratory diseases, depression, and among the general community.
- Pro-active telephone counseling, where the counselor initiates one or more calls to provide support or help to avoid relapse, is an effective intervention.

INTRODUCTION

Tobacco is a major burden of disease, disability, and death in the world. Currently, smoking causes the death of one in 10 adults, globally (1). This is more than any other cause of mortality and more than the projected death tolls from pneumonia, diarrheal diseases, tuberculosis, and the complications of childbirth combined (1). Tobacco kills smokers at the height of their productivity in middle age, losing 20 to 25 years of life and depriving families of, breadwinners and nations of, a healthy workforce. The use of tobacco has been estimated to cause an annual global net loss of US $200 thousand million, with a third of this loss in developing countries (1). Even a modest breakthrough in developing and implementing interventions with greater impact on populations of smokers could prevent millions of premature deaths and billions of lost years of life (2).

This chapter comprises four sections. In the first section, the prevalence of smoking within subpopulations is described with emphasis on those groups at high risk. The second section explores the health effects of smoking and details the main diseases caused by smoking with an emphasis on cardiovascular conditions. As tobacco use is associated with poverty and low socioeconomic status, so are its damaging effects on health (1). Smoking contributes heavily to the widening of the survival gap, over time, between affluent and disadvantaged men in developed countries (1). The nicotine pharmacology, nicotine dependence, and effects of involuntary tobacco smoke are described, ending on a positive note with benefits gained from quitting.

There are many tobacco control measures that can be used in different settings that have a significant impact on tobacco use. In the third section of this chapter, a range of strategies are described including public health initiatives such as increasing tobacco tax and price, decreasing tobacco advertising, encouraging smoke-free environments in public and work settings, and warnings on tobacco packaging. The physician has a key role to play in reducing smoking prevalence among smoking patients and this is the focus of the fourth section. Guidelines for assisting smokers to quit, pharmacotherapies and behavioral methods used in cessation, and case studies are described in this section of the chapter.

PREVALENCE OF SMOKING RATES

Globally one in three adults or 1.1 billion people are smokers, representing 47% of men and 12% of women (1). Of these, around 80% live in low- and middle-income countries; and it is these populations that have been increasing their tobacco consumption since 1970 (3).

The total number of smokers is expected to reach about 1.6 billion by 2025 due to the growth in adult population and increase in tobacco consumption. In developing countries, there are around 48% of men and 12% of women who smoke, whereas in developed countries, 42% of men and 24% of women smoke (1,3). This indicates that different countries are at different stages of the tobacco epidemic (discussed below).

The Death Toll from Smoking

The World Health Organization (WHO) has estimated that in 2001 there were four million deaths per year caused from tobacco (3). If current smoking patterns continue, it will cause 10 million deaths each year by 2030 with 70% of these deaths occurring in developing countries. Tobacco will then be the leading cause of fatal disease in the world, responsible for one in every eight deaths (4). Half the people who smoke today, which is, about 650 million people, will eventually die from tobacco-related diseases.

Adding to the tragic scene, is the estimation that if current smoking patterns continue, 250 children alive today will eventually die from tobacco-related diseases (4). In the United States, on average, among 1000, 20-year-olds who smoke cigarettes regularly, about six will die from homicide, about 12 will die in motor vehicle accidents, and about 500 will be killed by smoking (250 in middle age, 35 to 69 years, and 250 more in older age). In the United Kingdom in this group, about one will die from homicide, six from motor vehicle accidents, and the same 500 from smoking (5).

The main adverse effect of nicotine in tobacco is its addictive properties (discussed below), which sustains the tobacco use among smokers. Nicotine dependent smokers continue to expose themselves to toxins in tobacco and these are responsible for most of the adverse health effects (6–8). In the United States, 92% of smokers think that their habit is addictive, and 70% want to quit (9).

Smoking related deaths were once largely confined to men in the high-income countries, but have now spread to women in high-income countries and men throughout the world (1). Back in 1990, two out of every three smoking related deaths were in either the high-income countries or the former socialist states of Eastern Europe and Central Asia. However, by 2030 seven out of every 10 deaths from tobacco use will be in low- and middle-income countries. Of the half-billion deaths expected among people alive today, about 100 million will be among Chinese men (1).

In 2000, an estimated 4.83 million premature deaths globally were attributable to smoking, 2.41 million in developing countries and 2.43 million in industrialized countries. There were 3.84 million male deaths and 1.00 million female deaths attributable to smoking; 2.69 million smoking attributable deaths were between the ages of 30 to 69 years, and 2.14 million were 70 years of age and above (10). The leading causes of death from smoking in developed regions are cardiovascular diseases (CVD), lung cancer, and chronic obstructive pulmonary disease (COPD), and in the developing world, CVD, COPD, and lung cancer (10).

Regional Patterns of Smoking

Prevalence of tobacco use varies around the world, with developed countries typically displaying high or moderate rates in men and women, and developed nations having high rates in men and very low rates in women. Table 1 shows that there are wide variations between World Bank regions. In particular, there is a great difference between the prevalence of smoking among women in different regions. For example, in Eastern Europe and Central Asia (mainly the former socialist economies), 59% of men and 26% of women smoked in 1995, which is more than in other regions (10). Yet in East Asia and in the Pacific regions, male smoking prevalence was 59%, but the female smoking rate was low at 4% (10). These variations in tobacco use can be explained by the Model of the Tobacco Epidemic described below. Table 2 demonstrates the variability in adult and youth smoking rates by selected countries and youth exposure to involuntary smoking in the home.

The Model of the Tobacco Epidemic

The model of the tobacco epidemic describes the evolution of tobacco use and follows the curve of an epidemic in stages rather than a series of isolated events (12,13). This is a theoretical model that applies to some but not all countries. The situation of the tobacco epidemic is complicated and this useful framework enables an understanding of the complexity in a simplified form (Fig. 1).

In Stage 1 smoking prevalence is below 20% in men, with minimal smoking among women. Countries that exemplify Stage 1 of the tobacco epidemic include Nigeria (smoking prevalence is 15% among males and 2% among females), Swaziland (smoking prevalence is 25% among males and 2% among females), Malawi (smoking prevalence is 20% among males and 9% among females), Ghana (smoking prevalence is 28% among males and 3.5% among

TABLE 1 Patterns of Smoking in World Health Organization Regions

	Smoking prevalence (%)		
World bank region	Males	Females	Total
East Asia and Pacific	59	4	32
Eastern Europe and Central Asia	59	26	41
Latin America and Caribbean	40	21	30
Middle East and North Africa	44	5	25
South Asia (cigarettes)	20	1	11
South Asia (bidis)	20	3	12
Sub-Saharan Africa	33	10	21
Low/middle income	49	9	29
High income	39	22	30
World	47	12	29

Source: From Ref. 11.

females), and the Democratic Republic of the Congo (smoking prevalence is 24% among males and 5.5% among females) (12).

These countries have not yet been drawn into the global tobacco economy, and represent a major untapped market for the multinational tobacco industry and are ready for expansion. In the words of a public affairs manager of Rothmans Ltd: "It would be stupid to ignore a growing market" (15). The first stage of the tobacco epidemic is characterized by low uptake of tobacco and low cessation rates.

In Stage 2 of the continuum there are increases in smoking rates to above half for men, and an increase in smoking rates among women, with rising mortality rates from lung cancer among men, but little tobacco-related female mortality. This pattern occurs in China, Japan, North Africa, and Latin America. Smoking prevalence in the Philippines is 75% among males and 18% among females, in China the smoking prevalence among men is as high as 63% and for socioeconomic and cultural reasons, prevalence among women is still low at 4%. In North Africa, smoking prevalence in Yemen is 60% among males and 29% among females, and in Mexico is 56% among males and 20% among females (12). As incomes rise within populations, the number of people that smoke also rises. In the early stages of the tobacco epidemic, smoking is more likely to occur among the affluent than among the poor. In this stage, smoking is used to signal wealth and upward mobility and physicians have high smoking rates in these countries, e.g., among Chinese physicians, 61% of males and 12% of females smoke (12).

Already in several African countries, the acreage devoted to tobacco growing has increased 10-fold since 1970. Women are being actively targeted by tobacco companies in countries where there are improvements in economic, social, and educational status, with cigarettes being marketed as the key to emancipation, independence, and success (16). In Stage 2, the health risks of smoking are not widely known, tobacco control activities are not

TABLE 2 The Demographics of Tobacco Use (Selected Countries)

Country	Population (millions)	Adult smoking (%)			Youth smoking (%)			Youth exposure to passive smoke at home (%)
		Total	Male	Female	Total	Male	Female	
Australia	19	19.5	21	18	–	–	–	–
Brazil	140	34	38	29	–	–	–	–
China	1282	36	67	4	11	14	7	53
India	1008	16	29	2.5	–	–	–	34
Indonesia	212	31	59	4	22	38	5	63
United Kingdom	59	26.5	27	26	–	–	–	–
United States of America	283	24	26	21.5	26	27.5	24	42

Source: From Ref. 11.

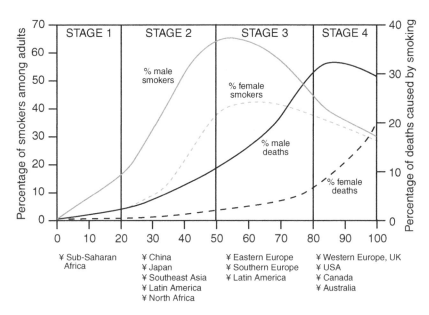

FIGURE 1 Model of the tobacco epidemic: the four stages of the tobacco epidemic. *Source*: From Ref. 14 with permission of BMJ Publishing Group.

well developed, and there is low public and political support for the implementation of tobacco control measures.

With Stage 3 there is a marked downturn in smoking prevalence among men, and a gradual decline in women, and continued increases in mortality from smoking (12). The gender-specific difference in smoking prevalence in developed countries narrowed between 1965 and 1985. Smoking attributable deaths are 10% to 30% of all deaths, with about three-quarters of these being in men. Many countries in Eastern and Southern Europe are at this stage of the tobacco epidemic. For example, the prevalence of smoking in Luxembourg is 39% (males) and 27% (females); in Turkey is 51% (males) and 49% (females), and in Switzerland is 38% (males) and 27% (females) (12).

In Stage 3, health education and media coverage erode public acceptance of tobacco use, and the educated population views smoking as undesirable.

Stage 4 is marked by further declines in smoking rates among men and women, with numbers of new smokers starting to decrease. Deaths attributable to smoking among men peak at 30% to 35% of all deaths and subsequently decline. Among women, smoking attributable deaths rise to about 20% to 25% of all deaths. Countries at this stage include the United States, Australia, and Northern and Western Europe. In Australia daily smoking prevalence is 21% (males) and 18% (females) (17); in Canada smoking prevalence among males is 27% and females, 23% (11); in the United Kingdom smoking rates among males have fallen from more than 50% in 1974 to 26% in 2000 and from 40% to 27% among females over the same period (18). Smoking rates among subpopulations in the United States are described below.

While overall smoking rates are declining during Stage 4, the decline in smoking rates among the poor and unskilled are very much less (18). In high-income countries affluent men have increasingly abandoned smoking, whereas men from disadvantaged groups continue to smoke. For example, in Norway, the proportion of males with high incomes who smoked declined from 75% in 1955 to 28% in 1990. Over the same time, the percent of men on low incomes who smoked declined much less steeply, from 60% in 1955 to 48% in 1990. In most high income countries today there are significant differences in prevalence of smoking between different socioeconomic groups. In the United Kingdom, for example, only 10% of females and 12% of males in the highest socioeconomic group smoke. However, in the lowest socioeconomic group, 35% of females and 40% of males continue to smoke (1). More than three-quarters of women want to quit smoking and nearly a half, report having tried to quit during the previous year (19).

The four stages of the tobacco epidemic provide a valuable understanding of where countries are in relation to evolution in the tobacco epidemic and engagement in tobacco control activities (described below). It offers an explanation for the variation in uptake of the tobacco habit, and highlights the pattern in developing countries, which reflects that of developed countries 50 to 60 years earlier.

Tobacco Use in the United States

The United States is an example of a country in Stage 4 of the tobacco epidemic. However, a closer look among specific subpopulations reveals a more complex situation showing some groups at an earlier stage of the tobacco epidemic. Overall in the United States there are 24% of men and 19% of women who smoke (i.e., 45.4 million). Prevalence of tobacco use for women of various ages is: 18 to 24 years (25%), 25 to 44 years (23%), 45 to 64 years (21%), and 65 years or older (9%) (20). For the second consecutive year, more adults had quit smoking than had continued to smoke; half of those who had ever smoked were former smokers (21). This was the first time since 1965 that the prevalence of tobacco use by women had dropped below 20% (21). Table 3 presents the prevalence of tobacco use among various U.S. demographic groups over the past 50 years. Smoking rates among the groups identified in Table 3 (males, females, whites, and blacks) have significantly decreased over this period, exemplifying a country in Stage 4 of the Tobacco Epidemic.

The prevalence of tobacco use was lower in older people (9% in those aged 65 years and older vs. 26% in those aged 25–44 years). During 1983 to 2003, a sustained decline in cigarette smoking prevalence occurred in all age groups except persons aged 18 to 24 years. It was lower in those with a higher level of educational attainment (7.5% among those with masters, professional, and doctoral degrees vs. 44% in those who had attained a General Educational Development diploma). The prevalence of tobacco use was higher among those living in poverty (30.5%) compared to 22% living at or above the poverty level (21).

The prevalence of tobacco use among subpopulations in the United States is described. Rates are lowest among Asians (12%) and Hispanics (16%) and highest among American Indians/Alaska Natives (40%), (the latter group an example of smokers in an earlier stage of the tobacco epidemic) (21).

African Americans

In the United States the prevalence of smoking among African American adults is similar to that of white adults (Table 3) (22). Compared to other Americans, African Americans are more likely to prefer mentholated cigarettes; approximately 75% smoke mentholated cigarettes compared to 25% of all smokers; mentholated cigarettes may be more harmful than other cigarettes (23).

Most African Americans smokers (70%) report that they want to quit smoking, and are more likely than white smokers to have quit for at least one day during the previous year (30% compared with 26%) (23).

American Indians and Alaska Natives

Approximately 2 million American Indians and Alaska Natives live in the United States (23). In 1997, smoking was more prevalent between American Indian and Alaska Native men than

TABLE 3   Percentage of Smoking Prevalence Among U.S. Adults, 18 Years of Age and Older, 1955–2003

Year	Overall population (%)	Males (%)	Females (%)	Whites (%)	Blacks (%)
1955		57	28		
1965	42	52	34	42	46
1970	37	44	31.5	37	41
1974	37	43	32	36	44
1978	34	38	31	34	38
1980	33	38	29	33	37
1985	30	33	28	30	35
1990	25.5	28	23	26	26
1995	25	27	23	26	26
2000	23	26	21	24	23
2003	22	24	19	23	21.5

Source: From Ref. 21.

among white men (38% vs. 27%) (23). The prevalence of smoking between American Indian and Alaska Native women was higher than that of white women (31% vs. 23%) (22).

American Indians and Alaska Natives smoke fewer cigarettes each day than white smokers; in 1994 to 1995, half of American Indians and Alaska Natives reported that they smoked less than 15 cigarettes per day, compared to 35% of whites (23). Pipe smoking and the use of chewing tobacco or snuff appeared to be more common in American Indian and Alaskan Natives than in other groups (23).

Tobacco is used as a traditional medicine and during religious ceremonies by many tribes, with use varying by tribe; chronic use of smoked or spit tobacco contributes to many chronic diseases.

Asian Americans and Pacific Islanders

In 1997, the prevalence of smoking was lower among Asian Americans and Pacific Islanders (17%) than for all other ethnic or racial groups (22). Both Asian American and Pacific Islander men and women were less likely to smoke compared with white men and women (22% vs. 27% and 12% vs. 23%, respectively) (22).

Hispanics

Approximately 31 million (11%) Americans are of Latin American descent (23). In 1997, the prevalence of smoking among Hispanic adults was 20% (20), i.e., lower than all other groups except Asian Americans and Pacific Islanders. The smoking rate among Hispanic men was comparable to that of white men (26% vs. 27%) but the rate among Hispanic women was much lower than that of white women (14% vs. 23%) (22).

High Risk Groups

Several subgroups that are at high risk from smoking are described. They include: women, adolescents, those who have a mental illness, those who misuse substances, and prisoners.

Women and Smoking

Smoking prevalence has always been lower among women than men. However, the difference in prevalence between the genders narrowed in the 1960s and 1970s in developed countries particularly, as countries progressed through the stages of the tobacco epidemic.

The prevalence of tobacco use is rising among young women. In some nations, for example, the United States, Germany, and Denmark, more women aged 14 to 19 years, smoke compared to young men (5). Reasons for increased uptake include concerns about body image, beliefs that smoking causes weight loss, and peer pressure. In some Asian and Pacific countries, smoking is seen as a symbol of freedom from traditional gender roles and thus desirable.

Women smokers potentially face greater health effects from tobacco than male smokers, and may be more susceptible to carcinogens (5). When smoking the same number of cigarettes, women display higher rates of lung cancer than men.

In the United States smoking is more common among women with lower levels of education: 33% in women with 9 to 11 years of education versus 11% in those with 16 or more years of education (20). Smoking is more common among the poor women (30% of those below the poverty level vs. 22% of those above it). Of concern, is the increase in the prevalence of tobacco use that occurred among United States schoolgirls in the 1990s; the prevalence of schoolgirls who reported smoking in the last month increased from 26% in 1992 to 35% in 1997 (20). Similarly, the prevalence of tobacco use by young women aged 18 to 24 also increased. Among U.S. women, the prevalence of tobacco use is highest among American Indians or Alaska Natives (41%), followed by whites (22%), African Americans (19%), Hispanics (11%), and Asians (7%) (20).

In the United States around 17% of pregnant women aged 15 to 44 years smoke compared to 31% of nonpregnant women, with a higher prevalence of smoking among young women (17% among women aged 18 vs. 10.5% among women aged 25–49), women of lower levels of educational attainment, and was higher among American Indian and Alaskan native women compared to other ethnic groups (24).

Only 18% to 25% of all women quit smoking once they become pregnant (25). Women who quit smoking before or during pregnancy reduce the risk for adverse reproductive outcomes.

Adolescents

Tobacco use by adolescents appears to be increasing; there is some evidence of earlier uptake of tobacco use by children and adolescents. The majority of smokers start before age 25 years, often in childhood (1). In high-income countries, eight in 10 begin in adolescence; in middle- and low-income countries, most smokers start by their early 20s, but the trend is toward young ages (1).

Those with a Mental Illness

People with a psychotic illness have consistently been shown to have much higher smoking rates than members of the general population (26,27). With at least 70% of people with schizophrenia smoking cigarettes (28), there is cause for concern, because of the serious financial and health costs. It has been estimated that smokers with schizophrenia in the United States spend just over a third of their weekly income on cigarettes (29). People diagnosed with a mental illness are about twice as likely to smoke as the general population (29). In a meta-analysis of 42 studies conducted around the world across 20 nations, an association between schizophrenia and current smoking was found. Those diagnosed with schizophrenia were more likely to be heavy smokers and more highly dependent on nicotine when compared to the general population. Those with schizophrenia were less likely to cease smoking, when compared with the general population (30).

In the National Comorbidity Survey conducted in the United States, the prevalence of smoking among those with current mental illness was 41%, compared to 35% of those who had ever suffered a mental illness, and 22.5% in controls (29).

Smokers with psychiatric illnesses are less likely to quit smoking compared to people without psychiatric illnesses, probably because of higher levels of nicotine dependence (26). In addition to smoking for many of the same reasons as smokers without a psychiatric illness (27), smokers with a psychotic illness may do so in order to alleviate negative symptoms, cognitive dysfunction, and/or medication side-effects (31). Smokers with a psychotic illness experience increased psychiatric symptoms, number of hospitalizations, and a need for higher medication doses (32).

People Who Use Other Drugs

The prevalence of tobacco use among those who misuse alcohol and other drugs is high; prevalence of tobacco use ranges from 74% to 100% (33–37). Tobacco use is associated with alcohol dependence (38), cannabis use (39), heroin use (40), and cocaine use (41). There appears to be a synergistic effect of the combination of tobacco and other substances; it is estimated that the combined health risks of smoking and alcohol use are 50% higher than the sum of their individual risks (42). Those with alcohol and drug dependence are more likely to die from tobacco-related causes, such as CVD and cancer, than from other effects of their drug misuse (43).

Prisoners

Most inmates in correctional facilities are smokers. Two surveys of prisoners conducted in jails in NSW, Australia reported prevalence of smoking at 88% in 1996 and 79% in 2001 (44). A meta-analysis of 62 prison mental health surveys reported that inmates were more likely to have a psychotic illness, major depression, and a personality disorder than the general population (45). Lifetime use of illicit drugs was reported to be 80% among male prisoners in NSW, with 48% having used illicit drugs in prison (46). Cannabis and heroin were the most commonly consumed drugs in prison. Smoking is particularly common among those with substance-use disorders (47). These studies raised the need for prison-based health promotion programs.

Health Effects of Smoking

In the second section of this chapter the health consequences of tobacco use are described. The main diseases resulting from smoking are discussed with an emphasis on cardiac conditions. This is followed by an exploration of nicotine pharmacology and addiction. Then a discussion of the effects of involuntary or passive smoking ensues. This section ends on a positive note in which the health benefits of quitting are elucidated.

Diseases Caused by Smoking

Tobacco is a cause of at least 25 diseases that include:

- CVD
- respiratory diseases
- cancers including lung and oral cavity
- menstrual function and menopause
- reproductive outcomes
- gastrointestinal disease
- arthritis
- eye disease
- depression and other psychiatric disorders
- neurological diseases

The focus of this section is on the first five listed: cardiovascular including cerebrovascular diseases, respiratory diseases, cancers, menstrual function, menopause, and reproduction is summarized in Table 4.

On average, lifelong smokers have a 50% chance of dying from a tobacco-related disease, and half of these deaths occur in middle age (45–54 years). For example, tobacco use was responsible for 35% of deaths in middle aged men (50).

In developed countries, smoking is the cause of 40% of heart disease deaths among people less than age 65 years, 21% of all heart disease deaths, 87% of lung cancer deaths, 82% of emphysema deaths, 33% of all cancers, and 10% of infant deaths (51).

Before the widespread use of cigarettes, lung cancer was a rare disease; in 1990 smoking caused 29% of all cancer deaths among men and 6% among women (52). However, the toll of death and disease from tobacco use in low and middle-income countries is expected to significantly rise. This is because the diseases caused by smoking take between 25 and 30 years to develop.

Atherosclerosis

Coronary heart disease (CHD) and cerebrovascular disease caused by tobacco use are the most common causes of mortality in developed countries. Overall, 30% to 40% of the annual death toll is related to coronary artery disease attributable to smoking (53). Tobacco use contributes to the development of atherosclerosis, which in turn causes ischemic heart disease (25). Smoking is strongly related to myocardial infraction and cardiac death in the general population (54–56). Smokers who are in their 30s and 40s have five times the chance of suffering a heart attack as nonsmokers of the same age, and switching to low tar cigarettes does little to alter the risk (57). Among those in their 30s, the heart attack rate in smokers is 6.3 times that of nonsmokers; for those in their 40s, the rate was 4.7 times higher, for those in their 50s, it was 3.1 times higher, and for those in their 60s and 70s, it was 2.5 and 1.9 times that of nonsmokers (57). In the United States there are about 40,000 heart attacks caused by smoking among people in their 30s and 40s. Smokers between the ages of 45 and 64 years triple their risk of dying from heart disease compared to nonsmokers (58). Cigarette smoking accounts for 45% in men and 41% in women of the total risk for CHD, for those under age 65 years (59). Cigarette smoking increases the risk of sudden cardiac death, suggesting that it increases myocardial vulnerability to ventricular fibrillation, a fatal rhythm disturbance (60). A smoker's chance of having a heart attack falls steeply after quitting, and in two years approximates that of someone who has never smoked (57).

In 2003 an estimated 1.1 million Americans had a new myocardial infarct (25). The presence of ischemic heart disease also contributed to the development of congestive heart failure. Cigarette smoking is associated with sudden cardiac death (25). It is associated with increases in serum low-density lipoprotein cholesterol and triglycerides (58). Smoking causes higher levels of serum-free fatty acids. In particular, this exposure causes higher levels of very low-density lipoproteins. Smoking interferes with the normal metabolism of cholesterol and triglycerides. U.S. smokers are three times more likely to die in middle age of vascular diseases, including heart attacks, strokes, and other diseases of the arteries or veins (1). As ischemic heart disease is common in high-income countries, the smoker's excess risk translates into a very

TABLE 4 Health Effects of Smoking

Health system	Relationship with smoking	Possible mechanisms
Cardiovascular system		
Ischemic heart disease	Causal relationship inferred with ischemic heart disease and with atherosclerosis	Nicotine increases risk of atherosclerosis, thrombosis, and arrhythmia. It impairs plasma lipid profile (increases low-density lipoproteins, d ecreases high density lipoproteins), and increases blood clotting by enhancing platelet reactivity and inhibiting prostacyclin. It increases circulating cate-cholamines. It decreases endothelial NO content. It pro-duces endothelial injury, leading to development of atherosclerotic plaque Carbon monoxide increases blood carboxyhemo-globin levels, reduces oxygenation of hemoglobin, and inhibits mitochondrial cytochrome oxidase Smoking also leads to the irreversible inhibition of the activity of NO synthase leading to low levels of NO
Cerebrovascular disease	Causal relationship inferred	Thromboxane A2 induced by cigarette smoke causes cerebral vasoconstriction. Alters platelet aggre-gation and survival, resulting in thrombosis
AAA	Causal relationship inferred	AAA occur secondary to the development of atherosclerosis (see above)
PVD	Causal relationship inferred	PVD occurs due to the development of atherosclerosis (see above)
Hypertension		Possibly due to the development of atherosclerosis
Respiratory system		
Lung cancer	Causal relationship inferred. Tobacco smoking increases risk dose dependently	Numerous carcinogens contained in tobacco smoke
COAD	Causal relationship inferred. Tobacco smoking increases risk dose dependently	Smoking inhibits anti-proteases and stimulates release of proteases by neutrophils. Smoking causes smooth muscle constriction leading to airway obstruction
Pneumonia	Causal relationship inferred in those without COAD, but insufficient evidence to infer a causal relationship in those with preexisting COAD	Smoking impairs ciliary movement, inhibits alveolar macrophages, causes hypertrophy of mucus-secreting glands, and stimulates submucosal irritant receptors
Chronic bronchitis	Causal relationship inferred	As for pneumonia
Emphysema	Tobacco smoking increases risk dose dependently	Inhibits antiproteases; stimulates release of proteases by neutrophils
Asthma	Insufficient evidence to infer a causal relationship. Children passively exposed to environmental tobacco smoke have higher risk of developing asthma	Smoking increases airway obstruction and increases production of cysteinyl leukotrienes
Other systems		
Pancreatic cancer	Causal relationship inferred	Carcinogens contained in tobacco
Stomach cancer	Causal relationship inferred	Carcinogens contained in tobacco
Peptic ulcer	Causal relationship inferred	Smoking impairs healing, inhibits pancreatic bicarbonate secretion, decreases the pressure of esophageal and pyloric sphincters (thus promoting reflux), and interferes with H2-receptor antagonist treat-ment
Perinatal effects	Lower birthweight by 200 to 250 g. Increased stillbirth rate. Increased rate of SIDS (48)	Nicotine may cause constriction in blood vessels of the umbilical cord and uterus, thus reducing fetal oxygenation
Osteoporosis	Tobacco smoking is a risk factor	Impairs calcium metabolism

Abbreviations: NO, nitrous oxide; AAA, abdominal aortic aneurysm; PVD, peripheral vascular disease; COAD, chronic obstructive air-ways disease; SIDS, sudden infant death syndrome.
Source: From Refs. 25, 49.

large number of deaths, making heart disease the most common smoking-related cause of death in these countries.

Cigarette smoking is equivalent to an additional two decades of ageing in terms of the risk of damage to the carotid arteries in the neck (61). Smoking is the most significant risk factor for carotid artery atherosclerosis. Smokers have a 50% increase in the rate of plaque accumulation in the carotid arteries, former smokers, a 25% increase, and those exposed to environmental tobacco smoke (ETS), a 20% increase (59).

In women who smoke and use oral contraceptives, the risk of acute myocardial infarction is increased by 20.8 times (53). The risk of myocardial infarction is increased 41-fold in women who smoke and have a history of toxemia in pregnancy compared to only 4.5-fold among smoking women without a history of toxemia. In women, 30 to 55 years old who smoke 25 cigarettes per day, the relative risk for fatal CHD is 5.5 times that of a nonsmoker; the relative risk for nonfatal myocardial infarction is 5.8, and for angina pectoris is 2.6 (62).

Cerebrovascular disease (e.g., stroke) is the third leading cause of death in the United States, with an estimated 600,000 cases per year (25,63). Tobacco use also causes aortic aneurysms (23). The prevalence of cerebrovascular disease is twice as high among African Americans men than among white men (53 per 100,000 vs. 26 per 100,000) and twice as high among African Americans women as among white women (41 per 100,000 vs. 23 per 100,000) (23). CVD is the leading cause of death among American Indians, Alaska Natives, and Hispanics living in the United States (23). Whereas Asian Americans and Pacific Islanders had lowest of death rate from CHD compared to all other U.S. populations (23). The relative risk of stroke among hypertensive smokers is five times that of smokers without hypertension, and 20 times that of normotensive nonsmokers (64). The risk of stroke decreases steadily after smoking cessation. Smoking cessation reduces the risk of cerebrovascular disease; exsmokers have the same risk of stroke as never-smokers after 5 to 15 years (25,63).

Respiratory Diseases

Tobacco use is linked to the development of lung cancer, pneumonia, and chronic obstructive airways disease. Ninety percent of all lung cancer deaths are attributed to smoking. Since 1950 lung cancer deaths among women have increased by more than 600%. Smokers in the United States are 20 times more likely to die of lung cancer in middle age than nonsmokers (1). Development of lung cancer is affected more strongly by the duration of smoking and quantity of daily use. A threefold increase in the duration of smoking is associated with a 100-fold risk of lung cancer, whilst a threefold increase in number of cigarettes smoked per day is only associated with a threefold risk of lung cancer (1). African Americans men are at least 50% more likely to develop lung cancer than white men (23) and are more likely to die from cancer of the lung and bronchus. Smoking-attributable deaths from cancers of the lung, trachea, and bronchus were slightly more common among American Indian and Alaska Native men and women than among Asian–American and Pacific Islander and Hispanic men and women, but lower than rates among African Americans men and women and white men and women (23). Lung cancer is the most common cause of cancer death among Asian Americans and Pacific Islander. Lung cancer is the leading cause of cancer deaths among Hispanics and occurs at a rate that is three times higher for Hispanic men than for Hispanic women (23).

In 1912, only 374 cases of lung cancer were reported. Now more than 150,000 deaths from cancer of the lung and bronchus each year are reported in the United States. Lung cancer has surpassed breast cancer as the leading cause of cancer deaths in U.S. women (19). In fact, more women in the United States died of lung cancer in 2000 than of cancers of the breast, uterus, and ovary combined (19). Globally, smoking caused 29% of all cancer deaths among men and 6% among women (4,65). The important point about this fact is that those who start smoking in adolescence, which is the case for most smokers, face the biggest risks.

Nicotine is not a significant cause of cancer among those who smoke. Other tobacco smoke constituents such as polycyclic aromatic hydrocarbons, tobacco-specific nitrosamines, aldehydes, and aromatic amines, are responsible for the induction of cancers caused by smoking (66).

COPD is a leading cause of disability, hospital admission, and premature mortality in men and women (67). Tobacco smoking is the major cause of COPD. It is estimated that 15% to 20% of smokers will develop clinically significant COPD (68,69). Although there is a physiological decline in lung function over time due to aging, this decline is increased by exposure to tobacco smoke; however, following cessation reverts to the rate observed in nonsmokers (70,71).

Reproduction and Pregnancy

Cigarette smoking has clinically significant effects on reproduction (19). Women who smoke have increased risks for the following:

- infertility and conception delay
- ectopic pregnancy and spontaneous abortion
- preterm premature rupture of membranes, abruption placenta, placenta previa, and preterm delivery
- prenatal mortality both stillbirth and neonatal deaths, and sudden infant death syndrome (SIDS)
- infants with lower average birth weight and small for gestational age (18).

Effects on Unborn Babies and Infants

Women who smoke are at an increased risk for infertility and premature menopause (25). Nicotine is a potential fetal teratogen and may contribute to obstetrical complications in pregnant women and may lead to SIDS (6). Nicotine may cause constriction in blood vessels of the umbilical cord and uterus, thus reducing fetal oxygenation (25). Maternal smoking is also linked to a reduction in the lung function of infants (25). The infants of women who smoke are, on average, 200 to 250 g lower in birthweight than of those who do not smoke (72,73). Placenta praevia is twice as common in smokers and placental abruption is 1.4 to 2.4 times as common in smokers (25). Premature rupture of membranes, leading to premature delivery is also more common. The infants of women who smoke are also more likely to be stillborn, to die as neonates, or from SIDS (48). The children of smoking mothers are more likely to be admitted to hospital with respiratory illness (74). However, smokers are less likely to suffer from preeclampsia (25).

The effects of smoking continue into the postnatal period; breastfeeding is more likely to be of shorter duration in women who smoke. Despite the knowledge of the health effects of smoking during pregnancy, many pregnant women and girls continue to smoke. In the United States, approximately 12% to 22% of pregnant women, and only 18% to 25% of these quit once they became pregnant (25).

Effects on Children and Adolescents

Children and adolescents who smoke are less physically fit. The prevalence of respiratory illness is greater than that of nonsmokers and is related to impaired lung growth, chronic coughing, and wheezing (25).
In adolescence, smoking is related to increased susceptibility to, and severity of (75):

- respiratory infections
- reduced lung function and rate of lung growth
- increased likelihood of coughing spells and coughing up phlegm or blood
- increased likelihood of wheezing and gasping
- increased likelihood of shortness of breath when not exercising
- decreased physical activity and endurance.

Menstrual Function and Menopause Related to Smoking

The prevalence of dysmenorrheal is around 50% higher among current smokers than among former smokers or women who have never smoked (19,76,77). There is increasing prevalence of dysmenorrheal with increasing amount smoked and duration of smoking (77).

There is evidence that age of onset of menopause is earlier among smokers. In the Framingham study the mean age at menopause was 0.8 years earlier among smokers than nonsmokers (78). In the U.S. Nurses' Health Study the effect of smoking was greater with the age at menopause among women who smoked 35 cigarettes or more per day being two years earlier than among those who had never smoked (79). In Scotland, a dose response relationship with pack years of smoking was found to strongly increase the risk of menopause among women aged 45 to 49 years (80). The risk for menopause among former smokers was similar to that of women who had never smoked suggesting that the effect of smoking is largely reversible with cessation (81).

In studies conducted in Australia and England smokers were more likely than nonsmokers to experience more menopausal symptoms (82,83). Women who smoke have increased risk for hot flashes after hysterectomy and oophorectomy (84).

Other Health Effects

Smoking is associated with cancers of other organs including the bladder, kidney, larynx, mouth, pancreas, and stomach (1). Smokers' illnesses last longer (25). Smokers spend more money on medical care, and are admitted to hospital more frequently and for longer periods of time than nonsmokers (25). Smokers have a high mortality following surgery because of reduced immune response, slower wound healing, and higher rates of wound infections, and pneumonia (25).

Smokers are more likely to suffer from periodontitis (25). Those with helicobacter colonization are more likely to develop peptic ulcers (25).

Oral Cancers and Chewing Tobacco

Around 6.9 million Americans use smokeless tobacco (85). Smokeless tobacco products contain nitrosamines and other carcinogens that are known to produce oral cancer. Smokeless tobacco, and especially snuff-dipping, induces gingival recession, precancerous lesions of the oral cavity, and oral cavity cancer (86). Smokeless tobacco products contain carcinogens, such as nitrosamines, formaldehyde, crotonaldehyde, benzo [a] pyrene, and polonium-210 (87). Among these, the tobacco-specific nitrosamines N'-nitrosonornicotine (NNN) and 4-(methylnitrosamino)-1-(3-pyridyl)-1-butanone (NNK) are clearly the most prevalent. Strong carcinogens in smokeless tobacco are likely to play a significant role in oral cancer. Levels of NNN and NNK in smokeless tobacco products sold in the United States range from 3 to 10 mcg/g and are far greater than nitrosamine levels in any other consumer product (87,88). Amounts of tobacco-specific nitrosamines in some Swedish snuff products are lower than those sold in the United States, but the levels of these carcinogens—approximately 5 mcg/g—are still unacceptably high (89). Users of smokeless tobacco may experience heightened energy or strength that are really elevations in heart rate and blood pressure.

Longitudinal Studies of the Health Effects of Smoking

There are several notable longitudinal studies that have provided continued knowledge of the health effects of tobacco use over very considerable time periods. Two are described: the 50-year study of male British doctors (51,90), and the Framingham Heart Study (91).

U.K. Study of Male Doctors

The 50 years observations of male British doctors consisted of a series of surveys over many time periods (50,90). This study monitored 34,439 male doctors born between 1900 and 1930. They were monitored by questionnaires about their smoking habits in 1957, 1966, 1971, 1978, 1991, and 2001. Sir Richard Doll, Sir Richard Peto and colleagues have reported that among this cohort of men born around 1920, cigarette smoking tripled age-specific mortality rates. Among British men born between 1900 and 1909, cigarette smoking approximately doubled age-specific mortality rates both in middle and old age. Longevity improved rapidly for nonsmokers, but not for men who continued to smoke cigarettes. They reported that cessation of smoking at age 50 years halved the likelihood of developing a cigarette related disease, and that cessation at 30 years, avoided almost all of the harms resulting from tobacco use. They found that on average, cigarette smokers died about 10 years younger than nonsmokers. But that stopping at ages 60, 50, 40, or 30 years gained, respectively, about 3, 6, 9, or 10 years of life expectancy.

Framingham Heart Study

For over 50 years the Framingham Heart Study has produced major discoveries that have helped the understanding of the development and progression of heart disease and its risk factors. The Framingham Heart Study recruited 5209 men and women between the ages of 30 and 62 in 1948 (91) and subsequently enrolled a further two generations of study participants that comprised 5124 of the original participants': adult, their spouses, and children. With more than 1000 scientific publications of research findings, appearing first in 1957 and regularly thereafter, the Framingham Heart Study has demonstrated the significance of CHD risk factors, including smoking, high blood pressure, high blood cholesterol, and overweight. The

Framingham Heart Study found that multiple risk factors in the same person increased the risk much above the sum of the individual risk factors. Before the Framingham Heart Study, physicians believed that atherosclerosis was an inevitable part of the aging process; they were taught that blood pressure was supposed to increase with age, and the notion that risk factors for heart disease could be identified and modified was not part of standard medical practice. At that time also, physicians did not understand the relationship between high levels of serum cholesterol and heart attacks.

Health Effects of Passive Smoking

Breathing other people's smoke is referred to as passive, involuntary or secondhand smoking. The nonsmoker breathes sidestream smoke from the burning tip of the cigarette as well as the mainstream smoke that is inhaled and then exhaled by the smoker. ETS is a major source of indoor air pollution (51). In United States, even with an adult smoking prevalence rate of 25%, almost 90% of nonsmokers had some exposure to ETS (92). Passive smoking is a risk factor (93,94) for the following:

- Low birthweight
- Cot or crib death (SIDS)
- Middle ear infection in children
- Asthma (induction and exacerbation) in children and adults
- Bronchitis (induction and exacerbation) in children and adults
- Pneumonia (induction and exacerbation) in children and adults
- Heart disease
- Stroke
- Lung cancer
- Nasal cancer
- Spontaneous abortion (miscarriage)
- Meningococccal infections in children
- Cancers and leukaemia in children
- Decreased lung function
- Cervical cancer

Passive Smoking and Atherosclerosis

Heart disease caused by passive smoking is the third leading preventable cause of death in the United States, ranking behind active smoking and alcohol abuse. Nonsmokers living with smokers have an increased risk of heart disease of between 20% and 30% (95–97). This 20% risk accounts for an estimated 35,000 to 40,000 heart disease deaths in the United States each year (95). Exposure to ETS causes the blood to thicken, and platelet aggregation, which adversely affects cells lining the coronary arteries. The dysfunction of these endothelial cells contributes to the narrowing of arteries and reduction in blood flow (98).

Nonsmokers have a 23% to 25% increased risk of CHD when living or working with a smoker compared with nonsmokers that are not exposed (99,100). Damage caused to arteries by passive smoking can be reversed in healthy adults if further tobacco smoke exposure is avoided for at least a year (101). Passive smoking increases the risk of stroke by 82% (102).

Passive Smoking and Lung Cancer

Meta-analyses of studies show a significant risk of lung cancer among nonsmokers who live with smokers; risk is 20% for women and 30% for men (103). Nonsmokers exposed to ETS at work have an increased risk of lung cancer of 16% to 19%. A review of studies of the risk of lung cancer in nonsmokers reported that the excess risk in lifelong nonsmokers who lived with a smoker was 24% (104). Tobacco specific carcinogens in the blood of nonsmokers were clear evidence of the effect of passive smoking. There was a dose response relationship between a nonsmoker's risk of lung cancer and exposure to quantity and duration of ETS (104). A study carried out in seven European countries of nonsmokers' exposure to ETS also found an increased risk of lung cancer of 10% to 30% among nonsmokers who work in a smoky environment or who live with a spouse who is a smoker (105). Others have reported similar findings in the order of 20% to 30% increased risk of lung cancer in nonsmokers (93,94).

Passive Smoking and Respiratory Diseases

Passive smoking affects the respiratory health of nonsmokers causing increased coughing, phlegm production, chest discomfort, and reduced lung function (93,94). Among asthmatics, ETS causes serious problems by triggering asthma attacks. ETS causes respiratory difficulties in up to 80% among people with asthma.

Nonsmokers exposed to ETS either at home or in the workplace have a 40% to 60% increase in the risk of asthma compared to adults who are not exposed. Passive smoking causes COPD in nonsmokers (106).

Impact of Passive Smoking on Children

Almost half of the world's children (700 million) are exposed to tobacco smoke by the 1.2 billion adults who smoke (107). According to the WHO, passive smoking causes in children: bronchitis, pneumonia, coughing and wheezing, asthma attacks, middle ear infection, cot death, and possibly cardiovascular and neurobiological impairment (107). In the United Kingdom, 17,000 children under the age of five years are admitted to hospital every year as a result of illnesses resulting from passive smoking (108).

In young children, the major source of tobacco smoke is smoking by parents and other household members, with maternal smoking the largest source of ETS due to the cumulative effect of exposure during pregnancy and close proximity to the mother during early life. Maternal smoking during pregnancy is a major cause of low birth weight, spontaneous abortion and reduced lung function, and a major cause of SIDS in babies.

Other Effects of Passive Smoking

Passive smoking by nonsmoking adults is associated with many health effects including: nasal sinus cancer (93,94), meningococcal infections in children, cancers and leukemia in children, and discomforts such as eye irritation, headache, cough, sore throat, dizziness, and nausea.

Pharmacology and Nicotine Dependence

Pharmacology

Tobacco smoke is a complex mixture that contains more than 4000 different chemicals. More than 40 are carcinogenic, and nine of these (including benzene, cadmium, and nitrosamines) have been classed as group 1 carcinogens (7). The chemicals in cigarettes include: acetone used in paint stripper, ammonia used in floor cleaner, arsenic, which is a poison, butane, which is in lighter fluid, cadmium, which is used in batteries, formaldehyde, which is a preservative used in the morgue, hydrogen cyanide, which was used in the gas chambers, methanol used in rocket fuel, naphthalene, which is in moth balls, and polonium-210, which is radioactive. The majority of tobacco smoke components are divided into nicotine, carbon monoxide, tar, and gases, including oxidizing and irritant gases. The tar, oxidizing gases, and carbon monoxide are the main causative factors in tobacco related diseases (6,7). Polycyclic aromatic hydrocarbons and nitrosamines are the causative agents for lung and other cancers. Oxidant and irritant gases are responsible for pulmonary disease; oxidant gases and carbon monoxide are implicated in CVD (88).

Tobacco smoke also contains carcinogens that have the potential to alter genes and stimulate the growth of cancer cells (25). Oxidative stress may potentially cause mutation of DNA and promote atherosclerosis; smokers have lower levels of antioxidants in their blood than do nonsmokers. Exposure to tobacco smoke also may result in chronic inflammation (25).

Nicotine is inhaled in tobacco smoke and absorbed into the bloodstream where it travels through the human body, for example, reaching the brain only 10 seconds after inhaling. It travels to every part of the body, including breast milk (25). The average nicotine intake from a single cigarette is about 1 mg. But sometimes may exceed 3 mg (49). The typical pack-a-day smoker obtains 20 to 40 mg of nicotine daily.

Nicotine has a plasma half-life of one to three hours; so daily smoking results in a plateau after six to eight hours, which continues until the last cigarette (49). During sleep, nicotine levels fall and acute tolerance is lost. Nicotine is widely distributed into tissues, crossing the placenta and mammary gland. When tobacco burns during smoking, nicotine is distilled and carried into the lungs where it is absorbed rapidly through the pulmonary alveoli (19). After absorption, nicotine is then distributed into various body organs and tissues; those with the highest affinity for nicotine include the kidney, liver, lung, brain, and heart (19).

The pharmacological processes relevant to nicotine addiction include absorption, distribution, elimination, and dosing of nicotine in the body (pharmacokinetics), pharmacological effects on target organs (pharmacodynamics), and behavioral manifestations of the pharmacological effects (109–111).

Another ingredient of tobacco smoke, carbon monoxide, prevents full oxygenation of the hemoglobin in red blood cells.

Nicotine Tolerance, Dependence, and Withdrawal Tolerance

Repeated use of nicotine results in neuronal adaptations that are reflected in nicotine tolerance, sensitization, and withdrawal. In smokers, tolerance to the behavioral and cardiovascular effects of nicotine develops. The first cigarette produces euphoria and tachycardia (49). Smokers lose a substantial degree of tolerance while sleeping but regain it upon commencement of smoking the next day. Metabolic tolerance to nicotine develops with repeated daily smoking.

Nicotine Dependence

Most smokers become dependent on nicotine, which is the addictive drug found in all tobacco products. Nicotine addiction has been classified as a substance disorder by the WHO ICD-10 disease classification system, which lists the disorder as tobacco dependence, and by the American Psychiatric Association DSM-4 classification system, which lists the disorder as nicotine dependence (109).

Primary criteria for addiction (1,112,113) include:

- psychoactive effects that involve alterations in mood, behavior, and/or cognition
- reinforcing effects that maintain self-administration of nicotine
- highly controlled or compulsive use driven by strong urges to smoke
- development of physical dependence on nicotine, which is characterized by tolerance and withdrawal symptoms
- continued use despite negative consequences
- difficulty in maintaining abstinence or in reducing quantity smoked
- recurrent cravings to smoke.

The extent of nicotine addiction is clear in the proportion of smokers who have tried to quit, those who suffer withdrawal symptoms, and the successful quitting rate. Around 90% of cigarette smokers, smoke on a daily basis (114). Of those who smoke one packet of cigarettes each day, 80% of them have unsuccessfully tried to reduce the number of cigarettes smoked. About half of those who stop smoking experience nicotine withdrawal symptoms. Of those making a serious attempt to quit, fewer than 3% have long-term success.

Nicotine dependence is also supported by stimuli that become associated with tobacco use through learning and conditioning. Stimuli that are repeatedly paired with smoking (triggers such as speaking to particular people, drinking alcohol, or ashtrays) are cues to smoking (115). Similarly, stimuli that are associated with abstinence from tobacco can elicit withdrawal symptoms (being in settings where smoking is banned or restricted) (116).

Withdrawal

Physical dependence on nicotine refers to the development of withdrawal symptoms on quitting. Withdrawal symptoms after cessation are associated with the development of tolerance, a decreased effect after repeated exposure to nicotine, or the need for increased nicotine administration to obtain a specific effect (19).

Nicotine is like cocaine, it affects the brain dopamine reward system. Part of the reinforcement of tobacco use comes from the relief of withdrawal symptoms (negative reinforcement) (49). Nicotine produces several pleasurable effects that are important for positive reinforcement. It has both stimulant and depressant-like actions. The smoker feels alert, yet there is also muscular relaxation. Nicotine activates the reward system in the brain that includes the pathways from the ventral tegmental area to the nucleus accumbens (49). Increased extracellular dopamine has been found in the nucleus accumbens after nicotine ingestion (49).

Many people who use tobacco regularly become physically, behaviorally, and psychologically dependent on continued smoking and have great difficulty stopping smoking even when seriously motivated to quit (117). Unlike other drug use, most smokers are addicted to nicotine. The main adverse effect of nicotine in tobacco products is addiction, which sustains tobacco use. As most smokers are nicotine dependent, they continue to expose themselves to toxins from tobacco.

Most people do not realize that nicotine is a highly addictive drug, as addictive as heroin or cocaine. Nicotine is used to modulate mood and arousal, as well as for pleasure. When tobacco use is terminated, such as during sleep or when the smoker quits altogether, withdrawal symptoms develop which can disrupt daily life and are a strong motivator for continuing smoking. Withdrawal symptoms start within a few hours of cessation and for most smokers, peak around 24 to 72 hours after the last cigarette (49).

Diagnostic criteria for nicotine withdrawal according to the DSM-IV classification includes at least four of the eight symptoms and signs listed occur within 24 hours of stopping smoking (113):

- dysphoria or depressed mood
- insomnia
- irritability, frustration, or anger
- anxiety
- difficulty concentrating
- breathlessness
- decreased heart rate
- increased appetite or weight gain.

The Benefits of Stopping Smoking

Most smokers know that smoking is damaging their health, but they may have limited understanding of the various adverse effects. In particular, they may not be aware that most of the negative health effects from smoking decline rapidly after stopping smoking. There is plenty of good news for smokers of all ages who quit their smoking habit. There are many health benefits when smoking is ceased, with health benefits existing even for cessation at an advanced age. Former smokers live longer than continuing smokers; no matter what age they stop smoking. The excess risk of death from smoking begins to decrease shortly after cessation and continues to decrease for at least 10 to 15 years (50,118). Those who quit smoking before the age of 50 years, have half the risk of dying within the next 15 years compared to those who continue to smoke (118). The famous British doctors study found that male doctors who stop smoking before the age of 35 years survived about as well as those who had never smoked. Those who quit between the ages of 35 and 44 years also gain great benefits, and there are benefits at older ages as well (50,90).

Tables 5 and 6 highlight the health benefits of cessation related to time from last cigarette (Table 5) and change in disease process (Table 6). These can be used in a clinical setting to motivate smokers to make a quit attempt.

Mortality Risk Reduction Associated with Smoking Cessation in Patients with CHD

The causative relationship between tobacco use and CHD is well established with the relative risks or odds ratios (OR) estimated between 1.5 and 3 or higher in the large-scale longitudinal studies of the British Doctors Study (50), British Regional Heart Study (120), and the Framingham Study (91), respectively. Quitting smoking results in significant reductions in risk for all-cause mortality among patients with CHD. Observational studies have reported that quitting smoking reduces the risk of subsequent death and further cardiac events among patients with CHD by as much as 50% (118,121). A systematic review of 20 studies was carried out and the risk reduction among those who had quit was consistent regardless of age, sex, index cardiac event, and country (122). The review found a 36% reduction in relative risk of mortality for patients with CHD who quit compared with those who continued to smoke. However, the rapidity and magnitude of the risk reduction of mortality when a smoker quits is still under debate (122).

Patients who cease smoking after coronary artery bypass graft surgery had a substantial lower risk of coronary events and lower mortality rate compared to those who continue smoking (55,123). Additionally, those who continued to smoke also underwent repeat revascularization procedures more frequently than those who quit (55). Further, cessation of smoking after

TABLE 5 Health Benefits of Cessation Related to Time from Last Cigarette

Time since last cigarette	Health benefits of cessation
12 hours	Almost all the nicotine has been metabolized
24 hours	Blood levels of carbon monoxide have dropped dramatically
5 days	Most nicotine by-products have been removed. Sense of taste and smell improve
6 weeks	Risk of wound infection after surgery is substantially reduced
3 months	Cilia begin to recover and lung function improves
1 year	Risk of coronary heart disease is halved after one year compared to continuing smokers
10 years	Risk of lung cancer is less than half that of a continuing smoker and continues to decline
15 years	Risk of coronary heart disease is the same as a nonsmoker. About 10 to 15 years after quitting the all-cause mortality in former smokers declines to the same level as people who have never smoked

Source: From Refs. 63, 119.

percutaneous coronary angioplasty has an important beneficial effect on the clinical course after the procedure (124). Those who continue smoking are at greater risk for atherosclerosis of vein grafts compared to nonsmokers (125). Physicians are encouraged to recommend patients to stop smoking either on their own or with the aid of a smoking cessation program and pharmacotherapy in order to reduce the risk after coronary artery bypass graft (CABG).

PUBLIC HEALTH APPROACHES TO REDUCING TOBACCO USE

In this section, the variety of public health approaches to reduce tobacco use are described including evidence for their effectiveness. Although it is difficult to disaggregate the individual effects of each strategy, the growing body of knowledge suggests that each have a significant impact. They consist of:

- increasing taxes and the price of tobacco products
- raising awareness of the health effects of smoking by education
- banning advertising and promotion of tobacco products
- restricting smoking in public places and in the workplace
- positioning health warnings on cigarette packs
- counter-advertising in the mass media
- assisting smoking cessation with interventions and pharmacotherapies

Increasing Taxes and the Price of Tobacco Products

The first type of public health approach is based on increasing the price of tobacco products. Raising taxes significantly reduces the consumption of tobacco (1). The impact of higher taxes

TABLE 6 Health Effects of Smoking Cessation

Disease process	Effect of cessation
Stroke	Risk reduces to that of nonsmoker after 5 to 15 years
Coronary heart disease	Risk halves after one year of quitting, and is almost the same as a nonsmoker after 15 years
Peripheral vascular disease	Reduces after quitting
Cancer of the mouth, throat, and esophagus	Risk halves after 5 years
Cancer of the larynx	Risk reduces after quitting
Cervical cancer	Risk reduces a few years after quitting
Bladder cancer	Risk reduces after quitting
Chronic obstructive airways disease	Risk of death reduces after quitting
Lung cancer	Risk halves after 10 years
Stomach ulcer	Risk reduces after quitting
Low birthweight baby	Risk reduces to normal if a mother quits before pregnancy or in the first trimester

Source: From Refs. 63, 119.

mainly affects young people who are more responsive to price rises than older smokers (126). The amount of tax charged is different across countries, with high-income countries levying taxes that are two-thirds or more of the retail price of a cigarette pack, while lower-income countries tax at no more than half the retail price (1). Smokers' demand for tobacco is strongly affected by its price. For example, an increase in the price of cigarettes resulted in substantial falls in consumption in Canada, South Africa, Australia, and the United Kingdom (1,127,128).

Many countries use the taxes raised on tobacco for antismoking activities and health promotion foundations, e.g., Australia, United States, and selected regions in China.

Raising Awareness of the Health Effects of Smoking by Education

Providing information about the health effects and addictive nature of smoking can lead to reduction in cigarette consumption. The decline in smoking prevalence in most high-income countries over the past three decades (Stage 4 of the tobacco epidemic) is related to the increase in smokers' knowledge about the harmful health effects of their habit. For example, in 1950 in the United States, only 45% of adults knew that smoking caused lung cancer, but by 1990, 95% knew smoking was a major cause (1). Over the same period smoking rates in the United States fell from 40% to 25%. Young people are less responsive to information about the health effects of tobacco than older people and more educated people respond more quickly to new information than those with minimal education.

The Surgeon General's reports have had a great influence on raising awareness of the health consequences of smoking (19,23,25,51,63,109,118). Parents' awareness of the health effects, their smoking has on their children has increased through these important publications.

Although antismoking programs in schools are widespread, particularly in high-income countries, they are less effective than other types of information that is disseminated. Adolescents are generally present oriented and are not motivated to change by learning about the health effects of smoking that may occur sometime in the distant future. They are also rebellious and less convinced by authority figures that present the information.

Banning Advertising and Promotion of Tobacco Products

Cigarette advertising and promotion affect consumption. Surveys of young people's recall of advertising messages have reported that they affect demand for cigarettes, remember the messages, and attract new recruits to smoking. Bans on advertising and promotion are effective only if they are comprehensive, and cover several media. Partial bans on advertising have very little effect on smoking rates. However, a comprehensive approach, which includes multiple restrictions on advertising in all media and on promotional activities such as sponsorship of sports and other events, can reduce smoking by more than 6% in high income countries (129). A study of 100 countries, comparing consumption trends found that in those with complete bans there was a downward trend in tobacco use compared to those countries that had no bans (1).

Restricting Smoking in Public Places and in the Workplace

Many countries have implemented restrictions on smoking in public places, such as in restaurants and transport facilities, and in the workplace. The benefits of restricting smoking include those to nonsmokers who are spared exposure to the health risks of environmental smoke, and for smokers, who reduce their consumption of cigarettes, and some quit. In the United States, restrictions on smoking in public places have reduced tobacco consumption by between 4% and 10% (1).

Smoking restrictions or bans with increased taxation of tobacco products increase motivation to quit, number of quit attempts, and lead to higher quit rates (126,130–132).

Positioning Health Warnings on Cigarette Packs

Many tobacco manufacturers have called their cigarettes "lights" and their promotion leads many smokers to the false information that this brand is safer. Light cigarettes are not safer than smoking regular ones; in fact they are virtually identical. Light cigarettes have more chemical additives as cigarette makers often add extra chemicals to hide the harsh taste of the smoke. The lighter cigarettes make it easier to inhale the smoke deeper into the lungs. The illusion that light cigarettes are safer for the smoker comes from the nearly invisible vent holes that are drilled in the filter. Light cigarettes have vent holes in the filter, so they score lower on smoking machines that measure tar and nicotine. However, these holes are covered by the smoker's fingers during smoking and are therefore clogged during smoking. The size and number of vent holes changes the way people smoke: the bigger the vents, the deeper the puffs taken by the smoker.

Since the 1960s many governments have required cigarette manufacturers to print health warnings on cigarette packs. By 1991, 77 countries required health warnings that were often rotated on packs. Health warnings on cigarette packs in Australia include the following messages: Smoking causes lung cancer; smoking is addictive; smoking kills; smoking causes heart disease; smoking when pregnant harms your baby; and your smoking can harm others.

Health warnings cause consumption to fall that has been documented in Turkey and South Africa. A weakness of warning labels is that they may not reach poor smokers and adolescents. In high-income countries the size of warning labels on cigarette packs have increased considerably in order for them to have an effect on smokers. Evidence shows that warning labels can still be effective in motivating smokers to make a quit attempt if they are large (1) (by occupying 60% of the cigarette pack as in Canada; 50% as in Australia; 44% as in United Kingdom, and 30% as in United States), and are prominently placed with hard-hitting content.

Counter-Advertising in the Mass Media

Negative messages about the harms caused by smoking used in counter-advertising have been found to reduce overall tobacco consumption. These messages are usually funded by governments and health promotion organizations in North America, Australia, Israel, and European countries such as Finland, Norway, and Turkey. For example, in Switzerland, adult tobacco consumption reduced by 11% over the period because there was antismoking publicity in the mass media (1).

Antitobacco mass media campaigns can reduce tobacco consumption and increase cessation rates when implemented in conjunction with other public health interventions such as community education and tax increases (126,130–132).

Assisting Smoking Cessation with Interventions and Pharmacotherapies

In addition to raising taxes and price of cigarettes and the nonprice measures described above (bans, restrictions, education, etc.), there is a third set of measures to reduce tobacco consumption. These consist of various programs designed to assist smokers to stop smoking including hospital outpatient smokers clinics, counseling programs conducted in various settings such as primary care, and training in tobacco control and smoking cessation such as teaching medical students, and training primary care physicians in smoking cessation methods. There is also a growing range of pharmacological products used to aid cessation such as nicotine replacement therapies, and antidepressant drugs (bupropion and nortriptyline). This third public health approach is very important and is described in section 4 of this chapter.

Potential Impact of Public Health Measures on Tobacco Consumption

When the price of tobacco rises, smokers in low-income countries cut back their cigarette consumption compared to those on in high-income countries. For example, in the United States, a price rise of 10% for a cigarette pack decreases the demand by about 4%, whereas in China, Brazil, and South Africa, a similar price rise will decrease the demand by 6% (1). Therefore, even a modest price rise has a striking impact on the rates of smoking and on the number of tobacco-related premature deaths among smokers. A real rise in the price of cigarettes of 10% would result in 40 million people globally who would quit smoking, and many others who might have taken up smoking would be deterred from doing so (1). Thus with a modest price rise, a huge number of premature deaths would be avoided: nine million premature deaths would be avoided in developing countries (1).

The combined impact of the public health measures that are not price measures such as those are described above would persuade between 2% and 10% of smokers to quit (1). These nonprice measures could reduce the number of smokers by 23 million worldwide resulting in 5 million lives saved (133).

Based on the effectiveness of smoking cessation therapies when used by only 6% of smokers, would result in six million smokers who are enabled to quit, resulting in one million deaths from cigarette related diseases that would be averted (1). However, if 25% of smokers sought help from smoking cessation therapies, this would mean that 29 million smokers would be enabled to quit, and thus averting seven million deaths.

The cost effectiveness of different public health interventions can be evaluated by estimating the expected gain in years of healthy life that each will achieve in return for the public costs, needed to implement that intervention. Tobacco control strategies are considered cost effective and worthy of inclusion in a package of healthcare measures. Public health programs cost about $20 to $80 per discounted year of healthy life saved (135). High-income countries with comprehensive public health programs spend between 50 cents and $2.50 per capita each year on these programs. However, to deliver a package of public health interventions that include tobacco control, governments would need to spend $4 per capita in low-income countries and $7 in middle-income countries (1). Any way that one looks at it, implementing multipronged public health strategies have a significant impact on reducing smoking rates in a population, which in turn reduces the number of premature deaths for cigarette related diseases. A comprehensive approach to tobacco control is likely to prove the most successful; that is, combining economic, legislative, educative, and clinical approaches (63). Sustained funding for program delivery is likely to be a major factor in determining outcomes.

Global Public Health Initiatives for Tobacco Control

There are several global public health initiatives that are designed to raise awareness of the dangers of smoking and reduce tobacco use. Two of these are briefly described: The WHO Framework Convention on Tobacco Control (FCTC), and the WHO World No Tobacco Day.

The World Health Organization Framework Convention on Tobacco Control

The WHO initiated the development of the framework convention for tobacco control that was unanimously adopted by WHO's 191 Member States in May 2003. The FCTC is an international legal instrument designed to circumscribe the growth of the global tobacco pandemic, especially in developing countries. It is the first multilateral convention focusing on a public health issue: tobacco. The negotiation and implementation of the WHO FCTC is designed to help curb tobacco use by mobilizing national and international awareness as well as technical and financial resources for effective national tobacco control measures. The FCTC aims at strengthening global cooperation on aspects of tobacco control that transcend national boundaries and includes global marketing and promotion of tobacco products and smuggling (1). It sets standards and guidelines for tobacco control in the following areas:

- tobacco advertising, promotion, and sponsorship;
- packaging and labeling;
- regulation and disclosure of contents of tobacco products and smoke;
- illicit trade;
- price and tax measures;
- sales to and by minors;
- government support for tobacco
- manufacturing and agriculture;
- treatment of tobacco dependence;
- passive smoking and smoke-free environments;
- surveillance, research, and exchange of information;
- and scientific, technical, and legal cooperation.

The WHO FCTC entered into force on 27 February 2005.

World No Tobacco Day

World No Tobacco Day (WNTD) is promoted by the WHO's Tobacco Free Initiative to promote a tobacco-free world, and is celebrated around the world each year on May 31. WNTD informs the public on the dangers of using tobacco, the business practices of tobacco companies, what WHO is doing to fight the tobacco epidemic, and what people around the world can do to claim their right to health and healthy living and to protect future generations (134).

TREATING TOBACCO DEPENDENCE
The Role of the Physician

Physicians in both primary care and specialty practice are well placed to treat tobacco dependence and increase rates of smoking cessation. It is estimated that 70% of smokers see a physician each year (117). Physicians are perceived as a credible source of information on risks of smoking and as a source of information on smoking cessation (135). Though physicians are especially well placed to intervene, other health professionals, such as physician assistants, nurse practitioners, nurses, physical and occupational therapists can also have a role in smoking cessation (117).

The opportunities provided to physicians by this contact to identify and counsel smokers are not, however, being fully realized. In Australia family physicians identify only two thirds of their patients who smoke (136,137). The situation is similar in the United States where smoking status was identified in only 67% of office visits and cessation counseling provided in 21% of smokers' clinic visits (138).

Barriers to greater involvement by physicians to greater activity in smoking cessation include: perception of lack of effect (139,140); lack of physician time (141); lack of skills (136) reluctance to raise the issue due to patient sensitivity about smoking (136); perceived lack of patient motivation (136); and physicians not using effective strategies or using ineffective strategies (140).

Evidence of Efficacy of Advice from Physicians

There is evidence from a number of meta-analyses of randomized trials that physician advice on smoking cessation is effective. The Cochrane Review on the effect of physician advice on smoking cessation examined evidence from 39 trials involving over 31,000 smokers (142). The most common setting for advice was primary care. The outcomes used were abstinence from smoking after at least six months follow-up, using the most rigorous definition of abstinence in each trial, and biochemically validated rates were available. Pooled data from 17 trials of brief advice versus no advice (or usual care) showed a significant increase in the OR of quitting [OR 1.74, 95% confidence interval (CI) 1.48–2.05], equating to an absolute difference in quit rates of 2.5%. The Cochrane Review found evidence of a small advantage of intensive advice (OR 1.44, 95% CI 1.24–1.67).

The meta-analysis conducted for the U.S. Clinical Practice Guidelines (118) was more positive about the effects of more intensive advice. This review concluded that minimal duration counseling (up to three minutes) results in an abstinence rate at six months of 13% (2.5% higher than control); low intensity (3–10 minutes) in an abstinence rate of 16% (5% higher than controls); and higher intensity (more than 10 minutes) in an abstinence rate of 22% (11% higher than controls). The number of person-to-person treatment sessions also influenced the outcome. Treatments lasting more than eight sessions were significantly more effective than interventions over three or less sessions.

The benefits of smoking cessation for patients with CVD are dramatic with a systematic review showing a 36% reduction in crude relative risk of mortality for patients with CHD, who quit compared with those who continued smoking (123). Although the majority of smokers quit when admitted for myocardial infarction or cardiac surgery up to 70% start smoking again within a year (143).

One of the barriers for greater involvement of physicians in smoking cessation is time pressure; so one option is to delegate this responsibility to other clinicians. There is a lack of evidence on the effect of advice to quit, from nonphysician clinicians but the U.S. Clinical Practice Guideline took the view that it is reasonable to believe that such advice is effective in increasing long-term quit rates. A Cochrane Review of nursing interventions concluded that nurse advice could be effective. Nurses' advice to quit, to hospitalized patients with CVD was more effective than for inpatients with other conditions (144). The pooled estimate of effect from four trials in hospitalized smokers with CVD was 1.44 (95% CI 1.16–1.78) Three trials that included a smoking cessation intervention from a nurse as part of cardiac rehabilitation showed more than double the cessation rate (OR 2.14, 95% CI 1.39–3.31).

Hospitalized Smokers

Hospitalized smokers are an important group for intervention as they may be more motivated to quit and are temporarily in a smoke-free environment. Motivation is likely to be higher if patients are in hospital with a smoking related disease such as CVD. There is evidence that augmented in-hospital interventions for smoking cessation are more effective than usual care (117,145). The Cochrane Review concluded that at least one month of follow-up after discharge is necessary to achieve an increase in abstinence at six months after the start of the intervention compared to usual care. Although the area has not been intensively researched, there is evidence that relatively intensive interventions can help acute cardiac patients to quit but that brief intervention during hospital admission is not superior to routine care (146).

Clinical Practice Guidelines for Smoking Cessation

Guidelines for smoking cessation that are based on evidence have been developed and disseminated in many countries including the United States, United Kingdom, Canada, Australia, and New Zealand. The majority use or have adapted the 5 As approach of the U.S. Clinical Practice Guideline (117). It has been demonstrated in a randomized trial that this approach when implemented leads to increased cessation (147).

Providing Smoking Cessation Advice

Table 7 from the U.S. Clinical Practice Guideline summarizes the 5 As for brief intervention.
Figure 2 summarizes in the form of a flow chart the identification and treatment process for smokers using the 5 As approach for brief intervention.

Step 1: Ask—Identifying Tobacco Use

Asking about tobacco use is a key step to effective intervention. All patients should be asked about tobacco use at every visit. The exception to this is adult patients who have never used tobacco or have not used tobacco for many years. The U.S. Clinical Practice Guideline recommends recording tobacco use as a vital sign along with blood pressure, pulse, weight, temperature, and respiratory rate (117).

If the patient is a smoker, the physician should take a brief history as follows (119)

■ Number of cigarettes (or other form of tobacco) smoked per day or per week and the year of starting smoking.
■ Previous quit attempts and their results.
■ Presence of smoking related disease.

Smoking status should be documented as current smoker, former, or never smoked. For current smokers the frequency should be categorized as daily, weekly, or irregular. The amount (number per day) and year of commencement of smoking should also be documented. For exsmokers the quit date should be recorded.

The meta-analyses conducted for the development of the U.S. Clinical Practice Guideline (117) found that having a screening system in place to identify smoking status leads to a substantially higher rate of clinician intervention and a small increase in the abstinence rate at six months follow-up. Instituting such a system in practice is therefore highly recommended.

Step 2: Advise Tobacco Users to Quit

All tobacco users should be advised to quit in a way that is clear, strong, personalized, supportive, and nonjudgmental (117,148). Linking the need to quit to the patient's current health or illness can help the tobacco user to recognize the salience of the cessation message. The remarkable health benefits of quitting such as the rapid fall in risk of CVD can also be highlighted.

TABLE 7   The 5 A's for Brief Intervention

Ask about tobacco use	Identify and document tobacco use status for every patient at every visit
Advise to quit	In a clear, strong, and personalized manner urge every tobacco user to quit
Assess willingness to make a quit attempt	Is the tobacco user willing to make a quit attempt at this time?
Assist in quit attempt	For the patient willing to make a quit attempt, use counseling and pharmacotherapy to help him or her quit
Arrange follow-up	Schedule follow-up contact, preferably the first week after the quit date

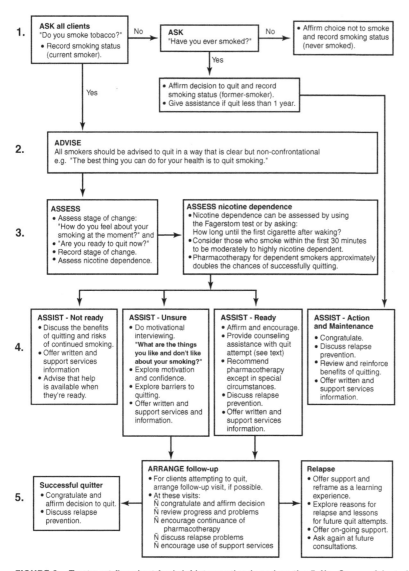

FIGURE 2   Treatment flowchart for brief intervention based on the 5 A's. *Source*: Adapted from Ref. 119.

There is evidence from qualitative research that advising smokers repeatedly that they should quit, especially in consultations unrelated to smoking, can damage patient-doctor rapport (149). Strategies to avoid this are establishing rapport in the consultation and asking permission to discuss the subject of smoking (150).

Where possible, personalize the benefits of cessation. Examples are improvement in other illnesses, importance of smoking as a risk factor for future illness, not exposing others (including children) to environmental smoke, importance as a role model to children and adolescents, and saving money.

All smokers should be offered written information about smoking and smoking cessation and the option of further assistance from support services such as referral to a telephone quit line.

Step 3: Assess

The majority of smokers report wanting to quit and in the United States approximately 46% have made a quit attempt in the preceding year (151). However, the patient's willingness to make a quit attempt varies. The Transtheoretical Model of Change, developed by American psychologists Prochaska and DiClemente (152) remains a useful way for physicians to assess a patient's

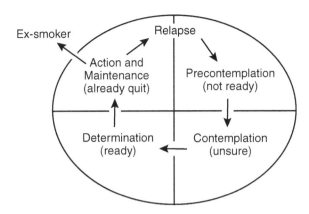

FIGURE 3   Stages of readiness to stop smoking.
Source: From Refs. 152,154,155.

readiness to quit. Cessation is explained as a process, rather than a single discrete event and smokers cycle through the stages of being ready, quitting, and relapsing on an average of three to four times, before achieving long term success (119). Large studies in the United States involving 18,500 smokers found approximately 40% of smokers are Not Ready, 40% are Unsure, and 20% are in the Ready group (153). Percentages are the same for male and female smokers and for all ages, but vary with the educational level (people with lower educational levels of achievement are more likely to be Not Ready or Unsure). Smokers will be in different stages of readiness when the physician sees them at different times, so readiness needs to be periodically reevaluated (Fig. 3).

Key Questions for the Physician to Ask Smoking Patients

Willingness to quit can be assessed using a nonjudgmental question (156). The key question to facilitate assessment is *"How do you feel about your smoking at the moment? "* Where needed, clarify the response by asking the patient whether they are willing to make a quit attempt at this time or in the near future (e.g., the next 30 days). For example ask *"Are you ready to quit now?"* It is important to express concern/interest, and not criticism when assessing the smoking patient's stage of readiness to quit.

Assessment also includes examining barriers to quitting, triggers for smoking (e.g., social situations, stress, and negative emotions), social support, and the smoker's experiences in previous quit attempts. Assessing previous use of pharmacotherapy is helpful to determine if it was used optimally and what problems occurred. The implications of other physical health, mental health, and other drug dependencies also need to be assessed.

Assessing Nicotine Dependence

Assessment of nicotine dependence will help predict whether the smoker is likely to experience nicotine withdrawal on stopping smoking. The American Psychiatric Association's Diagnostic and Statistical Manual of Mental Disorders (DSM-IV) states that nicotine dependence and withdrawal can develop with all forms of tobacco. Features of nicotine dependence include: smoking more heavily, smoking soon after waking, smoking when ill, difficulty refraining from smoking, reporting the first cigarette of the day to be the most difficult to give up, and smoking more in the morning than in the afternoon.

The modified Fagerström Test for Nicotine Dependence can be used to assess nicotine dependence (157).

Fagerström Test for Nicotine Dependence

Questions	Answers	Score
1. How soon after waking up do you smoke your first cigarette?	Within 5 min	3
	6–30 min	2
	31–60 min	1
2. Do you find it difficult to abstain from smoking in places where it is forbidden?	Yes	1
	No	0
		(*Continued*)

3. Which cigarette would you hate to give up?	The first one in the morning	1
		0
	Any other	
4. How many cigarettes a day do you smoke?	10 or less	0
	11–20	1
	21–30	2
	31 or more	3
5. Do you smoke more frequently in the morning than in the rest of the day?	Yes	1
	No	0
6. Do you smoke even though you are sick in bed for most of the day	Yes	1
	No	0

Score: 1–2, very low dependence; 3–4, low dependence; 5, medium dependence; 6–7, high dependence; 8+, very high dependence.

Patients who are nicotine dependent tend to smoke soon after waking. So if time is limited, asking "How long until the first cigarette after waking?" can provide a good indication of the level of dependence. Consider those who smoke within the first 30 minutes to be moderately to highly dependent (158).

Step 4: Assist

The assistance provided is based on the assessment process described above in Step 3. The deliverable components for each readiness group (*not ready, unsure,* and *ready to quit now*) come from the Smokescreen Program (154,155).

> *Not ready* smokers are not seriously considering quitting in the next six months. Smokers like these, who are unwilling to try to quit smoking, should be provided with brief advice to increase their motivation, such as pointing the benefits of quitting and the risks of continued smoking. They can be offered written information and the offer of further help at future visits.
>
> *Unsure* smokers are uncertain or ambivalent about their smoking and are seriously considering quitting in the next six months. They should be offered a motivational intervention. Motivational interventions are most likely to be effective when the physician is empathic, promotes patient autonomy, avoids arguments, and supports the patient's self-efficacy (117). Smokers who are unsure about quitting can be motivated to change by helping them to weigh up the pros and cons of smoking (154). These smokers should be encouraged to think about the discrepancy between smoking and personal goals such as health, fitness, improved appearance, and saving money. Asking patients to rate their motivation and confidence in quitting on a scale of 1 to 10 can be a helpful addition to motivational interviewing. Distinguishing motivation and confidence can provide an insight into barriers to quitting and can be used to initiate a discussion on how to enhance motivation or confidence (159).
>
> *Ready* smokers are willing to quit in the next 30 days and have usually made a quit attempt within the last year. These patients can be assisted with their quit attempt. This involves the clinician helping the patient develop problems-solving skills and providing social support (117).

Specific counseling strategies to assist are:

- Helping the patient to select a quit date within the next two weeks
- Reviewing past quitting experiences
- Identifying challenges such as fear of failure, coping with stress, and concern about weight gain
- Addressing alcohol use and the presence of other smokers in the household

Most patients attempting to quit should be encouraged to use effective pharmacotherapies except in special circumstance (160). These medications increase smoking cessation success and reduce withdrawal symptoms (see Smoking Cessation Pharmacotherapy).

Step 5: Arrange Follow-up

Follow-up visits after advice to quit has been shown to increase the likelihood of successful long-term abstinence (161,162). Most relapse occurs early in the quitting process (117) and follow-up contact should occur soon after the quit date, preferably during the first week. A second follow-up contact is recommended within the first month (117). During follow-up contact the suggested actions are:

- Congratulate success and affirm decision not to smoke, and remind patient of benefits of being a nonsmoker
- Review progress and problems, if tobacco use has occurred review circumstances and elicit commitment to total abstinence
- Assess pharmacotherapy use including adherence, any problems and encourage continuation
- Discuss early relapse prevention—awareness of coping strategies for high risk situations such as stress, negative emotional states, alcohol, and social environment
- Encourage social support and use of support services.

Relapse Prevention

Relapse is a return to regular smoking. The risk of relapse is highest in the first week after a quit attempt (163,164). Seventy five percent of relapses occur in the first six months. Even after being abstinent for a year, about one third of exsmokers may relapse. After two years the probability of relapse decreases to about 4% (165). Relapse can occur because people have not planned how to cope with cravings, do not recognize triggers, or decide to "just have one." Common triggers for relapse are alcohol and negative emotional states such as interpersonal conflict, anger, frustration, and anxiety.

Strategies to prevent relapse are:

- Identify high-risk smoking situations and important smoking triggers
- Plan coping strategies in advance
- Consider lifestyle changes that may reduce the number of high-risk situations encountered, e.g., stress management, abstinence from alcohol, or reduction in alcohol consumption
- Encourage patients to have a plan for how to deal with a slip to prevent it becoming a full relapse.

Quit Smoking Methods

Despite the availability of counseling support and pharmacotherapies many attempts to cease tobacco use occur without the use of evidence-based aids to cessation. Most quit attempts are unsupported and have a high rate of relapse. In the United States of the 17 million adults who attempted cessation in 1991 only 7% were still abstinent one year later (117).

Evidence-Based Quit Approaches

There are a number of pharmacological and nonpharmacological approaches that have been shown to increase success rates for quitting smoking. These include:

- Smoking cessation pharmacotherapy
- Individual behavioral counseling
- Group counseling
- Telephone quit lines

Smoking Cessation Pharmacotherapy

Pharmacological treatments to assist first become available with the licensing of 2 mg nicotine gum in Switzerland in 1978. Since then there has been an extensive research and development on pharmacotherapies for tobacco dependence. Currently available forms of pharmacotherapy for which there is evidence of efficacy are nicotine gum, patch, nasal spray, lozenge, tablet, bupropion, nortriptyline, and clonidine. These treatments approximately double success rates at one year compared to placebo (139,140,168). Most patients attempting to quit should be encouraged to use effective pharmacotherapies for smoking cessation except in the presence of special circumstances (117). Special circumstances include medical contraindications, those smoking fewer than 10 cigarettes per day, pregnant/breastfeeding women, and adolescent smokers (117).

Nicotine replacement therapy (NRT) and bupropion are current first line options for pharmacotherapy while nortriptyline and clonidine are second line agents due to their adverse effects

TABLE 8 Summary of Efficacy of Currently Available Pharmacotherapies

Drug	Number of comparisons	Percent abstinent active arm	Percent abstinent control arm	Odds ratio (95% confidence interval)
Nicotine replacement therapy (139)	103	17	10	1.77 (1.66, 1.88)
Bupropion (140)	21	20	11	1.99 (1.73, 2.30)
Nortriptyline (140)	7	17	11	2.14 (1.49, 3.06)
Clonidine (168)	6	23	14	1.89 (1.3, 2.74)

profile (117). A summary of the evidence for effectiveness from the Cochrane Library systematic reviews placebo (139,140,166) is shown in Table 8. Given that the currently available first line medications are equally efficacious, choice should be based on clinical suitability and patient preference.

A number of medications are in development phase. These act in new ways on parts of the brain and neurotransmitters involved in nicotine dependence and withdrawal. A common site of action of a number of these medications is the release of dopamine triggered by the action of nicotine on nicotinic acetylcholine receptors. Varenicline is a selective partial nicotine agonist, which blocks the action of nicotine on the alpha-4 beta-2 nicotinic acetyl choline receptor. The theoretical mode of action is twofold, to reduce nicotine withdrawal by partial activation of the receptor and to occupy the receptor site and therefore block other agonists such as nicotine itself. Another drug in development is rimonabant, a selective cannabinoid-1 receptor antagonist. Animal studies have suggested that activation of the cannabinoid system may participate in the motivational and dopamine releasing effects of nicotine (167). This drug has also shown favorable effects in weight loss and improving insulin sensitivity, independent of its use in smoking cessation.

Also in development are nicotine vaccines, which are designed to block the action of nicotine by formation of antigen-antibody complexes that are too large to cross the blood-brain barrier. There is concern however, that because the vaccines so far studied reduce but do not eliminate nicotine reaching the brain, some smokers increase tobacco consumption to overcome the effects of vaccination (167). Figure 4 is a flowchart to assist selection of currently available first line medications.

Nicotine Replacement Therapy

The aim of NRT is to replace some of the nicotine from cigarettes without the harmful constituents found in tobacco smoke. NRT reduces withdrawal symptoms associated with nicotine addiction, allowing the smoker to focus on the psychosocial aspects of quitting smoking. The best results are achieved when combined with behavioral advice and follow-up.

Meta-analyses of the evidence on efficacy of NRT were carried out by the Cochrane Library (139) and by the U.S. Guidelines Panel (117). Both concluded that NRT is effective. The Cochrane review looked at 103 studies and found an overall OR of 1.77 (95% CI 1.66, 1.88) when comparing cessation rates at 12 months of various forms of NRT to placebo or nonNRT control group. The effect sizes (difference in abstinence rate between intervention and control groups) for different forms of NRT ranged from 5% to 12% but no form was significantly better than another. In the meta-analysis of 47 studies by Fiore et al., the OR ranged from 1.6 to 2.7 and effect sizes from 7% to 17% comparing various forms of NRT to placebo at six months follow-up.

Plasma nicotine levels have been found to be lower in subjects using NRT than when they were smoking (168). This means that some patients will be under-replaced when on standard doses of NRT, leading to persistent withdrawal symptoms that may make relapse to smoking more likely. Smokers using NRT to quit may confuse withdrawal symptoms with nicotine toxicity from the NRT (a rare occurrence). Treatment with NRT has been found to delay the weight gain commonly associated with smoking cessation.

Nicotine Patch

The nicotine transdermal patch has the advantage of simplicity of use (169). Use of the 21 mg nicotine patch produces blood levels approximately half those of smoking (170). There is no difference in effectiveness of 16 hour versus 24 hour patches (139). Eight weeks of patch therapy is as effective as longer courses and there is no evidence that tapered therapy is better than abrupt withdrawal (139,171).

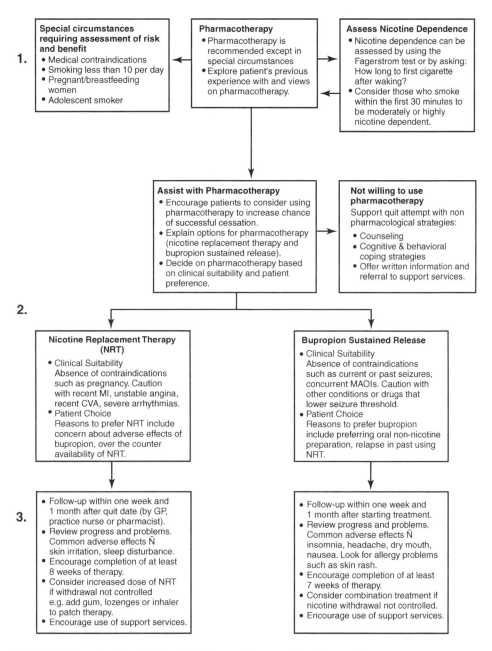

1.

Special circumstances requiring assessment of risk and benefit
- Medical contraindications
- Smoking less than 10 per day
- Pregnant/breastfeeding women
- Adolescent smoker

Pharmacotherapy
- Pharmacotherapy is recommended except in special circumstances
- Explore patient's previous experience with and views on pharmacotherapy.

Assess Nicotine Dependence
- Nicotine dependence can be assessed by using the Fagerstrom test or by asking: How long to first cigarette after waking?
- Consider those who smoke within the first 30 minutes to be moderately or highly nicotine dependent.

Assist with Pharmacotherapy
- Encourage patients to consider using pharmacotherapy to increase chance of successful cessation.
- Explain options for pharmacotherapy (nicotine replacement therapy and bupropion sustained release).
- Decide on pharmacotherapy based on clinical suitability and patient preference.

Not willing to use pharmacotherapy
Support quit attempt with non pharmacological strategies:
- Counseling
- Cognitive & behavioral coping strategies
- Offer written information and referral to support services.

2.

Nicotine Replacement Therapy (NRT)
- Clinical Suitability
  Absence of contraindications such as pregnancy. Caution with recent MI, unstable angina, recent CVA, severe arrhythmias.
- Patient Choice
  Reasons to prefer NRT include concern about adverse effects of bupropion, over the counter availability of NRT.

Bupropion Sustained Release
- Clinical Suitability
  Absence of contraindications such as current or past seizures, concurrent MAOIs. Caution with other conditions or drugs that lower seizure threshold.
- Patient Choice
  Reasons to prefer bupropion include preferring oral non-nicotine preparation, relapse in past using NRT.

3.

- Follow-up within one week and 1 month after quit date (by GP, practice nurse or pharmacist).
- Review progress and problems. Common adverse effects Ñ skin irritation, sleep disturbance.
- Encourage completion of at least 8 weeks of therapy.
- Consider increased dose of NRT if withdrawal not controlled e.g. add gum, lozenges or inhaler to patch therapy.
- Encourage use of support services.

- Follow-up within one week and 1 month after starting treatment.
- Review progress and problems. Common adverse effects Ñ insomnia, headache, dry mouth, nausea. Look for allergy problems such as skin rash.
- Encourage completion of at least 7 weeks of therapy.
- Consider combination treatment if nicotine withdrawal not controlled.
- Encourage use of support services.

FIGURE 4 Flow chart for selection of first line smoking cessation pharmacotherapy.

Local adverse effects include transient itching, burning, and tingling at the application site, which may affect up to 47% of patch users, but they are usually mild and rarely lead to withdrawal of patch use (172). Skin erythema can also occur but usually does not persist for more than 24 hours. Hydrocortisone cream can be effectively used for this reaction. Allergic contact dermatitis can occur uncommonly (in 2%–3% of people) and requires cessation of transdermal therapy. Patients should be instructed to apply the patch to dry nonhairy skin above the waist. Rotating the patch site decreases the likelihood of skin reactions. Sleep disturbance including insomnia and vivid dreams can occur. If sleep disturbance is a problem, the patch can be removed at night. After removal, nicotine absorption continues for up to two hours from nicotine already in the skin.

Nicotine Gum

The blood levels achieved by use of the nicotine chewing gum are 1/3 (2 mg), and 2/3 (4 mg) those of smoking (173). There is evidence that in more dependent smokers (smoking more than 20 cigarettes per day) 4 mg gum results in higher cessation rates than 2 mg gum. Correct chewing technique is important as nicotine is absorbed through the oral mucosa. The patient should be instructed to chew slowly (about 15 chews) until a peppery taste or tingling sensation is noticed. Then park the gum in the cheek or under the tongue for one to two minutes or until the taste disappears. Repeat this cycle for 30 minutes.

Recommend the use of at least 8 to 12 pieces per day initially, or a fixed schedule such as one piece per hour, as the gum is more effective if used regularly. A common problem is the under-use of the gum. Three months use is recommended by the manufacturers followed by a period of tapering.

Adverse effects include gastrointestinal disturbances, dyspepsia, nausea, hiccups, and occasionally headache if the gum is chewed too rapidly. Other common adverse effects are jaw pain and dental problems (172,174). People who wear dentures cannot use the gum. Dependence on the gum can occur. Although this is not ideal, it is safer than smoking. A study of safety of nicotine gum used by 3094 participants in the Lung Health Study found no evidence of increase in rates of hospitalization for cardiovascular conditions among nicotine gum users during the five years of the study (175).

Nicotine Sublingual Tablet

With this form of NRT a small sublingual tablet is held under the tongue where it slowly disintegrates within 30 minutes and nicotine is absorbed sublingually. Like the lozenge it has the advantage of not requiring chewing. The levels of nicotine obtained by use of the 2 mg sublingual tablet are similar to those from the same dose of gum and lozenge (176). In a randomized trial there was an approximate doubling of quit rates at six months compared to placebo, which is comparable to other forms on NRT (177).

Nicotine Lozenge

This form of NRT has advantages for people who prefer an acute onset oral form of replacement but who do not wish to use or have problems with use of nicotine gum. In a 12-month follow-up study, OR for abstinence for the 2 mg dose was 2.10 (95% CI 1.59, 2.79) and for the 4 mg dose was 2.69 (95% CI 1.69, 4.29) (178). The choice of dose in this study was based on the time of day of the first cigarette. If the patient smoked their first cigarette within half an hour of waking then the 4 mg dose is suggested. Absorption of nicotine from the lozenge is through the oral mucosa.

Nicotine Inhaler

This device consists of a plastic mouthpiece and cartridge containing 10 mg of nicotine. Although the device is called inhaler, nicotine is absorbed through the oral mucosa, not through the respiratory tract. The inhaler produces nicotine concentrations that are about one third of those achieved with cigarette smoking. The inhaler is aimed at those smokers who miss the hand to mouth action of smoking. The more common side effects include: coughing, headache, heartburn, nausea, hiccups, throat irritation, rhinitis and occasionally, taste disturbance, and sinus irritation (179).

Nicotine Nasal Spray

Nasal spray is the most rapidly acting form of nicotine replacement. It is absorbed locally by the nasal mucosa. It should not be swallowed or deeply inhaled. Initial dosing is one to two sprays per hour. Nasal irritation is very common and transient changes can occur in sense of smell and taste. The nasal spray can cause airway reactions, so is not recommended for people with reactive airways disease (117). One study that directly compared four of the six NRT products found no difference in abstinence rates or withdrawal discomfort, although compliance was lower for inhaler and nasal spray (180).

Higher Dose and Combination Nicotine Replacement Therapy

Highly dependent smokers (20 or more cigarettes per day) benefit more from 4 mg than 2 mg gum and there may be a small benefit of higher dose patches across the range of 15 mg to 42 mg in 16 hours or 24 hours patches (139,181).

More rapid onset and slower onset nicotine delivery systems have been combined in a number of studies such as the transdermal patch for a steady background level of nicotine, supplemented by gum for immediate relief of craving (182,183). A meta-analysis of combination therapies (117) showed that combination therapy almost doubles cessation rates at 12 months compared to one form of therapy. Like other patients on NRT, patients on high dose and combination therapy should be monitored for symptoms of under or overdosing.

Nicotine Replacement Therapy and Cardiovascular Disease

Although it would be expected that use of NRT would have some of the same hemodynamic effects as smoking, use of NRT has not been associated with an increased risk of acute cardiovascular events (184–186) in patients including those who continue to smoke intermittently while on the nicotine patch (117,187). Reviews of safety have concluded that NRT is safe in patients with stable CVD (184).

The safety of NRT in patients with recent acute cardiovascular events has not been well studied, and in many countries the approved product information for NRT specifies that NRT is contraindicated for patients who have had a recent myocardial infarct, unstable angina, or a cerebrovascular accident. In a randomized trial of nicotine patch for patients with CVD (186) no difference was found in cardiac outcomes. A recent case control study concluded that transdermal nicotine therapy is safe in smokers admitted with acute coronary syndromes (188). Clinical practice guidelines in both the United States (117) and other countries (147) state that NRT should be used with caution in the immediate (within two weeks) post myocardial infarction period, in those with serious arrhythmias, and those with serious or worsening angina. Advice from a cardiologist can assist other physicians in deciding whether to advise NRT, and the patient should be informed of its risks and benefits.

Nicotine Replacement Therapy and Pregnancy

Nonpharmacological methods of smoking cessation are preferred in pregnant women. However, pharmacotherapy should be considered when a pregnant woman is otherwise unable to quit and when the likelihood and benefits of cessation outweigh the risks of NRT and potential continued smoking (117). Delivery systems should be considered that yield intermittent, rather than continuous nicotine exposure (i.e., inhaler, gum, lozenge, or sublingual tablet, rather than transdermal patch) due to potential neurotoxicity in the fetus of continuous exposure to nicotine (117,189,190).

Bupropion

Bupropion sustained release is an oral nonnicotine oral therapy to assist smoking cessation, which affects neuronal re-uptake of noradrenaline and dopamine. Use of bupropion sustained release approximately doubles cessation rates compared with placebo at six months follow-up (30.5% vs. 17.3%) when used as part of a comprehensive program of regular follow up and brief behavioral strategies (117). A review of bupropion for smoking cessation concluded that this medication is efficacious in a range of patient populations including those with cardiac and respiratory diseases, depression and among the general community (191).

The initial dose is 150 mg to be taken once daily for three days, increasing to 150 mg twice daily with an interval of at least eight hours between successive doses. Treatment with bupropion should be initiated while the patient is still smoking, quitting should occur during the second week, and the medication continued for at least seven weeks. Treatment with bupropion has been found to delay the weight gain commonly associated with smoking cessation. Safety considerations with bupropion are shown in Table 9.

In a randomized controlled trial by Jorenby et al. (192) the combination of bupropion with nicotine patch was significantly more effective than patch alone (point prevalence abstinence at twelve months combined 35.5% vs. 16.4%) but was not significantly better than bupropion alone (30.3%). In this study elevated blood pressure was noted in some patients on bupropion and nicotine patch treatment, which was more common in those with pre-existing hypertension. If bupropion and NRT are being used in combination, the blood pressure should be monitored.

Other Forms of Pharmacotherapy

The U.S. Clinical Practice Guideline recommends both nortriptyline and clonidine as second-line agents to treat tobacco dependence.

TABLE 9 Safety Considerations When Advising Use of Bupropion

Contraindications	Allergy to bupropion, past or current seizures, known CNS tumors, abrupt withdrawal from alcohol or benzodiazepines, current or previous bulimia or anorexia nervosa, concomitant use of MAOI's or use within the last 14 days. The safety of bupropion in pregnancy has not been established. Small amounts of bupropion and its metabolites are excreted in breast milk
Seizure risk	Patients with predisposing risk factors for seizure must not be prescribed bupropion unless the potential benefit of smoking cessation outweighs the increased risk of seizure. Predisposing risk factors for seizure include: concomitant use of medications known to lower seizure threshold; alcohol abuse; history of head trauma; diabetes treated with hypoglycemic or insulin; the and use of stimulants or anorectic products
Other precautions	Concern has been expressed in use of bupropion in people with schizophrenia because of the possibility of precipitating a psychotic episode
Adverse effects	Most common adverse effects are insomnia (42%), headache (26%), dry mouth (11%), nausea (10%), dizziness (11%), and anxiety (9%). The risk of seizures is 0.1% (1/1000) and patients need to be made aware of these potentially serious adverse effects. Hypersensitivity reactions occur at a rate of about 3%. The most common reaction is pruritis, urticaria, and/or angioedema. Serum-sickness-like reactions of arthralgia, myalgia, and fever can occur in association with skin rash and these can be delayed 10 to 20 days after starting bupropion

Source: From Ref. 119.

Nortriptyline

In a meta-analysis of three studies of nortriptyline for smoking cessation abstinence rates were 30.1% (95% CI 18.1, 41.6) versus 11.7% in the placebo group. The Cochrane systematic review of antidepressants for smoking cessation (141) concluded that there was evidence of effect for nortriptyline. In smoking cessation studies treatment has been initiated at 25 mg/d and increased gradually up to 75 to 100 mg/d. The drug has been initiated 10 to 28 days prior to the quit date and continued for 12 weeks. Nortriptyline is limited in its application by its adverse effects that include sedation, dry mouth, and light-headedness. There is also a risk of arrhythmia in patients with CVD. The efficacy of nortriptyline does not appear to be affected by a past history of depression (140).

Clonidine

Clonidine is a centrally acting adrenergic agonist that has been used to reduce nicotine withdrawal symptoms especially cravings. In a meta-analysis of five studies for the U.S. Clinical Practice Guideline (117) clonidine was found to double smoking cessation abstinence at five months compared to placebo. The adverse effects of clonidine, in particular postural hypotension, greatly limit its use for smoking cessation.

Individual Behavioral Counseling

This form of intervention involves individual face to face assistance from a trained counselor outside the normal clinical care. Behavioral approaches used include, developing coping and relapse prevention skills and health belief models. There is evidence of efficacy with an OR of 1.7 (95% CI 1.4–2.0) and an estimated abstinence rate of 16.8% at six months in the meta-analysis for the U.S. Clinical Practice Guideline. A Cochrane Review (193) identified 21 trials with over 7000 participants and concluded that individual counseling was more effective than control with an OR for successful cessation of 1.56 (95% CI 1.32–1.84).

The elements of counseling and behavioral therapy include (117,193):

- Review of smoking history and motivation to quit
- Help in the identification of high risk situations
- Generation of problem solving strategies to deal with high risk situations
- Providing social support as part of treatment
- Helping smokers obtain social support outside of treatment.

The U.S. Clinical Practice meta-analysis (117) also examines aversive smoking techniques and found evidence of some effect from rapid smoking at six months follow-up (OR 2.0, 95% CI 1.1–3.5). There was no significant effect from cigarette fading however (OR 1.1, 95% CI 0.8–1.5).

Group Counseling

Group techniques, which focus on skills training and provide mutual support can also be effective in assisting smoking cessation. The meta-analysis for the U.S. Clinical Practice Guideline found an OR of 1.3 (95% CI 1.1–1.6) with an abstinence rate of 13.9% at six months follow-up (117). Group programs are not appealing to all smokers but are likely to be helpful for those that do (194).

Telephone Quitlines

Telephone counseling provided through state or national services is available in many countries. Evidence on effectiveness has been reviewed by both the Cochrane Library (195) and as part of the development of the U.S. Clinical Practice Guideline (117). Both reviews found evidence that proactive telephone counseling, where the counselor initiates one or more calls to provide support or help avoid relapse is an effective intervention. The meta-analysis for the U.S. Clinical Practice Guideline included 26 arms and found an OR of 1.2 (95% CI 1.1–1.4) and an estimated abstinence rate of 13% at six months follow-up (1). Pro-active counseling has been shown to be more effective than provision of self-help materials in a randomized study (196). The evidence for reactive counseling, where the smoker initiates the call for assistance, is less clear and there is a lack of randomized studies. Fiore concluded that the impact of such a "self help" intervention is smaller and less certain than proactive counseling (117).

Nonevidence-Based Approaches

Acupuncture

Two meta-analyses have reviewed the results of controlled studies of acupuncture (117,197). There was no significant difference between "active" acupuncture and "inactive" or sham acupuncture procedures. Positive expectations of the effect of acupuncture may, therefore be the factor responsible for benefit rather than any effect of the acupuncture itself.

Hypnotherapy

Hypnotherapy as an aid to smoking cessation has been the subject of a number of studies, including some controlled trials. The Cochrane Collaboration on reviewing the controlled studies in 1998 (198) concluded that there was such heterogeneity between methods and results that a meta-analysis of the literature was not possible at that time. The review concluded that hypnotherapy does not show a greater effect on six month quit rates than other interventions or no treatment.

Harm Reduction

Harm reduction is the strategy of tobacco users altering, rather than eliminating the use of nicotine or tobacco to reduce or avoid its harmful consequences (117). Harm reduction strategies include reducing tobacco use including through concomitant use of pharmacotherapy; use of less hazardous forms of tobacco; and use of less addictive forms of tobacco. The health benefits of harm reduction strategies for smoking remain unproven and further research is needed (117). It has been argued however that the potential for health gain in less harmful forms of tobacco products such the Swedish tobacco product snus needs to be further explored (199).

Application of the Clinical Approach to Two Patients Cases

The application of the smoking cessation approach in clinical practice is highlighted in the following two cases that a physician may encounter in medical practice.

▪ Case Study: Sam Lee

Sam Lee is a 40-year-old man, who presents for a life insurance medical examination. He has not seen a physician for two years. He has been employed as a security officer for 22 years. He smokes one packet of cigarettes per day and has done so for the last 20 years. He lives with his wife who is a nonsmoker. Both his parents are alive and have no history of CHD. He is overweight (BMI 29kg/m2) and does not exercise regularly. His blood pressure is 140/90 mmHg. His total cholesterol level is 220mg/dL (normal range 140–200), and triglycerides level 145mg/dL (normal range 30–150). Framingham Risk Score for CHD in next 10 years 11%.

When asked "How do you feel about your smoking?" he replies he wants to quit but is concerned about how he will manage cravings and weight gain. He has made several unsuccessful attempts to quit "cold turkey" in the past, but found that he recommenced smoking during the "debriefing" sessions with fellow security officers over a few beers at the local bar. Most of his work mates drink alcohol and smoke.

Discussion

This is an important opportunity to intervene with a patient who does not often attend a physician. A health professional should:

- Ask about tobacco use: This should be documented for each visit, along with a record of previous quit attempts, and tobacco consumption.
- Advise to quit: This advice should be personalized, for example to emphasis the health benefits of cessation (improved fitness, a reduction in risk of CVD, or cancer), the health benefits to his wife (reduced risk of lung cancer of ETS) and financial gains associated with cessation.
- Assess willingness to quit: He is motivated to quit, but there are a number of barriers that need to be addressed. These include managing his nicotine dependence and minimizing weight gain.
- Assist in a quit attempt: With him, develop a quit plan including setting a quit day (within the next two weeks), mobilizing social support, and avoiding alcohol. He could be given health promotion materials and encouraged to use pharmacotherapies, for example nicotine patches and/or bupropion sustained release. In addition, he could be referred to specialist quit services. Weight gain with smoking cessation is common. Although the majority of patients gain less than 10 pounds, as many as 10% gain as much as 30 pounds. Weight gain is less of a health threat than continued smoking. He should be given advice on avoidance of weight gain, by reducing food intake, increasing exercise, and avoidance of environments that may trigger him to recommence smoking. While using pharmacotherapy, both NRT and bupropion sustained release delay weight gain (118). Discuss options for avoiding work situations where Sam might be tempted to smoke, for example changing the time and venue of the "debriefing" sessions at work.

Note that becoming a nonsmoker, cessation greatly reduces the Framingham Risk Score—a nonsmoker with the same blood pressure and lipid parameters has a risk score of 3%. Arrange follow-up: He should be encouraged to return to discuss progress with cessation.

■ Case Study: Lola Bryant

Lola Bryant is a 56-year-old African American woman with a history of type 2 diabetes for the last five years controlled with diet, exercise, and oral hypoglycemic medication. She also has hypertension for which she is taking an angiotensin converting enzyme inhibitor. She has recently commenced aspirin 100 mg/day. Lola works part-time in a grocery store. She lives with her husband, who also smokes and suffers from emphysema, and two of her adult children smoke. Lola started smoking at age 19 and has smoked about 15 cigarettes per day since with periods of abstinence during her two pregnancies. At previous visits she simply laughed when you suggested she might consider quitting.

She is obese (BMI 31kg/m2) and does not exercise regularly. Her blood pressure is 130/80mmHg. Her total cholesterol level is 165mg/dL (normal range 140–200), and triglycerides level 120mg/dL (normal range 30–150). Her HbA1C is 7.2% (normal range 4.0–6.0).

She presented to hospital two months ago with chest pain. Angiography revealed significant blockage in the left anterior descending coronary artery. She underwent angioplasty and stent placement. She did not smoke in hospital but since discharge she has had family stresses and she says this prompted a relapse to smoking. She relapsed to smoking 15 cigarettes per day, with her first cigarette within 30 minutes of waking. Her husband reports that she continues to smoke even when she is sick enough to stay in bed all day.

You discuss a plan for cessation with her, and discuss the use of pharmacotherapy. At her next visit, she is still smoking, although she reports ceasing for ten days since she last saw you. She laughs and says, "I'm too old to give up smoking. I don't care if I die soon—I'm an old woman. I got too many other things to worry about."

Discussion

Patients commonly stop smoking while in hospital but relapse on returning to their home environment. Emotional stress is a common trigger to relapse, as is the presence of other smokers. However, a new diagnosis of CVD may provide an important trigger for smokers to quit.

Health professionals should:

- Ask about tobacco use: This should be documented for each visit, along with a record of previous quit attempts, and tobacco consumption.

- Advice to quit: Smoking has adverse hemodynamic and vascular effects and this woman is at substantially increased risk of further cardiovascular events if she continues to smoke (200). Quitting smoking would make a major contribution to decreasing her risk (122). Her smoking is therefore an issue of major importance. For people in lower socioeconomic groups, smoking cessation brings substantial financial gains; continued smoking has a strong link to poverty.
- Assess willingness to quit: Lola is starting to smoke early in the day and when she is unwell, and this indicates that she has moderate to high level of nicotine dependence. This is confirmed by administering the Fagerstrom test for nicotine dependence. Knowing her level of dependence will assist in deciding whether to use pharmacotherapies for cessation. While Lola may report being willing to quit, this may be moderated by the effect of her environment—for example that her husband and children are also smokers. They also are likely to benefit from support to quit.
- Assist in a quit attempt: Lola should be helped to develop a quit plan including setting a quit day. NRT can be used to help Lola to stop smoking, as there is no evidence that use of NRT increases the risk of cardiovascular events (185–187). Use of NRT for the normal duration of treatment will not have a significant adverse effect on her diabetes (201,202). Choice of NRT product is dependent on the patient preference and physician familiarity. Options include patch, gum, lozenge, sublingual tablet, inhaler, and nasal spray. Whatever form of NRT is used, the patient should be encouraged to use it for at least six weeks to achieve best results. It is recommended that medication be combined with supportive behavioral counseling. Relapse prevention strategies include discussing other ways of dealing with stress such as structured problem solving and relaxation exercises.
- Another option for pharmacotherapy is bupropion sustained release. This could be considered if she prefers a nonnicotine medication. This drug should be used with caution in this patient as her diabetes and oral hypoglycemic medication lower her seizure threshold and therefore, the risk of seizures if she is prescribed bupropion may be increased. The risk of using bupropion needs to be weighed up against the risk of continued smoking.
- At admission to hospital, all smokers should be encouraged to quit, and be supported by pharmacotherapies as inpatients, where appropriate. At discharge, a formal plan to support continued abstinence should be set in place, for example through a cardiac rehabilitation program.
- Arrange follow-up: Lola should be encouraged to return to assess her progress. She could be praised for trying to quit and be given advice to overcome any lapses; she should be encouraged to keep trying. Health professionals should offer cessation support at every future visit.

CONCLUSION

The world is in the throes of an epidemic of tobacco related diseases (203). It is a very sad fact that more people die from smoking than from illicit drug abuse, motor vehicle accidents, suicides, homicides, drowning, in fact all other external causes of death combined. Over the past decades we have seen a decline in smoking prevalence particularly in developing countries in Stage 4 of the tobacco epidemic. Thousands of studies have expanded our knowledge of the health effects of smoking on health, and our understanding of the many factors that influence commencement of tobacco use, maintenance, and cessation. Unless the use of tobacco is curbed further, the health effects of tobacco use will continue to be significant. Smokers are at increased risk of CVD, cancers, and pulmonary diseases. In addition, women also experience risks related to menstrual cycle, reproduction, and pregnancy. Although there have been many improved health outcomes from a range of diseases, it is tragic that smoking, which is an entirely preventable lifestyle habit, continues to claim so many lives.

To be successful in reducing smoking rates a multipronged approach is necessary including public health and clinical strategies. These include increasing taxes and price of cigarettes, anti-smoking media campaigns, promotion of nonsmoking in public places and in the workplace, bans and restrictions on tobacco advertising, promotion and sponsorship, enforcement of legislation to reduce adolescents' access to tobacco products, and use of effective evidence-based treatment programs, which consist of combinations of behavioral advice and pharmacotherapy. The role of physicians in providing smoking cessation advice is critical as they see a large proportion of the smoking population.

The challenges ahead are to establish comprehensive tobacco control programs in each state of every country, and this endeavor is being fostered by the WHO's Tobacco Free Initiative.

REFERENCES

1. World Bank. Curbing the Epidemic: Governments and the Economics of Tobacco Control. Washington DC: The World Bank, 1999.
2. Peto R, Lopez A, Boreham J, Thun M, Heath C. Mortality from tobacco in developed countries: indirect estimation from national vital statistics. Lancet 1992; 339:1268–1278.
3. World Health Organization. Tobacco or Health: A Global Status Report. Geneva, Switzerland, 1997.
4. Murray CJL, Lopez AD. Global Health Statistics: A Compendium of Incidence, Prevalence and Mortality Estimates for over 200 Conditions. Geneva: World Health Organization, 1996.
5. Peto R et al. Mortality from Smoking in developed Countries, 1950–2000. Oxford University Press, 1994.
6. Benowitz NL. Summary: risks and benefits of nicotine. In: Benowitz NL, ed. Nicotine Safety and Toxicity. New York (NY): Oxford University Press, 1998.
7. Smith CJ, Livingston SD, Doolittle DJ. An international literature survey of "IARC Group I Carcinogens" reported in mainstream cigarette smoke. Food Chem Toxicol 1997; 35:1107–1130.
8. Centers for Disease Control and Prevention. Indicators of nicotine addiction among women—United States-1991–1992. Morbidity and Mortality Weekly Report 1995; 44(6):102–105.
9. Koop CE. Lecture at Walter Reed, 2000.
10. Ezzati M, Lopez AD. Regional, disease specific patterns of smoking-attributable mortality in 2000. Tob Control 2004; 13(4):388–395.
11. World Health Organization. The Tobacco Atlas. World Health Organization, 2003.
12. Corrao MA, Guindon GE, Sharma N, Shokoohi DF, eds. Tobacco Control Country Profiles. American Cancer Society, Atlanta, GA, 2000.
13. Richmond R. You've come a long way baby: women and the tobacco epidemic. Editorial. Addiction 2003; 98:553–557.
14. Lopez AD, Collishaw NE, Piha T. A descriptive model of the tobacco epidemic in developed countries. Tobacco Control 1994; 3:242–247.
15. Sweeney J. On selling cigarettes to the Africans. The Independent Magazine (UK), 1988:16. 29 october
16. Amos A, Haglund M. From social taboo to "torch of freedom": the marketing of cigarettes to women. Tobacco Control 2000; 9:3–8 (Spring).
17. Australian Institute of Health and Welfare 2001 National Drug Strategy Household Survey First Results Drug Statistics, Series No. 9, 2002. http://www.aihw.gov.au/publications/
18. Crofton J, Simpson D. Tobacco: A Global Threat. Oxford: Macmillan Publishers Ltd., 2002.
19. United States Surgeon General. Women and Smoking: A Report of the Surgeon General, 2001.
20. Centers for Disease Control. Cigarette smoking among adults-United States, 2002. Morbidity and Mortality Weekly Report 2004; 53(20):427–431.
21. Centers for Disease Control and Prevention. Cigarette smoking among adults-United States, 2003. Morbidity and Mortality Weekly Report 2005; 54(20):509–513.
22. Centers for Disease Control and Prevention. Cigarette smoking among adults-United States, 1997. Morbidity and Mortality Weekly Report 1999; 48:993–996.
23. U.S. Department of Health and Human Services. Tobacco Use Among US Racial/Ethnic Minority Groups–African Americans, American Indians and Alaska Natives, Asian Americans and Pacific Islanders, and Hispanics. A Report of the Surgeon General. Atlanta, GA: Centers for Disease Control and Prevention, 1998.
24. Substance Abuse and Mental Health Services Administration. Results from the 2002 National Survey on Drug Use and Health: National Findings, Tobacco Use. Rockville, Substance Abuse and Mental Health Services Administration, 2003.
25. United States Surgeon General. The Health Consequences of Smoking: A Report of the Surgeon General. Centers for Disease Control, 2004.
26. Hughes JR, Hatsukami DK, Mitchell JE, Dahlgren LA. Prevalence of smoking among psychiatric outpatients. Am J Psychiatry 1986; 143:993–997.
27. Reichler H, Baker A, Lewin T, Carr V. Smoking among in-patients with drug–related problems in an Australian psychiatric hospital. Drug Alcohol Rev 2001; 20:231–237.
28. de Leon J. Smoking and vulnerability for schizophrenia. Schizophr Bull 1996; 22:405–409.
29. Lasser K, Boyd JW, Woolhandler S, Himmelstein DU, McCormick D, Bor DH. Smoking and mental illness: a population-based prevalence study. JAMA 2000; 284(20):2606–2610.
30. de Leon J, Diaz F. A meta-analysis of worldwide studies demonstrates an association between schizophrenia and tobacco smoking behaviors. Schizophr Res 2005; 76(203):135–157.
31. Dalak GW, Healy DJ, Meador-Woodruff JH. Nicotine dependence in schizophrenia: clinical phenomena and laboratory findings. Am J Psychiatry 1998; 115:1490–1501.
32. Williams JM, Ziedonis D. Addressing tobacco among individuals with a metal illness or an addiction. Addict Behav 2004; 29:1067–1083.
33. Batel P, Pessione F, Maitre C, Rueff B, et al. Relationship between alcohol and tobacco dependencies among alcoholics who smoke. Addiction 1995; 90:977–980.
34. Clarke JG, Stein MD, McGarry KA, Gogineni A. Interest in smoking cessation among injection drug users. Am J Addict 2001; 10:159–166.
35. Richter KP, Gibson CA, Ahluwalia JS, Schmelzle KH. Tobacco use and quit attempts among methadone maintenance clients. Am J Public Health 2001; 91(2):296–299.

36. Shakeshaft AP, Bowman JA, Sanson-Fisher RW. Community-based drug and alcohol counseling: who attends and why? Drug Alcohol Rev 2002; 21(2):153–162.
37. John U, Hill A, Rumpf H-J, Hapke U, Meyer C. Alcohol high risk drinking, abuse and dependence among tobacco smoking medical care patients and the general population. Drug Alcohol Dependence 2003; 69(2):189–195.
38. Drobes D. Concurrent alcohol and tobacco dependence. Alcohol Res Health 2002; 26:136–142.
39. Highet G. The role of cannabis in supporting young people's cigarette smoking: a qualitative exploration. Health Educ Res 2004; 6:635–643.
40. Frosch DL, Shoptaw S, Nahom D, Jarvik ME. Associations between tobacco smoking and illicit drug use among methadone-maintained opiate-dependent individuals. Exp Clin Psychopharmacol 2000; 8:97–103.
41. Roll J, Higgins S. Cocaine use can increase cigarette smoking: evidence from laboratory and naturalistic settings. Exp Clin Psychopharmacol 1997; 3:263–268.
42. Bien T, Burge R. Smoking and drinking: a review of the literature. Int J Addict 1990; 25:1429–1454.
43. Hurt RD, Offord KP, Croghan IT, et al. Mortality following inpatient addiction treatment: role of tobacco use in a community-based cohort. JAMA 1996; 275:1097–1103.
44. D'Souza RM, Butler T, Petrovsky N. Assessment of cardiovascular disease risk factors and diabetes in Australian prisons: is the prisoner population unhealthier than the rest of the Australian population? Aust N Z J Public Health 2005; 29(4):318–323.
45. Fazel S, Danesh J. Serious mental disorder in 23,000 prisoners: a systematic review of 62 surveys. Lancet 2002; 359:545–550.
46. Hockings B, Young M, Falconer A, O'Rourke PK. Queensland Women Prisoners' Health Survey. Brisbane, Department of Corrective Services, 2002.
47. Degenhardt L, Hall W. The relationship between tobacco use, substance-use disorders and mental health: results from the National Survey of Mental Health and Well-being. Nicotine Tobacco Res 2001; 3:234.
48. Dwyer T, Ponsonby AL, Couper D. Tobacco smoke exposure at one month of age and subsequent risk of SIDS: a prospective study. Am J Epid 1999; 147:960–968.
49. McLean S, Richmond R, et al. Management of alcohol and drug problems. In: Hulse G, White J, Cape G, eds. Melbourne: Chapter on Tobacco. Oxford University Press, 2002:100–123.
50. Doll R, Peto R, Wheatley K, Gray R, Sutherland I. Mortality in relation to smoking: 40 years observation on male British doctors. BMJ 1994; 309:901–911.
51. U.S. Department of Health and Human Services. Reducing the Health Consequences of Smoking: 25 years of progress. A Report of the Surgeon General. Rockville, MD: US Department of Health and Human Services. Centers for Disease Control and Prevention, 1989.
52. Centers for Disease Control and Prevention. Tobacco use-United States, 1990–1999. Morbidity and Mortality Weekly Report, 1999; 48:986–993.
53. Moyer D. Cardiovascular disease. The Tobacco Reference Guide. UICC Global Link, 2000.
54. Rosenberg L, Kaufman DW, Helmrich SP, Miller DR, Stolley PD, Shapiro S. Myocardial Infarction and cigarette smoking in women younger than 50 years of age. JAMA 1985; 253:2965–2969.
55. van Domburg RT, Meeter K, van Berkel DFM, Veldkamp RF, van Herwerden LA, Bogers A. Smoking cessation reduces mortality after coronary artery bypass surgery: a 20-year follow-up study. J Am Coll Cardiol 2000; 36(3):878-883.
56. Mulcahy R, Hickey N, Graham IM, Mac Airt J. Factors Affecting the five-year survival rate of men following acute coronary heart disease. Am Heart J 1977; 93:556–559.
57. Parish S, Collins R, Peto R, et al. Cigarette smoking, tar yields, and non-fatal myocardial infarction: 14000 cases and 32000 controls in the United Kingdom. BMJ 1995; 311:471–477.
58. Shah PK, Helfant RH. Smoking and coronary artery disease. Chest 1988; 94:449–452.
59. Caralis DG, Deligonul U, Kern MJ, Cohen JD. Smoking is a risk factor for coronary spasm in young women. Circulation 1992; 85:905–909.
60. Hallstrom AP, Cobb LA, Ray R. Smoking as a risk factor for recurrence of sudden cardiac arrest. NEJM 1986; 314:271–275.
61. Howard G, Burke GL, Szklo M, et al. Active and passive smoking are associated with increased carotid wall thickness. The Atherosclerosis Risk in Communities Study. Arch Internal Med 1994; 154:1277–1282.
62. Willett WC, Green A, Stampfer MJ, et al. Relative and absolute excess risks of coronary heart disease among women who smoke cigarettes. NEJM 1987; 317(21):1303–1309.
63. U.S. Department of Health and Human Services. The Health Benefits of Smoking Cessation: A Report of the Surgeon General. Atlanta GA: US Department for Health and Human Services, Centers for Disease Control and Prevention, National Center for Chronic Disease Prevention and Health Promotion. Office on Smoking and Health, 2004.
64. Aldoori MI, Rahman SH. Smoking and stroke: a causative role BMJ 1998; 317:962–963.
65. Greenlee RT, Murray T, Bolden S, Wingo PA. Cancer Statistics. CA Cancer J Clin 2000; 50:7–33.
66. Hecht SS. Tobacco smoke carcinogens and lung cancer. J Natl Cancer Inst 1999; 91:1194–1210.
67. Frith P, McKenzie D, Pierce R. Management of chronic obstructive disease in the twenty-first century. Internal Med J 2001; 31:508–511.
68. Fletcher C, Peto R. The natural history of chronic airflow limitation. BMJ 1977; 1:1645–1648.

69. Burrows B, Knudson RJ, Cline MG, Lebowitz MD. Quantitative relationships between cigarette smoking and ventilatory function. Am Rev Respir Dis 1977; 115:195–205.
70. Anthonisen NR, Connett JE, Murray RP. Smoking and lung function of lung health study participants after 11 years. Am J Respir Crit Care Med 2002; 166:675–679.
71. Anthonisen NR, Connett JE, Kiley JP, et al. Effects of smoking intervention and the use of an inhaled anticholinergic bronchodilator on the rate of decline of FEV1. The Lung Health Study. JAMA 1994; 272:1497–1505.
72. Wilcox A. Birth weight and perinatal mortality: the effect of maternal smoking. Am J Epidemiol 1993; 137:104–109.
73. Lieberman E, Gremy I, Lang JM, Cohen AP. Low birthweight at term and the timing of fetal exposure to maternal smoking. Am J Public Health 1994; 84:1127–1131.
74. Harlop S, Davies A. Infant admissions to hospital and maternal smoking. Lancet 1974; 1:529–532.
75. Arday DR, Giovino GA, Schulman J, Nelson DE, Mowery P, Samet JM. Cigarette smoking and self reported health problems among US high school seniors, 1982–1989. Am J Health Promotion 1995; 10:111–116.
76. Sundell G, Milsom I, Andersch B. Factors influencing the prevalence and severity of dysmenorrhoea in young women. Br J Obstetrics Gynaecol 1990; 97(7):588–594.
77. Parazzini F, Tozzi L, Mezzopane R, Luchini L, Marchini M, Fedele L. Cigarette smoking, alcohol consumption, and risk of primary dysmenorrhea. Epidemiology 1994; 5(4):469–472.
78. McNamara PM, Hjortland MC, Gordon T, Kannel WB. Natural history of menopause: the Framingham Study. J Continuing Educ Obstetrics Gynecol 1978; 20:27–35.
79. Willett W, Stampfer MJ, Bain C, et al. Cigarette smoking, relative weight, and menopause. Am J Epidemiol 1983; 117(6):651–658.
80. Torgerson DJ, Avenell A, Russell IT, Reid DM. Factors associated with onset of menopause in women aged 45–49. Maturitas 1994; 19(2):83–92.
81. Midgette AS, Baron JA. Cigarette smoking and the risk of natural menopause. Epidemiology 1990; 1(6):474–480.
82. Greenberg G, Thompson SG, Meade TW. Relation between cigarette smoking and use of hormonal replacement therapy for menopausal symptoms. J Epidemiol Community Health 1987; 41(1):26–29.
83. Dennerstein L, Smith AM, Morse C, et al. Menopausal symptoms in Australian women. Med J Australia 1993; 159(4):232–236.
84. Langenberg P, Kjerulff KH, Stolley PD. Hormone replacement and menopausal symptoms following hysterectomy. Am J Epidemiol 1997; 146(10):870–880.
85. Berigan TR, Deagle EA. Treatment of smokeless tobacco addiction with bupropion and behavior modification. JAMA 1999; 281:233.
86. International Agency for Research on Cancer. Tobacco habits other than smoking: Betel quid and areca nut chewing and some related nitrosamines. IARC Monograph on the Evaluation of the Carcinogenic Risks of Chemicals to Humans. Vol. 37. 1985.
87. Hecht SS. Biochemistry, biology, and carcinogenicity of tobacco-specific N-nitrosamines. Chem Res Toxicol 1998; 11:559–603.
88. Hoffmann D, Hoffmann I. The changing cigarette 1950–1995. J Toxicol Env Health 1997; 50:307–364.
89. Osterdahl B-G. Occurrence of and exposure to N-nitrosamines in Sweden: a review. In: O'Neill IK, Chen JS, Bartsch H, eds. Relevance to Human Cancer of N-Nitroso Compounds, Tobacco Smoke, and Mycotoxins. 1991:235–237.
90. Doll R, Peto R, Boreham J, Sutherland I. Mortality in relation to smoking: 50 years' observations on male British doctors. BMJ 2004; 328;1519–1527.
91. Kannel WB, McGee DL, Catelli WP. Latest perspective on cigarette smoking and cardiovascular disease: the Framingham experience. J Cardiac Rehab 2000; 4:267–277.
92. Pirkle JL, Flegal KM, Bernert JT, Brody DJ, Etzel RA, Maurer KR. Exposure of the US population to environmental tobacco smoke: the Third National Health and Nutrition Examination Survey. JAMA 1996; 275:1233–1240.
93. Environmental Protection Agency. Respiratory Health Effects of Passive Smoking: Lung Cancer and Other Disorders. Washington, DC: Environmental Protection Agency, Office on Air and Radiation, 1992.
94. Health Effects of exposure to environmental tobacco smoke. The report of the California Environmental Protection Agency. Smoking and Tobacco Control. Monograph 10, National Cancer Institute, 1999.
95. Steenland K, Thun M, Lally C, Heath C. Environmental tobacco smoke and coronary heart disease in the American Cancer Society, CPS-II Cohort. Circulation 1996; 94:622–628.
96. Glantz SA, Parmley WW. Passive smoking and heart disease epidemiology, physiology and biochemistry. Circulation 1991; 83:1–12.
97. Glantz SA, Parmley WW. Passive smoking and heart disease. JAMA 1995; 273(13):1047–1053.
98. Otsuka R, Watanabe H, Hirata K, et al. Acute effects of passive smoking on the coronary circulation in healthy young adults. JAMA 2001; 286:436–441.
99. Law MR, Morris JK, Wald NJ. Environmental tobacco smoke exposure and ischemic heart disease: an evaluation of the evidence. BMJ 1997; 315:973–980.
100. He J, Vupputuri S, Allen K, Prerost MR, Hughes J, Whelton PK. Passive smoking and the risk of coronary heart disease – a meta-analysis of epidemiological studies. NEJM 1999; 340:920–926.

101. Raitakari OT, et al. Atherial endothelial dysfunction related to passive smoking is potentially reversible in healthy young adults. Ann Internal Med 1999; 130:578–581.
102. Bonita R, Duncan J, Truelsen T, Jackson RT, Beaglehole RT. Passive Smoking as well as active smoking increases the risk of acute stroke. Tobacco Control 1999; 8:156–160.
103. International Agency for Research on Cancer. Tobacco Smoke and Involuntary Smoking. IARC Monograph on the Evaluation of Carcinogenic Risks to Humans, Vol 83, 2002.
104. Hackshaw AK, Law MR, Wald NJ. The accumulated evidence on lung cancer and environmental tobacco smoke. BMJ 1997; 315:980–988.
105. Boffetta P, et al. Multicentre case-control study of exposure to environmental tobacco smoke and lung cancer in Europe. J National Cancer Inst 1998; 90:1440–1450.
106. Coultas DB. Passive smoking and risk of adult asthma and COPD: an update. Thorax 1998; 53:381–387.
107. World Health Organization. Making a Difference. World Health Report, 1999. Geneva, Switzerland, 1999.
108. Smoking and the Young Summary of a Report of a Working Party of the Royal College of Physicians, 1992.
109. U.S. Department of Health and Human Services. The Health Consequences of Smoking: Nicotine Addiction. A Report of the Surgeon General. Washington DC: Government Printing Office, 1988.
110. Le Houezec J, Benowitz NL. Basic and clinical psychopharmacology of nicotine. Clin Chest Med 1991; 12(4):681–699.
111. Henningfield JE, Schuh LM, Jarvik ME. Pathophysiology of tobacco dependence. In: Bloom FE, Kupfer DJ, eds. Psychopharmacology: The Fourth Generation of Progress. New York: Raven Press, 1995:1715–1729.
112. British Journal of Addiction: Nomenclature and classification of drug- and alcohol-related problems: a shortened version of a WHO memorandum. Br J Addict 1982; 77(1):3–20.
113. American Psychiatric Association. Diagnostic and Statistical Manual of Mental Disorders, 4th ed. DSM-IV. Washington: American Psychiatric Association, 1994.
114. U.S. Department of Health and Human Services. An analysis regarding the food and drug administration's jurisdiction over nicotine-containing cigarettes and smokeless tobacco products, 60 Fed. Reg. 41453, 1995.
115. Stewart J, de Wit H, Eikelboom R. Role of unconditioned and conditioned drug effects in the self administration of opiates and stimulants. Psychol Rev 1984; 91(2):251–268.
116. Wikler A. Conditioning factors in opiate addiction and relapse. In: Wilner DM, Kassebaum GG, eds. Narcotics. New York: McGraw-Hill 1965:85–100.
117. Fiore MC, Bailey WC, Cohen SJ, et al. Treating Tobacco Use and Dependence. Clinical Practice Guideline. Rockville, MD: US Department of Health and Human Services. Public Health Service, 2000.
118. U.S. Department of Health and Human Services. The Health Benefits of Smoking Cessation: A Report of the Surgeon General. Rockville, MD: US Department for Health and Human Services. Centers for Disease Control and Prevention, 1990.
119. Zwar N, Richmond R, Borland R, Stillman S, Cunningham M, Litt J. Smoking Cessation Guidelines for Australian General Practice. Commonwealth Dept of Health and Aging, 2004.
120. Shaper AG, Pocock SJ, Walker M, Phillips AN, Whitehead TP, Macfarlane PW. Risk factors for ischemic heart disease: the prospective phase of the British Regional Heart Study. J Epidemiol Community Health 1985; 39:197–209.
121. Sato I, Nishida M, Okita K, et al. l. Beneficial effect of stopping smoking on future cardiac events in male smokers with previous myocardial infarction. Jpn Circ J 1992; 56:217–222.
122. Critchley JA, Capewell S. Mortality risk reduction associated with smoking cessation in patients with coronary heart disease. A systematic review. JAMA 2003; 290:86–97.
123. Ramanathan KB, Vander Zwang R, Maddock V, Kroetz FW, Sullivan JM, Mirvis DM. Interactive effects of age and other risk factors on long-term survival after coronary artery surgery. J Am Coll Cardiol 1990; 15:493–499.
124. Hasdai D, Garratt KN, Grill DE, Lerman A, Holmes DR. Effect of smoking status on the long-term outcome after successful percutaneous coronary revascularisation. N Eng J Med 1997; 336:755–761.
125. FitzGibbon GM, Leach AJ, Kafka HP. Atherosclerosis of coronary artery bypass grafts and smoking. Can Med Assoc J 1987; 136:45–47.
126. Centers for Disease Control and Prevention. Response to increases in cigarette prices by race/ethnicity, income, and age groups–United States, 1976–1993. Morbidity and Mortality Weekly Report 1998; 47:605–609.
127. Saloojee Y. Price and income elasticity of demand for cigarettes in South Africa. In: Slama K, ed. Tobacco and Health. New York, NY: Plenum Press, 1995.
128. Townsend J. The role of taxation policy in tobacco control. In: Abedian I et al., eds. The Economics of Tobacco Control. Cape Town, South Africa: Applied Fiscal Research Centre, University of Cape Town, 1998.
129. Safer H. The control of tobacco advertising and promotion. In: The World Bank: Curbing the Epidemic: Governments and the Economics of Tobacco Control. Washington DC: The World Bank, 1999.
130. Hopkins DP, Briss PA, Ricard CJ, et al. Reviews of evidence regarding intervention to reduce tobacco use and exposure to environmental tobacco smoke. Am J Prev Med 2001; 20:16–66.

131. Centers for Disease Control and Prevention. Strategies for reducing exposure to environmental tobacco smoke, increasing tobacco-use cessation, and reducing initiation in communities and health-care systems. A report on recommendations of the Task Force on Community Prevention Services. Morbidity and Mortality Weekly Report 2000; 49:1–11.

132. Chaloupka FJ. Macro-social influences: the effects of prices and tobacco-control policies on the demand for tobacco products. Nicotine Tob Res 1999; 1:S105–S109.

133. Ranson K, Jha P, Chaloupka F, Yurekli A. Effectiveness and cost effectiveness of price increases and other tobacco control policy interventions. In: The World Bank: Curbing the Epidemic: Governments and the Economics of Tobacco Control. Washington DC: The World Bank, 1999.

134. World Health Organization. Why is Tobacco a Public Health Priority? Tobacco Free Initiative, World Health Organization, 2005.

135. Richmond RL. The physician can make a difference with smokers: evidence based clinical approaches. Int J Tub Lung Dis 1999; 3(2);100–112.

136. Young JM, Ward JE. Implementing guidelines for smoking cessation advice in Australian general practice: opinions, current practices, readiness to change and perceived barriers. Family Practice 2001; 18(1):14–20.

137. Wiggers JH, Sanson-Fisher RW. Practitioner provision of preventive care in general medical consultations: association with patient educational and occupational status. Social Sci Med 1997; 44:13–146.

138. Thorndike AN, Rigotti NA, Stafford RS, Singer DE. National patterns in the treatment of smoking by physicians. JAMA 1998; 279:604–608.

139. Silagy C, Lancaster T, Stead L, Mant D, Fowler G. Nicotine replacement therapy for smoking cessation (Review). The Cochrane Database of Systematic Reviews, 2004, Issue 3.

140. Hughes JR, Stead LF, Lancaster T. Antidepressants for smoking cessation (Review). The Cochrane Database of Systematic Reviews, 2004, Issue 4.

141. Richmond RL, Anderson P. Research in general practice for smokers and drinkers. Part 3: dissemination of interventions. Addiction 1994; 89:49–62.

142. Lancaster T, Stead L. Physician advice for smoking cessation. The Cochrane Database of Systematic Reviews, 2004, Issue 4.

143. Rigotti NA, Singer DE, Mulley AG Jr, Thibault GE. Smoking cessation after admission to a coronary care unit. J Gen Intern Med 1991; 6:305–311.

144. Rice VH, Stead LF. Nursing interventions for smoking cessation. The Cochrane Database of Systematic Reviews, 2004, Issue 1.

145. Rigotti NA, Munalfo MR, Murphy MFG, Stead LF. Interventions for smoking cessation in hospitalized smokers. The Cochrane Database of Systematic Reviews, 2002, Issue 4.

146. Hajek P, Taylor TZ, Mills P. Brief intervention during hospital admission to help patients give up smoking after myocardial infraction and bypass surgery: randomized controlled trial. BMJ 2002; 324:1–6.

147. Katz DA, Muehlenbruch DR, Brown RL, Fiore MC, Baker TB. AHRQ Smoking Cessation Guideline Study Group. Effectiveness of implementing the agency for healthcare research and quality smoking cessation clinical practice guideline: a randomized, controlled trial. J National Cancer Inst 2004; 96(8):594–603.

148. Guidelines for Smoking Cessation. National Advisory Committee on Health and Dissability. Wellington, New Zealand 2002.

149. Butler CC, Rollnick S, Cohen D, Bachmann M, Russell I, Stott N. Motivational consulting versus brief advice for smokers in general practice: A randomized trial. Br J General Practice 1999; 49(445):11–616.

150. Butler CC, Rollnick S. Treatment of tobacco use and dependence. (Letter) New England J Med 2002; 347(4):294–295.

151. Centers for Disease Control and Prevention. Cigarette smoking among adults–United States. 1995. Morbidity and Mortality Weekly Report, 1997; 46(51):1217–1220.

152. Prochaska JO, DiClemente CC. Stages and processes of self-change in smoking: towards and integrative model of change. J Consulting Clin Psychol 1983; 51:390–395.

153. Velicer WF, Fava JL, Prochaska JO, Abrams DB, Emmons KM, Pierce JP. Distribution of stages of change in three representative samples. Preventive Med 1995; 24:401–411.

154. Richmond R, Webster I, Elkins L, Mendelsohn C, Rollnick S. Smokescreen for the 1990s: a stop smoking programme for General Practitioners to use with Smokers. NSW Department of Health. 2nd ed., 1991.

155. Richmond RL, Mendelsohn CP. Physicians' views of programs incorporating stages of change to reduce smoking and excessive alcohol consumption. Am J Health Promotion 1998; 12(4):254–257.

156. Richmond RL, Kehoe L, de Almedia Neto AC. Three year continuous abstinence in a smoking cessation study using the nicotine transdermal patch. Heart 1997; 78(6):617–618.

157. Heatherton TF, Kozlowski LT, Frecker RC, Fagerstrom KO. The Fagerstrom test for nicotine dependence: a revision of the Fagerstrom Tolerance Questionnaire. Br J Addict 1991; 86:1119–1127.

158. NSW Department of Health. "Let's take a moment" quit smoking brief intervention–a guide for all health professionals, 2005.

159. Rollnick S, Butler CC, Stott N. Helping smokers make decisions: the enhancement of brief intervention for general medical practice. Patient Educ Counseling 1997; 31(3):191–203.

160. Fiore MC, Hatsukami DK, Baker TB. Effective tobacco dependence treatment. JAMA 2002; 288(14):1768–1771.

161. Richmond RL, Austin A, Webster IW. Three year evaluation of a program by general practitioners to help patients stop smoking. BMJ 1986; 292:803–806.

162. Richmond RL, Makinson RJ, Kehoe LA, Giugni AA, Webster IW. One year evaluation of three smoking cessation interventions administered by general practitioners. Addict Behav 1993; 18:187–199.

163. Kenford SL, Fiore MC, Jorenby DE, Smith SS, Wetter D, Baker TB. Predicting smoking cessation. Who will quit with and without the nicotine patch. J Am Med Assoc 1994; 21:589–594.

164. Hughes JR. Nicotine withdrawal, dependence and abuse. In: Widiger T, Frances A, Pincus H, et al., eds. DSM-IV Sourcebook. Vol. 1. Washington DC: American Psychiatric Association, 1994:19–116.

165. Guidelines for Smoking Cessation. New Zealand National Advisory Committee on Health and Disability, 1999.

166. Gourlay SG, Stead LF, Benowitz NL. Clonidine for smoking cessation. The Cochrane Database of Systematic Reviews, 2004, Issue 3.

167. Henningfield JE, Fant RV, Buchhlater AR, Stitzer ML. Pharmacotherapy for Nicotine dependence. CA Cancer J Clin 2005; 55:282–299.

168. Hurt RD, Dale LC, Fredrickson PA, et al. Nicotine patch therapy for smoking cessation combined with physician advice and nurse follow-up. One-year outcome and percentage of nicotine replacement. JAMA 1994; 21:95–600.

169. Raw M, McNeill A, West R. Smoking cessation guidelines for health professionals. A guide to effective smoking cessation interventions for the public health system. Thorax 1998; 53(suppl 5):S1–S38.

170. Benowitz N. Pharmacodynamics of nicotine: implications for rational treatment of nicotine addiction. Br J Addict 1991; 86:495–499.

171. Fiore MC, Smith SS, Jorenby DE, Baker TB. The effectiveness of the nicotine patch for smoking cessation: a meta-analysis. JAMA 1994; 27(124):1940–1947.

172. Fiore MC, Jorenby DE, Baker TB, Kenford SL. Tobacco dependence and the nicotine patch. Clinical guidelines for effective use. JAMA 1992; 268:2687–2694.

173. McNabb ME, Ebert RV, McCusker K. Plasma Nicotine levels produced by chewing nicotine gum. JAMA 1982; 248:865–868.

174. Palmer KJ, Buckley MM, Faulds D. Transdermal nicotine. A review of its pharmacodynamic and pharmacokinetic properties, and therapeutic efficacy as an aid to smoking cessation. Drugs 1992; 44:498–529.

175. Murray RP, Bailey WC, Daniels K, et al. Safety of nicotine polacrilex gum used by 3094 participants in the Lung Health Study. Chest 1996; 109:438–445.

176. Molander L, Lunnell E. Pharmacokinetic investigation of a nicotine sublingual tablet. Eur J Clin Pharmacol 2001; 56:813–819.

177. Wallstrom M, Nilsson F, Hirsch JM. A randomized double-blind, placebo controlled clinical evaluation of a nicotine sublingual tablet in smoking cessation. Addiction 2000; 95:1161–1171.

178. Shiffman S, Dresler CM, MD, Hajek P, Gilburt SJA, Targett DA, Strahs KR. Efficacy of a nicotine lozenge for smoking cessation. Arch Intern Med 2002; 162:1267–1276.

179. Schneider NG, Olmstead R, Nilsson F, Mody FV, Franzon M, Doan K. Efficacy of a nicotine inhaler in smoking cessation: a double-blind, placebo controlled trial. Addiction 1996; 91:1293–1306.

180. Hajek P, West R, Foulds J, Nilsson F, Burrows S, Meadow A. Randomised comparative trial of nicotine polacrilex, a transdermal patch, nasal spray and an inhaler. Arch Internal Med 1999; 159(17):2033–2038.

181. Hughes JR, Lesmes GR, Hatsukami DK, et al. Are higher doses of nicotine replacement more effective for smoking cessation? Nicotine Tobacco Res 1999; 1:169–174.

182. Kornitzer M, Bousten M, Dramaix M, Thijs J, Gustavsson G. Combined use of nicotine patch and gum in smoking cessation: placebo controlled trial. Preventive Med 1995; 24:41–47.

183. Puska P, Korhonen HJ, Vartianinen E, Urjanheimo EL, Gustavsson G, Westin A. Combined use of nicotine patch and gum compared with gum alone in smoking cessation: a clinical trial in North Karelia. Tobacco Control 1995; 4:231–235.

184. Benowitz N, Gourlay S. Cardiovascular toxicity of nicotine: implications for nicotine replacement therapy. J Am Coll Cardiol 1997; 56:460–464.

185. Joseph AM, Norman SM, Ferry LH, et al. The safety of transdermal nicotine as an aid to smoking cessation in patients with cardiac disease. New England J Med 1996; 335:1792–1798.

186. Mahmarian JJ, Moye LA, Nasser GA, et al. Nicotine patch therapy in smoking cessation reduces the extent of exercise-induced myocardial ischemia. J Am Coll Cardiol 1997; 30:125–130.

187. Working Group for the study of transdermal nicotine in patients with coronary artery disease. Nicotine replacement therapy for patients with coronary artery disease. Arch Int Med 1994; 154:989–995.

188. Meine TJ, Patel MR, Washam JB, Pappas PA, Jollis J. Safety and effectiveness of transdermal nicotine patch in smokers admitted with acute coronary syndromes. Am J Cardiol 2005; 95:976–978.

189. Benowitz NL. Nicotine replacement therapy during pregnancy. JAMA 1991; 266:3174–3177.

190. Dempsey DA, Benowitz NL. Risks and benefits of nicotine to aid smoking cessation in pregnancy. Drug Safety 2001; 24:277–322.

191. Richmond R, Zwar N. Therapeutic review of bupropion slow release. Drug Alcohol Rev 2003; 22:203–220.

192. Jorenby DE, Leischow SJ, Mides MA. A controlled trial of sustained-release bupropion, a nicotine patch, or both for smoking cessation. New England J Med 1999; 340(9):685–691.

193. Lancaster T, Stead LF. Individual behavioral counseling for smoking cessation. The Cochrane Database of Systematic Reviews, 2005, Issue 2.

194. Stead LF, Lancaster T. Group behaviour therapy programmes for smoking cessation. The Cochrane Database of Systematic Reviews, 2005, Issue 2.
195. Stead LF, Lancaster T, Perera R. Telephone counseling for smoking cessation. The Cochrane Database of Systematic Reviews, 2003, Issue 1.
196. Borland R, Segan CJ, Livingstone PM, Owen N. The effectiveness of callback counseling for smoking cessation: a randomised trial. Addiction 2001; 96:881–889.
197. White AR, Resch KL, Ernst E. A meta-analysis of acupuncture techniques for smoking cessation Tobacco Control 1999; 8:393–397.
198. Abbott NC, Stead LF, White AR, Barnes J. Hypnotherapy for smoking cessation (Cochrane Review). In: The Cochrane Library, Issue 4, 2002. Oxford: Update Software.
199. Gray N. Mixed feelings on snus. Lancet 2005; 366(9490):966–967.
200. Benowitz NL. Cigarette smoking and cardiovascular disease: pathophysiology and implications for treatment. Prog Cardiovasc Dis 2003; 46:91–111.
201. Epifano L, Di Vincenzo A, Fanelli C, et al. Effect of cigarette smoking and of a transdermal nicotine delivery system on glucoregulation in type 2 diabetes mellitus. Eur J Clin Pharmacol 1992; 43:257–263.
202. Assali AR, Beigei Y, Schreibman R, Shafer Z, Fainaru M. Weight gain and insulin resistance during nicotine replacement therapy. Clin Cardiol 1999; 22:357–360.
203. Howard G, Wagenknecht LE, Burke GL, et al. Cigarette smoking and progression of atherosclerosis: the atherosclerosis risk in communities (ARIC) Study. JAMA 1998; 279:119–124.

20 | Women and Coronary Heart Disease

Vera Bittner

Department of Medicine, Division of Cardiovascular Disease,
University of Alabama at Birmingham, Birmingham, Alabama, U.S.A.

KEY POINTS

- Coronary heart disease (CHD) is the leading cause of death among women and men.
- Many gender differences in anatomical and physiological aspects of CHD have been described, but mechanisms remain poorly understood.
- While most women will present with typical chest discomfort and accompanying symptoms, clinicians should be alert to atypical symptom constellations among women (and men), interpret symptoms in the context of the overall risk profile, and follow up with appropriate diagnostic testing.
- Diabetes disproportionately increases CHD risk among women compared to men, while other CHD risk factors seem to affect both sexes to a similar degree.
- When assessing CHD risk and making treatment decisions, both 10-year CHD risk and lifetime risk should be considered.
- The CVD Prevention Guidelines for Women provide an evidence-based framework for primary and secondary prevention of CHD.

EPIDEMIOLOGY OF CORONARY HEART DISEASE IN WOMEN

Coronary heart disease (CHD) is the leading cause of death among women in most industrialized countries and is becoming increasingly important in the developing world. In its 2005 report on the global burden of chronic diseases, the World Health Organization estimated that 3.6 million women will die from CHD in 2005; 8 out of 10 of these deaths will occur in low-and middle-income countries (1). CHD is also a major cause of disability among women worldwide accounting for 5.3% of disability-adjusted life-years lost in 2002 (2). Trends in CHD mortality rates in recent years differ by country: in Western industrialized countries rates have declined in both genders, while rates in Eastern Europe and the Russian Federation have increased (Fig. 1) (3).

CHD mortality is consistently lower among women than men whether assessed in regions with high or low CHD mortality rates (Fig. 2) (4). The ratio of male to female deaths due to CHD is greater than one throughout life, but this gender gap is most pronounced in the younger age groups (e.g., 3.5- to 4.5-fold excess of deaths among men in the 45 to 54 year age groups in the United States and the United Kingdom) (5). CHD mortality increases with advancing age in both genders. Although the more favorable outlook among women compared to men has been widely attributed to protective effects of endogenous estrogens, there is no evidence of a marked increase in CHD mortality rate among women at the time of menopause (6) and prospective studies of the impact of endogenous sex hormone levels on subsequent CHD have not been able to document a protective relationship (7). This lack of association does not disprove the hypothesis, but suggests that more sophisticated methods of investigation are needed (see below).

PATHOLOGY, PATHOPHYSIOLOGY, AND SYMPTOMS

In both genders, coronary atherosclerosis starts in early childhood, increases with age, and closely correlates with the number and severity of traditional risk factors (8). Autopsy studies show that girls and young women tend to have less extensive atherosclerotic involvement than age-matched boys and young men (9). Coronary calcification is less extensive among young women compared to age-matched men (10). It increases with age in both genders, but women lag behind men by 10 to 15 years (11). Angiographic studies consistently show lesser degrees of epicardial coronary artery disease among women than among similarly aged men even after stratification by

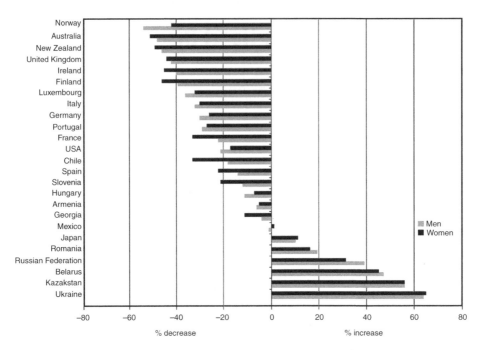

FIGURE 1   Change in coronary heart disease rates by country 1990–2000. *Source*: From Ref. 3.

symptoms (typical angina, atypical angina, nonanginal chest pain) (12) and in populations with-out CHD symptoms who undergo coronary angiography in preparation for valvular surgery (13).

Women have smaller coronary arteries than men even after correcting for body surface area (14,15). Coronary remodeling in response to increasing atherosclerotic plaque burden

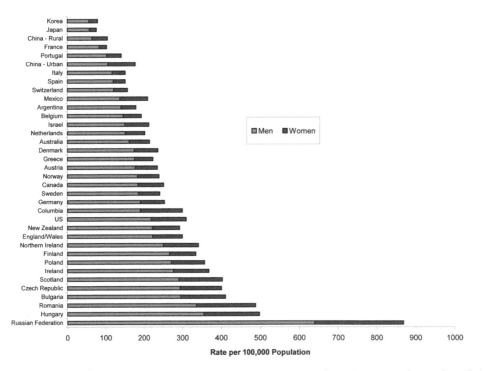

FIGURE 2   Death rates from coronary heart disease among women and men by country. *Source*: From Ref. 4.

appears to be similar in both genders (16). Whether plaque composition differs by gender is less clear. Advanced lesions slated for percutaneous intervention have similar ultrasound characteristics in women and men (17), but the overall proportion of hard plaques may be greater among men than women (18). In an autopsy study of women and men above 40 years of age who died more than one year after coronary artery bypass grafting, investigators found greater amounts of cellular fibrous tissue and lesser amounts of dense fibrous tissue in both native coronary arteries and saphenous vein grafts among women, while the amount of intracellular lipid, the degree of inflammatory infiltration, and the severity of obstruction were similar in both genders (19). Plaques among younger women have been reported to contain large amounts of lipid-containing foam cells with a relative lack of acellular scar tissue (20). Among victims of fatal myocardial infarction (MI), culprit lesions among women are more likely to manifest plaque erosion while culprit lesions among men are more likely to show frank plaque rupture (21). Among women who died suddenly, plaque erosion was more common among younger women and was strongly associated with smoking. Among older women, plaque rupture with superimposed thrombus and stable plaque with healed infarction were the predominant findings; plaque rupture was associated with high total cholesterol, and stable plaque with healed infarct was associated with glycosylated hemoglobin and hypertension (22). It is unknown whether changes in plaque that precipitate nonfatal acute coronary syndromes and MIs also differ by gender. Intravascular ultrasound or other imaging modalities used in the acute setting may provide such data in the future and may indicate prevention strategies.

MI incidence increases with age in both genders and, as is the case for CHD mortality, women have lower rates than men. Whether case fatality rate is higher among women than men remains controversial. Most of the seemingly adverse in-hospital outcomes in women are explained by their older age at presentation and their greater comorbidity burden (23,24). However, two analyses, one from the National Registry of Myocardial Infarction and a retrospective review of MI mortality in 15 Connecticut hospitals, suggest that there is a sex/age interaction with poorer outcomes among younger but not older women compared to their age-matched male counterparts (25,26). It is possible that the greater in-hospital mortality among women seen in some but not all studies may be counterbalanced by a greater prehospital mortality among men (27,28). Sudden death is indeed more common among men than women in all age groups, among those with known angina, those with prior MI, and among individuals without a history of CHD (29). In both genders, individuals with a history of CHD have a higher risk of sudden death than those without such a history. However, among women, over 60% of sudden deaths occur in individuals without a history of CHD; among men the proportion is lower at 44% (29). Sudden death as the first manifestation of CHD among women reinforces the importance of identifying these women earlier in the course of their disease and providing them with appropriate preventive care. Data from the Nurses' Health Study indeed suggest that identification of women at risk for sudden death should be feasible: although 69% of women in this cohort who suffered sudden death had no history of CHD, 94% of them had at least one major coronary risk factor and smoking, hypertension, and diabetes were all potent predictors of subsequent sudden death; obesity and family history of premature CHD had moderate predictive value (30). Although crude mortality rates among survivors of MI are often higher among women than men, long-term survival after MI appears to be better among women than men when analyses are adjusted for baseline differences between the two groups (31–33).

Although most patients with myocardial ischemia or evidence of MI will have angiographically demonstrable obstructive coronary lesions, there is a subset of patients who have either "nonobstructive" coronary disease or angiographically normal coronary arteries. In such patients, symptoms can be due to a demand/supply mismatch (e.g., decreased coronary perfusion due to hypotension), epicardial coronary spasm (Prinzmetal's angina), abnormal endothelial function in the conduit vessels, microvascular disease, or to a combination of these factors (34). Myocardial ischemia or infarction in the setting of normal coronary angiography or nonobstructive coronary disease appears to be more common in women than in men (35). Although normal coronary angiograms in general indicate a good prognosis, there appears to be a subset of women with abnormal responses to intracoronary acetylcholine who continue to suffer from recurrent episodes of chest pain for years and develop angiographic coronary disease long term (36).

Much has been written about the lack of specificity of typical ischemic symptoms among women and about the greater probability of atypical presentations (37–42). This literature is very difficult to interpret for many reasons. First, causes of chest discomfort are very heterogeneous ranging from noncardiac chest pain to cardiac chest pain not due to CHD, to symptoms of ischemia with or without demonstrable coronary obstruction. Second, we lack a universally accepted gold-standard for the diagnosis of myocardial ischemia and/or coronary artery disease and studies have thus correlated symptoms with a wide variety of diagnostic methods, some anatomical, some physiological, which differ greatly in sensitivity and specificity. Patients may thus be classified as having "noncardiac chest pain" by one diagnostic method and as having "ischemia" by another. Third, most studies suffer from considerable selection bias by virtue of the study setting (e.g., recruitment in the emergency room vs. in the hospital cardiology ward vs. in the cardiac catheterization laboratory). Furthermore, many studies are conducted in tertiary care referral centers which tend to attract patients with more complex clinical presentations. Fourth, disease prevalence is an important determinant of diagnostic test performance, making it even difficult to compare results across studies which use the same diagnostic test methodology. Fifth, women tend to get coronary disease at a more advanced age than men and it is often difficult to disentangle differences in symptom presentation due to gender from differences in symptom presentation due to advanced age and/or its associated comorbidities (e.g., diabetes) (43). Sixth, we lack a good understanding of physiological and psychological determinants of symptom perception and symptom attribution. Awareness of disease risk is one determinant of symptom attribution which is particularly relevant among women. Although serial surveys in the United States suggest that women have become more aware of being at risk for CHD, these same surveys point out that such knowledge is still not universal and is particularly lacking among minority women who tend to have poorer CHD outcomes (44). Seventh, results can differ greatly depending on how symptoms are assessed (e.g., check lists vs. spontaneous description of symptoms), when symptoms are assessed (e.g., before a diagnostic procedure or event vs. after a patient has been appraised of the procedure results or has been given a diagnostic label), and by whom symptoms are assessed (e.g., whether the clinician has a low or high degree of suspicion of disease). Despite all these study limitations, there appears to be a consensus that there are indeed gender differences in symptom presentation. While most women will present with typical chest discomfort and accompanying symptoms, clinicians should be alert to atypical symptom constellations among women (and men), interpret symptoms in the context of the overall risk profile, and follow up with appropriate diagnostic testing.

DIAGNOSIS

Selection of appropriate candidates for diagnostic workup is based on Bayesian principles in women and men. As Gibbons et al. summarized in their 2002 guidelines for exercise testing, Bayes theorem states that the probability of a patient (man or woman) of having the disease after a test is performed will be the product of the disease probability before the test and the probability that the test provided a true result (the latter is a function of the test result and the diagnostic characteristics of the test) (45). The application of these principles is more challenging in women than in men because disease prevalence among women is lower, thus increasing the probability of "false positive" test results (Table 1). Most asymptomatic women below the age of 70 without a history of CHD tend to fall into the "very low" risk category and most women aged 70 or over will be at "low risk" for CHD. Routine screening of such women is unlikely to be helpful. It is clear, however, that diagnostic testing should not be withheld solely on the basis of risk stratification by gender and age. Using Framingham equations or other risk prediction tools discussed in more detail below, we can distinguish women who are at low, intermediate, and high risk. While screening of asymptomatic women who are at low risk is not recommended, selective screening of higher risk asymptomatic women (e.g., women with diabetes or other CHD risk equivalents) may be reasonable, although convincing clinical trial data for such a strategy are lacking (46). "Not screening" should not be confused with "not treating." Such women should be closely monitored for the onset of symptoms. Symptoms of chest discomfort, anginal equivalents, and more subtle signs of CHD such as diminishing exercise capacity beyond that expected with advancing age should be actively sought during clinic visits. More importantly, modifiable risk factors should be identified and addressed through lifestyle modifications and pharmacologic therapy as recommended by current guidelines (47).

TABLE 1 Pretest Probability of Coronary Artery Disease by Age, Gender, and Symptoms[a]

Age (yr)	Typical/definite angina pectoris	Atypical/probable angina pectoris	Nonanginal chest pain	Asymptomatic
30–39				
Men	Intermediate	Intermediate	Low	Very low
Women	Intermediate	Very low	Very low	Very low
40–49				
Men	High	Intermediate	Intermediate	Low
Women	Intermediate	Low	Very low	Very low
50–59				
Men	High	Intermediate	Intermediate	Low
Women	Intermediate	Intermediate	Low	Very low
60–69				
Men	High	Intermediate	Intermediate	Low
Women	High	Intermediate	Intermediate	Low

[a]No data exist for patients below 30 or above 69 years, but it can be assumed that prevalence of CAD increases with age. In a few cases, patients with ages at the extremes of the decades listed may have probabilities slightly outside the high or low range. High indicates above 90%; intermediate, 10% to 90%, low, below 10%; and very low, below 5%.
Abbreviation: CAD, coronary artery disease.
Source: From Ref. 45.

Strategies for the evaluation of symptomatic women are outlined in detail in the recent Consensus Statement on the role of noninvasive testing in the clinical evaluation of women with suspected coronary artery disease (46). Among women who are symptomatic, disease probability is very low if they are otherwise at very low or low risk. In such women, the probability of a false positive test is higher, and routine screening is thus not generally recommended (46). Clinical judgment is critical, however, and the value of reassurance by a negative test with its high negative predictive value should not be underestimated. Among symptomatic intermediate and higher risk women, noninvasive testing has two purposes: diagnosis and prognostication. For diagnosis, provocative testing is most helpful among women at intermediate risk. Testing for prognostication is useful in both intermediate and high-risk women. Selection of the test modality should be based on patient and test characteristics. Among women who are able to exercise and have a normal baseline electrocardiogram (ECG), graded exercise testing is recommended as the initial test modality (45,46). The Duke Activity Status Index questionnaire can be very helpful to the clinician when trying to determine whether a given woman will be able to exercise to a sufficient degree to provoke myocardial ischemia (48). False positive ECG responses with graded exercise testing are more common in women than men, suggesting that test interpretation should not be solely limited to the presence or absence of ST segment depression. Interpretation of exercise test data can be improved by taking into account functional capacity, heart rate recovery, and/or integrative test scores such as the Duke Treadmill Score, which all provide valuable prognostic information (46).

Noninvasive imaging (echocardiography or gated radionuclide perfusion imaging) in conjunction with exercise or pharmacologic stress has higher sensitivity and specificity for the detection of ischemia than treadmill exercise testing alone, provides additional information about left ventricular size and function, and provides a wealth of prognostic data. A detailed discussion of pros and cons of either imaging modality is beyond the scope of this chapter. For practical purposes, choice of imaging modality should be determined by the level of expertise available in a given clinical setting. Selection of women for stress cardiac imaging and interpretation of results as proposed by the 2005 Consensus Statement are outlined in the algorithm in Figure 3 (46). The role of newer imaging modalities such as positron-emission tomography, cardiovascular magnetic resonance imaging, or X-ray computed tomography is the subject of active investigation.

RISK FACTORS LEADING TO THE DEVELOPMENT OF CHD

Risk factors can be broadly categorized into nonmodifiable and modifiable risk factors, lifestyle risk factors, and emerging risk factors as suggested by the Third Adult Treatment Panel of the National Cholesterol Education Program (Table 2) (49). The prevalence of traditional risk factors among American women, such as obesity, physical inactivity, and diabetes mellitus is

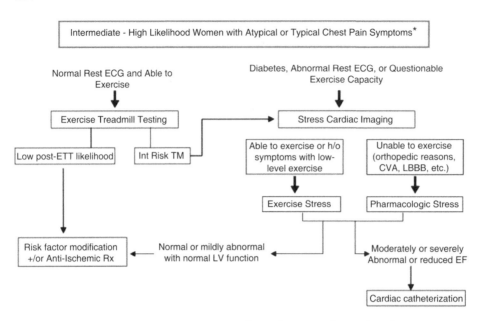

FIGURE 3   Algorithm for the diagnosis of coronary disease in women. *Source*: From Ref. 46.

high, and for some, prevalence has been increasing over the last decade (Fig. 4) (50). Prevalence rates of hypertension, obesity, physical inactivity, and diabetes are higher among African-American women than among whites and are higher among women with lower levels of education and lower socioeconomic status (50,51).

Smoking

Each year at least 4.9 million people die worldwide as a result of tobacco use, many of them women (1). In the United States, smoking prevalence among women varies by ethnicity: Native American women and Alaskan natives are the most likely to smoke (37%), followed by white women (21%), African-American women (19%), Hispanic women (13%), and Asian women (6.9%) (50). Smoking has increased among middle and high school children as well as college students in recent years (50,52). The percentage of female high school students who smoked in 2003 was 22% (50). There are strong gradients by socioeconomic status, with higher smoking rates among the less affluent and less educated (50,51). The prevalence of smoking among women is even higher in parts of Europe (53). Although there has been a decrease in recent years, exposure to second hand smoke in the United States remains high (approximately 60% for U.S. adults and 64% for U.S. children) (50).

The adverse impact of smoking on cardiovascular morbidity and mortality is well documented in all age, gender, and ethnic subgroups studied (54). Smoking has a particularly adverse impact on the risk of CHD among younger women with a very steep dose-response curve: in a case-control study of women below the age of 44 (mean age 41 years), women smoking as few as one to five cigarettes per day had 2.47-fold greater odds of a MI (95% CI 1.12–5.45), while women smoking 40 or more cigarettes had 75-fold greater odds (95% CI 33–169) (55). The population-attributable risk for smoking and MI among middle-aged and younger women was estimated to be 73% (55). In the Nurses' Health Study, the adjusted relative risk of incident CHD for a former smoker relative to a lifelong nonsmoker was 1.55 compared with 3.12 for a woman smoking 1 to 14 cigarettes, and 5.48 for a woman smoking 15 or more cigarettes per day (56).

The benefits of smoking cessation are also well established. A meta-analysis of cohort studies that measured the effect of smoking cessation on mortality after having a MI, for example, reported a 46% lower risk of death among quitters compared to continued smokers without heterogeneity by age, gender, or country in which the study was conducted (57). In the Nurses' Health Study, 13% of the decline in CHD incidence between 1980 and 1994 was attributed to concurrent reductions in smoking (58).

TABLE 2   Classification of Selected Risk Factors and Risk Markers

Nonmodifiable	Modifiable risk factor	Emerging risk factor	Subclinical disease
Age	Major risk factors	Nonlipid	Ankle brachial index
Sex	Total cholesterol	Inflammatory markers	Left ventricular hypertrophy
Family history	LDL cholesterol/	Thrombogenic/hemostatic	Tests for myocardial ischemia
of premature CHD	non-HDL cholesterol	factors	
	Low HDL Cholesterol	Impaired fasting glusoce	Carotid intimal medial
			thickening
	Smoking	Homocysteine	Coronary calcium
	Hypertension		
	Diabetes		
	Lifestyle risk factors	Lipid	
	Sedentary lifestyle	Triglycerides	
	Obesity	Remnants	
	Atherogenic	Lipoprotein (a)	
		Small LDL particles	
		HDL subspecies	
		Apolipoproteins	
	Psychosocial risk factors		
	Low income		
	Poor education		
	Depression/anger		
	Enviromental factors		

Abbreviations: LDL, low-density lipoprotein; HDL, high-density lipoprotein; CHD, coronary heart disease.
Source: From Ref. 49.

Passive smoking has similar adverse effects (59). A 1994 analysis estimated that over 12,000 women who never smoked died in 1985 due to CHD as a consequence of spousal tobacco exposure and an additional 13,000 due to background environmental tobacco smoke (60). The true impact of passive smoking is far greater, since nonfatal events are believed to outnumber fatal events by a factor of three (59). In a case-control study from Argentina, 18% of MI cases among women who had never smoked were attributed to passive smoking at home (61).

Evidence-based guidelines for treating tobacco dependence were published by the American College for Chest Physicians in 2002 (62). The guideline promotes a systematic approach to ascertainment of smoking status and treatment of tobacco dependence referred to as the "5 As" (Table 3). A motivational intervention labeled as the "5 Rs" is suggested for smokers who do not wish to quit (Table 3). Many aspects of tobacco dependence differ by gender and should be taken into consideration during smoking cessation counseling. Women appear to be more sensitive to the effects of nicotine, may have less physical dependence on nicotine, but report greater withdrawal symptoms, and may smoke for different reasons than men. Alleviation of stress, moderation of negative affect, and weight control may be particularly important reasons for smoking among women, suggesting that smoking interventions beyond

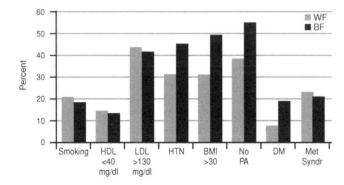

FIGURE 4   Risk factor prevalence among U.S. women. *Abbreviations*: BF, black female; BMI, body mass index; DM, diabetes mellitus; HDL, high density lipoprotein; HTN, hypertension; LDL, low density lipoprotein; Met Syndr, metabolic syndrome; PA, physical activity; WF, white female. *Source*: From Ref. 50.

TABLE 3 Treating Tobacco Use and Dependence—The
"5 A's" and "5 R's"

Ask about tobacco use and document status for every patient visit
Advise the patient to quit in a clear personalized manner
Assess willingness to make an attempt to quit
Assist patient to make an attempt to quit
Arrange for follow-up
Relevance: Identify factors that are personally relevant to the smoking behavior
Risks: Emphasize risks pertinent to the smoker
Rewards: Identify potential benefits of smoking cessation
Roadblocks: Identify real and perceived barriers to smoking cessation
Repetition: Repeat the motivational intervention at each clinic visit

Source: From Ref. 62.

treatment of physical nicotine dependence are required to improve cessation rates (63). Future research on gender-specific intervention strategies is clearly needed.

Physical Activity and Physical Fitness

Physical inactivity is more prevalent among U.S. women than men, varies by ethnic group (white women: 38%, African-American women: 55%, Hispanic women: 57%, Asian women: 43%, native American women: 55%, and native Hawaiian/Pacific islander women: 27%), and becomes increasingly prevalent with age (50). Over 70% U.S. women do not meet the physical activity goal of walking 30 minutes on most days of the week (64). As with other risk factors, there are steep gradients by socioeconomic status, with greater prevalence of inactivity among the less educated and the less affluent. Particularly worrisome is the increasing rate of inactivity among children and adolescents (50).

Physical inactivity and lack of physical fitness strongly relate to cardiovascular events and mortality in both genders (65). Worldwide estimates suggest that 1.9 million people die annually as a result of physical inactivity (1). Optimal frequency, duration, and intensity of exercise remain controversial because the definition of "optimal" may vary by the endpoint studied, and because efficacy and feasibility have to be balanced to achieve the best possible outcomes. Two reports from the Nurses' Health Study showed that walking for as little as one hour per week at a moderate pace was associated with up to 50% reduction in ischemic stroke and CHD in women (66,67). Bouts of activity as brief as 10 minutes may improve cardiovascular risk factors among sedentary women (68), but cardiovascular endpoints with such an exercise regimen have not been reported in women. Although lifelong physical activity should be strongly encouraged, even increases in physical activity level late-in-life result in lower cardiovascular mortality among women (69). Physical activity counseling is thus important in all age and gender subgroups in the clinical setting. Even brief counseling activities (three to four minutes) as used in the multicenter Activity Counseling Trial helped patients to become more active (70). The "Call To Action" recently published by Manson et al. provides a blueprint for such counseling activities (71).

For healthy individuals, the 2005 U.S. Dietary Guidelines recommend 30 minutes of moderate physical activity beyond usual activity at home or at work on most days of the week for the prevention of chronic illness, but acknowledge that greater health benefits can be achieved with more vigorous activity or activity of longer duration (72). For weight management, at least 60 minutes of moderate to vigorous activity is recommended and the guidelines suggest that 60 to 90 minutes of such activity on most days of the week may be necessary for maintaining the achieved weight loss (72). Individuals are encouraged to incorporate cardiovascular conditioning, flexibility exercises, and strength training into their routine (72).

For women with established CHD, cardiac rehabilitation is recommended (47). A recent review summarizes available gender-specific data for women in cardiac rehabilitation including referral and enrollment patterns, baseline characteristics, and sex-specific outcomes reported within each core component of care, and concludes that women are less likely to be referred to cardiac rehabilitation, but seem to benefit as much as their male counterparts with improvements in clinical, psychosocial, and behavioral domains (73). Among clinical trials included in the 2004 Cochrane review of morbidity and mortality, women only made up 4.4% of the patients enrolled in the exercise intervention trials and 11% of the patients enrolled in comprehensive cardiac rehabilitation studies; benefits of cardiac rehabilitation on hard CHD endpoints and survival among women could thus not be estimated (74). A recent community-based observational study, however, documented improved six-year survival and decreased recurrence of myocardial infarction in a large cohort of MI survivors (42% women) in Olmsted County, Minnesota, even after adjustment for factors known to affect participation in cardiac rehabilitation and factors known to influence prognosis after MI (75). Among women, the attributable risk of death for nonparticipation in cardiac rehabilitation was estimated at 39% (95% CI 33–45%) (75). As documented in prior studies, enrollment rates for women were lower than among men: women were less than half as likely to enroll in cardiac rehabilitation as their male counterparts (multivariate RR 0.45, 95% CI 0.34–0.60) (75). Among those enrolled, risk factor and comorbidity burden tends to be high and drop-out rates are substantial, especially among women who are obese or depressed (76). Studies to determine whether gender-specific interventions can improve enrollment and adherence rates are ongoing.

Obesity, Metabolic Syndrome, and Diabetes

Global estimates for 2005 suggest that over one billion people are overweight [body mass index (BMI) ≥ 25], including 805 million women, and that over 300 million people are obese (BMI ≥ 30) (1). Overweight and obesity are increasing in prevalence worldwide, among children and adults of both sexes and all ethnic groups (1). Worldwide 2.6 million people die annually as a result of being overweight or obese (1). In the United States, prevalence of overweight and obesity among girls, female adolescents, and adult women vary significantly by ethnic background, being highest among African-Americans and lowest among the U.S. whites (Table 4) (50).

Obesity relates to CHD risk directly and indirectly. Adipose tissue is an active endocrine organ and secretes a multitude of mediators with known adverse effects on insulin sensitivity, endothelial function, blood pressure, and atherosclerosis such as tumor necrosis factor alpha, interleukin 6, plasminogen activator inhibitor, monocyte chemoattractant protein 1, and angiotensinogen, to name a few (77). Obesity promotes development of diabetes, dyslipidemia, and hypertension which then, in turn, also increase cardiovascular risk. In Framingham, percentage of desirable weight based on the Metropolitan Relative Weight nomogram, predicted 26-year incidence of coronary disease, stroke, heart failure, and coronary and cardiovascular death among women and demonstrated that weight gain after the young adult years conveyed an increased risk of cardiovascular death independent of baseline weight and change in risk factors due to weight gain (78). In the Nurses' Health Study, BMI was related to coronary events after eight years of follow-up and total mortality after 16 years of follow-up (79,80). An increase of CHD risk in middle-aged women is even seen within the normal weight range (81). Fat distribution may be an even better predictor of outcome than relative weight or BMI. In the

TABLE 4 Prevalence of Overweight and Obesity Among U.S. Women and Children

Ethnic group	Overweight and obesity (%)	Obese (%)
Adults		
Whites	57.2	30.7
African-Americans	77.2	49
Mexican Americans	71.7	38.4
Adolescents (age 12–19)		
Whites	12.7	
African-Americans	23.6	N/A
Mexican Americans	19.9	
Girls (age 6–11)		
Whites	13.1	
African-Americans	22.8	N/A
Mexican Americans	17.1	

Note: Overweight in adults is body mass index (BMI) 25 and higher. Obesity in adults is BMI 30.0 or higher. Overweight in children is BMI 95th percentile or higher of the Centers for Disease Control and Prevention 2000 growth chart.
Source: From Ref. 50.

Nurses' Health Study, waist-hip ratio and waist circumference were independently associated with incident CHD in the overall cohort as well as in a subgroup analysis of women of normal weight (82). In the Iowa Women's Health Study, the waist-hip ratio was an independent predictor of coronary death and total mortality as well as diabetes and hypertension (83). In this cohort, the risk of incident diabetes was particularly high among women who had both BMI and waist-hip ratios in the top quintile (83). Some authors have suggested that differences in abdominal fat distribution are a major explanation for disparity in the incidence of MI between the sexes (84). Interestingly, BMI and abdominal girth were significant predictors of total mortality and CHD death in white, but not in African-American women in the Charleston Heart Study (85). The lower predictive value among African-Americans may be related to ethnic differences in the distribution of superficial and visceral fat (86). The impact of intentional weight loss on mortality may vary by the presence or absence of obesity-related health conditions, with greater reductions in mortality among individuals who have such obesity-related health conditions (87).

Although it is clear that risk factors such as abdominal obesity, hypertension, dyslipidemia, and abnormalities in glucose metabolism cluster together, there is controversy whether this clustering of risk factors constitutes a "syndrome" and, if it is a syndrome, how to define it (88,89). In the Third National Health and Nutrition Survey (1988–1994), the prevalence of metabolic syndrome [defined as three or more of the Adult Treatment Panel (ATP) III criteria (49)] was 22.8% among white women, 25.7% among African-American women, 35.6% among Mexican American women, and 19.9% among other ethnic groups (90). In the National Health and Nutrition Examination Survey (NHANES) II follow-up study ($n = 6255$, 54% women, follow-up 13.3 years), age- and gender-adjusted analyses showed that metabolic syndrome in the absence of diabetes doubled CHD mortality; gender-specific analyses were not reported (91). In the European DECODE study, the prevalence of metabolic syndrome, using the World Health Organization (WHO) definition, was 14.2% among women and was associated with a 38% higher risk of all-cause mortality and a 2.78-fold increased risk of cardiovascular mortality at a median follow-up of 8.8 years; risks among women were similar to those among men in the study (92). An analysis from the Diabetes Prevention Program, which included 3234 participants (67% women) with impaired glucose tolerance and a fasting blood sugar between 95 and 125 mg/dL suggests that intensive lifestyle modification can reduce the prevalence of metabolic syndrome among those with metabolic syndrome at baseline and reduce the incidence of metabolic syndrome in those who do not meet the criteria initially (93).

Diabetes' incidence and prevalence have markedly increased in recent years in developing and developed nations. In 2003, world-wide prevalence of diabetes was estimated at 5.1% with substantial regional differences: WHO African region: 2.4%, Eastern Mediterranean region and the Middle East: 7%, Europe: 7.8%, and South and Central American region: 5.6% (3). In the United States, 4.7% of the U.S. white women, 12.6% of the African-American women, and 11.3% of the Mexican American had physician diagnosed diabetes in 2002, and 2.7%, 6.1%, and 1.8%, respectively, had undiagnosed diabetes (50). The overall annual incidence among women was estimated at 1.3 million and annual mortality was estimated at 73,200 deaths (50).

Diabetes closes the gender gap in cardiovascular disease as the relative risks of coronary and cardiovascular disease associated with diabetes among women are higher than men. In a meta-analysis, Kanaya et al. concluded that the gender differences in the odds ratios for fatal and nonfatal CHD due to diabetes were abolished after adjusting for classic CHD risk factors (94), but this is not seen in all studies. In a Finnish population-based study with 13 years of follow-up, for example, the hazard ratios for CHD adjusted for age and place of residence were 2.9 (95% CI 2.2–3.9) for men and 14.4 (95% CI 8.4–24.5) for women; after adjustment for cardiovascular risk factors, the hazard ratio remained more than three-fold higher among women than men [9.5 (95% CI 5.5–16.9) vs. 2.8 (95% CI 2.0–3.7)] (95).

Among women, diabetes is a more potent prognostic factor for future CHD than is established CHD. In the Framingham Study, the hazard ratio for CHD death over 20 years was 3.8 (95% CI 1.1–3.4) among women with diabetes and 1.9 (95% CI 1.1–3.4) for women with established CHD; among men, the hazard ratio for death was higher for those with established CHD [4.2 (95% CI 3.2–5.6)] than for those with diabetes [2.1 (95% CI 1.3–3.3)] (96). It could be argued that this gender gap is due to the inclusion of angina pectoris in the "established CHD" definition, which is known to have a better outcome among women than men, at least in part due to lower prevalence of angiographic coronary disease among women (97,98). An analysis from the NHANES Epidemiology Follow-up Study, however, suggests otherwise at least for women with longstanding diabetes (99). Among women, the risk of CHD death associated with diabetes exceeded that of prior MI [multivariate hazard ratio 4.9 (95% CI 3.2–7.5) for long-term diabetes, 2.6 (95% CI 1.6–4.2) for history of MI; women with neither diabetes nor history of MI were the referent group] while the hazard ratio for diabetes of shorter duration [1.6 (95% CI 1.0–2.6)] was similar to that of prior MI (99). Treating women with long-term diabetes merely as "having a CHD risk equivalent" may thus underestimate their true risk of future CHD mortality.

Clinical trials of lifestyle interventions, pharmacologic hypoglycemic therapy, blood pressure control, and treatment of dyslipidemia suggest that women and men respond equally to vigorous risk modifications, at least in those trials that provide gender-specific estimates (100). A detailed discussion of diabetes therapy is beyond the scope of this chapter and readers are referred to the guidelines of the American Diabetes Association (101).

Hypertension

Hypertension is defined as systolic blood pressure of 140 mmHg and above and/or diastolic blood pressure of 90 mmHg and above (102). In Europe, the prevalence of hypertension among 35- to 64-year-old women varies between 30.6% in Italy and 50.3% in Germany; in Canada, 23.8% of women in this age range are hypertensive (103). In the United States, 31% of white women, 45.4% of African-American women, and 28.7% of Mexican American women have hypertension (50). Many other women have pre-hypertension (systolic blood pressure between 120 and 139 or diastolic blood pressure between 80 and 89): 23.1% of white women, 24.5% of African-American women, and 20.3% of Mexican American women (104). Prevalence of hypertension among women increases steeply with age. Among younger adults, hypertension is more prevalent among men than women, but in older age groups, hypertension is more common among women than men (50). Among women who are not hypertensive at the age of 55, the lifetime risk of developing hypertension is 86%, for those at age of 65, the probability is still 83% (105). Many women with hypertension have coexisting risk factors or target organ damage (106).

Systolic and diastolic blood pressure are strong independent predictors of future cardiovascular morbidity (stroke, CHD, left ventricular hypertrophy, heart failure, peripheral vascular disease, renal failure) and mortality in both sexes (107). Measurement of pulse pressure (systolic blood pressure minus diastolic blood pressure) and ambulatory recordings may provide additional prognostic information (108–110). In the United States, almost 50,000 deaths among women were due to hypertension in 2002 (50). Worldwide, 7.1 million people die annually as a result of hypertension, many of them women (1).

Despite greater awareness about hypertension and higher treatment rates among U.S. women than men, data from the National Health and Examination Survey 1999 to 2000 indicate that women are less likely to achieve blood pressure treatment goals than men (111). Among the 98,705 postmenopausal women examined at baseline in the Women's Health Initiative study, 37.8% were hypertensive, 64.3% of hypertensive women were on drug therapy, but only 36.1% had their blood pressure controlled (112). There was a striking gradient by age with blood pressure control rates from 41.3% among the 50- to 59-year-old subgroup to 29.3% in the 70 to 79-year-old subgroup. Interestingly, blood pressure control is better among African-Americans (40.5%) than among whites (35.9%), Hispanics (30.2%), or Asians (27.4%) (112).

Such undertreatment, especially among older individuals, may relate to past reports of a J- or U-shaped relationship between systolic blood pressure and mortality in older individuals with higher mortality among women and men at both blood pressure extremes. Closer analysis of these relationships reveals, however, that the apparent increase in mortality at the lower end of the blood pressure range is attributable to preexisting cardiovascular disease rather than to lower blood pressure per se (113). Clinical trials amply document reductions in cardiovascular and coronary morbidity and mortality in both genders; older women may benefit to a greater degree than older men (114–116). Choice of antihypertensive agent may be less critical than degree of blood pressure lowering (117). For detailed information on treatment options, the reader is referred to current treatment guidelines for hypertension (102,118).

Dyslipidemia

Over half the women in the U.S. population have total cholesterol levels above 200 mg/dL, over 40% have low density lipoprotein cholesterol (LDL-C) levels above 130 mg/dL, and 15% have high density lipoprotein cholesterol (HDL-C) levels below 40 mg/dL (50). Prevalence rates of dyslipidemia are lower among African-American women than among white women (50). Dyslipidemia is increasing in prevalence globally as lifestyles become more westernized, and as obesity and diabetes are increasing worldwide. Estimates by the World Health Organization suggest that 4.4 million people die annually as a result of elevated total cholesterol levels (1).

The impact of dyslipidemia in women has recently been reviewed in detail and will only be briefly summarized here (119). Levels of LDL cholesterol and non-HDL cholesterol are lower in young and middle-aged women than in age-matched men, but the reverse is true after menopause, even though LDL particle number remains lower in women than men throughout life (120–122). Lipoprotein(a) [Lp(a)] increases with age among women, but not men (123). Beginning at puberty, girls have higher HDL-C levels than boys and this gender difference in HDL-C is maintained throughout the lifespan, including among individuals with CHD (120,124–127). Although a HDL-C of 60 mg/dL or higher is considered protective for CHD (49), about one in five women with documented CHD enrolled in the Heart and Estrogen/progestin Replacement Study (HERS) had HDL-C above this threshold without a greater prevalence of other lipid and nonlipid risk factors that could have explained the development of CHD (128). In premenopausal women, lipoprotein concentrations vary throughout the menstrual cycle, with substantial heterogeneity in the degree of variation among individuals and studies (129). Effects of oral contraceptives on lipid and lipoprotein levels also vary widely between preparations and by phase of therapy (130–132). Phase of menstrual cycle should thus be considered when evaluating a premenopausal woman for dyslipidemia and when following serial lipid levels during treatment. Oral contraceptives should be considered a potential cause of secondary dyslipidemia. Serial empiric trials of different preparations may be necessary to find a formulation that is well tolerated metabolically.

Lowering of LDL-C and increasing of HDL-C with oral hormone therapy in postmenopausal women has not translated into lower event rates in the primary or secondary prevention setting (133–137). Use of hormone therapy is thus no longer recommended for cardiovascular disease prevention (47). Oral hormone therapy, especially unopposed estrogen therapy, can significantly increase triglyceride levels and should not be used in women with hypertriglyceridemia for fear of precipitating pancreatitis. Use of transcutaneous therapy is preferable among such women who require hormone therapy for noncardiovascular indications (49). Women with metabolic syndrome and diabetes tend to manifest so-called "atherogenic dyslipidemia" characterized by low HDL-C, dense LDL-particles, and elevated triglycerides, often in the absence of significant LDL-C elevations. It is important to remember that non-HDL-C is a secondary treatment target in these women and that titration of lipid-lowering agents should not be foregone just because the LDL-C is technically "at goal" (49).

Elevations in total and LDL-C and lower levels of HDL-C are strongly associated with higher CHD rates in both genders while triglyceride elevations appear to be stronger predictors of CHD among women than men (138,139). Non-HDL-C also appears to be a stronger predictor in women than in men (140). It is important to remember that risk attributable to hypercholesterolemia is higher among older than younger women even though relative risk decreases with age (138). Age may also modify the relationship between small dense LDL particles and CHD with a stronger relationship among younger than among older women (141,142). Elevated Lp(a) levels strongly predict incident myocardial infarction (MI) and recurrent events among women with CHD (143,144). Although a post hoc subgroup analysis from the HERS study suggested potential benefit of hormone therapy among women with high Lp(a) levels, such therapy is not recommended in the absence of prospective randomized trials confirming benefit (47,144).

Lifestyle modification should be recommended to all women with dyslipidemia even in the absence of randomized clinical trials documenting direct effects on atherosclerosis, cardiovascular endpoints, or mortality (47,49). Women and men with CHD (acute or chronic), diabetes, or otherwise at increased cardiovascular risk seem to benefit equally from intensive lipid lowering with statins (145–149). A report prepared for the Agency for Healthcare Research and Quality in 2003 concluded that there was insufficient evidence to determine whether lipid-lowering therapy among lower risk women affected cardiovascular endpoints (150). A meta-analysis published subsequently in 2004 concluded that lipid-lowering therapy among women without established cardiovascular disease reduced CHD events by 23%, but did not affect mortality endpoints (149). Detailed recommendations for treatment of dyslipidemia are available in the ATP III report and the cardiovascular disease prevention guidelines for women summarized later in this chapter (Table 5) (47,49). Undertreatment of dyslipidemic women remains a significant concern, although awareness, and treatment and control rates have improved in recent years (119).

Psychosocial Risk Factors

Personality traits and environmental stressors contribute to the development of CHD and subsequent morbidity and mortality in women, but the mechanisms are not well understood and there is considerable heterogeneity in study results. Among the personality traits, hostility appears to have the strongest association with subsequent CHD events, even after adjustment for standard CHD risk factors (151). Suarez et al. suggested that adverse changes in the lipid profile could be in the causal pathway (152). The role of anxiety is less clear. In the Women's Ischemia Syndrome Evaluation (WISE) Study, anxiety was associated with a lower probability of angiographically significant coronary disease among women referred for diagnostic angiography (153). Others have reported an increase in carotid atherosclerosis among women with sustained anxiety who were followed over years (154). Socioeconomic factors not only correlate with risk factor prevalence but are also powerful predictors of prognosis. In the WISE study, income was a powerful independent predictor of five year cardiovascular death or nonfatal MI even after adjustment for age, ethnicity, CHD risk factors, and severity of angiographic coronary disease (155). Low job control has been shown to have an adverse impact of CHD in women (156). Marital stress and being a caregiver for a disabled spouse also adversely affect cardiovascular outcomes (157,158). Further research is needed to better understand the interplay between personality traits, environment, health behaviors, and cardiovascular outcomes.

Depression is common, especially among older adults and strongly relates to cardiovascular events and mortality in both genders. In the NHANES I Study, for example, 17.5% of the 5007 women and 9.7% of the 2886 men were depressed (159). Depressed men and women had a 1.7-fold increased risk of nonfatal CHD after adjustment for other CHD risk factors. Among men but not women, there was also a statistically significant increased risk of CHD mortality and total mortality (159). In the Study of Osteoporotic Fractures, a cohort of 7518 women aged 67 years or older, seven year mortality was strongly related to the number of depressive symptoms at study entry (no depression: 7%, 3–5 symptoms: 24%, ≥ 6 symptoms: 24%; $p < 0.001$) (160). In another population-based study of older individuals, the Cardiovascular Health Study, depression was an independent risk factor for mortality even after adjustment for sociodemographic factors, prevalent clinical disease, subclinical disease indicators, and biological and behavioral risk factors (161). Increase in depressive symptoms over time was highly prognostic in the Systolic Hypertension in the Elderly Program, suggesting that clinicians should be alert to such changes when following patients over time (162). Whether the adverse impact of depression is mediated predominantly via adverse physiological changes (e.g., high stress hormone levels, enhanced platelet reactivity) or predominantly via adverse behavioral changes (e.g., poor adherence to therapy, adverse lifestyle) remains unclear, but is the subject of active investigation (163). Trials of behavioral interventions in women after MI have been disappointing (164,165). Although pharmacologic treatment of depression with sertraline in the post MI setting appears to be safe, CHD endpoint data for such a treatment approach are lacking (166). Since women may be more susceptible to QT prolongation and torsades de pointes ventricular tachycardia, caution is advised in the use of older antidepressants known to prolong the QT interval (167).

Sex Hormones, Menopause, and CHD

As reviewed above, CHD in premenopausal women in the absence of diabetes and smoking is unusual, even in the presence of dyslipidemia, hypertension, or other risk factors. This low incidence of CHD has been attributed to the protective effects of endogenous estrogens. Presence of estrogen receptors in coronary arteries correlates with absence of coronary atherosclerosis in premenopausal women (168). Variants of the estrogen receptor have been linked to increased risk of MI (169,170). Polymorphisms in the estrogen receptor alpha may also partially account for risk of restenosis after coronary stenting (171). Although there is some heterogeneity in study results, many investigators have demonstrated favorable effects of estrogens on

TABLE 5   Clinical Recommendations for Women with CVD

Lifestyle interventions

Cigarette smoking

    Consistently encourage women not to smoke and to avoid environmental tobacco. (Class I, Level B)$_{GI=1}$

Physical activity

    Consistently encourage women to accumulate a minimum of 30 min of moderate-intensity physical activity (e.g., brisk walking) on most, and preferably all, days of the week. (Class I, Level B)$_{GI=1}$

Cardiac rehabilitation

    Women with a recent acute coronary syndrome or coronary intervention, new onset or chronic angina should participate in a comprehensive risk-reduction regimen such as cardiac rehabilitation or a physician-guided home- or community-based program. (Class I, Level B)$_{GI=2}$

Heart-healthy diet

    Consistently encourage an overall healthy eating pattern that includes intake of a variety of fruits, vegetables, grains, low-fat or nonfat dairy products, fish, legumes, and sources of protein low in saturated fat (e.g., poultry, lean meats, plant sources). Limit saturated fat intake to <10% of calories, limit cholesterol intake to <300 mg/dL, and limit intake of *trans* fatty acids. (Class I, Level B)$_{GI=1}$

Weight maintenance/reduction

    Consistently encourage weight maintenance/reduction through an appropriate balance of physical activity, caloric intake, and formal behavioral programs when indicated to maintain/achieve a BMI between 18.5 and 24.9 kg/m^2 and a waist circumference <35 in. (Class I, Level B)$_{GI=1}$

Psychosocial factors

    Women with CVD should be evaluated for depression and refer/treat when indicated. (Class IIa, Level B)$_{GI=2}$

Omega 3 fatty acids

    As an adjunct to diet, omega 3 fatty-acid supplementation may be considered in high-risk[a] women. (Class IIb, Level B)$_{GI=2}$

Folic acid

    As an adjunct to diet, folic acid supplementation may be considered in high-risk[a] women (except after revascularization procedure) if a higher-than-normal level of homocysteine has been detected. (Class IIb, Level B)$_{GI=2}$

Major risk factor interventions

Blood pressure

    Lifestyle

        Encourage an optimal blood pressure of <120/80 mmHg through lifestyle approaches. (Class I, Level B)$_{GI=1}$

    Drugs

        Pharmacotherapy is indicated when blood pressure is ≥140/90 mmHg or an even lower blood pressure in the setting of blood pressure-related target-organ damage or diabetes. Thiazide diuretics should be part of the drug regimen for most patients unless contraindicated. (Class I, Level A)$_{GI=1}$

Lipid, lipoproteins

    Optimal levels of lipids and lipoproteins in women are LDL-C <100 mg/dL, HDL-C >50 mg/dL, triglycerides <150 mg/dL, and non–HDL-C (total cholesterol minus HDL cholesterol) <130 mg/dL and should be encouraged through lifestyle approaches. (Class I, Level B)$_{GI=1}$

Lipids

    Diet therapy

        In high-risk women or when LDL-C is elevated, saturated fat intake should be reduced to <7% of calories, cholesterol to <200 mg/d, and *trans* fatty acid intake should be reduced. (Class I, Level B)$_{GI=1}$

    Pharmacotherapy

        High risk[a]

        Initiate LDL-C–lowering therapy (preferably a statin) simultaneously with lifestyle therapy in high-risk women with LDL-C ≥100 mg/dL (Class I, Level A)$_{GI1}$, and initiate statin therapy in high-risk women with an LDL-C <100 mg/dL unless contraindicated (Class I, Level B)$_{GI=1}$

        Initiate niacin[b] or fibrate therapy when HDL-C is low, or non–HDL-C is elevated in high-risk women. (Class I, Level B)$_{GI=1}$

        Intermediate risk[c]

Initiate LDL-C-lowering therapy (preferably a statin) if LDL-C level is ≥130 mg/dL on lifestyle therapy (Class I, Level A)GI=1, or niacin[b] or fibrate therapy when HDL-C is low or non–HDL-C is elevated after LDL-C goal is reached. (Class I, Level B)GI=1

Lower risk[d]

Consider LDL-C-lowering therapy in low-risk women with zero or one risk factor when LDL-C level is ≥190 mg/dL or if multiple risk factors are present when LDL-C is ≥160 mg/dL (Class IIa, Level B) or niacin[b] or fibrate therapy when HDL-C is low or non–HDL-C is elevated after LDL-C goal is reached. (Class IIa, Level B)GI=1

Diabetes

Lifestyle and pharmacotherapy should be used to achieve near normal HbA1$_C$ (<7%) in women with diabetes. (Class I, Level B)GI=1

Preventive drug interventions

Aspirin

High risk[a]

Aspirin therapy (75–162 mg), or clopidogrel if patient is intolerant to aspirin, should be used in high-risk women unless contraindicated. (Class I, Level A)GI=1

Intermediate risk[c]

Consider aspirin therapy (75–162 mg) in intermediate-risk women as long as blood pressure is controlled and benefit is likely to outweigh risk of gastrointestinal side effects. (Class IIa, Level B)GI=2

Beta-blockers

Beta-blockers should be used indefinitely in all women who have had a myocardial infarction or who have chronic ischemic syndromes unless contraindicated. (Class I, Level A)GI=1

ACE inhibitors

ACE inhibitors should be used (unless contraindicated) in high-risk[a] women. (Class I, Level A)GI=1

ARBs

ARBs should be used in high-risk[a] women with clinical evidence of heart failure or an ejection fraction <40% who are intolerant to ACE inhibitors. (Class I, Level B)GI=1

Atrial fibrillation/stroke prevention

Atrial fibrillation

Warfarin

Among women with chronic or paroxysmal atrial fibrillation, warfarin should be used to maintain the INR at 2.0–3.0 unless they are considered to be at low risk for stroke (<1%/yr) or high risk of bleeding. (Class I, Level A)GI=1

Aspirin

Aspirin (325 mg) should be used in women with chronic or paroxysmal atrial fibrillation with a contraindication to warfarin or at low risk for stroke (<1%/yr). (Class I, Level A)GI=1

Class III interventions

Hormone therapy

Combined estrogen plus progestin hormone therapy should not be initiated to prevent CVD in postmenopausal women. (Class III, Level A)

Combined estrogen plus progestin hormone therapy should not be continued to prevent CVD in postmenopausal women. (Class III, Level C)

Other forms of menopausal hormone therapy (e.g., unopposed estrogen) should not be initiated or continued to prevent CVD in postmenopausal women pending the results of ongoing trials. (Class III, Level C)

Antioxidant supplements

Antioxidant vitamin supplements should not be used to prevent CVD pending the results of ongoing trials. (Class III, Level A)GI=1

Aspirin—lower risk[d]

Routine use of aspirin in lower-risk women is not recommended pending the results of ongoing trials. (Class III, Level B)GI=2

[a]High risk is defined as CHD or risk equivalent, or 10-year absolute CHD risk 20%.
[b]Dietary supplement niacin must not be used as a substitute for prescription niacin, and over-the-counter niacin should only be used if approved and monitored by a physician.
[c]Intermediate risk is defined as 10-year absolute CHD risk 10% to 20%.
[d]Lower risk is defined as 10-year absolute CHD risk 10%.
Abbreviations: GI, generalizability index; LDL-C, low-density lipoprotein cholesterol; HDL-C, high-density lipoprotein cholesterol; ACE, angiotensin-converting enzyme; ARB, angiotensin receptor blocker.
Source: From Ref. 47 with permission Lippincott, Williams, and Wilkins.

endothelial function, vasomotor tone, and the renin-angiotensin system; estrogens also favorably modify lipid and glucose metabolism and have antioxidant properties (172).

Changes in the hormonal environment in premenopausal women may be associated with adverse cardiovascular consequences. Kawano et al., for example, reported an increased frequency of ischemic episodes between the end of the luteal phase to the beginning of the menstrual phase in women with variant angina, i.e., increased symptoms during the portion of the menstrual cycle when estrogen levels were the lowest (173). Others have reported greater susceptibility to QT prolongation during the first half of the menstrual cycle (174). Among premenopausal women undergoing coronary angiography for suspected myocardial ischemia in the WISE study, hypoestrogenemia of hypothalamic origin characterized by low estradiol levels in the setting of low levels of follicle stimulating and luteinizing hormone was a powerful independent correlate of angiographic coronary disease (multivariate OR 7.4, 95% CI 1.7, 33.3) (175). In a study of women undergoing hysterectomy for benign reasons, thickened or sclerotic arterial intima of the uterine arteries was more commonly seen in women who had irregular menstrual cycles preceding the surgery (176). Cross-sectionally, premenopausal women with CHD have lower levels of estradiol than premenopausal women without CHD, even when matched for other cardiovascular disease (CVD) risk factors (177). It is clear that women with polycystic ovary syndrome have a greater burden of cardiovascular risk factors, but studies that convincingly link this risk factor burden to greater cardiovascular morbidity and mortality are lacking (178). Although these results are intriguing, they do not prove a causal link between disruptions in the premenopausal hormonal environment and subsequent CHD. Further studies, both mechanistic and clinical, are clearly needed.

The metabolic changes seen during the peri-menopausal transition are reminiscent of the metabolic syndrome with adverse changes in lipids and lipoproteins, impaired endothelial function, insulin resistance, and abnormal glucose metabolism, redistribution of body fat with increased visceral adiposity, shift toward a more pro-coagulant environment, and increase in blood pressure, at least in some if not all studies (179,180). Despite the adverse changes in the cardiovascular risk profile of women at the time of menopause, the relationship between menopause and cardiovascular morbidity and mortality remains controversial (6,181).

CHD prevalence is higher among postmenopausal compared to premenopausal women, but postmenopausal women are also older and such cross-sectional investigations are thus not suitable to determine any effect of menopause. CHD mortality rates do not accelerate at or after natural menopause and the apparent increase in CHD risk among women with premature natural menopause appears to be due to confounding by smoking (6,181,182). Endogenous estrogen and testosterone levels do not correlate with severity of atherosclerosis or coronary events (6). A study by California Seventh-Day Adventists found a U-shaped relationship between menopause and CHD mortality with higher risks for those with early (age 35–40 years) and very late (age >55 years) menopause without any apparent biologic explanation (183). Some authors have suggested a link between progressive postmenopausal bone loss and progression of aortic calcification (184). The relationship between hormonal changes in the peri-menopausal transition and CHD is vastly more complex than can be appreciated by correlating levels of circulating sex hormones or age at cessation of menses with CHD prevalence and incidence. Future studies should carefully delineate the multitude of changes in the hypothalamic-pituitary-ovarian axis that occur in the menopausal transition, measure changes in tissue sensitivity to circulating sex hormones, and determine whether changes in hormone levels or hormone sensitivity alter the impact of known CHD risk factors on development of atherosclerosis and subsequent events.

Newer Risk Factors: Homocysteine and hs–CRP

Homocysteine levels are higher in the follicular than the luteal phase, increase with age, and may be adversely affected by menopause (185,186). Two meta-analyses suggest an association between homocysteine levels and CHD and stroke and polymorphisms in methylene tetrahydrofolate reductase and CHD, respectively (187,188). Only the former provided sex-specific estimates and suggested a similar association in women and men (187). Elevated homocysteine as a risk factor for CHD may be more important among diabetic individuals and among younger women with elevated Lp(a) (189,190). Low folate levels have been linked to greater cardiovascular disease mortality among women while high vitamin B6 and folate intakes are associated with lower levels of CHD (191,192). Folate and vitamin B6 supplementation can reduce homocysteine levels, but to date there is no convincing evidence that such reductions in homocysteine levels lead to reduced CHD or stroke morbidity or mortality (193,194). Current cardiovascular disease prevention guidelines for women classify folate supplementation as a Class IIb intervention among high-risk women (47).

Inflammation appears to play an important role in the development of atherosclerosis. Among the inflammatory markers under investigation, "high sensitivity C-reactive protein" (hs-CRP) has shown the most consistent relationship with subsequent events. In a recent meta-analysis, the odds ratio for CHD was 1.45 (95% CI 1.25–1.68) for individuals in the top third of hs-CRP levels compared to those in the bottom third; point estimates were similar in women and men (195). Whether hs-CRP is a risk marker or a risk factor is the subject of intense debate (196). CRP levels correlate with other risk factors, especially with adiposity, diabetes, lipoprotein levels, coagulation factors, and smoking (196). Elevations in CRP with oral hormone replacement therapy may explain, in part, the lack of benefit of such therapy among women with CHD (197). Statins reduce CRP levels and it is believed that this anti-inflammatory, pleiotropic effect may contribute to the benefits of statins on incident and recurrent CHD (198–200). The 2003 Statement for Health Professionals from the Centers for Disease Control and Prevention and the American Heart Association endorsed selective screening with hs-CRP in intermediate risk individuals without known cardiovascular disease when a physician desires additional information to guide further evaluation and therapy (196).

ASSESSMENT OF RISK

For any given risk factor, absolute rates of CHD events are higher among men than women, but the relative impact of risk factors on CHD events is similar in women and men with the exception of diabetes mellitus and left ventricular hypertrophy where relative risk among women appears to be greater (Table 6) (201). Clustering of risk factors is common in both genders and is associated with a markedly increased risk of CHD. The impact of such clustering may be greater among women than men: in Framingham, for example, clusters of three or more risk factors were associated with a 2.4-fold increase in CHD risk among men and a 5.9-fold increase in risk among women (202). Absence of risk factors, in contrast, confers a substantial survival advantage in both genders. Stamler et al. estimated that middle-aged, nonsmoking women with normal serum cholesterol (<5.17 mmol/L, <200 mg/dL), blood pressure of 120/80 mmHg or lower, and no diabetes had a greater life expectancy of almost six years (203).

Because CHD is often fatal, and because nearly two-thirds of women who die suddenly have no previously recognized symptoms, it is essential to identify women at risk and match the intensity of interventions to the baseline level of cardiovascular risk (29). Cardiovascular risk in a given woman can be estimated by multivariable gender-specific risk prediction equations. These equations are based on prospective follow-up studies in the United States and Europe. Risk prediction instruments variously target populations with or without cardiovascular disease or other CHD equivalents, differ by type of endpoint, include different variables, and predict over different time frames. Selected instruments are shown in Table 7 (47,49,204–210). Among individuals without cardiovascular disease, a risk above 20% of a hard CHD endpoint equates to a risk of more than 25% when softer endpoints such as unstable angina and stable angina are included; the corresponding values for intermediate risk are 10% to 20% versus 15% to 25%, and for low risk, below 10% versus below 15%, respectively (49).

Applicability of a prediction algorithm for a population not represented in the original cohort used to generate the data is a significant concern. The Framingham algorithm which is based on a U.S. Caucasian population has been validated and appears to be robust for use among African-American women (211). While relative risks for a given risk factor are similar among white U.S. women and African-American women, the fraction of CHD deaths in the population differs significantly between ethnic groups (212). In Stamler's five-cohort study, 58% of the CHD deaths among African-American women were attributable to hypertension compared to 27% among white women; the impact of hypercholesterolemia and diabetes was also somewhat greater among black women than white women, while smoking played a greater role among white women (203). The Framingham CHD equations tend to overestimate risk among native American women, Chinese and German populations, while overall cardiovascular risk among

TABLE 6 Impact of Cardiovascular Risk Factors in Women and Men in Framingham

Risk factors	Age-adjusted rate/1000		Risk ratio	
	Men	Women	Men	Women
Age: 35–64 yr				
Elevated cholesterol	45	23	1.7	1.4
Hypertension	65	35	2.2	2.5
Diabetes	76	65	2.2	3.7
Smoking	45	21	1.7	1.2
Left ventricular hypertrophy	164	135	4.7	7.4
Age: 65–94 yr				
Elevated cholesterol	91	63	1.1	1.0
Hypertension	125	81	1.8	1.8
Diabetes	138	102	1.7	1.8
Smoking	95	84	1.2	1.5
Left ventricular hypertrophy	234	235	2.8	4.1

Source: From Ref. 201.

South Asians and Africans living in the United Kingdom may be underestimated (211,213–215). The Framingham equations have not been validated in U.S., Hispanic, or Asian women (211).

The "accuracy" of the Framingham equations for women has been questioned because the equations focus on 10-year absolute risk and thus have a propensity to undertreat young people at high relative risk (e.g., premenopausal women with multiple risk factors) and to overtreat older people at lower relative risk (e.g., older men) (216). Indeed, most women under the age of 70 years in the Framingham cohort are at low or moderate 10-year absolute risk while the majority of men are in the intermediate or high-risk category by age 60 (217). The ATP III panel thus suggested that lifetime risk be considered in addition to absolute 10-year risk before making treatment decisions (Table 8) and the risk calculator on the National Heart Lung and Blood Institute website provides not only absolute but also relative risk compared to an average woman and a woman with optimal risk factors (49,218). Furthermore, women with diabetes are automatically assigned to the high-risk group by virtue of having a "CHD risk equivalent" (49). To overcome the undertreatment of individuals of high relative risk and overtreatment of older individuals with low relative risk, the latest Joint British Societies charts have been modified so that anyone below age 50 years is assessed on the basis of their risk factors as if they were aged 49 years and all those aged 60 years and above are assessed as if they were 69 years of age (216). The current Evidence-Based Guidelines for Cardiovascular Disease Prevention in Women, endorsed by many U.S. organizations and the World Heart Federation, add chronic kidney disease as another CHD risk equivalent, further refining risk stratification among women (47).

At this time, there is no consensus on whether newer risk factors such as high sensitivity CRP should be included in the risk prediction algorithms or whether evidence of subclinical disease (e.g., coronary calcium assessment, measurements of carotid intimal thickness) should be systematically sought. Having this additional information may be most useful among individuals at intermediate risk by the Framingham algorithm (219). On the other hand, the traditional major CHD risk factors appear to explain most CHD events. Among women under the age of 60, elevation of at least one major CHD risk factor was present in 90% to 100% of the individuals who died from CHD in the Chicago Heart Association Project and the Framingham Study and in 69% to 87% of those who suffered a nonfatal MI in the Framingham Study (220). When risk factors at "higher than favorable levels" where considered, 96% to 100% of women under the age of 60 who died of CHD and 85% to 99% who suffered a nonfatal MI had at least one such risk factor (220). Smoking appears to play a particularly prominent role among women between age 18 and 39 with a prevalence between 80% and 100% among those who die of CHD and 62% of those who suffer a nonfatal MI (220). The importance of traditional and lifestyle risk factors was most recently highlighted by the INTERHEART study and extends observations in Western societies to Asia, the Middle East, Africa, and South America (221). Abnormal lipids, smoking, hypertension, diabetes, abdominal obesity, psychosocial factors, lack of consumption of fruits, vegetables, and alcohol, and lack of regular physical activity accounted for most of the risk of MI worldwide in both sexes and at all ages in all geographic regions (221).

TABLE 7   Comparison of Selected Multivariable Risk Prediction Equations for Women

Instrument	Target population	Reference cohort	Variables included	Time frame of prediction (yr)	Endpoints
Framingham (1998) (204)	Women without CVD	Framingham	Age, total cholesteril (or LDL cholesterol), HDL cholesterol, systolic and diastolic BP, diabetes, smoking	10	Hard CHD (nonfatal MI or CHD death)
Framingham (2000) (205)	Women without CVD	Framingham	Age, menopause,l HDL-C, diabetes, alcohol, smoking, TG, systolic BP	2	CHD (MI, coronary insuffi-ciency, angina pectoris, CHD death)
New Zealand (2000) (206)	Womwen without CVD, LVH by ECG, or diabetic nephropathy	Framingham	Age, smoking, diabetes, systolic and diastolic BP, total cholesterol to HDL-C ratio	5	CVD events (death related to CHD, non fatal MI, new angina, fatal or non fatal stroke or TIA, development of heart failure or peripheral vascular disease)
ATP III (2001) (49)	Women without CVD and without diabetes	Framingham	Age, total and HDL-C, smoking, systolic BP, treatment for HTN	10	Hard CHD (nonfatal MI or CHD death)
CVD Prevention Guidelines for Women (2004) (47)	Women without CVD, diabetes or chronic kidney disease	Framingham	Age, total and HDL-C smoking, systolic BP, treatment for HTN	10	Hard CHD (nonfatal MI or CHD death)
SCORE Project (2003) (207)	Women without prior MI	12 European Cohort Studies	Age, total cholesterol, systolic BP, smoking	10	Fatal CVD (can calculate separately for fatal CHD and non-CHD endpoints and for low and high-risk regions)
Joint British Societies (2004) (208)	Women without CVD and without diabetes	Framingham	Age (3 categories), total cholesterol to HDL ratio, systolic BP, smoking	10	Cardiovascular Disease risk (combined fatal and nonfatal stroke and CHD)
Framingham (2000) (205)	Women with a history of ischemic stroke or CHD	Framingham	Age, HDL-C, smoking, diabetes, systolic BP	2	CHD (MI, coronary insuffi-ciency, angina pectoris, CHD death)
UKPDS Risk Engine (2001) (209)	Women with Type II Diabetes	UKPDS Database	Age, ethnicity, smoking, total to HDL cholesterol ratio, hemoglobin A1C, systolic BP	Variable	Fatal or nonfatal MI, sudden cardiac death
GISSI Algorithm (2001) (210)	Women after myocardial infarction	GISSI Prevenzione Cohort	Age, ischemia, LV dysfunction, HTN, DM, HR, smoking, HDL-C, fibrinogen, leukocytes, claudication	4	Death

Abbreviations: LDL, low-density lipoprotein; HDL, high-density lipoprotein; CHD, coronary heart disease; BP, blood pressure; HTN, hypertension.

PREVENTION GUIDELINES

In 2004, cardiovascular disease prevention guidelines specific to women were published (47). These guidelines outline an evidence-based cardiovascular disease prevention strategy with the intensity of the intervention matched to the risk level of a given woman. The expert panel dif-ferentiated four risk categories based on use of the Framingham risk algorithm and provided some clinical examples for each category: optimal risk (optimal levels of risk factors, heart healthy lifestyle), less than 10% 10-year CHD risk (e.g., women with multiple risk factors, meta-bolic syndrome, or one or no risk factors), 10% to 20% 10-year CHD risk [e.g., subclinical cardio-vascular disease, metabolic syndrome, multiple risk factors, markedly elevated levels of a single

TABLE 8 Short-Term and Lifetime Risk of Coronary Heart Disease (%) by Cholesterol Levels Obtained at Various Ages

	Men			Women		
	<200[a]	200–239[a]	240+[a]	<200[a]	200–239[a]	240+[a]
Age 40						
10-yr risk	3	5	12	1	2	5
40-yr risk	31	43	57	15	26	33
Age 50						
10-yr risk	8	10	15	2	4	8
40-yr risk	40	42	63	19	30	39
Age 60						
10-yr risk	16	15	21	5	8	11
Lifetime risk	34	41	51	20	24	36
Age 70						
10-yr risk	18	22	28	5	7	13
Lifetime risk	27	36	42	14	20	29
Age 80						
10-yr risk	14	23	29	14	16	17
Lifetime risk	17	23	34	17	18	21

[a]Total cholesterol level in mg/dL.
Source: From Ref. 49.

risk factor, first-degree relative(s) with early-onset atherosclerotic disease], and above 20% 10-year CHD risk (e.g., CHD and CHD risk equivalents such as cerebrovascular disease, peripheral arterial disease, abdominal aortic aneurysm, diabetes mellitus, chronic kidney disease). These guidelines are not meant to supersede clinical judgment and encourage the clinician to take into account frailty, life expectancy, and regional and cultural preferences as appropriate.

Treatment recommendations are grouped by usefulness and strength of the evidence (Class I: Intervention is useful and effective, Class IIa: Weight of evidence/opinion is in favor of usefulness/efficacy; Class IIb: Usefulness/efficacy is less well-established by evidence/opinion, Class III: Intervention is not useful/effective and may be harmful; A: designates sufficient evidence from multiple randomized trials, B: limited evidence from single randomized trial or other nonrandomized studies, C: based on expert opinion, case studies, or standard of care) and are assigned a generalizability index (1: Very likely that results generalize to women; 2: somewhat likely that results generalize to women; 3: Unlikely that results generalize to women; 4: Unable to project whether results generalize women). As shown in Tables 5 and 9, there are recommendations for "lifestyle interventions," "major risk factor interventions," "atrial fibrillation/stroke prevention," "preventive drug interventions," and a Class III category, i.e., interventions for cardiovascular disease that are not recommended.

Class III interventions include postmenopausal hormone therapy for cardiovascular disease prevention, antioxidant therapy, and aspirin therapy for low risk women. Since the publication of the HERS study and the estrogen only and estrogen/progestin arms of the Women's Health Initiative (133–137), it is clear that use of hormone therapy for treatment of dyslipidemia or cardiovascular disease prevention can no longer be advocated. Risk benefit ratios are less clear among much younger women who are severely symptomatic from postmenopausal symptoms. A 2004 report from the American College of Obstetricians and Gynecologists reaffirms prior recommendations that hormone therapies are appropriate for the relief of vasomotor symptoms, so long as a woman has weighed the risks and benefits with her doctor, takes the smallest effective dose for the shortest possible time, and annually reviews the decision to take hormones with her physician (222).

Clinical decision making will be illustrated with three case examples.

■ Case 1

M.J. is a 60-year-old accountant. She has been healthy all her life. One of her cousins aged 50, suffered a heart attack three weeks ago and she thus decided to participate in a Health Fair. Based on an on-site ultrasound exam, she was told that "her arteries looked beautiful." She was encouraged to see her doctor because her cholesterol was "very high" (she recalls a total cholesterol of 250) and that her blood pressure was elevated (she thinks that the "top number" was 150). Her parents are in their 80s and have no cardiac disease. She is an only child. She has never smoked. She drinks an occasional glass of wine. She walks to work every day (about 1.5 miles one way), is able to do all her house work and yard work, and has no symptoms suggestive of cardiovascular disease. She "watches her salt and fat." On exam, she is 158 cm tall and weighs 70 kg (BMI: 28); her waist circumference is 80 cm. Blood pressure in both arms is 136/88 mmHg. The remainder of the exam is benign. Lab data—TC: 248, HDL-C: 90, LDL-C: 146, TG: 60, fasting glucose: 92, creatinine: 0.6.

Clinical decision making: She does not have any CHD or CHD risk equivalent. She is overweight, but does not have an increased waist circumference suggestive of metabolic syndrome. She is moderately active. Her kidney function and fasting glucose are in the normal range. Her LDL-C is higher than desirable and she has "pre-hypertension" by Joint National Committee (JNC) VII criteria. Her 10-year CHD risk calculates to 2%, i.e., in the low risk category. She does not require any pharmacologic therapy for her risk factors at this time, but should receive dietary counseling with particular attention to weight management and restriction of saturated fat and salt intake, and should get regular follow-up blood pressure checks. An increase in her physical activity level would be desirable. Hormone therapy should not be used to lower her LDL cholesterol.

Should she be counseled to take an aspirin daily for prevention of MI and stroke? The guidelines suggested a conservative approach (i.e., no therapy) in a low risk woman, pending results of ongoing clinical trials. In March of 2005, Ridker et al. published the results of the Women's Health Study (223). In this trial, 39,876 initially healthy women 45 years or older were randomized to receive 100 mg of aspirin on alternate days, or placebo and followed for 10 years with a composite endpoint of "first major cardiovascular event" (i.e., nonfatal MI, nonfatal stroke, or death from cardiovascular causes). Overall, there was an insignificant reduction in risk with aspirin therapy of 9% ($p = 0.13$), but there was a 17% reduction in the

TABLE 9   Priorities for Prevention in Practice According to Risk Group

High-risk women (>20% risk)
Class I recommendations
■ Smoking cessation
■ Physical activity/cardiac rehabilitation
■ Diet therapy
■ Weight maintenance/reduction
■ Blood pressure control
■ Lipid control/statin therapy
■ Aspirin therapy
■ Beta-Blocker therapy
■ ACE inhibitor therapy (ARBs if contraindicated)
■ Glycemic control in diabetics
Class IIa recommendation
■ Evaluate/treat for depression
Class IIb recommendations
■ Omega 3 fatty-acid supplementation
■ Folic acid supplementation
Intermediate-risk women (10% to 20% risk)
Class I recommendations
■ Smoking cessation
■ Physical activity
■ Heart-healthy diet
■ Weight maintenance/reduction
■ Blood pressure control
■ Lipid control
Class IIa recommendations
■ Aspirin therapy
Lower-risk women (<10% risk)
Class I recommendations
■ Smoking cessation
■ Physical activity
■ Heart-healthy diet
■ Weight maintenance/reduction
■ Treat individual CVD risk factors as indicated
Stroke prevention among women with atrial fibrillation
Class I recommendations
High-intermediate risk of stroke
■ Warfarin therapy
Low risk of stroke (<1%/yr) or contraindication to warfarin
■ Aspirin therapy

Abbreviations: ACE, angiotensin-converting enzyme; ARB, angiotensin receptor blocker.
Source: From Ref. 47 with permission of Lippincott, Williams, and Wilkins.

risk of stroke which reached statistical significance ($p = 0.04$). Such benefit came at a price: gastrointestinal bleeding requiring transfusion was increased by 40% in the aspirin group ($p = 0.02$). The authors tried to determine whether subgroups of women had more or less favorable risk benefit ratios and concluded that women 65 years and older who were treated with aspirin had significantly reduced risk of major cardiovascular events, ischemic stroke, and MI. For the patient in our case example, risks of therapy likely outweigh benefits and aspirin therapy for cardiovascular disease prophylaxis should not be used.

■ Case 2

AT is a 39-year-old woman who comes to the office for her annual physical and says that she is feeling fine. She works as a cashier at a 24-hour restaurant and eats all her meals at the restaurant. Her knees have been hurting for some time and she avoids walking whenever possible to minimize the discomfort. She has been smoking since she was a teenager; over the last year she has cut down from 1 to 1.5 packs per day to 0.5 pack per day. She takes her birth control pills regularly and recent gynecologic checkups have been normal. On exam, she is 170 cm tall and weighs 95 kg (BMI: 32.9); her waist circumference is 92 cm. Her blood pressure is 142/82 mmHg. Her physical exam is benign except for her obesity. Lab data: Her fasting blood sugar is 112 mg/dL. Her TC is 248, HDL-C: 46, LDL-C: 146, TG: 168, creatinine: 0.9.

Clinical decision making: AT has metabolic syndrome with abdominal obesity, hypertension, impaired fasting glucose, low HDL-C, and elevated triglycerides. The oral contraceptives may be contributing to her dyslipidemia and abnormal blood pressure. Her diet is high in fat and calories; she is physically inactive and smokes. The combination of oral contraceptive therapy and smoking is particularly worrisome. Her 10-year Framingham CHD risk calculates to only 6%. Although she technically falls into a "low risk category," her lifetime risk of CHD is at least 33% (Table 8), even without taking into account her metabolic syndrome, her lifestyle risk factors, and her contraceptive use on a smoking background. She is also at very high risk of developing diabetes. This is thus not a "low risk patient" who can be scheduled for a routine annual appointment. She needs intensive lifestyle modification including cessation of smoking, regular physical activity, and weight and diet management. Given her advancing age, abnormal lipids, and elevated blood pressure, alternatives to oral contraceptive therapy should be explored, especially if she finds it difficult to quit smoking or is unwilling to do so. Pharmacologic therapy for her dyslipidemia and hypertension can be deferred at this initial visit, but should be considered on subsequent visits, if lifestyle modifications do not have the desired effect.

■ Case 3

SB is a 45-year-old smoker who has a several-year history of "borderline diabetes" and multiple relatives with diabetes and coronary disease below the age of 60. She comes to the office after a recent hospitalization for chest pain which had been bothering her for several months without a change in severity or frequency. She underwent cardiac catheterization and was told that she had multiple artery blockages, but that none were severe enough to require revascularization at this time. She was discharged on aspirin and nitrates, and told to watch her fat intake because her cholesterol was a little high. She was told to stop smoking and that exercise is very important, but she has been afraid to exert herself for fear of recurrent chest pain and says that she is under too much stress to quit smoking. On exam, she is 160 cm tall, weighs 60 kg, her blood pressure is 120/70 mmHg in both arms. She has a soft right carotid bruit, but no other abnormal physical findings. Lab data obtained in the hospital include two fasting sugars of 126 and 128, a TC of 220, HDL-C of 35, LDL-C of 125, and TG of 300. Her creatinine is normal at 0.8. Follow-up fasting sugar on the morning of the office visit was 127.

Clinical decision making. This patient is clearly in a very high-risk category with established CHD, smoking, diabetes, and dyslipidemia. She should be referred to a cardiac rehabilitation program, counseled to quit smoking, counseled regarding a therapeutic lifestyle, change her diet, and should receive statin therapy for her dyslipidemia with a goal LDL-C below 70 mg/dL and non-HDL-C below 100 mg/dL. Treatment targeted at her low HDL-C should also be considered (although there is no clinical trial data in women to date to support HDL-C directed therapy). Aspirin therapy should be prescribed unless contraindicated; she should receive beta-blocker therapy, and she should be placed on an angiotensin converting enzyme inhibitor.

Awareness of and adherence to cardiovascular risk prevention guidelines in the U.S. remain suboptimal. This "treatment gap" was most recently documented in a web-based survey, which utilized a standardized questionnaire as well as case studies (224). Over 90% of the primary care providers and cardiologists were aware of the current guidelines for lipid-lowering therapy and treatment of hypertension, while only around 60% and 45%, respectively, of obstetricians/gynecologists (OBGYN) were aware of the lipid-lowering and hypertension guidelines. Only 60% of the primary care providers and OBGYN physicians and 80% cardiologists were aware of the cardiovascular disease prevention guidelines in women. Among those who were aware of these guidelines, only around 40% reported that they applied them in practice. For the case examples, physicians' perceptions of patient risk were compared with actual risk calculated by the Framingham algorithm. Misclassification of risk was very common (Table 10) and was more pronounced for women than men: intermediate-risk women were significantly less likely to be assigned to a higher-risk category than men with similar risk profiles (OR 0.62; 95% CI

TABLE 10 Misclassification of Cardiovascular Risk

	Percent correct responses		
	Primary care provider	OBGYN physician	Cardiologist
Low-risk man	34	19	29
Intermediate-risk man	47	41	51
High-risk man	59	43	58
Low-risk woman	43	17	36
Intermediate-risk woman	47	38	53
High-risk woman	55	37	56

Source: From Ref. 224.

0.49–0.78) by primary case physicians, with similar but insignificant trends for OBGYN and cardiologists. This observation is important as perception of intermediate or high-risk strongly predicted adherence to guideline recommendations and gender disparities in recommendations for preventive therapy were largely explained by the lower perceived risk despite similarly calculated risk for women versus men. The authors concluded that educational interventions for physicians were needed to improve the quality of cardiovascular disease preventive care and lower morbidity and mortality from cardiovascular disease for men and women (224).

CONCLUSIONS

CHD is common among women and is a major cause of morbidity and mortality among women worldwide. Although there are many similarities among men and women in the pathogenesis and pathophysiology of CHD, important differences clearly exist and have major implications for prevention, diagnosis, and treatment. Due to past and present under-representation of women in clinical trials and inconsistent reporting of gender-specific subgroup analyses, many recommendations for therapy are based on data extrapolated from clinical trial results among men (47). A 2001 report from the Institute of Medicine recommended the study of sex differences "from womb to tomb," concluding that much is to be learned by seeking out potential sexual dimorphisms at all levels of research, be it at the cellular level, in animal models, in epidemiologic research, or in clinical trials (225). Evidence-based medicine is only as good as the evidence it is based on. A systematic expansion of research attuned to potential gender differences will improve health care and health outcomes among women and men.

REFERENCES

1. World Health Organization. Preventing Chronic Diseases: A Vital Investment. World Health Organization Global Report, 2005, ISBN 92 4 156300 1.
2. World Health Organization Atlas of Heart Disease and Stroke, 2004; Section 12: Women: A special case? downloaded from: www.who.int/cardiovascular_diseases/resources/atlas/en/ (accessed 11/26/05).
3. Petersen S, Peto V, Scarborough P, Rayner M. British Heart Foundation Health Promotion Research Group, Department of Public Health, University of Oxford. Coronary Heart Statistics—2005 ed. Downloaded from: www.heartstats.org (accessed 11/26/05).
4. American Heart Association. Statistical Fact Sheet—Populations. International Cardiovascular Disease Statistics. American Heart Association, Dallas, TX, 2004. downloaded from: www.americanheart.org (accessed 1/22/05) .
5. Khaw KT. Epidemiology of coronary heart disease in women. In: Wenger NK, Collins P, eds. Women & Heart Disease. 2nd ed. London and New York: Taylor & Francis, 2005.
6. Barrett-Connor E. Sex differences in coronary heart disease. Why are women so superior? The 1995 Ancel Keys Lecture. Circulation 1997; 95:252–264.
7. Barrett Connor E, Goodman-Gruen D. Prospective study of endogenous sex hormones and fatal cardiovascular disease in post-menopausal women. BMJ 1995; 311:1193–1196.
8. Berenson GS, Srinivasan SR, Bao W, Newman WP III, Tracy RE, Wattigney WA. For the bogalusa heart study. Association between multiple cardiovascular risk factors and atherosclerosis in children and young adults. N Engl J Med 1998; 338:1650–1656.
9. McGill HC Jr., McMahan A, Zieske AW, et al. For the pathobiological determinants of atherosclerosis in youth (PDAY) research group. Arterioscler Thromb Vasc Biol 2000; 20:1998–2004.

10. Mahoney LT, Burns TL, Stanford W, et al. Coronary risk factors measured in childhood and young adult life are associated with coronary artery calcification in young adults: the muscatine study. J Am Coll Cardiol 1996; 27:277–284.

11. Hoff JA, Chomka EV, Krainik AJ, Daviglus M, Rich S, Kondos GT. Age and gender distribution of coronary artery calcium detected by electron beam tomography in 35,246 adults. Am J Cardiol 2001; 87:1335–1339.

12. Chaitman BR, Bourassa MG, Davis K, et al. Angiographic prevalence of high-risk coronary artery disease in patient subsets (CASS). Circulation 1981; 64:360–367.

13. Enriquez-Sarano M, Klodas E, Garratt KN, Bailey KR, Tajik AJ, Holmes DR Jr. Secular trends in coronary atherosclerosis: analysis in patients with valvular regurgitation. N Engl J Med 1996; 335:316–322.

14. Dodge JT Jr., Brown BG, Bolson EL, Dodge HT. Lumen diameter of normal human coronary arteries: influence of age, sex, anatomic variation, and left ventricular hypertrophy or dilation. Circulation 1992; 86:232–246.

15. Sheifer SE, Canos MR, Weinfurt KP, et al. Sex differences in coronary artery size assessed by intravascular ultrasound. Am Heart J 2000; 139:649–653.

16. Clarkson TB, Prichard RW, Morgan TM, Petrick GS, Klein KP. Remodeling of coronary arteries in human and nonhuman primates. JAMA 1994; 271:289–294.

17. Kornowski R, Lansky AJ, Mintz GS, et al. Comparison of men versus women in cross-sectional area luminal narrowing, quantity of plaque, presence of calcium in plaque, and lumen location in coronary arteries by intravascular ultrasound in patients with stable angina pectoris. Am J Cardiol 1997; 79:1601–1605.

18. Rasheed Q, Nair R, Sheehan H, Hodgson JM. Correlation of intracoronary ultrasound plaque characteristics in atherosclerotic coronary artery disease patients with clinical variables. Am J Cardiol 1994 73:753–758.

19. Mautner SL, Lin F, Mautner GC, Roberts WC. Comparison in women versus men of composition of atherosclerotic plaques in native coronary arteries and in saphenous veins used as aortocoronary conduits. J Am Coll Cardiol 1993; 21:1312–1318.

20. Dollar AL, Kragel AH, Fernicola DJ, Waclawiw MA, Roberts WC. Composition of atherosclerotic plaques in coronary arteries in women <40 years of age with fatal coronary artery disease and implications for plaque reversibility. Am J Cardiol 1991; 67:1223–1227.

21. Arbustini E, Dal Bello B, Morbini P, et al. Plaque erosion is a major substrate for coronary thrombosis in acute myocardial infarction. Heart 1999; 82:269–272.

22. Burke AP, Farb A, Malcom GT, Liang Y, Smialek J, Virmani R. Effect of risk factors on the mechanism of acute thrombosis and sudden coronary death in women. Circulation 1998; 97:2110–2116.

23. Becker RC, Terrin M, Ross R, et al. and the thrombolysis in myocardial infarction investigators. Comparison of clinical outcomes for women and men after myocardial infarction. Ann Intern Med 1994; 120:638–645.

24. Malacrida R, Genoni M, Maggioni AP, et al. A comparison of the early outcome of acute myocardial Infarction in women and men. N Engl J Med 1998; 338:8–14.

25. Vaccarino V, Parson L, Every NR, Barron HV, Krumholz HM. For the National Registry of Myocardial infarction 2 participants. Sex differences in early mortality after myocardial infarction. N Engl J Med 1999; 341:217–225.

26. Vaccarino V, Horwitz RI, Meehan TP, Petrillo MK, Radford MJ, Krumholz HM. Sex differences in mortality after myocardial infarction. Arch Intern Med 1998; 158:2054–2062.

27. Sonke GS, Beaglehole R, Stewart AW, Jackson R, Stewart FM. Sex differences in case fatality before and after admission to hospital after acute cardiac events: analysis of community based coronary heart disease register. BMJ 1996; 313:853–855.

28. White AD, Rosamond WD, Chambless LE, et al. For the atherosclerosis risk in communities (ARIC). Sex and race differences in short-term prognosis after acute coronary heart disease events: the atherosclerosis risk in communities (ARIC) study. Am Heart J 1999; 138:540–548.

29. Kannel W, Wilson PWF, D'Agostino RB, Cobb J. Sudden coronary death in women. Am Heart J 1998; 136:205–212.

30. Albert CM, Chae CU, Grodstein F, et al. Prospective study of sudden cardiac death among women in the United States. Circulation 2003; 107:2096–2101.

31. Brett KM, Madans JH. Long-term survival after coronary heart disease. Comparisons between men and women in a national sample. Ann Epidemiol 1995; 5:25–32.

32. Goldberg RJ, Gorak EJ, Yarzebski J, et al. A communitywide perspective of sex differences and temporal trends in the incidence and survival rates after acute myocardial infarction and out-of-hospital deaths caused by coronary heart disease. Circulation 1993; 87:1947–1953.

33. Fiebach NH, Viscoli CM, Horwitz RI. Differences between women and men in survival after myocardial infarction. Biology or Methodology? JAMA 1990; 263:1092–1096.

34. Kern MJ. Coronary blood flow and myocardial ischemia. In: Zipes DP, Libby P, Bonow RO, Braunwald E, eds. Braunwald's Heart Disease. A Textbook of Cardiovascular Medicine. 7th ed. Philadelphia: Elsevier; Saunders, 2005:1103–1127.

35. Bugiardini R, Bairey–Merz CN. Angina with "normal" coronary arteries. A changing philosophy. JAMA 2005; 293:477–484.

36. Buigardini R, Manfrini O, Pizzi C, et al. Endothelial function predicts future development of coronary artery disease. Circulation 2004; 109:2518–2523.
37. Douglas PS, Ginsberg GS. The evaluation of chest pain in women. N Engl J Med 1996; 334:1311–11315.
38. McSweeney JC, Cody M, O'Sullivan P, Elberson K, Moser DK, Garvin BJ. Women's early warning symptoms of acute myocardial infarction. Circulation 2003; 108:2619–2623.
39. Goldberg RJ, Goff D, Cooper L, et al. Age and sex differences in presentation of symptoms among patients with acute coronary disease: the REACT trial. Coronary Artery Disease 2000; 11:399–407.
40. Goldberg RJ, O'Donnell C, Yarzebski J, et al. Sex differences in symptom presentation associated with acute myocardial infarction: a population-based perspective. Am Heart J 1998; 136:189–195.
41. Sheps DS, Kaufmann PG, Sheffield D, et al. Sex differences in chest pain in patients with documented coronary artery disease and exercise induced ischemia: results from the PIMI study. Am Heart J 2001; 42:864–871.
42. Milner KA, Vaccarino V, Arnold AL, Funk M, Goldberg RJ. Gender and age differences in chief complaints of acute myocardial infarction (Worcester Heart Attack Study). Am J Cardiol 2004; 93:606–608.
43. Solomon CG, Lee TH, Cook EF, et al. Comparison of clinical presentation of acute myocardial infarction in patients older than 65 years of age to younger patients: the multicenter chest pain study experience. Am J Cardiol 1989; 63:772–776.
44. Mosca L, Ferris A, Fabunmi R, Robertson M. Tracking women's awareness of heart disease. An American Heart Association National Study. Circulation 2004; 109:573–579.
45. Gibbons RJ, Balady GJ, Bricker JT, et al. ACC/AHA 2002 guideline update for exercise testing. A Report of the American College of Cardiology/American Heart Association Task Force on Practice Guidelines (Committee on Exercise Testing). Circulation 2002; 106:1883–1892.
46. Mieres JH, Shaw LJ, Arai A, et al. Role of noninvasive testing in the clinical evaluation of women with suspected coronary artery disease. Circulation 2005; 111:682–696.
47. Mosca L, Appel LJ, Benjamin EJ, et al. Evidence-based guidelines for cardiovascular disease prevention in women. Circulation 2004; 109:672–693.
48. Von Dras DD, Siegler IC, Williams RB, Clapp-Channing N, Haney TL, Mark DB. Surrogate assessment of coronary artery disease patients' functional capacity. Soc Sci Med 1997; 44:1491–1502.
49. Expert Panel on Detection, Evaluation, and Treatment of High Blood Cholesterol in Adults. Third report of the National Cholesterol Education Program (NCEP) Expert Panel on Detection, Evaluation, and Treatment of High Blood Cholesterol in Adults (Adult Treatment Panel III): final report. Circulation 2002; 106:3143–3421.
50. American Heart Association. Heart Disease and Stroke Statistics—2005 Update. American Heart Association. Dallas, TX, 2004.
51. Centers for Disease Control and Prevention. Behavioral Risk Factor Surveillance System http://www.cdc.gov/brfss/ (accessed 9/14/05).
52. Wechsler H, Rigotti NA, Gledhill-Hoyt J, Lee H. Increased levels of cigarette use among college students. A cause for National concern. JAMA 1998; 280:1673–1678.
53. Kesteloot H. Queen margrethe II and mortality in danish women. Lancet 2001; 357:871–872.
54. The health consequences of smoking: a report of the Surgeon General. Cardiovascular Diseases. Washington, DC: Department of Health and Human Services, Centers for Disease Control and Prevention, National Center for Chronic Disease Prevention and Health Promotion, Office on Smoking and Health, 2004.
55. Dunn NR, Faragher B, Thorogood M, et al. Risk of myocardial infarction in young female smokers. Heart 1999; 82:581–583.
56. Stampfer MJ, Hu FB, Manson JE, Rimm EB, Willett WC. Primary prevention of coronary heart disease in women through diet and lifestyle. New Engl J Med 2000; 343:16–22.
57. Wilson K, Gibson N, Willan A, Cook D. Effect of smoking cessation on mortality after myocardial infarction: meta-analysis of cohort studies. Arch Int Med 2000; 160:939–944.
58. Hu FB, Stampfer MJ, Manson JE, et al. Trends in the incidence of coronary heart disease and changes in diet and lifestyle in women. New Engl J Med 2000; 343:530–537.
59. Glantz SA, Parmley WW. Passive smoking and heart disease. Mechanisms and risk. JAMA 1995; 273:1047–1053.
60. Wells AJ. Passive smoking as a cause of heart disease. J Am Coll Cardiol 1994; 24:546–554.
61. Ciruzzi M, Pramparo P, Esteban O, et al. For the argentine FRICAS investigators. Case control study of passive smoking at home and risk of acute myocardial infarction. J Am Coll Cardiol 1998; 31:797–803.
62. Anderson JE, Jorenby DE, Scott WJ, Fiore MC. Treating tobacco use and dependence: an evidence based clinical practice guideline for tobacco cessation. Chest 2002; 121:932–941.
63. Apacible MAF, Martin K, Froehlicher ESS. Other risk interventions: smoking. In: Wenger NK, Collins P, eds. Women & Heart Disease. 2nd ed. London and New York: Taylor & Francis, 2005.
64. Schoenborn CA, Barnes PM. Leisure time physical activity among adults: United States, 1997-1998. Advance Data from Vital and Health Statistics No. 325. Hyattsville, MD: National Center for Health Statistics, 2002.
65. Williams PT. Physical fitness and activity as separate heart disease risk factors: a meta-analysis. Med Sci Sports Exerc 2001; 33:754–761.
66. Hu FB, Stampfer MJ, Colditz GA, et al. Physical activity and risk of stroke in women. JAMA 2000; 283:2961–2967.

67. Lee IM, Rexrode KM, Cook NR, Manson JAE, Buring JE. Physical activity and coronary heart disease in women. JAMA 2001; 285:1447–1454.
68. Jakicic JM, Wing RR, Butler BA, Robertson RJ. Prescribing exercise in multiple short bouts versus one continuous bout: effects on adherence, cardiorespiratory fitness, and weight loss in overweight women. Int J Obes Relat Metab Disord 1995; 19:893–901.
69. Gregg EW, Cauley JA, Stone K, et al. Relationship of changes in physical activity and mortality among older women. JAMA 2003; 289:2379–2386.
70. Writing Group for the Activity Counseling Trial Research Group. Effects of physical activity counseling in primary care: the activity counseling trial: a randomized controlled trial. JAMA 2001:286:677–687.
71. Manson JE, Skerrett PJ, Greenland P, VanItallie TB. The escalating pandemics of obesity and sedentary lifestyle: a call to action for clinicians. Arch Intern Med 2004; 164:249–258.
72. Dietary Guidelines for US Adults. U.S. Department of Health and Human Services, U.S. Department of Agriculture www.healthierus.gov/dietaryguidelines (accessed 10/30/05).
73. Bittner V, Sanderson BK. Women in cardiac rehabilitation. JAMWA 2003; 58:227–235.
74. Taylor RS, Brown A, Ebrahim S, et al. Exercise-based rehabilitation for patients with coronary heart disease: systematic review and meta-analysis of randomized controlled trials. Am J Med 2004; 116:682–692.
75. Witt BJ, Jacobsen SJ, Weston SA, et al. Cardiac rehabilitation after myocardial infarction in the community. J Am Coll Cardiol 2004; 44:988–996.
76. Sanderson BK, Bittner V. Women in cardiac rehabilitation: outcomes and identifying risk for dropout. Am Heart J 2005; 150:1052–1058.
77. Berg AH, Scherer PE. Adipose tissue, inflammation, and cardiovascular disease. Circ Res 2005; 96:939–949.
78. Hubert HB, Feinleib M, McNamara PM, Castelli WP. Obesity as an independent risk factor for cardiovascular disease: a 26 year follow-up of participants in the Framing Heart Study. Circulation 1983; 67:968–977.
79. Manson JAE, Coldlitz GA, Stampfer MJ, et al. A prospective study of obesity and risk of coronary heart disease in women. N Engl J Med 1990; 322:882–889.
80. Manson JAE, Willett WC, Stampfer MJ, et al. Body weight and mortality among women. N Engl J Med 1995; 333:677–685.
81. Willett WC, Manson JAE, Stampfer MJ, et al. Weight, weight change, and coronary heart disease in women. JAMA 1995; 273:461–465.
82. Rexrode KM, Carey VJ, Hennekens CH, et al. Abdominal adiposity and coronary heart disease in women. JAMA 1998; 280:1843–1848.
83. Folsom AR, Kushi LH, Anderson KE, et al. Associations of general and abdominal obesity with multiple health outcomes in older women. The Iowa Women's Health Study. Arch Intern Med 2000; 160:2117–2128.
84. Larsson B, Bengtsson C, Bjoerntorp P, et al. Is abdominal body fat distribution a major explanation for the sex difference in the incidence of myocardial infarction? The Study of Men Born in 1913 and the Study of Women, Goteborg, Sweden. Am J Epidemiol 1992; 135:266–273.
85. Stevens J, Keil JE, Rust PF, et al. Body mass index and body girths as predictors of mortality in black and white women. Arch Intern med 1992; 152:1257–1262.
86. Lovejoy JC, Smith SR, Rood JC. Comparison or regional fat distribution and health risk factors in middle-aged white and African American women: the healthy transitions study. Obes Res 2001; 9:10–16.
87. Williamson DF, Pamuk E, Thun M, Flanders D, Byers T, Heath C. Prospective study of intentional weight loss and mortality in never smoking overweight US white women aged 40–64 years. Am J Epidemiol 1995; 141:1128–1141.
88. Grundy SM, Brewer B, Cleeman JI, Smith SC, Lenfant C. For the conference participants. Definition of Metabolic Syndrome. Report of the National Heart, Lung, and Blood Institute/American Heart Association Conference on Scientific Issues Related to Definition. Circulation 2004; 109:433–438.
89. Kahn R, Buse J, Ferrannnini E, Stern M. The metabolic syndrome: time for a critical appraisal. Joint Statement from the American Diabetes Association and the European Association for the Study of Diabetes. Diabetes Care 2005; 28:2289–2304.
90. Ford ES, Giles WH, Dietz WH. Prevalence of the metabolic syndrome among US adults. Findings from the Third National Health and Nutrition Examination Survey. JAMA 2002; 287:356–359.
91. Malik S, Wong ND, Franklin SD, et al. Impact of the metabolic syndrome on mortality from coronary heart disease, cardiovascular disease, and all causes in United States adults. Circulation 2004; 110:1245–1250.
92. Hu G, Qiao Q, Tuomilehto, J, et al. For the DECODE study group. Prevalence of the metabolic syndrome and its relation to all cause and cardiovascular mortality in nondiabetic European men and women. Arch Intern Med 2004; 164:1066–1076.
93. Orchard TJ, Temprosa M, Goldberg R, et al. For the diabetes prevention program research group. The effect of metformin and intensive lifestyle intervention on the metabolic syndrome: the diabetes prevention program randomized trial. Ann Intern Med 2005; 142:611–619.
94. Kanaya AM, Grady D, Barrett-Connor E. Explaining the sex difference in coronary heart disease mortality among patients with Type 2 diabetes mellitus. Arch Intern Med 2002; 162:1737–1745.

95. Juutilainen A, Kortenlainen S, Lehto S, Roennemaa T, Pyorala K, Laakso M. Gender difference in the impact of Type II diabetes on coronary heart disease risk. Diabetes Care 2004; 27:2898–2904.

96. Natarajan S, Liao Y, Cao G, Lipsitz SR, McGee DL. Sex differences in risk for coronary heart disease mortality associated with diabetes and established coronary heart disease. Arch Intern Med 2003; 163:1735–1740.

97. Orencia A, Bailey K, Yawn BP, Kottke TE. Effect of gender on long-term outcome of angina pectoris and myocardial infarction/sudden unexpected death. JAMA 1993; 269:2392–2397.

98. Chaitman BR, Bourassa MG, Davis K, et al. Angiographic prevalence of high-risk coronary artery disease in patient subsets. The Collaborative Study in Coronary Artery Surgery (CASS). Circulation 1981; 64:360–367.

99. Natarajan S, Liao Y, Sinha D, CaoG, McGee DL, Lipsitz SR. Sex differences in the effect of diabetes duration on coronary heart disease mortality. Arch Intern Med 2005; 165:430–435.

100. Kanaya AM, Barrett-Connor E. The A, B, C, D, and E of diabetes and heart disease in women. The A, B, C, D, and E of diabetes and heart disease in women. In: Wenger NK, Collins P, eds. Women & Heart Disease. 2nd ed. London and New York: Taylor & Francis, 2005.

101. American Diabetes Association. Standards of medical care in diabetes. Diabetes Care 2005; 28: S1-S79 (also accessible at: http://care.diabetesjournals.org/content/vol28/suppl_1/; accessed 11/14/05).

102. Chobanian AV, Bakris GL, Black HR, et al. Seventh report of the joint national committee on prevention, detection, evaluation, and treatment of high blood pressure. Hypertension 2003; 42:1206–1252.

103. Wolf-Maier K, Cooper RS, Banegas JR, et al. Hypertension prevalence and blood pressure levels in 6 European countries, Canada, and the United States. JAMA 2003; 289:2363–2369.

104. Wang Y, Wang QJ. The prevalence of prehypertension and hypertension among US adults according to the new joint national committee guidelines. New challenges of the old problem. Arch Intern Med 2004; 164:2126–2134.

105. Vasan RS, Beiser A, Seshadri S, et al. Residual lifetime risk for developing hypertension in middle-aged women and men. The Framingham Heart Study. JAMA 2002; 287:1003–1010.

106. Lloyd-Jones DM, Evans JC, Larson MG, O'Donnell CJ, Wilson PWF, Levy D. Cross-classification of JNC VI blood pressure stages and risk groups in the Framingham heart study. Arch Intern Med 1999; 159:2206–2212.

107. Stamler J, Stamler R, Neaton JD. Blood pressure, systolic and diastolic and cardiovascular risks. US population data. Arch Intern Med 1993; 153:598–615.

108. Glynn RJ, Chae CU, Guralnik JM, Taylor JO, Hennekens CH. Pulse pressure and mortality in older people. Arch Intern Med 2000; 160:2765–2772.

109. Verdecchia P, Porcellati C, Schillaci G, et al. Ambulatory blood pressure. An independent predictor of prognosis in essential hypertension. Hypertension 1994; 24:793–801.

110. Staessen JA, Thijs L, Fagard R, et al. For the systolic hypertension in europe trial investigators. Predicting cardiovascular risk using conventional vs. ambulatory blood pressure in older patients with systolic hypertension. JAMA 1999; 282:539–546.

111. Hajjar I, Kotchen TA. Trends in prevalence, awareness, treatment and control of hypertension in the United States, 1988-2000. JAMA 2003; 290:199–206.

112. Wassertheil-Smoller S, Anderson G, Psaty BM, et al. Hypertension and its treatment in postmenopausal women: baseline data from the women's health initiative. Hypertension 2000; 36:780–789.

113. Kannel WB, D'Agostino RB, Sibershatz H. Blood pressure and cardiovascular morbidity and mortality rates in the elderly. Am Heart J 1997; 134:758–763.

114. Gueyffier F, Boutitie F, Boissel J-P, et al. Effect of antihypertensive drug treatment on cardiovascular outcomes in women and men: a meta-analysis of individual patient data from randomized, controlled trials. The INDANA Investigators. Ann Intern Med 1997; 126:761–767.

115. Lonn E, Roccaforte R, Yi Q, et al. Effect of long-term therapy with ramipril in high-risk women. J Am Coll Cardiol 2002; 40:693–702.

116. Dahlöf B, Devereux RB, Kjeldsen SE, et al. Cardiovascular morbidity and mortality in the losartan intervention for endpoint reduction in hypertension study (LIFE): a randomised trial against atenolol. Lancet 2002; 359:995–1003.

117. Blood Pressure Lowering Treatment Trialists' Collaboration. Effects of different blood-pressure-lowering regimens on major cardiovascular events: results of prospectively-designed overviews of randomised trials. Lancet 2003; 362:1527–1535.

118. World Health Organization, International Society of Hypertension Writing Group. 2003 World Health Organization (WHO)/International Society of Hypertension (ISH) statement on management of hypertension. J Hypertens 2003; 1983–1992.

119. Bittner V. State of the art paper: perspectives on dyslipidemia and coronary heart disease in women. J Am Coll Cardiol 2005; 46:1628–1635.

120. Expert Panel on Detection, Evaluation, and Treatment of High Blood Cholesterol in Adults. Second Report of the Expert Panel on Detection, Evaluation, and Treatment of High Blood Cholesterol in Adults. NIH Publication No. 93–3095, September 1993.

121. Gardner CD, Winkleby MA, Fortmann SP. Population frequency distribution of non-high density lipoprotein cholesterol (Third National Health and Nutrition Examination Survey NHANES III, 1988-1994). Am J Cardiol 2000; 86:299–304.

122. Schaefer EJ, Lamon-Fava S, Cohn SD, et al. Effects of age, gender, and menopausal status on plasma low density lipoprotein cholesterol and apolipoprotein B levels in the Framingham offspring study. J Lipid Res 1994; 35:779–792.

123. LaRosa JC. Lipoproteins and CAD risk in women. J Myocardial Ischemia 1991; 3:35–42.

124. National Heart, Lung, and Blood Institute. The Lipid Research Clinics Population Studies Data Book: Volume 1—The Prevalence Study. Bethesda, MD: U.S. Department of Health and Human Services, Public Health Service, National Institutes of Health, NIH Publication No. 80-1527, July 1980.

125. Freedman DS, Bowman BA, Srinivasan SR, Berenson GS, Otvos JD. Distribution and correlates of high-density lipoprotein subclasses among children and adolescents. Metabolism 2001; 50:370–376.

126. Gardner CD, Tribble DL, Young DR, Ahn D, Fortmann SP. Population frequency distributions of HDL, HDL(2), and HDL(3) cholesterol and apolipoproteins A-I and B in healthy men and women and associations with age, gender, hormonal status, and sex hormone use: the stanford five city project. Prev Med 2000; 31:335–345.

127. The Bezafibrate Infarction Prevention (BIP) Study Group, Israel. Lipids and lipoproteins in symptomatic coronary heart disease: distribution, intercorrelations, and significance for risk classification in 6,700 men and 2,500 women. Circulation 1992; 86:839–846.

128. Bittner V, Simon JA, Fong J, Blumenthal RS, Newby K, Stefanick ML. Correlates of high HDL cholesterol among women with coronary heart disease. Am Heart J 2000; 139:288–296.

129. Gosland IF, Wynn V, Crook D, Miller NE. Sex, plasma lipoproteins and atherosclerosis: prevailing assumptions and outstanding questions. Am Heart J 1997; 114:1467–1503.

130. Greenlund KJ, Webber LS, Srinivasan S, Wattigney W, Johnson C, Berenson GS. Associations of oral contraceptive use with serum lipids and lipoproteins in young women: the bogalusa heart study. Ann Epidemiol 1997; 7:561–567.

131. Godsland IF, Crook D, Simpson R, et al. The effects of different formulations of oral contraceptive agents on lipid and carbohydrate metabolism. N Engl J Med 1990; 323:1375–1381.

132. Foulon T, Payen N, Laporte F, et al. Effects of two low-dose oral contraceptives containing ethinylestradiol and either desogestrel or levonorgestrel on serum lipids and lipoproteins with particular regard to LDL size. Contraception 2001; 64:11–16.

133. Hulley S, Grady D, Bush T, et al. Randomized trial of estrogen plus progestin for secondary prevention of coronary heart disease in postmenopausal women. Heart and Estrogen/Progestin Replacement Study (HERS) research group. JAMA 1998; 280:605–613.

134. Grady D, Herrington D, Bittner V, et al. Cardiovascular disease outcomes during 6.8 years of hormone therapy: heart and estrogen/progestin replacement study follow-up (HERS II). JAMA 2002; 288:49–57.

135. Rossouw JE, Anderson GL, Prentice RL, et al. Risks and benefits of estrogen plus progestin in healthy postmenopausal women: principal results from the women's health initiative randomized controlled trial. Writing group for the Women's Health Initiative investigators. JAMA 2002; 288:321–333.

136. Manson JE, Hsia J, Johnson KC, et al. Estrogen plus progestin and the risk of coronary heart disease. Women's Health Initiative investigators. N Engl J Med 2003; 349:523–534.

137. The Women's Health Initiative Steering Committee. Effects of conjugated equine estrogen in postmenopausal women with hysterectomy. The Women's Health Initiative Randomized Controlled Trial. JAMA 2004; 291:1701–1712.

138. Manolio TA, Pearson TA, Wenger NK, Barrett-Connor E, Payne GH, Harlan WR. Cholesterol and heart disease in older persons and women. Review of an NHLBI workshop. Ann Epidemiol 1992; 2:161–176.

139. Hokanson JE, Austin MA. Plasma triglyceride level is a risk factor for cardiovascular disease independent of high-density lipoprotein cholesterol level: a meta-analysis of population-based prospective studies. J Cardiovascular Risk 1996; 3:213–219.

140. Cui Y, Blumenthal RS, Flaws JA, et al. Non-high-density lipoprotein cholesterol level as a predictor of cardiovascular disease mortality. Arch Intern Med 2001; 161:1413–1419.

141. Kamigaki AS, Siscovick DS, Schwartz SM, et al. Low density lipoprotein particle size and risk of early-onset myocardial infarction in women. Am J Epidemiol 2001; 153:939–945.

142. Mykkänen L, Kuusisto J, Haffner SM, Laakso M, Austin MA. LDL size and risk of coronary heart disease in elderly men and women. Arterioscler Thromb Vasc Biol 1999; 19:2742–2748.

143. Bostom AG, Gagnon DR, Cupples LA, et al. A prospective investigation of elevated lipoprotein (a) detected by electrophoresis and cardiovascular disease in women: the framingham heart study. Circulation 1994; 90:1688–1695.

144. Shlipak MG, Simon JA, Vittinghoff E, et al. Estrogen and progestin, lipoprotein(a), and the risk of recurrent coronary heart disease events after menopause. JAMA 2000; 283:1845–1852.

145. Heart Protection Study Collaborative Group. MRC/BHF Heart Protection Study of cholesterol lowering with simvastatin in 20 536 high-risk individuals: a randomized placebo-controlled trial. Lancet 2002; 360:7–22.

146. LaRosa JC, Grundy SM, Waters DD, et al. For the treating to new targets (TNT) investigators. Intensive lipid lowering with atorvastatin in patients with stable coronary disease. N Engl J Med 2005; 352:1425–1435.

147. Cannon CP, Braunwald E, McCabe CH, et al. For the pravastatin or atorvastatin evaluation and infection therapy-thrombolysis in myocardial infarction 22 investigators. Intensive versus moderate lipid lowering with statins after acute coronary syndromes. N Engl J Med 2004; 350:1495–1504.

148. Colhoun HM, Betteridge DJ, Durrington PN, et al. On behalf of the CARDS investigators. Primary prevention of cardiovascular disease with atorvastatin in type 2 diabetes in the Collaborative Atorvastatin Diabetes Study (CARDS): multicentre randomised placebo controlled trial. Lancet 2004; 364:685–696.
149. Walsh JME, Pignone M. Drug treatment of hyperlipidemia in women. JAMA 2004; 291:2243–2252.
150. Grady D et al. Diagnosis and Treatment of Coronary Heart Disease in Women: Systematic Reviews of Evidence on Selected Topics. Report Number 81. AHRQ Publication No. 03–E037, May 2003.
151. Lahad A, Heckbert SR, Koepsell TD, Psaty BM, Patrick DL. Hostility, aggression and the risk of nonfatal myocardial infarction in postmenopausal women. J Psychosomatic Research 1997; 43:183–195.
152. Suarez EC, Bates MP, Harralson TL. The relation of hostility to lipids and lipoproteins in women: evidence for the role of antagonistic hostility. Ann Behav Med 1998; 20:59–63.
153. Rutledge T, Reis SE, Olson M, et al. History of anxiety disorders is associated with a decreased likelihood of angiographic coronary artery disease in women with chest pain: the WISE study. J Am Coll Cardiol 2001; 37:780–785.
154. Paterniti S, Zureik M, Ducimetiere P, Touboul PJ, Feve JM, Alperovitch A. Sustained anxiety and 4-year progression of carotid atherosclerosis. Arterioscler Thromb Vasc Biol 2001; 21:136–141.
155. Shaw L, Johnson BD, Cooper-DeHoff R, et al. Importance of socioeconomic status as a predictor of cardiovascular outcome in women [abstr 3746]. Circulation 2005; 112:II-808.
156. Marmott MG, Bosma H, Hemingway H, Brunner E, Stansfeld S. Contribution of job control and other risk factors to social variations in coronary heart disease incidence. Lancet 1997; 350:235–239.
157. Orth Gomez K, Wamala SP, Horsten M, Schenck-Gustafsson K, Schneiderman N, Mittleman MA. Martial stress worsens prognosis in women with coronary heart disease. The Stockholm Female Coronary Risk Study. JAMA 2000; 284:3008–3014.
158. Schulz R, Beach SR. Caregiving as a risk factor for mortality. The Caregiver Health Effects Study. JAMA 1999; 282:2215–2219.
159. Ferketich AK, Schwartzbaum JA, Frid DJ, Moeschberger ML. Depression as an antecedent to heart disease among women and men in the NHANES I Study. Arch Intern Med 2000; 160:1261–1268.
160. Whooley MA, Browner WS. For the study of osteoporotic fractures research group. Association between depressive symptoms and mortality in older women. Arch Intern Med 1998; 158:2129–2135.
161. Schulz R, Beach SR, Ives DG, Martire LM, Ariyo AA, Kop WJ. Association between depression and mortality in older adults. The Cardiovascular Health Study. Arch Intern Med 2000; 160:1761–1768.
162. Wassertheil-Smoller S, Applegate WB, Berge K, et al. for the SHEP Cooperative Research Group. Change in depression as a precursor of cardiovascular events. Arch Intern Med 1996; 156:553–561.
163. Sheps DS, Rozanski A, eds. Depression and heart disease: epidemiology, pathophysiology and treatment. Psychosom Med 2005; 67(suppl 1):S1–S73.
164. Frasure Smith N, Lesperance F, Prince RH, et al. Randomized trial of home-based psychosocial nursing intervention for patients recovering from myocardial infarction. Lancet 1997; 350:473–479.
165. Writing Committee of the ENRICHD Investigators. Effects of treating depression and low perceived social support on clinical events after myocardial infarction. The Enhancing Recovery in Myocardial Infarction Patients (ENRICHD) Randomized Trial. JAMA 2003; 289:3106–3116.
166. Glassman AH, O'Connor CM, Califf RM, et al. Sertraline treatment of major depression in patients with acute MI or unstable angina. JAMA 2002; 288:701–709.
167. Makkar RR, Fromm BS, Steinman RT, Meissner MD, Lehmann MH. Female gender as a risk factor for torsades de pointes associated with cardiovascular drugs. JAMA 1993; 270:2590–2597.
168. Losordo DW, Kearney M, Kim EA, Jekanowski J, Isner JM. Variable expression of the estrogen receptor in normal and atherosclerotic coronary arteries of premenopausal women. Circulation 1994; 89:1501–1510.
169. Shearman AM, Cupples LA, Demissie S, et al. Association between estrogen receptor alpha gene variation and cardiovascular disease. JAMA 2003; 290:2263–2270.
170. Schuit SCE, Oei HH, Witteman JCM, et al. Estrogen receptor alpha gene polymorphisms and risk of myocardial infarction. JAMA 2004; 291:2969–2977.
171. Ferrero Va, Ribichini F, Matullo G, et al. Estrogen receptor alpha polymorphisms and angiographic outcome after coronary artery stenting. Arterioscler Trhomb Vasc Biol 2003; 23:2223–2228.
172. Herrington DA, McClain BP. Sex hormones and normal cardiovascular physiology. In: Wenger NK, Collins P, eds. Women & Heart Disease. 2nd ed. London and New York: Taylor & Francis, 2005.
173. Kawano H, Motoyama T, Ohgushi M, Kugiyama K, Ogawa H, Yasue H. Menstrual cyclic variation of myocardial ischemia in premenopausal women with variant angina. Ann Intern Med 2001; 135:977–981.
174. Rodriguez I, Kilborn MJ, Liu XK, Pezzullo JC, Woosley RL. Drug-induced QT prolongation in women during the menstrual cycle. JAMA 2001; 285:1322–1326.
175. Bairey Merz CN, Johnson BD, Sharaf BL, et al. For the WISE study group. Hypothalamic hypoestrogenemia and coronary artery disease in premenopausal women: a report from the NHLBI–sponsored WISE study. J Am Coll Cardiol 2003; 41:413–419.
176. Punnonen R, Jokela H, Aine R, Teisala K, Salomaeki A, Uppa H. Impaired ovarian function and risk factors for atherosclerosis in premenopausal women. Maturitas 1997; 27:231–238.
177. Hanke H, Hanke S, Ickrath O, et al. Estradiol concentrations in premenopausal women with coronary heart disease. Coron Artery Dis 1997; 8:511–515.

178. Wild RA. Polycystic ovary syndrome: a risk for coronary artery disease? Am J Obstet Gynecol 2002; 186:35–43.
179. Godsland IF. The metabolic syndrome in postmenopausal women. In: Stimpel M, Zanchetti A, eds. Hypertension After Menopause. Berlin/New York: De Gruyter, 1997:43–51.
180. Carr MC. The emergence of the metabolic syndrome with menopause. J Clin Endocrinol Metab 2003; 88:2404–2411.
181. Tunstall-Pedoe H. Myth and paradox of coronary risk and the menopause. The Lancet 1998; 351:1425–1427.
182. Hu FB, Grodstein F, Hennekens CH, et al. Age at natural menopause and risk of cardiovascular disease. Arch Intern Med 1999; 159:1061–1066.
183. Jacobsen BK, Knutsen SF, Fraser GE. Age at natural menopause and total mortality and mortality from ischemic heart disease: The Adventist Health Study. J Clin Epidemiol 1999; 52:4:303–307.
184. Hak AE, Pols HAP, van Hemert AM, Hofman A, Witteman JCM. Progression of aortic calcification is associated with metacarpal bone loss during menopause. A population-based longitudinal study. Arterioscler Thromb Vasc Biol 2000; 20:1926–1931.
185. Tallova J, Tomandl J, Bicikova M, Hill M. Changes of plasma total homocysteine levels during the menstrual cycle. Eur J Clin Invest 1999; 29:1041–1044.
186. Hak AE, Polderman KH, Westendorp ICD, et al. Increased plasma homocysteine after menopause. Atherosclerosis 2000; 149:163–168.
187. The Homocysteine Studies Collaboration. Homocysteine and risk of ischemic heart disease and stroke. A meta-analysis. JAMA 2002; 288:2015–2022.
188. Klerk M, Verhoef P, Clarke R, Blom HJ, Kok FJ, Schouten EG. And the MTHFR studies collaboration group. MTHFR 677C→T polymorphism and risk of coronary heart disease. A meta-analysis. JAMA 2002; 288:2023–2031.
189. Hoogeveen EK, Kostense PJ, Jakobs C, et al. Hyperhomocysteinemia increases risk of death, especially in Type 2 diabetes. 5-year follow-up of the Hoorn Study. Circulation 2000; 101:1506–1511.
190. Foody JAM, Milberg JA, Robinson K, Pearce GL, Jacobsen DW, Sprecher DL. Homocysteine and lipoprotein(a) interact to increase CAD risk in young men and women. Arterioscler Thromb Vasc Biol 2000; 20:493–499.
191. Loria CM, Ingram DD, Feldman JJ, Wright JD, Madans JH. Serum folate and cardiovascular disease mortality among US men and women. Arch Intern Med 2000; 160:3258–3262.
192. Rimm EB, Willett WC, Hu FB, et al. Folate and vitamin B6 from diet and supplements in relation to risk of coronary heart disease among women. JAMA 1998; 279:359–364.
193. Brouwer IA, van Dusseldorp M, Thomas CMG, et al. Low-dose folic acid supplementation decreases plasma homocysteine concentrations: a randomized trial. Am J Clin Nutr 1999; 69:99–104.
194. Wald DS, Bishop L, Wald NJ, et al. Randomized trial of folic acid supplementation and serum homocysteine levels. Arch Intern Med 2001; 161:695–700.
195. Danesh J, Wheeler JG, Hirschfield GM, et al. C-reactive protein and other circulating marker of inflammation in the prediction of coronary heart disease. N Engl J Med 2004; 350:1387–1397.
196. Pearson TA, Mensah GA, Alexander RW, et al. Markers of inflammation and cardiovascular disease. Application to clinical and public health practice. A Statement for Healthcare Professionals From the Centers for Disease Control and Prevention and the American Heart Association. Circulation 2003; 107:499–511.
197. Cushman M, Legault C, Barrett-Connor E, et al. Effect of postmenopausal hormones on inflammation-sensitive proteins. The Postmenopausal Estrogen/Progestin Intervention (PEPI) Study. Circulation 1999; 100:717–722.
198. Ridker PM, Rifai N, Clearfield M, et al. Measurement of C-reactive protein for the targeting of statin therapy in the primary prevention of acute coronary events. N Engl J Med 2001; 344:1959–1965.
199. Ridker PM, Cannon CP, Morrow D, et al. C-reactive protein levels and outcomes after statin therapy. N Engl J Med 2005; 352:20–28.
200. Nissen SE, Tuzcu EM, Schoenhagen P, et al. Statin therapy, LDL cholesterol, C-reactive protein, and coronary artery disease. N Engl J Med 2005; 352:29–38.
201. Kannel WB. Risk factors for cardiovascular disease in women. Cardiol Rev 2001; 18:11–16.
202. Wilson PWF, Kannel WB, Silbershatz H, D'Agostino RB. Clustering of metabolic factors and coronary heart disease. Arch Intern Med 1999; 159:1104–1109.
203. Stamler J, Stamler R, Neaton JD, et al. Low risk-factor profile and long-term cardiovascular and noncardiovascular mortality and life expectancy. Findings for 5 large cohorts of young adult and middle-aged men and women. JAMA 1999; 282:2012–2018.
204. Wilson PWF, D'Agostino RB, Levy D, Belanger AM, Silbershatz H, Kannel WB. Prediction of coronary heart disease using risk factor categories. Circulation 1998; 97:1837–1847.
205. D'Agostino RB, Russell MW, Huse DM, et al. Primary and subsequent coronary risk appraisal: new results from the Framingham study. Am Heart J 2000; 139:272–281.
206. Jackson R. Updated New Zealand cardiovascular disease risk-benefit prediction guide. BMJ 2000; 320:709–710.
207. Conroy RM, Pyorala K, Fitzgerald AP, et al. Estimation of ten-year risk of fatal cardiovascular disease in Europe: the SCORE project. Eur Heart J 2003; 24:987–1003.

208. British Cardiac Society, British Hyperlipidaemia Association, British Hypertension Society, endorsed by the British Diabetic Association. Joint British recommendations on prevention of coronary heart disease in clinical practice. Heart 1998; 80:1–29.

209. Stevens RJ, Kothari V, Adler AI, Stratton IM. The UKPDS risk engine: a model for the risk of coronary heart disease in Type II diabetes (UKPDS 56). Clin Sci (Lond) 2001:101:671–679.

210. Marchioli R, Avanzini F, Barzi F, et al. Assessment of absolute risk of death after myocardial infarction by use of multiple-risk-factor assessment equations. GISSI Prevenzione mortality risk chart. Eur Heart J 2001; 22:2085–2103.

211. D'Agostino RB, Grundy S, Sullivan LM, Wilson P. For the CHD risk prediction group. Validation of the Framingham Coronary Heart Disease Prediction Scores. JAMA 2001; 286:180–187.

212. Liao Y, McGee DL, Cooper RS. Prediction of coronary heart disease mortality in blacks and whites: pooled data from two national cohorts. Am J Cardiol 1999; 84:31–36.

213. Liu J, Hong Y, D'Agostino RB, Wu Z, et al. Predictive value for the Chinese population of the Framingham CHD risk assessment tool compared with the Chinese multi–provincial cohort study. JAMA 2004; 291:2591–2599.

214. Hensea HW, Schulte H, Loewel H, Assmann G, Keila U. Framingham risk function overestimates risk of coronary heart disease in men and women from Germany—results from the MONICA Augsburg and the PROCAM cohorts. Eur Heart J 2003; 24:937–945.

215. Cappuccio FP, Oakeshott P, Strazzullo P, Kerry SM. Application of Framingham risk estimates to ethnic minorities in United Kingdom and implications for primary prevention of heart disease in general practice: cross sectional population based study. BMJ 2002; 325:1271–1276.

216. Williams B, Poulter NR, Brown MJ, et al. British Hypertension Society Guidelines. Guidelines for management of hypertension: report of the fourth working party of the British Hypertension Society, 2004—BHS IV. J Human Hypertension 2004; 18:139–185.

217. Pasternak RC, Abrams J, Greenland P, Smaha LA, Wilson PWF, Houston-Miller N. Task force #1 – identification of coronary heart disease risk: is there a detection gap? J Am Coll Cardiol 2004; 41:1863–1874.

218. National Heart Lung and Blood Institute. http://hin.nhlbi.nih.gov/atpiii/riskcalc.htm (accessed 12/10/05).

219. Greenland P, LaBree L, Azen SP, Doherty TM, Detrano RC. Coronary artery calcium score combined with Framingham score for risk prediction in asymptomatic individuals. JAMA 2004; 291:210–215.

220. Greenland P, Knoll MD, Stamler J, et al. Major risk factors as antecedents of fatal and nonfatal coronary heart disease events. JAMA 2003; 290:891–897.

221. Yusuf S, Hawken S, Ôunpuu S, et al. On behalf of the INTERHEART study investigators. Effect of potentially modifiable risk factors associated with myocardial infarction in 52 countries (the INTERHEART study): case-control study. Lancet 2004; 364:937–952.

222. ACOG Task Force on Hormone Therapy. Hormone Therapy. Obstetrics & Gynecology 2004; 104(suppl):S1–S129.

223. Ridker PM, Cook NR, Lee IM, et al. A randomized trial of low-dose aspirin in the primary prevention of cardiovascular disease in women. N Engl J Med 2005; 352:1293–1304.

224. Mosca L, Linfante AH, Benjamin EJ, et al. National study of physician awareness and adherence to cardiovascular disease prevention guidelines. Circulation 2005; 111:499–510.

225. Wizemann TM, Pardue ML, eds. Exploring the Biological Contributions to Human Health: Does Sex Matter? Committee on Understanding the Biology of Sex and Gender Differences. Board on Health Sciences Policy, Institute of Medicine. Washington, DC: National Academy Press, 2001.

21 | Cardiovascular Disease in Racial and Ethnic Minorities

Keith C. Ferdinand
Association of Black Cardiologists, Atlanta, Georgia, U.S.A.

Annemarie Armani
Critical Pathways in Cardiology, Boston, Massachusetts, U.S.A.

KEY POINTS

- Cardiovascular disease (CVD) and associated risk factors such as hypertension, dyslipidemia, diabetes, and obesity disproportionately affect certain racial/ethnic populations in the United States. There is evidence of distinct variations of CVD morbidity and mortality based on racial/ethnic status, potentially related to social and environmental factors.
- African Americans have the highest rates of coronary heart disease (CHD) death, more premature death, including sudden death, stroke, hypertension, type 2 diabetes, and obesity.
- CVD data for Hispanics, defined based on ethnicity versus a racial characteristic, are accumulating, which is clinically important as they are the largest and perhaps fastest growing racial/ethnic minority in the United States. High rates of obesity and cardiometabolic syndrome suggest a potential increase in CHD prevalence in the future.
- Recent data indicate that American-Indian groups may be at high risk for CVD. More data are needed on the rates of cardiovascular morbidity and mortality in Asian and Pacific Islander groups.
- Although the United States is defined as a melting pot of diversity, there remain unacceptable health care disparities in risk factor prevalence, disease states, and cardiovascular outcomes.

INTRODUCTION

Cardiovascular disease (CVD) is the leading cause of death in the United States and other industrialized societies. Specifically, coronary heart disease (CHD), stroke, and associated risk factors such as hypertension, dyslipidemia, diabetes, and obesity disproportionately affect certain racial/ethnic populations in the United States. Race itself is not a scientific category, but a demographic term utilized by social scientists, historians, statisticians, and others. Indeed, the Human Genome Project demonstrates that, to a large extent, there is greater variation within previously described racial categories versus across self-identified groupings. Nevertheless, potentially related to social and environmental factors, including socioeconomic status (SES), there appears to be distinct variations of cardiovascular morbidity and mortality based on racial/ethnic status. African Americans, or blacks, have the highest rates of CHD death, more premature death, including sudden death, stroke (fatal and nonfatal), hypertension, type 2 diabetes and obesity (especially black females), when compared to whites. There are more data available for the degree and severity of CVD in African Americans versus other described racial/ethnic groups. Hispanics are defined based on ethnicity versus a racial characteristic, per se. Data are accumulating, documenting this group, which is defined as the largest and perhaps fastest growing racial/ethnic minority in the United States. Recent data indicate that American-Indian groups may be at high risk for CVD. More data are needed on the rates of cardiovascular morbidity and mortality in Asian and Pacific Islander groups. Nevertheless, it is clear that these are markedly heterogeneous populations in whom racial/ethnic characteristics should be determined with caution, if at all.

Perhaps the most compelling argument for documenting cardiovascular morbidity and mortality in various racial/ethnic groups is the unfortunate reality that although the United States and most western societies are defined as melting pots of diversity, there remain unacceptable health care disparities in risk factor prevalence, disease states, and cardiovascular outcomes. Furthermore, because minority groups in the United States are antic-ipated to grow in size, and may become almost 50% of the U.S. population by the year 2050, it is imperative that the collection of data and the reporting of clinical trials appropriately reflect potential differences in drug response or disease manifestation in various groups.

EPIDEMIOLOGY OF RACE

Of the more than 285 million people counted by the 2004 Census (1) as U.S. residents, over 216 million are classified as white, comprising 75.6% of the population (Fig. 1). Of the racial groups, 12.2% are defined as black (34,772,381), 4.2% as Asian (12,097,281), 0.8% as American-Indian or Alaska Natives (2,151,322) and 0.1% as Native Hawaiian (403,832). Over 14 million people, or 5.2%, consider themselves as "some other race" and 5.4 million, or 1.9%, classify themselves as two or more races. Those classified as Hispanic or Latinos of any race comprise 14.2% of the population (40.4 million people) and are listed separately, because Hispanic is not a racial category but an ethnicity. The federal government has since realized that race and Hispanic origin are two separate and distinct concepts. Therefore, the Office of Management and Budget (OMB)'s federal standard for self-designation includes race: American Indian or Alaska Native, Asian, black or African American, Native Hawaiian or other Pacific Islander, and white, some other race, two or more races; and for ethnicity: Hispanic or Latino; not Hispanic or Latino.

The race categories presently used are defined as: "White" refers to people having origins in any of the original peoples of Europe, the Middle East, or North Africa. "Black or African-American" refers to those having origins in any of the black racial groups of Africa. Although this group is predominantly comprised of descendants of Africans brought to the United States during the slave era, it also includes more recent migrants primarily from Africa and the Caribbean. "American-Indian and Alaska Native" refers to those having origins in any of the native or original peoples of North and South America (including Central America), and who maintain tribal affiliation or community attachment. "Asian" refers to those having origins in any of the original peoples of the Far East, Southeast Asia, or the Indian subcontinent, includ-ing for example, Cambodia, China, India, Japan, Korea, Malaysia, Pakistan, the Philippine Islands, Thailand, and Vietnam. "Native Hawaiian and Other Pacific Islander" refers to those having origins in any of the original peoples of Hawaii, Guam, Samoa, or other Pacific Islands. The term Native Hawaiian does not include individuals native to the state of Hawaii by virtue of being born there. "Some other race" was added for respondents who felt unable to identify with the five OMB race categories, and include for example write-in entries such as Moroccan, South African, or a Hispanic origin (for example, Mexican, Puerto Rican, or Cuban).

"Hispanic or Latino" refers to a person of Cuban, Mexican, Puerto Rican, South or Central American (non-indigenous), or other Spanish culture or origin, regardless of race. They are also asked to report the race or races they considered themselves to be. Although grouped together, *Hispanic* actually refers to those who derive from the mostly white Iberian Peninsula

(A)

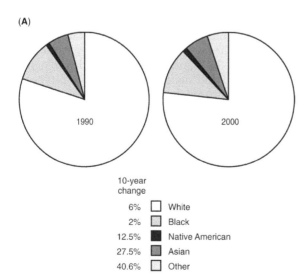

10-year change		
6%	☐	White
2%	☐	Black
12.5%	■	Native American
27.5%	▨	Asian
40.6%	☐	Other

FIGURE 1 (**A**) U.S. population trends by race and ethnicity. *On facing page*: (**B**) U.S. demographic prevalence by all race and Hispanic or Latino origin. (**C**) U.S. demo-graphic minority prevalence by all race and Hispanic or Latino origin. *Source*: Courtesy of U.S. Census Bureau.

(B)

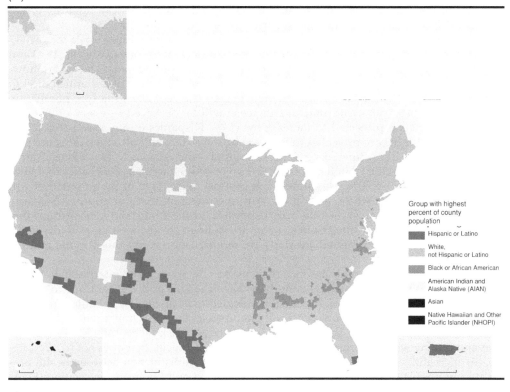

Group with highest
percent of county
population

Hispanic or Latino

White,
not Hispanic or Latino

Black or African American

American Indian and
Alaska Native (AIAN)

Asian

Native Hawaiian and Other
Pacific Islander (NHOPI)

(C)

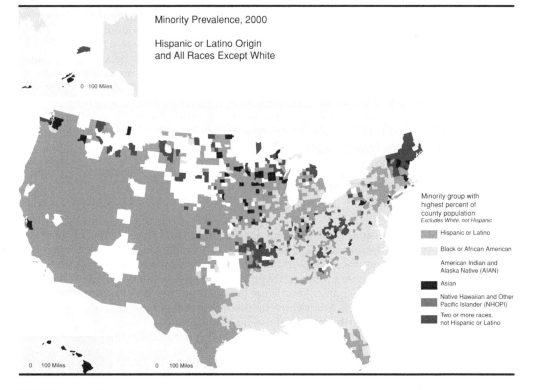

Minority Prevalence, 2000

Hispanic or Latino Origin
and All Races Except White

0 100 Miles

Minority group with
highest percent of
county population
Excludes White, not Hispanic

Hispanic or Latino

Black or African American

American Indian and
Alaska Native (AIAN)

Asian

Native Hawaiian and Other
Pacific Islander (NHOPI)

Two or more races,
not Hispanic or Latino

0 100 Miles   0 100 Miles

FIGURE 1   (*Continued*)

that includes Spain and Portugal (i.e., European), and *Latino* derives from the brown indigenous people of the Americas (Mexico, Central America, and South America). Interestingly, in 2000, 9 out of 10 Hispanics or Latinos self-reported "white" or "some other race."

Because of the recent addition of "some other race" having multiple totals for racial/ethnic categories portends that comparisons of population growth rates between 1990 and 2000 will vary, and have made meaningful population trends problematic. One point, however, is becoming increasing clear. The minority groups in this country are anticipated to continue to increase. The census bureau predicts that by the year 2050, the U.S. population will increase by almost 50%, and that this increase will be observed in every ethnic and racial group: Asians are projected to increase by 213%, Hispanics of any race projected to increase by 188%, blacks are projected to increase by over 70%, and all other races are predicted to increase by 217% (including American-Indian and Alaska Native alone, Native Hawaiian and Other Pacific Islander alone, and Two or More Races), as compared to whites who will only increase by 30%. Therefore, each groups' percentage of the population will rise, except for the whites who will decline. With the direction that our country is clearly headed, the fact that there exists health- care disparities for the ethnic and racial groups that comprise the mosaic of the United States, a country defined by its "melting pot" diversity, is entirely unacceptable and immediate steps are required to remedy this chronic and yet acute problem.

Clearly, researchers and clinicians face challenges in the writing and interpreting of medical literature about race and ethnicity: definitions have changed and will continue to change as fast as the populations do, although probably doomed to be always steps behind, nonetheless making meaningful comparisons practically impossible; the sheer limitations in race/ethnicity data itself; differentiating between race/ethnicity as a risk factor rather versus a risk marker; and finding ways to write-in medicine about race/ethnicity that does not (i) overcategorize, (ii) stigmatize, and (iii) even oversuggest some sort of distinction between health professionals and populations of color. Most recently, the Food and Drug Administration (FDA) released their guidance (2) recommending the use of a standardized approach for collecting and reporting race and ethnicity information in clinical trials. This recommended standardized approach was that which had been developed by the OMB, and its suggested categories for race and ethnicity. For the sake of this chapter, the terminology used to define racial/ethnic groups is consistent with that of the FDA's guidance. Although unfortunately there appears to be undeniable health and health care issues for minority, racial and ethnic groups across innumerable disease states, for the purposes of this chapter, we will restrict ourselves to those of cardiovascular risk, health and disease. Additionally, this chapter may appear as though it is more detailed or complete with regard to information regarding African Americans, which only further attests to the marked paucity in good data regarding the other racial and ethnic groups. This chapter intends to assemble all existing data to date, but also to call attention to the areas where the knowledge base is still drastically lacking.

CARDIOVASCULAR MORBIDITY AND MORTALITY
IN RACIAL/ETHNIC GROUPS
Mortality

CVD persists as the leading cause of death in the United States, and this remains particularly true among each of the different racial/ethnic populations (Fig. 2). There are, however, important differences between the racial/ethnic groups with regard to cardiovascular morbidity and mortality. Among these groups, African Americans experience the highest rate of mortality from heart disease. Hispanic Americans face double the risk of dying of diabetes compared to all others and Native Americans die disproportionately from diabetes as well. Furthermore, cardiovascular death impacts these minority groups at younger ages (Fig. 3) (4). In 2001, the number of premature deaths (<65 years) due to CVD was highest among American-Indians or Alaska Natives (36%) and blacks (31.5%) and lowest among whites (14.7%). Hispanics' rate of premature death was higher (23.5%) than non-Hispanics (16.5%), and among them, Hispanic blacks were shown to have higher rates (27.5%) than Hispanic whites (23.3%). Similarly, non-Hispanic blacks were also shown to have higher premature death rates (31.5%) than non-Hispanic whites (14.4%) (5). Yearly totals of out-of-hospital deaths due to cardiovascular disease in people ages 15 to 34 were also shown to be higher

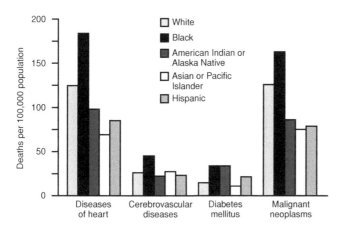

FIGURE 2 Age-adjusted death rates for selected causes of death by ethnicity, United States, 1950–1998. *Source*: From Ref. 3. © 2002 by the National Academy of Sciences, courtesy of the National Academics Press, Washington, D.C.

among young African Americans than among Caucasians (6). Although there has fortunately been a steady decline in years of potential life lost to CVD over the last two decades among blacks and whites, years lost among black men and women remain considerably greater than years lost among their white counterparts (Fig. 4) (7). Asians, attesting to the marked heterogeneity of this designation, experience differing rates of CHD death, as shown in (Fig. 5).

For the most part, Asian groups, such as the Vietnamese and Japanese, experience relatively low rates of CHD death, but emerging is information regarding South Asians and their incredibly increased risk of cardiovascular death. There are limited data available in the United States as of yet, but one American study (8) suggests that Asian Indians in California have the highest proportional mortality ratios for CHD, reflective of the higher percentage of CHD deaths compared with all cause deaths in this group, as compared with non-Hispanic white, Hispanic, non-Hispanic black, Chinese, Japanese, and Asian Indian Americans. Most South Asian cardiovascular data is attained from the United Kingdom, where it is known that South Asians living in the United Kingdom are also 50% more likely to die from heart disease than the general population (9).

Stroke is the third leading cause of death in the United States and a foremost cause of severe, long-term disability. African Americans (10,11), American-Indians or Alaska Natives (12) and Mexican-Americans (13), have a higher than average stroke risk. Compared with whites, young African Americans face three times the risk of ischemic stroke and four times the risk of stroke death (14). The death rate due to stroke is significantly high in the southeastern United States for the general population, and notably for blacks (15), earning 23 states the designation of the "Stroke Belt" from the National Heart, Lung, and Blood Institute (NHLBI) (16). The Center for Disease Control's report maintained that a greater proportion

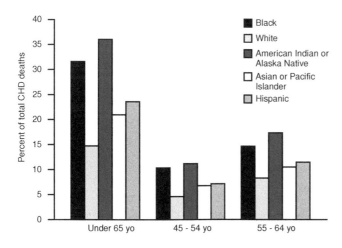

FIGURE 3 Premature death from coronary heart disease varies between ethnicities. *Source*: From Ref. 4 with permission of Lippincott, Williams, and Wilkins.

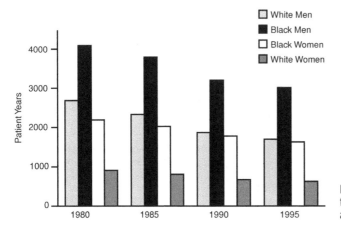

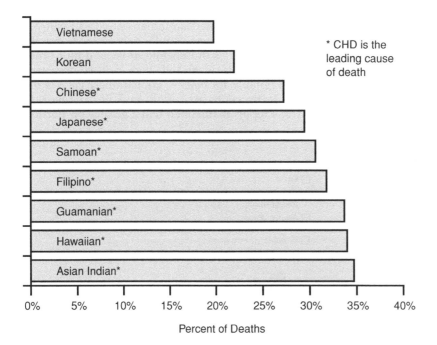

FIGURE 4 Years of potential life lost to total heart disease before age 75, by race and sex. *Source*: From Ref. 7.

of African- Americans live in these southeastern states, more so than elsewhere in the country (Fig. 1C) as well as acknowledged that variations in socioeconomic characteristics and risk factors were also associated with disparities in stroke, and these variations have been associated with region and race (17).

In women, CVD is the leading cause of death, although in an American Heart Association survey (18), only 13% of women were found to consider heart disease their greatest health risk. Unfortunately, racial disparity may become even more remarkable when specifically considering gender. Despite declining death rates from heart disease over the past 50 years, diseases of the heart remain the major cause of death for all females, except Asian and Pacific Islander females, for whom they are the second major cause of death. The largest disparity can clearly be seen between white women and black women. Whereas age-adjusted mortality due to heart disease is 19% greater for black men compared with white men, black women are one third more likely to die from heart disease than white women (19). In comparison to the 2002 overall death rate from CVD of 320.5, death rates were 265.6 for white females and yet 368.1 for

FIGURE 5 Coronary heart disease as cause of death in Asians. *Source*: Courtesy of National Vital Statistics System, CDC, NCHS.

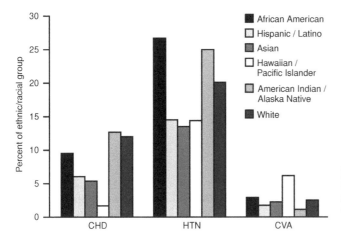

FIGURE 6 Cardiovascular disease across racial and ethnic groups. *Abbreviations*: CHD, coronary heart disease; HTN, hypertension; CVA, cardiovascular accident. *Source*: From Ref. 20.

black females (20). Using Cox proportional hazards models from the 2699 women enrolled in the Heart and Estrogen/progestin Replacement Study (HERS) study, it was shown that black women with coronary artery disease were twice as likely to sustain a CHD event and had higher mortality than white women, 16% (34 deaths) versus 8% (205 deaths) ($p < 0.001$) (21).

Morbidity

Amongst African Americans, 9.6% have heart disease, 26.7% have hypertension and 2.9% have had a stroke. Among Hispanics or Latinos, 6.1% have heart disease, 14.5% have hypertension and 1.8% has had a stroke. Among Asians, 5.4% have heart disease, 13.5% have hypertension and 2.2% have had a stroke. Among Native Hawaiians or other Pacific Islanders, 1.6% has heart disease, 14.5% have hypertension and 6.3% have had a stroke. Among American-Indians or Aleutian Islanders Alaska Natives, 12.6% have heart disease, 25.0% have hypertension and 1.1% has had a stroke. Among whites only, 12.2% have heart disease, 20.1% have hypertension and 2.4% have had a stroke (Fig. 6) (22).

African Americans and CVD

African Americans have the highest overall CHD mortality rate and rate of sudden cardiac death as an initial manifestation of CHD of any ethnic group in the United States, particularly at younger ages. The 2002 overall preliminary death rate from CVD was 320.5. The rates were 373.8 for white males and 492.5 for black males; 265.6 for white females and 368.1 for black females (20). In addition, African Americans are more likely to be at high risk for CHD because of a greater prevalence of multiple or "clustering" of CHD risk factors. Hypertension is a particularly powerful risk factor for CHD in blacks, especially in black women. In contrast, diabetes is a weaker predictor of CHD in blacks than in whites (23). The rate of hypertension in blacks in the United States is among the highest in the world. Compared with whites, blacks are much more likely to be hypertensive, less likely to be physically active, more likely to be overweight or obese, and more likely to have diabetes (20). Death rates per 100,000 due to CHD are 272 and 193 for African American men and women, compared with 249 and 153 for white men and women, claiming the lives of 36.4% of all U.S. deaths in blacks each year. In fact, death rates due to CHD in African Americans are the highest in the world (24). Figure 2 demonstrates the marked contrast in cardiovascular death rates among blacks versus all other racial and ethnic groups. These differences reflect a black/white mortality ratio of 1.6 times, which is disturbingly unimproved from that of, for example, the black/white mortality ratio in 1950 in the United States (25).

Over 40% of non-Hispanic black adults have CVD[a] (41.1% of black men/44.7% of black women) (26). There is clear separation between black and white men and between black and white women with regard to rates of first myocardial infarction by age, as shown in (Fig. 7).

---

[a]Including CHD, hypertension and/or stroke. Estimates are age-adjusted.

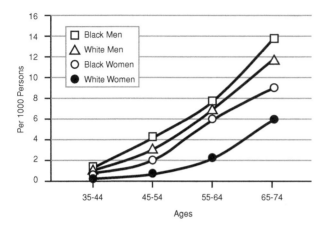

FIGURE 7 Annual rate of first myocardial infarction by age, race, and sex. *Source*: From Ref. 27.

African Americans experience almost twice the risk of first-ever stroke compared with whites (10,11). Between 1980 and 1999, African Americans were shown to be at more than 70% greater risk for a stroke hospitalization as compared with whites (28). In 2002, the overall death rate for stroke was 56.2, and yet for blacks were 81.7 for males and 71.8 for females. Furthermore, when compared with the non-Hispanic whites, non-Hispanic blacks have higher risk of stroke earlier; four times higher risk of stroke at ages 35 to 54, three times higher at ages 55 to 64 and still almost two times higher at ages 65 to 74. Only at ages 75 and older, does the risk of stroke begin to assimilate to that of the white population (17). Even in children, compared to the stroke risk of white children, black children have an increased relative risk of 2.12, and this increased risk among blacks has been shown not to be explained by their increased risk for sickle cell disease (29).

The racial disparities between black and white Americans are even more pronounced among women. Whereas age adjusted mortality due to heart disease is 19% greater for black men compared with white men, black women are one third more likely to die from heart disease than white women (19). Black women have higher CVD risk factors than white women, even of comparable SES (30). The HERS study recently confirmed that black women with CHD have 50% higher adjusted risk for nonfatal myocardial infarction as well as CHD death as compared with white women (21).

American Indians/Alaskan Natives and CVD

CVD is the leading cause of death among American-Indians/Alaskan Natives and has been for decades. Previous reports have suggested that CVD mortality for American-Indians and Alaska Natives was considerably lower than the general U.S. population. These results, however, have been in disaccord with their significantly high prevalence rates of important cardiovascular risk factors such as smoking, diabetes, and obesity. In addition, mortality rates appeared to rise significantly during the 1990s, unlike for those of the other racial and ethnic groups. It was also realized that previous data might have been be faulty due to possible racial and/or event misclassification. Therefore, the Strong Heart Study (SHS), was created and has been supported by the NHLBI since 1988, and is the largest epidemiological study of American-Indians to date. The SHS has confirmed that CVD incidence and mortality rates are as bad as or worse than those in comparable general populations (12). A recent study of American-Indians and whites from Montana (31) has confirmed that American Indians have significantly higher heart-disease (283/100,000 vs. 216/100,000) and stroke (81/100,000 vs. 60/100,000) death rates as compared to whites. It was also reported that despite the fact that heart-disease and stroke mortality has been declining in whites over the past 10 years, there has been no such decline in the American-Indian population. Among American-Indians/Alaska Natives, over 60% of adults (63.7% of men/61.4% of women) have one or more CVD risk factors, including hypertension, cigarette smoking, hypercholesterolemia, obesity or diabetes. It is noted that had data on physical activity been included in the analysis, the prevalence of risk factors in all probability would have been significantly higher (32). Of 100 American-Indian men aged 45 to 74, it is thought that 17 to 25 of them have some evidence of heart disease (12).

American-Indians/Alaska Natives increased risk of stroke is apparent in all the three stroke subtypes than whites (33) (ischemic stroke, subarachnoid hemorrhage and intracerebral hemorrhage). They have higher relative risk of stroke death; almost two times higher at ages 35 to 44; 1.3 times higher at ages 45 to 54; and 1.5 times higher at ages 55 to 64. After the age of 65, the risk actually appears to be lower; 0.9 at ages 65 to 84 and 0.4 at age 85 and older (17).

ASIAN OR PACIFIC ISLANDERS AND CVD

Unfortunately, epidemiological information for this heterogeneous group remains problematic. Most U.S. epidemiological data group together all Asians, ranging from the Japanese at low cardiovascular risk to Southeast Asians with remarkably high cardiovascular risk. The rates of CHD as cause of death in the various Asian populations are shown in Figure 5. Furthermore, the international data set available for each population is very difficult to be extrapolated, as these groups' cardiovascular risk, morbidity and mortality seem particularly vulnerable to "westernization," thereby suggesting their rates of heart disease reflects a disease of migration. The Honolulu Heart Program was designed to investigate the disparities in the rates of heart disease and stroke among Japanese men living in Japan, Hawaii, and the U.S. mainland. Japanese- American men appeared to have higher rates of CHD and lower rates of stroke than did their counterparts living in Japan. The average annual incidence rate of CHD (per 1000) in middle-aged Japanese-American men is 4.6 for ages 45 to 49, 6.0 for ages 50 to 54, 7.2 for ages 55 to 59, 8.8 for ages 60 to 64, and 10.5 for ages 65 to 68 (34), while their stroke rate declined; by 5% for total stroke, 3.5% for thromboembolic stroke, and 4.3% for hemorrhagic stroke.

Although the 2002 overall CHD death rate was 170.8 and the 1999 CHD death rate for Asian/Pacific Islanders was 115.5 (20), it is becoming increasingly clear that South Asians are at high risk for coronary artery disease (CAD) compared to the general population. South Asians are a rapidly growing population in the United States. Their very high CHD prevalence, evident early in life, is worth noting as it does not appear to necessarily be associated with traditional risk factors. This elevated CAD risk may reflect higher prevalence rates of insulin resistance, metabolic syndrome, or diabetes, or even elevated C-reactive protein (CRP) and/or lipoprotein (a) levels (35,36).

Hispanics/Latinos and CVD

CVD claims the lives of 29.3% of more than 117,000 Hispanics or Latinos who die each year. Among Mexican-American adults, 29.2% of men and 29.3% of women have CVD. Mexican-Americans are more likely to be overweight or obese, and are more likely to have diabetes. Mexican-American men are more likely to have high blood cholesterol and Mexican-American women have higher CVD risk factors than white women, even of comparable SES (30). Hispanic American women are less likely to be physically active. They are also afflicted younger. In 2001, the number of premature deaths (<65 years) from heart disease was higher for Hispanics (23.5%) than non-Hispanics (16.5%), although important to note that Hispanic blacks had higher rates of the premature death (27.5%) than Hispanic whites (23.3%) (17).

Yet despite their increased risk factors, Hispanics have historically profited from a lower age-adjusted CHD death rate than the general population (For every 100,000 persons in the United States in 2002, 170.8 people died from CHD compared with 138 for Hispanics*) (20), contributing to the phenomenon known as the "Hispanic paradox." CVD death rates from 1990 to 1998 were shown to decline the most for Hispanics, at 17% as compared to 15% for non-Hispanic whites, 14% for Asian/Pacific Islanders, 11% for non-Hispanic blacks, and 8% for American Indians/Alaska Natives (37). The concept of the Hispanic paradox, however, is ultimately deteriorating as data suggests that it is in all probability not valid. More recent data suggests that the Hispanic paradox theory may have arisen because of, once again, the use of data (from the U.S. Census and the National Death Index) that had probable biases in the data. The San Antonio Heart Study attempted to conclusively resolve these potential biases by following 1700 individuals for almost 14 years. Eight hundred and forty five were U.S.-born Mexican Americans; 182 were Mexican-Americans born in Mexico, and 678 were non-Hispanic whites from the United States. This study concluded that Mexican-Americans born in the United States were 1.7 times more likely to die from CVD than non-Hispanic whites (38).

Mexican-Americans were shown in the Brain Attack Surveillance in Corpus Christi project to have an increased incidence of stroke (168/10,000 in Mexican-Americans as compared to 136/10,000 in non-Hispanic whites). Specifically, Mexican-Americans have an increased incidence of intracerebral hemorrhage and subarachnoid hemorrhage, as well as an increased incidence of ischemic stroke and transient ischemic attack at younger ages when compared with whites (13). Nonetheless, for the collective Hispanic population, the 2002 overall death rate for stroke was 40.0, as compared to the overall rate of 56.2 for the general population (20).

DISEASE CHARACTERISTICS AND RISK FACTORS
Atherosclerosis

Data exists suggesting that patterns of atherosclerotic disease differ between racial/ethnic groups. In the Bogalusa Heart Study, a long-term epidemiological study following black and white children for over 30 years, adolescent blacks were shown to have more aortic fatty streaks as compared to whites of similar age. Even after controlling for levels of risk factors, the post-mortems of the African American adolescents were shown to have an additional 16% surface involvement with aortic fatty streaks compared with whites ($p < 0.001$) (39). As compared with whites, several studies have shown blacks and Hispanics to have significantly lower prevalence of coronary artery calcium (CAC) and obstructive coronary disease (40–44), although results (45) from the Dallas Heart Study had suggested that population estimates of the frequency of a positive scan for CAC were in fact not statistically different between blacks and whites. The Multi-Ethnic Study of Atherosclerosis (MESA) was analyzed to definitively determine the relative prevalence and quantity of coronary calcification across ethnic groups and to determine whether ethnic differences persist after controlling for concurrent traditional CHD risk factors (46). Through use of computed tomography, of the 6814 white, black, Hispanic and Chinese men and women aged 45 to 84 years with no clinical CVD who participated in the MESA, the prevalence of coronary calcification in these four ethnic groups was determined to be 70.4%, 52.1%, 56.5%, and 59.2%, respectively, in the men ($p < 0.001$) and 44.6%, 36.5%, 34.9%, and 41.9%, ($p < 0.001$) in the women of these groups, substantiating the higher rate of CAC in Caucasians (Fig. 8). South Asians, however, have been shown to experience high rates of CAC (47), and consequently, a greater plaque burden than Asians, Hispanics, or African Americans, although the data is only beginning to emerge.

Hypertension

In the United States, African Americans bear the greatest burden of hypertension with 41.8% of African American men and 45.4% of African American women afflicted. Comparatively, hypertension occurs in 30.6% of white men and 31.0% of white women; 27.8% and 28.7% of Mexican men and women, respectively (26).

African Americans

The prevalence of hypertension in blacks in the United States is among the highest in the world. Compared with whites, blacks develop hypertension at an earlier age and their average

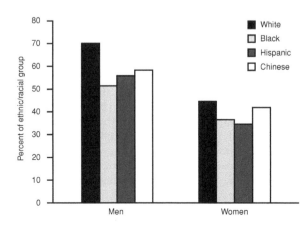

FIGURE 8 Prevalence of coronary calcification: Multi-Ethnic Study of Atherosclerosis. *Source*: From Ref. 46.

blood pressures are much higher. The higher prevalence of hypertension in African Americans is also accompanied by a worse disease severity. The prevalence of stage 3 hypertension (>180/110 mmHg) is 8.5% for African Americans as compared with 1% for whites. For hypertensive African Americans, the mean difference in blood pressure in hypertensives versus their normotensive counterparts, is 30/20 mmHg in African Americans whereas for hypertensive whites, the difference is 23/15 mmHg (30). As irrefutable consequence of this hypertension, compared with whites, blacks have a 1.3 times greater rate of nonfatal stroke, 1.8 times greater rate of fatal stroke, 1.5 times greater rate of heart disease death, 4.2 times greater rate of end-stage kidney disease (48), and a 50% higher frequency of heart failure (49), overall, mortality due to hypertension and its consequences is four to five times more likely in African Americans than in whites (50). The racial divergence is apparent even in childhood, as the Bogalusa Heart Study confirmed more reported elevations in the blood pressures prior to the age of 10 years in black children as compared with white children (51).

Hypertension is associated with serious sequelae, particularly in African Americans. Left ventricular hypertrophy is common sequelae of hypertension and is a separate risk factor for coronary events and sudden death. The coronary artery risk development in young adults (CARDIA) study confirmed that African Americans have greater left ventricular mass, shown to be independently correlated with their systolic blood pressure (52). Hypertension-related end stage renal disease, another common and critical consequence of hypertension, is also more prevalent in African Americans. The racial disparity is most striking in young African Americans, ages 25 to 44, who are 20 times more likely than whites of that age group to develop kidney failure caused by high blood pressure (53).

The pathophysiology for the increased risk for hypertension in African Americans is complex and not entirely elucidated. Studies have shown both increases in vascular resistance (54–56) and/or disturbances in both endothelial dependent and independent vasodilation (57–62). A cohort from the Atherosclerosis Risk in Communities (ARIC) study (63) demonstrated that 268 African Americans had stiffer common carotid arteries than the Caucasian population, leading the authors to suggest that stiffening either occurs earlier or progresses more rapidly in African Americans. Other studies (57–61,64) have found important racial differences in vasoreactivity, including a higher minimum forearm vascular resistance, depressed vasodilation and/or increased peripheral vasoconstriction in response to (β-adrenergic stimulation, attenuation in cyclic nucleotide-mediated vascular smooth muscle relaxation, depressed postischemic vasodilation, and an increased median effective concentration in response to acetylcholine among African American subjects. Furthermore, blacks have been shown to have lower levels of plasma renin activity, more salt-sensitive (salt- or NaCl-dependent) hypertension, and a delayed ability to excrete a sodium load compared with whites, despite comparable levels of renal function (65). So although therapeutic blockade of the renin-angiotensin system appears to be less effective for lowering blood pressure and preventing kidney disease in blacks compared with whites, salt restriction leads to a greater reduction in systolic blood pressure in African Americans (approximately 12 mmHg) than in whites (66).

There are no clinical trial data at present to suggest that lower-than-usual blood pressure targets should be set for high-risk demographic groups such as African Americans. Although the use of diuretics in African American patients may be a logical first-line choice for blood pressure reduction, in order to reach appropriate blood pressure goals most patients will require combination therapy. Although certain combinations have been shown to be effective in non-African American patients, the choice of drugs for combination therapy in African-American patients may be different. Angiotensin-converting enzyme (ACE) inhibitors and angiotensin receptor blockers both reduce angiotensin-II–mediated stimulation of transforming growth factor β_1, which may be of clinical significance in the treatment of hypertension in African Americans (67). Although data suggests a solid association between visceral obesity in African American women and sympathetic nervous system activity (68), beta blockers have been shown to be somewhat less effective as monotherapy for hypertension in African-Americans (69).

The African American Study of Kidney Disease and Hypertension prospectively addressed the impact of three antihypertensive drug classes on the progression of hypertensive renal disease. It was noted in this study that African American patients with hypertension uniformly required a multidrug regimen to achieve adequate blood pressure control (53). African American patients treated with the ACE inhibitor ramipril had a significantly lower incidence of the primary composite end point (glomerular filtration rate reduction, end-stage renal disease, or death) than African Americans treated with either a calcium channel blocker or beta blocker. Moreover, the study suggested that lower levels of proteinuria than previously thought may be important for identifying those at higher risk for kidney disease progression, particularly relevant in the African American population. The recent Antihypertensive and Lipid-Lowering Treatment to Prevent Heart Attack Trial (ALLHAT) was the first study to test the effectiveness of ACE inhibitors and calcium channel blockers in preventing the cardiovascular complications of hypertension in black hypertensive patients (70). In ALLHAT, comprised of over 42,000 participants, it was demonstrated that after five years of follow-up, patients taking lisinopril, an ACE inhibitor, had a 2 mmHg higher systolic blood pressure and a similar diastolic blood pressure compared to those taking the diuretic chlorthalidone. The difference in blood pressure lowering was smaller between those receiving amlodipine, a calcium channel blocker, and chlorthalidone, with a 1 mmHg higher systolic blood pressure and yet 1 mmHg lower diastolic blood pressure compared to those on chlorthalidone. Of the over 15,000 black participants (approximately 35% of the study size), black hypertensive patients were shown to have similar results with the amlodipine versus chlorthalidone experience; however, the differences between the lisinopril and chlorthalidone groups were greater in the black ALLHAT participants. Compared to those taking chlorthalidone, Black participants on lisinopril had a 4 mmHg higher systolic blood pressure, a 19% higher risk of all cardiovascular events, including 40% higher risk of stroke, and a 32% greater risk of heart failure. It is uncertain how much the blood pressure difference accounted for the difference in outcomes. ALLHAT did not permit combination therapy with ACE inhibitors plus diuretics, therefore, the benefits of such regimens in this patient population could not be assessed, but again, of note, by the completion of the trial, patients received on average of two medications in order to lower blood pressures to 140/90 mmHg. In the Losartan Intervention For Endpoint reduction in hypertension study (71), in contrast to the overall study population, 533 black patients with left ventricular hypertrophy treated with atenolol were at lower risk of experiencing the primary composite end point (death, myocardial infarction, and stroke) than African Americans treated with losartan, with or without diuretics.

Within the African American group, the responsiveness to monotherapy with ACE inhibitors, angiotensin receptor blockers, and beta blockers may be less than the responsiveness to diuretics and calcium channel blockers, but these differences are corrected when diuretics are added to the neurohormonal antagonists. The International Society on Hypertension in Blacks has crafted guidelines (72) and an algorithm (Fig. 9) to guide ideal management of high blood pressure in African Americans. But of note, African American patients with systolic BP $\geq$15 mmHg or a diastolic BP $\geq$10 mmHg above goal should be treated with first-line combination therapy.

Hispanic Americans

The prevalence of hypertension in Hispanic Americans is lower than in the general population, although it does vary by specific country of origin. Data regarding hypertension in Hispanic Americans has been problematic as the standard for defining the prevalence of hypertension in this country has relied on the National Health and Nutrition Examination Survey (NHANES). NHANES, however, classified their survey into four groups, including non-Hispanic whites, non-Hispanic African Americans, Mexican-Americans, and other groups. Therefore, reliable information has been captured for Mexican-Americans but not in actuality for other Hispanic Americans, despite the fact that Hispanic Americans are the fastest-growing segment of the U.S. population. Nonetheless, Hispanic Americans experience low levels of hypertension (14.5%), despite elevated levels of diabetes and obesity. Among Mexican Americans, NHANES reports 27.8% of men and 28.7% of women to have hypertension (26).

The San Antonio Heart Study was one of the few studies to systematically examine the prevalence of hypertension and related diseases in Hispanics, although again comparing Mexican-Americans with whites (73). Despite the fact that the Mexican-Americans were more obese and experienced markedly higher prevalence of type 2 diabetes, the prevalence of hypertension was slightly lower in Mexican-Americans (74), of which where the so-called "Hispanic paradox" gets its name.

Information about hypertension in Asian Americans and American-Indians/Alaskan natives is even more problematic. Prevalence appears to be low as estimated by NHANES

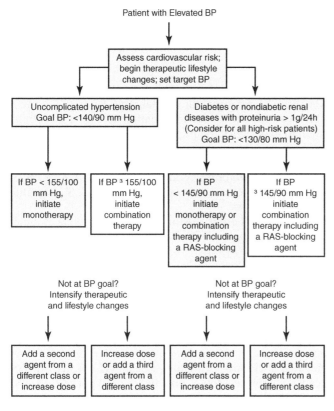

Patient with Elevated BP

Assess cardiovascular risk;
begin therapeutic lifestyle
changes; set target BP

Uncomplicated hypertension
Goal BP: <140/90 mm Hg

Diabetes or nondiabetic renal
diseases with proteinuria > 1g/24h
(Consider for all high-risk patients)
Goal BP: <130/80 mm Hg

If BP < 155/100 mm Hg, initiate monotherapy

If BP ³ 155/100 mm Hg, initiate combination therapy

If BP < 145/90 mm Hg initiate monotherapy or combination therapy including a RAS-blocking agent

If BP ³ 145/90 mm Hg initiate combination therapy including a RAS-blocking agent

Not at BP goal?
Intensify therapeutic
and lifestyle changes

Not at BP goal?
Intensify therapeutic
and lifestyle changes

Add a second agent from a different class or increase dose

Increase dose or add a third agent from a different class

Add a second agent from a different class or increase dose

Increase dose or add a third agent from a different class

Not at BP goal with 3 agents?
Consider factors that may decrease compliance or efficacy with current regimen.
Consider referral to a BP specialist.

FIGURE 9 International Society on Hypertension in Blacks Treatment Algorithm for African Americans with Hypertension. *Source*: From Ref. 72. Copyright © 2003 American Medical Association. All rights reserverd.

(1999–2002) (75), and is 16.7% and 21.2%, respectively, but it is widely known from non-American epidemiological studies (76) that South Asians experience high rates of hypertension, is a significant concern in the Indian subcontinent and is an important cardiovascular risk for South Asians worldwide. The World Health Organization (WHO) has reported that Indian men in the age range of 40 to 55 years have the highest blood pressure among populations from 20 other developing countries (77). As quickly as our population is changing, the onus is on the U.S. medical community to obtain and stratify better hypertension epidemiological data.

Diabetes Mellitus

Native Americans have the highest rates of diabetes at 16%, having increased 33.2% between 1994 and 2002. Mexican-Americans and African Americans also have elevated prevalence rates double that of their Caucasian counterparts. The overall age-adjusted prevalence for American Indian or Alaska Native adults was more than twice that of U.S. adults overall (78). The NHANES III reported the prevalence of diabetes in whites, blacks, and Hispanics living in the United States, reporting an overall diabetes prevalence of 5.3% in persons living in the United States aged ≥20 years of age. They found a higher prevalence of diabetes in Hispanics (9.3%) and blacks (8.2%) compared with whites (4.8%) in the ≥20 years age group. South Asians were not categorized separately in this study. One recent community-based survey attempted to be one of the first to evaluate the prevalence of diabetes mellitus in South Asians living in the United States. Of 1046 South Asian immigrants living in a community in the Southeast United States, an overall prevalence of diabetes mellitus of 18.3% (22.5% in men and 13.6% in women) was revealed (78), possibly suggesting a much higher prevalence of diabetes in Asian Indians than in whites, blacks, and Hispanics living in the United States, although much more data is required.

Mortality rates due to diabetes, however, are highest in African Americans (80). This is most probably due to the presence of concomitant risk factors, and most likely comorbid hypertension.

Metabolic Syndrome

Using the National Cholesterol Education Program (NCEP) Third Adult Treatment Panel (ATP III) criteria (81) applied to the NHANES III database, the incidence of the metabolic syndrome is 1 in 5 for American adults but was shown to also be elevated across racial/ethnic groups. Hispanic Americans were shown to experience the highest incidence of the metabolic syndrome, at 31.9% overall and 35% of Hispanic-American women. Age-adjusted prevalence figures estimate that 35.6% of Mexican-American women and 28.3% of Mexican-American men have criteria satisfying the diagnosis of metabolic syndrome followed by 25.7% of African American women and 16.4% of African American men, as compared to 22.8% of white women and 24.8% of white men in the United States.

The SHS, however, based on the NCEP ATPIII criteria estimated the prevalence of metabolic syndrome among Native Americans to be as high as 55% (82). The attainment of accurate epidemiological data in ethnic or racial groups is always challenging in itself, but epidemiological reports of metabolic syndrome face their own interpretative challenges, as differing definitions or criterion might be used. The WHO's definition (83), when applied to the above NHANES data, produced even higher metabolic syndrome prevalence rates in Mexican-Americans and African Americans. Although among Pima Indians who did not have diabetes, the prevalence of the metabolic syndrome was 31% under both definitions (84), in the San Antonio Heart Study the WHO definition produced a lower estimate among white and Mexican-American women and a higher estimate among Mexican-American men (85). As mentioned previously, despite the elevated incidence of insulin resistance, obesity and/or metabolic syndrome, Hispanic Americans experience a lower prevalence of hypertension, and therefore the metabolic syndrome in this population does not appear to impart as significant CVD risk for Hispanic ethnicity (86).

Data continues to materialize regarding South Asians and their nontraditional, or emerging risk factors, including metabolic syndrome. Again, data from the United Kingdom suggest that the prevalence of the metabolic syndrome is highest in South Asians (WHO, men 46%, women 31%; NCEP, men 29%, women 32%) and lowest in European women (WHO, 9%; NCEP, 14%) (87).

The International Diabetes Federation (IDF) has most recently released their IDF Consensus Worldwide Definition of Metabolic Syndrome (88). This definition suggests criteria, not unlike the existing criteria in use put forth by NCEP ATPIII (81), but placing emphasis on waist circumference and insulin resistance. These guidelines go one step further by providing ethnic specific values on waist circumference, with different measurement for Europids, South Asians, Chinese, Japanese, Ethnic South and Central Americans, Sub-Saharan Africans, Eastern Mediterranean and Middle East (Arab) Populations (Table 1).

Obesity

The prevalence of both overweight and obesity is higher in African Americans and Hispanic Americans than in whites and it has been disproportionately rising in these groups as well. The mean body mass indexes (BMI) for African Americans, Hispanic Americans, and whites are 29.2, 28.6, and 26.3, respectively. This remains especially true in women, where as compared with white women, the prevalence of obesity is much higher in both African American and Mexican-American women. African American women are on average 17 pounds heavier than their white contemporaries. The highest prevalence of obesity is in African American women (44%) (89) and rises in the Southeastern United States to as high as 71% (90). This remains true among children and adolescents as well, where the prevalence of obesity is also greater in African Americans and Mexican-Americans compared with Caucasians. Furthermore, overall, 22% of the U.S. population is physically inactive, but almost double that rate (40%) of African-American women is physically inactive. Data taken from the CARDIA study demonstrate that African American women have higher BMI, higher caloric intake, less physical activity and physical fitness than white women (91). Obesity and overweight is also prevalent among Pacific Islanders. Native Hawaiians and Samoans are among the most obese people in the

TABLE 1 International Diabetes Federation: Ethnic Specific Values for Waist Circumference for Diagnosis of Metabolic Syndrome

Country/ethnic group	Waist circumference[a]		
Europids			
In the USA, the ATP III values (102 cm male; 88 cm female) are likely to continue to be used for clinical purposes	Male	≥94 cm	
	Female	≥80 cm	
South Asian			
Based on a Chinese, Malay and Asian-Indian population	Male	≥90 cm	
	Female	≥80cm	
Chinese	Male	≥90 cm	
	Female	≥80 cm	
Japanese	Male	≥85 cm	
	Female	≥90 cm	
Ethnic south and Central Americans	Use South Asian recommendations until more specific data are available		
Sub-saharan Africans	Use European data until more specific are available		
Eastern Mediterranean and Middle East (Arab) populations	Use European data until more specific are available		

[a]In future epidemiological studies of populations of Europid origin, prevalence should be given using both European and North American cut-points to allow better comparisons.
Source: From Ref. 88.

world. The Molokai Heart Study demonstrated a 64% prevalence of obesity in Native Hawaiians (92).

There is evidence that excess adiposity may have greater effect on African Americans. Data from the Bogalusa Heart Study have shown that the effect of a high BMI is strongly correlated with later manifestation of multiple risk factors in African Americans (93). There are racial/ethnic effects on the relationship of visceral adipose tissue (VAT) with metabolic risk factors that have been reported (94), apparent as early as childhood (95,96). Higher VAT has been shown in Caucasians compared with African Americans (97), despite greater total fat in African American women (98). VAT has been demonstrated to be strongly associated with other cardiovascular risk factors in Caucasian women; these relationships were not present in African American women (99). Upon analysis of examined data from NHANES III (100), it was shown that waist circumference values that correspond to both overweight and obesity were significantly lower in African Americans and Hispanic Americans compared with those in Caucasians.

Dyslipidemia

There do not appear to be significant differences in low-density lipoprotein (LDL) cholesterol and total cholesterol levels across race/ethnic groups. Among Americans of age 20 and older, the following have a LDL cholesterol of 130 mg/dL or higher: 49.6% of white men and 43.7% of women; 46.3% of black men and 41.6% of black women; 43.6% of Mexican-American men and 41.6% of Mexican-American women. Of these, an LDL cholesterol of 160 mg/dL or higher is found in non-Hispanic whites, 20.4% of men and 17.0% of women; non-Hispanic blacks, 19.3% of men and 18.8% of women; Mexican-Americans, 16.9% of men and 14.0% of women. Differences noted by the NCEP's ATP III between African American and white patients in CHD-risk-associated lipid levels include a somewhat lower mean LDL-C and higher mean high-density lipoprotein cholesterol (HDL-C) levels in African American men compared with white men (81). Triglyceride (TG) levels are also lower in African American men and women (81). It remains unclear whether the relatively higher HDL-C levels observed in African-American men and women are protective against CHD.

Small, dense LDL particle size is another emerging risk factor for CVD. LDL size was also investigated as a possible explanation for differences in CVD rates among African Americans, Hispanics, and non-Hispanic whites in the Insulin Resistance Atherosclerosis Study (101). The study suggests that LDL size differed significantly ($p < 0.001$) by ethnic group, as did HDL-C and TG levels. A comparison of the three ethnic groups revealed that reduced LDL size was associated with lower HDL-C levels and higher TG levels. African Americans had higher HDL-C and lower TG levels than non-Hispanic whites. Hispanics had the opposite pattern, with lower HDL-C and higher TG levels than non-Hispanic whites.

Lipoprotein (a), which is currently emerging as another risk factor for CHD, has been shown to be two to three times higher in African Americans than in whites (102–105), however the significance of this in African Americans has not been confirmed. Recent trials in African-Americans that assessed possible relationships of Lp(a) levels and atherosclerosis were unable to identify one. The lack of atherogenicity of Lp(a) in African Americans may be due to the presence differing isoforms of apolipoprotein A, most liskely less amounts of small apolipoprotein A isoforms, which has been associated with CHD (106). Data from the Study of Women's Health Across the Nation, a prospective multiethnic study of menopausal women (1368 Caucasians, 808 African Americans, 220 Chinese, 216 Hispanic, and 251 Japanese) also demonstrated that African American women had twofold higher mean Lp(a) values than women of the other four race/ethnic groups (106).

Although African Americans may not be at elevated risk for hyperlipidemia, they were still the only ethnic group with which the 2002 NCEP ATP III report had sufficient data and rationale to develop alternate guidelines for lipid evaluation as appropriate (81). The report recognized that risk factor patterns among African Americans were different enough from those of the general population to warrant consistent adaptations in NCEP ATP III risk categorizations and recommended treatment options. Because of the higher rates of type 2 diabetes mellitus and multiple risk factors in African Americans, many more patients in this population are likely to meet the criteria for a high-risk LDL-C goal (Table 2). With respect to lipid evaluations, the report found that among black males, although mean LDL-C levels are slightly lower than in whites, elevated levels are more common, so that the overall relationship of total cholesterol to CAD risk is similar among males in both groups. Evaluation of LDL-C in black women does not differ from whites. Although lipoprotein (a) levels are higher in both black men and women, the impact of this risk for CAD among African Americans/Blacks is not known.

The ALLHAT trial was also the first clinical outcome trial of the efficacy of statin therapy in a large population of African Americans (108). African Americans comprised 33% to 34% of the study population of >10,000 patients with moderate hypercholesterolemia (with or without CHD) and controlled hypertension (as mentioned earlier, see African Americans and Hypertension). In this trial, patients were randomized to receive 40 mg of pravastatin or usual care for a mean follow-up period of 4.8 years. African Americans in the pravastatin group experienced a significantly reduced risk for CHD events compared with non-black patients (relative risk, 0.73 vs. 1.02; $p = 0.03$). However, this may have been because of the underuse of treatment in the usual care cohort of black patients. Analysis of stroke showed a significantly less favorable effect of statin treatment in black patients (relative risk, 1.12 vs. 0.74). Most other available data, limited but becoming increasingly available suggest that lipid response to statins in African American patients is similar to that in white patients,

TABLE 2 National Cholesterol Education Program Third Adult Treatment Panel: Special Considerations for Cholesterol Management in African Americans

Risk level	Special consideration in Blacks/African Americans
CAD and CAD risk equivalents 10-yr risk >20%	High risk for cardiac death
LDL-C goal < 100 mg/dL	No charge in recommended LDL-C goal
Multiple (2+) risk factors 10-yr risk 10–20%	Hypertension is a powerful risk factor in this population, when present, check for LVH
LDL-C goal <130 mg/dL	Risk factor clustering more common
Multiple (2+) risk factors 10-yr risk 10%	Drug therapy warranted if TLC does not lower LDL-C below 130 mg/dL within 3 mon
LDL-C goal < 130 mg/dL	Pay particular attention to detection and control of hypertension
0–1 risk factor 0-2 10-yr risk <10%	No change in recommended LDL-C goal
LDL-C goal <160 mg/dL	No change in recommended LDL-C goal

Abbreviations: LDL-C, low-density lipoprotein-cholesterol; CAD, coronary artery disease; LVH, left ventricular hypertrophy; TLC, total lymphocyte Count.
Source: From Ref. 81.

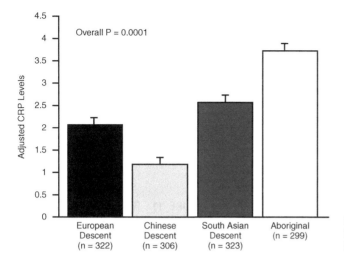

FIGURE 10 Ethnic variations in C-reactive protein levels. *Abbreviation*: CRP, C-reactive protein *Source*: From Ref. 112.

except for an apparently smaller increase in HDL-C levels (109–111). With respect to safety, the NCEP ATPIII report (81) recommends that because of relatively high-normal creatine kinase (CK) levels observed, CK levels should be documented before initiation of lipid-lowering therapy in black men. Studies such as U.S. demographic trials African American Rosuvastatin Investigation of Efficacy and Safety, Study Assessing Rosuvastatin in the Hispanic population, and Investigation of Rosuvastatin in South Asian subjects, among others are investigating lipid effects of statins in specific ethnic populations.

C-REACTIVE PROTEIN

Data describing distribution of CRP in different race/ethnic groups within the United States are beginning to emerge. One study (112) of 1250 adults of South Asian, Chinese, European, and Aboriginal ancestry were randomly sampled from four communities in Canada. The mean CRP was the highest among Aboriginals, followed by South Asians, intermediate among people of European origin, and lowest among the Chinese. The age- and sex-adjusted mean CRP was 3.74 mg/L among Aboriginals, 2.59 mg/L among South Asians, and 1.18 mg/L among Chinese compared with 2.06 mg/L among Europeans (overall $p < 0.0001$) (Fig. 10). Analysis of CRP collected from 28,345 participants in the Women's Health Study (113) indicates that baseline CRP levels vary according to self-reported race/ethnic groups, and that black women have significantly higher CRP levels and Asian women have lower CRP levels than their white and Hispanic counterparts. CRP levels were determined to be similar among white and Hispanic women. Specifically, median CRP levels were 2.96 mg/L among black women, 2.06 mg/L among Hispanic women, 2.02 mg/L among white women, and 1.12 mg/L among Asian women. Although BMI was a significant confounder of CRP levels in all women, the effect was most striking among black women. But again, in contrast to Asian women, South Asians have been reported to have high CRP concentrations (114–116), although this finding has not always been consistent (117).

It is also important to remember that the gender specific CRP data cannot simply be extrapolated, as plasma levels of CRP vary considerably between men and women. Recent CRP data collected from the Dallas Heart Study (118) demonstrated median CRP levels to be higher among black subjects than whites (3.0 mg/L vs. 2.3 mg/L, $p < 0.001$) and among women compared with men (3.3 mg/L vs. 1.8 mg/L, $p < 0.001$). The proportions of subjects with CRP levels suggestive of high risk were 29.1% for white men, 42.3% for black men, 50.4% for white women and 63.4% for black women.

RISK FACTOR CLUSTERING

Indeed, the increased cardiovascular risk among blacks appears to be related to clustering of risk factors. Studies, such as the Dallas Heart Study (45) and ARIC Study (11), suggest that clustering

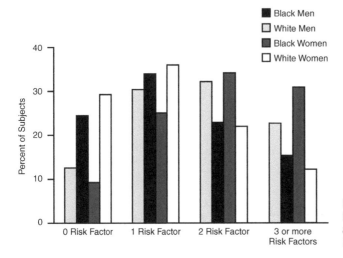

FIGURE 11 Risk factors for coronary heart disease cluster and increase in black and white men and women. *Source:* From Ref. 11.

of risk factors (such as obesity, hypertension, diabetes, smoking, hypercholesterolemia, hypertriglyceridemia, and low HDL-C) is markedly greater in black men and women (Fig. 11).

RISK ASSESSMENTS

Current guidelines all strongly stress that for primary prevention of CVD, an individual's personal cardiovascular risk must be calculated. This approach guides the intensity and focus on individual CV risk factors. The most widely known and frequency used risk assessment method derives from the Framingham Heart study, for prediction of 10-year development of CHD. Despite being derived from a predominately white New England population, the method has already been shown to reproducibly and somewhat accurately predict events in other major American studies (119–122). The validity of this method, however, in racial/ethnic groups has been questioned, and therefore was further analyzed (123) to investigate its utility in predicting cardiovascular outcome in six prospective studies from ethnically diverse cohorts.

Framingham risk equations were shown to perform well for white and black men and women. A systematic overestimate of events was found when applying the equations to Japanese-American and Hispanic men and Native American women, for whom the authors were then able to "re-calibrate" to significantly improve the performance. Unfortunately it is unclear at this time whether the Framingham risk is valid for South Asian population. Thus, further work on ethnic groups other than white Caucasians is needed.

RACIAL DISPARITY IN HEALTH CARE

Although different racial and ethnic groups have different and evidently higher rates of cardiovascular risk, differing genetics, pathophysiologies and perhaps even subtle differences in the way that members of different racial and ethnic groups respond to treatment, the majority of studies still consistently find disparities in the health care itself, which adds to the complexity of this issue. The disparities in health care are evident across a wide range of disease areas and clinical services. Disparities are found even when clinical factors, such as stage of disease presentation, co-morbidities, age, and severity of disease are taken into account. Furthermore, it has been demonstrated that even when insurance and income are the same, minorities often receive fewer tests and less sophisticated treatment for most diseases, including heart disease. In 1999, Congress requested that the Institute of Medicine assess the extent of racial and ethnic disparities in health care (124). The study committee itself was "struck by the consistency of research findings.... even among the better-controlled studies, the vast majority indicated that minorities are less likely than whites to receive needed services, including clinically necessary procedures." These disparities are found steadily across the United States, in procedures, practices, in all clinical settings, including outpatient and inpatient, public and private hospitals,

TABLE 3 Black and White Differences in Specialty Procedure Utilization Among Medicare Beneficiaries Age 65 and Older, 1993

	Black	White	Black-to-white ratio
Angioplasty (procedures per 1,000 beneficiaries per year)	2.5	5.4	0.46
Coronary artery bypass graft surgery (procedures per 1,000 beneficiaries per year)	1.9	4.8	0.40
Mammography (procedures per 100 women per year)	17.1	26.0	0.66
Hip fracture repair (procedures per 1,00 beneficiaries per year)	2.9	7.0	0.42
Amputation of all or part of limb (procedures per 1,00 beneficiaries per year)	6.7	1.9	3.64
Bilateral orchiectomy (procedures per 1,00 beneficiaries per year)	2.0	0.8	2.45

Source: From Ref. 125.

even teaching and non-teaching hospitals. Note the differences between African Americans and whites in specialty procedure utilization among Medicare beneficiaries (Table 3) (126). Even examples such as lack of good relationships with primary care providers and less access to private physicians result in increased utilization of emergency rooms and therefore less comprehensive care for minorities, even when they are shown to be insured at the same level as whites. Disparity in health care has been shown to be associated with higher mortality among minorities (127–129). Of 81 studies specifically investigating racial/ethnic differences in cardiac care from 1984 to 2001, 68 found racial/ethnic differences in cardiac care for at least one of the minority groups analyzed. Of them, two-thirds found differences in cardiac care for all of the procedures and treatments investigated, and only 1/3 of them found differences in some cardiac procedures and treatments and not others (130).

PROCEDURES

Studies have shown that African Americans are less likely than whites to receive cardiac catheterization, angioplasty, and bypass surgery (Fig. 12) even after adjustment for clinical and socioeconomic factors (130). In the 21 studies that found a statistically significant difference, African Americans were shown to be only 26% to 68% as likely as whites to receive bypass surgery (130). Furthermore, a recent study (131) has confirmed for the first time that this differential use of revascularization contributes to worse long-term patient outcomes, and moreover another recent study suggests that post-coronary artery bypass graft follow-up care and repeat revascularizations may also be at racial risk (132). New Center for Disease control and Prevention statistics (133) indicate that African Americans are also less likely than whites to receive drug-eluting stents. Differences in these procedures, such as cardiac catheterization rates in white versus black patients persist regardless of the race of the treating physician. Unfortunately similar data regarding the racial disparity in cardiac procedures in Latinos, Asians and Native Americans is currently very limited.

HOSPITALS

A recent retrospective observational study (134) discovered that of those hospitalized with ST-segment elevation, myocardial infarction or left bundle-branch block and receiving acute reperfusion therapy, that time from hospital entry to reperfusion therapy is 7.3 minutes longer for African Americans receiving thrombolytic therapy and 18.9 minutes longer for those receiving percutaneous transluminal coronary angiography. This study, however, did also reveal that the racial/ethnic disparity in time to treatment was also attributable to the specific hospital to which the patients were admitted, rather than simply differential treatment by race within the given hospital. For example, it was also documented that an observed mean difference in "door-to-balloon times" between Hispanic patients and white patients was reduced by nearly 75% after accounting for differences between the hospitals in

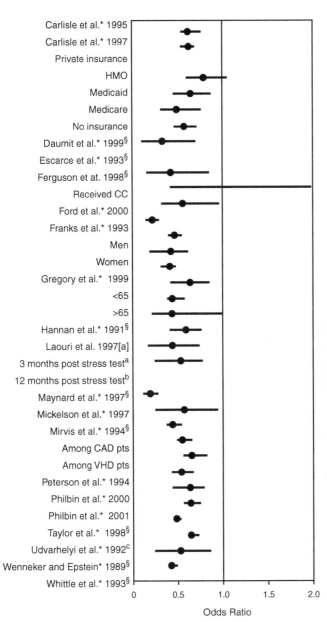

FIGURE 12 Odds ratios for selected strong studies CABG (African Americans/whites). *Study analyzes more than one procedure or treatment and appears in more than one table. §Odds ratio findings taken from Kressin and Petersen. *Annals of Internal Medicine*, 2001. ᵃOdds ratio: AA/W 1.05 (0.54–2.06). ᵇOdds ratio: AA/W 1.24 (0.64–2.40). ᶜThe authors computed relative risks, which are comparable to odds ratios when the events are rare. Both measure the strength of an association between a factor and an outcome. *Note*: Studies selected for this figure were all strong studies that used odds ratios for analyzing statistical differences between African Americans and whites. An odds ratio of 1.0 means there is an equal likelihood of receiving the procedure or treatment. An odds ratio of <1.0 means African Americans are less likely to receive the procedure or treatment. *Abbreviation*: CABG, coronary artery bypass graft. *Source*: From Ref. 130 with permission from the Henry J. Kaiser Family Foundation.

which they were treated. Furthermore, one must also consider who the patients' admitting attending and/or primary care physicians may be, as they are instrumental in overseeing and orchestrating their patients' inpatient care. According to a cross-sectional analysis (135) of 150,391 visits by black and white patients 65 years of age or older for medical "evaluation and management," the physicians treating black patients were less likely to be board certified (77.4% vs. 86%) and reported being less able to access high-quality specialists, high-quality diagnostic imaging, nonemergency hospital admissions, adequate number of inpatient days, and high-quality ancillary services. Thus, the choice of hospitals and the continuity of care between physician and hospital contribute to an extremely complex issue. Although, there are many epidemiological examples of racial/ethnic disparity in cardiac care in U.S. hospitals, it is of interest to note, that only 12% of cardiologists thought disparities existed in their own hospital (136).

Diagnosis

Obviously, the provision of adequate cardiovascular risk factor treatment can only begin with awareness. But evidence exists that suggests that racial and ethnic groups are less likely to be aware of their risk factors. As an example, regardless of age, blacks and Mexican Americans are consistently less likely than whites to have their cholesterol levels tested, with an average screening rate at 70% of that for whites. Only 63% of all Americans >25 years of age have undergone ≥1 lipid screenings. Overall, covariate-adjusted estimates from NHANES III indicate that as compared to 71% of whites, only 52% of blacks, and 42% of Mexican Americans have lipid levels tested. In the ARIC study (11), only 25% of African American men and 27% of African American women with hypercholesterolemia were aware of their condition. One NHANES survey determined among adults with hypertension, that half of Mexican Americans are unaware of their diagnosis, as compared to 29.7% among non-Hispanic blacks and 37.1% among non-Hispanic whites (137).

RACIAL VARIATIONS IN DRUG USE

Despite the armamentarium of new therapies to manage and/or prevent cardiovascular risk factors, and disease, disparity in health care persists into trends in drug use. African Americans were shown to use less statins (black 27%, white 37%; $p = 0.003$) and less aspirin (black 72%, white 80%; $p = 0.01$), two of the safest and most efficacious tools available today in the primary and secondary prevention of CVD (21). Data from the National Registry of Myocardial Infarction III showed that black patients were less likely than white patients to receive lipid-modifying medication at hospital discharge after acute myocardial infarction (138). Asian/Pacific Islanders were also shown to receive less of any secondary prevention treatment. A study of over 19,000 elderly stroke survivors living in nursing homes revealed that variability in use of anticoagulation therapy ranged from 58% of American-Indians to only 39% of Asian/Pacific Islanders, and that Asian/Pacific Islanders, blacks, and Hispanics were all less likely than non-Hispanic whites to receive warfarin (139). Again, it is always remarkable to realize that these groups are less likely to receive the appropriate therapy although they have greater burden of disease (21).

THERAPEUTIC GOALS

With less screening, and less use of existing therapy, it may come as little surprise that minorities are less likely to reach most measured therapeutic goals in the medical literature to date. Joint National Committee VII reports that BP control rates vary in minority populations and are lowest in Mexican Americans and Native Americans (69). In the 1999 to 2000 NHANES, rates of blood pressure control were 17.7% in Mexican-Americans compared with 33.4% in non-Hispanic whites and 28.1% in non-Hispanic blacks (28.1%) (140). Low rates of hypertension control in Hispanic individuals have also been reported in other studies (48,141–143) although the data on blood pressure control in blacks have been inconclusive (141,144–147). An ongoing national hypertension quality improvement initiative being conducted by 10 health plans in the United States enrolls 1.9 million people, of which 292,996 were identified as having hypertension. Despite the incidence, prevalence and severity of hypertension in African Americans, Joint National Committee-VI goals were met in less than half in the African Americans in the group, and patients with diabetes were three times more likely to have their blood pressure uncontrolled (148).

Fewer blacks were shown to be at NCEP ATP III lipid goals (81), with the relatively high attainment of lipid targets by the youngest age group of blacks progressively declining to approximately two-thirds that of white patients by age ≥60 years. In the previously mentioned ARIC study, of the small percentage even aware of their hypercholesterolemia, only 32% and 45%, men and women respectively, achieved treatment goals (149). In the Lipid Treatment Assessment Project, African Americans receiving lipid-lowering therapy achieved ATP II low-, medium-, and high-risk LDL-C level goals less frequently than white patients, and they had a lower overall goal achievement rate than did white or Hispanic patients (150). Overall, LDL-C level goals were achieved in 29% of African American patients, compared with 39% of white patients and 40% of Hispanic patients.

TABLE 4   Poor Inclusion of Blacks in Lipid-Lowering Therapy Trials

Trial	Drug	No. of total patients	No. or % of blacks
WOSCOPS	Pravastatin	6595	N/A
AFCAPS/TEXCAPS	Lovastatin	6605	206
4S	Simvastatin	4444	N/A
CARE	Pravastatin	4159	Others, 7–8%
LIPID	Pravastatin	9014	N/A
HPS	Simvastatin	20,536	N/A
ASCOT	Atorvastatin	10,305	Others, 5–5.5%
ALLHAT	Pravastatin	10,355	2491

Abbreviations: WOSCOPS, West of Scotland coronary prevention study; AFCAPS/TEX CAPS, The Air Force/Texas Coronary Atherosclerosis Prevention study; CARE, cholesterol and recurrent events; LIPID, long-teem intervention with pravastatin in ischemic disease; HPS, Health Protection Study; ASCOT, Anglo-Scandinavian Cardiac Outcomes Trial; ALLHAT, Antihypertensive and Lipid-Lowering Treatment to Prevent Heart Attack Trial; 4S, Scandinavian Simvastatin Survival study.
Source: From Refs. 24, 108, 153–158.

TABLE 5   Association of Black Cardiologists: Barriers to Eliminating Disparities in Cardiovascular Care and Outcomes

Barriers to eliminating disparities in CV care and outcomes
Access and utilization of low and high-tech diagnostics
Access and utilization of cardiac procedures and therapies
Patient education
Adherence to guidelines for CV care
Inequities in health care system/infrastructure
Ineffective physician-patients communication
Health disparities research
Awareness and monitoring of health care disparities

Abbreviation: CV, cardiovascular.
Source: Courtesy of Association of Black Cardiologists Working Group.

UNDER-REPRESENTATION IN CLINICAL TRIALS

In addition, ethnic and racial groups have been grossly under-represented in major cardiovascular clinical trials (151,152). One review indicates that black patients accounted for 5.1% of a total of >450,000 patients enrolled in major trials in the past three decades (151). Recent studies of antihypertensive therapy have included more African Americans than in the past (53,70,71), but despite the recent surge of lipid-lowering trials in CVD prevention, African-Americans have been severely overlooked (Table 4).

In the Cholesterol and Recurrent Events trial (159), approximately 92% of the patients in the active treatment and placebo groups were white, whereas in and the Air Force/Texas Coronary Atherosclerosis Prevention Study (153), black patients accounted for only 3% of patients in the active treatment and placebo groups. Neither study reported subgroup analyses of outcomes in black patients.

BARRIERS

The evidence is clear that there exists major disparity in health care in the United States today, across races and ethnic groups. Identification of barriers to eliminating this disparity is the first critical step (Table 5).

Lower Socioeconomic Status

Although there is much advance in cardiovascular health, it is unfortunately well accepted if not admitted aloud that most of these improvements have occurred among wealthier, better-educated Americans, whereas progress among groups with lower SES has always lagged behind. Furthermore, the gap between high-SES and low-SES populations continues to widen. And despite all advances, SES remains strongly associated with race and ethnic groups in this country. The Conference on SES and Cardiovascular Health and Disease, sponsored by the NHLBI convened to review data on SES–CVD relationships and to explore possible biological, psychosocial, and lifestyle-related pathways by which SES may relate to CVD from specific U.S. population strata, including blacks, whites, Hispanics, Asians and Pacific Islanders, Native Americans, rural populations,and employed groups. Their report (160), in agreement with national data, suggested that specific U.S. population groups generally show an inverse relationship between SES and CVD (i.e., higher CVD rates with lower SES). Two major associations were made linking SES and CVD: (i) less favorable patterns of established major lifestyle and biomedical risk factors (smoking, adverse diet, sedentary lifestyle, hypercholesterolemia, hypertension, obesity, and diabetes) in lower- than in higher-SES strata and (ii) less favorable patterns of psychosocial factors (hostility, depression, low social support, social isolation, racism, job instability/insecurity/strain/powerlessness, unemployment) in lower- than in higher-SES strata. Both of these major associations could be found common to cultures and races. Although data are sparse on possible SES-related biological mediators of relationships between psychosocial factors and CVD and on social-environmental mechanisms whereby lower SES leads to development of more adverse behavioral and psychosocial patterns, racial and ethnic groups would always be at considerable risk.

CULTURAL BARRIERS
Educational

In a country where patient education and autonomy play a major role in health care decisions, patient awareness, education, and belief must be additional factors. A report accompanying the American Heart Association's Guidelines in the Primary Prevention of Cardiovascular Disease in Women (161) suggested that black and Hispanic women were less likely to realize that heart disease was the #1 killer of women than white women. Similarly, in a joint American Diabetes Association/American College of Cardiology survey (162) revealed that Hispanics were most "in the dark" about diabetes and awareness of risk for CVD. In a new prospective study showing that among patients deemed appropriate for such a procedure, rates of coronary revascularization were lower among South Asians in the United Kingdom than among whites (163), researchers had adjusted for and ruled out both SES and physician bias, and felt that it was in fact patient understanding and preference at play.

Language Barriers

It is not difficult to imagine that if patients cannot communicate with their health care providers, that this would provide yet another although immense obstacle to access of optimal care. For example, according to the U.S. Census Bureau, 20% of Spanish-speaking Latinos had not visited a doctor in the previous two years, as compared with <10% of non-Latino whites and blacks. Furthermore, another study showed that nearly half (45%) of the Spanish-speaking Latino population without insurance reported problems in communicating with their doctors, as compared with fewer than one third of uninsured whites (28%) and blacks (30%) (164). This can only be more problematic in Asian and other populations with the multitude of different languages.

Diet and Other Cultural Behaviors

Along with culture goes diet. Ethnic groups are virtually defined by their cuisines that may add benefit or harm to cardiovascular risk. As the Mediterranean diet is surfacing as one with verified cardiovascular benefit, other diets and customs are being shown to contribute to the obesity, metabolic syndrome and diabetes epidemic occurring in the United States today. As an example, the Mexican diet has been implicated as partially responsible for their incidence of metabolic syndrome as it includes foods saturated in fats, flours and carbohydrates, as well as of large quantities of carbonated and sugared soft drinks.

According to tobacco use surveys, African Americans, American-Indian/Alaska Natives, Asian American/Pacific Islanders, as well as Hispanics are smoking at increased rates. For example, American-Indians/Alaska Natives have the highest rates of tobacco use, and African American and South Asian men also have a high prevalence of smoking. Asian American women and Hispanic women have the lowest levels of smoking. The U.S. Surgeon general reports that, in general, smoking rates among Mexican-American adults increase as they learn and adopt the values, beliefs, and norms of American culture (165). Minorities also perform less physical activity. NHANES III found that while 18% of whites do not exercise, 35% of African- Americans and 40% of Mexican-Americans remain inactive. Several reasons have been hypothesized as to why minorities do not get enough exercise, including living in less safe neighborhoods, more family and work obligations, and the inability to afford gym memberships or exercise equipment. However, even when adjusting for socioeconomic background, they found even at higher education and income levels, minorities still exercised less frequently than whites of comparable background. Needless to say, increased smoking, less physical exercise, and even higher levels of alcohol intake (166), all contribute in varying amounts to further increasing cardiovascular risk.

HEALTH CARE PROVIDERS

How could well-meaning and highly educated health professionals, working in their usual environs with diverse populations of patients, create a pattern of care that appears to be discriminatory? The Institute of Medicine's report (124) suggested three mechanisms that might be at play in health care disparities from the health care provider's side of the exchange: bias (or prejudice) against minorities; greater clinical uncertainty when interacting with minority patients; and beliefs (or stereotypes) held by the provider about the behavior or health of minorities. The Institute of Medicine examined these three issues extensively determining that no clear evidence exists to suggest that providers are more likely than the general public to express biases, although some evidence suggests that unconscious biases may perhaps exist. They felt that uncertainty might be a possible factor, particularly when providers treat patients that are dissimilar in cultural or linguistic background. But they found extensive evidence (124,167–169) suggesting that physicians "like everyone else," do, in fact stereotype, calling them "cognitive shortcuts." One study they specifically recounted, found that physicians referred white male, black male, and white female hypothetical "patients" (actually videotaped actors who displayed the same symptoms of cardiac disease) for cardiac catheterization at the same rates (approximately 90% for each group), but were significantly less likely to recommend catheterization procedures for black female patients exhibiting the same symptoms (167). Interesting, another study they detailed found similar results in medical students with their tendency to diagnosis white male "patients" with "definite" or "probable" angina with symptoms of cardiac disease, relative to black female "patients" with objectively similar symptoms (168). The report included various other unfortunate examples of physician stereotyping, such as one suggesting that health care professionals were more likely to evaluate patients more negatively after being "primed" with words associated with African American stereotypes (169).

Eliminating Disparities in Cardiovascular Care and Outcomes

The American Heart Association held a Minority Health Summit and the report of the Outcomes Writing Group (170) highlighted important findings from several of the key observational studies of CVD in order to make recommendations about future direction and effort in CVD health, disease and risk identification and management in racial/ethnic minority populations. The studies included the National Health and NHANES, the Honolulu Heart Program, the SHS, and the MESA as well as many other epidemiological observational studies. Their recommendations are as follows:

> *Research.* The scientific community must support efforts to increase minority participation in scientific studies, broaden the racial/ethnic groups included, and increase the validity of the studies. Although it would not be economically feasible for all studies to achieve the objectives that follow, investigators should ask themselves whether they have addressed the inclusion of racial/ethnic minorities appropriately. Grant applications should be evaluated by the integrity of their plans to include partnerships with racial/ethnic minority groups that are involved in the studies and should include a community outreach and education program. The scientific community must increase the number of qualified minority investigators by increasing the training, recruitment, and retention of such investigators. Research bodies, including the American Heart Association (AHA) should strongly encourage disclosure of the ages, sexes, races/ethnicities, and SESs of study participants. The AHA, National Institutes of Health, and other organizations should encourage research on racial/ethnic disparities in CVD risk factors, outcomes, and access to health care.

Advocacy. The AHA and other organizations should advocate for federal funding for the identification of gaps in access to and the quality of health care and services offered to racial/ethnic minorities; the identification of ways to improve quality; and an increased focus on environmental, systems-level, and policy-level research. The AHA should commit to crafting a mission statement dedicated to eliminating racial/ethnic and SES disparities in CVD and its attendant health behaviors and risk factors, and post the mission statement and minimal standards of care on the AHA's web site. The AHA and health care provider should advocate for the following changes. The AHA should advocate for universal access to high-quality health care. The AHA should target their advocacy efforts to promote child and adult health across races/ethnicities in schools, families, and communities.

Education. The AHA should issue an annual report on disparities in CVD. The AHA and other organizations should develop web-based downloadable health education materials on CVD for racial/ethnic minorities and low-SES communities, including slides and pamphlets. The AHA should pursue culturally and linguistically appropriate public education on CVD prevention and disparities; the message should include that CVD occurs disproportionately in racial/ethnic minorities and low-SES populations.

—Minority Health Summit 2003: Report of the Advocacy Writing Group

CVD persists as the leading cause of the death in the United States and most industrialized society regardless or race or ethnicity. Nevertheless, African Americans experience the highest rates of cardiovascular mortality and increased rates of stroke, both fatal and nonfatal when compared to whites. Hispanic-American is an ethnic categorization versus a racial distinction. This population is expected to have increased rates of CVD in the future because of disproportionate numbers of type 2 diabetes and metabolic syndrome and obesity. Asian populations are markedly heterogeneous but emerging information indicates an increased rate of CVD and death in South Asians. Recent data have indicated American-Indians may also be at an increased risk for cardiovascular events. Conventional risk factors do not explain, to a large extent, disparate rates of CVD in ethnic minorities. For instance, LDL cholesterol is not significantly elevated in non-Hispanic blacks when compared to whites and HDL levels actually appear somewhat higher versus other populations, with lower TG. Higher rates of hypertension may potentially override the lack of excess dyslipidemia in this population. Hispanics on the other hand have lower HDL and higher TG than non-Hispanic whites, along with higher rates of type 2 diabetes. Furthermore, novel risk factors such as CRP appear to be higher in certain racial/ethnic populations including blacks, Hispanics, and south Asians. Risk factor clustering, SES and other clinical factors may explain much of the disparities noted in cardiovascular outcomes. Furthermore, utilization of procedures, including technologic diagnostic and cardiovascular interventions, appear to have variations in use based on race and ethnicity. Disparities in cardiovascular medications also may increase the burden of CVD outcomes. In the future, the application of evidence-based medicine, including appropriate inclusion of racial/ethnic groups in clinical trials may minimize or even reverse health care disparities.

REFERENCES

1. U.S Census Bureau. Available at http://www.census.gov/population/www/socdemo/race.html
2. U.S. Department of Health and Human Services. FDA Guidance for Industry-Collection of Race and Ethnicity Data in Clinical Trials. September 2005. http://www.fda.gov/cber/ guidelines.htm.
3. Smedley BD, Stith AY, Nelson AR, et al., eds. Unequal treatment: confronting racial and ethnic disparities in health care. The Institute of Medicine. Washington, D.C.: National Academies Press, 2002:83.
4. Oh SS, Croft JB, Greenlund KJ, et al. Disparities in premature deaths from heart disease: 50 states and the District of Columbia, 2001. Morb Mortal Wkly Rep 2004; 53:121–125.
5. Centers for Disease Control. Behavioral Risk Factor Surveillance System, CDC/NCHS. Morb Mortal Wkly Rep 2004; 53(6).
6. Centers for Disease Control. Sudden Cardiac Death in U.S. Young Adults, 1989–96, CDC, 2001.
7. Clark LT, Ferdinand KC, Flack JM, et al. Coronary heart disease in African Americans. Heart Dis 2001; 3:97–108; National Vital Statistics System, Health, United States, 1996–1997.
8. Palaniappan L, Wang Y, Fortmann SP. Coronary heart disease mortality for six ethnic groups in California, 1990–2000. Ann Epidemiol 2004; 14(7):499–506.
9. British Heart Foundation: Accessed at http://www.bhf.org.uk/

10. Kissela B, Schneider A, Kleindorfer D, et al. Greater Cincinnati/Northern Kentucky Stroke Study (GCNKSS). Stroke in a Biracial Population The Excess Burden of Stroke Among Blacks. Stroke 2004; 35:426.
11. Hutchinson RG, Watson RL, Davis CE, et al. Racial differences in risk factors for atherosclerosis. The ARIC Study. Atherosclerosis Risk in Communities. Angiology 1997; 48:279–290.
12. National Institute of Health, NHLBI. Strong Heart Study Data Book. A Report to American Indian Communities. NIH Publication No. 01-3285 November, 2001.
13. Morgenstern LB, Smith MA, Lisabeth LD, et al. Excess stroke in Mexican Americans compared with non-hispanic whites: the Brain Attack Surveillance in Corpus Christi Project. Am J Epidemiol 2004; 160:376–383.
14. Centers for Disease Control and Prevention. Health Disparities Experienced by Black or African Americans—United States. Morb Mortal Wkly Rep 2005; 54(1):1–35.
15. Pickle LW, Mungiole M, Gillum RF. Geographic variation in stroke mortality in blacks and whites in the United States. Stroke 1997; 28(8):1639–1647.
16. Centers for Disease Control and Prevention. Regional and Racial Differences in Prevalence of Stroke. MMWR Weekly 2005; 54(19):481–484.
17. Centers for Disease Control. Racial/Ethnic and Socioeconomic Disparities in Multiple Risk Factors for Heart Disease and Stroke – United States, 2003. Morb Mortal Wkly Rep 2005; 54(05):113–117.
18. Mosca L, Ferris A, Fabunmi R, Robertson RM. Tracking Women's Awareness of Heart Disease: An American Heart Association National Study. Circulation 2004; 109:573–579.
19. Minino AM, Arias E, Kochanek KD, et al. Deaths: final data for 2000. National Vital Statistics Reports. Hyattsville, MD: National Center for Health Statistics, 2002; 20 (15).
20. American Heart Association. Heart Disease and Stroke Statistics—2005 Update. Dallas, Texas: American Heart Association, 2005.
21. Jha AK, Varosy PD, Kanaya AM, et al. Differences in medical care and disease outcomes among black and white women with heart disease. Circulation 2003; 108:1089.
22. Centers for Disease Control, NHIS [2001], CDC/NCHS. Vital Health Stat 2004; Series 10(219).
23. Jones DW, Chambless LE, Folsom AR, et al. Risk factors for coronary heart disease in African Americans the atherosclerosis risk in communities study. Arch Intern Med 2002; 162:2565–2571.
24. Gillum RF. The epidemiology of cardiovascular disease in black Americans. N Engl J Med 1996; 335(21):1597–1599.
25. Williams DR, Jackson PB. Social sources of racial disparities in health. Health Affairs 2005; 24:325–334.
26. Centers for Disease Control. National Center for Health Statistics. National Health and Nutrition Examination Survey 1 999–2002.
27. American Heart Association. Heart Disease and Stroke Statics Update 2004. Dallas, Texas: American Heart Association, 2005.
28. Kennedy BS, Kasl SV, Brass LM, et al. Trends in hospitalized stroke for blacks and whites in the United States, 1980–1999. Neuroepidemiology 2002; 21(3):131–141.
29. Fullerton HJ, Wu YW, Zhao S, Johnston SC. Risk of stroke in children: ethnic and gender disparities. Neurology 2003; 61:189–194.
30. Winkleby MA, Kraemer HC, Ahn DK, Varady AN. Ethnic and socioeconomic differences in cardiovascular disease risk factors: findings for women from the Third National Health and Nutrition Examination Survey, 1988–1994. JAMA 1998; 280:356–362.
31. Harwell TS, Oser CS, Okon NJ, et al. Defining disparities in cardiovascular disease for American Indians. Circulation 2005.
32. Centers for Disease Control. National Center for Health Statistics (NCHS). Behavioral Risk Factor Surveillance System [BRFSS, 1997]: Press release. http://www.cdc.gov/OD/OC/MEDIA/pressrel/r2k0602.htm
33. Ayala C, Greenlund KJ, Croft JB, et al. Racial/ethnic disparities in mortality by stroke subtype in the United States, 1995–1998. Am J Epidemiol 2001; 154:1057–1063.
34. Curb JD, Reed D. Fish consumption and mortality from coronary heart disease [Lett]. N Eng J Med 1985; 313:821–822.
35. McKeigue P, Sevak L. Coronary Heart Disease in South Asian Communities. London: Health Education Authority, 1994.
36. Anand SS, Yusuf S, Vuksan V, et al. Difference in risk factors, atherosclerosis, and cardiovascular disease between ethnic groups in Canada: the Study of Health Assessment and Risk in Ethnic groups (SHARE). Lancet 2000; 356:279–284.
37. Centers for Disease Control. Healthy People 2000, Statistical Notes, No. 23, CDC/NCHS, Jan 2002.
38. Hunt KJ, Resendez RG, Williams K, et al. All-cause and cardiovascular mortality among Mexican-American and non-Hispanic White older participants in the San Antonio Heart Study-evidence against the "Hispanic paradox". Am J Epidemiol 2003; 158(11):1048–1057.
39. Freedman DS, Newman WP III, Tracy RE, et al. Black-white differences in aortic fatty streaks in adolescence and early adulthood: the Bogalusa Heart Study. Circulation 1988; 77(4):856–864.
40. Budoff MJ, Yang TP, Shavelle RM, et al. Ethnic differences in coronary atherosclerosis. J Am Coll Cardiol 2002; 39(3):408–412.
41. Tang W, Detrano RC, Brezden OS, et al. Racial differences in coronary calcium prevalence among high-risk adults. Am J Cardiol 1995; 75:1088–1091.

42. Newman AB, Naydeck BL, Whittle J, et al. Arterioscler Thromb Vasc Biol 2002; 22:424–430.
43. Lee T, O'Malley P, Feuerstein I, Taylor A. The prevalence and severity of coronary artery calcification on coronary artery computed tomography in black and white subjects. J Am Coll Cardiol 2003; 41:39–44.
44. Reaven PD, Thurmond D, Domb A, et al. Comparison of frequency of coronary artery calcium in healthy Hispanic versus non-Hispanic white men by electron beam computed tomography. Am J Cardiol 2003; 92(10):1198–1200.
45. Jain T. African Americans and Caucasians have a similar prevalence of coronary calcium in the Dallas Heart Study. J Am Coll Cardiol 2004; 44(5):1011–1017.
46. Bild DE, Detrano R, Peterson D, et al. Ethnic differences in coronary calcification the multi-ethnic study of atherosclerosis (MESA). Circulation 2005; 111:1313–1320.
47. Hatwalkar A. Comparison of prevalence and severity of coronary calcium determined by electron beam tomography among various ethnic groups. Am J Cardiol 2003; 91(10):1225–1227.
48. Hicks LS, Fairchild DG, Horng MS, et al. Determinants of JNC VI guideline adherence, intensity of drug therapy, and blood pressure control by race and ethnicity. Hypertension 2004; 44:429.
49. Yancy CW. Heart failure in African Americans: a cardiovascular enigma. J Card Fail 2000; 6:183.
50. Rahman M, Douglas JG, Wright JT. Pathophysiology and treatment implications of hypertension in the African American population. Endocrinol Metab Clin North Am 1997; 26:125.
51. Berenson GS, Voors AW, Webber LS, et al. Racial differences of parameters associated with blood pressure levels in children: The Bogalusa Heart Study. Metabolism 1979; 28:1218.
52. Gardin JM, Wagenknecht LE, Anton-Culver H, et al. Relationship of cardiovascular risk factors to echocardiographic left ventricular mass in healthy young black and white adult men and women: The CARDIA study. Circulation 1995; 92:380.
53. Wright JT, Bakris G, Green T, et al. Effect of blood pressure lowering and antihypertensive drug class on progression of hypertensive kidney disease. Results from the AASK Trial. JAMA 2002; 19:2421.
54. Murphy JK, Alpert BS, Moes DM, Somes GW. Race and cardiovascular reactivity: a neglected relationship. Hypertension 1986; 8:1075–1083.
55. Light KC, Turner JR, Hinderliter AL, Sherwood A. Race and gender comparisons, I: hemodynamic responses to a series of stressors. Health Psychol 1993; 12:354–365.
56. Saab PG, Llabre MM, Hurwitz BE, et al. Myocardial and eripheral vascular responses to behavioral challenges and their stability in black and white Americans. Psychophysiology 1992; 29:384–397.
57. Stein CM, Lang CC, Nelson R, et al. Vasodilation in black Americans: attenuated nitric oxide-mediated responses. Clin Pharmacol Ther 1997; 62:436.
58. Li R, Lynd D, Lapu-Bula R, et al. Relation of endothelial nitric oxide synthase gene to plasma nitric oxide level, endothelial function, and blood pressure in African Americans. Am J Hypertens 2004; 17(7):560–567.
59. Hinderliter AL, Sager AR, Sherwood A, et al. Ethnic differences in forearm vasodilator capacity. Am J Cardiol 1996; 78: 208–211.
60. Cardillo C, Kilcoyne CM, Cannon RO III, Panza JA. Attenuation of cyclic nucleotide-mediated smooth muscle relaxation in blacks as a cause of racial differences in vasodilator function. Circulation 1999; 99:90–95.
61. Perragaux D, Chaudhuri A, Rao S, et al. Brachial vascular reactivity in blacks. Hypertension 2000; 36:866–876.
62. Jones DS, Andrawis NS, Abernethy DR. Impaired endothelial-dependent forearm vascular relaxation in black Americans. Clin Pharmacol Ther 1999; 65:408–412.
63. Din-Dzietham R, Couper D, Evans G, et al. Arterial stiffness is greater in African Americans than in whites: evidence from the Forsyth County, North Carolina, ARIC cohort. Am J Hypertens 2004; 17(4):304–313.
64. Lang CC, Stein CM, Brown RM, et al. Attenuation of isoproterenol-mediated vasodilation in blacks. N Engl J Med 1995; 333:155–160.
65. Weinberger MH. Salt sensitivity of blood pressure in humans. Hypertension 1996; 7:481–490.
66. Sacks FM, Svetkey LP, Vollmer WM, et al. Effects on blood pressure of reduced dietary sodium and the Dietary Approaches to Stop Hypertension (DASH) diet. DASH-Sodium Collaborative Research Group. N Engl J Med 2001; 344:3.
67. August P, Levental B, Suthanthiran M. Hypertension-induced organ damage in African Americans: transforming growth factor-β1 excess as a mechanism for increased prevalence. Curr Hypertension Rep 2000; 2:184–191.
68. Nesbitt S, Victor RG. Pathogenesis of hypertension in African Americans. Congest Heart Fail 2004; 10:24.
69. Hobanian AV, Bakris GL, Black HR, et al. The Seventh Report of the Joint National Committee on Prevention, Detection, Evaluation and Treatment of High Blood Pressure. The JNC 7 report. JAMA 2003; 289:2560.
70. Wright JT Jr., Dunn JK, Cutler JA, et al., for the ALLHAT Collaborative Research Group. Outcomes. JAMA 2005; 293:1595–1607.
71. Lindholm LH, Ibsen H, Dahlof B, et al. Cardiovascular morbidity and mortality in patients with diabetes in the Losartan Intervention for Endpoint reduction in hypertension study (LIFE): a randomised trial against atenolol. Lancet 2002; 359:1004–1010.
72. Douglas JG, Barkis GL, Epstein M, et al, for the Hypertension in African Americans Working Group. Management of high blood pressure in African Americans: consensus statement of the Hypertension in African Americans Working Group of the International Society on Hypertension in Blacks. Arch Intern Med 2003; 163:525–541.

73. Haffner SM, Mitchell BD, Valdez RA, et al. Eight-year incidence of hypertension in Mexican-Americans and non-Hispanic whites. The San Antonio Heart Study. Am J Hypertens 1992; 5(3):147–153.

74. Haffner SM, Mitchell BD, Stern MP, et al. Decreased prevalence of hypertension in Mexican-Americans. Hypertension 1990; 16(3):225–232.

75. Fields LE, Burt VL, Cutler JA, et al. NHANES (1999–2002), The Burden of Adult Hypertension in the United States 1999 to 2000: a rising tide hypertension. Hypertension 2004; 44:398–404.

76. Burden AC. Blood pressure control and cardiovascular risk in patients of Indo-Asian and African-Caribbean descent. Int J Clin Pract 1998; 52:388–394.

77. The World Health Organization. Surveillance of Major Noncommunicable Diseases in the South East Region Report of an Intercountry Consultation WHO/SEARO, 2000.

78. Centers for Disease Control. Diabetes Prevalence Among American Indians and Alaska Natives and the Overall Population—United States, 1994–2002. Morb Mortal Wkly Rep 2003; 52(30), CDC/NCHS.

79. Venkataraman R, Nanda NC, Baweja G, et al. Prevalence of diabetes mellitus and related conditions in Asian Indians living in the United States. Am J Cardiol 2004; 94(7):977–980.

80. Centers for Disease Control. National Center for Health Statistics (NCHS): Fast stats 2002. http://www.cdc.gov/nchc/fastats/

81. Third Report of the National Cholesterol Education Program (NCEP) Expert Panel on Detection, Evaluation, and Treatment of High Blood Cholesterol in Adults (Adult Treatment Panel III) final report. Circulation 2002; 106:3143–3421.

82. Resnick HE. Strong Heart Study Investigators: metabolic syndrome in American Indians. Diabetes Care 2002; 25(7):1246–1247.

83. Alberti KG, Zimmet PZ. Definition, diagnosis and classification of diabetes mellitus and its complications. Part 1: diagnosis and classification of diabetes mellitus: provisional report of a WHO consultation. Diabet Med 1998; 15:539–553.

84. Hanson RL, Imperatore G, Bennett PH, Knowler WC. Components of the "metabolic syndrome" and incidence of type 2 diabetes. Diabetes 2002; 51(10):3120–3127.

85. Meigs JB, Wilson PW, Nathan DM, et al. Prevalence and characteristics of the metabolic syndrome in the San Antonio Heart and Framingham Offspring Studies. Diabetes 2003; 52(8):2160–2167.

86. Ferrannini E, Natali A, Capaldo B, et al. Insulin resistance, hyperinsulinemia and blood pressure. Hypertension 1997; 30:1144.

87. Tillin T, Forouhi N, Johnston DG, et al. Metabolic syndrome and coronary heart disease in South Asians, African-Caribbeans and white Europeans: a UK population-based cross-sectional study. Diabetologia 2005; 48(4):649–656.

88. Alberti KG, Zimmet P, Shaw J. International Diabetes Federation. The metabolic syndrome—a new worldwide definition. IDF Epidemiology Task Force Consensus Group. Lancet 2005; 366(9491): 1059–1062.

89. Must A, Spadano J, Coakley EH. The disease burden associated with overweight and obesity. JAMA 1999; 282:1523.

90. Hall WD, Ferrario CM, Moore MA. Hypertension related morbidity and mortality in the southeastern United States. Am J Med Sci 1997; 313:195.

91. Flack JM, Ferdinand KC, Nasser SA. Epidemiology of hypertension and cardiovascular disease in African Americans. J Clin Hypertens 2005:; 5(1 suppl 1):5.

92. National Heart Lung and Blood Institutes. Molokai Heart Study. From "Addressing Cardiovascular Health in Asian Americans and Pacific Islanders: A Background Report" NIH Publication No. 00-3647.

93. Wattigney WA, Webber LS, Srinivasan SR, Berenson GS. The emergence of clinically abnormal levels of cardiovascular disease risk factor variables among young adults: the Bogalusa Heart Study. Prevent Med 1995; 24:617–626.

94. Despres JP, Couillard C, Gagnon J, et al. Race, visceral adipose tissue, plasma lipids, and lipoprotein lipase activity in men and women. The Health, Risk Factors, Exercise Training, and Genetics (HERITAGE) family study. Arterioscler Thromb Vasc Biol 2000; 20:1932–1938.

95. Goran MI, Gower BA. Relation between visceral fat and disease risk in children and adolescents. Am J Clin Nutr 1999; 70:149S–156S.

96. Gower BA, Nagy TR, Goran MI. Visceral fat, insulin sensitivity, and lipids in prepubertal children. Diabetes 1999; 48:1515–1521.

97. Conway JM, Yanovski SZ, Avila NA, Hubbard VS. Visceral adipose tissue differences in black and white women. Am J Clin Nutr 1995; 61:765–771.

98. Lovejoy JC, de la Bretonne JA, Lemperer M, Tulley R. Abdominal fat distribution and metabolic risk factors: effects of race. Metabolism 1996; 45:1119–1124.

99. Perry AC, Applegate EB, Jackson ML, et al. Racial differences in visceral adipose tissue but not anthropometric markers of health-related variables. J Appl Physiol 2000; 89:636–643.

100. Okosun IS, Tedders SH, Choi S, Dever GEA. Abdominal adiposity values associated with established body mass indexes in white, black and Hispanic Americans. A study from the Third National Health and Nutrition Examination Survey. Int J Obesity 2000; 24:1279–1285.

101. Haffner SM, D'Agostino R, Goff D, et al. LDL size in African Americans, Hispanics, and non-Hispanic whites. The Insulin Resistance Atherosclerosis Study. Arterioscler Thromb Vasc Biol 1999; 19:2234–2240.
102. Moliterno DJ, Jokinen EV, Miserez AR. No association between plasma lipoprotein(a) concentrations and the presence or absence of coronary atherosclerosis in African Americans. Arterioscler Thromb Vasc Biol 1995; (15):850–855.
103. Guyton JR, Dahlen GH, Patsch W. Relationship of plasma lipoprotein Lp(a) levels to race and to apolipoprotein B. Arteriosclerosis 1985; (5):265–272.
104. Sorrentino MJ, Vielhauer C, Eisenbart JD. Plasma lipoprotein(a) protein concentration and coronary artery disease in black patients compared with white patients. Am J Med 1992; 93:658–662.
105. Schreiner PJ, Heiss G, Tyroler HA. Race and gender differences in the association of Lp(a) with carotid artery wall thickness. The Atherosclerosis Risk in Communities (ARIC) study. Arterioscler Thromb Vasc Biol 1996; 16:471–478.
106. Watson KE, Topol EJ. Pathobiology of atherosclerosis: are there racial and ethnic differences? Rev Cardiovasc Med 2004; 5:S14–S21.
107. Sowers M, Crawford SL, Cauley JA, Stein E. Association of lipoprotein(a), insulin resistance, and reproductive hormones in a multiethnic cohort of pre- and perimenopausal women (The SWAN Study). Am J Cardiol 2003; 92(5):533–537.
108. The ALLHAT Officers and Coordinators for the ALLHAT Collaborative Research Group. Major outcomes in moderately hypercholesterolemic hypertensive patients randomized to pravastatin vs. usual care. The Antihypertensive and Lipid-Lowering Treatment to Prevent Heart Attack Trial (ALLHAT-LLT). JAMA 2002; 288:2998–3007.
109. Jacobson TA, Chin MM, Curry CL, et al. Efficacy and safety of pravastatin in African Americans with primary hypercholesterolemia. Arch Intern Med 1995; 155:1900–1906.
110. LaRosa JC, Applegate W, Crouse JR III, et al. Cholesterol lowering in the elderly results of the Cholesterol Reduction in Seniors Program (CRISP) pilot study. Arch Intern Med 1994; 154:529–539.
111. Prisant LM, Downton M, Watkins LO, et al. Efficacy and tolerability of lovastatin in 459 African Americans with hypercholesterolemia. Am J Cardiol 1996; 78:420–424.
112. Anand SS, et al. European, Chinese, South East Asian, aborigines. Arterioscler Thromb Vasc Biol 2004; 24:1509–1515.
113. Albert MA, Glynn RJ, Buring J, Ridker PM. C-Reactive protein levels among women of various ethnic groups living in the United States (from the Women's Health Study). Am J Cardiol 2004; 93(10):1238–1242.
114. Forouhi NG, Sattar N, McKeigue PM. Relation of C-reactive protein in body fat distribution of the metabolic syndrome in Europeans and South Asians. Int J Obes Relat Metab Disord 2001; 25:1327–1331.
115. Chambers JC, Eda S, Bassett P, et al. C-reactive protein, insulin resistance, central obesity and coronary heart disease risk in Indian Asians from the United Kingdom compared with European whites. Circulation 2001; 104:145–150.
116. Chandalia M, Cabo-Chan AV Jr., Devaraj S, et al., Elevated plasma high-sensitivity C-reactive protein concentrations in Asian Indians living in the United States. J Clin Endocrinol Metab 2003; 88:3773–3776.
117. Chatha K, Anderson NR, Gama R. Ethnic variation in C-reactive protein UK resident Indo-Asians compared with Caucasians. J Cardiovasc Risk 2002; 9:139.
118. Khera A, McGuire DK, Murphy SA, et al. Race and gender differences in C-reactive protein levels. J Am Coll Cardiol 2005; 46:464–469.
119. McGee D, Gordon T. Section 31. The results of the Framingham study applied to four other US-based epidemiological studies of cardiovascular disease. In: Kannel WB, Gordon T, eds. The Framingham Study. An Epidemiological Investigation of Cardiovascular Disease. DHEW Publications no. (NIH) 76–1083, Bethesda Public Health Service, National Institute of Health, 1986.
120. West of Scotland Coronary Prevention Study Group. Baseline risk factors and their association with outcome in the West of Scotland coronary prevention study. Am J Cardiol 1997; 79:756–762.
121. Ramachandran S, French JM, Vanderpump MPJ, et al. Using the Framingham model to predict heart disease in the United Kingdom: retrospective study. BMJ 2000; 230:676–677.
122. Schulte H, Assman G. CHD risk equations obtained from the Framingham Heart Study, applied to PROCAM Study. Cardiovasc Risk Factors 1991; 1:126–133.
123. D'Agostino RB, Grundy S, Sullivan LM, Wilson P, for the CHD Risk Prediction Group. Validation of the Framingham Coronary Heart Disease Prediction Scores: results of a multiple ethnic groups investigation. JAMA 2001; 286:180–187.
124. Institute of Medicine. Unequal Treatment: What Healthcare Providers Need to Know About Racial and Ethnic Disparities in Healthcare. March 2002.
125. Gornick et al. 1996.
126. Schneider EC, Zaslavsky AM, Epstein AM. Racial Disparities in the Quality of Care for Enrollees in Medicare Managed Care. JAMA 2002; 287:1288–1294.
127. Bach PB, Schrag D, Brawley OW, et al. Survival of Blacks and whites after a cancer diagnosis. JAMA 2002; 287:2106–2113.
128. Peterson ED, Shaw LK, DeLong ER, et al. Racial variation in the use of coronary-revascularization procedures—Are the differences real? Do they matter? N Engl J Med 1997; 336:480–486.

129. Bennett CL, Horner RD, Weinstein RA, et al. Racial differences in care among hospitalized patients with pneumocystis carinii pneumonia in Chicago, NY, Los Angeles, Miami, and Raleigh-Durham. Arch Inter Med 1995; 55:1586–1592.

130. Kaiser Family Foundation, American College of Cardiology Foundation. Racial/ethnic differences in cardiac care: the weight of the evidence. Menlo Park, CA: Henry J Kaiser Family Foundation, 2002.

131. Kaul P, Lytle BL, Spertus JA, et al. Influence of racial disparities in procedure use on functional status outcomes among patients with coronary artery disease. Circulation 2005; 111:1284–1290.

132. Konety SH, Vaughan Sarrazin MS, Rosenthal GE. Patient and hospital differences underlying racial variation in outcomes after coronary artery bypass graft surgery. Circulation 2005.

133. Centers for Disease Control. Use of stents among hospitalized patients undergoing coronary angioplasty, by race: United States, 2003. Morb Mortal Wkly Rep 2005; 54:310.

134. Bradley EH, Herrin J, Wang Y, et al. Racial and ethnic differences in time to acute reperfusion therapy for patients hospitalized with myocardial infarction. JAMA 2004; 292:1563–1572.

135. Bach PB, Pham HH, Schrag D, et al. Primary care physicians who treat blacks and whites. N Engl J Med 2004; 351:575–584.

136. Lurie, N, Fremont A, Jain AK, et al. Racial and ethnic disparities in care: the perspectives of cardiologists. Circulation 2005; 111:1264–1269.

137. Centers for Disease Control: Racial/Ethnic Disparities in Prevalence, Treatment, and Control of Hypertension-United States, 1999–2002. Morb Mortal Wkly Rep 2005; 54(01):7–9.

138. Fonarow GC, French WJ, Parsons LS, et al. Use of lipid-lowering medications at discharge in patients with acute myocardial infarction data from the national registry of myocardial infarction 3. Circulation 2001; 103:38–44.

139. Christian JB, Lapane KL, Toppa RS. Racial disparities in receipt of secondary stroke prevention agents among US nursing home residents. Stroke 2003; 34:2693.

140. Hajjar I, Kotchen T. Regional variations of blood pressure in the United States are associated with regional variations in dietary intakes: The NHANES-III Data. J Nutr 2003; 133:211–214.

141. Wolf-Maier K, Cooper RS, Kramer H, et al. Hypertension treatment and control in five European countries, Canada, and the United States. Hypertension 2004; 43:10.

142. Sudano JJ, Baker DW. Antihypertensive medication use in hispanic adults: a comparison with black adults and white adults. Med Care 2001; 39(6):575–587.

143. Crespo CJ, Loria CM, Burt VL. Hypertension and other cardiovascular disease risk factors among Mexican Americans, Cuban Americans, and Puerto Ricans from the Hispanic Health and Nutrition Examination Survey. Public Health Reports 1996; 111(suppl 2):7–10.

144. Hyman DJ, Pavlik VN. Characteristics of patients with uncontrolled hypertension in the United States. N Engl J Med 2001; 345:479–486.

145. Psaty BM, Manolio TA, Smith NL, et al. Time trends in high blood pressure control and the use of antihypertensive medications in older adults: the Cardiovascular Health Study. Arch Intern Med 2002; 162:2325–2332.

146. Berlowitz DR, Ash AS, Hickey EC, et al. Inadequate management of blood pressure in a hypertensive population. N Engl J Med 1998; 339:1957–1963.

147. Knight EL, Bohn RL, Wang PS. Predictors of uncontrolled hypertension in ambulatory patients. Hypertension 2001; 38:809.

148. Jackson JH IV, Bramley TJ, Chiang TH, et al. Determinants of uncontrolled hypertension in an African American population. Ethn Dis 2002; 12(4):S3-53–57.

149. Nieto FJ, Alonso J, Chambless LE, et al. Population awareness and control of hypertension and hypercholesterolemia. The Atherosclerosis Risk in Communities Study. Arch Intern Med 1995; 155:677–684.

150. Pearson T, Laurora I, Chu H, Kafonek S. The Lipid Treatment Assessment Project (L–TAP). Arch Intern Med 2000; 160:459–467.

151. Asher CR, Topol EJ, Moliterno DJ. Insights into the pathophysiology of atherosclerosis and prognosis of black Americans with acute coronary syndromes. Am Heart J 138(6 part 1):1073–1081.

152. Hall WD. Representation of blacks, women, and the very elderly (aged >80) in 28 major randomized clinical trials. Ethn Dis 1999; 9:333–340.

153. Downs JR, Clearfield M, Weis S, et al. Primary prevention of acute coronary events with lovastatin in men and women with average cholesterol levels: results of AFCAPS/TexCAPS. Air Force/Texas Coronary Atherosclerosis Prevention Study. JAMA 1998; 279:1616–1622.

154. WOSCOPS N Engl J Med 1998; 339:1349–1357.

155. 4S Lancet 1994; 344:1383–1389.

156. Care N Engl J Med 1995; 333:1301–1307.

157. HPS Lancet 2002; 360:7–22.

158. ASCOT Lancet 2003; 361:1149–1158.

159. Sacks F, Pfeffer M, Moye L, et al. For the Cholesterol and Recurrent Events Trial Investigators. The effect of pravastatin on coronary events after myocardial infarction in patients with average cholesterol levels. N Engl J Med 1996; 335:1001–1009.

160. Lenfant C. Conference on socioeconomic status and cardiovascular health and disease. Circulation 1996; 94:2041–2044.

161. Mosca L, Appel LJ, Benjamin EJ, et al. Evidence-based guidelines for cardiovascular disease prevention in women. Circulation 2004; 109:672–693.

162. American Diabetes Association and American College of Cardiology. The diabetes-heart disease link: surveying attitudes, knowledge and risk executive summary. Available at: http://www.diabetes. org/main/uedocuments/executivesummary.pdf. Accessed May 6, 2003.
163. Feder G, Crook AM, Magee P, et al. Ethnic differences in invasive management of coronary disease: prospective cohort study of patients undergoing angiography. BMJ 2002; 324:511–516.
164. Doty M. Hispanic patients' double burden: lack of health insurance and limited English. New York: The Commonwealth Fund, 2003.
165. Satcher D. Surgeon General Surgeon General's Report AT-A-GLANCE: Tobacco Use Among U.S. Racial/Ethnic Minority Groups A Report of the Surgeon General.
166. Galvan FH, Caetano R. Alcohol use and related problems among ethnic minorities in the United States. National Institute on Alcohol Abuse and Alcoholism of the National Institutes of Health. http://pubs.niaaa.nih.gov/publications/arh27–1/87–94.htm
167. Schulman KA, Berlin JA, Harless W, et al. The effect of race and sex on physicians' recommendations for cardiac catheterization. N Engl J Med 1999; 340:618–626.
168. Rathore et al. Race, quality of care, and outcomes of elderly patients hospitalized with heart failure. JAMA 2003; 289:2517–2524.
169. Abreu JM. Conscious and nonconscious African American stereotypes: impact on first impression and diagnostic ratings by therapists. J Consult Clin Psychol 1999; 67(3):387–393.
170. Benjamin EJ, Jessup M, Flack JM, et al. Discovering the full spectrum of cardiovascular disease minority health summit 2003 report of the outcomes writing group. Circulation 2005; 111:e124–e133.

Index

T - #0298 - 101024 - C0 - 254/178/42 [44] - CB - 9780849340666 - Gloss Lamination